LIST OF PROCEDURES

Fundamentals of Nursing Practice

Fundamentals of Nursing Practice

Second Edition

Barbara W. Narrow, R.N., ED.D
Professor Emerita
College of Nursing
Syracuse University
Syracuse, New York

Kay Brown Buschle, R.N., M.S.
Associate Professor
College of Nursing
Syracuse University
Syracuse, New York

A WILEY MEDICAL PUBLICATION
John Wiley & Sons
New York   ·   Chichester   ·   Brisbane   ·   Toronto   ·   Singapore

Photos from ''Of Faith and Fire,'' reprinted from *Syracuse Herald American,* appearing on pages 2, 4, 7, 8, 9, 11, 12, and 13 and as Figures 3.4, 7.4, 8.4, 8.5, 8.6, 9.1, 9.4, 9.6, 10.2, 10.3, 10.4, 12.4, 13.3, 15.3, 15.4, 16.1, 16.2, 23.4, 23.5, 23.6, 23.7, 26.11, 29.6, 30.6, 33.1, 35.2, 36.1, 37.1, 37.3, 37.4, 37.5, 38.1, 39.3, and 39.4 copyright 1985 by Seth Resnick.

Figures 1.1, 3.3, 5.1, 6.1, 10.1, 13.4, 23.1, 26.10, 27.10, 29.1, 29.37, and 29.44 courtesy of Health Science Center, State University of New York at Syracuse, New York.

Figures 3.2, 3.5, 7.1, 7.2, 7.3, 8.1, 9.5, 13.2, 15.2, 17.1, 18.30, 20.1, 21.2, 23.2, and 29.2 courtesy of Syracuse University College of Nursing.

Library of Congress Cataloging-in-Publication Data:

Narrow, Barbara W.
    Fundamentals of nursing practice.

    (A Wiley medical publication.)
    Includes bibliographies and index.
    1. Nursing. I. Buschle, Kay Brown. II. Title.
III. Series. [DNLM: 1. Nursing. WY 100 N234f]

RT41.N33   1987   610.73   86-28945
ISBN 0-471-81853-4

Printed in the United States of America

10 9 8 7 6 5 4 3 2 1

To our husbands,
Wilbur and Gabe,
whose encouragement, understanding, and support made this book possible

Barbara W. Narrow, friend, colleague, and dedicated nursing teacher

Dr. Narrow's creative ideas, perseverance, and deep commitment to beginning nursing students provided the constant energy for this project. Her sudden death just before publication of this second edition has made her messages and the example of her life even more vital, and left those of us who knew Barbara with reflections and memories about her creative ideas and multiple nursing talents. In our last conversation together she talked freely about the essence of nursing. She believed that we should value what we do in nursing and practice what it is we value. She herself did this and she helped others, beginning nurses and graduate students, to do that too. Her spirit and oneness of purpose never faltered throughout our work together. Barbara's inspiration and constant search for new meanings in nursing combined to make her a most unique individual. This book completes one of her dreams and goals.

Kay Brown Buescher

Contributors

Patricia Button-Dye, R.N., M.S.
Quality Assurance Coordinator
Department of Nursing
Mary Hitchcock Hospital
Hanover, New Hampshire

Patricia A. Duncan, R.N., M.S.
Assistant Professor
College of Nursing
Syracuse University
Syracuse, New York

Rosalinda T. Lagua, M.N.S., R.D.
Senior Nutrition Services Consultant
Office of Health Systems Management
New York State Department of Health (OHSM)
Syracuse Area Office
Syracuse, New York

MaryAnn Middlemiss, R.N., M.S.
Assistant Professor
College of Nursing
Syracuse University
Syracuse, New York

Cecilia F. Mulvey, R.N., M.S.
Associate Professor
College of Nursing
Syracuse University
Syracuse, New York
Past President (1983–1985), New York State Nurses
    Association

Nancy L. Noel, R.N., ED.D.
Assistant Professor
Adelphi University
Long Island, New York
Former Curator, Nursing Archives
Boston University

Pamela Forand Ryan, R.N., M.S.
Staff Nurse, Obstetrical Department
Community General Hospital
Syracuse, New York
Lecturer, Cazenovia College
Department of Nursing
Cazenovia, New York

Preface

The purpose of this second edition is to provide a philo-sophical, theoretical, and clinical basis for nursing. We have continued to present professional nursing as a discipline in which sensitive, skillful, and knowledge-able practitioners carry out a wide variety of inde-pendent actions as well as collaborate with members of other disciplines. Nursing as a component of culture and society reflects ongoing social changes. The in-crease in home health care, the complex technology of intricate acute care, and the ever-greater number of people with chronic health problems all place a variety of new demands upon the nurse. We are in a unique position in relation to the changing constellation of the health care delivery system because nursing has long stood for the values which the public now demands from health care. Nursing is a partnership with people who have a wide range of needs in illness and in health and who live in vastly different sociocultural situations. We are accountable to assist in providing conditions under which people become or remain well, achieve a higher potential of well being, or die peacefully. Nurs-ing in this context demands a broad view of the world around us, of ourselves, and of the evolving content of nursing.

working knowledge of those concepts. This book makes no such assumption and deliberately integrates into every section of the book ideas related to the nature of man, patient's rights, accountability of the nurse, need for excellence, importance of the family, and ethical con-cerns. This subtle, unobtrusive repetition and applica-tion of ideas enhances the slow process of attitudinal change and the development of a professional value system.

The concepts of self-care and holistic nursing are emphasized and integrated throughout. The book is de-signed to:

Introduce major concepts relevant to nursing

Provide an adequate base for students' initial clinical experiences

Begin to socialize the student into the profession of nursing

Emphasize the unique partnership of the nurse and patient

Excite the reader about the scope and potential of professional nursing practice

Stimulate curiosity and commitment to lifelong learning in nursing

FOCUS OF THE NEW EDITION

Fundamentals of nursing texts sometimes present sig-nificant theoretical concepts in their early chapters, with the assumption in later chapters that the learner has a

CHANGES IN THE NEW EDITION

This second edition has been reorganized, completely revised, and redesigned to provide carefully selected content in adequate depth for a sound introduction to nursing. It includes:

- Expansion, revision, and updating throughout all the chapters to reflect new ideas, suggestions from readers, and new trends in the evolution of health care delivery.
- Six new chapters:
  History of Nursing in the United States
  Perinatal Development
  Individual Development
  Family Development
  Care of the Surgical Patient
  Care of the Unconscious Patient
- New tables and figures to illustrate both theoretical and clinical concepts; to relate theory to practice; to make a point; to teach.
- Forty-two clinical nursing procedure summaries following thorough in-text discussion. Printed on the front endpaper is a checklist of essential nursing actions that must take place in order for any procedure to be deemed safe and effective. This should be referred to before reading or practicing any procedure described.
- Patient–family teaching and related student activities which can be used for study assignments and seminar discussion.
- Student-oriented suggested readings at the end of each chapter, carefully selected to supplement the text and to introduce students to the excitement and satisfaction of reading professional literature. Journal articles were included if they were current, nursing-oriented, and easily accessible.
- Prerequisite and/or suggested student preparation at the beginning of each chapter.
- A unique human interest story preceding Part One. The story, printed as it originally appeared, is about a six-year-old girl and her family and their relationship with the staff at a medical center. The photographs by a prize-winning photographer have captured many common human responses to the acute care and recovery phases, and are used to illustrate these responses throughout the text.

REORGANIZATION OF CONTENT

Part One, **Nursing Practice,** includes a new chapter on the historical perspective of nursing, introduces the student to nursing as a profession, and describes the role of the nurse within the health care system.

Part Two, **Concepts Basic to Nursing Practice,** expands upon the conceptual frameworks and nursing models, systems theory, values, health and illness with epidemiology, stress and coping, teaching and learning, communication, and selected pathophysiological concepts and principles of physics.

Part Three, **Individuals and Families,** is almost totally new and is devoted to human needs, prenatal, individual, and family development with a broad cultural focus.

Part Four, **Nursing Process,** has a revitalized overview and greater clarity in delineating and describing the five phases of nursing process. The chapter on assessment includes basic health assessment, vital signs, measurements, interviewing, frequently used tests, charting and recording.

Part Five, **Nursing Interventions Related to Psychological Needs,** discusses crisis intervention, the importance of self-image, sexuality, spiritual needs, desires and satisfactions, and the interdependence of the mind, emotions, and physical responses.

Part Six, **Nursing Interventions for Physical Care and Comfort,** is completely revised to include new and expanded content. The chapter on nutrition is enlarged and covers more detailed information on eating disorders. The chapter on sensory status reflects major additions in the areas of assessment, levels of consciousness, and variables which influence nursing. New guidelines for infection control are discussed.

Part Seven, **Nursing Interventions in Specific Situations,** places new importance on those areas which have been and continue to be the domain of nursing, such as pain, wound care, administration of drugs, and applications of heat and cold. There are new chapters on the surgical patient and the unconscious patient, including theory and clinical concerns. The chapter on care of the dying patient has been revised to more strongly reflect patient–family concerns and the role of the nurse.

The word *patient* is used in the text to denote the recipient of health care without reference to the person's state of health or degree of independence. While we continue to acknowledge and respect the diversity of opinion related to the use of the terms *patient* and *client,* we have chosen to use *patient* to indicate a participant in a specific interpersonal helping relationship unique to health care. As the scope and meaning of the words *nurse* and *nursing* expand, so should the scope and meaning of the word *patient.*

Men in nursing continue to contribute in important ways and in a variety of health care settings, and the text photographs show both men and women in the practice of nursing. However, in order to ensure consistency and clarity of sentence structure and grammar, we have referred to the nurse as *she* and the patient as *he*. For ease of expression the single word *family* is used to indicate those persons who are significant to the patient and to whom the patient is significant. The relationship between these persons may have been established by genetic background, adoption, marriage, proximity, necessity, or mutual consent.

The content of this book is appropriate for professional programs with differing curricula and differing conceptual frameworks. We have included concepts basic to many current models of nursing and have deliberately refrained from espousing a specific conceptual framework. The promotion of health and the prevention of illness underlie all content in this book, but many of the chapters are designed to help the beginning student acquire the knowledge, skill, and perspective needed for the successful completion of clinical assignments for a person with an identified health problem or illness. It is our hope that this book will be stimulating and effective in helping students begin their journey toward professional nursing. We welcome comments from students, instructors, and readers so that your ideas and suggestions can continue to make teaching and learning about nursing as challenging and dynamic as we have always found it to be.

B.W.N.
K.B.B.

Acknowledgments

No textbook is ever written in isolation. The help and support of many people combine to create the environment in which writing occurs. Family, friends, colleagues, and students all contributed either directly or indirectly to our preparation of this book.

We particularly appreciated the interest, suggestions, and support offered by the faculty at Syracuse University College of Nursing during the many months of manuscript preparation. The part the students played in the revision of this book deserves recognition. Their interest, ideas, and motivation served as our inspiration.

We gratefully acknowledge the special expertise of the following people:

Beverly B. Martin, Assistant Professor, College of Nursing, Syracuse University, for her assistance with Chapter 1.

Barbara Van Noy, Associate Professor, College of Nursing, Syracuse University, for her pertinent suggestions related to the psychosocial content in Chapters 9 and 23.

Julie White, Nurse Epidemiologist at New England Deaconess Hospital, Boston, for her additions to Chapter 27.

Kathleen Fitzgerald, faculty, St. Joseph's Hospital and Health Center School of Nursing, Syracuse, for her suggestions and help with the preparation of Chapter 37.

Linda DeVona, Dan DeVona, Patricia Apples, and Margaret De Rapps, our artists, whose original line drawings were carefully prepared.

Our photographer, Peter L. Taralli, for his excellent renditions of the skills we wanted to demonstrate.

Seth Resnick, photographer, for his creative ability to capture the poignant moments in the life of a child who had suffered facial and body burns.

The contributors to the book deserve special mention because they worked long hours to create, revise, and reformulate important content in their chapters.

We thank the staff of numerous departments of Syracuse University and the Health Science Center of the State University of New York at Syracuse for their assistance in countless ways throughout the preparation of the book.

Special recognition is reserved for two significant people who, without question, made this edition a reality. Many thanks to Jane de Groot, Nursing Editor at John Wiley & Sons, Inc., for her support, friendship, and encouragement throughout the whole effort and especially during the difficult times; and to Bernice Heller, Consultant and Development Editor, for her unique ability to share her talents and expertise in manuscript preparation. She helped to shape our efforts and never wavered in her quest for excellence.

We thank those at Wiley for their input and generous help, especially: Margery Carazzone, Production

Manager, Jean Morley, Design Manager, Denise Watov, Senior Production Supervisor, and Marie Saget, Editorial Assistant. And finally, we thank the nursing educators and nursing students who made the effort of writing this book all worthwhile!

B.W.N.
K.B.B.

I would like to give special thanks to the Narrow family for their love, devotion, and stability: Barbara's husband, Wilbur; her children, Pat, Mary, and Elizabeth; their husbands, Larry and Tom; and her grandchildren, Mathew, Julie, and Ann; Susan and Natalie.

K.B.B.

Contents

Detailed Contents

Fundamentals
of Nursing Practice

Of Faith and Fire:
The Story of Renee

Nursing has been confronted by many challenges throughout its long history, but none have been more significant than the one it now faces. This challenge is the task of providing sensitive holistic nursing care in situations which are likely to be technical, impersonal, and dehumanizing.

Medical technology has made many wonderful things possible, but it has also produced equipment and procedures which place extraordinary demands upon the nurse. In order for nursing to continue its rich heritage of giving care which is sensitive yet scientific, nurses must strive to keep technological advances in perspective, and to focus their attention on the patient more vigorously than ever.

It is to this end that we have used the story of Renee as an introduction of this book. Her story exemplifies the heart of nursing and its reason for being—the story describes how nurses in a large medical center helped Renee recover from a tragic accident, and equally important, to grow and develop as a person. Renee's story provides a basis for the clinical application of theories and principles throughout the book, and additional photographs are used to illustrate important concepts in subsequent chapters.

Renee's story was published in 1984 and is reprinted below as it originally appeared except that the names of her family and hometown have been changed to protect the family's privacy. The photo essay is by Seth Resnick, and the text was written by Jim Naughton, both of whom were employed at the time by the Syracuse Herald American.

Reprinted from *Syracuse Herald American*, April 22, 1984, with permission. Text by Jim Naughton. Photographs copyright 1985 by Seth Resnick.

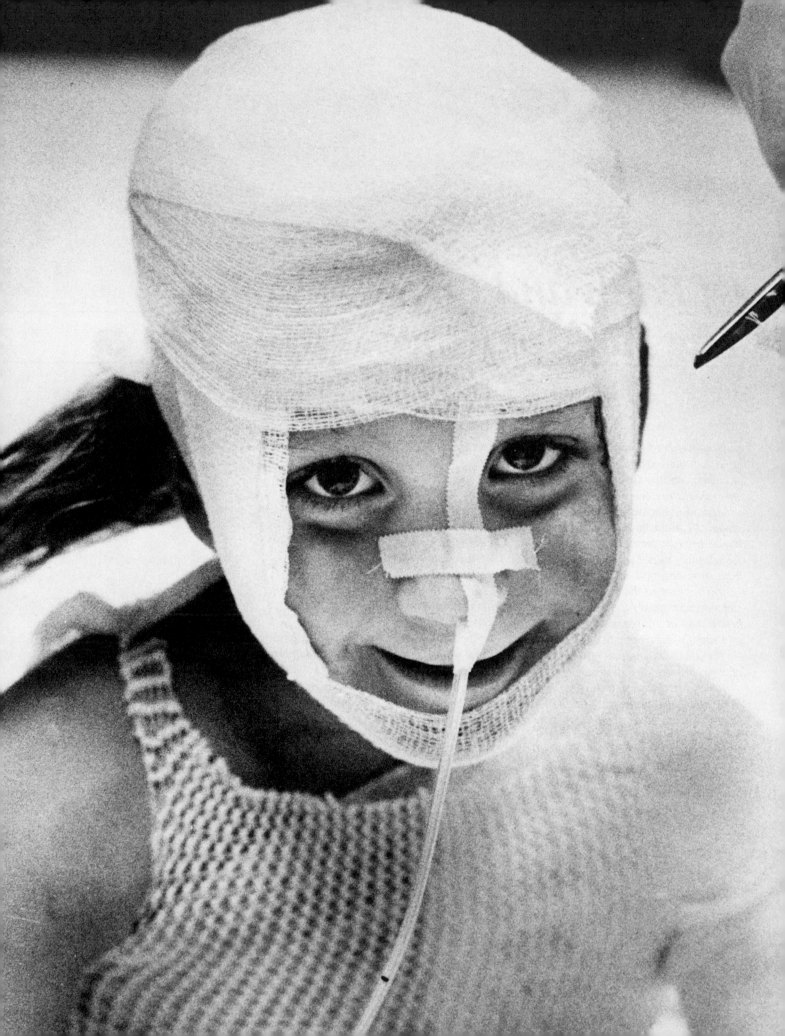

Paint me a kitchen in a two-story town just after nightfall in autumn. Use warm colors and whispering light.

The girl beside the stove has chestnut hair. She should be smiling the way she was in her first-grade class picture. The photographer must have told her that ponies grew on trees and her daddy had just ordered a sapling.

Leave the dough on the table where Renee and her brother can flatten it into shells. Turn the flame up and give the frying pan a good thick greasing.

Make the neighbor a motherly woman. Sketch her in beside the counter top with her back turned for a moment, reaching for the powdered sugar. The first batch of cookies should be sitting before her.

No one would blame you for leaving out the telephone, or the way Renee spun when she heard it ring.

"I went down and my head hit the handle and the grease just spilled all over me," she says now.

Her neighbor dug through her cabinets for baking soda and began pouring it all over Renee's head, left arm and back, but it didn't soothe her.

"She quickly took me outside and it was real cool outside and my brother ran over and got Daddy and Daddy came over and pulled my shirt off and carried me over to our house," Renee says.

"And then ran over to get the doctor and the doctor came over and he looked at me and said that he wanted me to go to the hospital. And Daddy carried me out to the car and Mommy sat in the car and Daddy gave me to Mommy and Daddy had to drive real fast and that's what happened."

On Oct. 18, 1982, 6-year-old Renee suffered burns, most of them third degree, to about 15 percent of her body. Her family took her first to a nearby hospital, but she was moved almost immediately to the Medical Center burn unit. For 22 days she suffered through perhaps the most excruciatingly painful procedures in modern medicine: burn surgery and rehabilitation.

Burn care is so intensely torturous that some victims choose to die. Others don't have that choice; they succumb to one of a myriad of complications ranging from infection of the burned skin, to heart, respiratory and kidney failure.

The doctors knew Renee would live. What they didn't know is that she would grow, that some blend of their tenderness and her courage would make the horrors of burn surgery one of the most meaningful experiences of her young life.

Thirteen days after her accident, the expression on Renee's face shows that she is recovering in body and in spirit.

On the morning of Oct. 19, she sat in the burn unit looking around what was known as the tubbing room. The walls were blue and a huge silver tub, surrounded by all sorts of lifts and pulleys, sat in the middle of the floor.

Renee couldn't know what a terror the room would become for her. But the doctors and nurses, who had already begun to pity her, could not know how beautifully she would handle her recovery or how deeply involved they would become in her whole pain-filled ordeal.

Dr. George Tremiti, a surgical resident, was in his second day without sleep when they brought Renee in that morning to have her head shaved and her wounds cleaned. The closer he shaved her, the more furious he became.

The burns were bigger and deeper than he thought.

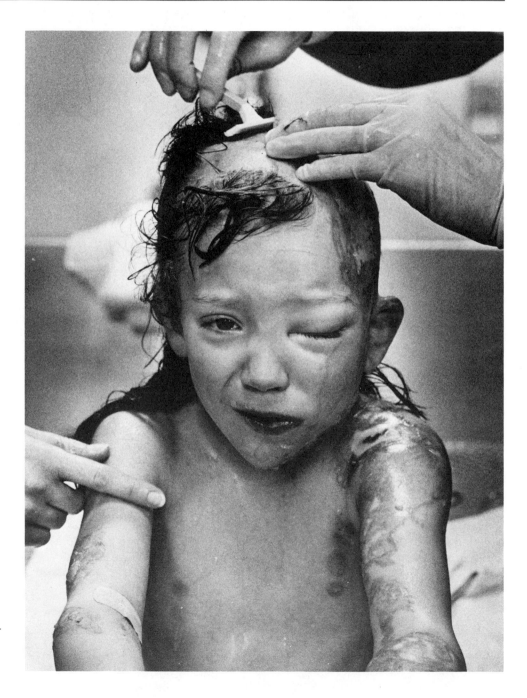

Dr. Tremiti uses a disposable razor to shave away Renee's hair so he can fully assess the extent of her burns.

4

Some of the wounds were leathery to touch. Those were third-degree burns where the nerve endings had been destroyed. Renee felt no pain as Tremiti ran the blade over them.

He threw away one disposable razor and the nurse handed him another.

The second-degree burns were less severe, but acutely sensitive. Renee shrieked as the blade scraped away her burnt skin. She twisted a towel into a ball, pressed it to her face and began to wail.

Tremiti would have calmed her with additional painkillers, but that would have slowed Renee's heart and lungs which were straining to keep blood flowing to her massive wounds. Unless her cardiovascular system continued to work unimpeded, Renee's wounds would get deeper.

Tremiti refastened his mask and took another razor. He came to the delicate parts.

Renee's left eye was swollen shut. The burns on her neck, back and left arm were filling with fluid.

Hideous as it looked, the swelling was a good sign. It meant the burns in those areas were not deep enough to destroy the nerve endings and blood vessels. Renee's body was pumping fluid to these wounds the way it would to any other.

Doctors kept her on a high protein, high calorie intravenous diet. In the eight days before her condition stabilized, the 41-pound 6-year-old used as many calories per day as an adult.

Like most burn victims, Renee's skin was so badly damaged that she had trouble regulating her body temperature. Even a slight chill would have been an additional strain on her respiratory system. The tubbing room is heated to 95 degrees.

Tremiti was slick with sweat.

Renee was convulsed by pain.

The tubbing room walls are soundproofed, but during treatment the screams of burn victims can be heard in the adjacent wing.

Tremiti kept swearing and throwing away the disposable razors.

*　　*　　*　　*　　*

The skin grafts for Renee's face would be taken from the backs of her thighs. In the operating room on the morning of Oct. 27, nurses washed and shaved both her legs.

They cleaned her "donor sites" with a scrub made from Betadine, a sterilizing agent, then coated both thighs with a Betadine solution. They wiped the sites dry with sterile towels, then reapplied the Betadine. In burn surgery, godliness is next to cleanliness.

It had taken eight days for Renee's burned skin to deteriorate completely. Now Dr. Margherite Bonaventura, her surgeon, could be sure which areas needed skin grafts. She would also be able to remove the burned skin more easily. If the grafts were laid correctly, on the fresh tissue beneath the burned skin, they would take hold. Slowly Renee's wounds would repair themselves.

Renee's parents arrived early that morning. They spent the day moving back and forth between the second floor waiting room and the first floor coffee shop, changing the props for their anxious drama every few hours.

Until Renee's accident, the family had led a quiet life in a quiet town. The father was a carpenter. He'd been out of work quite a bit during the worst of the recession, but the building trades had made a comeback around the area and he was doing pretty well now.

The mother was thinking about opening a little beauty parlor on the ground floor of the family's home.

Renee's accident had plunged them into another world: the Medical Center burn unit. For six and a half hours on the day of the operation, the inhabitants of that world would begin the arduous process of making their daughter well again.

The lamps in the operating room threw pale, hot light onto the table. The room was heated to 90 degrees. Renee lay on a thermal blanket.

The operating team listened to WKFM because Bonaventura liked easy listening music better than rock "n" roll during an operation. One of the male nurses sang along.

The first stage of burn surgery is called debridement. Bonaventura began by taking a weck blade, which looks like a small straight razor, and scraping away the burned skin on Renee's left arm and left cheek.

Debridement is like sculpting. Bonaventura had to cut away the charred skin until she reached the fresh layer underneath. She wanted to scrape away all the charred skin, but only the charred skin.

The truest sign of fresh tissue is profuse bleeding, not in rivulets, because that denotes a puncture, but in sheets. Bonaventura sculpted Renee's face and neck until the fresh tissue, slick with blood, shone beneath the heat lamps.

As she worked, her attendants stepped away, one by one, to suck orange juice up a straw through the holes in their masks. They took turns rubbing each other down with alcohol, hoping to stay cool.

Bonaventura's only breaks came when she changed her bloody gloves and surgical garments. She had to do that a dozen times.

After four hours and 30 new weck blades, the doctor had finished debriding Renee's face, left arm and shoulder. Bonaventura and her assistants then lifted the little girl onto a separate gurney so a nurse could change the blood-soaked dressings on the operating table. When she finished, the team turned Renee onto her stomach and delicately placed her back on the table, so Bonaventura could debride her neck, back and head.

When she had finished removing the thick layers of dead skin from Renee's back, Bonaventura began the second stage of the operation, harvesting the skin for grafts.

The harvesting tool is called a dermatome and it works like a sophisticated cheese slicer. While Bill Myers, a registered nurse who served as wound technician, held the skin taut, Bonaventura ran the dermatome across Renee's thighs. The skin peeled off in long thin strips. Surgeons prefer long strips because they reduce scarring.

Bill took the strips from Bonaventura, handling them gingerly and placing them beneath the skin mesher. The mesher looks like a credit card press and works much the same way. It meshes the skin so there are no air bubbles in the grafts. While being perforated, the skin is also stretched so it can cover a greater area. The grafts for Renee's face were not meshed because meshing increases scarring.

While Bill laid the harvested skin on plastic sheets, Bonaventura began to wrap the donor sites in a fine mesh gauze dressed with a weak solution of thrombin, which aids clotting.

The final and most delicate stage of the operation was laying the skin grafts. This was more difficult in Renee's case because there were burns on her face which had to be grafted precisely to keep scarring to a minimum.

Bonaventura studied Renee's face, judging which grafts would best follow the contours of the little girl's cheek and jaw. She had to determine how to cover the area with as few grafts as possible, then cut each graft to fit perfectly. Her tools in this delicate endeavor were a pair of scissors and a sure eye.

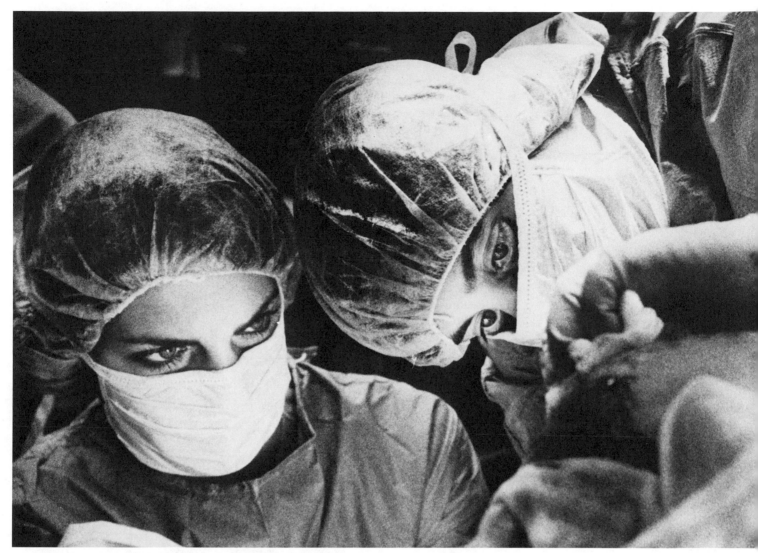

Dr. Bonaventura concentrates on the task of following the contours of Renee's face as she positions each carefully shaped graft.

She laid the grafts gently on Renee's face with a scissors tip, applying just the slightest pressure to keep the new skin in place and smooth the edges where grafts overlapped.

The operation lasted six and a half hours. When it was over, the grafted areas were bandaged with gauze dressed with a saline solution to keep the skin moist.

Renee was wrapped in gauze from head to foot. The bandages weighed six pounds. They not only kept her warm, but also kept the grafts from moving by serving as a cushion against accidental contact. Lying on the operating table, she appeared to be the size of a full-grown adult.

When a patient is moved from burn surgery to recovery, the security guards close the elevators on the floors involved so no one will see the temporary mummy.

A janitorial crew comes in almost immediately to clean the blood-puddled floor.

*   *   *   *   *

Renee awoke in her own room the next morning around 7:30. She had been either sedated or asleep for 27 hours.

*   *   *   *   *

"What's a matter, peach? You just scared of what's gonna go on here?"
"Yes, I'm scared. I wish I was back in my room."
"You won't even know I'm here, I'm gonna do it sooo light."
"I'm colder than a polar bear being soaked."
"A polar bear being soaked?"
"Yeah."
From a sitting position she couldn't see out of the tub without craning her neck. It was a long shiny tunnel where she played with a Smurf in a row boat and waited for her ordeal to start. "Bridge Over Troubled Waters" played on the radio that morning and pain was all around.

The washing was not so bad, but because burns must heal from the inside out, Bill Myers had to pick off Renee's scabs, too. From her thighs he peeled layers of gauze that were caked in dried blood and clung like second skin.

When Bill began to pick at the wounds with the forceps Renee would moan "Caaare-ful." "Caaare-ful."

"Come on," he said as she gripped his hand. "Squeeze that thumb until it turns blue."

When the pain is really bad, it helps to be able to squeeze the strong thumb of nurse Bill Myers.

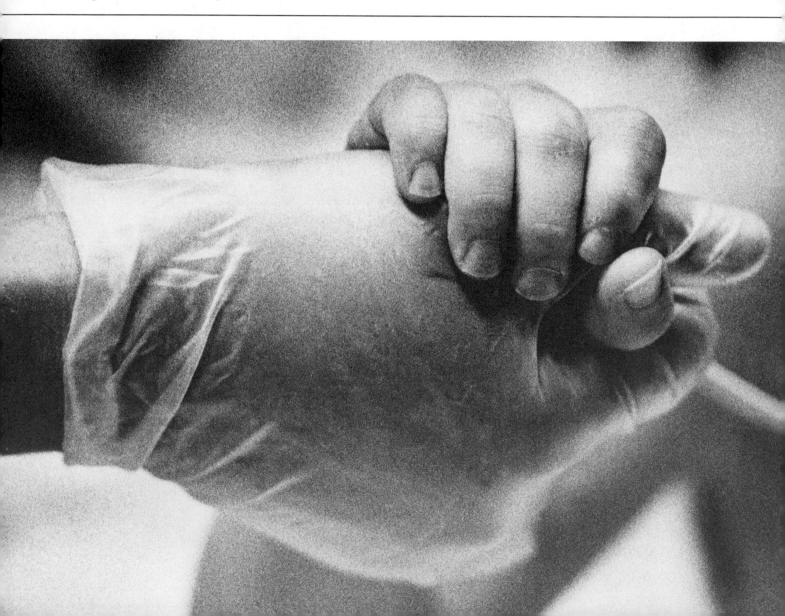

Renee's shrieks came in short bursts as though her breath was being pumped out of her.

"Come on, I can't feel it. Squeeze that thumb."

Shrieking.

"Squeeze it."

More shrieking.

"I can feel it now."

"It stings. It stings. It stings."

"Sorry peach. We have one thing left."

"Can we have a long break then?"

"Very long. Until the black hand gets to the seven."

He'd only been at it a few days when Bill realized that something important was taking place in the tub each morning, something more important even than the slow rejuvenation of Renee's burned skin.

She had always been a shy little girl. All her relatives said so. But morning after morning in the tub, that shyness seemed to be melting away.

It may have been fear that drove her to trust Bill Myers and Debbie Nowack, who cleaned her wounds each morning. It may have been that she loved them for their gentleness when wound care was over. It may even have been pride, for she understood that she was getting better and that that was the right thing to do.

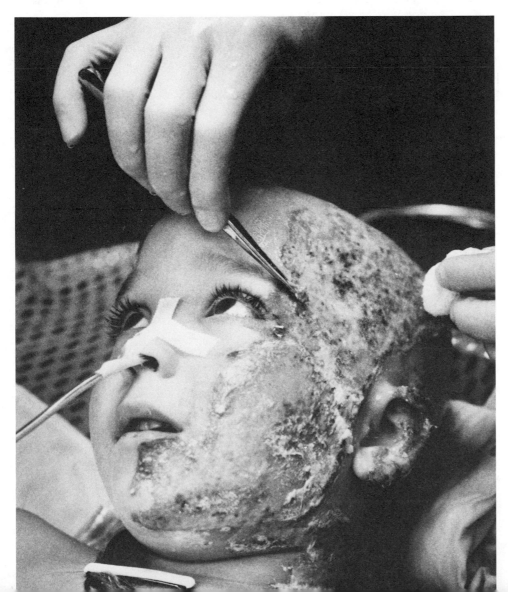

Renee's eyes reveal the depth of trust and rapport which has developed with nurse Bill Myers in spite of painful treatments.

9

Bill used to come in late in the morning and blow up surgical gloves until they looked like the undersides of cows. He and Renee would bat them around for a while, until she got tired. Then, when she was lying flat, he would build a tower of paper cups on the bandages on her forehead, higher and higher until it fell down all around her.

She became more talkative in the tub.

"Can we put on a tiny bandage, cause then it won't take so long?"

"We can't do that, peach."

"When my Mom makes me laugh too much, I hurt a lot."

"It hurts to laugh?"

"No, if I laugh too much. If I laugh when I'm walking or laugh in bed, I get lots of pain."

"Do you know any jokes?"

"Yeah, I hear 'em from my Sesame Street tape. What kind of a dog has no tail?"

"A hot dog. You know, a hot dog. That you eat."

"I should have known that."

"Why did the dodo bird throw the alarm clock out the window?"

"He wanted to see time fly. Want to hear another one?"

*   *   *   *   *

Bonaventura knew right after surgery that Renee would be all right physically. No matter how shrill her screams, Bill knew that the pain she endured each morning had not made her fearful, resentful or withdrawn.

Physical therapy was a problem. The skin on her donor sites stung intensely and the 41-pound, 6-year-old walked around like the hunchback of Notre Dame. But though she struggled with the plastic bowling set and heavy beach ball her therapists set out for her, it was clear that one day soon she would walk normally.

Only one obstacle remained.

On November 1, Bill brought a mirror into Renee's room. He propped it on a table where she could see it. Slowly, he unwrapped the bandages from her face while Renee stared straight ahead.

It was a foregone conclusion that she would cry. The only question was how best to help her get over it. Whether it was best to say it wasn't so bad, or to discuss plastic surgery, or tell her it would smooth out as she grew older.

Everyone in the room studied Renee's face. Nobody studied it more closely than she.

She was bald now, except for a shock of long hair on the back of her head. The left side of her face was enveloped in scars. The last flicker of impetuousness died in her eyes.

She raised her chin slowly to examine her neck, then bit by bit, turned her left cheek to the mirror, then stopped and turned her right cheek to the mirror. She repeated that ritual, as though mesmerized by the movement of her unbandaged face. Suddenly she stopped, and stared vacantly into the reflections of her eyes.

She poked her tongue from the left side of her mouth, trying in vain to lick the corner of her new skin. Withdrawing her tongue, she glanced at nurse Cindy Horton, then back at the mirror.

Her grin took them by surprise. So did the way she lurched forward, thrust a gleeful finger at the mirror and smiled as though seeing this face of hers was a better break than discovering that ponies grew on trees.

*   *   *   *   *

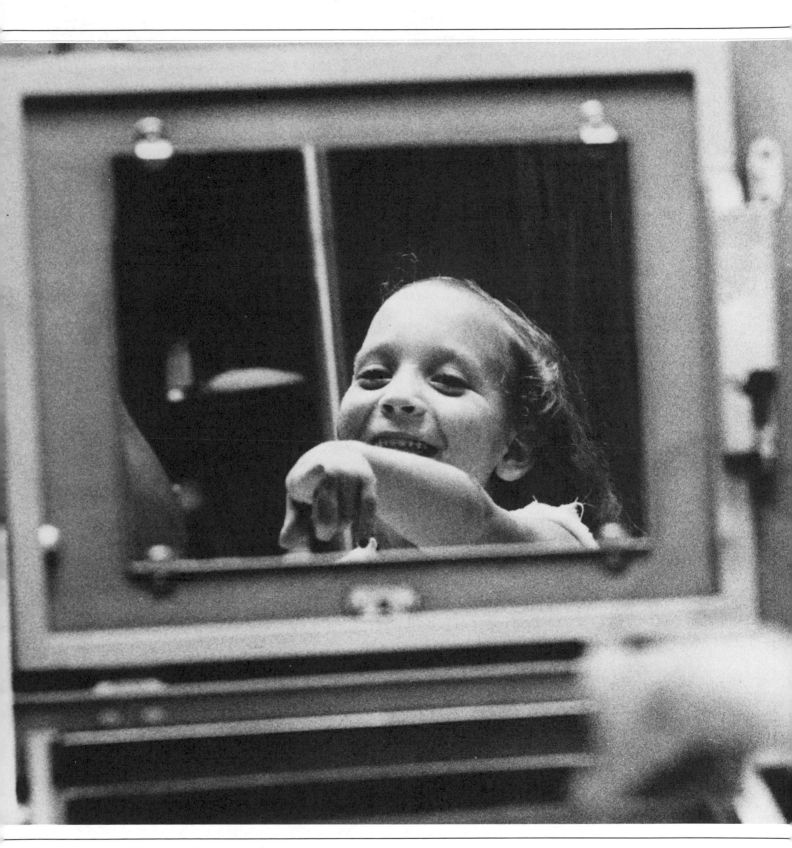

Renee's acceptance of her appearance is the result of the loving support she has received from her family and the hospital personnel.

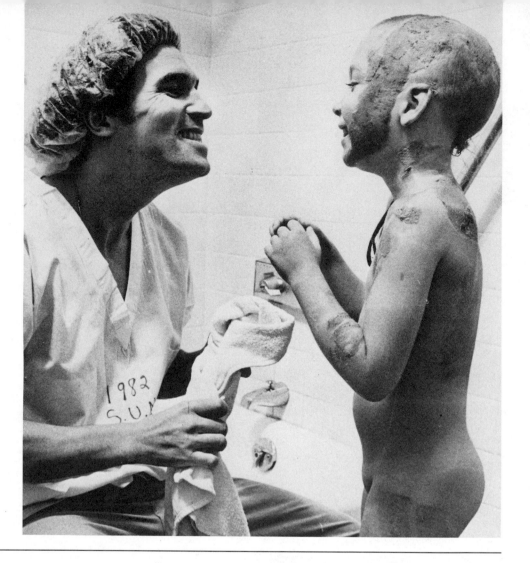

A deal is a deal, and Renee has not forgotten.

On November 9, Renee woke up knowing that she was going home. She knew that after her bath she would put on her best long dress and hurry out to say goodbye to everyone. Under the dress she would wear a Jobst, a nylon body stocking with a mask, that looks like a spider-man costume and helps to control scarring. The Jobst is highly flammable, but she wasn't thinking about worrisome things like that.

She didn't like the idea of taking a wheelchair to the hospital door, but she already knew she could bring Oscar the Grouch along for company.

Her parents were going to take her to her favorite restaurant—McDonald's. But before that, there was one last order of business to be taken care of. On her second day in the hospital Renee had made a deal with Bill that after her final bath, she could push him into the tub where she had withstood so much pain. She had been transferred to the pediatrics ward four days before her release, but she decided that the shallow, standard issue tub she bathed in there would do just fine.

She was quiet through her bath and Bill thought perhaps she had forgotten their deal, but it was the first thing she mentioned when she stepped from the tub.

Bill tried clowning his way out of it, but Renee wasn't about to be distracted. She thrust her hands into his chest and Bill sunk back into the shallow water.

He was drenched by the time he pulled himself from the tub and his hospital whites were matted to his skin. Renee laughed and ran from the room. She thought he looked funny. Like a polar bear being soaked.

Turnabout is fair play!

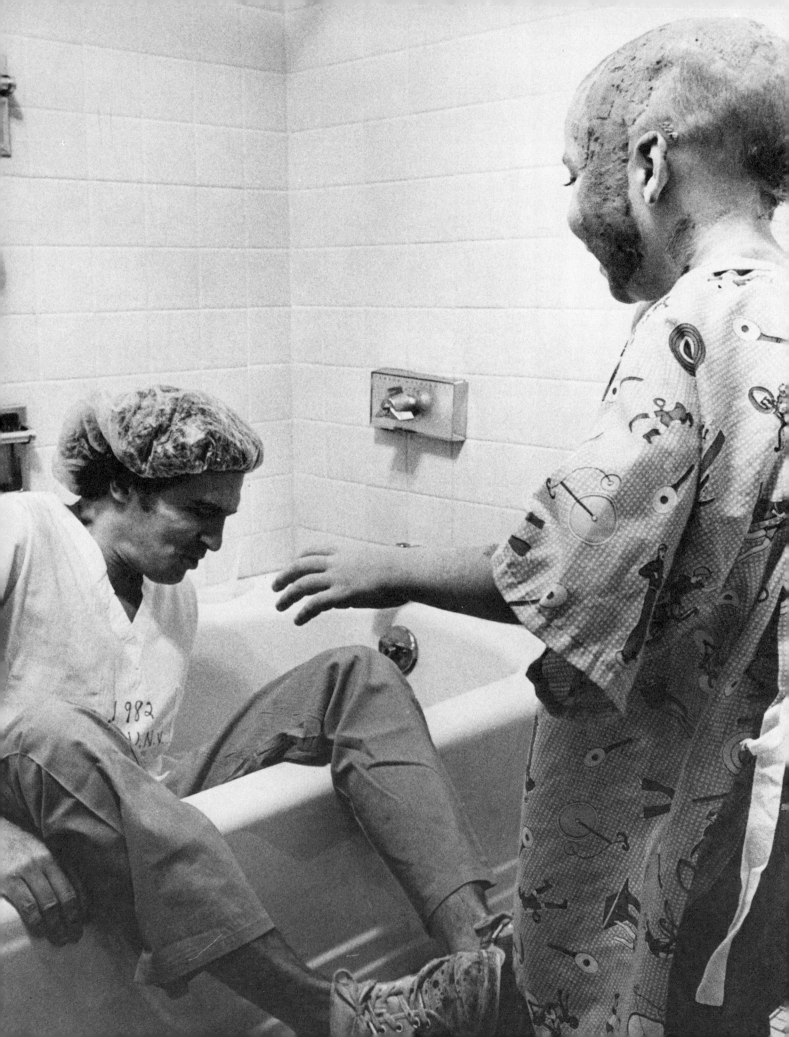

EPILOGUE

On June 7, 1983, Renee gave a lecture to her first-grade classmates.

She'd been planning the big day for more than a month.

Although she'd been back in school since January, Renee hadn't really talked to anyone about her burns. On the last day of school she broke her silence.

That morning she came to school accompanied by her mother and Gabby Liddard, her physical therapist.

First, Gabby showed the class a film strip about fire prevention and let the children handle a doll wearing a Jobst, much like Renee's.

Then Renee talked about fire safety. She told her classmates that if their clothes ever caught on fire, there were three things to remember: Stop, drop, and roll.

When her lecture was over she talked about her experiences at the burn unit. Then, for the first time in public, Renee took off her bandages.

The adults in the room—Gabby, Renee's teacher and photographer Seth Resnick—were expecting the class to gape and gasp, but the children barely seemed to notice. They had accepted Renee's burns months ago.

It has been 15 months since she was burned by boiling grease and Renee is still wearing her Jobst to minimize scarring. Her parents have already contacted plastic surgeons at Shriners Hospital in Boston to discuss the restorative surgery she will need. But because Renee is still growing, and her facial features are still developing, she is not likely to have plastic surgery for six or seven years.

Renee will always be bald on the spots of the third-degree burns. Her hair grows in thickly on the rest of her head and can be styled to minimize the effect.

She returns to the hospital every three months for checkups and to visit her friends in the burn unit.

Her family says the little girl is more personable than ever, probably because of her contact with the burn unit staff.

Visiting the New York State Fair last summer with photographer Seth Resnick, she said that she was glad she made a lot of new friends at the hospital, but she wished she could have done it without getting burned.

Part One

Nursing Practice

1

Nursing as a Profession

Prerequisites and/or Suggested Preparation
There are no prerequisites for this chapter.

THE NATURE OF NURSING

Nursing is without a doubt one of the most *varied, demanding, fulfilling,* and *challenging* of all professions. The nature of nursing has changed over the centuries in response to the needs and conditions of each new era, and it is both frightening and thrilling to contemplate the challenges which will be presented to nursing in the 21st century.

Nursing Is Varied

Nursing is one of the most varied of all professions because the opportunities for practicing nursing are limited only by the interests and dreams of the individual. A nurse may choose to care for a specific group of patients such as premature infants, trauma victims, or the mentally ill. Some individuals use nursing as a mode of entry into foreign service or missionary work. Specialized training makes it possible for a person to become a nurse midwife or nurse anesthetist. Graduate study and a Master's or Doctoral degree makes it possible to combine nursing and an interest in law, politics, or research. Advanced clinical preparation enables a nurse or group of nurses to set up an office and establish a private nursing practice just as a physician sets up a private medical practice.

Nursing Is Demanding

Nursing is a difficult profession; it makes four types of demands upon its members. These demands are clinical

---

Example of an Early Standard for Nursing Practice

THE FLORENCE NIGHTINGALE PLEDGE

I solemnly pledge myself before God and in the presence of this assembly to pass my life in purity and to practice my profession faithfully.

I will abstain from whatever is deleterious and mischievous and will not knowingly take or administer any harmful drug.

I will do all in my power to maintain and elevate the standard of my profession and will hold in confidence all personal matters committed to my keeping and family matters coming to my knowledge in the practice of my calling.

With loyalty will I endeavor to aid the physician in his work, and devote myself to the welfare of those committed to my care.

---

expertise, academic achievement, physical stamina, and personal integrity. *Clinical expertise* is required in order to function safely and effectively in one's chosen field of practice, whether it be at the site of an industrial disaster, on board a hospital ship, or in a highly technical medical center.

Academic achievement provides the theoretical base for a nurse's clinical skills, and makes it possible for the nurse to interact on an equal basis with members of other professions such as law, political science, education, and medicine. *Physical stamina* is important because jobs such as nursing in a trauma center, summer camp, or rehabilitation unit are physically demanding.

Nursing demands *personal integrity* because the nurse receives confidential information from the patient and family, has access to a variety of drugs, must monitor the performance of her peers, and is involved in making increasingly complex ethical decisions.

Nursing Is Challenging

Nursing will be an even more *challenging* profession in the 21st century because of the nursing problems created by medical phenomena such as the increased use of artificial hearts, and breakthroughs in the treatment of mystifying conditions such as AIDS and Alzheimer's disease.

Nurses will need to be assertive, accountable, and willing to take risks as they move into these as yet uncharted dimensions of nursing while continuing to function in traditional and timeless roles. Nursing will make significant contributions toward helping people reach as yet undreamed of levels of wellness, and will continue to strive for a holistic approach to health which will protect the individuality of each person in a health care system which is often impersonal and dehumanizing.

Nursing Is Satisfying

Regardless of the time and place, nursing will always be satisfying, rewarding, and fulfilling to the majority of nurses. The impact of significant experiences does not change over the centuries even though the circumstances may be dramatically different. The thrill of a baby's first cry, and the good feeling of helping a person die in comfort, peace, and dignity are never diminished by the passing of time. Stress, burnout, and frustration will continue to be serious occupational hazards, but they somehow seem less urgent whenever a patient or family member whispers "Thank you, nurse. Thank you."

DEFINITIONS OF NURSING

What is nursing? What is a nurse? Answers to these questions are as elusive today as they were a hundred years ago when Florence Nightingale was overturning the centuries-old concepts of a nurse as either substitute mother, religious worker, or low-paid servant.

Defining nursing is as difficult as defining justice, law, or any other abstract term. It is difficult to define *justice* in such a way that the definition applies equally to both neighborhood and international grievances, and it is difficult to define nursing in a manner that describes nursing both in a developing nation and in the aerospace program. Any definition of nursing is influenced by a number of variables such as geographic location and setting, numbers and functions of nurses in the area, and the perceptions of the person doing the defining. A patient, for example, will define nursing differently than will a nurse, legislator, lawyer, or physician.

For a definition of nursing to be helpful to nurses, it must meet the following criteria:

- *It describes what is unique about nursing and differentiates it from other endeavors.* (Some definitions of nursing sound scholarly but are not very useful because they are equally applicable to other types of helping professions.)

- *It is consistent with current practices and laws relevant to nursing.* (A definition that contradicts or fails to consider legal, ethical, and professional constraints is not useful.)

- *It reflects the beliefs and philosophy of the person or group that wrote it.* (A definition of nursing set forth by the American Nurses' Association, for example, must be endorsed by that group, and a definition by a nursing leader should capture and express the beliefs and philosophy of that person.)

It is not possible to include in this book even a representative sample of the scores of definitions of nursing that have been written over the years. Because definitions of nursing reflect both the writer's personal convictions and the status of nursing at the time of writing, many definitions have become less relevant with the passage of time and have been replaced by more current ones.

One of the most timeless definitions or descriptions of nursing was written by Virginia Henderson, a noted nursing educator, author, researcher, and lecturer. She was asked by the International Council of Nurses in 1958 to describe her concept of basic nursing. Her statement, originally published in pamphlet form in 1961, has won international recognition and acceptance. Some of the currently popular emphases are implied rather than expressed, but her definition is as comprehensive and eloquent today as when it was written a quarter of a century ago.

This classic definition of nursing is printed below, and selections from it are used throughout this chapter as introductions to its various sections.

The unique function of the nurse is to assist the individual, sick or well, in the performance of those activities contributing to health or its recovery (or to peaceful death) that he would perform unaided if he had the necessary strength, will or knowledge. And to do this in such a way as to help him gain independence as rapidly as possible. This aspect of her work, this part of her function, she initiates and controls; of this she is master. In addition she helps the patient to carry out the therapeutic plan as initiated by the physician. She also, as a member of a medical team, helps other members, as they in turn help her, to plan and carry out the total program whether it be for the improvement of health, or the recovery from illness or support in death. No one of the team should make such heavy demands on another member that any one of them is unable to perform his or her unique function. Nor should any member of the medical team be diverted by nonmedical activities such as cleaning, clerking, and filing, as long as his or her special task must be neglected. All members of the team should consider the person (patient) served as the central figure, and should realize that primarily they are all "assisting" him. If the patient does not understand, accept, and participate in the program planned with and for him, the effort of the medical team is largely wasted. The sooner the person can care for himself, find health information, or even carry out prescribed treatments, the better off he is. This concept of the nurse as a substitute for what the patient lacks to make him "complete," "whole," or "independent," by the lack of physical strength, will or knowledge, may seem limited to some. The more one thinks about it, however, the more complex the nurse's function as so defined proves to be. Think how rare is "completeness," or "wholeness" of mind and body: to what extent good health is a matter of heredity, to what extent it is acquired, is controversial but it is generally admitted that intelligence and education tend to parallel health status. If then each man finds "good health" a difficult goal, how much more difficult is it for the nurse to help him reach it: she must, in a sense, get "inside the skin" of each of her patients in order to know what he needs. She is temporarily the consciousness of the unconscious, the love of life for the suicidal, the leg of the amputee, the eyes of the newly blind, a means of locomotion for the infant, knowledge and confidence for the young mother, the "mouthpiece" for those too weak or withdrawn to speak, and so on. (Henderson, 1964).

THE UNIQUENESS OF NURSING

The unique function of the nurse is to assist the individual, sick or well, in the performance of those activities contributing to health or its recovery (or to peaceful death) that he would perform unaided if he had the necessary strength, will or knowledge.

The unique function of the nurse consists of those activities that *differentiate* nursing from the activities of other members of the health care team. Some activities that nurses ascribe to themselves, such as coordination, planning, leading, delegating, and teaching, are common to *all* members of the health care team and therefore do not differentiate nursing from medicine, physical therapy, or social work.

The activities which distinguish nursing from other health professions are determined and defined in three ways: by law, by professional nursing organizations, and by current local practice.

Legal Definitions of Nursing

The first Nurse Practice Act in the United States was passed in 1903, and since that time the practice of nursing has been defined by law in each of the 50 states. The following definition of nursing practice was enacted into law in New York State in 1972 and is an example of a state Nurse Practice Act.

Section 6902
Definition of the Practice of Nursing

The practice of the profession of nursing as a registered professional nurse is defined as diagnosing and treating human responses to actual or potential health problems through such services as case finding, health teaching, health counseling, and provision of care supportive to or restorative of life and well-being, and executing medical regimens prescribed by a licensed or otherwise legally authorized physician or dentist. A nursing regimen shall be consistent with and shall not vary any existing medical regimen.

Nurse practice acts vary from state to state and from country to country, and each nurse is responsible for knowing the legal limits of nursing practice wherever she is employed. Other determinants of nursing practice can be more, but not less, restrictive than state law. *No person, group, or agency can grant the nurse permission to do something that is forbidden by law.*

In addition to differentiating between nursing and other groups of health care workers, legal definitions of nursing form the basis for determining both the independent and dependent aspects of nursing. *Independent* nursing actions are those actions that can be legally ordered and directed by *nurses.* *Dependent* nursing actions are those activities that must be ordered and directed by a *physician.*

Nursing as Described by Its Professional Organizations

The actions of nurses in the United States are guided by two codes: The code of the International Council of Nurses (ICN) and the code of the American Nurses' Association.

ICN Code

The first international code for nurses was adopted in 1953 and was revised in 1965 and again in 1973. The process of developing the code was lengthy and difficult, and the final product was of necessity general in nature so that it would be useful both in the developing nations of the world and in the highly industrialized nations.

ANA Code

In the United States the most specific guidelines for nurses have been developed by the American Nurses' Association. The ANA Code for Nurses was adopted in 1950, just 3 years before the ICN code was accepted, and has been revised periodically. The latest revision was done in 1976. Every nurse has an obligation to learn and follow the ANA code of ethics because any nurse who violates the code can be reprimanded, censored, suspended, or expelled from ANA membership. Such sanctions are serious but they are necessary to ensure the highest quality of nursing care and professional standards.

The ANA code is printed in its entirety below because it is essential that each nurse understand the professional guidelines which are basic to all aspects of nursing practice. Questions related to the use of the code in a specific situation can be addressed to the ANA or to any state nurses' association office.

ANA CODE FOR NURSES WITH INTERPRETIVE STATEMENTS

1. THE NURSE PROVIDES SERVICES WITH RESPECT FOR HUMAN DIGNITY AND THE UNIQUENESS OF THE CLIENT UNRESTRICTED BY CONSIDERATIONS OF SOCIAL OR ECONOMIC STATUS, PERSONAL ATTRIBUTES, OR THE NATURE OF HEALTH PROBLEMS.

1.1 SELF-DETERMINATION OF CLIENTS. Whenever possible, clients should be fully involved in the planning and implementation of their own health care. Each client has the moral right to determine what will be done with his/her person; to be given the information nec-

---

ICN Code for Nurses—Ethical Concepts Applied to Nursing

The fundamental responsibility of the nurse is fourfold: to promote health, to prevent illness, to restore health and to alleviate suffering.

The need for nursing is universal. Inherent in nursing is respect for life, dignity and rights of man. It is unrestricted by considerations of nationality, race, creed, color, age, sex, politics or social status.

Nurses render health services to the individual, the family and the community and coordinate their services with those of related groups.

NURSES AND PEOPLE

The nurse's primary responsibility is to those people who require nursing care.

The nurse, in providing care, promotes an environment in which the values, customs and spiritual beliefs of the individual are respected.

The nurse holds in confidence personal information and uses judgment in sharing this information.

NURSES AND PRACTICE

The nurse carries personal responsibility for nursing practice and for maintaining competence by continual learning.

The nurse maintains the highest standards of nursing care possible within the reality of a specific situation.

The nurse uses judgment in relation to individual competence when accepting and delegating responsibilities.

The nurse when acting in a professional capacity should at all times maintain standards of personal conduct which reflect credit upon the profession.

NURSES AND SOCIETY

The nurse shares with other citizens the responsibility for initiating and supporting action to meet the health and social needs of the public.

NURSES AND CO-WORKERS

The nurse sustains a cooperative relationship with co-workers in nursing and other fields.

The nurse takes appropriate action to safeguard the individual when his care is endangered by a coworker or any other person.

NURSES AND THE PROFESSION

The nurse plays the major role in determining and implementing desirable standards of nursing practice and nursing education.

The nurse is active in developing a core of professional knowledge.

The nurse, acting through the professional organization, participates in establishing and maintaining equitable social and economic working conditions in nursing.

---

essary for making informed judgments; to be told the possible effects of care; and to accept, refuse, or terminate treatment. These same rights apply to minors and others not legally qualified and must be respected to the fullest degree permissible under the law. The law in these areas may differ from state to state; each nurse has an obligation to be knowledgeable about and to protect and support the moral and legal rights of all clients under state laws and applicable federal laws, such as the 1974 Privacy Act.

The nurse must also recognize those situations in which individual rights to self-determination in health care may temporarily be altered for the common good. The many variables involved make it imperative that each case be considered with full awareness of the need to provide for informed judgments while preserving the rights of clients.

1.2 SOCIAL AND ECONOMIC STATUS OF CLIENTS. The need for nursing care is universal, cutting across all national,

ethnic, religious, cultural, political, and economic differences, as does nursing's responses to this fundamental need. Nursing care should be determined solely by human need, irrespective of background, circumstances, or other indices of individual social and economic status.

1.3 PERSONAL ATTRIBUTES OF CLIENTS. Age, sex, race, color, personality, or other personal attributes, as well as individual differences in background, customs, attitudes, and beliefs, influence nursing practice only insofar as they represent factors the nurse must understand, consider, and respect in tailoring care to personal needs and in maintaining the individual's self-respect and dignity. Consideration of individual value systems and lifestyles should be included in the planning of health care for each client.

1.4 THE NATURE OF HEALTH PROBLEMS. The nurse's respect for the worth and dignity of the individual human being applies irrespective of the nature of the health problem. It is reflected in the care given the person who is disabled as well as the normal; the patient with the long-term illness as well as the one with the acute illness, or the recovering patient as well as the one who is terminally ill or dying. It extends to all who require the services of the nurse for the promotion of health, the prevention of illness, the restoration of health, and the alleviation of suffering.

The nurse's concern for human dignity and the provision of quality nursing care is not limited by personal attitudes or beliefs. If personally opposed to the delivery of care in a particular case because of the nature of the health problem or the procedures to be used, the nurse is justified in refusing to participate. Such refusal should be made known in advance and in time for other appropriate arrangements to be made for the client's nursing care. If the nurse must knowingly enter such a case under emergency circumstances or enters unknowingly, the obligation to provide the best possible care is observed. The nurse withdraws from this type of situation only when assured that alternative sources of nursing care are available to the client. If a client requests information or counsel in an area that is legally sanctioned but contrary to the nurse's personal beliefs, the nurse may refuse to provide these services but must advise the client of sources where such service is available.

1.5 THE SETTING FOR HEALTH CARE. The nurse adheres to the principle of non-discriminatory, non-prejudicial care in every employment setting or situation and endeavors to promote its acceptance by others. The nurse's readiness to accord respect to clients and to render or obtain needed services should not be limited by the setting, whether nursing care is given in an acute care hospital, nursing home, drug or alcoholic treatment center, prison, patient's home, or other setting.

1.6 THE DYING PERSON. As the concept of death and ways of dealing with it changes, the basic human values remain. The ethical problems posed, however, and the decision-making responsibilities of the patient, family, and professional are increased.

The nurse seeks ways to protect these values while working with the client and others to arrive at the best decisions dictated by the circumstances, the client's rights and wishes, and the highest standards of care. The measures used to provide assistance should enable the client to live with as much comfort, dignity, and freedom from anxiety and pain as possible. The client's nursing care will determine to a great degree how this final human experience is lived and the peace and dignity with which death is approached.

2. THE NURSE SAFEGUARDS THE CLIENT'S RIGHT TO PRIVACY BY JUDICIOUSLY PROTECTING INFORMATION OF A CONFIDENTIAL NATURE.

2.1 DISCLOSURE TO THE HEALTH TEAM. It is an accepted standard of nursing practice that data about the health status of clients be accessible, communicated, and recorded. Provision of quality health services requires that such data be available to all members of the health team. When knowledge gained in confidence is relevant or essential to others involved in planning or implementing the client's care, professional judgment is used in sharing it. Only information pertinent to a client's treatment and welfare is disclosed and only to those directly concerned with the client's care. The rights, well-being, and safety of the individual client should be the determining factors in arriving at this decision.

2.2 DISCLOSURE FOR QUALITY ASSURANCE PURPOSES. Patient information required to document the appropriateness, necessity, and quality of care that is required for peer review, third party payment, and other quality assurance mechanisms must be disclosed only under rigidly defined policies, mandates, or protocols. These written guidelines must assure that the confidentiality of client information is maintained.

2.3 DISCLOSURE TO OTHERS NOT INVOLVED IN THE CLIENT'S CARE. The right of privacy is an inalienable right of all persons, and the nurse has a clear obligation to safeguard any confidential information about the client acquired from any source. The nurse-client relationship is built on trust. This relationship could be destroyed and the client's welfare and reputation jeopardized by injudicious disclosure of information provided in confidence. Since the concept of confidentiality has legal as well as ethical implications, an inappropriate breach of confidentiality may also expose the nurse to liability.

2.4 DISCLOSURE IN A COURT OF LAW. Occasionally, the nurse may be obligated to give testimony in a court of law in relation to confidential information about a client. This should be done only under proper authorization or legal compulsion. Privilege in relation to the disclosure of such information is a legal right that only the patient or his representative may claim or waive. The statutes governing privilege and the exceptions to them vary from state to state, and the nurse may wish to consult legal counsel before testifying in court to be fully informed about professional rights and responsibilities.

2.5 ACCESS TO RECORDS. If, in the course of providing care, there is need for acccess to the records of persons not under the nurse's care, as may be the case in relation to the records of the mother of a newborn, the person should be notified and permission first obtained whenever possible. Although records belong to the agency where collected, the individual maintains the right of control over the information provided by him, his family, and his environment. Similarly, professionals may exercise the right of control over information generated by them in the course of health care.

If the nurse wishes to use a client's treatment record for research or nonclinical purposes in which confidential information may be identified, the client's consent must first be obtained. Ethically, this ensures the client's right to privacy; legally, it serves to protect the client against unlawful invasion of privacy and the nurse against liability for such action.

3. THE NURSE ACTS TO SAFEGUARD THE CLIENT AND THE PUBLIC WHEN HEALTH CARE AND SAFETY ARE AFFECTED BY INCOMPETENT, UNETHICAL, OR ILLEGAL PRACTICE OF ANY PERSON.

3.1 ROLE OF ADVOCATE. The nurse's primary commitment is to the client's care and safety. Hence, in the role of client advocate, the nurse must be alert to and take appropriate action regarding any instances of incompetent, unethical, or illegal practice(s) by any member of the health care team or the health care system itself, or any action on the part of others that is prejudicial to the client's best interests. To function effectively in the role, the nurse should be fully aware of the state laws governing practice in the health care field and the employing institution's policies and procedures in relation to incompetent, unethical, or illegal practice.

3.2 INITIAL ACTION. When the nurse is aware of inappropriate or questionable conduct in the provision of health care, concern should be expressed to the person carrying out the questionable practice and attention called to the possible detrimental effect upon the client's welfare. When factors in the health care delivery system threaten the welfare of the client, similar action should be directed to the responsible administrative person. If indicated, the practice should then be reported to the appropriate authority within the institution, agency, or larger system.

There should be an established mechanism for the reporting and handling of incompetent, unethical, or illegal practice within the employment setting so that such reporting can go through official channels and be done without fear of reprisal. The nurse should be knowledgeable about the mechanism and be prepared

to utilize it if necessary. When questions are raised about the appropriateness of behaviors of individual practitioners or practices of health care systems, documentation of the observed behavior or practice must be provided in writing to the appropriate authorities. Local units of the professional association should be prepared to provide assistance and support in reporting procedures.

3.3 FOLLOW-UP ACTION. When incompetent, unethical, or illegal practice on the part of anyone concerned with the client's care is not corrected within the employment setting and continues to jeopardize the client's care and safety, additional steps need to be taken, The problem should be reported to other appropriate authorities such as the practice committees of the appropriate professional organizations or the legally constituted bodies concerned with licensing of specific categories of health workers or professional practitioners. Some situations may warrant the concern and involvement of all these groups. Reporting should be both factual and objective.

3.4 PEER REVIEW. In addition to the role of advocate, the nurse should participate in the planning, establishment, and implementation of other activities or procedures which serve to safeguard clients. Duly constituted peer review activities in employment agencies directed toward the improvement of practice are one example. This ongoing method of review is based on objective criteria, it includes a mechanism for making recommendations to administrators for correction of deficiencies, it facilitates the improvement of delivery services, and it promotes the health, welfare, and safety of clients.

4. THE NURSE ASSUMES RESPONSIBILITY AND ACCOUNTABILITY FOR INDIVIDUAL NURSING JUDGMENTS AND ACTIONS.

4.1 ACCEPTANCE OF RESPONSIBILITY AND ACCOUNTABILITY. The recipients of professional nursing services are entitled to high quality nursing care. Individual professional licensure is the protective mechanism legislated by the public to ensure basic and minimum competencies of the professional nurse. Beyond that, society has accorded to the nursing profession the right to regulate its own practice. The regulation and control of nursing practice by nurses demands that individual professional practitioners of nursing bear primary responsibility for the nursing care clients receive and be individually accountable for their practice.

4.2 RESPONSIBILITY. Responsibility refers to the scope of functions and duties associated with a particular role assumed by the nurse. As nursing assumes functions, these functions become part of the responsibilities or expectations of performance of nurses. Areas of responsibilities expected of nurses include: data collection and assessment of the health status of the client; determination of the nursing care plan directed toward designated goals; evaluation of the effectiveness of nursing care in achieving the goals of care; and subsequent reassessment and revision of the nursing care plan as defined in the ANA Standards of Nursing Practice. By assuming these responsibilities, the nurse is held accountable for them.

4.3 ACCOUNTABILITY. Accountability refers to being answerable to someone for something one has done. It means providing an explanation to self, to the client, to the employing agency, and to the nursing profession. Over and above the obligations such accountability imposes on the individual nurse, there is also a liability dimension to accountability. The nurse may be called to account to be held legally responsible for judgments exercised and actions taken in the course of nursing practice. Neither physician's prescriptions nor the employing agency's policies relieve the nurse of ethical or legal accountability for actions taken and judgments made. Accountability, therefore, requires evaluation of the effectiveness of one's performance of nursing responsibilities.

4.4 EVALUATION OF PERFORMANCE

Self-evaluation. The nurse engages in ongoing evaluation of individual clinical competence, decision-making abilities, and professional judgments. The nurse also engages in activities that will improve current practice. Self-evaluation carries with it the responsibility for the continuous improvement of one's nursing practice.

Evaluation by peers. Evaluation of one's performance by peers is a hallmark of professionalism, and it is primarily through this mechanism that the profession is held accountable to society. The nurse must be willing to have practice reviewed and evaluated by peers. Guidelines for evaluating the appropriateness, effectiveness, and efficiency of nursing practice are emerging in the form of revised and updated nurse practice acts, ANA's Standards of Nursing Practice, and other quality assurance mechanisms. Participation in the development of objective criteria for evaluation that provide valid and reliable data is the responsibility of each nurse.

5. THE NURSE MAINTAINS COMPETENCE IN NURSING.

5.1 PERSONAL RESPONSIBILITY FOR COMPETENCE. Nursing is concerned with the welfare of human beings, and the nature of nursing is such that inadequate or incompetent practice may jeopardize the client. Therefore, it is the personal responsibility and must be the personal commitment of each individual nurse to maintain competence in practice throughout a professional career. This represents one way in which the nurse fulfills accountability to clients.

5.2 MEASUREMENT OF COMPETENCE IN NURSING PRACTICE. Competence is a relative term, and an individual's competence in any field may be diminished or otherwise affected by the passage of time and the emergence of new knowledge. This means that for the client's optimum well-being and for the nurse's own professional development, nursing care should reflect and incorporate new techniques and knowledge in health care as these develop and especially as they relate to the nurse's particular field of practice.

Measures of competence are developing; they include peer review criteria, outcome criteria, and ANA's program for certification.

5.3 CONTINUING EDUCATION FOR CONTINUING COMPETENCE. Nursing knowledge, like that in the other health disciplines, is rendered rapidly obsolete by mounting technological advances and scientific discoveries, changing concepts and patterns in the provision of health services, and the increasing complexity of nursing responsibilities. The nurse, therefore, should be aware of the need for continuous updating and expansion of the body of knowledge and skills current. The nurse should assess personal learning needs, should be active in finding appropriate resources, and should be skilled in self-directed learning. Such continuing education is the key to maintenance of individual competence.

5.4 INTRAPROFESSIONAL RESPONSIBILITY FOR COMPETENCE IN NURSING CARE. All nurses, be they practitioners, educators, administrators, or researchers, share responsibility for quality nursing care. Therefore all nurses need thorough knowledge of the current scope of professional nursing practice. Advances in theory and practice made by one professional must be disseminated to colleagues. Since individual competencies vary in relation to educational preparation, experience, client population and setting, when necessary, nurses should refer clients to and/or consult with other nurses with expertise and recognized competencies, e.g. certified nurses and clinical specialists.

6. THE NURSE EXERCISES INFORMED JUDGMENT AND USES IN-DIVIDUAL COMPETENCE AND QUALIFICATIONS AS CRITERIA IN SEEKING CONSULTATION, ACCEPTING RESPONSIBILITIES, AND DELEGATING NURSING ACTIVITIES TO OTHERS.

6.1 CHANGING FUNCTIONS. Because of the increased complexity of health care, changing patterns in the delivery of health services, continuing shortages in skilled health manpower, and the development acceptance of evolving nursing roles, nurses are being requested or expected to carry out functions that have formerly been performed by physicians. In turn, nurses are assigning some nursing functions to variously prepared ancillary personnel. In this gradual shift of functions, as the scope of practice of each profession changes, the nurse must exercise judgment in seeking consultation, accepting responsibilities, and assigning responsibilities to others to ensure that clients receive quality care at all times.

6.2 JOINT POLICY STATEMENTS. Nurse practice acts are usually expressed in broad and general language in order to provide the necessary freedom for interpretation of the law so that future developments, new knowledge, and changing roles will not necesssitate constant revision of the law. The nurse must not engage in practice prohibited by law or delegate to others activities prohibited by practice acts of other health care personnel or by other laws.

Recognition by nurses of the need for a more definitive delineation of roles and responsibilities, however, has resulted in collaborative efforts to develop joint policy statements. These statements may involve other health care providers or associations and usually specify the functions that are agreed upon as appropriate and proper for the nurse to perform. Such statements represent a body of expert judgment that can be used as authority where responsibilities are not definitively outlined by legal statute.

6.3 SEEKING CONSULTATION. The provision of health and illness care to clients is a complex process that requires a wide range of knowledge and skills. Interdisciplinary team effort with shared responsibility is the most effective approach to provision of total health services. Nurses, whether practicing in clearly defined or new and emerging roles, must be aware of their own individual competencies. When the needs of the client are beyond the qualifications and competencies of the nurse, consultation must be sought from qualified nurses or other appropriate sources.

Discretion must be exercised by the nurse before intervening in diagnostic or therapeutic matters that are not recognized by the nursing profession as established

nursing practice. Such discretion should be based on education, experience, legal parameters, and professional guidelines and policies.

6.4 ACCEPTING RESPONSIBILITIES OR DELEGATING ACTIVITIES. The nurse should look to mutually agreed upon policy statements for guidance and direction; but even where such statements exist, personal competence should be carefully assessed before accepting responsibility or delegating activities. Decisions in this area call for knowledge of and adherence to joint policy statements and the laws regulating medical and nursing practice as well as for the exercise of informed nursing judgments.

6.5 ACCEPTING RESPONSIBILITY. If the nurse does not feel personally competent or adequately prepared to carry out a specific function, the nurse has the right and responsibility to refuse. In so doing, both the client and the nurse are protected. The reverse is also true. The nurse should not accept delegated responsibilities that do not utilize nursing skill or competencies or that prevent the provision of needed nursing care to clients. Inasmuch as the nurse is responsible for the client's total nursing care, the nurse must also assess individual competence in assigning selected components of that care to other nursing service personnel. The nurse should not delegate to any member of the nursing team a function for which that person is not prepared or qualified to perform.

7. THE NURSE PARTICIPATES IN ACTIVITIES THAT CONTRIBUTE TO THE ONGOING DEVELOPMENT OF THE PROFESSION'S BODY OF KNOWLEDGE.

7.1 THE NURSE AND RESEARCH. Every profession must engage in systematic inquiry to identify, verify, and continually enlarge the body of knowledge which forms the foundations for its practice. A unique body of verified knowledge provides both framework and direction for the profession in all of its activities and for the practitioner in the provision of nursing care. The accrual of knowledge promotes the advancement of practice and with it the well-being of the profession's clients. Ongoing research is thus indispensable to the full discharge of a profession's obligation to society. Each nurse has a role in this area of professional activity, whether involved as an investigator in the furthering of knowledge, as a participant in research, or as a user of research results.

7.2 GENERAL GUIDELINES FOR PARTICIPATING IN RESEARCH.

Before participating in research the nurse has an obligation:

1. To ascertain that the study design has been approved by an appropriate body.
2. To obtain information about the intent and nature of the research.
3. To determine whether the research is consistent with professional goals.

Research involving human subjects should be conducted only by scientifically qualified persons or under such supervision. The nurse who participates in research in any capacity should be fully informed about both nurse and client rights and responsibilities as set forth in the publication *Human Rights Guidelines for Nurses in Clinical and Other Research prepared by the ANA Commission on Nursing Research.*

7.3 THE PROTECTION OF HUMAN RIGHTS IN RESEARCH. The individual rights valued by society and by the nursing profession have been fully outlined and discussed in *Human Rights Guidelines for Nurses in Clinical and Other Research*; namely, the right to freedom from intrinsic risks of injury and the rights of privacy and dignity. Inherent in these rights is respect for each individual to exercise self-determination, to choose to participate, to have full information, to terminate participation without penalty.

It is the duty of both the investigator and the nurse participating in research to maintain vigilance in protecting the life, health, and privacy of human subjects from unanticipated as well as anticipated risks. The subjects' integrity, privacy, and rights must be especially safeguarded if they are unable to protect themselves because of incapacity or because they are in a dependent relationship to the investigator. The investigation should be discontinued if its continuance might be harmful to the subject.

7.4 THE PRACTITIONER'S RIGHTS AND RESPONSIBILITIES IN RESEARCH. Practitioners of nursing providing care to clients who serve as human subjects for research have a special need to clearly understand in advance how the research can be expected to affect treatment and their own moral and legal responsibilities to clients. Here, as in other problematic situations, the practitioner has the right not to participate or to withdraw under the circumstances described in paragraph 1.4 of this document. More detailed guidance about the rights and responsibilities of nurses in relation to research activities may be found in *Human Rights Guidelines for Nurses in Clinical and Other Research.*

8. THE NURSE PARTICIPATES IN THE PROFESSION'S EFFORTS TO IMPLEMENT AND IMPROVE STANDARDS OF NURSING.

8.1 RESPONSIBILITY TO THE PUBLIC. Nursing has the responsibility to admit to the profession only those who have demonstrated a capacity for those competencies believed essential to the practice of nursing. Areas of concern for nursing competence should include adequate performance of nursing skills, academic achievement, humanitarian concern for others, acceptance of responsibility for individual actions, and the desire to improve nursing practice. Nurses involved in the evaluation of student attainment carry a primary responsibility for ensuring that the profession's obligation(s) to the public relative to entry qualifications for practice are met.

The nursing profession exists to give assistance to those persons needing nursing care. Standards of nursing practice provide guidance for the delivery of quality nursing care and are a means for evaluating that care received by clients. The nurse has a responsibility to the public for personally implementing and maintaining optimal standards.

8.2 RESPONSIBILITY TO THE DISCIPLINE. The professional practice of nursing is founded on an understanding and application of a body of knowledge reflected in its standards. As the profession's organization for nurses, ANA had adopted standards for nursing practice, nursing service, and nursing education. The nurse has the responsibility to monitor these standards in everyday practice and through voluntary participation in the profession's ongoing efforts to implement and improve standards at the national, state, and local levels.

8.3 RESPONSIBILITY TO NURSING STUDENTS. The future of nursing rests with new recruits to the profession. Nursing has a responsibility to maintain optimal standards of nursing practice and education in schools of nursing and/or wherever students engage in learning activity. This places a particular responsibility on all nurses whose services are concerned with the educational process.

9. THE NURSE PARTICIPATES IN THE PROFESSION'S EFFORTS TO ESTABLISH AND MAINTAIN CONDITIONS OF EMPLOYMENT CONDUCIVE TO HIGH QUALITY NURSING CARE.

9.1 RESPONSIBILITY FOR CONDITIONS OF EMPLOYMENT. The nurse must be concerned with conditions of economic and general welfare within the profession. These are important determinants in the recruitment and retention of well-qualified personnel and in assuring that each practitioner has the opportunity to function optimally.

The provision of high quality nursing care is the responsibility of both the individual nurse and the nursing profession. Professional autonomy and self-regulation in the control of conditions of practice are necessary to implement standards of practice as established by organized nursing.

9.2 COLLECTIVE ACTION. Defining and controlling the quality of nursing care provided to the client is most effectively accomplished through collective action. Collective action may include assistance and representation from the professional association in negotiations with employers to achieve employment conditions in which the professional standards of practice can be implemented and which are commensurate with the qualifications, functions, and responsibilities of the nurse.

The Economic and General Welfare program of the professional association is the appropriate channel through which the nurse can work constructively, ethically, and with professional dignity. This program, encompassing commitment to the principle of collective bargaining, promotes the right and responsibility of the individual nurse to participate in determining the terms and conditions of employment conducive to high quality nursing practice.

9.3 INDIVIDUAL ACTION. A nurse may enter into an agreement with individuals or organizations to provide health care, provided that the agreement is in accordance with the Standards of Nursing Practice of the American Nurses' Association and the nurse practice law of the state and provided that the agreement does not permit or compel practices which are in violation of this Code.

10. THE NURSE PARTICIPATES IN THE PROFESSION'S EFFORT TO PROTECT THE PUBLIC FROM MISINFORMATION AND MISREPRESENTATION AND TO MAINTAIN THE INTEGRITY OF NURSING.

10.1 ADVERTISING SERVICES. A nurse may make factual statements that indicate availability of services through means that are in dignified form, such as:

- A professional card identifying the nurse by name and title, giving address, telephone number, and other pertinent data.
- Listing name, title, and brief biography in reputable directories and reputable professional publications. Such published data may include the following: Name, address, phone, field of practice or concentrates; date and place of birth; schools attended, with dates of graduation, degrees, and other scholastic distinctions; offices held; public or professional honors; teaching positions; publications; memberships and activites in professional societies; licenses; names and addresses of references.

A nurse shall not use any form of public or professional communication to make self-laudatory statements or claims that are false, fraudulent, misleading, deceptive, or unfair.

10.2 USE OF TITLES AND SYMBOLS. The right to use the title "Registered Nurse" is granted by state governments through licensure by examination for the protection of the public. Use of that title carries with it the responsibility to act in the public interest. The nurse may use the title "R.N." and symbols of academic degrees or other earned or honorary professional symbols of recognition in all ways that are legal and appropriate. The title and other symbols of the profession should not be used, however, for personal benefit by the nurse or by those who may seek to exploit them for other purposes.

10.3 ENDORSEMENT OF COMMERCIAL PRODUCTS OR SERVICES. The nurse does not give or imply endorsement to advertising, promotion, or sale of commercial products or services because this may be interpreted as reflecting the opinion or judgment of the profession as a whole. Since it is a nursing responsibility to engage in health teaching and to advise clients on matters relating to their health, it is not unethical for the nurse to utilize knowledge of specific services and/or products in advising individual clients. In the course of providing information or education to clients or other practitioners about commercial products or services, however, a variety of similar products or services should be offered or described so that the client or practitioner can make an informed choice.

10.4 PROTECTING THE CLIENT FROM HARMFUL PRODUCTS. It is the responsibility of the nurse to advise clients against the use of dangerous products. This is seen as discharge of nursing functions when undertaken in the best interest of the client.

10.5 REPORTING INFRACTIONS. Not only should the nurse personally adhere to the above principles, but alertness to any instances of their violation by others should be maintained. The nurse should report promptly, through appropriate channels, any advertisement or commercial which involves a nurse, implies involvement, or in any way suggests nursing endorsement of a commercial product, service, or enterprise. The nurse who knowingly becomes involved in such unethical activities negates professional responsibility for personal gain, and jeopardizes the public confidence and trust in the nursing profession that have been created by generations of nurses working together in the public interest.

11. THE NURSE COLLABORATES WITH MEMBERS OF THE HEALTH PROFESSIONS AND OTHER CITIZENS IN PROMOTING COMMUNITY AND NATIONAL EFFORTS TO MEET THE HEALTH NEEDS OF THE PUBLIC.

11.1 QUALITY HEALTH CARE AS A RIGHT. Quality health care is mandated as a right to all citizens. Availability and accessibility to quality health services for all citizens require collaborative planning by health providers and consumers at both the local and national levels. Nursing care is an integral part of quality health care, and nurses have a responsibility to help ensure that citizens' rights to health care are met.

11.2 RESPONSIBILITY TO THE CONSUMER OF HEALTH CARE. The nurse is a member of the largest group of health providers, and therefore the philosophies and goals of the nursing profession should have a significant impact on the consumer of health care. An effective way of ensuring that nurses' views regarding health care and nursing service are properly represented is by involvement of nurses in political decision making.

11.3 RELATIONSHIPS WITH OTHER DISCIPLINES. The complexity of the delivery of health care service demands an interdisciplinary approach to delivery of health services as well as strong support from allied health occupations. The nurse should actively seek to promote collaboration needed for ensuring the quality of health services to all persons.

11.4 RELATIONSHIP WITH MEDICINE. The interdependent relationship of the nursing and medical professions requires collaboration around the need of the client. The evolving role of the nurse in the health delivery system requires joint practice as colleagues, deliberations in determining functional relationships, and differentiating areas of practice between the two professions.

11.5 CONFLICT OF INTEREST. Nurses who provide public service and who have financial or other interests in health care facilities or services should avoid a conflict of interest by refraining from casting a vote on any deliberation affecting the public's health care needs in those areas.

Nursing Defined by Current Local Practice

In addition to the guidelines provided by legal definitions of nursing and by professional codes, nursing practice is further defined by the practice setting. In remote rural areas, where the nurse is the only health care worker within hundreds of square miles, she may be expected to assume responsibilities that would not be required in a medical center. She might, for example, be expected to report her observations of an acutely ill patient by radio to a physician many miles away, help establish a working diagnosis, and carry out his prescribed therapy without the protection and benefit of written orders and a documented medical diagnosis. The responsibilities of a nurse who has a private practice of her own will differ from those of a nurse in a physician's office or hospital, though both are bound by state law and professional codes.

Advanced, specialized education and training often enable a nurse to assume additional responsibilities. A few states in the United States, for example, now permit nurses with special certification to prescribe medications, although this has long been recognized almost universally as the privilege and responsibility of the physician. New roles for nurses such as primary care provider and clinical nurse specialist influence local practice and eventually lead to changes in both professional and legal definitions of nursing.

Individual Definitions of Nursing

Legal and professional definitions of nursing tend to describe an optimal level of *current nursing practice*, whereas individual nurses often describe nursing in terms of their perception of *what nursing could or should be*. Such definitions are frequently abstract and idealistic or visionary. They are inspirational and provide a goal toward which nurses can strive. Individual definitions are sometimes controversial because they often reflect the definer's strong preference for a holistic, humanistic, scientific, or other approach to nursing. Such definitions are often used by a group of like-minded people as a basis for a conceptual framework for nursing practice and the development of nursing curricula.

AUTONOMY AND ACCOUNTABILITY IN NURSING

This aspect of her work, this part of her function, she initiates and controls; of this she is master.

Nursing is emerging from its sheltered and subservient position as a subbranch of medicine and is moving toward a position of autonomy and equality. The transition from "handmaiden of the physician" to colleague of the physician has been slow and has often been both risky and painful. It is difficult to alter the traditional relationships between nursing and medicine and to change some long-established male-female interdisciplinary relationships.

In the past, the adjectives used to describe the stereotype of an "ideal nurse" have included: clean, healthy, hard-working, devoted, willing, and cheerful. While such attributes are undeniably important in nursing, nursing is now placing greater emphasis on qualities such as intelligence, education, leadership, independence, assertiveness, confidence, and creativity.

Whenever nurses view themselves, their role, and their accomplishments in a positive light, their perceptions of nursing itself change. Whenever nurses demand and receive enlarged and expanded roles within the health care system, the higher status which results enhances their sense of identity, and the cycle of progress continues. At times the progress of nursing seems discouraging because change is slow and there is indecision and disagreement within the profession about the nature and future of nursing. This period can be likened to an adolescent search for identity from which nursing shall surely emerge as a mature profession. To participate knowledgeably and effectively in the process of achieving professional maturity and autonomy, every nurse should be aware of significant events in the history of nursing and should keep abreast of current developments in both nursing and the contemporary women's rights movement.

Nursing is unique with respect to the number of agencies and groups that intentionally and deliberately influence the effectiveness of nursing practice. Physicians determine in part what nurses can or cannot do. Insurance companies often designate (indirectly) which patients can be taught by stating the conditions under which a community health nurse, for example, can be paid for home visits. Some hospitals influence nursing by advocating a form of *institutional* licensure by which an institution sets the standards for employment in that setting. The federal government influences the quality of nursing care by arbitrarily raising or lowering standards for nursing homes. Year in and year out, nurses attend countless committee meetings and legislative sessions in an effort to protect the progress that nursing has made to date and to increase nursing's control over its own functions in the future.

Professional Organizations

The two major nursing organizations are the ANA and the National League for Nursing (NLN). The ANA was founded in 1896 and was a charter member of the ICN, which was founded 3 years later. The NLN was founded when three smaller organizations merged in 1952.

American Nurses' Association

The American Nurses' Association (ANA) is nursing's *professional* organization, with membership open only to registered professional nurses. As such, it is the most significant of all organizations to which nurses may belong because it is the organization through which nurses themselves decide upon the functions, activities, and goals of their profession. The ANA serves as spokesman and agent for nurses and nursing, acting in accordance with the expressed wishes of its membership. ANA membership is voluntary and in mid 1986 totaled 188,728 nurses.

Functions of the American Nurses' Association

- Establish and enunciate standards of nursing practice, nursing education and nursing service and to implement them through appropriate channels.
- Establish a code of ethical conduct for nurses.
- Stimulate and promote research in nursing, disseminate research findings, and encourage the utilization of new knowledge as a basis for nursing.
- Provide for continuing education for nurses.
- Promote and protect the economic and general welfare of nurses.
- Assume an active role as consumer advocate in health.
- Analyze, predict, and influence new dimensions of health practices and the delivery of health care.
- Act and speak for the nursing profession in regard to legislation, governmental programs, and national health policy.
- Represent and speak for the nursing profession with allied health, national and international organizations, government bodies, and the public.
- Serve as the official representative of the United States nurses as a member of the International Council of Nurses.
- Promote relationships and collaboration with the National Student Nurses' Association.
- Ensure a national archive for the collection and preservation of documents and other materials which have contributed and continue to contribute to the historical and cultural development of nursing.

Excerpted from American Nurses' Association *Bylaws*, Kansas City, MO., The Association, 1980

MEMBERSHIP. The ANA is a federation of state and territorial associations. The latter, in turn, are made up of district nurses' associations, the number within each state varying with its geography, population distribution, and other factors.

PURPOSES AND FUNCTIONS. Throughout ANA's existence, its functions and activities have been adapted or expanded in accordance with the changing needs of the profession and the public. As a changed or changing major function becomes crystallized, it is incorporated in the bylaws by vote of the ANA membership. Thus the purposes of ANA, as expressed in the current bylaws, are

to work for the improvement of health standards and the availability of health care services for all people, and foster high standards of nursing and stimulate and promote the professional development of nurses and advance their economic and general welfare. These purposes shall be unrestricted by considerations of nationality, race, creed, life-style, color, sex or age.

National League for Nursing

The NLN is an organization for both nurses and non-nurses. It was founded in 1952 with the merging of the National League of Nursing Education, the National Organization for Public Health Nurses, and the Association of Collegiate Schools of Nursing. The NLN is a coalition of people involved in nursing education, and social agencies interested in health planning and action. Through the various councils of the league, nurses, members of allied professions, and citizen consumers of nursing services can work toward the development and improvement of nursing services in hospitals, public health agencies, schools, industries, and education for nursing.

Professional Competency

Nursing promotes professional competency by setting standards for the *preparation* of nurses and standards for the *performance* of nurses. Measures taken to ensure adequate preparation include the periodic accreditation of schools of nursing to make sure each educational program meets established standards, and the periodic revision of licensing laws and examinations.

Measures designed to promote high-quality performance include the establishment of standards of care (Chapter 22), the evaluation of nursing care in terms of established standards (nursing audit), and the evaluation of nurses' performance by fellow nurses (peer review). In addition, some states require proof of ongoing continuing education for renewal of a nurse's license.

Ethical Considerations

Rapid advances in medical technology have made it possible to save lives by means of organ transplantation, chemotherapy, kidney dialysis, and extraordinary measures involving complex life-support systems. As a result, nurses and physicians are now confronted with ethical questions about the quality of the life which could be saved or prolonged. An example of such a question is: Is it right to keep a person alive if he has suffered massive, irreversible brain damage and is unlikely ever to regain consciousness?

Part of a nurse's professional competency lies in her ability to examine the ethical aspects of a given situation and then take action that does not violate her beliefs about right and wrong. Many colleges and universities offer one or more courses on medical or nursing ethics, which are helpful in learning to deal with such complex questions as those related to genetic engineering, adolescent suicide, and the use of extraordinary means to prolong life. Much material is being published on nursing ethics, and each nurse should read widely as she strives to develop a basis for the ethical decisions she must make.

Legal Aspects of Nursing

Each nurse, whether student or graduate, is responsible for her own acts. Other people, such as employers or instructors, may also be held responsible, but this in no way lessens the accountability of the individual nurse.

The two major categories of law are criminal law and civil law. An act which is *forbidden by law* is a crime, and the offender will be dealt with in criminal court. Civil law is concerned with offenses by one person against the person or property of another, and an act that causes harm is referred to as a tort. These offenses are wrong and harmful, but are not illegal. For example, it is wrong to let a patient fall out of bed, and the nurse can be held liable, but there is no law against it.

General categories of torts include such acts as assault and battery, defamation of character, false imprisonment, and fraud, all of which have specific application in the context of health care. Charges of *battery* may result from unwarranted and inappropriate physical contact, while charges of *assault* involve some degree of force. The harmed person is usually awarded a sum of money for damages.

A basic element of the laws of torts is called the standard of reasonableness, and a person is usually *not* held liable for any behavior which is reasonable. With regard to nursing and health care, reasonable care is defined as *that degree of skill and knowledge customarily used by a competent health practitioner of similar education and experience in treating and caring for the sick and injured in the community in which the individual is practicing or learning his profession. (Hemelt and Mackert, 1982, p. 11)*

The concept of reasonableness applies to acts committed in the line of duty and also provides the basis for Good Samaritan laws that are designed to protect those who give aid and assistance in an emergency from subsequent lawsuits. Such laws vary from state to state with respect to their applicability to physicians, nurses, and all others. In general, a nurse is expected to ascertain that an emergency exists, that she is the person most qualified to take action, and then do what any other nurse of similar education and experience would do under similar circumstances.

Most torts involving nurses are torts of negligence. Every person is responsible for conducting himself in a reasonable and prudent manner at all times, and *failure to do so* constitutes negligence. The negligence of a professional person is often referred to as *malpractice*. Negligent behavior is more inclusive than careless behavior because carefully considered behavior is negligent if it is beyond the scope of the person's training or experience (Hemelt and Mackert, 1978). A nurse can be held liable, therefore, if she does something for which she has not had adequate training or experience.

There is an increasing tendency for patients to sue for damages if they have been, or think they have been, harmed or wronged by health care workers; and many nurses, both student and graduate, carry malpractice insurance. Each educational institution and health care facility carries insurance, but both the individual practitioner and the institution can be sued by a single patient.

The bases for malpractice suits are varied and too numerous to list, but examples include the following types of harm or damage: falls, medication errors, loss of personal property, improper use of physical restraints, failure to communicate essential information, failure to exercise reasonable judgment, use of defective supplies or equipment, burns, infection, falls, overlooked surgical sponges or instruments, inadequate identification of the patient, and the revelation of confidential information.

Avoidance of Malpractice

Nurses protect themselves against possible malpractice by: (1) becoming and remaining clinically competent, (2) understanding relevant laws and codes, and (3) accepting the legal doctrine of personal liability. *Clinical competence* is achieved through extensive study and practice in an accredited educational program and is maintained through a lifetime commitment to contin-

uing education. Clinical competence includes the ability to foresee any potential dangers and to *predict* the likely outcomes of a given course of action. If there is a reasonable possibility that physical or psychological harm could come to the patient, the nurse is negligent if she fails to take measures to protect the patient.

An *understanding of relevant laws and codes* is essential because *ignorance is not defensible* in court. Every nurse should read and understand the nurse practice act of the state in which she is practicing, and this understanding should be updated each time the law is amended. This information is essential because, for instance, if the law mandates patient teaching as a nursing responsibility, a nurse can be held liable if harm befalls a patient as a result of her failure to teach him. Nurses also need to study the ANA code and keep up with the changes as they are made. The number of laws and court decisions related to nursing is increasing rapidly, and no text on the legal aspects of nursing can be current and comprehensive enough to serve as an adequate resource to the practicing nurse. It is imperative, therefore, that each nurse make sure that each nursing action is consistent with the current ANA code and relevant nurse practice act. Finally, nurses need to study carefully the Patient's Bill of Rights, which follows later in this chapter, and determine the nursing implications of each right accorded the patient.

Adherence to the legal doctrine of personal liability is an integral part of professional nursing. A nurse is liable for her actions whether she initiates them or is following the orders or directions of another person. If a patient is harmed, the fact that the nurse was following the suggestions, directions, or orders of a supervisor, physician, instructor, or other person does not relieve her of responsibility for her action. The nurse is held responsible if it is reasonable to expect that she should have known or suspected that the action could cause harm to the patient. The nurse also is responsible for the outcome of care given by any other person to whom she has delegated a task. If harm comes to a patient because the task exceeded the known capability and preparation of that worker, the nurse is responsible as well as the worker.

RECORDING AND REPORTING. If an accident or adverse reaction occurs, the situation should be reported *immediately* to the appropriate person so that any necessary steps can be taken either to treat the patient or to protect the patient from possible harm. Failure to report an accident or incident is an act of negligence, and a nurse is liable for any damage caused by such an omission.

All charting must be accurate, complete, and current. This is especially critical if a patient refuses a medication, treatment, or test; when a reasonable request cannot be met; when the patient is upset or angry over an incident, real or alleged; and when a mistake or an accident has occurred. A written description of the situation is a more reliable form of evidence than a verbal recollection, in the event that legal action is taken at some later date.

In the event of legal action, a nurse should *seek legal counsel at once*. Laws related to professional practice are complex and subject to change, and a nurse should obtain and follow the advice of a competent lawyer whenever a question of legality and legal action is raised. Legal counsel and support for a nursing student is usually available from the college or university involved, and from the local or state nurses' association.

Development of a Body of Nursing Knowledge

One of the hallmarks of a profession is the existence of a substantial body of knowledge that has been developed over a long period of time and that can be transmitted to students (Flexner, 1915). Nursing has long been considered an applied science because much of the knowledge on which it is based is derived from physical and social sciences such as chemistry, microbiology, and psychology. Nursing theorists and researchers have contributed to the development of nursing theories which, though not yet fully formulated and tested, provide the basis for the substantial body of knowledge that characterizes a profession. Increasing numbers of nurses are pursuing graduate study at both the master's and the doctoral levels and as a result, the number of competent nurse-researchers is increasing steadily.

Sigma Theta Tau is the national honor society of nursing; it was founded in 1922 at Indiana University. Membership is open to people who have earned a baccalaureate or higher degree in nursing and to selected students in baccalaureate and higher degree programs.

Political Action

The ANA has long been politically active in efforts to improve the status of nursing and the health care of all citizens. Increasing numbers of nurses are serving on federal, state, and local committees dealing with aging, pollution, mental health, nutrition, and a wide variety of other health-related concerns.

Many documents have outlined and described the nurse's *responsibilities*, but it has been only recently that nurses have addressed the issue of their own professional *rights*. Nurses have begun to participate in strikes, either for better working conditions or to promote bet-

ter patient care; and nurses have won a number of lawsuits against discrimination and unfair labor practices. Claire Fagin, a nurse, developed the following list of nurses' rights:

1. The right to find dignity in self-expression and self-enhancement through the use of our special abilities and educational background
2. The right to recognition for our contribution through the provision of an environment for its practice, and proper, professional economic rewards
3. The right to a work environment which will minimize physical and emotional stress and health risks
4. The right to control what is professional practice within the limits of the law
5. The right to set standards for excellence in nursing
6. The right to participate in policy making affecting nursing
7. The right to social and political action in behalf of nursing and health care (Fagin, 1975, p. 84)

Fagin believes that nurses must set the highest possible standards for delivering quality nursing care because subsequent consumer acceptance and demand for that quality of nursing care will clearly affect nurses' rights.

PATIENT RIGHTS AND NURSING

In addition, she helps the patient to carry out the therapeutic plan as initiated by the physician.

This statement recognizes that the patient should be an active participant in his own care whenever possible. Newborn infants and unconscious people are obviously unable to participate in decisions about themselves, but all other patients are, to a greater or lesser degree, able to contribute to the plan of care. Even small children can make requests, state preferences, and share their reactions to both the illness and the treatment of it (Fig. 1.1).

The degree of patient participation in decision making is influenced by the *psychological climate* of the nursing unit. Participation is likely to be high when nurses respect each patient as a person with a fundamental right to make decisions related to his own care. Participation in decision making will be low when nurses imply that they know what is best for the patient, disregard suggestions and requests from patients, or give

A Patient's Bill of Rights

The American Hospital Association presents a Patient's Bill of Rights with the expectation that observance of these rights will contribute to more effective patient care and greater satisfaction for the patient, his physician, and the hospital organization. Further, the Association presents these rights in the expectation that they will be supported by the hospital on behalf of its patients, as an integral part of the healing process. It is recognized that a personal relationship between the physician and the patient is essential for the provision of proper medical care. The traditional physician-patient relationship takes on a new dimension when care is rendered within an organizational structure. Legal precedent has established that the institution itself also has a responsibility to the patient. It is in recognition of these factors that these rights are affirmed.

1. The patient has the right to considerate and respectful care.

2. The patient has the right to obtain from his physician complete current information concerning his diagnosis, treatment, and prognosis in terms the patient can be reasonably expected to understand. When it is not medically advisable to give such information to the patient, the information should be made available to an appropriate person in his behalf. He has the right to know, by name, the physician responsible for coordinating his care.

3. The patient has the right to receive from his physician information necessary to give informed consent prior to the start of any procedure and/or treatment. Except in emergencies, such information for informed consent should include but not necessarily be limited to the specific procedure and/or treatment, the medically significant risks involved, and the probable duration of incapacitation. Where medically significant alternatives for care or treatment exist, or when the patient requests information concerning medical alternatives, the patient has the right to such information. The patient also has the right to know the name of the person responsible for the procedures and/or treatment.

4. The patient has the right to refuse treatment to the extent permitted by law, and to be informed of the medical consequences of his action.

5. The patient has the right to every consideration of his privacy concerning his own medical care program. Case discussion, consultation, examination, and treatment are confidential and should be conducted discreetly. Those not directly involved in his care must have the permission of the patient to be present.

6. The patient has the right to expect that all communications and records pertaining to his care should be treated as confidential.

7. The patient has the right to expect that within its capacity a hospital must make reasonable response to the request of a patient for services. The hospital must provide evaluation, service, and/or referral as indicated by the urgency of the case. When medically permissible a patient may be transferred to another facility only after he has received complete information and explanation concerning the needs for and alternatives to such a transfer. The institution to which the patient is to be transferred must first have accepted the patient for transfer.

8. The patient has the right to obtain information as to any relationship of his hospital to other health care and educational institutions insofar as his care is concerned. The patient has the right to obtain information as to the existence of any professional relationships among individuals, by name, who are treating him.

9. The patient has the right to be advised if the hospital proposes to engage in or perform human experimentation affecting his care or treatment. The patient has the right to refuse to participate in such research projects.

10. The patient has the right to expect reasonable continuity of care. He has the right to know in advance what appointment times and physicians are available and where. The patient has the right to expect that the hospital will provide a mechanism whereby he is informed by his physician or a delegate of the physician of the patient's continuing health care requirements following discharge.

11. The patient has the right to examine and receive an explanation of his bill regardless of source of payment.

12. The patient has the right to know what hospital rules and regulations apply to his conduct as a patient.

No catalogue of rights can guarantee for the patient the kind of treatment he has a right to expect. A hospital has many functions to perform, including the prevention and treatment of disease, the education of both health professionals and patients, and the conduct of clinical research. All these activities must be conducted with an overriding concern for the patient, and above all, the recognition of his dignity as a human being. Success in achieving this recognition assures success in the defense of the rights of the patient.

(Approved by the House of Delegates of the American Hospital Association, February 6, 1973) the impression that patients who are passive and compliant receive more care and attention.

Patients are more likely to assume an active role in health care when they realize that they have rights and understand the nature of those rights. In 1973, the American Hospital Association (AHA) developed the Patient's Bill of Rights, and a copy is usually presented to each patient admitted to a hospital or other health care facility. Nurses must understand it fully, because any action, intentional or unintentional, that deprives a patient of his stated rights could constitute malpractice.

Patient Advocacy. Some nurses consider patient advocacy to be an important aspect of nursing. Others believe that, although many patients do indeed need someone to protect their rights or to help them speak up for themselves, such as a person need not be a nurse. If a patient advocate is someone other than a nurse,

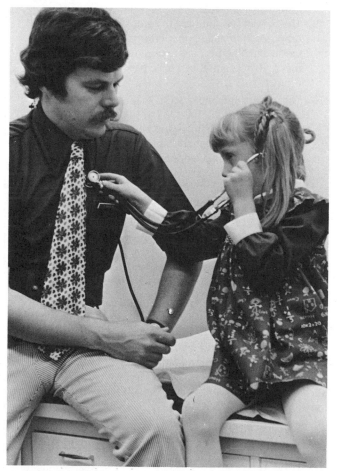

Figure 1.1 *Patient involvement is an integral aspect of nursing and contributes to the development of a trusting relationship.*

the nurse must make sure that the patient knows the role of a patient advocate, how to contact him, and how to use his services.

COLLEGIAL RELATIONSHIPS IN NURSING

She also, as a member of a medical team, helps other members, as they in turn help her, to plan and carry out the total program whether it be for the improvement of health, or the recovery from illness, or support in death.

This portion of Henderson's definition focuses on the *interdependent* functions of nursing whereby nurse and patient collaborate with other workers such as the nutritionist, social worker, psychiatric nurse, physical therapist, chaplain, and physician for the good of the patient. All these people, who were initially called a medical team but are now called the health care team, may serve as resources for the nurse or they may work directly with the patient.

The relative contribution of each member of the health care team should depend on the *needs of the patient*, as explained by Henderson (1964):

If we put total medical care in the form of a pie graph we might assign wedges of different sizes to members of what we now refer to as "the team." The wedge must differ in size for each member according to the problem facing the patient; in some situations certain members of the team have no part of the pie at all. The patient always has a slice, although that of a newborn infant or the unconscious adult is only a sliver; his very life depends upon others, but most particularly the nurse.

In contrast, where an otherwise healthy adult is suffering from a skin condition such as acne, he and his physician compose the team and they can divide the whole pie between them. If the problem is an orthopedic disability, the largest slice may go to the physical therapist; when a sick child is cared for at home by the mother, then the latter's share may be by far the largest. But of all the members of the team, excepting the patient and the physician, the nurse has most often a piece of the pie, and next to theirs, hers is usually the largest share. (p. 66)

In addition to these interdependent professional relationships, the nurse delegates responsibilities and tasks to other people such as licensed practical nurses, orderlies, or nurse's aides.

As a member of the health care team, the nurse is often expected to plan, lead, administer, delegate, organize, and coordinate. Such activities are an essential part of nursing, but they are activities shared by many other professional people and are, therefore, not unique to nursing.

SUGGESTED READINGS

—— Male nurses: What they think about themselves and others. *RN* 1983 Oct; 46(10):61–64.

—— Nurses today—a statistical portrait. *Am J Nurs* 1982 March; 82(3):448–451.

Bullough, Bonnie (ed.): *The Law and the Expanding Nursing Role*. New York, Appleton-Century-Crofts, 1980.

Daria, Joan, and Sally Moran: Nursing in the 90's. *Nursing 85* 1985 Dec; 15(12):26–29.

Diers, Donna: Nursing reclaims its role. *Nurs Outlook* 1982 Sept/Oct; 30(8):459–463.

Doheny, Margaret O'Bryan, Christina Benson Cook, and Sr. Mary Constance Stopper: *The Discipline of Nursing*. Bowie, MA, Brady, 1982.

Dossey, Larry: Consciousness and caring: Retrospective 2000. *Top Clin Nurs* 1982 Jan; 3(4):75–83.

Dunn, Jeanne M: Warning: Giving telephone advice is hazardous to your professional health. *Nursing 85* 1985 Aug; 15(8):40–41.

Edmunds, Linda: Computer-assisted nursing care. *Am J Nurs* 1982 July; 82(7):1076–1079.

Elmore, Joyce Ann: Black nurses: Their service and their struggle. *Am J Nurs* 1976 March; 76(3):435–438.

Fagin, Claire M: Nurses' Rights. *Am J Nurs* 1975 Jan; 75(1):82–85.

Fenner, Kathleen M: *Ethics and Law in Nursing*. New York, VanNostrand, 1980.

Gray, Peggy L: Gerontological nurse specialist: luxury or necessity? *Am J Nurs* 1982 Jan; 82(1):82–85.

Hemelt, Mary Dolores, and Mary Ellen Mackert: *Dynamics of Law in Nursing and Health Care*. Reston, VA, Reston Publishing Co, 1978.

Hemelt, Mary Dolores, and Mary Ellen Mackert: Steering clear of legal hazards. *Nursing 84* 1984 May; 14(5):81–86.

Henderson, Virginia: The nature of nursing. *Am J Nurs* 1964 Aug; 64(8):62.

Kallish, Philip A, and Beatrice J Kallish: *The Advance of American Nursing*. ed.2. Boston, Little, Brown and Company, 1985.

Kelly, Lucie Young: *Dimensions of Professional Nursing*. ed.3. New York, Macmillan, 1985.

Kohnke, Mary F: The nurse as advocate. *Am J Nurs* 1980 Nov; 80(11):2038–2040.

Marshall-Burnett, Syringa: Socio-economic power—the role of the professional organization. *Int Nurs Rev* 1981 May/June; 28(3):75–78.

Masson, Veneta: International nursing: What is it and who does it? *Am J Nurs* 1979 July; 79(7);1242–1245.

Mauksch, Ingeborg: *Implementing Change in Nursing*. St. Louis, Mosby, 1980.

McCloskey, Joanne Comi: The professionalization of nursing: United States and England. *Int Nurs Rev* 1981 March/April; 28(2):40–47.

McCloskey, Joanne Comi, and Helen K Grace: *Current Issues in Nursing*. Boston, Blackwell Scientific Publications, 1981.

Nightingale, Florence: *Notes on Nursing—What It Is and What It Is Not*. New York, Dover Publications, 1969.

Newton, Lisa H: In defense of the traditional nurse. *Nurs Outlook* 1981 June; 29(6):348–354.

Schlotfeldt, Rozella M: Nursing in the future. *Nurs Outlook* 1981 May; 29(5):295–301.

Smith, Gloria R: Nursing beyond the crossroads. *Nurs Outlook* 1980 Sept; 28(9):540–545.

Ulin, Priscilla: International nursing challenge. *Nurs Outlook* 1982 Nov/Dec; 30(9):531–535.

Watson, Jean: Nursing's scientific quest. *Nurs Outlook* 1981 July; 29(7):413–416.

Watson, Jean: Professional identity crisis — is nursing finally growing up? *Am J Nurs* 1981 Aug; 81(8):1488–1490.

Welch, Martha J: Dysfunctional parenting of a profession. *Nurs Outlook* 1980 Dec; 28(12):724–727.

Whitman, Maureen: Toward a new psychology for nurses. *Nurs Outlook* 1982 Jan; 30(1):48–52.

REFERENCES

American Hospital Association: *Statement on Patient's Rights*. Chicago, The Association, 1973.

American Nurses' Association: *Code for Nurses With Interpretive Statements*. Kansas City, American Nurses' Association, 1976.

American Nurses' Association: *Standards for Nursing Practice*. Kansas City, American Nurses' Association, 1973.

2

History of Nursing in the United States

Nancy L. Noel

The Oldest Art, The Youngest Profession
  Origin of Nursing
  Judeo-Christian Influences
  Nursing in Colonial United States
  Nursing During the Industrial Revolution
  Nursing and the Civil War
  Nursing Education in the United States
  The Rise of Nursing Organizations
  Nursing at the Turn of the Century
  World War I
  Coping With the Shortage of Nurses
  Nursing and the Depression
  World War II
  Nursing After World War II
  Moving Into the 21st Century

Prerequisites and/or Suggested Preparation
There are no prerequisites for this chapter.

THE OLDEST ART, THE YOUNGEST PROFESSION

Nursing has been called the oldest art and the youngest profession. Anyone who has experienced the gentleness and skill of a compassionate nurse will agree that nursing is truly an art. Anyone who has traced the evolution of nursing, through its bad times and good, from its "dark days" in Dickens's time to the outstanding research, academic achievement, and leadership of today's nurses will agree that nursing is truly a profession.

Persons joining any profession are curious about it, and nursing is no different. We seek answers to questions such as: "Where did we come from?" "What are we like now?" and "Where will we be as we enter the 21st century?" Specifically, nurses ponder questions such as "What happened to us between the Crimean War and the Korean War, between Florence Nightingale and today's military nurse. We also wonder "what forces made it possible for the likes of Sairy Gamp to be replaced by Dr. Carolyne Davis?"

Sairy Gamp was a central character in Charles Dickens's novel *Martion Chuzzlewit* and represents accurately the status of nursing in England in the 1840's. Nurses were "illiterate, rough, and inconsiderate, oftentimes immoral and alcoholic . . . Nurses were drawn from among discharged patients, prisoners, and the lowest strata of society . . . There was little organization with nursing and certainly no social standing. No one would enter nursing who could possibly earn a living some other way" (Donahue, 1985). Given this blot on our history, it is truly remarkable that only 140 years later, Carolyne Davis, R.N., Ph.D., was appointed Administrator of the Health Care Financing Administration by President Reagan and thereby became responsible for one of the largest federal budgets. How could such change come about so quickly?

History is so vast and complex that any historical perspective can give only a partial view of the past. This limited view may be biased by the interests and knowledge of the historian who has selected the data to be included, the points to be emphasized, and the conclusions to be drawn. The history of nursing is no exception.

A complete history of nursing would cover a span of many thousands of years, because the sick have been cared for in one way or another since the dawn of civilization. A complete history of nursing would have to include an accurate account of the chronological changes of every nation on earth because nursing has always been affected by and responded to each significant event in the life of a nation, whether that change be related to war, prosperity, famine, or an industrial revolution. Given the limitations of the average book on nursing history, some portion of the content will be considered incomplete by virtually every scholar and practitioner within the profession because the significance of any event in nursing is judged from the perspective of an individual nurse or group of nurses. If, for example, a large group of nurses was asked to review the manuscript for a new text on the history of nursing, their critical comments might vary as follows:

- Public health nurses—"needs a more detailed description of the work of Lillian Wald, and also more detailed information about the development of Visiting Nurse Associations"
- Nurse educators—"inadequate treatment of the development of a process for accrediting schools of nursing"
- Nurse midwives—"must include more coverage of medical and legal barriers encountered by midwives who try to set up a private practice in the 1980s"
- Nurse administrators—"material related to union representation and strikes by nurses must be added"

The list of perceived criticisms and suggestions would be endless!

This chapter makes no attempt to cover the history of nursing in general, or of the United States in particular. It is designed, instead, to provide a brief introduction to the ways in which nursing has been influenced by some of the significant changes in American life. This overview provides the basis for a beginning awareness of the impact on nursing of the changes which are occurring as we approach the end of the 20th century.

Origin of Nursing

Societies have consistently valued wellness and health because healthy people are able to create, build, and protect their communities. Individuals with health-preserving or healing powers have always been valuable to society. This value increases during times of war or epidemics; history is filled with examples of both.

There has always been a relationship among healing, health, and religion. Ancient religious figures such as priests, priestesses, and gods were thought to be endowed with healing powers. Conversely, early superstition suggested that sick people were cursed with illness because they had sinned. To be healthy, to have health, has always been the ideal. Ancient healers were empiricists who used what observation and history had taught them as the basis for treating and caring for their patients. Their healing tools were drugs, manipulations, and other methods of treatment, prayers, and religious practices. If healers were successful, all was well; if additional problems developed the care providers may have been punished.

Most nursing care was given in the home by the women of the household, but patients with serious health problems might be taken to a local religious or healing center.

Judeo-Christian Influences

Many early cultures were based on slave labor and the value of the individual depended upon his station or position in life. This concept began to change with the Judaic emphasis on justice and the individual. Although the Jews had been enslaved at times, they were able to develop strong community and family ties. The value placed on the individual, family, and community coupled with sanitary practices which they developed during the exodus from Egypt were influences that raised their level of wellness and helped them survive as a nation.

The teachings of Christ stressed the inherent value of each individual man, woman, and child. The followers of this religious leader were held responsible for the care of the sick, the helpless, and the poor, and early Christians were taught that salvation in another life could depend on their good treatment of each other in this life. This emphasis on the care of the poor, the hungry, and the sick fostered the development of nursing as never before.

During the early Christian period, women, particularly the deaconesses of the early church, were the primary care providers for the sick. During the anarchy which followed the breakdown of the Roman Empire some remarkable women like Fabiola and Saint Paula set up hospitals and later monasteries which became refuges for the poor and sick. At this time, poverty and the diseases associated with it, particularly infectious diseases, were the most prevalent nursing and public health problems. Women continued to work toward making societies well, and what they were able to accomplish in any given era was influenced by the degree of social freedom which the women were currently experiencing. The contribution of a Roman matron or a medieval abbess might range from creating a hospital to giving direct care to patients.

During the Crusades, men nursed the sick and wounded as members of military nursing orders such as the Order of St. John of Jerusalem, the Teutonic Knights, and the Knights Hospitaliers. After the Crusades, parts of the Western world settled into a monastic way of life. Monasteries were self-contained and

protected, and since these monastic communities offered education, opportunity, and a good way of life to probationers, many young people left their families to join a monastery. Nursing was an integral part of the education and practice of the community member. The probationer would learn how to care for the sick and infirm, and would progress through various areas of the community learning new things such as the use of medieval pharmaceuticals. The monastic educational system later became an important influence on the development of formal nursing education in hospital diploma programs in the United States even though the monastery itself remained a European phenomenon.

Nursing in Colonial United States

Early settlers in the U.S. lived in large nuclear families in an agrarian economy. Nursing was done by the women of the house as were all other housekeeping tasks and some farming responsibilities. Colonial cookbooks invariably included recipes for various home remedies. Some women earned reputations as skillful healers, nurses, and midwives. Their responsibilities included delivering babies, caring for children (many of whom suffered and died from childhood disease), and treating injuries from accidents and war. They began to extend their practices beyond their immediate families to their communities and they often received payment of some kind for the services they provided. As women began to provide their services to other households, they began to earn exchangeable commodities, and gradually they began to be paid in currency. The payment for nursing care depended on the economics and level of development of the particular society.

There were no formal educational programs for these women who nursed the sick, but nursing knowledge was valued because a developing nation needed a large, healthy, strong population. Women probably passed this knowledge on to their children and to apprentices.

Nursing During the Industrial Revolution

Although the Industrial Revolution in the United States occurred later than it did in Europe, the impact was equally great. Families, the basic unit of society, were fragmented when members began to migrate to urban areas where there were jobs and new opportunities. Problems resulting from the disintegration of families, massive immigration of foreigners, and exploitive factory work situations were compounded by poverty and by unhealthy, crowded living conditions. The poor, foundlings, orphans, and the sick were cared for in charitable institutions such as the poor house at public or philanthropic expense. The nurses in these charitable or public institutions were often not "respectable" women. They were very often of low moral and ethical character. They might even have been serving time in jail for criminal offenses, but released to work for hire. Nursing was considered a very menial occupation and the status of women who nursed in institutions had diminished markedly. Paradoxically, when society probably needed nurses most, the *trained nurse* had not yet become a reality. During this time there were few opportunities for middle class women to live and work outside of family life. Educational opportunities for women were still undeveloped; women who worked for wages did so as self-educated nurses, teachers, factory workers, and as domestic servants in other people's homes.

Eventually, women began to organize and they tried to develop new and different approaches to social reform. They began to agitate for the right to vote, the abolition of slavery, for better health. They tried to open new opportunities for women in education and the work place. The efforts of these women were intensified by the Civil War. War always focuses a country's attention on nursing because it seems right and reasonable that men who are battling for their country deserve to be cared for when they are injured. At this time in England, Florence Nightingale was using her experiences during the Crimean War and her consequent public image to set forth a new model for nursing. She opened her training school for nurses in 1850 at St. Thomas's hospital in London, England. There had been earlier attempts by others to formalize nursing education but it was the Crimean War and the gratitude of the English people which set the stage for Miss Nightingale's efforts and the emergence of modern nursing in the middle of the 19th century.

Nursing and the Civil War

The tragedy of the Civil War proved to be the impetus for many changes in the United States. The wounded and dying in both Confederate and Union armies needed nursing care, and many women left home to nurse the wounded as private citizens without government sanction or support. Clara Barton and Louisa May Alcott were among the Northern volunteers. Kate Cummings was a volunteer Confederate nurse. Their families had mixed reactions to the activities of these women. It was probably more difficult for Southern women to work as volunteer nurses because the public, particularly in the South, believed that women belonged in the home.

Army physicians, accustomed to dealing with army medics who followed commands and did not "coddle" their patients, were not enthusiastic about these volunteer female nurses, many of whom had little if any

experience. Dorothea Dix, an early reformer from the northeast, had been placed in charge of the Union nurses, and the need for some kind of training for the volunteer nurses prompted a group led by Louisa Schuyler to organize a month-long training program at Bellevue Hospital in New York. The committee was disgusted by the conditions within the hospital and resolved to return after the war to reform the hospital and the nursing care.

Infectious disease and malnutrition were major health problems both in hospitals and on the battlefield. The germ theory and antisepsis were in their infancy and there were no antibiotics to treat the sick and dying. Nurses kept fevers down as best they could by bathing and sponging patients. They dressed wounds, fed those who could not feed themselves, applied leeches, assisted surgeons in amputating limbs, and wrote letters for the invalids. Nurses often became ill themselves and many died.

The war ended, slaves were freed, and black men were given the right to vote. Reconstruction began and people realized there was a necessity for change in the care of the sick in peace as well as war.

Nursing Education in the United States

During the later part of the 19th century, a few colleges for women were established. College curriculums were different for men and women, with the programs for women being less rigorous. There were not many career opportunities for women who were college graduates, and homemaking was still considered the most important role. Educated women were often in a double-bind situation, because although they had been educated to participate in the public sphere, they were in reality confined to a private role in the home.

Some women sought fulfillment in the community as social reformers. The experiences encountered by women during the Civil War coupled with higher levels of education prompted them to work toward necessary social reform. These middle and upper class reformers were concerned about a variety of social problems, but some of them focused their attention on the public hospital. They believed that training nurses in a hospital-based school such as Miss Nightingale's would improve hospital care. Formal educational programs to train nurses would also give women a socially worthwhile career opportunity.

During the 1870's, groups of women in New York, Connecticut, Massachusetts, Illinois, and elsewhere overcame the resistance of some hospital administrators, physicians, and others and established training schools for nurses. Their accomplishments were remarkable because they had to raise the money, find nurse educators, and operate these schools in sometimes hostile institutions. This was accomplished primarily by women long before women had been granted the right to vote. The success of those first nursing schools was phenomenal. Beleaguered public institutions were profoundly changed by the advent of the trained nurse; hospitals began to provide care for those people *who could afford to pay* and who formerly had been cared for at home. Trained nurses and nurses in training had made the difference.

Unfortunately, the success of these schools led to a host of problems because the late 19th century was one of rugged individualism with few controls against the exploitation of an idea. An idea as successful as the training of nurses was vulnerable, and the women who had started these schools soon lost control to the hospitals and their administrators. By the turn of the century there was marked proliferation of hospital-owned training schools for nurses, but problems developed rather rapidly as the schools increased in size and number.

Early schools of nursing had very little in common with one another. A school might be large and run by a public charitable institution or it might be part of a small cottage hospital owned and operated for profit. In some hospitals students learned to care for patients suffering from a variety of health problems, while educational opportunities were limited in other hospitals which were designed to care exclusively for those who were mentally ill, had tuberculosis, or suffered from another specific illness. Hospitals were staffed almost entirely by student nurses who sometimes worked without the guidance and direction of a trained nurse, teacher, or superintendent. The student nurse served as an apprentice as did most physicians at the time. The patients and their health problems were the only curriculum for many students—a form of the case method of learning.

Some of the better teaching hospitals offered classes. The nursing superintendent taught classes such as nursing ethics, bandaging, and massage while physicians or physicians in training taught anatomy, physiology, surgery, medicine, and obstetrics. Physicians taught the nursing student for two reasons: (1) Physicians were better educated than nurses and (2) there was not yet a body of nursing knowledge which could be clearly distinguished from medical knowledge. Nurses were expected only to attend to the patient's hygiene, food, elimination, and comfort, and to follow the physician's directions. Therefore, it seemed appropriate for doctors to teach student nurses.

Classes were generally held in the evening after both students and teachers had already worked their 12-hr day. The labor unions which had been formed to protect factory workers from long hours and unhealthy conditions had little impact on working conditions for nurses. Nurses, both students and graduates, frequently became ill through the combination of exposure to infection, long hours of hard work, and inadequate nutrition, rest, exercise, and diversion.

Graduates of these 1- or 2-year training programs worked primarily in patients' homes as private duty nurses. They usually were employed through a referral from their superintendent of nurses, a physician, or an alumni registry. There were no licensing examinations or legislative protection for the public, and some of those working as nurses were actually lay people with no training whatsoever. Nursing was not a financially lucrative career; but, compared to most other career opportunities, it had a certain dignity and importance. It was socially acceptable and familiar because it represented the institutionalization of tasks which women had performed in their homes for generations.

The Rise of Nursing Organizations

At the turn of the century, nursing was beset by many problems. The lack of even minimal standards for nursing education and the subsequent confusion about who was entitled to practice nursing were at the center of a tangled group of problems and issues. Some of these issues were: economic security, a lack of control of the job market, a need for protection of the public from untrained and unqualified nurses, a dearth of opportunities for formal education for nursing leadership, a lack of nursing literature, and ignorance about the current focus and future goals of the nursing profession.

At the Chicago World's Fair in 1893, Isabel Hampton spearheaded the effort which resulted in the founding of the country's first organization of nurses. It was clear that the issues and problems facing the nursing community could not be solved by individual nurses, and the American Society of Superintendents of Training Schools was organized in 1894. Its goals were to standardize and improve nursing education and to further the best interests of the nursing profession. Over the years, this organization evolved into the present day National League for Nursing (NLN), which continues to focus much of its attention on nursing education.

A second organization was needed which would focus on improving working conditions for nurses and securing legislation to differentiate the trained nurse from the untrained. In 1896, the Nurses' Associated Alumnae of the United States and Canada was formed. Isabel Hampton (now Mrs. Isabel Hampton Robb) served as the organization's president from its founding in 1896 to 1901. This organization evolved into what we now know as the American Nurses' Association.

Nursing has referred to itself as a profession since the beginning of the century; those two organizations provided guidance and direction for nursing as it expanded to become the largest body of health care professionals in the United States.

At that time, black nurses were not admitted to the existing organizations, and they formed their own nursing association in 1908.

Nursing at the Turn of the Century

By the end of the 19th century, two nursing organizations had been formed. The *American Journal of Nursing* began publication in October 1900. Educational opportunities were increasing and the Superintendents' Society made arrangements for graduate nurses to attend Teachers College, Columbia University, for a course in Hospital Economics. In the aftermath of the brief Spanish-American War, American nurses gained legislative support for military nursing and the permanent Army Nurse Corps came into being. States began to pass legislation to regulate the practice of nursing and nurses began to be licensed. New opportunities for nursing practice, particularly in the field of public health, became available for graduate nurses in visiting nurse services and settlement houses around the country.

Nursing organizations were being developed around the world; the International Council of Nurses held its first formal meeting in Buffalo, New York, in 1901. Most nurses were not in the mainstream of the women's suffrage movement but there were exceptions like Lavinia Lloyd Dock, who exhorted nurses to work for women's right to vote.

The National League for Nursing Education (the former Superintendents' Society and presently the NLN) organized a volunteer curriculum committee whose members were scattered throughout the United States. This committee tried to develop an ideal nursing curriculum which would address the problems related to improving and standardizing nursing education. Since American nursing was controlled by hospitals and physicians, it was hampered by the lack of an independent financial base for nursing education. It continued to be plagued with problems of low salaries, little remuneration for personal experience and/or additional education, long hours, and heavy responsibility. The salary problem was not unique to nursing, however, and was shared by most women who worked outside the home during this era.

World War I

War causes social upheaval and radically alters the roles of the military and civilian population. It also focuses public attention on the importance of, and need for, nursing care. During World War I, waves of nationalism and patriotism in various countries caused women of the leisure classes to volunteer as nurses.

The International Red Cross, which had been founded in the middle of the 19th century, was firmly established by 1917, and had developed a brief training course for nurses aides. Aristocrats and upper class women in Europe were able to nurse the wounded as Red Cross Aides, and American socialites began to volunteer as nurses aides and in order to care for the US troops in Europe.

American nurses and their professional organizations believed that *trained* nurses would be the most effective care providers for both the military and civilian sectors. As a result, several innovations in recruitment and nursing education were developed to increase the available numbers of trained nurses. An Army Training School was established by an act of Congress, with Annie Goodrich as its dean. It was based on the newly completed curriculum developed by the National League for Nursing Education. There were branches of the Army Training School throughout the country which provided a free education to young women who were then expected to nurse for the war's duration. Subjects such as pediatrics, which students could not learn in military hospitals, were learned by experiences in affiliating civilian hospitals.

The Vassar Training Camp was another innovation. College educated women came to Vassar to take an intensive pre-nursing course, and after its completion, they moved into a hospital-based accelerated program. The Vassar College Alumni Association was instrumental in recruiting candidates for this program. Members of this Rainbow Division (named for the color and variety of the uniforms of their different schools) were also expected to serve for the war's duration. Graduates of the program became leaders in nursing during the year following.

It was fortunate that the nurses who served with the military forces abroad had received prior training because the method of warfare of World War I demanded more of nurses than any previous war. New weapons, including toxic gases, gave rise to problems which demanded new techniques in medical and nursing care. Trench warfare resulted in high infection rates, creating an urgent problem. Wound debridement and Dakin's solution were used to treat infections, and the technique of transfusing blood was developed. Nurses had to assume many roles formerly filled by military physicians because the number of patients who needed care was so great.

Persons responsible for the health of the civilians were also heavily burdened, caring for a society which had been mobilized to fight a war, and the war's end brought a new and unexpected menace. Although the war had been responsible for many American deaths, including those of some 300 nurses, the influenza epidemic that followed killed five times as many people. People who cared for the victims of the "flu" were naturally at risk, and many nurses and physicians, some still in training, died. The epidemic was an international calamity.

Coping With the Shortage of Nurses

Single women moved beyond the confines of family life to a greater extent than ever before, and their new freedom and choices made recruitment into nursing more difficult than ever. Many individuals living in the 1920's saw nursing education as archaic, with the result that there was an acute shortage of nurses.

The diploma-granting hospital programs for nurses had retained the military and monastic influences of the past, and the nursing profession was out of step with the times. Nursing wanted to maintain its respectable image; an oppressive moral climate in nursing education was considered necessary. Graduate nurses worked long hours (often working split shifts from 7 to 12 am, and 3 to 7 pm) and received low salaries compared to other working and professional women. There was little variety in graduate nurse roles although there were some exceptions like the Frontier Nursing Service in the Appalachian Mountains which was begun by Mary Breckenridge. Society needed competent nurses in sufficient numbers, but it was difficult to interest people in nursing as a career.

Nursing had sought funding to study itself ever since the turn of the century. After World War I, the Rockefeller Foundation funded and later published a study of nursing and nursing education. This study was headed by Josephine Goldmark; it was hoped that the Goldmark report on nursing would be as effective as the 1910 Flexner report on medical education had been in compelling the closing of poor medical schools and bringing improvements to the better ones.

Josephine Goldmark and her committee discovered that nurses were leaving their profession and others were not entering because dependence upon hospital finances made it impossible to provide education of high quality. Students and graduates were often exploited, poorly paid, and overworked. Graduate nurses lacked autonomy and power. Nurses felt that they were not receiving an adequate education on which to base their practice, and this was one of the main contributors to the recruitment problem. The Goldmark Committee stated that nurses needed a liberal education obtained in an institution of higher learning as well as an understanding of public health, in order to be able to develop innovative roles for delivering health care.

After the Goldmark report, and based on its findings, the Rockefeller Foundation provided funds to develop a nursing program with a sound theoretical and clinical basis at Yale University. The experiment proved so successful that it was later endowed and became a prototype for excellence in nursing education. During the 1920's, a few colleges and universities began to develop basic nursing programs which granted a Bachelor of Science degree in Nursing. Nurses who graduated from collegiate programs of nursing often chose to work in the public health area, and were in great demand as the country faced the Depression.

Nursing and the Depression

The Depression brought about many changes in nursing. There were fewer opportunities to do private duty nursing because people could no longer afford to hire nurses. Many graduate nurses moved into the hospital and replaced student nurses as care providers. This was the beginning of large scale employment of graduate nurses by hospitals.

For nurses, the misery of the Depression was offset to a degree by some interesting developments within nursing. The American Nurses' Association grew in numbers and power as it responded to the needs of its members. Sometimes the organization provided graduate nurse members with shoes and other articles they needed so they could work. The organization understood its constituency and was responsive to their problems.

The trend for women to work outside of the home grew. Many citizens believed that if a choice had to be made between giving employment to men and to women, the men should be given the opportunity because they had families to support. In reality, many trained nurses supported their families since they were the only ones who could find employment during the Depression. Poverty brought increasing illness and death. The federal government was forced to intervene through the Federal Emergency Relief Administration, which paid for nursing and medical care. This legislation provided funds through which the preparation of public health nurses was expanded and jobs were made available.

The Civil Works Administration and Works Progress Administration (WPA) put millions of people, including nurses, to work. The Social Security Act of 1935 expanded opportunities for nurses by its provisions for the public's health and by underwriting the cost of public health nursing education. Health insurance programs, developing technology, and larger hospitals were all products of the Depression.

World War II

In the late 1930's Europe was engaged in World War II, while the United States was preparing legislation to permit the drafting of young men into the Army. The Red Cross developed mobile hospital units for military purposes. A group of nurses formed a Nursing Council for National Defense in 1940 with a goal of preparing nurses to serve in a war which seemed inevitable. The Japanese attack on Pearl Harbor marked the entrance of the United States into the war, and once more there was a need for more nurses.

The funding for the federally funded Cadet Nurse Corps was one response to that need. Sponsored by Congresswoman Frances Payne Bolton, it provided a free education for young nursing students. Thousands of young women entered the field of nursing. The number of black nurses also increased.

There was a great need for many types of nursing services. For example, these efforts created new opportunities such as flight nursing in the military sector and industrial nursing in the civilian sector. The demand for public health nurses was high, and nurses were held in considerable public esteem.

Civilian hospitals were understaffed, so once again nursing students became the primary care providers. Auxiliary helpers and volunteers, such as the Red Cross Gray Ladies, became an important component of hospital service.

The experience of World War II focused attention and resources on the nursing needs of psychiatric patients. Psychiatric nurses increased in numbers, skill, and educational preparation. Their prestige was enhanced as society recognized the importance of their work.

Nursing After World War II

Following World War II, society was faced with another acute nurse shortage, few military nurses returned to the hospitals in which they had been employed before the war. During the war nurses had hired household help to enable them to work, but after the war it became financially impractical to retain such help because nurses' salaries were lower than those of secretaries and accountants, for example. In addition, their hours were long and often inconvenient because of weekend and split-shift assignments. Thus, some nurses retired; others took advantage of their veteran's benefits and returned to school. The resulting shortage of nurses was paradoxical, considering the amount of federal financial support for nursing education which had been provided only a few years earlier.

In 1948, Esther Lucille Brown, a researcher at the Russell Sage Foundation, completed a study of nursing. She learned that recruitment into nursing continued to be a problem because of the inferior quality of hospital-based nursing education. In no other profession was education based in a service institution, such as a hospital. Nursing schools needed to move into colleges and universities with qualified teachers, good libraries, and research facilities. Nursing provided a service which was *essential* to society and it could not continue to do so based on a frugal apprentice form of education. Dr. Brown's findings were reminiscent of the Goldmark report of 25 years earlier. A committee to implement the Brown report was established and developed a plan for the accreditation of nursing programs by the National League for Nursing.

The post-World War II years were as challenging as the decades of the turn of the century had been with regard to nursing and health care. During the 1940's President Truman recommended the establishment of a National Health Insurance Plan which would provide health care to all who needed it. Among other things the plan would have opened new opportunities for nursing practice and established more equitable incomes for the various types of health care providers. Nurses were solidly in favor of the plan, while physicians were vehement in their opposition to it. Opposition came from other quarters also, and it was broad, well organized, and effective. There is as yet no truly broad, effective, and universal health care system in the United States.

During the late 1940's nurses began to focus on their own economic and general welfare through their nursing associations. In time, these concerns led to collective bargaining, with many nurses represented by the various professional associations. Nurse negotiating teams understood nursing practice and learned to bargain effectively on issues of practice as well as of economics.

Nursing organizations were restructured in 1952, to unify the smaller specialty groups into larger, more powerful organizations. The Black Nurses Association that had been founded in 1908 became a part of the ANA, and the National Student Nurse Association was formed in 1952.

There was healthy growth in nursing literature at this time as a number of new nursing journals appeared, including *Nursing Outlook* and *Nursing Research.* An expansion of the literature was inevitable as nurses accepted the need for more advanced academic preparation for the work they were doing and began to be involved in nursing research. Initially, nurses themselves were the subjects of research by social scientists, but soon nurses began to use research methodology to benefit nursing education and practice, and eventually to design studies of their own which were related to nursing theory.

Also, in the 1950's many women left the work force when this was financially possible. Predictably, the return to home life led once more to a nurse shortage; innovative programs became necessary to meet the need for nurses. R. Louise McManus and Mildred Montag envisioned and developed a 2-year college program which would prepare technical nurses who could prac-, tice at the bedside under the direction of professional nurses. The community college movement was in its infancy and welcomed the new programs. The phenomenal growth, development, and acceptance of Associate Degree nursing education was reminiscent of the status of diploma nursing schools at the turn of the century. But unexpected problems emerged, because the nursing profession was unprepared for the success of the Associate Degree program. Graduates of 2-year Associate Degree, 3-year Diploma, and 4-year Baccalaureate programs all took the same licensure examination, in most instances received the same salary, and were perceived by the public to be practicing alike. The public was confused about who the nurse was and what to expect of her. The profession was divided by controversy over the titles *professional nurse* and *technical nurse*, and the roles and functions of each.

The explosive development of scientific and technologic advances including mankind's quest of space had made patient care and its organization more complex and expensive than ever before, but low salaries for nurses coupled with rising costs for a college education created a critical problem of recruitment into nursing, particularly at the Baccalaureate level. Many diploma schools were closing because hospitals found them unprofitable. In response to the shortage, the government provided some financial aid through the Nurse Training Act of 1964.

The nursing profession became convinced that nurse education should occur in a college or university environment, and in 1965 the American Nurses' Association adopted a position paper which stated that the "minimum preparation for beginning *professional* nursing should be the Baccalaureate degree." It was "the shot heard round the [nursing] world" and the struggle over entry into *professional* nursing practice intensified.

During the 1960's the United States was heavily involved in the Viet Nam War, students on campuses were in revolt, and a strong militant women's movement emerged once again. American nurses served in Viet Nam, nursing students demonstrated along with other students on campuses around the country, and a nurse, Wilma Scott Heidi, was elected the first president of the National Organization for Women.

Moving Into the 21st Century

The 1980's are providing remarkable opportunity and challenge for nurses, individually and collectively. Empowered by their movement into the mainstream of higher education, their hard-won political sophistication, and their developing knowledge base, nurses are ready to assume a greater role in providing health care for the country's people—despite the continuing problems related to economics, entry into practice, and curriculum standards.

Nurses have freed themselves from the stereotypic role as the physician's handmaiden, and have established a healthy collegial relationship with members of the medical profession. They have shown themselves to be fully equal to the challenges of the 21st century.

SUGGESTED READINGS

Carnegie, M Elizabeth: Nurses and war: Black nurses at the front. *Am J Nurs* 1984 October; 84(10):1250–1252.

Curtis, Dorothy E: Nurses and war: the way it was. *Am J Nurs* 1984 October; 84(10):1253–1254.

Dolan, Josephine, ML Fitzpatrick, and EK Herrmann: *Nursing in Society: A Historical Perspective.* ed. 15. Philadelphia, Saunders, 1983.

Donahue, M Patricia: *Nursing: The Oldest Art—An Illustrated History.* St. Louis, Mosby, 1985.

Hine, Darlene Clark (ed): *Black Women in Nursing: An Anthology of Historical Sources.* New York, Garland Publishing, 1984.

Kalisch, Philip A, and Beatrice J Kalisch: *The Advance of American Nursing.* ed.2. Boston, Little, Brown and Co, 1986.

———— Dressing for success (History of uniforms). *Am J Nurs* 1985 Aug; 85(8):887–893.

———— Improving the image of nursing. *Am J Nurs* 1983 Jan; 83(1):48–52.

———— The image of nurses in novels. *Am J Nurs* 1982 Aug; 82(8):1220–1224.

———— The image of the nurse in motion pictures. *Am J Nurs* 1982 April; 82(4):605–611.

———— Nurses on prime-time television. *Am J Nurs* 1982 Feb; 82(2):264–270.

Nutting, Adelaide, and Lavinia Dock: *A Short History of Nursing.* New York, Putnam, 1912.

Palmer, Irene Sabelberg: Nightingale revisited. *Nurs Outlook* 1983 July/Aug; 31(4):229–233.

Parsons, Margaret: Mothers and matrons. *Nurs Outlook* 1983 Sept/Oct; 31(5):274–276.

Smith, Frances T: Florence Nightingale: early feminist. *Am J Nurs* 1981 May; 81(5):1020–1024.

Thompson, John D: The passionate humanist: from Nightingale to the new nurse. *Nurs Outlook* 1980 May; 28(5):290–295.

3

Nursing and the Delivery of Health Care

Patricia Button-Dye

Prerequisites and/or Suggested Preparation
Introductory concepts related to the history of nursing and the profession of nursing (from Chapters 1 and 2 or another source) are prerequisite to understanding this chapter.

Every society in every nation has a system for delivering health care to its people, and nursing care is an integral part of the system. A health care system represents the way in which a society organizes its efforts to deliver or provide health care, and the system may range in complexity from an informal network of neighbors who care for the sick in conjunction with the local doctor, to a highly organized system of socialized medicine.

The components of a health care system include the individuals who work in the system, the types of services provided, the facilities and resources, the sources of financing, and, of course, the people who receive the health care. The larger systems include hospitals, clinics, nursing homes, state and federal departments of health, blood banks, hospitalization, insurance companies, medical centers, and other facilities. A health care delivery system includes patients, nurses, doctors, physical therapists, Red Cross workers, x-ray technicians, paramedics, dentists, and many other people. In the United States, the health care delivery system constitutes one of the most extensive networks of agencies and organizations in the world in terms of physical facilities, equipment, money, and personnel.

SOCIETAL INFLUENCES ON HEALTH CARE SYSTEMS

The main influences on the characteristics of a health care system are the values of the society, the knowledge available to or generated by the members of the society, the society's level of technology and economic development, and its political structure.

Values

The values of a society are derived from its philosophical framework or belief system about the nature of humanity and human priorities. The behavior of a person, group, or nation is determined by these values and beliefs. A dramatic example is the US Bill of Rights, which resulted from the values and beliefs that prompted the colonists to reject English society and government, fight a war, and establish a new society based on the values of equality and the inalienable rights of all people. Much of US history since the Revolutionary War reflects the struggle to implement these values. The Civil War, labor union activity, women's fight for voting privileges, civil rights, and the feminist movement are examples of this struggle. Similarly, the development of the US health care system reflects the values and beliefs of its people about health, disease, and health care.

Knowledge

The knowledge that members of a society possess, or the knowledge that they generate, influences the systems they develop. In health care systems the methods that are used to care for people are in large part *determined by what is known* about ways to keep people healthy, the causes of disease, and ways to treat disease. Knowledge in these areas directly influences health care practice and the system needed for the practice. For example, prior to general knowledge of the germ theory, it was standard practice for more than one patient to occupy a hospital bed at the same time, for each bed to be used by a series of patients without changing the sheets, and for physicians and nurses to move from one patient to another without washing their hands. Knowledge of the germ theory dramatically influenced these practices. It is now taken for granted that every hospitalized patient will have a separate bed and that he will have clean, disinfected sheets.

Technology

The level of technological development of a society has always been a significant influence on its health care systems, but it is only in the past century that the knowledge of disease causation and technology have been sufficient to allow the development of complex diagnostic and treatment methods. Much of modern medical practice is dependent on complicated machines and equipment, but in those countries or areas where advanced technology is not possible for economic or political reasons, medical care tends to be less complex and the health care system needed to deliver that care is thus less complex. In such areas, it may be impossible to diagnose and treat some health problems. For example, without sophisticated x-ray and surgical equipment, it is not possible to locate and treat blocked cerebral or coronary arteries.

Economics

The economic status of a society greatly influences its health care system because the components of health care systems, such as equipment, drugs, and trained personnel, cost money. In societies where there is general poverty, health care systems tend to be basic and simple, whereas complex facilities and techniques characterize health care systems in wealthy countries.

The *source* of wealth in a society is another economic factor. The individuals and groups who have control of the economic resources of a society influence the way that money is used. Therefore, the amount of money available to a health care system is related to the sources of wealth in that society. For example, the sophisticated treatment modalities and buildings of many health care facilities in the US are possible because wealthy people have given of their wealth and because the government has allocated funds for health care. Without access to economic resources, a health care system's development is limited.

Power and Politics

The power structure of a society is the manner in which that society chooses to assign authority and control to individuals and groups for the purpose of governing. Many individuals and groups are assigned authority because they possess wealth, while others have authority because of their knowledge or skills. The degree to which those in authority perceive health care as a societal priority influences the amount of time, energy, and money the society devotes to its health care system. In the US, for example, whenever the Democratic Party gains control of a majority of seats in Congress, there is typically an increase in funding available for developing new health care programs. This is because Democrats have traditionally encouraged government support of health care. When the Republican Party is in control, the reverse is likely to happen.

Complex Interactions

An understanding of how society's values, knowledge, technology, economics, and politics affect its health care system as well as other systems is of importance when one considers the current health care system of the US. The systems of government, law, education, transportation, communication, and health in the US are extremely complex, interrelated, and interdependent. When a change occurs in one of the major systems of the society, there is often a change in the health care system.

An interesting example is the impact of technology on two systems in the US. Both the transportation and the health care systems in this country have responded to what has been termed the *technological imperative,* a powerful drive to incorporate advanced technology into every aspect of living. The transportation system has sought to develop automobiles, airplanes, and other transportation devices with primary focus on the use of advanced technology, *regardless of cost.* Mechanic (1978) has expressed well a similar effect of the technological imperative on health care: "Physicians have been trained to pursue the 'technological imperative'— that is, the tendency to use any intervention regardless of cost if there is any possibility of benefit for the patient" (p. 329).

Significantly, the issue of cost of both transportation

and health care has received more and more attention in the past decade. This attention is not related to anything unique to either system but rather to another of the societal influences discussed in this chapter: the economy. In the past decade, our society's economy has undergone major changes because of wide variations in the cost of energy. Health care and its delivery have changed tremendously in the past because of technology, and now, as the economic situation changes, the health care system is being affected in many different ways.

HISTORICAL INFLUENCES ON HEALTH CARE

It is beyond the scope of this chapter to consider the historical development of health care systems in depth, but it is possible to highlight historical events particularly significant for an understanding of the current US health care system which are related to the societal influences discussed.

In ancient times the level of knowledge of disease causation was extremely limited. Disease and the suffering related to it were considered to be natural phenomena, like sun, wind, earthquakes, and storms. Like these other natural phenomena, disease was perceived as a work of the evil spirits and the gods. Treatment was therefore directed at using magic or medicine men to drive out evil spirits and to intervene with the gods.

Hippocrates lived in ancient Greece (460 BC to 370 BC) and has been called the father of medicine. He understood that disease was not inflicted by the gods, but was a natural process and therefore should be treated rationally. He recognized that making accurate observations of, and drawing general conclusions from, actual phenomena form the basis of sound medical reasoning, and also formulated the Hippocratic oath, which is still in use after 24 centuries.

Empedocles of Acragas, who lived at the same time as Hippocrates, put forth another theory of disease causation, the doctrine of the four humors. This doctrine stated that the body had four humors: blood, yellow bile, black bile, and phlegm. These four humors corresponded to the four elements of the world: fire, air, water, and earth. According to this doctrine, disease was determined by the particular humor that was predominant in a person's body. The doctrine also stated that treatment consisted of application of some combination of the four worldly elements in hot, cold, wet, and dry forms. The particular combination of worldly elements depended on the change needed in the body's humors. Interestingly, Empedocles's doctrine of four humors dominated medical practice for centuries while the more rational approach of Hippocrates was less influential. In the Dark Ages, nearly all the medical writings of ancient times were lost as a result of barbarian invasions.

In the eleventh, twelfth, and thirteenth centuries, the Crusades and the growth of monasteries significantly affected health care systems. Religious orders with the primary function of providing nursing care were developed to care for military casualties of the Crusades. These religious nursing orders and the monasteries founded hospitals to provide health care to a group of sick people who, for economic, geographical, or technical reasons, could not get the care elsewhere.

During the Middle Ages, the doctrine of four humors was generally rejected, and different theories of disease causation were proposed. The Renaissance (1400–1600), which followed the Middle Ages, was a period of major development of knowledge related to disease causation. Paracelsus (1493–1591) made an important contribution by suggesting that disease might be related to a chemical imbalance in the body rather than to the four humors. This period culminated with the work of Francis Bacon (1561–1626) and his statement of the scientific method.

Despite promising advances in the knowledge of disease causation, there was very little application of this knowledge to health care practice during the seventeenth, eighteenth, or early nineteenth centuries. Hospitals during this time were maintained for the care of the poor or those with infectious diseases. Wealthy people who became ill were still cared for in their homes. Regardless of the location of the care, there was little attention to cleanliness or to the prevention and transmission of disease. There were few effective measures for the disposal of sewage and garbage or contaminated food. The major treatments used by physicians during this time were bleeding, emetics, and purgatives. It is clear from some case studies that patients died from the treatment rather than the disease.

It was in the second half of the nineteenth century that advances in knowledge, technology, and health care practices occurred that provided the basis for modern medicine. For example, in 1864, Louis Pasteur validated the germ theory by proving that bacteria were living microorganisms that could be destroyed by heat and chemical action. Other scientists who are well known for the practical applications of this theory include Ignaz Philipp Semmelweiss, for his work with patients with puerperal (childbirth) fever, and Joseph Lister, for his use of carbolic acid to disinfect wounds. The germ theory and its clinical application (antisepsis) had a pervasive impact on all aspects of health care practice. It provided the basis for the identification of specific microorganisms and the diseases they cause and

eventually for appropriate prevention or curative treatments.

Of equal significance were the introduction of anesthetics (around 1850) and the discovery of four blood groups (1900) which provided the basis for compatible blood transfusions. These three developments—antisepsis, anesthesia, and transfusion—particularly affected the practice of surgery, and surgical treatment became safe as a result. Diagnostic aids developed in the late 1800s and the early 1900s include the thermometer, stethoscope, and microscope. These aids extended the physician's ability to assess patients and make accurate diagnoses. Another important technique developed in the late nineteenth century was the technique of psychoanalysis, developed by Sigmund Freud for the treatment of mental illness.

Simultaneous with these advances in medical knowledge and techniques, there were significant changes in hospital practice. Florence Nightingale played a major role in these changes; and as a result of her work in army hospitals in Scutari during the Crimean War, hospital care and the role of female nurses underwent marked changes. The focus of Nightingale's work was on developing the nurse's role and providing cleanliness, good food, and social services for soldiers. Her publications, *Notes on Matters Affecting the Health, Efficiency, and Hospital Administration of the British Army* (1858), *Notes on Hospitals* (1858), and *Notes on Nursing* (1859), represent the core of her work. As Dolan (1978) stated:

Miss Nightingale stressed the importance of primary prevention as well as health maintenance. Her definition of health was ''not only to be well, but to be able to use well every power we have.''

She taught that there were two major components of nursing— health nursing and sick nursing. Health nursing was identified as ''to keep or put the constitution of a healthy person in such a state as to have no disease,'' that is, retaining or regaining one's health. Sick nursing was described as ''to help the person suffering from disease to live''; that is, not merely to survive but live as full and satisfying a life as possible. She stated that ''both kinds of nursing are to put a person in the best possible condition for nature to restore or to preserve health, to prevent, or to cure disease or injury.

She was appalled at the criminal wastefulness caused by inadequate preventive and restorative practices as well as lack of emphasis on health in nursing practice. In maintaining that the whole person should be understood and treated, she advocated a holistic approach. She insisted that prevention was better than cure. This philosophy predated the theories of microbiologists and psychologists. (p. 165)

Florence Nightingale also applied the scientific method and statistics to the problems of health care. The combination of systematic problem solving with preventive measures such as cleanliness, sound nutrition, and attention to the emotional needs of patients, plus adequate education for nurses, provided the basis not only for modern professional nursing but the improvement of all health care practice.

Around 1900, the advances in knowledge of the late 1800s and the work of Nightingale began to come together. New sciences, such as pathology, microbiology, and immunology, promoted the advancement of scientific medicine and more complex technology. These developments increased the need for hospitals where equipment would be available for more sophisticated diagnosis and treatment. Facilities were developed for the treatment of bacterial infections and the promotion of antisepsis, pathology laboratories were founded, and casebooks began to be used to record the patient's previous history and the course of his disease.

It was at this time that changing patterns in the use of hospitals emerged. The advances in diagnosis and treatment made it increasingly difficult to care for patients at home, and as a result, more and more hospitals were built, usually including facilities for private paying patients separated from the traditional ward facilities for the poor. Wealthy patients were charged enough to provide funds for the care of the poor as well as for their own.

The remainder of the twentieth century has been characterized by phenomenal increases in knowledge and technology in all aspects of life. Dolan (1978) wrote:

This century has encompassed the transition from candlelight to satellite, from the horse and buggy era to the space age, from the laying on of hands to impersonal electronic monitoring. The struggle for freedom and independence of new nations, the trauma of international tensions and threat to survival itself have all played a part in writing current history.

The twentieth century has also witnessed a phenomenal improvement in the general standard of living, lengthening of the span of life, the identification of the causes of many diseases, the ability to conquer most bacterial diseases and the provision for a scientific plan of care for the patient and his family. In this century, the center of health care has been the hospital; the prevention and rehabilitative as well as the curative aspects of patient care have received increasing attention. The exigencies of war, the marked progress in transportation and communication, the remarkable inventions, along with scientific achievements have had an influence on keeping individuals healthy, on initiating changes in the care of the sick, on the expansion of the health care field in general. (pp. 242–243)

These events provided the basis for our current health care system, because it is only as a result of the advances in knowledge and technology that it has been possible and necessary to develop the complex system for delivering health care that exists today. If so much were not known, health care might still consist of magic or medicine men.

CURRENT INFLUENCES ON UNITED STATES HEALTH CARE

The health care delivery system in the US today reflects the complexity of society in general because the country's values, level of knowledge, economy, technology, and politics interrelate to produce strong and sometimes conflicting influences on how health care is delivered.

Effect of Values

Values that influence health care delivery include the belief that health care is a right and not a privilege, the belief that health care should be holistic, a commitment to examination of the moral and ethical issues that are raised by increased sophistication of treatment, a belief in consumerism, and the capitalistic belief in the profit motive.

Belief in Health Care as a Right

The belief that health care is a right and not a privilege was the basis for much of the health care legislation of the 1960s and early 1970s. This legislation created the Medicare and Medicaid systems, which are intended to provide health care for those who would be unable to obtain it because of their economic status. Medicare is a federally financed program that provides uniform medical benefits to elderly people who are covered by the social security retirement program. One part of the program is a *hospital insurance* plan for people over 65 years of age, and another part is a voluntary *medical insurance* plan for physicians' services and other benefits. In the second part, the federal government shares the costs of medical expenses with the recipient. Periodically, the specifics of these provisions are changed by new federal legislation.

Medicaid (Title 19 of the Social Security Act) is a different program. Medicaid provides federal *subsidies to states* that provide health care to people who are unable to pay. Each state has the authority to define who is eligible, and there are great differences from state to state. In the years since these programs were legislated, there has been much study of their effectiveness in providing high-quality care to those unable to obtain it otherwise. Several problem areas have been identified. First, the provisions regarding deductible have made it difficult for those who are least able to afford health care to get it. Second, there has been substantial fraud in the use of funds. The degree of fraud was a major factor in the establishment of the *Professional Standards Review Organization* (PSRO) in 1972. The PSRO has become one of the major national quality assurance programs in health care today, although initially it was created primarily to monitor the use of Medicare and Medicaid funds.

Another problem of Medicare and Medicaid is the inequalities in providing services to the elderly and the poor. It is well documented that these programs have not effectively delivered health care to all of the population for which they were created. In addition, the cost of these programs has become unacceptably high. In the 1980s these high costs are a challenge to a continued commitment to the value of health care as a right.

Belief in Holistic Health Care

Another value which significantly influences the health care system today is the belief that health care should be holistic. The proponents of holistic health care believe that all aspects of the person—mental, emotional, spiritual, and physical—must be considered if the health care system is to be effective. Much of the sickness and death in the United States today is caused by stress-related health problems. There have been significant research studies as well as individual stories that document the relationship between lifestyle and disease. The current focus of the health care system is on the disease rather than on the person who happens to have the disease. Those who advocate a holistic approach to health care suggest that the system must provide, in addition to the current highly technical acute care, an expansion of health education, an increase in care during the early

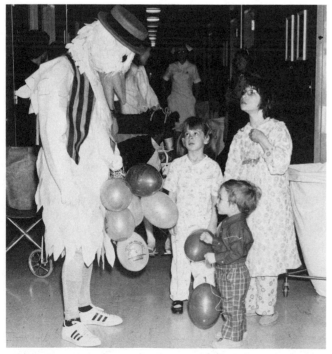

Figure 3.1 *An unexpected visitor complete with balloons can be an important part of holistic care in a pediatric unit.*

stages of illness, better coordination of all aspects of health care, and support for patients who are experiencing stress-related disease. All these efforts must be based on a redefined concept of health and illness that includes the whole person, not just one or two organs of the body at any one time (Fig. 3.1).

Moral and Ethical Issues

A third important value influencing health care systems is the commitment to examine the moral and ethical issues raised by increasingly sophisticated treatment. One hundred years ago one would have laughed at a series of articles which attempted to define death. In the past 15 years, however, an untold number of hours have been spent by physicians, nurses, theologians, lawmakers, patients, and family members struggling to clarify exactly what it now means to say a human being is dead and also what it now means to say that a human being is alive. The advances in medical care which have improved our ability to maintain physiological functions using mechanical devices and drugs have created situations that boggle the mind. Issues involving the prolongation of life, euthanasia, abortion, artificial insemination, sterilization, and experimental treatment now challenge the health care system to address serious moral-ethical dilemmas.

Consumerism

A fourth value of significance is the belief in consumerism. Traditionally, consumers of health care have been passive. They have played a minimal role in the organization, implementation, and evaluation of their own health care and of health care services in general. Because of their need for care and their vulnerability in the face of illness, consumers have thought they had little ability or right to take part in health care decisions. Pavalon (1980) described this phenomenon as follows:

There is the reality of the hospitalization process and the attitude of the patient and toward the patient that has existed for a long time. Much of the treatment for sickness takes place in the hospital, which many persons view as confinement. The person is confined to his bed, a wheelchair, or a hospital for a certain length of time until released by the physician and the hospital. The use of the terms confinement and release in themselves indicate a person's loss of control and subsequent loss of rights.

The hospitalized patient is under the almost total control of the doctors and staff. He or she is told what to wear, what to eat, when to sleep, when to rise, and when visitors are allowed. Often, patients need assistance in bathing, eliminating, and walking. As one writer put it, ''A stay in a hospital exposes an individual to a condition of passivity and impotence unparalleled in adult life.'' In such a setting where nearly all control is placed in the hands of the doctors and staff, it is no wonder that people forget their rights, if they ever knew them. (p. 5)

Experiences such as those, coupled with the trust that society has habitually placed in physicians, have resulted in patients being slow to make demands about the care they receive.

The current increased consumer activity is very much related to the increased concern for human rights which developed in the 1960s in this country. The emphasis on human rights initially focused on schooling, jobs, and pay for minorities, but has expanded to include adequate health care for all. It was during the 1960s that the value of health care as a right rather than a privilege became significant in health care decision making.

Other factors which have influenced consumer activities are the media and the women's movement. Through the media of television, radio, popular magazines, and newspapers, the consumer is provided with vast amounts of information about the health care delivery system, the effectiveness and cost of specific health care practices, and alternatives to traditional services. For example, the topic of unnecessary surgery has been widely discussed in the media. The response of consumers has been to seek a second opinion more frequently when a physician recommends a surgical procedure. Consumer pressure in this area has been so great that now physicians often suggest to patients that they get a second opinion, and some health insurance plans, such as Blue Cross/Blue Shield, will pay for second opinions.

The women's movement has contributed to consumer activism. Varying degrees of male domination and its counterpart, female subordination, have been found to be fundamental characteristics of the majority of systems in the US today, including the health care delivery system. The health care system has been particularly affected by sexism because not only are female clients exposed to sexist attitudes of male physicians but the hierarchy of the system itself has developed according to the traditional perceptions of male-female roles. Physicians and hospital administrators, those with control and power and high salaries in the hierarchy, have typically been men, while nurses, who have been expected to follow orders and receive lower pay, have typically been women. As women within and outside the health care system have become aware of the effects of sexism on the quality of care, they have become increasingly vocal about the need for changes in the system.

Many of the current changes in aspects of the health care delivery system are a reflection of the influence of consumerism. Health planning boards and boards of health care agencies now often include seats for nurses and for the consumers of health care. Specific groups of patients often request and receive health care in the manner they wish. A significant example of this is the change in obstetrical care. As couples expressed their preferences for family-centered care in a homelike atmosphere, some hospitals designed informal birthing rooms as alternatives to the traditional delivery room and allowed mothers to go home a few hours after a normal delivery.

Professional organizations have explicitly acknowledged the rights and role of the consumer of health care. The American Hospital Association published in 1973 *A Patient's Bill of Rights* for hospitalized patients (see Chapter 1). The American Nurses' Association (ANA), in its *Standards of Practice* (1973), stated that the inclusion of the consumer in health care decisions is a basic component of nursing practice. Standard 5 reads, "Nursing actions provide for client/patient participation in health promotion, maintenance, and restoration."

Other examples of the impact of consumerism are the increased emphasis on ethical and moral aspects of patient care and efforts to individualize care, as evidenced by primary care practice and primary nursing.

Profit Motive

Another value that influences the health care system is the capitalistic belief in the profit motive. The economy of the US is a capitalist system. Increasingly, health care delivery has become a commercial industry, similar to other US businesses. As a result, the influence of the goal of profit from participation in health care activities may be observed in a variety of situations. Manufacturers of highly technical equipment, which is very expensive and produces a large profit, exert great influence in treatment choices. Treatment that involves the use of costly, highly technical equipment is often considered the best alternative without thorough consideration of the benefits of the treatment. The basis for the choice is the unfounded belief that a treatment that is expensive and highly technical is best.

Another example of the influence of the profit motive is the economic gains which various health care personnel reap from their activities. Some people choose the field of medicine partly because of the social and economic status that our society grants to physicians. Physicians have traditionally received the permission of our society to make life-and-death decisions for their patients, often without consulting the patient, and to be paid very well for doing so. This situation is currently changing, but many physicians continue to expect to be paid well, and a significant proportion of society continues to expect to have to pay them well. The desire of some physicians to maintain their social and economic status affects both the choices of treatment for individual patients and the development of health care policies, as evidenced by documented cases of unnecessary surgery and decisions to fund highly expensive but questionably effective crisis care programs rather than preventive care programs.

Effect of Knowledge and Technology

One result of the proliferation of knowledge during recent decades is a change in focus in concepts of disease causation. The most predominant concept at this time is that of multiple causation of illness. The concept maintains that illness is the result of a basic imbalance in a person's adaptation to multiple physical and emotional stresses within the environment (Shindell, Salloway, and Oberembt, 1976). The significance of this concept is its recognition of the role of both the individual and the environment in health and illness. More effective treatment of chronic and stress-related diseases has increased the life expectancy of those with these problems, and increased knowledge of ways to treat these diseases has stimulated extensive specialization and role proliferation. It is no longer possible for one physician to deal with all aspects of one illness; other people must often be included—physicians, nurses, x-ray and laboratory technicians, pharmacists, social workers, occupational therapists, physical therapists, cardiopulmonary technicians, to mention a few.

The implication for health care delivery systems is the need for services that can attend to the multiple aspects of disease, which of necessity increases the complexity of health care systems.

Effect of Economics and Politics

Finally, there are the influences of the economic and political status of the society of health care delivery. It is difficult to separate the economic and political issues. Shindul, Salloway, and Oberembt (1976) identify clearly the trends in the development of health care delivery which were evident at the national level in the last half of the 1970's:

1. The attempt to lower financial barriers to obtaining care, exemplified by the Medicare and Medicaid legislation and the proposals for national health insurance.
2. The attempt to increase manpower available to provide care, exemplified by the expansion of facilities to train physicians, primary care practitioners, and physician assistants.
3. The attempt to modify the current structure to give more efficient and effective care, exemplified by the fostering of group practice settings as opposed to individual practices.

4. The attempt to control unnecessary care or unnecessary proliferation of facilities for care as exemplified by the techniques of professional standard review and resource allocation via the comprehensive planning approach.
5. The attempt to modify behavior, by fostering the preventive approach rather than crisis intervention via the use of multiphasic screening and the health maintenance approach to care.
6. The attempt to protect the public from unnecessary risk through environmental protection.

In the 1980's under the Reagan administration, the economic priority of controlling the federal budget has resulted in the realization of some of these trends and the virtual disappearance of others. The value of health care as a right has taken a backseat to the value of economic recovery. The trends of lowering financial barriers to care, increasing health care manpower, increasing preventive care, and improving the environment have been dropped because of the costs associated with them, whereas the trends of modifying the structure of the health care system to increase efficiency, lower costs, and control unnecessary care have become specific programs.

UNITED STATES HEALTH CARE SYSTEMS

Types

The structure of a health care delivery system is determined by the types of agencies that exist and the roles that health care workers play in the agencies. Health care agencies can be categorized either by their ownership and source of funds or by the service they provide.

Categorization of health care agencies according to *ownership* yields three types of agencies: voluntary, governmental, and proprietary.

Voluntary, or nonprofit, agencies are run by a board of trustees who are responsible to the community which the agency serves. The board hires an administrator to be the agent in running the agency. An additional, important aspect of the voluntary system in hospitals is the autonomous role of the medical staff. In voluntary hospitals, the medical staff has traditionally governed and regulated itself.

Governmental agencies may be financed at the federal, state, county, or municipal level. The hospitals of the US Army, Navy, Air Force, Veterans' Administration, and Indian Service are examples of federal agencies. Most states finance state mental hospitals. County and municipal agencies are usually acute- and chronic-disease general hospitals as well as preventive outpatient agencies. Proprietary agencies are agencies run by interested people or groups to make a profit. These agencies may be owned by physicians, an individual, or a corporation. A profit-making nursing home is an example of a proprietary agency. Another example is a chain of hospitals run by a corporation such as the Hospital Corporation of America.

The second way of categorizing health care agencies is according to the *type of service* provided, which may be either ambulatory (outpatient) or inpatient care.

Ambulatory Care

Ambulatory care is health care of people who do not need to be hospitalized. The care may be preventive, diagnostic, or therapeutic. The most common traditional ambulatory care agency is the private physician's office. According to the categories used in this discussion, a private physician's office is a proprietary agency—that is, the physician has financial control of the office and operates it on a fee-for-service basis to yield a profit. Often, several physicians share office space and equipment, and this is called a *group practice* (Fig. 3.2).

CLINICS. Other traditional ambulatory care agencies include ambulatory clinics of hospitals and public health clinics. Large hospitals have often developed outpatient departments in the same geographical location as the hospital so that its diagnostic facilities such as the x-ray equipment and laboratory can be used by clinic patients.

Historically, however, it was not for the purpose of efficient use of facilities and equipment that hospital-based clinics were developed. The early hospitals served the poor almost exclusively, and the tradition of hospitals serving the poor has been maintained to a significant degree in ambulatory care. There are a variety of reasons for this. First, there is the strength of tradition. Poor people have been conditioned to view the hospital as the appropriate source of health care for them. Second, those who are poor often have difficulty obtaining access to private physicians' offices because of their inability to pay and physicians' unwillingness to care for them.

Public health clinics are usually part of local health departments, which are local or state governmental agencies. The term public health is used to describe those needs that arise as a result of people living in groups. Typical clinics are for maternal and infant preventive care, including immunizations for screening of such communicable diseases as venereal disease and tuberculosis, and for the provision of public health nursing. Public health nursing departments serve peo-

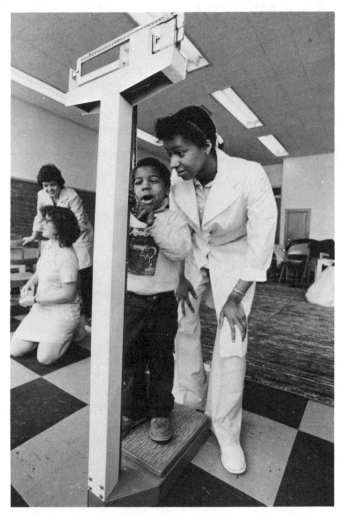

Figure 3.2 *This ambulatory care facility provides health supervision for a variety of patients.*

ple in their homes, either to prevent health problems or to provide nursing care for health problems.

The last traditional type of ambulatory care agency is the *voluntary agency* which is set up to provide a specific type of health care service. Examples include visiting nurse agencies, and clinics which have been developed to care for women's health problems, such as abortion clinics.

HEALTH MAINTENANCE ORGANIZATIONS. Another type of ambulatory care agency which became popular in the 1970s is a comprehensive prepaid group practice, which is called a *Health Maintenance Organization* (HMO). A comprehensive prepaid group practice has the following characteristics:

1. Physicians work as a team under a common organizational structure.
2. Physicians are paid by the group practice or-

ganization, *not by the patient* on a fee-for-service basis.

3. Patients pay a predefined enrollment or subscription charge that covers a broad range of benefits, usually defined as comprehensive health services. Each practice defines the specific details of services provided, but the intent is for the group practice to meet all health care needs and cover all expenses.

4. The practice serves a defined population; those who are enrolled in it.

An HMO is usually presented as an alternative to the more traditional fee-for-service care (Shindell, Salloway, and Oberembt, 1976). The intent of creating HMOs is to provide comprehensive health care in a way that is satisfying to consumers, is of high quality, is cost efficient, and includes more preventive health measures than traditional fee-for-service care. It is too early in the development of this method of providing care to assess its long-term effectiveness, but consumer reaction to HMOs is sometimes negative. Consumers appear to prefer traditional sources of care because such care tends to be more personalized, allowing for a one-to-one relationship between physician and patient. Some HMOs are reminiscent of large, impersonal institutions where consumers experience, or fear they will experience, a loss of personal identity.

IN-AND-OUT SURGERY. Two other ambulatory care services are *in-and-out surgery* (short-stay surgery) and *hospice care.* In short-stay surgery units, uncomplicated surgical procedures, such as the removal of tonsils or the repair of a simple hernia, are performed without the patient being hospitalized. Preoperative preparation is completed before the day of surgery. The patient arrives at the unit, usually located in a hospital, early in the morning. The surgery is performed and the patient remains in the unit for several hours to recover. He then returns home with specific instructions about his activity. The advantages of this approach are that the patient does not experience the trauma of separation from home and it is much less costly than overnight hospitalization.

HOSPICE CARE. Hospice care refers to care of terminally ill patients, often at home. In England, where the term *hospice* originated, hospice care referred to institutions that provided care for dying patients. In the US, more and more programs are developing to provide physical and emotional care for patients at home, so they may experience death more comfortably, with their families rather than in an impersonal hospital environment.

Inpatient Care

Patients who require care that cannot be provided in the home or in an ambulatory setting are placed in one of a variety of inpatient facilities. Short-term, *acute care hospitals* provide care to patients who are acutely ill and require sophisticated care for diagnostic or treatment purposes. Intermediate or *extended care facilities* provide convalescent or rehabilitation care to patients. Usually, patients are transferred from an acute care facility to an intermediate facility when their condition is no longer acute but they are not ready to go home because they still need treatment, care, or rehabilitation. *Long-term chronic care facilities* are those agencies that provide inpatient care to people who are chronically ill or disabled and are unable to receive the care they need in a home setting. This category includes nursing homes, which provide care for geriatric patients.

The specific definitions of acute, intermediate, and long-term care are, at this time, formulated mainly by those groups who reimburse for care. Insurance companies and federal programs (Medicare, Medicaid, and PSRO) set standards for the types of service for which they will pay, according to the type of facility where the service is provided. To be admitted to an acute care facility and have the care paid for, a patient must need the care that has been predefined as reimbursable acute care. When a patient no longer requires what has been labeled acute care, he must be discharged. The movement of patients among these levels of care in such a way that their care is of good quality and the insurance company or governmental agency will pay for the care is often problematic. The health care needs of patients do not always correspond with the payment sources' definitions of levels of care. In many situations, a patient may no longer require acute care but not meet the criteria for intermediate care or be able to manage at home.

Another aspect of inpatient facilities is the spectrum of services they provide. Hospitals may provide general care, which means that they provide basic medical, surgical, and emergency care to patients of all ages, usually including obstetric care. In addition, specialty services may be offered such as complex cardiovascular surgery; open heart surgery; complex surgery in any specialty; care of cancer patients including surgery, chemotherapy, and radiotherapy; psychiatric care; and high-risk obstetric and neonatal care.

Geographic location, financial resources, and proximity to educational facilities all influence the services offered by a particular hospital. The geographic location is significant in two ways: first, in relation to the size of the population served; and second, in relation to other hospitals in the same area and the type of services they offer. The federal government has been increasing its efforts to *equalize the availability* of all types of services throughout the country. In 1966, the Comprehensive Health Planning and Public Health Services Amendments was passed. This law provided for comprehensive health-planning agencies at the state level that were authorized to direct health-planning agencies at the local level. A significant requirement of the council of these agencies was the inclusion and participation of consumers of health care.

Health planning was further structured in 1974 with the enactment of the National Health Policy and Resources Development Act. This act revised health planning programs by requiring that a network of Health Systems Agencies (HSA) be created which divided the whole country into health planning areas. The act also revised programs related to construction and modernization of health care facilities. Among other activities, the HSA's review, and then approve or disapprove applications for construction, modernization, and obtaining new equipment. The intent of this is to equalize services and prevent unnecessary duplication, such as the concentration of several burn units or extraordinarily expensive pieces of equipment within a small geographical area (Fig. 3.3).

The type of specialty services a hospital offers depends upon its proximity to educational facilities. The presence of a university or medical school increases the likelihood of having personnel available who have special knowledge and skills.

Economics and Costs of Health Care

Historically, health care has been charged and paid for on a fee-for-service basis. This means that health care providers and health care institutions have charged a patient a fee for each service, such as an office visit, a test, or a surgical procedure, which the patient receives.

Under this fee-for-service framework, a large portion of health care costs have been paid for by third party payors, that is, the federal and state governments and private insurance companies. The combination of fee-for-service and the lack of visibility of actual costs to the consumer and provider because of third party payment resulted in minimal attention or concern regarding the cost of care. An overall attitude of "if some is good, more must be better" predominated the provision of health care. The provision of care characterized by this "ignore the cost attitude" resulted in huge increases in the overall cost of health care.

In the late 1970's, concern regarding health care costs grew. Politicians, economists, and some health care providers considered alternatives, including proposals for national health insurance. At the time of the writing of this chapter, national health insurance is not the

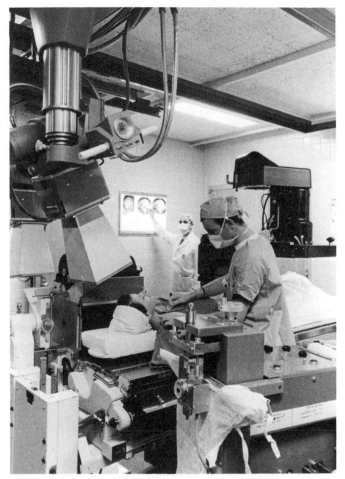

Figure 3.3 *Regional planning is needed to ensure an equitable geographical distribution of specialty services such as this computerized diagnostic unit.*

primary alternative under consideration. Rather, the federal government, consistent with its current priority to achieve control of government spending, has enacted legislation which target high cost government programs. Because health care costs have been such an increasingly large portion of both government spending and the gross national product, government health care programs have been changed significantly to decrease the amount of money allocated to these programs.

The most significant changes were accomplished by the Tax Equity and Fiscal Responsibility Act (TEFRA) of 1982 and the Social Security Amendments of 1983. This legislation significantly limited reimbursement for some services previously paid for by Medicare and Medicaid and then created a new type of reimbursement system called prospective pricing.

In a prospective pricing system, health care costs are charged very differently than under a fee-for-service system. Instead of the charges for care being based on an accumulation of fees for each service a patient receives, under prospective pricing, the charge for an episode of care is calculated prior to the provision of care. For example, when a patient is admitted to the hospital for an appendectomy under the fee-for-service system, the patient's total bill is an accumulation of charges for all the various services the patient received, such as the hospital room, tests, operating room time, and medications. Under the prospective pricing system, however, the amount the hospital can receive for the same hospital stay is predetermined based on the average cost of performing an appendectomy. The intent of prospective pricing is to challenge health care providers to provide care at a controlled, predefined cost. The expectation is that providers will be able to accomplish this by being more efficient in providing care and by omitting services which were previously done because they were interesting but did not actually impact the patient's overall outcome.

The current major prospective pricing system in effect impacts only hospital reimbursement by the federal government. In this system, Medicare patients are categorized into approximately 500 Diagnostic Related Groups, or DRG's. Each DRG has a predefined reimbursement rate based on the average cost of caring for a patient in that category. An example of a DRG is Coronary Bypass with Cardiac Catheterization. It is expected that the federal government will expand this type of reimbursement to physicians and extended and ambulatory care settings.

In the private sector, a similar type of reimbursement structure is more frequent in the form of Preferred Provider Organizations, or PPO's. In the PPO structure, an organization, often a corporation or company, contracts with a hospital for health care at a fixed price. The organization agrees that all employees requiring, for example, open-heart surgery will go to a certain hospital, and the hospital agrees to provide that service at a predefined price.

The concept of prospective pricing has expanded to some private health insurance companies. It is expected that this trend will continue.

The overall impact of prospective pricing is *competition*. The competition is focused on health care providers identifying means of providing care at reasonable, competitive costs while maintaining acceptable levels of quality. Health care providers are not accustomed to competing in this way with each other.

The Health Care Team

One hundred years ago, a description of the health care system would have consisted of a few sentences about the physician, the nurse, and the development of hospitals for the poor with no mention of a *health care team*

or its members and their roles. The proliferation of roles has been greatest in the past 40 years, as medical specialization has increased. Physicians, as they have narrowed the focus of their practices to specialized areas, have found it more and more difficult to continue to carry out the more general aspects of practice, and the health team has evolved as a result. The *health care team* refers to the groups of people who work together to provide a patient with all the services that are necessary for comprehensive health care. The physician is usually the leader of the health care team.

A health care team usually includes physicians, nurses, social workers, pharmacists, laboratory technicians, x-ray technicians, occupational therapists, physical therapists, speech therapists, dietitians, operating-room technicians, and professional medical administration personnel, such as hospital administrators, medical records librarians, and accounting personnel (Fig. 3.4). Each of these roles may have various levels of specialization within it. For example, nursing roles are increasingly specialized. Based on educational preparation, or sometimes on experience, nurses may specialize in critical care, cardiovascular care, oncology, rehabilitation, renal care, maternal-child care, community health, or mental health nursing, to mention a few.

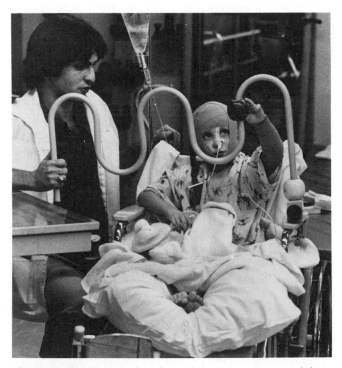

Figure 3.4 For Renee, the physical therapist was one of the most significant members of the health care team. Soon after surgery while she was still being fed via a nasogastric tube, Renee was encouraged to exercise in order to prevent contractions of her burned arm. Note her concentration as she exercises by moving the colored ball along the tubing.

Operating room technicians also specialize by becoming skilled in the operation of a particular piece of equipment, such as the open-heart pump, or in a particular surgical procedure.

Physicians' roles depend on their educational level and their area of medical specialization. On completion of medical school, physicians move through several years of on-the-job training. They are usually called interns during the first year of training and residents in the years thereafter. On completion of these years of training, they are ready to open their own practices and become attending physicians in hospitals, which means they are in charge of patients' medical care, and supervise interns and residents.

The exact composition of the health team in a specific agency varies according to the location and purpose of the agency and the population served. Urban teaching agencies and medical centers tend to have greater numbers of people on health teams. This is because of the availability of people educated and trained to give complex, specialized care. Rural community agencies tend to have fewer health care team members, and the general practitioner is more common in rural areas.

Regardless of the specific composition of the health care team at a particular time or in a particular place, the significance of the team itself is twofold. The team approach has great *potential* for increasing the quality of health care. A group of people, each with specialized preparation in a particular aspect of health care, working together to provide comprehensive care, is exciting. Unfortunately, this arrangement also includes potential problems of coordination and communication. There is the risk that a patient, as he receives care, will experience fragmentation and the results of poor communication. He may feel uncertain and lose trust in those caring for him, because it can appear that one team member does not know what the other is doing.

Coordination of the efforts of health care team members is certainly possible, but it does require time, motivation, good communication skills, and effective organization of the health care system. In addition, it is important for team members to clarify their areas of accountability.

Quality Assurance

An important aspect of the current US health care system is the increased development of formal quality assurance programs. *Quality assurance* is defined broadly as a process whereby the quality of health care is evaluated in terms of *predefined standards*. The standards include specific identification of how care should be given and the results that should be expected. The pur-

pose of this evaluation is the identification of problems, followed by solutions to the problems. The overall purpose of this process is to make certain that health care is consistently of high quality. The various quality assurance programs that have emerged represent the coming together of several strong forces that influence the health care system: professionalism, consumerism, and cost control.

Medicine was the first category of health care workers to become a profession. Among the criteria for acceptance as a profession are collegiality and autonomy. Collegiality includes (1) a professional organization that promotes and improves the quality of practice, and (2) peer evaluation to protect clients and assure high-quality care. Autonomy means responsibility for one's professional practice, including accountability for the quality of that practice. Donabedian (1966) described these characteristics of a profession as follows:

There is a "social contract" between society and the professions. Under its terms, society grants the profession authority over functions vital to itself and permits them considerable autonomy in the conduct of their own affairs. In return, the professions are expected to act responsibly, always mindful of the public trust. Self-regulation to assure quality in performance is at the heart of this relationship. It is the authentic hallmark of a mature profession. (p. 166)

Earlier in this chapter, consumerism was discussed as one of the important values influencing the health care system today. There is a direct relation between the increased role of the consumer in health care and quality assurance programs. As consumers have become increasingly assertive in stating what they do and do not want in health care, they also have expected the health care system to provide the desired level of care.

Cost control is also related to quality assurance. The cost of health care has increased tremendously because of increased technology and inflation. As this has happened, two major concerns about cost have emerged. First, there is the concern about fraudulent use of funds, particularly Medicare and Medicaid funds. Second, there is the concern about cost/benefit ratio. Many of the methods of diagnosis and treatment currently used or being developed are very expensive because of the complex equipment and trained personnel necessary for their use.

The *cost/benefit ratio* is a comparison of the benefit of a procedure in relation to its cost. For example, in order to evaluate a program of extensive care finding for cancer of the breast, the cost of the program must be analyzed in terms of its benefits. One question might be: Is the cost of routine mammography (x-ray examination of the breast) for all women over age 30 justified by any significant increase in the number of cases detected at an early stage? This concern with cost is related to quality assurance because more and more consumers, legislators, and insurance companies include cost as a criterion of quality.

In the 1980s, as mentioned earlier, cost controls have become formalized in programs such as *prospective pricing*. The competition which such cost control programs foster makes quality assurance programs more necessary than ever to carefully monitor the impact of competition on the *quality* of service.

Licensure

As the influence of consumers, legislators, and insurance companies has come together, the need for formalized processes whereby quality of care can be defined, measured, and systematically improved has become apparent. Historically, the earliest type of quality assurance program was the requirement of licenses for some health care professionals. Both physicians and nurses must have a license to practice. Licensing provides a mechanism whereby a member of a professional group submits evidence of competence in exchange for the legal permission to practice. Evidence of competence includes such things as documentation of graduation from an educational program, and of a passing grade on a licensing examination. The purpose of licensing is to assure that all who practice a particular profession have the necessary basic knowledge and skills.

Hospital Accreditation

Another early quality assurance effort was the Joint Commission on Accreditation of Hospitals (JCAH). The JCAH was created in 1951 as the result of nearly 35 years of cooperative work by the American College of Surgeons, the American College of Physicians, the American Hospital Association, the American Medical Association, and the Canadian Medical Association. These five groups had worked together to develop the Hospital Standardization Program to improve hospital care. When the program became too costly and complicated, the JCAH was formed as a voluntary, not-for-profit corporation for the purpose of "encouraging the voluntary attainment of uniformly high standards of institutional medical care" (Joint Commission on Accreditation of Hospitals, 1979).

The JCAH is a voluntary program whereby hospitals and other health-related facilities are evaluated in relation to the JCAH standards. An institution that meets the standards at an acceptable level receives JCAH accreditation. Although this accreditation process is voluntary, there are many pressures on an institution to obtain JCAH accreditation. For example, Blue Cross/Blue Shield and most insurance companies reimburse for care *only* if the care is provided in a JCAH-accredited facility. Also, most educational programs allow students to have clinical experience only in facilities with JCAH accreditation.

ANA Standards of Practice

More recently developed quality assurance activities include the American Nurses Association (ANA) Standards of Practice, the PSRO, and the increasing incidence of malpractice suits against health care professionals. The ANA, a recognized organization of professional nursing in the US, developed generic and specialty standards of practice in the 1970s. The ANA described the purpose of its standards as follows:

The standards of practice were developed to fulfill the profession's obligation to provide and improve nursing practice. Standards are tools, descriptive statements which reflect the dynamic nature of nursing practice and reflect the best current knowledge. The standards were intended to provide a means for determining the quality of nursing care which a client receives, regardless whether services are provided solely by a professional nurse or by a professional nurse and nonprofessional assistants.

The standards are based on the premise that the individual nurse is responsible and accountable to the client for the quality of nursing care the client receives. The standards are to be considered baseline for determining the quality of care (American Nurses Association, 1973).

There are now many sets of standards published, including the ANA Generic Standards of Practice which apply to nursing practice in any setting, Standards for Maternal-Child, Gerontological, Orthopedic, Rehabilitation, and Psychiatric-Mental Health Nursing Practice. The most recently developed standards are the Outcome Standards for Cancer Nursing Practice. There are also many other specialty standards. Having developed these standards, the ANA then defined a systematic process for their implementation, the ANA Model for Quality Assurance.

The ANA Standards of Practice and the ANA Model for Quality Assurance are being used increasingly in health care agencies as the basis for quality assurance programs of nursing care.

Professional Standards Review Organization

A second recently developed quality assurance program is the *Professional Standards Review Organization* (PSRO). The PSRO is different from the programs discussed so far in that it includes review of *cost* as well as quality of *care*. It is also different in that it is a federal government program, not associated with or developed by a professional organization such as the ANA or the AMA. The PSRO was enacted by the federal government in 1972 as an amendment to the Social Security

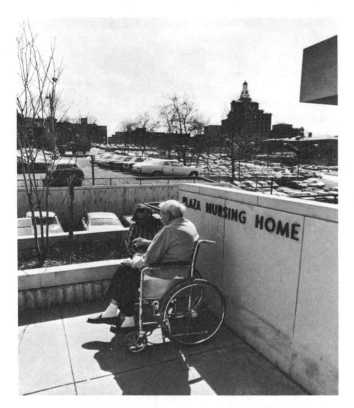

Figure 3.5 *No longer in need of acute care, this patient is in an extended care facility until he is able to return home. Warm sunshine and a friend help the time pass more quickly.*

Act. It mandates professional review of health care delivered to recipients of Medicare, Medicaid, and Maternal-Child Health programs. One of the major reasons for the enactment of the PSRO was the need to control the inappropriate use of funds from these programs.

The PSRO review process currently is required only in hospitals and nursing homes. It is intended to assure that the health care given is necessary, meets professional standards, and is provided economically in an appropriate health care setting. To accomplish these purposes, there are three components of the review process: (1) concurrent review, (2) medical care evaluation studies, and (3) hospital, practitioner, and patient profiles. *Concurrent review* refers to admission certification (review of patients at the time of admission to make sure they are being admitted to the right type of facility) and continued-stay review (review of patients while they are in a facility to make sure they are staying an appropriate length of time) (Fig. 3.5).

Medical care evaluation studies review the records of patients with a particular problem to determine if their care has met professional standards. *Hospital, practitioner,* and *patient profiles* involve the categorizing of information gathered in concurrent review and medical care evaluation studies according to hospitals, physicians, and patients. If a particular hospital's profile or a physician's profile reveals consistently inappropriate admissions or below-standard care, reimbursement by Medicare, Medicaid, or the Maternal-Child Health program may be withheld.

Malpractice Suits

A recent development related to quality assurance is the increasing incidence of malpractice suits. This is not a formal program but rather a reflection of consumers' increased participation in defining an acceptable quality of health care. When a consumer sues a person or institution for malpractice, two standards determine if malpractice has taken place: (1) a *legal standard,* constituting the relevant practice act or licensing requirements as well as decisions made in previous similar malpractice suits and (2) the *professional standard,* which is the expected level of performance as defined by the professional organization. An incident is evaluated in relation to these two standards, and a decision is made. Malpractice decisions are important to quality assurance because they provide very specific precedents of what is and what is not a legally expected quality of practice. As more and more malpractice cases are decided, the decisions provide a growing body of explicit directions for the expected and required quality of care.

Malpractice suits, like the other quality assurance activities, are directed at making certain that health care is safe, cost efficient, and good and, like the other activities, have done much for systematic evaluation and improvement of health care. Malpractice suits and the other quality assurance activities have also contributed to the cost of health care and the complexity of the health care delivery system, however. Some groups question whether the high cost is justified by the degree of improvement produced.

Alternative Health Care Approaches

Another significant characteristic of the current health care system is the development of alternative approaches and methods of health care. These alternatives are typically not part of the traditional health care delivery system. They tend to be based on commitment to the values of consumerism, holistic health, and individual responsibility for one's own health status. They perceive human adaptive capacity in a stressful work situation to be a major factor in disease causation. Some of the alternative approaches represent a rejection of the traditional system as inadequate and ineffective in dealing with health needs in the United States. They reject the traditional medical model in health care.

Mechanic (1978) discussed the trend toward alternative approaches in terms of medical sociology:

While the earlier literature assumed the correctness of the medical model, more recent literature attempts to examine cultural alternatives to medical care for dealing with many of the quasi-medical problems that doctors typically handle. Thus, while the older literature gives prominence to the physician's authority, more recent literature is likely to give more attention to patient responsibility, self-help groups such as Weight Watchers or Alcoholics Anonymous, new types of team practice, and consumer participation. While some of these new concerns are transient, others represent new ways of looking at man's adaptive ingenuity in coping with life problems. (p. 4)

Illich, in his strong statement against the traditional health care delivery system *Medical Nemesis* (1976) portrayed the US health care system as *antihealth*. He believes the system is antihealth because it has, in the process of its development and idealization of technology, transformed major life experiences, such as pain, impairment, and death, from personal challenges into technical problems.

A professional and physician-based health care system that has grown beyond critical bounds is sickening . . . it tends to mystify and to expropriate the power of the individual to heal himself and to shape his or her environment . . . The medical and paramedical monopoly over hygienic methodology and technology is a glaring example of the political misuse of scientific achievement to strengthen industrial rather than personal growth. Such medicine is but a device to convince those who are sick and tired of society that it is they who are ill, impotent, and in need of technical repair. (p. 9)

Many of the current alternative approaches to health care are an outgrowth of Illich's concern with the tendency of the traditional system to place the focus and control over a person's health with the physician, rather than with the person. Modern medicine has developed on the basis of the medical model, which focuses on disease. Disease has been diagnosed, treated, and sometimes cured *without consideration of the person* experiencing the disease or how that person interrelates with the disease.

The diagnosing and the treating have been done by the physician to the patient for the purpose of getting rid of the disease, specifically, getting rid of its symptoms and physiological cause. Believers in *holistic health and holistic health care* perceive well-being as a function of the harmonious interaction of the mind and body. Disease, to them, reflects disharmony or conflict among the various components of the total self. It is important to understand that traditional medicine perceives *disease as a thing,* which can be cut out or killed by a drug; whereas holistic medicine perceives *disease as a process.* There is increasing knowledge to support the holistic concept of disease. Relationships have been demonstrated among such factors as bottled-up emotion, disappointment, and cancer.

A holistic concept of health and disease requires that health care activities include (1) a search for patterns of disharmony in addition to specific physiological signs and symptoms and (2) a focus on healing through the use of alternative techniques as well as traditional medical interventions. The focus of alternative techniques is on the development and strengthening of all aspects of the person so that harmony is achieved. Such approaches as yoga, meditation, biofeedback, guided imagery, nutrition, self-help groups, exercise, music therapy, and folk healing are increasingly practiced.

Ferguson (1980), in her book *The Aquarian Conspiracy,* discussed this concept in relation, not only to health care, but to all aspects of life. Her premise is that many of society's systems are currently undergoing reexamination in light of dissatisfaction with material wealth and technological complexity as the ultimate goals of living. She pointed to the growing numbers of people concerned with individual growth and humanism. She specifically addressed the inadequacy of the medical model, high-technology health care system:

Like the foil wrap on a disappointing gift, the shiny technology has dealt stunningly with certain acute problems, as in inoculations and sophisticated surgical procedures, but its failures in chronic and degenerative disease, including cancer and heart disease, have driven practitioners and the public to look in new directions . . . Well-being cannot be infused intravenously or ladled in by prescription. It comes from a matrix; the body-mind. It reflects psychological and somatic harmony. As one anatomist put it, "the healer inside us is the wisest, most complex, integrated entity in the universe." In a sense, we know now, there is always a doctor in the house.

"You can't deliver holistic health," one practitioner said. It originates in an attitude: an acceptance of life's uncertainties, a willingness to accept responsibility for habits, a way of perceiving and dealing with stress, more satisfying human relationships, a sense of purpose . . . Health and disease don't just happen to us. They are active processes issuing from inner harmony or disharmony, profoundly affected by our states of consciousness, our ability or inability to flow with experience. This recognition carries with it implicit responsibility and opportunity.

If we are participating, however unconsciously, in the process of disease, we can choose health instead. (pp. 244–257)

The holistic concept of health and disease and its growing acceptance has serious implications for the current hospital-based, illness-oriented health care delivery system. In addition, the implementation of significant cost control programs will combine with the concerns for holistic care to significantly reshape the US health care delivery system.

SUGGESTED READINGS

Abdellah, Faye G: Nursing care for the aged in the United States of America. *J Gerontol Nurs* 1981 Nov; 7(11):657–660.

Aiken, Linda H: Nursing priorities for the 1980's. *Am J Nurs* 1981 Feb; 81(2):324–331.

Chaisson, G Maureen: Correctional health care—beyond the barriers. *Am J Nurs* 1981 April; 81(4):736–738.

Curtin, Leah L: Is there a right to health care? *Am J Nurs* 1980 Mar; 80(3):462–465.

Daniels, Mary Brett: A clinic for pregnant teens. *Am J Nurs* 1983 Jan; 83(1):68–71.

Dighton, Steve: Tough-minded nursing (prison nursing). *Am J Nurs* 1986 Jan; 86(1):48–51.

Fagin, Claire M: Nursing as an alternative to high-cost care. *Am J Nurs* 1982 Jan; 82(1):56–60.

Jamieson, Marjorie, and Ida Martinson: Block nursing: neighbors caring for neighbors. *Nurs Outlook* 1983 Sept/Oct; 31(5):270–273.

Johnston, Maxene: Ambulatory health care in the 80's. *Am J Nurs* 1980 Jan; 80(1):76–79.

Kendrick, Valen M: Nurse practitioner in a V N A *Am J Nurs* 1981 July; 81(7):1360–1362.

Lenehan, Gail P, et al: A nurses' clinic for the homeless. *Am J Nurs* 1985 Nov; 85(11):1237–1240.

Little, Liza: A change process for prison health nursing. *Am J Nurs* 1981 April; 81(4):739–742.

Marquis, Mary Jouppi: City streets—The public health ICU. *Am J Nurs* 1986 March; 86(3):362.

Moritz, Patricia: Health care in correctional facilities: a nursing challenge. *Nurs Outlook* 1982 April; 30(4):253–259.

O'Brien, Mary Elizabeth: Reaching the migrant worker. *Am J Nurs* 1983 June; 83(6):895–897.

Piper, Letty Roth: 10 ways to win the DRG game. *RN* 1985 Mar; 48(3):18–20.

Rinke, Lynn T: A VNA switches to primary nursing. *Am J Nurs* 1984 Oct; 84(10):1227–1229.

Robinson, Thelma: School nurse practitioners on the job. *Am J Nurs* 1981 Sept; 81(9):1674–1678.

Shimamoto, Yoshiko: Political factors influencing nursing practice. *Nurs Outlook* 1981 June; 29(6):355–357.

Smith, Carol E: DRGs: Making them work for you. *Nursing 85* 1985 January; 15(1):34–41.

Strasser, Judith A: Urban transient women. *Am J Nurs* 1978 Dec; 78(12):2076–2079.

Strauss, Anselm L, et al: Patient's work in the technologized hospital. *Nurs Outlook* 1981 July; 29(7):404–412.

Stuart-Burchardt, Sandra: Rural nursing. *Am J Nurs* 1982 April: 82(4):616–618.

Tisdale, Sallie: *The Sorcerer's Apprentice: Inside the Modern Hospital.* New York, McGraw-Hill, 1986.

Wald, Florence S, Zelda Foster, and Henry J Wald: The hospice movement as a health care reform. *Nurs Outlook* 1980 March; 28(3):173–178.

REFERENCES

Donabedian, Avedis: Evaluating the quality of medical care. *Millbank Memorial Fund Quarterly.* 1966:44(2):166.

Ferguson, Marilyn: *The Aquarian Conspiracy—Personal and Social Transformation in the 1980's.* Los Angeles, Tarcher, Inc, 1980.

Illich, Ivan: *Medical Nemesis—The Expropriation of Health.* New York: Bantam Books, 1976.

Joint Commission on Accreditation of Hospitals: *Accreditation Manual for Hospitals.* Chicago, Joint Commission on Accreditation of Hospitals, 1985.

Mechanic, David: *Medical Sociology.* New York, Free Press, 1978.

Pavalon, Eugene I: *Human Rights and Health Care Law.* American Journal of Nursing Co, 1980.

Shindell, Sidney, Jeffery C Salloway and Colette M Oberembt: *A Coursebook in Health Care Delivery.* New York, Human Sciences Press, 1979.

Tubesing, Donald A: *Wholistic Health—A Whole-Person Approach to Primary Health Care.* New York, Human Sciences Press, 1979.

Part Two

Concepts Basic to Nursing Practice

4

Conceptual Frameworks and Nursing

Conceptual Frameworks
Concepts
Principles
Theories

Models
Use of Models
Nursing Models
  Single versus Multiple Models
Nursing and Medical Models

Explanation of Nursing Process

Prerequisites and/or Suggested Preparation
Chapter 1 (Nursing as a Profession) or its equivalent from another source is prerequisite to this chapter.

Any endeavor, whether a game or a business deal, is more likely to be effective when it is organized and described in such a way that everyone understands what is going on. When neither the objectives nor the rules are clearly understood, the participants are likely to be working at cross purposes. The same is true in nursing. Unless the nurses in a given situation share a similar concept of what nursing is, what its goals are, and how those goals should be reached, there is likely to be considerable misunderstanding and much wasted energy. Such a situation is like a football game in which each team is composed of professional athletes, each of whom speaks a different language. Every player knows that the object of the game is to make a touchdown, but there is no way to devise and call the plays which would accomplish that goal *effectively*.

In professional and academic settings, a framework for effective action is referred to as the *conceptual model* or *conceptual framework* of that profession or school.

CONCEPTUAL FRAMEWORKS

A conceptual framework is a scheme or plan for organizing a group of ideas into a manageable whole. It describes the relationships between a variety of theories and facts, and provides a systematic way of unifying large amounts of information into a usable body of knowledge. A conceptual framework promotes effective and efficient action.

In nursing, the terms conceptual framework and model are sometimes used interchangeably, but in general, the first is used in reference to the curriculum of a school of nursing while the latter refers to the practice of nursing.

A *conceptual framework* consists of concepts, principles, theories, and laws that have been selected by the faculty. In each school, the faculty select from a number of current theories those that reflect their philosophies and beliefs about the practice of nursing. The most general or inclusive theory is usually designated as the major thread or focus of the conceptual framework while the lesser or more specific theories function as supporting ideas.

The conceptual framework of a school of nursing usually takes into account the liberal arts component of the curriculum and includes theories and concepts from many disciplines. The resulting organization of ideas makes it possible for students to integrate and understand large amounts of information which will provide the basis for effective nursing care.

A *nursing model* is usually developed by a nursing theorist or group of theorists, and is based both on research and on the theorist's own clinical experience

in nursing. Nursing acknowledges the value of a framework which can be described and understood by all persons involved, and is in the process of developing and testing a number of conceptual models.

Medicine has a well-established model (referred to as the *medical model* of health care) which has its own theories, protocol, organization, and authority, and as nursing separates itself from the medical profession and establishes itself as a separate discipline, it must develop a nursing model. The aims and practices of nursing are unique to nursing and must be described by nurses in a manner which can be communicated to a variety of people, both inside and outside of the nursing profession.

Concepts

The term *concept* is often used to refer to knowledge related to an academic subject, such as the concepts of mathematics or physics. This use of the term is convenient but imprecise. It is an easy way to refer *in general* to the basic information relevant to a particular area of study, but in many instances the term is no more useful than that.

More precisely, a concept is the result of a person's ability to categorize an object, characteristic, or phenomenon as belonging to a particular set of objects, characteristics, or phenomena. When a child, for example, calls a wide variety of two-legged creatures with beaks by the name *bird*, the child has acquired the *concept* of bird. When he regularly refers to the larger of two objects as the bigger, whether the objects be pencils, chairs, or candy, he understands the *concept* of size.

Concept formation or concept acquisition requires the ability to discriminate between objects or events, plus the ability to determine whether or not they belong to a given class or category. The child who possesses the concept of bird can discriminate between a beak and a mouth, and between two legs and four legs. Other concepts are based upon more complex discriminations, such as the difference between normal postoperative pain and the pain which would indicate a complication of surgery.

A concept has been defined as "a vehicle of thought" which makes it possible for a person to learn without the necessity of having to experience innumerable examples of a given event or object. The child who knows the *concept of bird* does not have to learn specifically that a robin is a bird, an owl is a bird, and so on. In similar fashion, once you have learned the concept of normal postoperative discomfort, you will not need to make a separate study of the discomfort to be expected for every example of a given type of surgery.

Concept learning is essential since it is not feasible to try to respond to each and every stimulus as a separate learning experience. The ability to recognize similarities and differences, and then make valid generalizations, is necessary for efficient learning. In addition, concept learning must precede more complex intellectual activities such as the learning of principles and problem solving.

Many instructors make a conscious effort to teach concepts while others expect their students to discover or formulate concepts for themselves. In either situation, it is important for you to *acquire concepts* rather than try to memorize a vast array of specific definitions which are often quickly forgotten.

Principles

A principle is a statement which shows the relationship between two or more concepts. Examples of a principle are: *round things roll* and *pain increases anxiety.* Relevant concepts must be learned before a principle can be learned. For example, a child must have acquired the concepts of both roundness and rolling in order to understand the relationship between round and roll. The learning of this principle is vastly different from the ability to merely parrot the words ''round things roll.''

At a more complex and abstract level, a nurse must have learned the concepts of both pain and anxiety in order to comprehend the *relationship* between pain and anxiety. Simply memorizing the definitions of each word does not result in the same degree of comprehension.

The learning of principles results in an understanding which is well retained. Strings of words (definitions, facts) are quickly forgotten since humans have a limited capacity to store and recall unrelated bits of information. Concepts and principles are resistant to forgetting and can be retained indefinitely.

Theories

A theory can be defined as a plausible or scientifically acceptable body of principles presented as an explanation of certain phenomena. A new theory can be developed by either the process of deduction or that of induction. The process of *deduction* involves the selection and use of existing theories to explain a certain event or phenomenon. The process of *induction* involves the observation and analysis of many instances of a similar event to arrive at a plausible explanation of that phenomenon.

Both deductive and inductive processes are used in nursing. Some nursing theorists select relevant concepts and theories from other bodies of knowledge such as anthropology, psychology, sociology, and other basic sciences, and then combine these concepts into an explanation for certain aspects of nursing. This is an example of the process of *deduction*.

Other theorists, using the process of *induction*, examine many instances of some occurrence in nursing and develop a reasonable explanation which can then be tested. The first step in this process is to identify the factors involved (What people, physical conditions, emotional responses, and so on seem to be present [or absent] in all instances of this event?). The next step is to determine the possible relationships among these factors. The third step is to make and test predictions about the cause and effect of the relationships. Finally, the theorist describes the situations which will either bring about the desired outcome or prevent an undesired event.

When a theory has been thoroughly analyzed and widely tested, it is generally accepted as true, and is often referred to as a law.

Nursing theory is an essential aspect of nursing practice because it gives direction to nursing practice, provides the rationale for many nursing actions, and indicates areas for further research and study. Nursing, as an emerging profession, is in the process of developing a body of knowledge which will be unique to nursing and not merely ''borrowed'' from other disciplines. Nursing theories are essential for the development of the nursing models which will shape the practice of nursing in the future.

MODELS

There are many times when an idea, a process, or an object is too large or abstract to be dealt with directly, and a model must be substituted for the real thing. It is not feasible, for example, for high school students to study the various forms of government by spending time in Washington, D.C., and in the capitals of foreign countries. It is not possible for an architect to build an unlimited number of homes from which each client can select the house that is right for him. Therefore, instead of actually experiencing each form of government, or of walking through scores of houses, the student must learn from, and the client must choose from, models that *represent* the real thing.

A model may be a verbal representation, such as a detailed description of an object or phenomenon. It may be a graphic representation such as a chart, diagram, or floor plan. It may be a three-dimensional structure, such as a model house, car, or plane. Whatever its form, a model facilitates both the study of, and communication about, an object or process.

Use of Models

The value of models can be illustrated by the use of models in the study of government. It is possible for a political scientist to examine the interactions of any group of people, from a primitive tribe to a highly developed nation, and then describe the nature of that group's government. The political scientist would ask questions such as "Who or what is the source of power and authority?" "How is this power and authority demonstrated and communicated to the people?" "How are rules, taboos, and laws developed?" "How are they enforced?"

Once the government being studied has been analyzed, it can be described verbally and represented by charts and diagrams. A *model* of that government is thus developed. The government in question can then be categorized as a democracy, a monarchy, a dictatorship, or some other recognized form of government and can be compared with other forms.

A composite representation of any form of government constitutes a model for that form. For example, the collective features of a number of democracies will yield a model of democracy. By examining the model of any form of government, a person can determine how laws are made and enforced, how justice is assured, how the rights of the individual are balanced against the needs of society, and so on. By using several models, it is possible to compare and contrast several forms of government.

A model of the US government enables a person to study the government without actually visiting Washington, without attending sessions of Congress or participating in nominating conventions, without observing the Supreme Court and the Cabinet in action, and without watching the President as he carries out his duties. The use of a model enables a person to acquire knowledge and understanding of the government without direct interaction with each phase of the governmental process. A model of a government, therefore, *represents reality* and permits people to understand the structure and function of that government without actually experiencing each and every part of it.

In similar fashion, a nursing model represents reality and permits us to examine the structure and function of nursing practice. A nursing model enables us to communicate in concrete terms about an abstract concept of nursing because the model helps us to answer such questions as:

What is nursing?

When and where does nursing take place?

What are the goals of nursing?

What are the functions of the nurse?

What is the relationship between patient and nurse?

What is the relationship between nursing and medicine?

What is the source of authority of the nurse's independent actions?

A comprehensive and useful nursing model addresses itself to these and similar questions and enables those nurses who understand and accept that model to discuss and practice nursing from the same frame of reference.

Nursing Models

Just as models enable a person to compare forms of government, so nursing models facilitate comparison of current concepts of nursing and also permit a person to compare the nursing of one era with that of another. For example, before the nineteenth century, the goal of nursing was to make the patient as comfortable as possible while waiting for nature to run its course or for the physician's treatment to take effect. Nursing was, in general, limited to the care of the sick; as a rule, nursing did not attempt to *actively* influence the outcome of a patient's illness.

A model of nursing during the latter part of the nineteenth century and the early part of the twentieth century would show that nursing had become increasingly attentive to Florence Nightingale's belief that the patient's condition could be improved by manipulating his environment. Nurses began to take the initiative and actively tried to influence the outcome of the patient's condition. This was done by providing light, warmth, fresh air, food, and proper sanitation. Gradually these factors came to be deemed important for everyone, not merely for the sick, and formed the basis for public health nursing.

As medical care became more complex, the physician delegated many of his responsibilities to the nurse. Activities that had once been the prerogative of the physician, such as taking the patient's temperature and blood pressure, were given to, and accepted by, nurses. Basic nursing interventions related to physical comfort, food, and sanitation were often superseded by procedures ordered by the physician, and the nurse came to be referred to as the "handmaiden" of the physician.

A model of nursing soon after World War II would indicate that nurses were still the handmaidens of physicians but that, in addition to caring for the sick, nurses were active in rehabilitation, and there was a growing interest in the prevention of illness. As a rule, patients were still passive recipients of medical and nursing care.

A current model of nursing reflects the many changes in the organization, philosophy, structure, and function of nursing. A current model indicates that (1) nursing and medicine are separate professions, and nursing has the potential for achieving a status comparable to that of medicine; (2) there is increasing interaction between nursing and other categories of health care workers; (3) patients are becoming active participants in matters related to their own health and well-being; and (4) nurses are committed to the promotion of health as well as to the prevention of illness and the treatment of disease.

A nursing model reflects a set of ideas and beliefs about nursing and organizes these ideas into a conceptual framework that enables us to examine and discuss the practice of nursing. Although leaders in nursing have long sought a definition and description of nursing that would effectively differentiate nursing practice from the practice of medicine, little formalized emphasis was placed on the development of distinctive nursing models until the late 1960s.

Because there is not yet a consensus about the nature and structure of nursing, numerous models have been and are being developed. Each model reflects the philosophy and beliefs of the person or group who developed it. Some models bear the name of the person or group who developed them; others are known by the predominant features of the model. Examples of a few of the *different concepts and beliefs about nursing* that form the basis for some of the various models being developed include:

1. *Nursing is a system* and can be described in terms of general systems theory, with nurse, patient, physician, therapist, and others as component parts of the system.
2. *Nursing is primarily a series of interpersonal relationships* and nursing can be described in terms of communication theory.
3. *Nursing is a process* similar to the process used in problem solving or the scientific method, and all activities of nursing can be categorized into the phases of nursing process.
4. *Nursing is the application of stress and adaptation theory* and is designed to help people adapt to the stresses of life and to reduce the incidence and severity of stress-related illnesses such as high blood pressure, ulcers, and rheumatoid arthritis.
5. *Nursing is a way of ensuring* that basic needs are met. The nurse is expected to identify and meet the basic needs of a person when he is unable to do so or to help him meet his needs until assistance is no longer necessary.

The preceding examples illustrate the diversity of approaches used by various theorists in the process of developing a nursing model. In addition to providing an overall view of the role of the nurse and the practice of nursing, a model should describe the theorist's concept of health, the patient, and the environment. The distinctive features of a number of current nursing models are shown in Table 4.1.

Each nursing model uses the vocabulary of the concepts on which it is based. This sometimes hampers communication when a group of nurses are trying to analyze and study a variety of models simultaneously; it often seems, and rightly so, that the proponents of each model are speaking a different language. For example, pain can be considered:

- A *component* in systems theory
- A *cue* during a patient-nurse interaction
- *Data* to be assessed and evaluated during nursing process
- An *adaptation* or a *stressor* in stress and adaptation theory
- An *indicator* of an unmet physiological need in a basic needs model
- A *symptom* in the medical model

Neither the nature of the pain nor the patient's perception of the pain is changed from model to model, but the way in which the pain is thought to be related to nursing depends on the perspective of each nursing theorist.

Single versus Multiple Models

There is considerable debate within the profession whether or not a single nursing model is, or ever will be, desirable. Some leaders believe that the use of only one model would decrease creativity in nursing, increase the structure and formalization of nursing care, and inhibit the growth and development of new and evolving roles in nursing.

Other leaders believe that the acceptance of a single model in nursing would enhance the development of nursing as a profession. A single model would give all nurses a common frame of reference and would facilitate communication and research. It would also define and delineate nursing's contribution to health care in general. Proponents of a single, unified nursing model suggest that, whereas there is little doubt or uncertainty about the role and functions of physician, lawyer, or teacher, there is confusion about what a nurse does when she is not caring for a sick person. A single nursing model might promote a greater understanding of nursing in areas such as private practice, research, and nontraditional settings such as HMOs and self-help clinics.

TABLE 4.1 COMPARISON OF SELECTED CONCEPTUAL MODELS FOR NURSING

Theorist	Nursing Model	Date Developed	Goals for Nursing Action
Florence Nightingale	Environmental Theory of Nursing	1859	Putting patient in best condition for nature to act to preserve/restore health; improving environment to assist process
Hildegard Peplau	Interpersonal Process for Nursing	1952	Utilizing interpersonal relationships in educating client/family and helping client achieve mature development
Virginia Henderson	Complementary-Supplementary Model	1966	Helping client maintain or restore independence in meeting 14 fundamental needs or achieve a peaceful death
Dorothy Johnson	Behavioral System Model	1968	Regulating and controlling behavioral system stability and equilibrium; reducing stress so client can move toward recovery
Martha Rogers	Principles of Homeodynamics	1970	Helping client achieve maximal wellness; promoting harmonious interaction between man and the environment
Dorothea Orem	Self-care Model	1971	Providing assistance to help client achieve an optimal level of self-care; determining client needs for self-care
Sister Callista Roy	Adaptation Model	1976	Assisting client to adapt in four modes in health or illness situations by manipulating stimuli

Nursing and Medical Models

Medicine has used a single model for centuries. The medical model is disease oriented, and the physician devotes himself to the diagnosis and treatment of pathological conditions. His attention is focused on the detection and treatment of abnormalities, dysfunction, and defects; and the majority of his activities, whether they are patient care, teaching, or research, are directed toward some aspect of disease and illness.

A nursing model, on the other hand, is focused on a *person or group of people* rather than on a disease or illness. A nursing model must be applicable to the needs of individuals, families, and communities and must be useful to nurses in a wide variety of roles and settings, and with all people, sick or well. It is probably fortunate that modern day nursing has not inherited a model from another era but has the opportunity to develop a model consistent with the health care needs of society in the twenty-first century.

The issue of single or multiple nursing models will not be decided for a number of years. In the meantime,

each nurse is obligated (1) to follow in professional journals the progress and trends in the development of models; (2) to test the usefulness of those models that seem valid; and (3) to give feedback to the appropriate people regarding the applicability and utility of any given proposed model.

EXPLANATION OF NURSING PROCESS

Nursing process is the term currently applied to a systematic and logical approach to nursing practice, and its concepts are an inherent part of every nursing theory. Nursing process refers to a series of activities by which the nurse collects information about the patient, uses that information to identify patient needs, makes a nursing care plan, implements the plan, and evaluates the effectiveness of the care given. These activities are not new; they have been carried out by skilled and scholarly nurses for many years, even though the activities were not then called nursing process.

Nursing process is explained in detail in Chapters 17

Beliefs About Nursing	Beliefs About Patient/Client	Beliefs About Health	Beliefs About Environment
Women's profession distinct from medicine; an art and science requiring formal education	Made up of physical, intellectual, social, emotional, and spiritual components	Opposite of disease but being able to use own powers to fullest	Physical elements external to and affecting the person, sick or well
Applied science and process which facilitates human health	Developing system of biochemical, physical, and psychological needs and characteristics	Linked to human development; energy directed to mature goals; relief from tension	External factors essential to human development
Function which assists individual to perform activities contributing to health	Biological being with mind and body inseparable; biological orientation	Individual's ability to function independently with respect to 14 needs	Not clearly defined; acts on client in positive or negative ways
Professional service discipline with both art and science components	Behavioral system made up of 7 interrelated subsystems; identified by actions and behavior	Elusive state decided by social, psychological, and physiological factors	All factors not part of the behavioral system of individual
Humanistic art and science that deals with the whole person	An open system, the whole of which is greater than the sum of the parts; unitary man	No specific definition; value defined by individuals and cultures	All outside any given human field; four-dimensional negentropic energy field
A personal, family, and community human service with primary emphasis on the individual	An integrated whole which functions biologically, symbolically, and socially	Integrity of the individual's being, parts, and functioning; a state of wholeness	Integrated system and subcomponent of man which is related to self-care
Theoretical system of knowledge which analyzes and reacts in relation to ill or potentially ill person	A living, open, adaptive system which is in constant interaction with environment; biopsychosocial being	Continuum of health and illness ranging from peak wellness to death; inevitable dimension of life	All things which surround and affect an organism's development, e.g., conditions, influences, and circumstances

to 22, but many references are made to nursing process in the chapters which precede that section; it is necessary, therefore, to understand the meaning of the terms which are used in the chapters which follow.

Explanation of Terms Related to Nursing Process

- *Assessment* The term applied to all the activities by which the nurse gathers necessary information about a patient or client. Areas to be assessed include the patient's condition, family, culture, environment, diagnosis, and treatment.

- *Diagnosis* The process of describing the patient's response to his present condition or situation. A nursing diagnosis describes a *nursing* problem which nurses are licensed to diagnose and treat; it is concerned with those areas of health care that are exclusively within the sphere of nursing. A nursing diagnosis may be related to the medical diagnosis, but it is separate and distinct.

    Individual nursing diagnoses make it possible for a nurse to plan personalized effective nursing care for each assigned patient.

- *Planning* The process by which the nurse decides upon a course of action which is to be helpful to the patient, and then organizes the necessary activities into a plan of action.

- *Implementation* The term applied to the activities by which the nurse carries out the nursing care plan. These activities are called nursing actions or *nursing interventions*.

- *Evaluation* The process of determining whether or not the nursing care given was effective and efficient. It is impossible to evaluate a product or performance unless the evaluator knows the characteristics which distinguish an excellent performance from a mediocre one. A judge must know exactly what he is looking for. In nursing, the standards used for evaluation are called *nursing standards, outcome criteria,* or *criteria for evaluation*.

If you find that you do not understand the way in which the above terms are used in Chapters 5 to 16, you will find a complete overview of nursing process in Chapter 17, and detailed descriptions of each phase of the process in Chapters 18 to 22.

RELATED ACTIVITIES

1. Communication problems are created when two people have different conceptions of a given word. For example, there is likely to be misunderstanding and confusion when a patient and a nurse have different concepts of terms such as *relief of pain* or *optimal health.* Some people refer to such a situation as "a problem in semantics" while others say "We don't speak the same language."

In order to avert such difficulties in nursing situations, especially with reference to theories and models, begin now to cultivate the habit of asking questions such as "What does that term mean to you?" or "How are you using that phrase?" Many problems can be avoided if each nurse tries to make sure that the concepts involved are clear to both parties.

2. When you are studying material that seems abstract, disjointed, or confusing, take time to look for *commonalities and similarities.* For example, if you are presented with several definitions of health, examine each one closely and determine what they have in common. As you do so, you will expand your understanding of health, and will acquire a *concept of health* which will be more useful than a series of separate definitions of health.

SUGGESTED READINGS

Bisch-Bryan, Sally Ann: Understanding international development models. *Nurs Outlook* 1983 Mar/Apr; 31(2):128.

Chin, Peggy L, and Maeona K Jacobs: *Theory and Nursing: A Systemic Approach.* St. Louis, Mosby, 1983.

Ellis, Rosemary: Conceptual issues in nursing. *Nurs Outlook* 1982 July/Aug; 30(7):406–410.

Field, Lucy, and Elizabeth Hahn Winslow: Moving to a nursing model. *Am J Nurs* 1985 Oct; 85(10):1100–1101.

Fitzpatrick, Joyce J, and Ann L Whall: *Conceptual Models of Nursing: Analysis and Application.* Bowie, Brady, 1983.

Meleis, Afaf Ibrahim: *Theoretical Nursing: Development and Progress.* Philadelphia, Lippincott, 1985.

Orem, Dorothea: *Nursing: Concepts of Practice.* ed.3. New York, McGraw-Hill, 1985.

Riehl, Joan P, and Callista, Roy: *Conceptual Models for Nursing Practice.* ed.2. New York, Appleton-Century-Crofts, 1980.

Walker, Lorraine, and Nicholson, Ruth: Criteria for evaluating nursing process models. *Nurse Educator* 1980 Sept/Oct; 5(5):8–9.

Williamson, Janet A: Mutual interaction: A model of nursing practice. *Nurs Outlook* 1981 Feb; 29(2):104–108.

5

Systems Theory

Prerequisites and/or Suggested Preparation
This chapter presumes no prior knowledge of systems theory, and no advance preparation is needed.

Over 300 years ago John Donne coined the now familiar phrase "No man is an island." This phrase is a poetic expression of modern systems theory, and indicates that Donne somehow felt and understood the basic concept even though the theory would not be developed for another three centuries. The following passage from his writing shows the extent to which he was able to put those ideas into words.

No man is an island, entire of itself; every man is a piece of the continent, a part of the main; if a clod be washed away by the sea, Europe is the less . . . Any man's death diminishes me, because I am involved in mankind. And therefore never send to know for whom the bell tolls. It tolls for thee.

Over the centuries, theorists have studied the interrelatedness of people, organizations, and objects, and about 25 years ago, systems theory was developed to explain these relationships. It has been widely used by many disciplines such as engineering, sociology, and political science for a number of years, and is currently used throughout the practice of nursing.

SYSTEMS THEORY AND NURSING PRACTICE

Skilled and sensitive nurses recognize the interrelatedness of the person's mind, body, family, and environment. They know, for example, that a patient's cardiovascular system affects and is affected by his nervous system, that a patient's health affects and is affected by his family, and that the family situation affects and is affected by the resources of the neighborhood. The term *interdependence* is applied to these reciprocal relationships; the concept of interdependence among cells, organs, systems, individuals, and groups of individuals is basic to both systems theory and effective nursing practice.

A very precise vocabulary is used to express the concepts of systems theory, and as a result, experts in all fields that use systems theory are able to share problems, solutions, and ideas because they all understand the language of systems theory. A working knowledge of systems theory enables the nurse to understand relationships between the physiological systems within the person's body as well as to understand the ways in which the patient, nurse, doctor, and family influence one another.

Furthermore, as nurses move into positions of power and leadership within local, state, and federal agencies, the ability to use systems theory becomes increasingly necessary.

Systems theory is basic to the concept of holistic nursing, and provides one way of examining the many influences on health and illness. Systems theory also facilitates the integration into nursing of relevant theories from psychology, physiology, and other sciences.

Basic Concepts

Systems theory states that:

1. A system, whether it be a digestive system, a political system, a heating system, or a family system, is composed of a number of identifiable, interrelated parts called *components*.
2. Because these parts or components are interrelated, whatever happens to one part affects one or more of the other parts and also affects the overall functioning of the system.
3. Each system is a component of a larger system, and whatever happens to one system affects one or more of the other systems and also affects the overall functioning of the larger system.
4. Because all systems are interrelated, the boundaries between systems are not rigid, and can be established arbitrarily and readjusted at any given time.
5. The functioning of a system depends on its input, output, feedback, equilibrium, and rate of entropy (see Table 5.1).

Application to the Health Care Delivery System

A theory, of course, is of little practical use until it is made operational, that is, until it can easily be applied to everyday situations. The paragraphs that follow are designed to explain briefly the basic concepts of systems theory within the context of the health care delivery system and to show how the theory can be used in nursing.

A system is composed of a number of identifiable, interrelated parts called components.

Nurses are familiar with the systems of the human body, with the parts of each of these systems, and with the relationships of one part of a system to the other parts. Usually, these parts or components are easily identified and described. For example, the mouth, esophagus, stomach, intestines, and rectum are all parts of the digestive system. In other types of systems, especially larger social systems, the components are less obvious. The hospital system, for example, is composed of many departments (components), some of which may not be known to the nurse or the patient. These components of the hospital system include the following depart-

TABLE 5.1 NURSING PROCESS, SCIENTIFIC METHOD, PROBLEM SOLVING: COMPARISON OF STEPS AND TERMINOLOGY USED

Activity	Nursing Process	Scientific Method	Problem Solving
Obtaining and organizing information	Assessment	Data collection; recognizing the problem situation	Data collection; studying the problem
Stating the problem	Making a nursing diagnosis	Making hypotheses; forming research questions	Defining problem; stating nature of the problem
Making plans	Planning	Choosing methodology	Making plan of action; finding possible solutions
Putting plan into action	Implementing	Testing hypothesis; conducting study	Carrying out plan Testing solutions
Reviewing the outcome	Evaluating	Interpreting the findings	Evaluating the results

ments: nursing, dietary, laundry, medical, laboratory, maintenance, bookkeeping, legal, public relations, and many others.

Because the parts of a system are interrelated, whatever happens to one part affects one or more of the other parts and also affects the overall functioning of the system.

For example, if a person has all his teeth extracted in preparation for getting dentures, the extraction affects all parts of his mouth, and his resultant inability to chew will affect the overall functioning of his digestive system.

Just so, whatever happens in the hospital laundry affects other parts of the hospital system. If the supply of hot water should fail, the laundry would be unable to supply fresh linen; nurses and aides would be delayed in meeting patient needs; the housekeeping department would be unable to make up fresh beds for new admissions to the hospital, and so on. As serious as these immediate and obvious effects might be, the *overall* effect on patient care would be even more serious. Such disruption in routines, procedures, and schedules would probably result in short tempers, frustration, and irritation among hospital personnel, which in turn could create anxiety, discomfort, and other negative responses in patients, families, and visitors. There is no way in which the effect of inadequate hot water can be confined to the laundry. Even if the hospital were able to secure an adequate supply of linen without delay from a commercial laundry in order to prevent the disruption of patient care, the unplanned expense of doing so would affect the budget, bookkeeping, and auditing departments.

Every system is a component of a larger system, and whatever happens to one system affects one or more of the other systems and also affects the overall functioning of the larger system.

Every clinic, nursing home, physician's office, and hospital is a system that is a component of the local health care delivery system (Fig. 5.1). This larger system is a component of a regional system, which in turn is part of the state health care delivery system; and some portions of the state system are parts of the federal Medicare system or the Department of Health and Human Services. The interrelationships are complicated and tend to become less obvious as the systems become larger. The individual patient and nurse may be unaware of the relationships, but both are vitally affected by them. For example, any new state regulation related to standards of care for premature infants will affect the size and type of newborn nurseries in local hospitals, which will affect the number and qualifications of nurses employed, which will in turn affect the rates paid by private citizens, welfare departments, and insurance companies.

Because all systems are interrelated, the boundaries between systems are established arbitrarily at any given time.

A boundary can be defined as a line which makes an imaginary circle around the components of a system, and which thereby determines what is within and what is outside the system. The setting of boundaries makes it possible for a person or group of people to work with a single system—to develop it, study it, evaluate it, treat it, or change it. Boundaries are set in accordance with

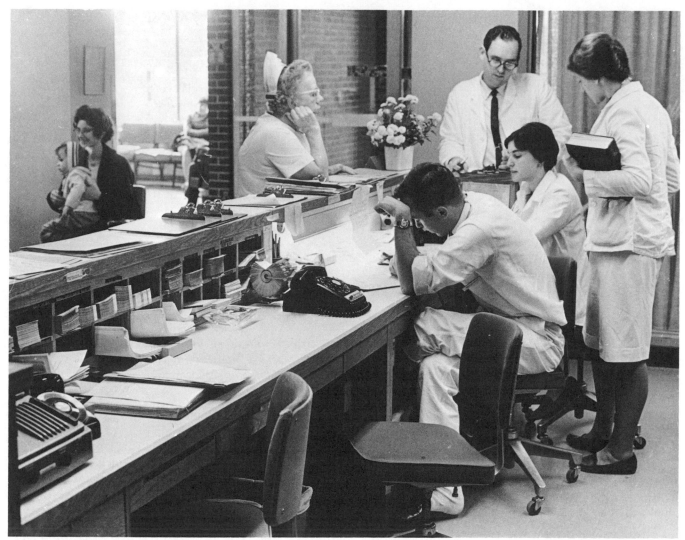

Figure 5.1 *Some of the components of this clinic system are patients, families, nursing service, medical staff, and the record keeping and communication systems.*

the purposes of those working with a system. For instance, the physician knows that the stomach is a component or subsystem of the digestive system, but if the stomach is the site of the problem for a given patient, he may choose arbitrarily to set narrow boundaries that enable him to focus only on the stomach. In another patient, he may extend the boundaries in order to study the interaction of enzymes within the entire digestive system.

To study the nursing care of surgical patients in hospital X, for example, an initial boundary would be set to *include* surgical patients and to *exclude* all other patients at hospital X. The boundaries could then be readjusted to either include or exclude orthopedic surgery, pediatric surgery, neurosurgery, and other specialties. The boundaries might be further adjusted to include only adult patients with abdominal, cardiac, or chest surgery.

One of the essential components of the system for delivering nursing care to these surgical patients is the nurses. If the nurses consider their nursing care to be adversely affected by inadequate staffing, the boundaries must be extended to include those people in nursing administration who are responsible for staffing the surgical units. If it seems that the quality of care is related to problems of chemotherapy, the boundaries of the system must be reset to include representatives of the pharmacy department and also the physicians who are writing the orders for the drugs in question.

Another study might be undertaken to examine the care of *all* surgical patients of *all* ages and *all* types of surgery in *all* hospitals in the county in order to find ways to reduce the incidence of postoperative infections. The boundaries of this large system would include the patients, nurses, infection control consultants, and possibly a statistician.

Such boundaries are, of course, intangible. They are probably unknown and of little concern to anyone except those working with the system, and these arbitrary boundaries do not usually affect the workings of the system in any noticeable way.

The functioning of a system depends on its input, output, feedback, equilibrium, and rate of entropy.

INPUT. Input consists of the information, materials, and energy that enter a system. Input may come from a component within the system or from outside the system. An *open system* receives a great deal of input, whereas a relatively *closed system* is receptive to very little input. The more open the system, the more varied and extensive is its input. All human systems are open systems.

The previously mentioned study of postoperative infections would be ineffective without extensive input. This input would be in the form of information that would include, among other items, a description of procedures and techniques currently in use in each hospital, an analysis of the degree to which nurses and patients are conforming with established procedures and policies, and statistics regarding the incidence and type of postoperative infections during a given period. Conversely, input related to the heating system of a small house would be much more limited because that system is relatively closed.

Nursing input may be in the form of information, materials, or energy. *Information* is supplied by giving directions, explanations, and patient teaching. *Materials* are involved when food, drugs, dressings, and so on are supplied. The *energy* supplied by the nurse can be either physical (helping the patient to move, turn over, feed himself), or psychic (giving hope, encouragement, and motivation). Energy is also transferred during some types of healing, such as the use of therapeutic touch.

OUTPUT. Output from a system is the end result of one or more processes of that system and may be in the form of information, materials, or energy. For example, output from the digestive system would be in the form of information related to waste materials, caloric energy, or sensations of hunger. Output from the study of the system for caring for surgical patients would be information such as statistics and recommendations.

FEEDBACK. Feedback is that portion of the output of a system which, when fed back into the system, enables that system to regulate itself. Feedback enables a system to compare *what is* with *what was expected* or needed. Feedback comes from a component that has been affected by some action of the system and is usually fed back to the component that initiated the action. It makes

a circle or loop commonly referred to as a feedback loop. One part of this loop consists of output from one component (usually the one affected by the system), and the other part of the loop becomes input back to the component that produced the effect.

Feedback, as a portion of the output of a system, will be in the form of information, material, or energy. The information may be verbal or nonverbal. If a person who is very hungry eats a single lettuce leaf, feedback from his digestive system will indicate that the lettuce leaf was not adequate to relieve his hunger. If a restless, uncomfortable patient falls asleep during a back rub, that behavior is feedback that enables the nurse to conclude that the back rub was effective. During range-of-motion exercises, resistance of a joint coupled with verbal or nonverbal indications of pain serves as feedback that causes the nurse to decide that the exercise should be discontinued until further evaluation of the joint has been made. Careful examination of vomitus, fecal matter, blood, and urine will give nurse and physician feedback on the functioning of various body systems.

Strictly speaking, *feedback describes the status of a portion of a system at a given point in time.* In many systems, feedback does not indicate whether the condition is good or bad, better or worse. It does give a nurse data with which to make a decision or a judgment. For example, a thermometer might indicate that a patient's body temperature is 101 degrees F. That feedback, that information by itself, cannot indicate the action to be taken. If a nurse were in the process of sponging the patient because of a previous temperature of 103.8 degrees F., the feedback of a body temperature of 101 degrees F. would indicate that the fever sponge bath had been effective and would be reassuring rather than a cause for concern. If, however, the patient was in his third day of postoperative recovery, had been having a normal temperature, and suddenly complained of a chill, the same feedback of a body temperature of 101 degrees F would give a nurse reason to suspect that something was wrong with one or more of the patient's physiological systems and that some intervention was needed.

A system needs feedback in order to regulate itself and grow more effective and efficient. For example, on a surgical unit, the procedure committee needs to receive feedback from the staff in order to evaluate its work. It is important to note that output does not automatically become useful feedback. Output from the staff in the form of muttering and sputtering that is never directed to the committee does not become feedback; it remains output and is of little value to the committee. Comments and/or complaints about a new type of dressing tray, for example, must actually reach the surgical procedure committee in order for the committee to learn that it made a poor choice of trays and for them to be able to make another selection.

Some type of feedback is present in every patient-nurse interaction because *the lack of a response is in itself a kind of feedback* about the patient. The absence of a palpable pulse may indicate that the patient is in deep shock; the patient's failure to respond to your questions is feedback which suggests that the patient either didn't hear you, chooses to ignore you, or is incapable of making a response.

A nurse consistently tries to get feedback from the individual, family, or community about the effectiveness of her nursing interventions. Since it is only through adequate feedback that a system can regulate itself, the nurse-patient interaction can correct itself, grow, and develop only when both patient and nurse obtain enough feedback to evaluate the system at frequent intervals.

EQUILIBRIUM. Every system is presumed to have a tendency to achieve a balance among the stresses and tensions exerted by its component parts. This balance is referred to by a variety of terms such as steady state, homeostasis, stability, and status quo. A stable system, such as a healthy, close-knit family, is able to tolerate a number of forces without losing its equilibrium, but an unstable family system is likely to be disrupted by a crisis of any sort.

ENTROPY. Every system requires energy to function and maintain the processes related to input and output. Additional energy is required when strain, stress, tension, or friction increases the normal work load of the system. Energy expended is lost, and therefore, every system tends to run down, wear out, or deteriorate. This tendency toward disorganization is called entropy; it will eventually destroy the system unless the energy loss is counteracted.

In machines, entropy results in parts wearing out, malfunction, and mechanical failures. In humans, entropy occurs as mental and physical fatigue, illness, aging, and death. Some forms of entropy can be slowed by measures such as rest, food, support, and therapy; but aging and death are inevitable.

Members of the helping professions are especially susceptible to a form of entropy currently referred to as professional burnout. It takes energy to support and care for other people, and the continued giving of oneself must be counteracted by measures that refresh, revitalize, and rejuvenate the individual.

Negentropy is the movement of a system toward integration, growth, and organization and is sometimes referred to as an evolutionary force. Examples of negentropy in humans include the growth and development of fetus and child, the acquisition of knowledge and skill, and the development of a satisfying interpersonal relationship or a cohesive group.

Systems as Recipients of Nursing Action

Three specific systems of concern to the nurse are the individual, the family, and the community. The individual is a complete system composed of many subsystems or components such as the circulatory and nervous systems. The individual in turn is a component of the family system. Every family, whether it be large or small, nuclear or extended, traditional or nontraditional, functions as a system capable of interacting with other systems. The family, in turn, is a component of the larger community system.

Individual Systems

In some acute care settings, such as the recovery room, emergency room, or an intensive care unit, the nurse must focus almost exclusively on the patient, *temporarily* excluding the family and community. Various systems of his body are threatened, and urgent physiological needs must be met. In some situations, a psychiatric nurse must interact with a single patient for an extended period of time. In each situation, the nurse is well aware that the individual is a component of a larger system of family and friends, but for the moment, top priority for nursing intervention belongs to the individual patient system.

Some nurses react negatively to the practice of referring to a person as a system or as a component of a system because they feel that such terms are dehumanizing. This terminology may be less objectionable if you understand that the terms *system* and *component* are applied to people only within the context of a theoretical framework, and never in a real life situation.

Family Systems

Whenever possible, the nurse extends the boundaries of the patient care system to include people who are significant to the patient. Because interactions within the family system influence a person's response to illness, therapy, and recovery, the nurse makes every effort to include the family when explanations are given, decisions are made, teaching is done, and feelings are explored. Failure to include the family may negate the effectiveness of patient teaching. For example, extensive teaching and planning with a newly diagnosed male diabetic may prove futile in the long run if the wife, who always prepares his meals, is not included.

The need for family involvement is quite obvious in some situations but is more covert in others. For instance, a married woman who has had a mastectomy may do well in the hospital environment. As a patient (a single system), she may seem to function well and adapt effectively to the removal of her breast. Upon discharge, however, she ceases to be an individual patient system and again becomes a more obvious component of the family system. Her mastectomy has affected her, and whatever affects her must of necessity affect her family in one way or another. Any teaching that focused entirely on the patient must be deemed incomplete and is likely to prove ineffective. If she was not taught to cope with her family's feelings, questions, and concerns, whether expressed or not, she may withdraw from them and resort to interactions that are not conducive to either family unity or good mental health.

Sometimes the nurse's interaction with the family system may be secondary to her interaction with one member of the family. At other times, the nurse's primary intervention will be with the family as a whole. A community health nurse may help a family prepare to receive a premature baby, an infant with birth defects, or an adult from a nearby psychiatric hospital. The nurse may never have seen the person about whom a family is concerned; the priority at the moment is the family system, of which that person will soon be a significant component.

Systems theory contributes to an understanding of the effect on the family of changes such as those created by birth, death, adoption, divorce, or remarriage. Furthermore, an understanding of systems theory contributes to the nurse's ability to help the patient move away from the health care system and back into the family during the course of an illness.

Community Systems

The nurse, especially the community health nurse, often interacts with the community as a system. This may occur for one of two reasons. First, an individual person or family may be the primary focus of the nurse's teaching, but because of the nature of the problem, the boundaries of that system must be set beyond the family to include all or part of the community. It may be that special transportation is needed for a handicapped schoolchild; volunteers may be needed in a crisis-ridden household; funds may be needed from a local organization to help a severely burned child; education may be needed to overcome the resistance of a small group of neighbors to the return of a young man from a drug detoxification facility. In each instance, effective nursing interaction recognizes that the individual and the family are components of the community system. The nurse may not be the one who actually interacts with the relevant segment of the community, but it is her assessment of the situation and her knowledge of systems theory that prompt the appropriate action.

The second reason for a nurse's interaction with the community as a system is that the nurse may be called on to teach a certain group or segment of the community. She may be asked to teach high school students about venereal disease, to promote better sanitation at a migrant camp, or to appear on a televised talk show to discuss the effects of stress with several businessmen. In each instance, the nurse will study the system and obtain input from those involved to determine what the group needs and wants.

Each of the groups to be taught is a small system that interacts with other systems within the larger system of the community. Inasmuch as whatever happens to one system affects the other systems to some degree, it is impossible to teach one group effectively without affecting a number of other groups. Only with a bland, easily forgotten presentation or program is the effect likely to be confined to the original system, and then only because *nothing* happened to that system. If a program on venereal disease, for instance, is effective for high school students, it will affect, in one way or another, the parents, younger brothers and sisters, the local newspaper, the school board, local church groups, and many others. Some of these effects will be desirable, and some will be undesirable; but the nurse who is knowledgeable about systems theory will anticipate these interactions between the component parts of the community system.

Systems Theory and Clinical Assignments

Once the nurse has identified the system with which she will be working (individual, family, or community), it is important that she identify or acknowledge the boundaries of that system. These boundaries may be, for instance, physical, temporal, psychological, or functional. For example, the physical and temporal boundaries for a nursing student might be the unit of an assigned patient, from 7 to 11 am. Four people might be included within that system in the functional roles of student, patient, instructor, and team leader. Each of these four people will function both as a separate system and as a component of the larger patient care system. Anything that happens to one of these four during the morning will affect the other three to a greater or lesser degree. Each one is receiving input from many sources into his own system, which in turn influences that person's input into the larger system.

Input from the patient into the system might be his reaction to pain and discomfort, his anger over his poor prognosis, and his anticipation of relaxation following a bath and back rub. Input from the student is likely to be her enthusiasm for nursing; her eagerness to please the patient, her instructor, and the team leader; and her apprehension about her ability to cope with the patient's pain and anger. The team leader's input is her insistence that all assignments be completed on time, and her concern for a beloved patient who is dying in the next room, while the instructor's input is support and assistance for the student.

Additional input from other sources intrudes on this system and affects the relationships within it. A late or cold breakfast tray, the unexpected arrival of the patient's clergyman, the frowns of a group of physicians making rounds, or the death of the patient next door—any such input will affect one or more of the component persons directly and the others indirectly. A working knowledge of systems theory enables the nurse to identify many of the various inputs into a given system and to anticipate the possible effects on the component parts as well as on the system as a whole. The nurse's knowledge of herself as a system enables her to recognize the variety of forces acting upon her and to acknowledge possible ways in which her responses to this input may influence her input into the health care system.

PATIENT TEACHING

An understanding of the concepts of systems theory gives individuals and families a basis for coping more effectively with the events in their lives. They do not need to know the terminology of systems theory, although some terms, such as input, output, and feedback, have become part of our everyday language as a result of the increased use of computers. The concepts of systems theory can be expressed very simply and directly in phrases such as:

- "Whatever affects you will affect the rest of your family"
- "Whenever there is a crisis in a family, it affects everyone, and it is important that everyone be able to participate in dealing with it"
- "No family can live in isolation—the things that are happening in your neighborhood will affect you and your children"

The basic concepts of systems theory will support the nurse's teaching related to the family's need for effective communication, the use of support groups in times of need and crisis, the advantages of family therapy over individual therapy, and the need for citizen involvement and consumerism with respect to health care.

RELATED ACTIVITIES

1. Make a visual aid for your own use or for patient teaching. Connect a number of paper clips (one for each member of the family or component of a system) with rubber bands and mount them by attaching a few of the rubber bands to a pegboard or bulletin board. Use large or small rubber bands to show loose or strong pulls and tensions, and attach as many rubber bands to a given person or component as needed to show the variety and number of relationships experienced by that person. Remove or add new paper clips and watch the effect on all the other clips. Use this visual aid to demonstrate the interdependency of all the clips, showing that it is impossible to change the position of one clip without affecting each of the others to some degree.

2. Analyze a situation in which you are currently involved by drawing a circle which contains all the significant components. Describe the input and output, and the nature and type of feedback. Then, change the boundaries, and by doing so, include or exclude certain people or other components. Adjust the description of the input, output, and feedback, and notice how your perception of the situation (the system) is altered by expanding or constricting its boundaries.

SUGGESTED READINGS

Auger, Jeanine Roose: *Behavioral Systems and Nursing.* Englewood Cliffs, NJ, Prentice-Hall, 1976.

Dossey, Larry: Care giving and natural systems theory. *Top Clin Nurs* 1982 Jan; 3(4):21–27.

Hall, Joanne E, and Barbara R Weaver: *Distributive Nursing Practice: A Systems Approach to Community Health.* ed.2. Philadelphia, Lippincott, 1985.

King, Imogene M, and M Jean Daubenmire: Nursing process models: A systems approach. *Nurs Outlook* 1973 Aug; 21(8):512–518.

Palmer, Irene Sabelberg: Nightingale revisited. *Nurs Outlook* 1983 July/Aug; 31(4):229–233.

Putt, Arlene M: *General Systems Theory Applied to Nursing.* Boston, Little, Brown and Co, 1978.

Robbins, Margaret, and Thomas Schacht: Family hierarchies. *Am J Nurs* 1982 Feb; 82(2):284–286.

6

Values

Prerequisites and/or Suggested Preparation
There are no prerequisites or suggested preparation for this chapter.

The terms values, ethics, and morals are sometimes used interchangeably, but they are not the same. *Ethics* is the branch of philosophy which deals with important questions of human conduct. Socrates has been called the 'patron saint of moral philosophy,' and succeeding generations of philosophers have continued to struggle with ethical concerns. In many instances, that which is right and good for an individual is not right and good for another individual or for society as a whole, and the resulting problem constitutes an *ethical dilemma*. Examples of ethical dilemmas include:

- The physician's obligation to treat a patient versus the patient's right to refuse treatment
- The use of heroin to relieve the pain of patients dying with cancer versus government regulation of all narcotic drugs
- The use of limited resources to provide extraordinary care to a small number of people versus using the same resources to provide at least minimal care to the greatest number of people possible

Ethical dilemmas and the need for moral decisions are increasing both in number and complexity because technological advances have made it possible to prolong life when there is no consensus that such actions are always desirable or beneficial. The urgency and diversity of such issues have given rise to specialization within the philosophical realm of ethics. These areas of study and practice are referred to as medical ethics, biomedical ethics, or bioethics.

The term *morals* usually refers to a set of standards or beliefs which enables people to determine what is right or wrong, good or bad. The source of a moral law may be the accumulated mores or norms of the group, or divine revelations such as the Ten Commandments or the teachings of Christ or Mohammed. Morals and moral standards are an integral part of ethical dilemmas and decision making because two or more moral rules can apply to a single situation, and the outcomes will be very different, depending upon which rule is chosen.

Values can be described as the outcome of an individual's efforts to apply universal moral laws to his everyday life. Every person, as well as every group and civilization, develops a value system of some sort which provides direction for the activities of daily life. There is no best or preferred definition of a value, but the following are representative of the many definitions currently available:

"Values are those assertions or statements that individuals make, either through their behavior, words, or actions, that define what they think is important and for which they are willing to suffer and even die—or perhaps continue living. Each person's character *is defined by the value choices he has made . . ." (Curtin, 1982, p. 8)*

"A value is an affective disposition towards a person, object, or idea. Values represent a way of life, and they give direction to life. Values are those things which make a difference in living." (Steele and Harmon, 1979, p.1)

"Values have to do with modes of conduct and end-states of existence. To say that a person "has a value" is to say that he has an enduring belief that a specific mode of conduct or end-state of existence is personally and socially preferable to alternative modes of conduct or end-states of existence. Once a value is internalized it becomes, consciously or unconsciously, a standard or criterion for guiding action, for developing and maintaining attitudes toward relevant objects and situations, for morally judging self and others, and for comparing self with others." (Rokeach, 1969)

These definitions vary in complexity, but each includes the concept that values are personal, and that they provide meaning and direction to life.

This chapter is designed to introduce concepts related to values and value systems in preparation for the subsequent study of ethics, ethical dilemmas and ethical decision making in future courses. The title of the chapter refers to the process by which a helping person such as a nurse or teacher can assist people to examine and develop their value systems.

IMPORTANCE OF VALUES

Values are important in nursing for two reasons. First of all, every nursing action should be congruent with the nurse's value system. For example, the manner in which a nurse gives an injection to a 6-year-old should be consistent with her values. If she values obedience highly and therefore believes that a child should do as he is told and that he should be disciplined if he refuses, then a no-nonsense approach would be consistent with those values; and the child would be physically restrained if he resisted the injection.

If a nurse values the concept of the child as a person with the right to some control over what is done to his body, then an entirely different approach is in order. The nurse might say to the child, "This is what needs to be done. What can I do to help? How can I help you control yourself so that you can lie still until it is over?" The child is not in a position to choose whether or not to receive the injection, but he can make significant choices about the manner in which he responds or behaves in the situation.

The nurse's value system will influence her actions in both simple and complex, routine and difficult situations; it will provide a rational basis for answers to questions such as: "Will I participate in the hospital

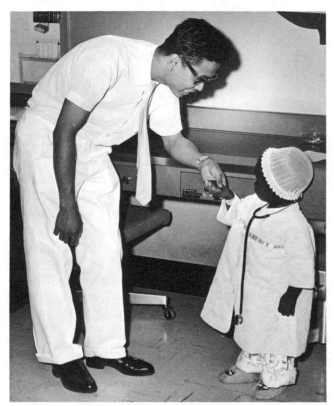

Figure 6.1 *The health care worker values the dignity of a young patient.*

strike?" "Do I approve of giving contraceptives to young adolescents without parental knowledge?" "How shall I deal with one of my staff nurses who calls in sick the day before each holiday?"

Nursing care based on well-defined values is likely to be more consistent, unified, and purposeful than nursing care that has no central focus or core. The process of examining and developing a value system is not easy, but only by doing so can a nurse build the internal supports that will provide some degree of stability as she makes decisions and takes action in complex and unpredictable situations. A well developed value system contributes to a greater correlation between what the nurse believes and what she does, and thereby increases job satisfaction, reduces stress, and promotes good mental health (Fig. 6.1).

Values are important in nursing for a second reason: many patients and families need help as they struggle with issues related to health and illness. They may or may not realize that values are involved as they try to make crucial choices and decisions; but in many situations, indecision is linked to the need to clarify certain underlying values. For example, the value placed on family relationships and the value placed on individual needs are basic to decisions on the possible placement of a grandparent in a nursing home. The value a person

places on his own identity and existence will influence that person's decision to accept or reject a physician's recommendation of radical and disfiguring facial surgery. A migrant worker who accepts illness as an inevitable aspect of life may not respond to the health teaching of a community health nurse because, to him, health is not a value to be actively pursued.

As the public gradually assumes an increasing responsibility for the quantity and quality of health care in this country, it becomes increasingly important for each person first to be a knowledgeable consumer of the health care provided by others and, second, to value highly his own pursuit of health. Many people will seek treatment for a specific disease or illness but expend little if any money, time, or energy on attaining a higher level of personal wellness. For this group of people, the nurse may be the primary catalyst in the clarification of values related to health and illness.

DEVELOPMENT OF VALUES

Values become important as a person develops his own lifestyle and begins to decide which things are right, desirable, and worthy. Some cultures and societies have tried to identify for themselves a uniform or universal set of values that could be taught or transmitted from one generation to another. Some basic concepts and tenets have endured for centuries, but many values have changed or are changing in response to changes in society. For example, not only do the values attributed to peace, sex, energy, old age, women, and material possessions vary from country to country; they vary from decade to decade within a given country. Values also vary from person to person, and the values of each person change and evolve as that person grows and matures.

Various researchers have suggested that values develop or result from a series of identifiable steps and stages. In 1978, Louis Raths and his colleagues proposed that values evolve from the choices a person makes, and they described seven steps in the process of developing a value. These steps in the process of valuing are also called the seven criteria for identifying a value. The seven steps are:

1. Choosing from alternatives
2. Examining the possible consequences
3. Choosing freely
4. Feeling good about the choice
5. Affirming the choice
6. Acting on the choice
7. Acting with a pattern

Choosing From Alternatives

For a value to develop or to be influential, a person must have more than one option. For example, if a person is arbitrarily isolated from all other humans, he cannot be said to value solitude; he has no choice in the matter. If a person is frugal, it should not be *assumed* that he values careful spending; he may shop cautiously because he is living on a fixed income, such as social security, and may have no other choice.

Examining the Possible Consequences

Even when there are alternatives, a value develops only when there is thoughtful consideration of the possible consequences of each alternative. The child who wants to earn money from a paper route instead of by doing chores around the house must be aware of the possible outcomes of each before he can make an informed choice. The person who is considering abortion as one alternative to an unwanted pregnancy must examine the possible physical, psychological, and social consequences of such an action. A specific action taken *without consideration of the consequences* is often based on a hunch, an idea, a conviction, or a feeling; it does not necessarily mean that the person values that course of action.

Choosing Freely

A crucial step in the process of developing a value is choosing freely. The choice must be made without coercion or pressure from parents, teachers, peers, or colleagues. Behavior determined by fear or directed by pressure, no matter how subtle, does not reflect the values of the person exhibiting the behavior.

Feeling Good About the Choice

Once a choice has been made freely from a number of alternatives, and with adequate knowledge of the likely consequences of each alternative, a person must be *satisfied* with his choice if it is going to contribute to his value system. Any choice of which he is not proud will certainly influence his behavior, but the choice cannot be considered a potential value.

Affirming the Choice

Given a choice of which a person is proud and satisfied, the person must then be willing to affirm that choice *when appropriate.* He must be willing to speak out and defend his position should the occasion arise.

Acting on the Choice

Action is critical to the process of developing a value because without action the process results in something more closely resembling a belief, an attitude, or a conviction. A value requires both an initial action and subsequent actions that follow a pattern. Depending on the nature of the choice that was made, the initial action might be a visit to a physician, a letter to a legislator, a brisk walk, a family conference, or a few minutes of prayer.

Acting With a Pattern

Initial action must be followed by a series of related actions over an extended period of time which indicate that the choice is valued enough to be integrated into many aspects of daily life. A single action that is never repeated is more likely to be the result of some type of problem solving than the result of value development. A nurse who writes a single letter to her congressman, but never again becomes involved in any aspect of political action, cannot be said to value the need for political action by nurses.

OTHER INFLUENCES ON BEHAVIOR

Many things other than values influence our behavior. They may approach values in importance and often indicate the presence of a value, but if they fail to meet the seven criteria, they are not considered true values. These influences include needs, goals, attitudes, interests and activities, feelings, and beliefs or convictions.

Needs

Although a person's unmet needs exert a powerful influence on his behavior, only a portion of them are likely to be related to his value system. The satisfaction of a basic physiological need is necessary for life, but it may be unrelated to a person's value system because he has no choice; he must eat, drink, and breathe. When these lower level needs have been met, higher level needs emerge; values can emerge or develop when a person begins to *make choices* related to meeting these needs.

Goals

Goals obviously influence our behavior, but they may or may not be directly related to our values. For example, a young mother may attend a nutrition workshop because she values the health of her family and because attention to nutrition is part of her overall commitment to health. On the other hand, she may attend because she is looking for ways to save money on food bills in order to be able to afford a longed-for vacation; her attendance at the nutrition workshop therefore cannot be presumed to indicate that she values good nutrition. Her attendance could, however, be based on a different value—family recreation—provided that meets all seven criteria.

Interests

A person's interest in a topic or activity may range from a passing fancy to the deep and abiding concern of a true value. Participation in an aluminum recycling project may be an attempt to earn a Boy Scout merit badge; it could be the result of pressure from one's club to be their representative on the recycling project; or it may be one of many activities undertaken as a result of a deep, long-lasting concern for and valuing of ecology.

Feelings

A person's feelings may be aroused by some aspect of his value system, but very often feelings are temporary reactions to some event or situation and may be precipitated by factors only remotely related to a value. For example, a person who values justice will feel outraged and angry when confronted by unfair personnel policies in a hospital, even though he himself may not be directly affected. Another person may also feel outraged and angry about the same unfair practice, but only because it seems to block his own career plans, *not* because he values justice.

Beliefs or Convictions

Many things believed on the basis of folklore, family tradition, indoctrination, or hearsay are not values. Yet, some of these same beliefs can and do represent a value if they have been carefully examined, freely chosen, and well integrated into a person's life. A parent, for example, might insist that a child eat everything on his plate. It may be that the parent values thrift and abhors waste, or it may be that the parent's demand is an almost involuntary response, a carryover from a childhood during the Depression when his own parents could ill afford any kind of waste.

One way to distinguish between those two possible interpretations is to examine the parent's responses to other stimuli. If the parent is *equally concerned* about conserving energy, saving money, and the careful use of tools and toys, that parent is likely to be responding to the child's failure to clean his plate on the basis of *valuing* thrift and conservation. The parent's response would reflect a value because the parent would be demonstrating the seventh stage of valuing, that of acting with consistency and repetition. If, however, the parent is wasteful and extravagant in other areas, then he is likely to be acting on the basis of some blindly accepted belief or conviction that cleaning one's plate is a virtue and somehow 'good' for one, despite nutritionists' warnings about overeating in childhood.

TRANSMISSION OF VALUES

Given that values help to provide meaning and direction for life, that values evolve and change over a period of time, and that values are deeply personal, the question arises of how children and adults can be helped to develop an effective set of values. The traditional approaches to teaching values have not been sufficient in our society, as evidenced by the indecision and controversy over such issues as care of the elderly, juvenile crime, care of street people, treatment of minorities and the future of marriage and the family. The traditional ways of imparting values include setting an example, persuading and convincing, limiting choices, imposing rules and regulations, cultural and religious teachings, and appeals to conscience.

Setting an Example

Because both children and adults tend to model certain aspects of their behavior after that of a person who typifies what they would like to become, the example set by such a person has the potential for influencing behavior in a very significant way. Before the advent of mass media, this role model was found in the family, the immediate neighborhood, or occasionally, in a book. Increased family mobility plus vastly expanded public communication, especially television, have presented a bewildering increase in the number of role models, all seeming to clamor for acceptance and imitation.

The adolescent girl, for example, is confronted with many would-be role models including her mother, Miss America, a teacher, the president's wife, an older sister, an Olympic champion, a television star, a female governor, a disco dancer, and a female construction worker. The list is endless; the choices seem almost infinite and overwhelming. In such a situation, reliance on the transmission of values through the use of an example is risky indeed because there can be no assurance that an appropriate role model will be selected and imitated.

Persuading and Convincing

Attempts to inculcate values on the basis of reason alone are almost certainly doomed to failure because a person's reason and intellect are only partially responsible for his behavior.

A person may "know in his head" that he should lose weight and yet continue to overeat. Another may know that prolonged high-level stress predisposes him to ulcers or hypertension, and yet he may persist in a frantic, stressful lifestyle. Arguments, rational explanations, and attempts to persuade and convince are likely to be ineffective motivators toward the valuing of a calmer, healthier way of life.

Limiting Choices

It is possible to *control the behavior* of a person to some degree by offering him a choice between two things that are equally acceptable to society in general. No matter which he chooses, his behavior will be socially acceptable in that situation, but such an approach leaves him without a basis for action in a situation where the alternatives are not specified and the choices have not been arbitrarily limited.

Imposing Rules and Regulations

Conformity to rules and regulations tends to produce behaviors that are socially acceptable now and in similar situations in the future. These behaviors may be long-lasting, especially if they are adequately rewarded, and may lead an observer to conclude that the person has a "correct" set of values. Unfortunately, the person who obeys all rules and regulations, perhaps without thinking, may be ill prepared to cope in a situation in which the rules and regulations have not yet been formulated or in a situation in which he knows that the rules cannot or will not be enforced. When rules and regulations have guided a person's behavior for many years, his moral and ethical decisions are probably rooted in a fear of being caught rather than in a conscious desire to do what is right.

Cultural and Religious Teachings

The tenets and practices of a person's tribe, society, or religious group will influence his behavior, even after he leaves that group of people. These teachings are likely to be very effective, especially in the setting in which they were taught. Because a person usually accepts cultural and religious teachings on faith, however, there may have been little or no choice involved. As a result, these *unquestioned teachings* can form the

basis for the development of values but often do not constitute values in and of themselves.

Appeals to Conscience

It is assumed by many that nearly everyone has an inner voice that directs him toward right and away from wrong. Failure to obey this inner voice or conscience usually results in feelings of guilt and remorse. Any action that fails to conform to a predetermined set of familial or societal norms has the potential for evoking guilt. Many individuals and groups have capitalized on this mechanism as a powerful method of influencing behavior.

THE CLARIFICATION PROCESS

The traditional approaches to the transmission of cherished values are usually employed in combination and have for centuries fostered the development of values in children and adults with varying degrees of success. It now seems that, *in addition to these approaches,* a process is needed which involves the person in the development of his own set of values. There is no set of values that can be simply transmitted from one person to another person. The *development of values is an internal process* that can be learned, but it is a task each person must do for himself.

Values clarification is a process by which a concerned and helping person, such as a parent, a teacher, or a nurse, intervenes when appropriate to help someone examine and clarify his behavior and values. Values clarification promotes the *process of valuing;* it does NOT attempt to teach a person what to value.

Some people are self-directed and highly motivated with a clear sense of purpose and identity. Such people do not need assistance in the form of value clarification but there are other easily identified people who do need help. Research has indicated that those whose values are unclear and to whom no one thing seems more important than any other living thing tend to lead aimless and unsatisfying lives. These people often exhibit one or more of the following attributes: apathy, marked inconsistency, considerable uncertainty, overconformity, unwarranted dissension, flightiness, and role playing. Such people are often helped by values clarification (Raths, 1978, pp. 7 and 248).

Behaviors That Suggest a Need for Values Clarification

In the context of nursing and health care, the attributes that may indicate an inadequate value system and a need for values clarification may be manifested as follows:

Apathy

The person does not really care about health issues such as nutrition, immunization, or pollution and may say, "It doesn't really matter to me, one way or another," or "I just can't get excited about it."

Inconsistency

The person does not seem to know when his beliefs and behaviors are incompatible with each other. For example, a chain smoker might state emphatically, "I think every person has a moral obligation to take care of his body" and not realize that his words and behavior are inconsistent.

Uncertainty

The person cannot seem to make a decision, take a stand, or state his opinion, and may verbalize his uncertainty with statements such as "I really think I ought to lose weight; but on the other hand, everyone knows that fat people are jolly and fun to be with."

Overconformity

The person may be committed to a variety of acceptable health practices, but the commitment is based on the *opinions of others* rather than on his own values. He usually justifies his behavior with remarks such as "The *nurse* says . . ." or "*They* say that . . ."

Dissension

The person may be lacking a strong personal value system and may compensate by persistent *unwarranted,* and often *unreasonable* dissension. He may argue against nonsmoking regulations, hospital policies, immunization requirements, or a multitude of other items. He often has strong convictions, none of which are true values, and he argues for the sake of arguing.

Flightiness

The person may focus intensely on first one concern and then another in fairly rapid succession, none of which become an integral part of his life. With respect to health, he may campaign for smoke abatement legislation for awhile, then do volunteer work at Planned Parenthood for a season, dropping it in favor of involvement with a nursing home. Another example would be the person who seeks better health first by diet, then by jogging and exercise, and later by meditation and a different diet, all within a short period of time.

Role Playing

The person may adopt a role that conceals the absence of adequate personal values. The person who is always jovial, the 'perfect' patient, or the apparently scatter-brained adolescent, may have found that such a *role* gives protection from the risks of trying to decide which things or causes are good and worth pursuing.

The Clarifying Response

There are many techniques used in values clarification, including games and group activities designed for use with children in the classroom. Similar activities would be useful in nursing with groups such as newly diagnosed diabetics or the parents of terminally ill children. But with an individual patient, the least time-consuming and probably the most effective technique is the clarifying response. This is a verbal response that stimulates another person to *examine what he is saying or doing.* It is the stimulus for a brief exchange that causes a person to examine various aspects of his thinking or behavior and thus begin to clarify his values.

There are no specific phrases or responses for the nurse or other helper to use. In general, a clarifying response may be any question that leads a person to focus his attention on one of the seven criteria of a value. For example, the second criterion of developing a value is choosing with knowledge of the likely consequences. A clarifying response might be "What do you think might happen if you did that?" There is no right or wrong answer; the clarifying response merely stimulates the person to consider the possible consequences of his proposed action. If a child or an adult is repeatedly asked to consider possible outcomes in a variety of situations and by a variety of people, this step of valuing is likely to become habitual, even in the absence of clarifying responses or other cues.

Characteristics of Clarifying Responses

The characteristics of a clarifying response and the interaction within which it occurs are as follows:

The clarifying interaction is brief. It often consists of only *two or three exchanges* between the nurse and patient or family member. It usually concludes with a nonjudgmental, noncommittal phrase from the nurse such as "Oh, I understand it better now" or "Let's talk about it again sometime."

One clarifying exchange will not produce a significant effect. A clarifying response is made to stimulate thought, and the major portion of this thinking will occur *after* the exchange is over. The effect of clarifying responses is *cumulative* and may not be evident for some time.

A clarifying response excludes all value judgments. There should be no hint of right or wrong, good or bad, acceptable or unacceptable in the response. The purpose of the interaction is to stimulate clarification; the purpose is not to advise, preach, teach, moralize, or evaluate.

The clarifying response is thought-provoking yet permissive. It is a nonthreatening *invitation* to examine some idea or action, but the person may not choose to do so.

The clarifying interaction does not seek information, the solution to a problem, or the resolution of a difficulty. There is no conclusion, finish, or summary; the only purpose is to stimulate thought.

Clarifying responses are used selectively. They are appropriate only in situations in which there are *no* right or correct answers, such as situations involving feelings, attitudes, beliefs, intentions, and aspirations. It is *not* feasible or appropriate to respond in this way to all or even a majority of the things said by others. Clarifying responses should be given to *selected* statements made by those patients, families, or colleagues who exhibit the attributes of people who seem to need help with values. These attributes, as indicated earlier, are apathy, uncertainty, inconsistency, overconformity, dissension, flightiness, and persistent role playing.

Clarifying responses cannot be memorized or formulated in advance. They are spontaneous and develop in response to a situation. They are, however, used consciously and with deliberation, and many nurses have a repertoire of possible responses for each of the steps of valuing. *Any response can be considered effective if it stimulates thought about one of the seven steps in developing a value.*

Examples of Clarifying Responses

As the nurse develops skill in value clarification, she will find she is able to formulate responses appropriate to the age, maturity, education, and culture of each patient. Some examples of clarifying responses for each of the seven stages of value development are given below.

1. *Choosing from alternatives.* The purpose of a clarifying response for step 1 would be either to (a) help the person to examine known alternatives, (b) identify or find alternatives if they are not known, or (c) discover that alternatives do exist. Possible clarifying responses for step 1 might be:

- What other things have you considered?
- Are there any other ways you might accomplish this?
- Where (or how) might you find out about alternatives?

Whenever the nurse offers choices or alternatives to another person, she should be sure that all alternatives are acceptable and have meaning for the person if she wants to promote development of a value. If only one choice is acceptable, or if neither choice is acceptable and the person has to choose the lesser of two evils, the choice makes no contribution to the development of a value because the fourth condition, that of feeling good about the choice, cannot be met. The child who is offered the choice of either turning off the television and doing his homework or going to bed may find neither choice acceptable. He will of necessity choose one or the other, but the decision will not help him learn much about setting priorities, being accountable, or the appropriate use of television.

Sometimes, a situation is such that no choice is possible. If an action is illegal, hurtful to another person, taboo, or forbidden, the person cannot be allowed to do it even though he may want to. A teacher can say, "I will not tolerate cheating in my classroom," can punish those who do cheat, and can still be free to engage in value clarification with her students about reasons for wanting to cheat, cheating in various circumstances, and so on.

2. *Examining the possible consequences.* The purpose of a clarifying response for step 2 is to help the person predict or anticipate the probable or possible outcomes of his behavior. Values do not develop easily if a person is often taken by surprise and frequently makes statements such as "If I had known that . . . might happen, I would have chosen to . . ." or "I wouldn't have done it if I had only known that . . . would result." Even a child can learn to predict some of the things that might happen, such as: "I might make a mess and Mother would get mad." "It might turn out nice and Mother would be glad." "My sister might get home in time to help me." Possible clarifying responses for step 2 might be:

- What do you think might happen if you do this?
- Where do you think this idea (or action) might lead?
- What do you think you will accomplish by doing this?
- What do you see as the advantages and disadvantages of each possibility?

3. *Choosing freely.* One of the most difficult tasks for the nurse as well as for the patient or family member

is to determine whether or not a choice was freely made. In some instances a person may have felt he had no choice in a matter, only to discover that choices were indeed possible. In other situations a person may believe that he has chosen freely, only to discover through values clarification that his apparent choice was dictated by peer pressure, guilt, family expectations, fear, or other constraints. Possible clarifying responses for step 3 might be:

- Is that something you chose or selected?
- What sorts of things influenced your choice?
- Do you have any choice in the matter?
- Is this a hard decision to make?

4. *Feeling good about the choice.* Because a person cannot value something of which he is ashamed, the purpose of a clarifying response in step 4 is to help the person evaluate his own reaction to his choice. Possible clarifying responses for step 4 might be:

- How do you feel about your decision?
- Will you be proud of what you have done?
- How do you think you will feel when it is all over?
- Are you pleased that it is turning out this way?

5. *Affirming the choice.* A true value requires that the person who holds it speak out in favor of his position or take action in support of that position, should the occasion arise. He may need to think about this behavior in advance. Possible clarifying responses for step 5 might be:

- If you are asked, what will you say about your decision?
- What do you see as the best way to make your position known?
- Will it be hard to tell others how you feel about this?

6. *Acting on the choice.* Unless a person embarks on a plan that translates his ideas into action, his choice will not contribute to his value system. He may need to learn to do a bit of brainstorming in which he thinks of many possibilities, some of which will be unrealistic or unfeasible, so that he can free his mind enough to identify some heretofore unconsidered ways of implementing his choice. Possible clarifying responses for step 6 might be:

- What steps will you take now to make this a reality?
- What will you do first?
- Where will you start in your efforts to make this work?
- What can you do to show how strongly you feel?

7. *Acting with a pattern.* Single actions or spurts of temporary enthusiasm have less impact on the direction of our lives than does a sustained involvement over a longer period of time. A person may need help in thinking of ways to keep his value alive by applying it to a variety of situations over an extended period of time, thereby integrating it into his lifestyle. Possible clarifying responses for step 7 might be:

- Was it worth it?
- Will you do it again?
- Is this action similar to others you are likely to take in the future?
- This action seems to be based on your belief that. . . . How might this belief influence choices you may make in the future?

Using Clarifying Responses

In nearly all clarifying interactions, the person being helped will not be aware of or concerned with the development of a value. In fact, a child may not even know what a value is. A person will only be aware that the clarifier has *asked a question that made him think* and that the clarifier is an accepting, nonjudgmental person to talk to.

The clarifying interaction is purposeful but brief, and might seem casual to an onlooker. Occasionally, especially with children, the interaction is done in passing as the clarifier attempts to capitalize on some behavior or statement he has just noted. In fact, these bits of dialogue have been called "one-legged conferences" because a nurse, parent, or teacher is sometimes almost literally standing on one leg en route to another task or activity (Raths, 1978, p. 57). Despite their brevity, these clarifying exchanges are significant because the person tends to ponder over them later on, when there is a lull in the day's activities or while falling asleep. The impact of a single clarifying response may be minimal, but the *cumulative* effect of numerous exchanges over an extended period can be of great benefit to people whose lives lack purpose and direction because of an unclear or poorly developed value system.

In nursing, maximum effectiveness is most likely in settings in which repeated patient-nurse contacts take place over an extended period, such as in public health nursing, a rehabilitation center, a well-baby clinic, a nursing home, or a physician's office. In an acute care setting, the nurse's clarifying responses may be beneficial to a patient or his family, but his stay may be so brief that the nurse will never know if her response was helpful.

It is important to note that, in nursing, the benefits of value clarification are not restricted to patients and families. All members of the health team are continually involved in moral and ethical decisions, some of which may be relatively minor, while others are matters of life or death. These decisions are more valid when they are based on accurate knowledge plus a strong value system rather than on a bias, an emotion, an attitude, a prejudice, or even apathy.

A clarifying response, being informal and spontaneous, can be made over coffee, in the elevator, during medical or nursing rounds, in the staff lounge, or during a team conference. Regardless of the setting or the position of the person to whom it is directed, the clarifying response is designed to stimulate thought. Because it is accepting, gentle, unobtrusive, and non-judgmental, a nurse can make a clarifying response without difficulty to almost any supervisor, aide, physician, therapist, student, or clinician. The hardest part of making a clarifying response is to *refrain from making the response one would ordinarily make.* The nurse's first impulse when listening to a person whose values seem to be unclear or poorly developed may be to teach, argue, reason, or persuade. These approaches are likely to produce a lively interaction but *no significant, long-term effect.* A quiet, clarifying response may seem to be a modest contribution to a given conversation, but it will stimulate considerable thought, possibly at a much later date.

VALUES CLARIFICATION AND COMMUNICATION

One benefit of values clarification is that it tends to keep the lines of communication open when a topic under discussion might otherwise provoke an emotional, moralistic response. Suppose, for example, that a patient's 14-year-old daughter asked, "What kind of birth control is cheap but safe?" A nurse's first impulse might be to say something such as "Do your parents know that you are asking me about this?"; "You'd better talk with your family doctor about it"; "I think it would be good if you talked with your pastor before you do anything"; or any of a dozen other remarks that would predictably stifle or squelch any further discussion.

If the nurse could, however, control her impulse to teach or moralize and take a minute to think of a clarifying response, the girl could talk with her without feeling trapped or defensive or needing to argue. Depending on the nurse's own values, she might or might not answer the girl's question briefly with a sentence or two of factual material similar to that available in newspapers and women's magazines. But, regardless

of whether or not the nurse feels she can give the girl the information she seeks at the time, the nurse can ask clarifying questions such as: "Have you been thinking about birth control quite a lot lately?", "What do you think would happen if you had a safe means of birth control?" or "How do you think you would feel if you had a safe contraceptive?" A few clarifying responses will stimulate the girl's thinking and open up new areas for her consideration.

At this point, the nurse does not know for sure *why* the girl is seeking the information, and this is *not* the time to quiz her. She may be asking for a friend, testing the nurse's reaction, or be desperately in need of help. Whatever the situation, the nurse has an opportunity to help the girl protect her own health and clarify her own values. Clarifying responses set the tone for an atmosphere of mutual inquiry, respect, and acceptance; and they will probably make it possible for the nurse to ask if there is an urgency to the question or if they can set a date to discuss the topic in greater detail.

The gentle, accepting manner in which the nurse interacts with this girl does *not* mean that the nurse approves of contraceptives for adolescents. It *does* mean that she accepts her as a person, respects her right to her own value system, and will not impose values on her. The process of values clarification does NOT in any way negate the nurse's right to her own strong convictions and strong values. Many people initially fear that values clarification implies a wishy-washy approach to questions of right and wrong, and a laissez-faire attitude toward all kinds of behavior. Such fears are unfounded because *people committed to the process of values clarification* are also *committed to the development of strong personal value systems,* both for themselves and for those they are trying to help.

There will probably come a time in the situation described above when the girl will ask the nurse what she thinks about birth control, and it will be important for the nurse to share her values *at that time.* A major difference between the process of values clarification and traditional methods of teaching values is the *timing* and *method* of professing one's values. In values clarification, the affirmation of the clarifier's values is *delayed and separated* from the clarifying responses. This separation is necessary because the person being helped is not free to explore all sides of an issue when the person helping him is assertively advocating a specific position. In values clarification, the helper's values are *shared* with the other person; they are not preached, imposed, impressed, taught, or forced on him. If the other person does not ask what the nurse believes or values with respect to the issue at hand, the nurse is still free to volunteer the information at a time when a statement of her position will not interfere with his thoughtful consideration of all sides of the question.

VALUES CLARIFICATION AND BASIC RULES

All people, children and adults alike, need firm guidelines for their behavior in many areas of life during the time when their own values are still unformed and when their behavior might pose a threat or hardship to other people. A family might, for example, use the values of the parents to establish two basic rules: (1) no one in this family may hurt another person, either physically or psychologically and (2) no one in this family may take, damage, or destroy another's property. Within this framework, other behavior may be negotiable. The two basic rules of this family can be used as follows to guide the children's behavior: "You may not use your brother's bike without permission." "You may not hit your sister." "I cannot permit you to upset the rest of the family with such noise."

When the rules or guidelines are based on a value, that *value should be made clear*, whenever appropriate, to those who are to follow the rule. An arbitrary rule has less validity than one based on values and reason. For example, a mother who yells, "I told you not to hit your sister," contributes little or nothing to the value system of her children; whereas another mother might contribute more by saying, "I can't permit you to hit your sister because I believe that violence is wrong. Hitting your sister isn't much different than a bully hitting someone in the playground or a robber hurting his victim." Firm adherence to basic rules does not preclude exploration and development of each family member's values. Issues such as minority rights, the use of alcohol, relations with an unpleasant neighbor, crimes of violence, lying for a good cause, and other topics can be examined from many angles despite the fact that parents or other family members may have well-developed values related to these topics. The same is true in other settings. Agency and institutional rules and policies need not detract from the process of values clarification.

THE IMPORTANCE OF AFFIRMATION

Taking action and acting with a pattern are important steps in the process of valuing, and one important action is the verbalization of values as they relate to be-

havior. For example, if a nurse's values will not permit her to participate in an abortion, to ignore the negligence of a colleague, or to restrain an elderly patient who wanders around at night, it is important for her to affirm the value that provides the basis for her decision. In a majority of instances, this affirmation of a value will be made only to the relatively small number of people involved in the situation, and the affirmation will be a quiet, nonjudgmental statement such as "I must do this because I believe that . . ." Occasionally, however, a more public affirmation may be appropriate.

The affirmation of a value is beneficial because it forces the reexamination of one or more values and it strengthens the value by using it as the basis for a given behavior. Affirmation is also important because those whose values are growing and evolving need the example of those whose values have proven to be an effective guide for their actions. In addition, in any era of moral indecision or uncertainty, nursing in particular and society in general become a bit stronger whenever one of its members is willing to take a stand on a fundamental issue.

PATIENT TEACHING

As health care systems become more complex and technology continues to advance, each man, woman, and child will be faced with increasing numbers of ethical dilemmas and problems which require moral decisions. And if the individual involved does not participate in resolving the issues, other people will make the decisions for him.

Individuals who are apathetic, indecisive, passive, or inconsistent with regard to their health would benefit from values clarification. If your contact with a given patient is extremely limited, you may be able to enlist the support and assistance of other nurses who are involved with the patient. (It may be necessary to teach them the process and explain the benefits.)

Some patients, whose contact with you is brief, realize that they need help with decision making and they are likely to follow your suggestion to check the book stores and local library for basic books on values clarification.

RELATED ACTIVITIES

During the next few weeks, try to identify at least *one* value which gives direction to some of your activities. Make sure that each value which you examine is a true value (in terms of the criteria used in this chapter), and not an attitude, belief, or conviction, by answering the following questions:

1. What alternatives did you choose from?
2. What were some of the possible consequences of each alternative?
3. How do you know that you chose freely? That you were not feeling pressured in any way?
4. Do you remember feeling proud and glad about your choice?
5. Are you willing to affirm your choice if appropriate?
6. What was your initial action in response to your choice?
7. What activities show that you are acting with a pattern and that you have incorporated the value into your life?

This is a difficult task indeed, and at this point in your life, you may be unable to identify a real value. If that is the case, post the seven steps in developing a value in a conspicuous place, and see if you can transform one of your beliefs or convictions into a value by the end of the semester. Refer to the seven criteria frequently and don't give up. It isn't easy, but the results are worth the effort.

SUGGESTED READINGS

Bayles, Michael: Betwixt and between: juggling ethical responsibilities on today's nursing scene. *Can Nurse* 1982 June; 78(6):36–40.

Bayles, Michael D: The value of life—by what standard? *Am J Nurs* 1980 Dec; 80(12):2226–2230.

Curtin, Leah, and M Josephine Flaherty: *Nursing Ethics: Theories and Pragmatics.* Bowie, MA, Brady, 1982.

Davis, Anne J, and Mila A Aroskar: *Ethical Dilemmas and Nursing Practice.* New York, Appleton-Century-Crofts, 1978.

Francoeur, Robert T: *Biomedical Ethics: A Guide to Decision Making.* New York, Wiley, 1983.

Ketefian, Shaki: Moral reasoning and moral behavior among selected groups of practicing nurses. *Nurs Res* 1981 May/June; 30(3):171–176.

Raths, Louis, et al: *Values and Teaching.* ed.2. Columbus, OH, Charles Merrill Books, 1978.

Smith, Sharon Jeanne, and Anne J Davis. Ethical dilemmas: conflicts among rights, duties and obligations. *Am J Nurs* 1980 Aug; 80(8):1463–1466.

Steele, Shirley M, and Vera M Harmon: *Values Clarification in Nursing.* New York, Appleton-Century-Crofts, 1979.

Uustal, Diane: Values clarification in nursing: Application to practice. *Am J Nurs* 1978 Feb; 78(2):2058.

Uustal, Diane: The use of values clarification in nursing practice. *J Cont Educ* 1977 Mar; 8(3):8–13.

7

Health and Illness

Cecilia F. Mulvey

Prerequisites and/or Suggested Preparation
Concepts related to the delivery of health care, systems theory, and values (Chapters 3, 5, and 6) are prerequisite to this chapter.

According to Greek mythology, Hygeia was a lovely goddess who watched over the health of the people of Athens. She was not involved in the treatment of the sick; she was the guardian of health and the symbol of a belief that people could remain well if they lived according to reason. She personified the virtues of a wise, sane life in a pleasant environment. Eventually, however, Hygeia was made subservient to Asclepius, the god of healing, who achieved fame, not by teaching wisdom, but by healing the sick through surgery and the use of curative plants (Dubos, 1979). The myth of Hygeia and Asclepius symbolizes the centuries-old conflict between those who believe that the most important function of the health professions is to discover and teach the natural laws that promote and sustain health, and those who believe that the chief function of the health professions is to treat disease and restore health when possible.

Nursing by history and philosophy has not focused exclusively on either of the above positions, but has moved toward a holistic approach to health. Nursing is "to have charge of the personal health of somebody." These words, from the preface of Florence Nightingale's *Notes on Nursing* (1858), identify health as the center and the purpose of nursing. Nursing's health orientation has remained constant throughout the intervening century and a half, and is clearly reflected in current nursing literature and many state nurse practice acts. The purpose of nursing is to promote, protect, and restore the health of individuals, families, and communities (Fig. 7.1).

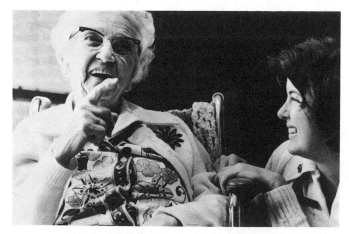

Figure 7.1 *"To heal does not necessarily imply cure. It can simply mean helping people to achieve a way of life compatible with their aspirations—to restore their freedom to make choices—even in the presence of disease"* (Dubos, 1978, p. 82).

CONCEPTS OF HEALTH

Various concepts of health have been linked to religion throughout history, and some early societies viewed health as proof of God's blessing and illness as God's punishment. Those people who have had miraculous recoveries were assumed to have had a close relationship to God or other spirits and were granted status and a role as an intercessor with God for the less fortunate (White, 1979). Such people became the first health care providers; it is important to note that this development transferred part of the responsibility for a person's health from himself to another person.

The ancient Greeks viewed health as a form of balance and harmony, and the person who possessed health was thought to be living in harmony with nature and fellow humans. The dissolution of a person's health was viewed as an indication of a life out of balance with nature. Ill health indicated that a person ate too much, drank too much, exercised too little—that the person was, in essence, intemperate.

Inherent in the classical view of health was a high degree of personal responsibility to live in harmony with self and nature, to be temperate, to care for one's own health, to have responsibility, authority, and control, to be sovereign over one's health.

Health referred to *both* body and soul. Plato tells us that Socrates cautioned:

Just as one should not attempt to cure the eyes apart from the head, nor the head apart from the body, so no one should attempt to cure the body apart from the soul. And this is the very reason why most diseases are beyond the Greek doctors, that they do not pay attention to the whole as they ought to do, since if the whole is not in good condition, it is impossible that the part should be.

Socrates's concept of a human as a holistic being was gradually discarded in favor of the "scientific" view of illness which indicated that something was wrong with an organ or some aspect of the person's body. The development of medical science has led to specialization on a single organ or aspect of the organ. It is unusual for a physician today to treat all of the patient's body, much less consider both the body *and* the soul. The patient's care is often fragmented as a result, and a person with a painful foot, for example, may be unable to decide whether to go to an orthopedist, a podiatrist, or a physician who treats arthritis.

Physicians have searched, and continue to search, for a *specific cause* for each specific disease condition and for the *specific cure* for each disease. The concept of harmony, balance, and the relations among mind, body, soul, and environment have been discounted by medicine in favor of scientific and technical advances.

Holistic Health

Given the cost, the depersonalization and the failure of the current system to deliver health, it is not surprising that some providers and informed consumers decided that there had to be a better, more humane way. The "better way," in the view of advocates of *holistic health,* is to: (1) focus on wellness, (2) place more responsibility on the individual for his or her own health, and (3) radically alter the role of the health care system.

Holistic health is a dynamic, harmonious equilibrium of body, mind, and spirit. Each aspect of the person is recognized and considered, and the individual is taught to live in a way which promotes health through holistic living.

Perhaps the best way to clarify the holistic approach to health is to contrast it with the current, dominant health care system approach.

The current medical model system identifies *symptoms* and diagnoses *disease.* The holistic approach assesses how the patient *views his situation* in addition to assessing his symptoms because a person generally moves toward better or worse health in accordance with his lifestyle, attitudes, and feelings.

The medical model directs a specialist's attention toward a *part* of the body or mind, while in the holistic approach, the *body, mind, and spirit* are *all* addressed, usually by a single health care worker in full partnership with the client.

The goal of intervention in traditional health care is to return the patient to a disease-free state. In holistic care, the goal is vibrant energy and higher self-awareness. In traditional health care, it is possible for the patient to remain a passive, unknowledgeable recipient of care, but in the holistic model, the individual is considered responsible for participating in the healing process.

Prevention, in the traditional medical sense, focuses on getting adequate rest, exercise, immunizations, and nutrition, avoiding substance abuse, and not smoking. Prevention in the holistic health sense takes all of these factors into consideration plus *internal serenity,* a feeling of "wholeness" in body, mind, and spirit.

Nursing and Holistic Health

Nurses have more opportunities to promote health and holistic living throughout the life-span than any other health professionals. Nurses have access to people at critical points in their lives, when they are more receptive to information related to health. Nurses are involved with expectant parents in childbirth classes, and they also work with new parents. Nurses work with children in schools and summer camps; adults in church groups, factories, and clinics; and elderly people in private homes, senior citizen clubs, and nursing homes. In each of these and other situations, nurses are in contact with people who are interested in learning how to maintain and improve their health.

"Nursing evolved as an intuitive response to the desire to keep people healthy as well as provide comfort, care, and assurance to the sick" (Dolan, 1978). A commitment to health promotion has always been an important focus of nursing, and nurses have recognized that the current complex, technological, and depersonalized system of delivering health services must be altered if health and wellness are to be an outcome of the system (Fig. 7.2). As a result, recent theory development in nursing has expanded to include research

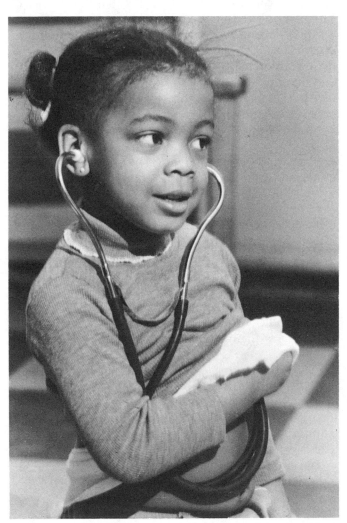

Figure 7.2 *One goal of society must be to make it possible for people to assume responsibility for their own health. This child's curiosity about her body indicates a readiness to learn and become involved in her own health care.*

in holistic living and health, and the use of new approaches to wellness such as therapeutic touch, humor and laughter, imagery, and inner dialogue.

DEFINITIONS OF HEALTH

The World Health Organization (WHO) struggled to formulate a universal definition of health and, in 1947, finally agreed on the following definition: "Health is a state of complete physical, emotional, and social well-being, and is not merely the absence of disease and infirmity." This definition embodies the WHO position that worldwide health is a fundamental human right, and it acknowledges three aspects of health: physical, emotional and social well-being. The statement is important because it refutes the belief that the absence of illness or infirmity is equivalent to health.

The WHO position on health remains an unrealized dream for most people in all parts of the world, and the definition has been criticized for being both utopian and limiting (Dubos, 1965). Not only is complete well-being considered unattainable, but the pursuit of well-being in a complex technological society is often beyond the control of the individual. Dubos views health as a *creative process* whereby people actively adapt to their changing environments. This view of health requires a person to have sufficient real income and resources for relevant action. Fuchs, a health economist (1974), concurs and states, "For most of man's history his health has depended upon his economic well-being. Adequate food supply, clean water, protection from the elements—these are historically critical factors affecting life expectancy and the avoidance of disability" (p. 144).

Some people believe the word *health* no longer has only a positive connotation because it has come to be used to indicate one of many personal attributes such as weight or mentality. Just as a person can be underweight or overweight, so a person can be said to be in good health or poor health. Some theorists suggest that levels of health can be plotted along a *single* continuum ranging from poor health (illness) to good health. Other theorists advance the idea that there is one distinct *health* continuum that is in dynamic interaction with another *illness* continuum.

Dunn (1961) has promoted the concept of wellness, and his definition of health (wellness) states:

Health level wellness for the individual is defined as an integrated method of functioning which is oriented toward the potential of which the individual is capable. It requires that the individual maintain a continuum of balance and purposeful direction within the environment where he is functioning. (p.11)

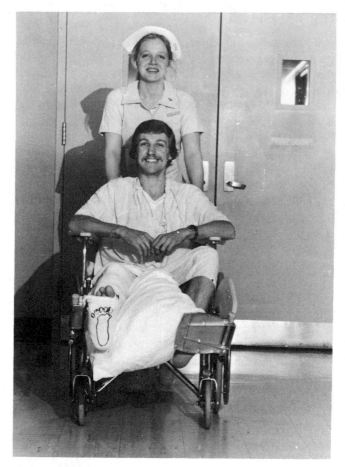

Figure 7.3 *This young man considers himself healthy despite a broken leg.*

Dunn's definition implies a *dynamic equilibrium* rather than the static, steady state of well-being implied by the WHO definition of health.

Dunn's definition does not require *complete* physical, emotional, and social well-being but, rather, suggests that in any conceivable circumstances, *there are ways in which a person can maximize his own health* (Fig. 7.3). Potential for health is continually changing and is affected both intrinsically by normal growth and development and extrinsically by, for example, a more abundant food supply. For Dunn's concept to be useful and workable, a person must have sufficient knowledge, resources, and authority to choose the behaviors that will maximize his potential for wellness. Thus far, societal resources have been too limited to allow this kind of personal responsibility and accountability.

Throughout recorded history, health, however defined, has been viewed as being essential to human progress and individual happiness. Health is integral to human freedom; it is necessary in order to do and be all that one aspires to. One recurring debate centers around the appropriate assignment of individual and societal responsibility for health promotion and protection.

Some theorists view the current medical establishment as a threat to health. In his book *Medical Nemesis* (1976), Illich described healthy people and healthy societies as follows:

The society which can reduce professional intervention to the minimum will provide the best conditions for health . . . Healthy people are those who live in healthy homes on a healthy diet, in an environment equally fit for birth, growth, work, healing, and dying, sustained by a culture which enhances the conscious acceptance of limits to population, of aging, of incomplete recovery and even imminent death . . . Man's consciously lived fragility, individuality and relatedness make the experience of pain, of sickness and of death an integral part of his life. The ability to cope with this trio autonomously is fundamental to his health. As he becomes dependent on the management of his intimacy he renounces his autonomy and his health must decline. (pp. 274–275)

There is congruence between Dunn's high-level wellness and Illich's prescription for health. They concur that the realization of health requires that informed people be able to function in a society that provides an environment conducive to well-being. Both theorists imply that there are healthy communities as well as healthy people, that people who live in healthy communities are healthy more often than people who live in unhealthy communities.

THE HEALTH FIELD CONCEPT

Even a cursory review of the literature, both popular and professional, indicates that there are profound differences between the health of various population groups with respect to such indicators as life expectancy, rates of hospitalization, hypertension, and infant mortality rates. Such evidence indicates that more than just human biology and individual genetic endowment help to determine health and its distribution; a commitment to holistic health requires a systematic approach that considers *all determinants* of health and sickness.

LaLonde (1974), Minister of National Health and Welfare of Canada, derived the concept of a *health field* that includes four elements—human biology, environment, lifestyle, and health care organization—from an examination of the determinants of sickness and death in Canada. The concept, although derived from a study of sickness, provides a useful framework for analyzing health.

Human Biology

The human biology element of the health field concept includes the physical organs and the complicated processes related to the biological functions of humankind. This element encompasses individual genetic makeup as well as structures and processes common to all people.

Human biology has many implications for health. For example, growth and development of the human organism is a major factor in the development of both health and illness. Intrinsic determinants of health and illness are those determinants which cannot be altered, such as age, sex, and genetic makeup. *Age* is the most dynamic intrinsic factor related to both biological and psychosocial health. The developing person has numerous age-specific needs that must be met to achieve and maintain health. An infant, for example, must have adequate human contact or he will develop a *maternal deprivation* or *failure-to-thrive syndrome* and will either die or fail to develop normally.

Human biology influences every type of ill health, including many chronic diseases such as diabetes, cancer, arthritis, and hypertension. Individual differences in human biology are responsible for variations in resistance and susceptibility to many illnesses. Research efforts are currently being directed toward altering human biology to make people more resistant to disease and illnesses. Such efforts include the development of new vaccines and attempts to eliminate certain hereditary defects through genetic engineering.

Environment

The second element of the health field concept refers to all health-related variables that are external to the human body (extrinsic). A person often has little control of his environments, which are physical, social, and political. The quality of the *physical* environment is determined by the quality of the air, the purity of the water supply, the level of noise, the climate, and the adequacy of sanitation. No person alone can control the quality of these factors that have so profound an effect on health.

The *social* environment refers to conditions related to a person's social and psychological needs. These needs vary with a person's age and developmental level and often cannot be separated from the physical environment. The social environment includes all health risks that a person is exposed to as a result of his milieu. For example, marijuana might be available in a person's physical environment; choosing whether to use it, or whether to use enough of it to cause detriment to health depends on his social environment. Research has demonstrated that there is a sequence of social experiences that must occur before a person exposed to marijuana becomes a habitual user. The presence of the drug in the *physical* environment is a necessary but insufficient condition for its use, because the *social* environment must also be conducive.

A positive social environment is essential for the promotion of health because a good physical environment alone (fresh air, pure water, ample food, adequate sanitation) is insufficient for health. Humans are social creatures and require human interaction and support to maintain and improve their health.

The *political* environment must be included in any consideration of health because political decisions determine the quality of the physical environment and influence the social environment. Political decisions determine whether or not a nation develops nuclear or solar energy, and whether pure water or a new chemical industry is more important for a community. Political decisions affect funding for educational programs and thereby influence their content. The length of a program, for example, might determine whether classes for expectant parents would include education about an infant's social as well as physical needs. Because of the importance of the political environment, any group that hopes to influence the level of health in a given society or community must first be aware of the impact of political decisions on health and health care and then be willing to take a public stand on issues that have an impact on health.

Lifestyle

The third element in the health field concept, *lifestyle,* is the result of the many daily decisions a person makes that affect his health. Such decisions include choice of diet and recreation, amount of sleep, and mode of handling stress—all of which influence level of health. Most of such decisions are related in a complex way to a person's physical, social, and political environment; and health care workers must be very careful not to blame a person for faulty decisions that were in fact imposed by these environments. For example, a person who works in a mine exposes himself to several lung diseases, including cancer of the lung and black lung disease. His occupation (part of his lifestyle) affects his level of health. If the miner is poorly educated or if there is no other industry in his community, his only alternative may be unemployment, followed by poverty and malnutrition for himself and his family. The miner's occupation carries a high risk of lung disease, but his social and political environments may have left him no viable alternative to mining.

The complex interaction between lifestyle and environment is illustrated in a vignette about a young mother who seemed to make decisions that could be detrimental to her own and her family's health. The children's immunizations were never up to date, for instance, despite the fact that they were free of cost. A public health nurse visited the home to learn why the mother was delinquent with regard to the immunizations of her 6-month-old infant and 2-year-old child.

The home was in a rural area. To reach the clinic, the mother and her children had to leave home several hours before the appointment and travel on two buses. The last time she went to the clinic, the young mother had said "The nurse yelled at me because the baby needed his diaper changed and Johnny's face was dirty." She explained that she could not change the baby's diaper en route, and the child's face was dirty because she had fed him in the bus while holding the baby. This woman's economic situation, limited amount of energy, geographic location, and treatment at the clinic influenced her decision not to return to the clinic despite the fact that the children should have been immunized, and she wanted to protect her children's health.

Health Care Organization

The fourth and final element of the health field concept, *health care organization,* determines the quantity, quality, and accessibility of resources and health care personnel. For any system of health care to be effective, it must be both acceptable and accessible to the people for whom it was organized. It must be *designed to meet the needs of the people,* and its services must be consistent with the health goals and values of the population. For example, in an undeveloped country where malnutrition is the major health problem, a different mix of health care workers, resources, and services is needed from that needed in the United States, where heart disease and cancer are the major health problems.

THEORY OF MULTIPLE CAUSATION

The health field concept is an excellent example of an organized, systematic way of assessing the health and risk factors of a group of people. The concept exemplifies the *multiple causation theory* of health and illness, which recognizes that many complex interactions promote health or foster illness. The theory of multiple causation negates the belief that one cause leads to one effect, and that a single agent can be responsible for a specific disease or illness.

When physicians accepted Pasteur's theory that diseases were caused by germs rather than by divine punishment, or by an imbalance of humors (phlegm, blood, "black" bile, and "yellow" bile) within the body, they began to search for *the* cause of each disease. Specific organisms were frequently identified as causative agents, but such information did not explain why one person exposed to a given organism contracted the disease and other people did not. It did not explain why only certain members of a household or a community became ill during an epidemic, for example.

Agent/Host/Environment Interrelationships

An important aspect of multiple causation is the interrelationship of agent, host, and environment. An *agent* is a substance or an organism that is capable of producing a reaction in a host. A *host* is the recipient of the agent, and in nursing and medicine, the host is a human being. *Environment* is the aggregate of all external conditions and influences affecting the life and development of the host. The agent and the host both affect and are affected by the environment.

Health care would be simpler if a disease process in humans was always the result of an agent acting upon a host. If that were the case, we might have solved all of our disease problems long ago. In reality, there are endless variations in the complex interactions between agent and host, host and environment, and agent and environment which complicate the process and validate the concept of multiple causation.

Agents of disease are ubiquitous. They may be biological, chemical, physical, psychological, or social. Given the multiplicity of these agents and their constant presence in our environment, it is a wonder that we are not ill all the time. The reason is that the mere *presence* of the agent is insufficient to cause disease.

Before an agent can cause a response in a human being, the agent must gain access to his body. Once access is gained and the agent has entered the body, disease will not occur unless the host is susceptible and the agent is potent enough to cause a reaction.

Origins of Health

The theory of multiple causation commonly refers to the origins of illness, but several researchers are exploring the *origins of health* in an effort to learn why some people stay well despite almost overwhelming odds.

Many current ideas about health and illness are related to stress theory. Hans Selye discovered that regardless of the kind of stressor, a person responds with a three stage *General Adaptation Syndrome* (GAS, Chapter 8). The three stages are: (1) alarm, (2) resistance, and (3) exhaustion, and these stages constitute the response of every person to every kind of stress. Selye emphasized that the first two stages (alarm and resistance) are essential responses to danger or change, and are not necessarily harmful to the organism. If the person's response to a stressor extends beyond these two stages, however, the person can enter the third stage of exhaustion, and illness is likely to result.

Aaron Antonovsky was curious about the reasons why some people stayed healthy despite repeated or prolonged exposure to virulent stressors. He is particularly interested in survivors—people who have lived through such horrors as concentration camps or prolonged child abuse without becoming mentally or physically ill.

Antonovsky's approach to health is in direct opposition to the approach of those who focus on the cause of disease, and he coined the term *salutogenesis* in contrast to the term *pathogenesis.*

Pathogenesis is the study of the origins of disease, and asks the question "Why and how did this person enter into a state of illness?" (There are over 1,040 diagnoses, or classified illnesses.)

Salutogenesis is the study of the origins of health, and asks the questions, "What are the factors which push persons *toward health?*" "Why do people stay healthy?" "Why is this person healthy *in spite of everything?*"

Antonovsky differentiated between stress, which could become harmful, and tension, which could be neutral or positive, depending upon the person's ability to resolve the tension in a satisfactory manner. He developed a theory of *general resistance resources* (GRR), and defined a GRR as any characteristic of a person, or group of persons, which promotes effective tension management. An example of a general resistance resource is the ability of some abused children to attach to whatever help is available, no matter how meager that help may be.

Health care professionals must be concerned with the commonalities among resistance resources so that they can be used as a means of promoting health. The mapping sentence in Table 7.1 shows one way of organizing these concepts.

EPIDEMIOLOGY

Epidemiologists study the distribution of health and disease in various populations. Epidemiologists are interested in identifying the factors which are associated with differences in health and disease, and any disease, illness, accident, or disability that is *prevalent in a human population* is of interest to epidemiologists. Epidemiology, therefore, studies the determinants of such various problems as communicable disease, automobile accidents, heart disease, and cancer.

TABLE 7.1 MAPPING-SENTENCE DEFINITION OF A GENERALIZED RESISTANCE RESOURCE (GRR)

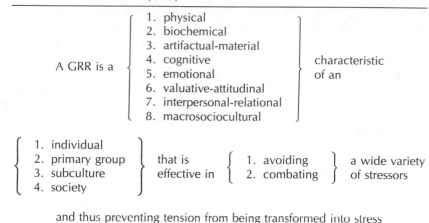

In the past, communicable diseases were the most terrifying of the health problems afflicting mankind. The development of vaccines and widespread immunization has reduced the threat of communicable disease with the exception of sexually transmitted diseases (STD) for which vaccines are not available. Recently, the incidence of acquired immune deficiency syndrome (AIDS) in the US population has reawakened fear and terror. Scientists do not completely understand the multiple factors involved in the transmission of AIDS, and epidemiologists are devoting considerable resources to identifying these factors in order to develop an effective prevention strategy.

Simultaneously, epidemiologists are studying other major health problems including accidents, heart disease, suicide, and teenage pregnancy.

Study of Populations

Epidemiology is concerned with the *mass phenomenon* of health and disease rather than the health status of an individual.

There are similarities between what a health professional does when he assesses an individual and what an epidemiologist does when he looks for signs and symptoms in the population as a whole. The epidemiologist looks at the symptoms and indicators in the *population* as a whole such as the kinds of disease, illness, accidents, and disabilities which are present, while the physician or nurse asks questions related to the symptoms which an *individual* presents.

In assessing an individual patient, the nurse or physician collects information related to age, family history, health history, medical history, occupation, residence, education, and other pertinent data. The data

collected about an individual case may or may not have a bearing on the condition of the population as a whole.

No conclusion concerning the disease or illness in a population can be drawn from *one case*. An epidemiologist who is studying a population will look not only at *how much* disease is present but also at who *is sick* and who *is not sick* with the disease/illness being studied. For example, he will try to learn if certain age groups are more affected by the disease than others, if one sex is more often affected by the disease than the other, if a given occupation seems to be more often related to this health problem than other occupations.

There are similarities between what an epidemiologist does in investigating a health problem and what a detective does when he investigates a crime. The detective looks for clues to solve a crime, with an ultimate goal of controlling crime. The epidemiologist also looks for clues such as common denominators of association between the disease and the environment, or factors prevalent within the population that may predispose to or influence the development of such disease.

It is possible to control a disease without possessing complete knowledge of its etiology. By identifying associations that recur consistently whenever a disease is present, control is possible by eliminating the factor or factors associated with it. The consistent link between cigarette smoking and lung cancer has been demonstrated, even though the precise mechanism by which tobacco causes cancer is not understood. It is possible to reduce the incidence of lung cancer by publicizing the risks of smoking and thereby influence people to stop or not start smoking.

Epidemiology is involved in establishing a relationship between factors that exist in the environment or in people and the disease processes to which they are heir. If enough factors can be identified and altered, disease can be prevented before the exact cause is identified.

Extrinsic/Intrinsic Factors

Factors or variables associated with patterns of health and disease are either *intrinsic* (part of the individual himself and therefore unalterable) or *extrinsic* (related to the individual's lifestyle or environment). Extrinsic factors are alterable and a person's predisposition to disease may be altered by changing one or more of the extrinsic factors.

Examples of intrinsic factors that might affect patterns of disease are: age, sex, genetic makeup. Examples of extrinsic factors that influence patterns of disease include: nutrition, smoking, drug use, occupation, response to stress, and family relationships.

Extrinsic factors influence the amount of disease in a population, and the identification and control of these extrinsic factors is essential to control of disease.

Incidence and Prevalence

Two rates used to measure the health of a community are incidence and prevalence. *Prevalence* describes the extent of a specific disease in a population at a given point in time. It is like a still picture. To take a hypothetical example, the prevalence of heart disease in New Town is the proportion of the *people with heart disease* in relation to the *population* of New Town as of the given date

$$\text{Prevalence Rate} = \frac{\text{Number of Existing Cases of a Disease (at a point in time)}}{\text{Total Population}}$$

Obviously, the accuracy of the prevalence rate is dependent on the accuracy of diagnosis, as well as the willingness and/or ability of people with a disease to be diagnosed.

Incidence is a measure of the probability that people without a given disease will develop that disease over a period of time. Incidence is like a moving picture of disease activity in a population.

$$\text{Incidence} = \frac{\text{Number of New Cases of a Disease (over a period of time)}}{\text{Population at Risk}}$$

Note that the denominator is different for incidence and prevalence. To compute the *prevalence* rate, the entire population in a community is involved because it is the extent of morbidity (sickness) from a given disease in a specific population that is being studied.

Incidence assesses the *risk* of illness due to a given disease and therefore the appropriate denominator is the population at risk. This ratio eliminates people who already have the disease, and those who are not at risk for the particular disease. For example, in computing an incidence rate for cervical cancer, males are eliminated from the denominator because cervical cancer is possible only in females.

THE HEALTH CARE DELIVERY SYSTEM IN THE UNITED STATES

Over the past half century the health care delivery system in the US has undergone drastic changes which can be attributed to (1) specialization, (2) technological advances, (3) predominance of the medical model in health care, and (4) health care expenditures.

Specialization

Medical specialties and subspecialties have multiplied, resulting in a lack of communication, fragmentation of services, and treatment of the patient's *disease* rather than the patient. The body, mind, and spirit of the patient are treated as separate and distinct entities.

Technological Advances

Technological advances have led to increased life expectancy and have had a positive impact on the treatment of disease. But technology has depersonalized health care because the patient is often forced to rely on a machine rather than on a health care worker.

Predominance of the Medical Model

The medical model of health care focuses on the diagnosis and treatment of pathology and often equates health with the absence of disease. This medical orientation has resulted in a health care delivery system that focuses on treatment and rehabilitation, and virtually ignores health promotion and illness prevention. In the US approximately 98% of health care expenditures is directed toward the treatment of illness and *only about 2%* is directed toward health promotion activities.

Cost of Health Care

National health expenditures have increased experientially throughout the past 50 years. In 1984 the cost of health care services in the US was 387.4 billion dollars,

80% more than in 1979, five times what it was in 1970, and over nine times what it was in 1965. The US spent 11 percent of its gross national product for health care in 1984.

RESPONSIBILITY FOR GOOD HEALTH

Two important outcomes of the current approach to health care have been: (1) *greater* control by health professionals and (2) *diminished* control by individuals over their personal health. As professionals assumed control and became the absolute authorities in all matters related to health and illness, individuals, families, and communities became dependent on the health professions, particularly medicine, to diagnose disease and prescribe treatment.

Health is a prerequisite of each and every society. If a society is to function effectively, illness must be controlled. Talcott Parsons (1951, 1978) defined the sick role and described ways in which it affects the control of illness in American society. This description is valid only in American society and is not helpful with respect to sickness behavior in other societies.

The American sickness role has four aspects:

1. The sick person is exempt from normal social responsibilities. The exemption depends on the nature and severity of the illness, and the exemption must be accepted as legitimate by the various other people who are affected. The physician is often the direct legitimizing agent. Legitimization protects society against malingerers.

2. The sick person is not expected to get well by himself. He must be taken care of and his condition must be changed so that he can resume his usual social roles.

3. The sick person has an obligation to get well. Illness is undesirable and the sick person should want to get well. This exemption from social roles carries with it an obligation as well as a right.

4. The sick person has an obligation to seek technically competent help (usually a physician), and to cooperate fully in getting well.

This aspect of the sick role identifies relationships between the sick person, now a patient, and the physician, the socially designated healer.

Parsons' conceptualization places the physician in the role of legitimizing agent for society. Friedsen (1979) sees the physician's role as even more powerful, because the physician has the authority to label one person's complaint an illness, and another's complaint not an illness. In Friedsen's view, medicine 'creates' illness

because, by being an authority on what illness "really" is, medicine creates the social possibility of a person acting sick.

There is clearly a distinction between biological disease and illness. An individual with a symptom has several options open to him. He can ignore the symptom, treat it himself, seek a family member's or other lay person's help, or seek professional help. If he chooses to seek professional help, usually from a physician, his symptoms can be diagnosed as a specific disease and treated—only then is he a patient with an illness.

Some aspects of health are under an individual's control, but in other fundamental ways, health rests with the community and the person's place in that community. A community that provides cohesiveness, social support, and a healthy physical environment is healthy for its *members,* but it may be unhealthy for those who are regarded as outsiders or who view themselves as outsiders.

It is important to recognize that individual choices and behaviors have a significant impact on health, but it is equally important to make sure that health care providers do not lay an unfair burden on people who seem to be making poor choices when in reality better choices are not possible. It would seem, for example, that most people could, if they wanted to, follow the health habits that have been proven by research to be significant but such is *not* the case.

Research studies by Breslow and Belloc (1972) of nearly 7,000 adults showed that life expectancy and health are significantly related to the following basic health habits:

- Three meals a day at regular times, with no snacks
- Breakfast every day, consisting of about half the caloric intake for the day
- Moderate exercise two to three times a week
- Adequate sleep (usually 7 to 8 hours a night)
- No smoking
- Moderate weight
- Alcohol used in moderation or not at all

SELF-CARE

The traditional pattern of an American sick role is changing and new ways of coping with problems of health and illness are emerging. The skyrocketing cost of health care, coupled with evidence that the *treatment of disease* will never be an effective way to *increase health,* has created an enormous interest in self-care and a return to individual control of personal health (see Fig. 7.4).

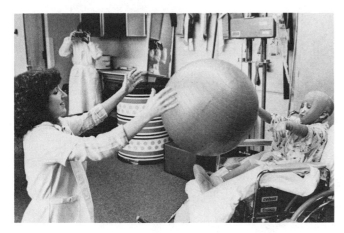

Figure 7.4 *Although she takes no pleasure in this ball game, Renee is accepting some of the responsibility for her own recovery. Despite her nasogastric tube, I.V., and bandages, Renee exercises as fully as she can. The pillows in the wheelchair help to reduce the pain from the donor sites on her back and thighs where the skin was removed for grafting.*

Self-care is not a new idea. Its roots go back to ancient times when the individual relied more heavily upon himself to keep healthy. This sense of responsibility was eventually undermined by an almost total dependency upon the medical profession, and has only recently begun to emerge once more. The resurgence is evidenced by the rapidly increasing numbers of self-help and mutual support groups as well as by an increase in health-related lay publications.

Nursing interest in self-care is increasing, and self-care has become an important part of nursing theory. Dorothea Orem (1971) defined self-care as "the practice of activities that individuals personally initiate and perform on their own behalf to maintain life, health and well being . . . It is an adult's personal contribution to his own health and well being."

At least part of the impetus for the current interest in self-care can be attributed to changes in the kinds of diseases that are seen. Major health problems have shifted from acute conditions to chronic conditions. Acute conditions are self-limiting; the diagnosis, treatment, and outcome take place within a limited time span. Chronic disease is a long-term illness, and the quality of the individual's life depends upon his ability to successfully live with the disease. Successful management of chronic disease requires *knowledge* of both the disease processes and the principles of healthy living, and a *willingness* to assume responsibility for making the necessary changes in attitude and life style.

Self-care is an integral part of holistic living, and requires full sovereignty of one's health and control of one's life.

PATIENT TEACHING

It is important for every individual, *regardless of age*, to learn to assume an appropriate degree of responsibility for his own health. Given adequate support and encouragement, children will assume an active role at a very early age, as evidenced by statements such as "No, that's not good for me!"

Active participation can be much more difficult to foster in adults who have assumed for many many years that the physician always "knows best," and who have passively followed the advice of doctors and nurses despite their personal reservations or doubts about the effectiveness of that advice.

The process of changing any attitude is long and difficult, and nurses must expect that *observable* changes in health practices will be slow to appear. It is essential for you to remember that, in most cases, the patient or family is not being difficult, stubborn, or uncooperative but that they are finding it difficult to change a personality and lifestyle in order to assume a new set of responsibilities.

RELATED ACTIVITIES

1. In preparation for helping others to assume self-care responsibilities, analyze your own health beliefs and practices. To what extent do you feel accountable for your own well being, and in what areas do you hold your parents, spouse, college, or society in general responsible for your current level of health, both physical and psychological? Furthermore, what do you plan to do about your situation?

SUGGESTED READINGS

———Motivating children to become assertive health-care consumers. *Nursing 82* 1982 Nov; 12(11):98–100.

Alford, Dolores M: Expanding older person's belief systems. *Top Clin Nurs* 1982 Jan; 3(4):35–44.

Anderson, Alan: Neurotoxic Follies. *Psych Today* 1982 July; 16(7):30–42.

Baranowski, Tom: Toward the definition of concepts of health and disease, wellness and illness. *Health Values: Achieving High Level Wellness* 1981 Nov/Dec; 5(6):246–256.

Birchfield, Marilyn M: *Stages of Illness: Guidelines for Nursing Care*. Bowie, MD, Brady, 1985.

Blattner, Barbara: *Holistic Nursing*. Englewood Cliffs, NJ, Prentice-Hall, 1981.

Fonesca, Jeanne D: On the side of the angels (editorial on self-care). *Nurs Outlook* 1980 Aug; 28(8):477.

Garrett, Sandra Sokolove, and Bruce Garrett. Humaneness and health. *Top Clin Nurs* 1982 Jan; 3(4):7–12.

Gulino, Claire K: Entering the mysterious dimensions of other: an existential approach to nursing care. *Nurs Outlook* 1982 June; 30(6):352–357.

Hazard, Merle Pabst, and Rosemarie Eagan Kemp: Keeping the well-elderly well. *Am J Nurs* 1983 April; 83(4):567–569.

Hill, Lyda, and Nancy Smith: *Self-Care Nursing: Promotion of Health.* Englewood Cliffs, NJ, Prentice-Hall, 1985.

Krieger, Dolores: *Foundations for Holistic Health Nursing Practices.* Philadelphia, Lippincott, 1981.

Moll, Janet A: High-level wellness and the nurse. *Top Clin Nurs* 1982 Jan; 3(4):61–67.

Natalini, John: The human body as a biological clock. *Am J Nurs* 1977 July; 77(7):1130–1132.

Riehl-Sisca, Joan: *The Science and Art of Self-Care.* Norwalk, CT, Appleton-Century-Crofts, 1985.

Rodgers, Janet A: Health is not a right. *Nurs Outlook* 1981 Oct; 29(10):590–591.

Rose, Michael: Shift work: How does it affect you? *Am J Nurs* 1984 April; 84(4):442–447.

Rubenstein, Carin: Wellness is all. *Psych Today* 1982 Oct; 16(10):28–37.

Smith, Frances B: Patient power. *Am J Nurs* 1985 Nov; 85(11):1260–1262.

Smitherman, Colleen: *Nursing Actions for Health Promotion.* Philadelphia, Davis, 1981.

Thompson, Marcia J, and David W Harsha: Our rhythms still follow the African sun. *Psych Today* 1984 Jan; 18(1):50–54.

Healing

Achterberg, Jeanne, and Frank Lawlis: Imagery and health intervention. *Top Clin Nurs* 1982 Jan; 3(4):55–60.

Boguslawski, Marie: The use of therapeutic touch in nursing. *J.Contin Educ Nurs* 1979 April; 10(4):9–15.

Clark, Carolyn Chambers: Inner dialogue: A self-healing approach for nurses and clients. *Am J Nurs* 1981 June; 81(6):1191–1193.

Goodykoontz, Lynne: Touch: Attitudes and practice: *Nurs Forum* 1979 Jan/Feb; 18(1):4–17.

Herth, Kaye Ann: Laughter: A nursing Rx. *Am J Nurs* 1984 Aug; 84(8);991–992.

Korn, Errol R, and Karen Johnson: *Visualization: The Uses of Imagery in the Health Professions.* Homewood, IL, Dow Jones-Irwin, 1983.

Krieger, Dolores, Erik Peper, and Sonia Ancoli: Therapeutic touch—searching for evidence of physiologic change. *Am J Nurs* 1979 April; 79(4):660–662.

Lamb, Michael: Second thoughts on first touch. *Psych Today* 1982 April; 16(4):9–11.

Miller, Judith Fitzgerald: Inspiring hope. *Am J Nurs* 1985 Jan; 85(1):22–25.

O'Connell, Anne L: Death sentence: An invitation to life *Am J Nurs* 1980 Sept; 80(9):1646–1649.

Osterland, Hob: Humor: A serious approach to patient care. *Nursing 83* 1983 Dec:13(12):46–47.

Sandroff, Ronni: A skeptic's guide to therapeutic touch. *RN* 1980 Jan; 43(1):24–31.

Scarf, Maggie: Images that heal. *Psych Today* 1980 Sept; 14(9):32–46.

Simonton, O Carl, Stephanie Matthews-Simonton, and James L Creighton: *Getting Well Again.* New York: Bantam Books, 1978.

Tobiason, Sarah Jane Bradford: Touching is for everyone. *Am J Nurs* 1981 April; 81(4):728–730.

Ujhely, Gertrud B: Touch: reflections and perceptions. *Nurs Forum* 1979 Jan/Feb; 18(1):18–32.

REFERENCES

———— *The Nation's Health.* American Public Health Association, March, 1986.

Antonovsky, Aaron: *Health, Stress and Coping.* San Francisco, Jossey-Bass, 1979.

Aiken, Linda H (ed.): *Health Policy and Nursing Practice.* New York, McGraw-Hill, 1981.

Belloc, Nedra B, and Breslow, Lester: Relationships of Physical Health Status and Health Practices. *Prev Med* 1972 1:409–422.

Dubos, Rene: Health and Creative Adaptation. *Hum Nature* 1978 1:74.

Dubos, Rene: *Man Adapting.* New Haven, CT, Yale University Press, 1965.

Dunn, Halbert: *High Level Wellness.* Arlington, VA, Beatty, 1961.

Friedson, Eliol: *Profession of Medicine.* San Francisco, Harper & Row, 1970.

Fuchs, Victor: *Who Shall Live.* New York, Basic, 1974.

Illich, Ivan: *Medical Nemesis; The Expropriation of Health.* New York, Pantheon, 1976.

LaLonde, Marc: *Perspectives on the Health of Canadians.* Ottowa, Lone Printing, 1974.

Nightingale, Florence: *Notes on Nursing—What It Is and What It Is Not.* New York, Dover Publications, 1969.

Orem, Dorothea: *Nursing: Concepts of Practice.* New York, McGraw-Hill, 1971.

Parsons, Talcott: *The Social System.* New York, Free Press, 1951.

Plato: *Laches and Charnides.* Sprague, RK (ed): Indianapolis, Bobbs-Merrill, 1973.

Selye, Hans: *The Stress of Life.* New York, McGraw-Hill, 1976.

Waldo, Donald R: *Health Care Financing Trends* vol.2, Washington, DC, Office of Research, Demonstration, and Statistics, 1980.

White, Robert L: *Right to Health: The Evolution of an Idea.* Iowa City, University of Iowa, 1971.

World Health Organization: *Health Aspects of Human Rights.* Geneva, World Health Organization, 1976.

8

Stress, Adaptation, and Coping

Prerequisites and/or Suggested Preparation
Chapter 5 (Systems Theory) is prerequisite to this chapter, and a basic knowledge of the endocrine system and the autonomic nervous system is necessary for understanding the physiological responses to stress.

Many people speak of stress as if it were a relatively new phenomenon, an unfortunate result of a rapidly changing, high technology society. It is true that stress was not studied and labeled until the 1920s, but stress has been present since the beginning of human life.

Life was stressful for cave men, sweatshop workers, Pilgrim settlers, explorers, slaves, and new arrivals at Ellis Island in the 1800s. These people did not know the term "stress," but their physiological responses to it were the same as those of today's tense air traffic controllers, or harried single parents.

Stress in humans is an abstract, subjective phenomenon. It is intangible and can be perceived only by the person experiencing it. It can be detected by others only through observation of that person's *response or reaction* to the stress he is experiencing. Dr. Hans Selye, who is usually considered the "father of stress theory," likened the abstract quality of stress to the wind, as he quoted Robert Louis Stevenson:

> *Who has seen the wind*
> *Neither you nor I*
> *But when the trees bow down their heads*
> *The wind is passing by.*

STRESS

Stress in humans is often equated with tension, anxiety, worry, and pressure. It has been described as the wear and tear of life. More often than not, stress has been considered potentially harmful, something to be avoided, and a threat to survival or well-being. At the same time, however, people accept the fact that stressing will strengthen certain substances. Steel, for example, is tempered to make it stronger, and muscles are strengthened by pulling against a weight. We intellectually accept the premise that hard times can "build character" and make an individual stronger in many ways.

Dr. Selye recognized the existence of both *distress* (potentially harmful stress) and *eustress* (beneficial stress). The word eustress is derived from the Greek "eu," meaning "good," as in euphoria. Theorists accept the fact that stress in humans is necessary for life, and capable of causing either beneficial or detrimental effects.

Definitions of Stress

Current definitions of stress are too numerous to list in this chapter, but several selected and representative definitions of stress include:

1. "Stress is always present in humans but is intensified when there is a change or threat with which a person must cope" (Byrne and Thompson, 1978, p. 66).
2. Stress is "that physical and emotional experience which results from a requirement to change from the condition of the moment to any other condition" (Hartl, 1979, p. 91).
3. Stress is "the common denominator of all adaptive responses of the body." It is a state manifested by the body's response to any demand placed upon it (Seyle, 1956, p. 54).
4. In the language of systems theory, stress can be defined as the internal condition that is created by any input which necessitates a change in the system, either to regain the system's equilibrium or to promote growth of the system.

In other words, *stress is a condition caused by the body's need to respond or adapt to either internal or external forces that have disturbed the body's equilibrium.*

Stressors

The agents or events that cause stress are called *stressors*. Any stimulus, either internal or external, that disturbs the equilibrium of an individual is a stressor. In systems theory, any input or feedback that necessitates a change in the system can be a stressor.

A stressor may be physical, social, psychological, cognitive, or physiological in nature. Examples of these categories of stressors include:

Physical stressors: heat, cold, pressure, chemicals, pollution, noise, and radiation.
Social stressors: peer pressure, the economy, and bureaucratic or political pressures.
Psychological stressors: the loss of a loved one, frustration, boredom, and loss of control over one's life.
Cognitive stressors: failing memory or the inability to grasp an idea or understand an abstract concept.
Physiological stressors: any condition such as hunger, fatigue, or disease that causes disequilibrium in one or more body systems.

The *condition of stress* itself can also be a stressor, and therefore a quick resolution of a stressful situation is sometimes needed to decrease the possibility of an escalating stress that could overwhelm the person experiencing it.

Effect of Multiple Stressors

Researchers have investigated the effect of multiple stressors and they have found that the potential for harm increases with the number of stressors acting on the person. The Social Readjustment Rating Scale

TABLE 8.1 SOCIAL READJUSTMENT RATING SCALE

Rank	Life Event	Life Change Units
1	Death of spouse	100
2	Divorce	73
3	Marital separation	65
4	Jail term	63
5	Death of close family member	63
6	Personal injury or illness	53
7	Marriage	50
8	Fired at work	47
9	Marital reconciliation	45
10	Retirement	45
11	Change in health of family member	44
12	Pregnancy	40
13	Sex difficulties	39
14	Gain of new family member	39
15	Business readjustment	39
16	Change in financial state	38
17	Death of close friend	37
18	Change to different line of work	36
19	Change in number of arguments with spouse	35
20	Mortgage over $10,000	31
21	Foreclosure of mortgage or loan	30
22	Change in responsibilities at work	29
23	Son or daughter leaving home	29
24	Trouble with in-laws	29
25	Outstanding personal achievement	28
26	Wife begins or stops work	26
27	Begin or end school	26
28	Change in living conditions	25
29	Revision of personal habits	24
30	Trouble with boss	23
31	Change in work hours or conditions	20
32	Change in residence	20
33	Change in school	20
34	Change in recreation	19
35	Change in church activities	19
36	Change in social activities	18
37	Mortgage or loan less than $10,000	17
38	Change in sleeping habits	16
39	Change in number of family get-togethers	15
40	Change in eating habits	15
41	Vacation	13
42	Christmas	12
43	Minor violations of the law	11

Adapted from: Holmes TH, Rahe RH: The Social Readjustment Rating Scale. *Journal of Psychosomatic Research,* 14:121, 1970.

(Table 8.1), for example, is a weighted list of commonly experienced life changes. It was developed to study the hypothesis that there is a connection between the number of life change units (LCUs) a person experiences within a given period and the likelihood that the person will become ill in the near future. It was found, for example, that a person with a total score of 300 points or more for the preceding 2 years had an 80 percent chance of developing a serious illness within the next year.

Such *scales must be adapted before use* to take into account such variables as age, personality, cultural bias, and changes which have taken place in society. Despite the need for ongoing study, the research findings have already documented the significance of change, and especially of multiple changes, as a stressor.

Stress And Energy

A stressor can be of external or internal origin, normal or pathological, physiological or psychological, and sudden or long-standing; but *any* stressor, regardless of type, causes the system to change or adapt in order to maintain its equilibrium. When there is a balance between all the forces (stressors) affecting the system, the system is said to be in a state of dynamic equilibrium, or in good working condition.

When a system in a state of equilibrium is upset by new or additional stressors, the system responds in whatever ways it can to restore its balance and equilibrium. The words used to designate this response are less important than the fact that the response occurs. The system can be said to change, respond, adapt, cope, or adjust; but regardless of the term used, the most important aspect of the process is that *the response takes energy*. Regardless of the nature of the stressor or the individual's perception of it, the system's efforts to restore its equilibrium always require energy, either physical or psychic energy. *This concept is basic to nursing*, because a person who is expending large amounts of energy in trying to cope with a powerful stressor such as terminal cancer or a multitude of small stressors may not have enough energy to meet his other needs. Many of a nurse's actions are designed to help a person meet his physiological and psychological needs until he has the energy to manage by himself.

There are two synonyms for equilibrium which are commonly used: homeostasis, and steady state. *Homeostasis* refers to a state of dynamic equilibrium of the internal environment of the body. *Steady state* has been defined as "that state existing when energy is allocated in such a way that man is freed to actualize himself according to his nature, maintained by effective and efficient activities at all behavioral levels" (Byrnes and Thompson, 1972, p. 9). This definition is useful because it emphasizes the allocation and use of available energy, the dynamic nature of human equilibrium, and the ultimate human goal of growth and self-actualization.

ADAPTATION

The response of any living system to a stressor is called its *adaptation*. In humans, responses to stress are generally described as falling into one or more of the following modes of adaptation: physiological, physical, intellectual, emotional, social, and spiritual.

Adaptation to a stressor may be voluntary or involuntary, conscious or unconscious, active or passive, overt or covert, but adaptation will always be reflected in some observable change in the system. In some instances, the changes will be small and difficult to detect, but they are discernible. In humans, *behavior* is one indicator of a person's adaptation to stress.

The outcome of any adaptation can be either positive or negative, adaptive or maladaptive. Because every adaptation is an *attempt* by a system to reduce stress and regain a steady state, some theorists believe that the concept of maladaptation is not logical, and that some adaptations are merely less effective than others.

Factors Affecting Adaptation

Human adaptation is affected by: (1) the characteristics of the person and (2) factors related to the stressor. Personal characteristics include age, state of health or illness (resistance), past history of successful adaptations, ability to problem solve, and the quantity and quality of available resources, both internal and external.

Factors related to the stressor which influence adaptation include the number of stressors acting on the system at one time and the intensity and duration of the stressor or stressors. The impact of the stress is often hard to predict because a multitude of seemingly minor or superficial stressors can produce greater stress than one or two major ones. Lay people express this concept in sayings such as: "It's the little things that get you down"; "It's not the mountain ahead that wears you out—it's the pebble in your shoe"; and "I'd rather be swallowed by a whale than nibbled to death by baby piranhas."

All of the above factors are important and must be taken into account when you assess a patient or family in preparation for helping to meet stress-related needs.

Physiological Adaptation

The human system makes both specific and nonspecific adaptation responses to a stressor.

Specific Adaptation

A *specific response* to a stressor is one which is uniquely designed to deal with that particular stressor. Examples of a specific response include pulling one's hand away from a hot object, sweating in a hot environment, the stimulation of antibody production to combat a specific antigen, and grieving over the loss of a loved one.

Nonspecific Adaptation

In addition to the system's specific response to a given stressor, *nonspecific responses* occur. These responses are described as nonspecific because they occur *regardless* of the exact nature of the stressor and they are *relatively uniform and consistent for all stressors* (Fig. 8.1). The body's general, nonspecific responses to a stressor are referred to as "stress responses" or "responses to stress." These responses are mediated through the hypothalamus and are evoked whenever the system senses that its homeostasis is disturbed or threatened. Although these general responses are *nonspecific with respect to the nature of the stressor,* they occur in a very precise, systematic fashion.

GENERAL ADAPTATION SYNDROME. In 1926 when he was a second-year medical student, Hans Selye became interested in the similarities of patient responses to illness. He observed that acutely ill people, whether suffering from a severe loss of blood, an infectious disease, or advanced cancer, tended to demonstrate similar stereotyped responses to "being sick": they looked "sick" and acted "sick." Each patient tended to lose his appetite, his muscular strength, and his interest and ambition. He tended to lose weight; his behavior changed; and his facial expression usually indicated that he was ill. Selye called this nonspecific response to stress the *general adaptation syndrome* (GAS). He wondered about the basis for this commonly encountered collection of

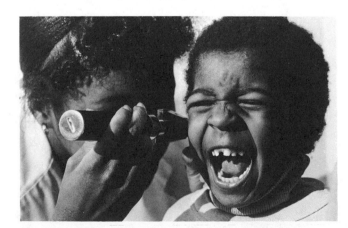

Figure 8.1 *It is not possible to tell whether this child is laughing or crying, but the initial stress is the same.*

symptoms—the syndrome of "being sick"—and devoted a lifetime of study to the phenomenon.

Selye's detailed experimental studies resulted in his theory of stress and adaptation, and provided a new basis for the understanding and treatment of stress-related diseases as well as a foundation for studies related to the avoidance of such disease and the promotion of health.

The process of physiological adaptation includes the endocrine responses described by Selye and the autonomic nervous system responses described by Cannon in 1939. The process consists of three phases: the alarm reaction, the resistance phase, and the stage of exhaustion.

The first indication of stress may be the physiological changes which characterize the body's initial reaction to a stressor, the *alarm reaction*. This reaction is often referred to as the "fight or flight response" because it represents man's most basic and primitive response to danger. For millions of years human survival depended upon the individual's ability to recognize a threat, and then to make a quick decision to flee from the threat or stay and fight it. The physiological changes which characterize this phase (the alarm reaction) are always the same, regardless of the final action taken (Fig. 8.2).

During the alarm phase, the sympathetic nervous system is stimulated to increase the efficiency of almost all of its functions. Blood pressure, heart rate, and respiratory rate are increased. The level of blood sugar is raised to make more glucose available to meet the need for increased energy. Blood clotting is increased, pupils are dilated, and mental acuity (alertness) increases. Additional changes occur in other physiological supportive processes, and as a result, the body's resources are mobilized for a brief, intense effort either to eliminate the stressor or to survive its initial attack.

These physiological changes are normal responses to stress, and do little harm when they are followed by the physical activity of "fighting or fleeing." For example, these responses are absolutely essential at times for athlete, cattleman, steeple jack, or jockey. Unfortunately, most people experience these stress responses in situations when it is socially inappropriate to take any kind of physical action, such as when angry over missing a promotion, being caught in traffic, failing a test, or being issued a ticket for speeding.

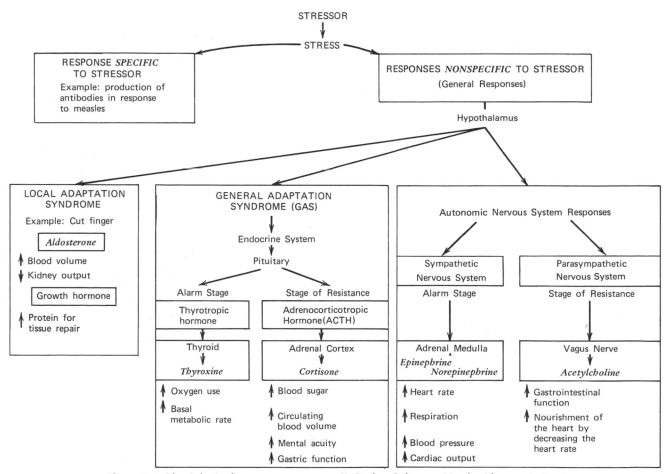

Figure 8.2 *Physiological responses to stress. (J. Evelyn Osborne. Used with permission.)*

According to Dr. O. Carl Simonton, in these circumstances when either "fighting" or "fleeing" would be socially unacceptable, people learn to override their reactions. Therefore, throughout the day, individuals constantly override their physiological responses to stress. When the physiological response to stress is not discharged, there is a negative cumulative effect on the body. This is *chronic stress,* stress that is held in the body and not released. And chronic stress, it is increasingly recognized, plays a significant role in many illnesses (Simonton, 1978, p.52). The hazards of unreleased physiological stress can be minimized by substituting *regular physical exercise* such as aerobic dancing, walking, jogging, or tennis for unusable "flight or fight" responses.

During the alarm phase, the pituitary gland is stimulated to release hormones that are stored either in that gland or in target glands such as the thyroid and the adrenals. The thyroid gland releases thyroxine which increases the metabolic rate. The adrenal gland releases ACTH which, through its stimulation of cortisone, increases blood volume, blood glucose, and muscular contraction. It also decreases unnecessary inflammatory responses in addition to many other actions.

If the body's responses are adequate and the person survives the alarm phase, he enters the second phase of the stress response, the *stage of resistance.* During this stage, the bodily responses that characterized the alarm reaction have subsided, and the resistance of the body increases and levels off above its normal level. The parasympathetic nervous system initiates a series of actions that enable the body to rebuild and restore the defenses used during the first phase. For example, digestion, which was slowed during the alarm phase, is now stimulated to provide the nutrients needed to rebuild the body's defenses.

A number of hormones are produced by the adrenal glands, but cortisone is usually considered the stress hormone, and experts generally agree that it is produced in higher than physiological doses during the period of resistance. Cortisone is tremendously beneficial in helping the body regain homeostasis provided the cortisone level is elevated for only a short-to-moderate period of time. If stress is intense, or the period of stress is prolonged, the effects of cortisone, though beneficial for a limited time, become potentially harmful to the system and lead to increased stress and dysfunction (diseases of adaptation) or death.

Some of the dysfunctional responses to a prolonged high level of cortisone include the development of diabetes mellitus (because of the prolonged high blood-glucose level); the development of peptic ulcers; hypertension; porous bones; decreased resistance to infection; increased risk of malignancies; and mental or emotional disturbances. These and other effects of prolonged stress (chronic stress) make it advisable to reduce high levels of stress (or shorten a period of prolonged stress) as quickly as possible.

The resistance stage, therefore, can lead to resolution of the stress, survival, and restoration of the system's equilibrium; or it can lead to a period of chronic stress with its potential for additional stress and disease. The resistance phase can also lead to a stage of exhaustion and death if the stress is severe enough or if the body's supply of energy or ability to use energy is inadequate. Death can also be caused by the lack of a will to live as a result of stress which seems overwhelming to the patient.

LOCAL ADAPTATION SYNDROME. In addition to the general adaptation syndrome (GAS), a *local adaptation syndrome* (LAS) occurs in response to certain physical and physiological stressors. Like the GAS, this response is mediated by the hypothalamus. An inflammatory process occurs at the site of injury, regardless of its cause, and healing eventually takes place (see Chapter 12 for a description of the inflammatory process). The GAS and LAS occur simultaneously and work together to help the body regain homeostasis.

Other Modes of Adaptation and Coping

The terms *coping* and *adapting* are sometimes used as if they were equivalent, but coping is more accurately used to indicate an intellectual mode of adaptation. A coping behavior or coping mechanism is usually a *deliberate, intentional* adaptation and is usually at least partly psychosocial in nature.

Adaptations to the existence of stress within the body are generally described as falling into one or more of the following modes of adaptation: physical (motor), cognitive (intellectual), affective (emotional), social, and spiritual (Fig. 8.3). These categories are somewhat arbitrary because many adaptations include a combination of modes, and because the mode of adaptation used may be unrelated to the specific nature of the stressor. For example, a physical stressor may call forth an emotional adaptation, and an emotional stressor may call forth a spiritual adaptation.

When the steady state (equilibrium) of an individual is altered by the demands of a stressor, the individual's energy must be directed toward an adaptive response which: (1) removes the stressor, (2) decreases the impact of the stressor, or (3) modifies the system's response to the stressor.

The *physical* mode of adaptation includes a variety of motor responses such as doodling on a piece of paper, fidgeting, jogging, cleaning, or nibbling and eating

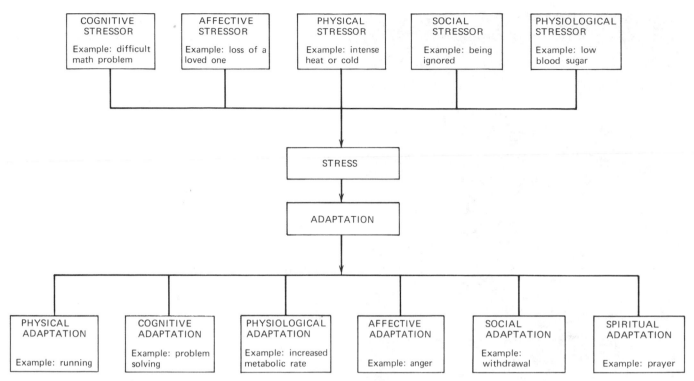

Figure 8.3 *Types of stressors and modes of adaptation. Note that stress can be the result of more than one stressor, and that more than one mode of adaptation can be used. There is no direct or necessary relationship between a type of stressor and a specific mode of adaptation. (J. Evelyn Osborne. Used with permission.)*

when not hungry (Fig. 8.4). The physical withdrawal of one's person from a stress-producing social situation is a form of physical adaptation related to Cannon's fight or flight response.

The *cognitive* mode of adaptation involves the use of specific intellectual activities that either decrease the amount of stress or modify a person's reaction to it. Such activities include reading, writing, reasoning, problem solving, and seeking information. Some people have learned to decrease their perception of pain by thinking about pleasant things. The will to live is a cognitive function, and few would deny its value in mobilizing the body's resistance to or recovery from stress. Spiritual adaptation is sometimes considered to be a cognitive mode.

Affective modes of adaptation are numerous and commonly used, especially in situations in which a person must tolerate a stressful condition that cannot be readily alleviated. Affective modes of adaptation are psychological or emotional in nature and behaviors such as laughing and crying often offer considerable relief from stress.

Some affective states, such as fear and anxiety, are such uncomfortable adaptations that the person experiencing them tries to change or move toward more satisfying and effective adaptations. Discomfort can be

growth producing if it leads to more effective adaptive or coping skills.

Psychological defense mechanisms such as denial, regression, sublimation, and compensation are all forms of affective adaptation that can lead to either increased function or dysfunction of the system, depending on the given situation. For example, at an early stage of extreme grief following the death of a loved one, *denial* is a useful and appropriate adaptation because it gives a person time to mobilize his resources enough to confront the crisis. If a person continues to deny the reality of the situation for an extended period of time, however, the denial will interfere with a healthy resolution of the loss. The research and writings of Dr. Elizabeth Kübler-Ross describe in detail how these and other affective adaptations are basic to the process of dying and death (Chapter 43).

Since many types of stress evoke an emotional response of some type (fear, guilt, joy, embarrassment, rage), the affective mode of adaptation is probably involved to some extent with most types of stress, and as with all other modes, a person must expend energy to continue the adaptation. Unless the adaptations are reducing the stress that is being experienced, they can deplete a person's energy reserves. Prolonged, unfocused anger, for example, is likely to be unproductive

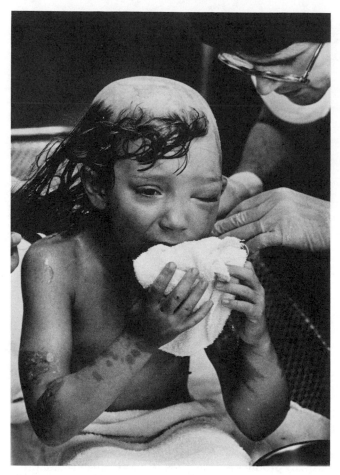

Figure 8.4 *For the moment, at least, biting a wash cloth helps Renee to cope with stress.*

and may almost literally "wear a person out." Such depletion of energy acts as a new and additional stressor in addition to decreasing a person's ability to cope with the existing stressors.

The *physiological* mode of adaptation to stress is designed to mobilize a person's physiological defenses to either destroy the stressor, escape the stressor, or develop an increased ability to survive the stress that is threatening to disrupt the individual's homeostasis. Physiological adaptations involve the responses made by the endocrine and autonomic nervous systems.

STRESS, HEALTH, AND ILLNESS

Dr. Simonton, a noted cancer specialist, has stated: "There is a clear link between stress and illness, a link so strong that it is possible to predict illness based on the amount of stress in people's lives." (Simonton, p. 46)

Physicians have noted for many years that illness is more likely to occur following highly stressful events in people's lives. They first noticed that diseases such

as ulcers, high blood pressure, heart disease, and headaches were susceptible to emotional influences. They now recognize that a relationship exists between stress and infectious diseases, backaches, accidents, and even cancer.

Holmes and Rahe were among the first researchers to study the relationship between stress and illness (Table 8.1). They discovered in one study that of the people with high scores related to recent life changes (300 points), 49 percent became ill within a year, while of the people with scores below 200, only 9 percent reported an illness (Table 8.1).

Implications for Health Care

By using scales such as the Holmes and Rahe scale and other research methods it is possible to predict the *probability* of illness based upon the number of stressful events in people's lives, but it is *not* possible to predict how an *individual* will react to a certain number of stressors. For example, in the Holmes and Rahe study, 49 percent of the high scorers became ill, *but* 51 percent of them did not! The important task for health care workers is to learn why some people under great stress do not get ill, and to use that knowledge to help other individuals.

STRESS AND HEALTH CARE

It is becoming increasingly evident that while stress may predispose to illness, the most significant factor in the development of illness may be an individual's ability to cope with stress. The ability to cope depends upon the nature of the stressors, the amount of stress, and the individual's techniques for managing stress. Each of these factors must be assessed before any type of nursing intervention can be contemplated.

Assessments Related to Stress

It is important for health care workers to remember that stress is omnipresent and necessary for life, that the effects of stress can be either harmful or beneficial, and that most humans have tremendous capabilities for successful resolution and management of stress (Fig. 8.5).

Because stress is an integral and essential component of life, it would be impractical and a waste of time to assess a given person or patient for signs of stress *in general* because every living person will exhibit evidence of stress of some sort. Nursing assessments, therefore, should be directed toward the detection of *unhealthy* levels of stress, such as sudden high stress that temporarily numbs and immobilizes a person;

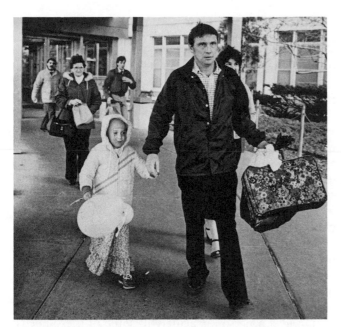

Figure 8.5 *According to Selye, even good things can be extremely stressful. The expression on the face of Renee's father reflects his concern about caring for Renee at home despite his happiness that she is able to leave the hospital. Note that Renee is wearing her jobst (a nylon body suit and mask) under her dress and jacket.*

multiple stressors that seem to surround a person, leaving him with no apparent escape and no place to turn; and stress that extends over a long period and gradually wears a person down. The physiological responses to such stress are relatively uniform from person to person, but the *behaviors that reveal the presence of stress are highly variable*.

Some important indicators of increased stress include:

- Accentuated use of *one* mode or pattern of behavior; behavior that is repetitive and seemingly purposeless
- Alteration in the variety of behaviors usually displayed
- Regression to a lower developmental level
- Increased sensitivity to the environment
- Behaviors that indicate alteration in usual physiological activity (such as patterns of eating and sleeping)
- Distortions of reality

Although the possible indicators of stress are numerous and varied, it is important to remember that *some people can be under great stress but display few, if any, overt cues* or behaviors that would reveal a stressful condition.

Effects of Prolonged Stress

SUBJECTIVE EFFECTS

Anxiety, aggression, apathy, boredom, depression, fatigue, frustration, guilt and shame, irritability and bad temper, moodiness, low self-esteem, threat and tension, nervousness, and loneliness.

BEHAVIORAL EFFECTS

Accident proneness, drug taking, emotional outburst, excessive eating or loss of appetite, excessive drinking and smoking, excitability, impulsive behavior, impaired speech, nervous laughter, restlessness, and trembling.

COGNITIVE EFFECTS

Inability to make decisions and concentrate, frequent forgetfulness, hypersensitivity to criticism, and mental blocks.

PHYSIOLOGIC EFFECTS

Increased blood and urine catecholamines and corticosteroids, increased blood glucose levels, increased heart rate and blood glucose levels, increased blood pressure, dryness of mouth, sweating, dilation of pupils, difficulty breathing, hot and cold spells, "a lump in the throat," numbness and tingling in parts of the limbs.

HEALTH EFFECTS

Asthma, amenorrhea, chest and back pains, coronary heart disease, diarrhea, faintness and dizziness, dyspepsia, frequent urination, headaches and migraine, neuroses, nightmares, insomnia, psychoses, psychosomatic disorder, diabetes mellitus, skin rash, ulcers, loss of sexual interest, and weakness.

ORGANIZATIONAL EFFECTS

Absenteeism, poor industrial relations and poor productivity, high accident and labor turnover rates, poor organizational climate, antagonism at work, and job dissatisfaction.

From Cox, T: *Stress*, Baltimroe, University Park, 1978, p. 92.

Assessments Related to Stressors

If a person's behavior indicates that his level of stress could be detrimental to his health, family life, career, or other relationships, it is appropriate for the nurse to try to identify the stressors that are responsible for the stressful condition.

When you seek to identify sources of stress, certain points are important. First, although it is useful and often necessary for the nurse to hypothesize about possible stressors, *the identification of specific stressors can be done only by the person under stress*. What is stressful for one person is not necessarily stressful for another. For example, three persons being led through a dark cave may be equally terrified, but for different reasons. One may be afraid of spiders, another of snakes, and the third of bats. In a hospital setting, three young women who are scheduled for the removal of a breast may all be afraid and under great stress, but the specific stressors may differ. One woman may fear the anesthesia and being out of control; the second may fear the pain; the third may fear the fantasized loss of her sexuality. Fear is the common stressor for these women, but it is the *nature of the specific stressor* (the source of the fear) that will determine the kind of help needed by each woman.

In many situations, much of the stress is perceived dimly or unconsciously, and a person is aware only of feelings of uneasiness, a sense of discomfort, or a feeling that "things are just not right." In such a situation, the process of identifying the sources of stress may be difficult and time consuming indeed. When the causes of stress are obscure, persistent and careful detective work will be necessary because unidentified stressors can range from unsuspected allergies to unresolved "oughts" and "shoulds" ("You ought to respect your boss," "You should be able to tolerate your mother's nagging"). If a stressor seems unacceptable to the person affected by it, his inability to acknowledge the existence of that stressor becomes an additional source of stress and an added stressor.

The manner and means by which stressors are identified depends on age, personality, condition, and situation of the person under stress and on his relationship with the person trying to help him. Possible approaches can range from a direct question such as "What's the matter?" through a permissive directive such as "Tell me about it," to an extensive analysis of the situation.

Management of Stress

A person can be helped to survive intense or prolonged stress by: (1) removing the stressor, (2) minimizing the effect of a stressor that cannot be removed, or (3) helping the person adapt to stressors that can be neither removed nor minimized.

Removal of Stressors

In some situations, it is possible to remove or eliminate an identified stressor. Examples of such actions include: elimination of certain foods or substances to which the person is allergic; minimizing contact with irritating or upsetting people; taking a different route to work to avoid frustrating delays due to road construction; the removal of unsightly blemishes, warts, or other skin lesions; reassigning household chores to avoid family conflicts; surgical repair of a hernia. In each of these examples, the stressor is removed and stress is relieved.

Increasing Resistance to the Stressor

If the identified stressor cannot be removed or eliminated, it is often possible to minimize the impact of the stressor by *increasing the person's ability to resist the stressor*. This increased resistance may be physical, psychological, or both.

MOBILIZATION OF THE BODY'S PHYSICAL RESOURCES. One of the foremost considerations for increasing resistance to stress is the production and efficient use of energy. Energy is required for every adaptation, and *inadequate energy, whether physical or psychic, is likely to result in inadequate adaptation.* The production of energy is enhanced by making certain that a person under stress obtains the food, rest, sleep, exercise, and oxygen he needs. Some people under stress will attend to these personal needs if reminded to do so and if the opportunity to do so is readily available. Others need much encouragement and sometimes guidance or supervision, and if a person is acutely ill some of these needs must be met with artificial aids such as IV fluids or a respirator. Attention to a person's need for energy is so basic that it would seem to be obvious, and yet many people under great stress are unable to cope effectively because they are tired, run down, undernourished, worn out, or exhausted.

In addition to increasing a person's ability to produce the energy needed for successful adaptation, it is helpful to reduce the demands on his available energy. Getting a person to cut back on outside engagements, seeing that a child is temporarily excused from some chores, or limiting the number of visitors to a sickroom are possible ways to reduce the drain on a person's available energy.

MOBILIZATION OF THE PERSON'S PSYCHOLOGICAL RESOURCES. In some situations, a person may be unable to handle his stress without the help of other people. This help may be needed for either of two reasons. First, the person may be able to handle most stressful situations effectively, but find the present stress overwhelming. Second, the person may lack the inner resources needed to handle stressful situations.

In the first instance, the person who is normally able to cope effectively may need extra psychological support and moral support to handle a time of unusually heavy stress. In many situations, the concern of a parent, or the understanding of a spouse or friend may be sufficient, but in other instances, the support of more than one person is needed. The resources of a medical center may be needed to help relieve the stress of a badly burned patient and his family. Flood victims will need the support of the Red Cross or other community agencies, while the family of a patient who is dying may need the support of other families who have had similar experiences.

In the second instance, the situation is very different indeed. The individual does not possess the skills needed to cope with even the basic stresses of everyday life. The help needed by such persons may take the form of counseling, assertiveness training, problem solving techniques, spiritual guidance, or relaxation techniques.

Development of Effective Adaptation and Coping Mechanisms

A person under stress should be helped to examine and understand his current modes of adaptation. If they are effective, they should be reinforced and maintained. If not, the person must be helped to develop more effective ways of dealing with the stress in his life. Short-term coping mechanisms such as snacking, drinking, smoking, using drugs, or excessive sleeping should be replaced by long-term approaches such as a program of regular exercise, talking about the stress, relaxation therapy, or counseling.

RELAXATION AS A COPING MECHANISM. Research has proven that relaxation can be an effective method of stress reduction, but it is imperative that the individual understand the difference between recreation and relaxation therapy. In a clinical context, relaxation cannot be equated with pleasurable activities such as watching television, playing cards, or attending a concert. These activities do *not* result in an adequate discharge of the physical effects of stress (Simonton, 1978, p. 137).

Relaxation therapy involves a series of conscious actions which are designed to reduce tension and completely relax all parts of the body. Relaxation techniques have been used for years to achieve childbirth without anesthesia, and to help people cope with pain. In 1975, Dr. Herbert Benson of Harvard University described his research on stress reduction in *The Relaxation Response,* and increasing numbers of nurses and doctors began to use relaxation therapy. There is no single best way to achieve a state of relaxation, and there are many techniques described in both professional journals and lay publications. One relaxation technique is described in the boxed material which follows. It is important for nurses to master a technique of relaxation both for their own personal use, and so that they can teach patients how to manage stress through a program of regular relaxation.

OTHER ASPECTS OF STRESS MANAGEMENT. Some people must be taught to recognize and avoid stressors that are harmful to them while others need to learn to reduce stress by establishing reasonable, attainable goals and

---

Technique for Progressive Relaxation

1. Go to a quiet room with soft lighting. Shut the door and sit in a comfortable chair with your feet flat on the floor and your eyes closed.

2. Become aware of your breathing.

3. Take in a few deep breaths, and as you let out each breath, mentally say the word, "relax."

4. Concentrate on your face and feel any tension in your face and eyes. Make a mental picture of this tension—it might be a rope tied in a knot or a clenched fist—and then mentally picture it relaxing and becoming comfortable, like a limp rubber band.

5. Experience your face and eyes becoming relaxed. As they relax, feel a wave of relaxation spreading through your body.

6. Tense your eyes and face, squeezing tightly, then relax them and feel the relaxation spreading throughout your body.

7. Apply the previous instructions to other parts of your body. Move slowly down your body—jaw, neck, shoulders, back, upper and lower arms, hands, chest, abdomen, thighs, calves, ankles, feet, toes—until every part of your body is relaxed. For each part of the body, mentally picture the tension, then picture the tension melting away; tense the area, then relax it.

8. When you have relaxed each part of the body, rest quietly in this comfortable state for 2 to 5 minutes.

9. Then let the muscles in your eyelids open up, become ready to open your eyes, and become aware of the room.

10. Now let your eyes open, and you are ready to go on with your usual activities.

From Simonton, O Carl, Matthews-Simonton, Stephanie, and James L Creighton: *Getting Well Again,* Bantam Books, New York, 1978, pp. 139–140.

---

priorities. Each person can be encouraged to evaluate the amount of control he already has over his life and destiny and to learn to accept and exert as much additional control as he can without adding to his existing stress. For some people, increased control will decrease their feelings of being helpless and powerless and thereby reduce their stress. For other people, the temporary transfer of control to someone else with knowledge and strength reduces stress. In each situation, the management of stress must be based on an accurate identification of stressors and a careful analysis of the person's current patterns of adaptation. Only then will it be possible to ascertain, for example, whether assertiveness training, relaxation therapy, or transfer to another department will be more likely to help a person who feels intimidated by his fellow employees.

STRESS AND NURSING

Knowledge of stress and adaptation theory and the ability to help people manage their stress are important in nursing because the ways people adapt to the stress they experience influence the extent to which they are able to achieve wellness, prevent illness, or regain some degree of health. In addition, nursing is a stressful profession, and the stressors encountered in settings such as an intensive care unit, the emergency room, or a hospice are tolerable only to those nurses who have adequate adaptation techniques and coping strategies (Fig. 8.6).

Everyone needs to learn that, though it may not be possible to change his situation and the stressors that accompany it, it is possible for him to modify his reaction to the situation and thereby minimize dangerous levels of stress and enhance his potential for growth.

The Assessment of Patterns of Coping With Stress

One of the goals of nursing is to reduce the incidence of stress-related illnesses through the prevention or management of excessive or prolonged stress. One way to reduce stress is to modify or eliminate the stressor. Although the manipulation of stressors is a logical approach when time permits, this is not always feasible in nursing. Some people are unable to describe or even identify the source of their stress without a time-consuming examination of their lifestyles and current situations. In other situations, the nature of the illness or treatment may preclude modification or removal of the stressor because *the illness or treatment itself may be the major stressor.*

An effective way to help some patients cope with stress is to focus less on the identification of stressors which often change from hour to hour and day to day, and focus more on the prompt recognition of the patient's manifestations of stress and the evaluation of his existing ability to cope with stress, regardless of its source. (See Related Activities at end of chapter.)

Therefore, whenever a patient-nurse interaction is likely to be relatively brief, an expedient approach to stress reduction is to help the patient assess and evaluate his general patterns of coping, with the intention of strengthening those which are effective and replacing those which are not effective. As a result, the patient develops an expanded repertoire of effective coping skills which could then be used in a variety of situations.

It is imperative for the nurse to be able to assess the patient's *current* patterns of coping because any pro-

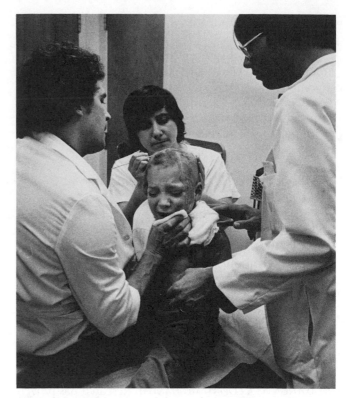

Figure 8.6 *During this initial assessment of Renee's burns, each person reveals his own stress in an individualized way. Note the tightened jaw and lips of Dr. Bonaventura, the intense facial expression and clenched hand of nurse Bill Myers, and the compassionate touch and holding of Renee's hand by the surgical resident. The personal stress of each adult is increased by his efforts to help Renee cope with her stress.*

posed changes in coping must be compatible with his age, personality, lifestyle, and present situation. It is not helpful to advocate a mode of coping which is unacceptable to the patient or incompatible with his present situation, and inappropriate suggestions may actually increase his stress.

Assessments of coping should identify the patterns and characteristics of the patient's existing coping skills, and to estimate the likelihood that those skills will be effective.

In a recent study (Narrow, Osborne, and Mac-Dermott, 1984), over 300 people, ranging in age from 7 to 59 years, were asked: "How do other people know when you are under stress? How can they tell?" Of this group, less than one third indicated that they would tell anyone, and well over half of them *expected other people to notice* that "I am not myself, that I look or act different." Approximately 20 percent felt that others could not tell and would not know when they were under stress. It is imperative, therefore, for nurses to learn ways of assessing patient manifestations of stress in order to learn which patients are "not themselves" so that help in coping with stress can be given quickly to those who need and want it.

The fact that approximately 60 percent of all groups expect other people to "notice that I am not myself, that I am acting different" places a heavy burden on members of any helping profession during their initial interactions with a new patient or client because the helper has no knowledge of the person's *usual* behavior. The need for the nurse to be able to assess a person's nonverbal indications of stress may be even greater when she is caring for adolescents since in this study only 19 percent of them indicated that they would tell anyone about their stress. The remaining 81 percent expected people to notice changes in their behavior and deduce that they were under stress.

The finding that close to 20 percent of the sample believed that other people did not know when they were under stress suggests that there may be a sizable number of persons who receive no help in coping with their stress simply because they exhibit no outward and visible manifestations of stress—they seem cool, calm, and collected. If such persons could be identified at the time, subsequent stress-related physical and psychological problems might be averted or minimized. Professional nurses, especially in high stress areas such as burn centers, trauma units, oncology units, or diagnostic centers, are in a position to contribute to the reduction of stress-related complications or illnesses in both patients and families.

There is evidence to indicate that ways of coping are age related, and therefore it is important to assess not only the current mode of coping of a given patient but also whether or not that patient might be in transition between established and new ways of coping. In such situations, the patients may need more assistance than usual in coping with stress.

Problem solving is not a preferred way of coping with stress for the children and adolescents in this study. The extensive use by adolescents of emotional release as a way of coping with stress could result in behaviors which might be considered inappropriate and unacceptable to adults, especially when the adolescent is hospitalized. For some children and teenagers, one of the nurse's most significant interventions might be to teach more acceptable and effective ways of coping with stress.

Nurses must know how to identify nonverbal signs of stress quickly and accurately, and how to recognize a potentially stressful situation and ask whether or not the person needs help in coping with it. The purpose of the initial evaluation of a patient's coping skills is to identify two groups of patients who are likely to need assistance in coping with stress. The first group includes those people whose current coping skills are deficient or inadequate. The second group includes people whose coping skills have been effective to date but who now either find themselves confronted with unusual stress which is beyond their means to cope, or who are suddenly deprived of their normal coping mechanisms. For example, if a person who normally uses physical activity for the reduction and release of stress is suddenly placed in traction or a full body cast, he is abruptly deprived of his preferred and customary way of coping with stress. If such a situation is promptly diagnosed by the nurse, the development of different coping strategies can become an integral part of the patient's nursing care.

PATIENT TEACHING

It has been reported that upwards of two-thirds of all persons who seek health care do so because of stress-related illnesses, and it seems likely that the management of stress may soon become one of the major means of preventing certain illnesses and promoting health.

Just as with all preventive health measures, *stress management should start in early childhood.* Whereas we would like to retain our concept of childhood as a carefree, happy time of innocence, today's children are beset by the threat of sexual assault, divorce, nuclear war, drug abuse, failure to achieve, and various forms of violence. The incidence of severe anxiety and depression in children is rising and the number of adolescent suicides is increasing at an alarming rate.

Some elementary school systems have initiated ongoing programs of stress education in which children are taught to recognize and cope with their own manifestations of stress. A few communities have instituted pilot programs directed toward the prevention of adolescent suicides. Health care workers must assume an active role in both promoting and assisting such programs, not only for young people but for people of all ages.

Every professional contact with an individual, family, or community should include an appraisal of the current and probable levels of stress, followed by plans for intervention whenever feasible and warranted.

RELATED ACTIVITIES

1. Nurses often ask, "Since nursing is a stressful profession, how can I help patients and families cope with stress when I am likely to be under great stress myself?" This question indicates the need for each nurse

to develop a set of effective coping techniques. A first step would be to examine your current patterns of coping by answering the questions below. Then, analyze your responses and decide whether you need to learn some additional ways of coping or merely strengthen the ones you now use.

(1) How do *YOU* know when you are under stress? What is your *first* or major indication?

    a. ____ I notice that I am *BEHAVING* or *ACTING* differently.

    b. ____ I notice a difference in my psychological, emotional, or mental reactions.

    c. ____ I experience some kind of *PHYSICAL* response.

    d. ____ Other (write in): _____

(2) How do people *who know you* know when you are under stress?

    a. ____ I tell them that I am under stress, or tell them how I am feeling.

    b. ____ They can figure it out because they know my situation.

    c. ____ They notice that I am not myself, that I look or act different.

    d. ____ They can't tell; they usually don't know when I am under stress.

    e. ____ Other (write in): _____

(3) How can people *who do not know you* tell that you are under stress? (Ex., a new roommate, instructor, nurse, neighbor)

_____

(4) What do you usually do to try to reduce your stress and try to make yourself more comfortable? (Check those responses which you use most often.)

    a. ____ *I become physically active.* (For example, I exercise, pace the floor, work, hit something, twist my hair, jog, play the piano, clean.)

    b. ____ *I try to find solutions or answers.* (Ask questions, seek advice, consult an expert, check reference books, ask my parents, problem solve.)

    c. ____ *I engage in some spiritual activity.* (Read devotional materials, pray, go to temple or church, meditate.)

    d. ____ *I seek the help and support of other people.* (Talk with my family, spouse or friends, join a support group, see a counselor.)

    e. ____ *I become emotional.* (Yell, cry, swear, giggle, pout, get angry, act moody, become irritable, get depressed.)

    f. ____ *I engage in some type of excessive or compulsive activity.* (Smoke or drink too much, overeat, sleep too much, clean unnecessarily, work too much.)

    g. ____ *I intentionally avoid the situation.* (Leave the room, refuse to talk about it, run away, stay home from work or school, avoid the other people involved.)

    h. ____ *I use drugs or other substances.* (Prescribed medicine, alcohol, tranquilizers, psychotropic drugs.)

    i. ____ *I distract myself with other thoughts or activities.* (Read, do puzzles, pursue a hobby, fantasize, listen to music, draw, knit, concentrate on pleasant thoughts.)

    j. ____ *I pay increased attention to my health.* (Get enough sleep, exercise, relaxation, good nutrition.)

    k. ____ *I feel or become abusive toward others.* (Am inclined to hit, bite, slap, spank, kick, or otherwise hurt another person.)

    l. ____ Other (write in): _____

(5) Which of the coping responses that you checked in question 4 is usually most helpful to you?

    a. ____ physical activity

    b. ____ solutions and answers

    c. ____ spiritual activity

    d. ____ support, help from others

    e. ____ emotional release

    f. ____ compulsive activity

    g. ____ intentional avoidance

    h. ____ drugs, other substances

    i. ____ distraction

    j. ____ attention to health

    k. ____ abusive behavior

    l. ____ other: _____

(6) How satisfied are you with your ability to cope with the stress in your life? Using the scale of 1–10 below, circle the number which most nearly represents your degree of satisfaction. (1 = very dissatisfied, 5 = neutral, 10 = very well satisfied)

    1 2 3 4 5 6 7 8 9 10

What is the basis for your satisfaction or dissatisfaction?

2. If you are a person who finds it difficult to communicate your need for support and help in coping with stress, make plans for learning to do so. Set some easily attainable goals that are relatively non-threatening. For example, ask for help of some kind at least

once a day. Start with simple requests at first, such as asking for directions or unimportant advice. As quickly as possible, begin to verbalize some minor concerns and ask for support, such as "I'm concerned about _____. Could I talk to you for a minute?"

By doing this on a *daily* basis, you will learn to deal with occasional unsatisfactory responses from other people, and you will gradually learn how to actively seek the support you will need to cope with some stressful aspects of professional nursing.

SUGGESTED READINGS

Antonovsky, Aaron: *Health, Stress and Coping.* San Francisco, Jossey-Bass, 1979.

Baldree, Kathleen Smith, Suzanne Pelletier Murphy, and Marjorie J Powers: Stress identification and coping patterns in patients on hemodialysis. *Nurs Res* 1982 March/April; 31(2):107–112.

Barry, Patricia D: Stress: its implications in physical illness (chap.9) in *Psychosocial Nursing: Assessment and Intervention.* Philadelphia, Lippincott, 1984.

Borkovec, Thomas D: What's the use of worrying? *Psych Today* 1985 Dec; 19(12):59–64.

Bryne, Marjorie L, and Thompson, L: DAF Key. *Concepts for the Study and Practice of Nursing,* Ed. 2., St. Louis, Mosby, 1978.

Cominskey-O'Flynn, Alice I: The type a individual. *Am J Nurs* 1979 Nov; 79(11):1956–1958.

Cunningham, Ann Marie: Is there a seismograph for stress? *Psych Today* 1982 Oct; 16(10):46–52.

DiMotto, Jean Wouters. Relaxation (six techniques). *Am J Nurs* 1984 June; 84(6):754–758.

Dossey, Barbara: A wonderful prerequisite. *Nursing 84* 1984 Jan; 14(1):42–45.

Duldt, Bonnie W: Anger: an occupational hazard for nurses. *Nurs Outlook* 1981 Sept; 29(9):510–518.

Elliott, Susan Marsh: Denial as an effective mechanism to allay anxiety following a stressful event. *JPN and Mental Health Services* 1980 Oct; 18(10):11–15.

Hardt, D.: Stress Management and the Nurse. *Advances in Nursing Science* 1(4): 91, 1979.

Jalowiec, Anne, and Marjorie J Powers: Stress and coping in hypertensive and emergency room patients. *Nurs Res* 1981 Jan/Feb; 30(1):10–15.

Miller, Thomas W: Life events scaling: clinical methodological issues. *Nurs Res* 1981 Sept/Oct; 30(5):316–320A.

Ostchega, Yechiam, and Joan Graetz Jacob: Providing "safe conduct": helping your patient cope with cancer. *Nursing 84* 1984 April; 14(4):42–47.

Pineo Maya: Psychological hardiness: the role of challenge in health. *Psych Today* 1980 Dec; 14(12):34.

Richter, Judith M, and Rebecca Sloan: A relaxation technique. *Am J Nurs* 1979 Nov; 79(11):1960–1964.

Saletta, Anne L, Donna M Behler, and Patricia A Chamings: Fit to fly. *Am J Nurs* 1984 April; 84(4):462–465.

Scully, Rosemarie: Stress in the nurse. *Am J Nurs* 1980 May; 80(5):912–914.

Simonton, O. Carl, Mattews-Simonton, Stephanie and James L. Crighton: Getting Well Again. Bantam Books, New York, 1978.

Smith, Marcy JT, and Hans Selye: Reducing the negative effects of stress. *Am J Nurs* 1979 Nov; 79(11):1953–1955.

Sparacino, Jack: Blood pressure, stress, and mental health. *Nurs Res* 1982 March/April; 31(2):89–94.

Thomas, Ellen G: Application of stress factors in gerontologic nursing. *Nurs Clin North Am* 1979 Dec; 14(4):607–620.

Tierney, Mary Jo Grace, and Lani Moskowitz Strom: Stress type a behavior in the nurse. *Am J Nurs* 1980 May; 80(5):915–918.

REFERENCES

Cannon, Walter B: *The Wisdom of the Body.* ed.2. New York, Norton Publishing Co, 1939.

Cox, Thomas: *Stress.* Baltimore, University Park Press, 1978.

Holmes, Thomas H, and Richard H Rahe: The social readjustment scale. *J Psychsom Res* 1967; 11:213.

Seyle, Hans: *The Stress of Life,* New York, McGraw-Hill, 1956.

Selye, Hans: *The Stress of Life.* New York, McGraw-Hill, 1976.

Selye, Hans: *Stress without Distress.* Philadelphia, Lippincott, 1974.

9

Communication

Prerequisites and/or Suggested Preparation
An understanding of feedback (Chapter 5, Systems Theory) is prerequisite to understanding parts of this chapter.

THERAPEUTIC VERSUS NONTHERAPEUTIC COMMUNICATION

Communication in nursing or any other helping profession differs from communication in a social or business setting in several ways. A social conversation is usually unplanned, leisurely, and satisfying to both persons. A business conversation is more purposeful and less leisurely, and is usually beneficial to both parties. In nursing, however, communication is not only purposeful, it is deliberately structured to accomplish a given purpose. There is usually a time limit, and the benefits to be derived are not mutual but one sided.

Communication which is designed to benefit the patient is called *therapeutic communication,* and differs from nontherapeutic communication in structure, time, and benefits.

Structural Differences

In the majority of interactions of everyday life, conversation is purposeful but unstructured. Transactions in a store, bank, or post office are purposeful, with a well-defined task to be accomplished. Social interactions are also purposeful, although the task—renewing a relationship or making a new friend—is less well-defined than a business task (Fig. 9.1). Though purposeful, the communication in these interactions is usually not *planned* by either party, and the direction and flow of the conversation are determined by the task at hand.

When one is shopping for shoes, for example, any conversation with the clerk is almost incidental; it is a

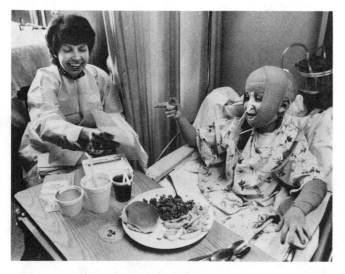

Figure 9.1 *A letter from a classmate can brighten even a difficult day in the hospital.*

means to an end. It is a necessary step in the acquisition of new shoes, but neither customer nor clerk consciously tries to direct the conversation itself. Both try to manipulate the transaction to a satisfactory result, but neither tries to analyze and direct the conversation.

In nursing, communication is often deliberately structured by the nurse because the *conversation is central* to the interaction, not incidental to it. Communication is often the primary concern because it may be the only tool by which you can relieve pain and suffering. The distress of bearing a deformed child or the psychological suffering that accompanies disfigurement cannot be relieved by a pill or procedure. In such situations, you have nothing to offer but yourself. Pain and suffering can be reduced by interaction with a helping person, and the degree of skill and sensitivity with which you can communicate with a person determines to a large extent the amount of relief and comfort you can give that person.

Time Differences

All human interactions are affected by the pressures of time, but in nursing, these constraints are often severe. The nurse's time with a patient may be limited by the length of his hospitalization, by his strength and energy, by the previously determined length of a home visit, or by other demands on the nurse's time.

In business, the length of a transaction is usually determined by the task to be accomplished; the sales clerk will stay with the customer until the purchase is completed. The nurse, however, must be able to initiate a conversation, move the conversation along toward its goal, and close the interaction within a specified period of time.

A community health nurse who has 1 hour to spend with a patient and his family has the responsibility of moving the conversation rather quickly from the opening pleasantries to communication that is likely to be significant and helpful. In a professional relationship, it is not appropriate to allow the conversation to drift, to plan to deal with a certain topic *if* it comes up, or to permit yourself to be sidetracked so extensively that you never quite get around to a therapeutic interaction.

Benefit Differences

Many human interactions are mutually beneficial. When buying a car, renting an apartment, or talking with a friend, both parties benefit from the transaction. In nursing and other helping interactions, the benefits are one sided and appropriately so, because the purpose of the conversation is to help the person who needs it. The interaction is focused on the needs of the patient or family member, not on the needs of the nurse. This is not to say that a nurse does not gain satisfaction from interactions with a patient. On the contrary, the rewards are great, and interactions are often fulfilling and satisfying. But regardless of any possible benefits to the nurse, the focus of the conversation must be the patient or client.

Although much communication in nursing is therapeutic in nature, there are also many social and business interactions. The social pleasantries of everyday life are important in nursing because they help to establish the identity of the patient as a unique and respected person. Brief questions such as "What's your opinion of that book you're reading?" "Is this a picture of your new grandchild?" or "Have you done any more of your needlepoint?" convey interest in the patient without detracting in any way from subsequent therapeutic communication. Some interactions in nursing are routine and businesslike; explanations of agency policy, directions, and requests for information are in this category. All types of conversation, whether social, business, or therapeutic, can be described in terms of general communication theory which follows.

GENERAL COMMUNICATION THEORY

Interpersonal communication is the process by which one person (the sender) transmits his thoughts and feelings to another person (the receiver). The process begins when a stimulus of some kind evokes a feeling or thought in a person and he decides to share that feeling or thought with someone else. The stimulus might be, for example, a promotion, a worry, a beautiful sight. The person who responds to this stimulus and who wants to share his response with others must first of all decide how he will communicate this response. He must choose an appropriate code or set of symbols. This process, called encoding, involves selecting a code that will facilitate the transfer of thoughts or feelings from one person to another (Fig. 9.2). The code may be verbal or nonverbal; possible codes range from words, facial expression, and gestures to music and painting. In selecting a code, the sender asks himself, "How can I best express my idea (or my feelings) to this other person?" The code must be able to convey the message as accurately as possible and must be appropriate in terms of both the message to be sent and the capabilities of the receiver. For example, facial expression and gestures may be adequate for the communication of feelings but are not likely to convey an abstract idea.

The receiver receives the message through one of his senses (usually sight, sound, or touch), which is referred to as the channel of communication. This channel must be *operating* and *compatible with the code* in order for the message to be received. This point seems obvious but it is frequently overlooked by senders. Examples of failure to use an appropriate and operating channel can be seen when a physician thoughtlessly gives printed instructions to a patient who has cataracts in both eyes, or a nurse carelessly stands to the side of a deaf patient who depends on lip reading for his messages.

Once the sender has selected the code for his message, he chooses the *medium*. If the code is verbal, the words may be written or spoken. The spoken word can be transmitted directly or indirectly via telephone, radio, television, or audiotape. A verbal message can also be transmitted by Morse code, sign language, semaphore, smoke signals, braille, jungle drums, or com-

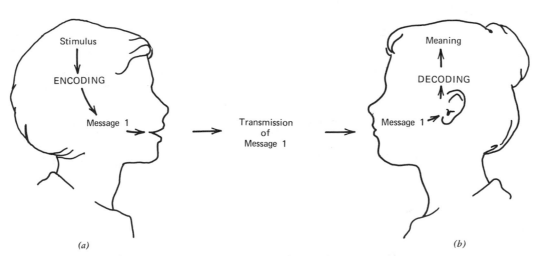

(a)   *(b)*

Figure 9.2 *The communication process: sending and receiving the initial message.*

puter. The choice of medium is affected by the distance between sender and receiver, the capabilities of the receiver, and the technology available.

Once the sender has encoded his message and selected a medium for its transmission, the message is transmitted to the receiver. The receiver must then decode the message to determine its meaning. This might involve a process of translation from one language to another or translation from flag positions or raised dots into letters and words. The speed of this process depends on the receiver's ability to use the code or codes involved.

The receiver must then put the message into context and interpret it in order for it to have meaning. The *meaning* of a given word or phrase will depend on the receiver's *perception* of it, e.g., spoken in anger, or meant as a joke.

Messages are subject to wide variations in meaning influenced by culture, age, sex, education, and so on.

The decoded message is a stimulus to the receiver, and he will respond to it in some way. He may get angry, ignore the message, mentally file it away for future reference, or any of a number of other possible responses. If the receiver chooses to reply to the message, he then becomes a sender, who encodes the reply into a second message, which is transmitted to the other person (Fig. 9.3). This response to the original message is often referred to as *feedback* and is a vital aspect of effective communication. Careful analysis of the receiver's response—the feedback—enables the sender to know whether or not the receiver understood the message and how he reacted to it. Failure to use feedback results in one-sided, ineffective communication in which a person sends messages but is unconcerned about their effect or impact.

VARIABLES THAT AFFECT COMMUNICATION

Communication between humans is an incredibly complex process subject to innumerable variables. Other forms of communication, such as computer-to-computer interactions, may seem to be more complicated, but the variables are usually technical and more easily adjusted and manipulated than are the variables involved in human interactions. The variables that influence the effectiveness of human interactions can be divided into three categories: general, nonverbal, and verbal.

General Variables

Nature of Message
Some messages are brief, noncontroversial, and factual, and hence can usually be transmitted without difficulty. On the other hand, messages that are long, complex, abstract, or ambiguous are subject to error or distortion.

Context of Message
Although a given message is simple, brief, clear, and therefore seemingly easy to understand, it may be part of a series of messages that have major implications for the receiver, and that are difficult for him to comprehend and accept. For example, a short one- or two-sentence message from the physician's office may seem incomprehensible to the receiver if it confirms his worst fears.

Timing
The commonplace statement "You caught me at a bad time" is often significant because stresses related to a

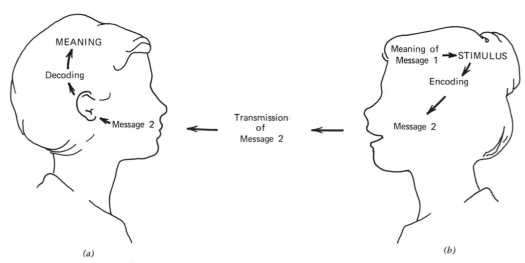

Figure 9.3 *Communication feedback: sending and receiving the reply.*

preceding or forthcoming event may interfere with the reception of a message. Physiological discomfort may also affect communication, and therefore, whenever feasible, it is good practice to ask, "Is this a good time to talk?"

Choice of Channel

If the intended receiver is confused, semiconscious, emotionally upset, or otherwise unresponsive, it may take considerable ingenuity to make any kind of meaningful contact with that person. While one agitated child might be calmed by being held and rocked, another might respond more quickly to a familiar music box. Food, odors, a gift, a gentle touch—any of these might prove to be the channel for communicating caring and concern. One nurse who was struggling to reach a semicomatose carpenter was successful when she placed some fresh cedar wood shavings where he could smell them. One young girl who was very much aware of her own responses stated, "If I am ever really out of it, just play the music from "Swan Lake." I'd respond to that, no matter what."

In those situations in which the patient can offer no clues to his own sensitivities, friends or members of the family may be able to suggest possible ways to communicate with him.

Feelings

Any strong emotion or intense feeling can block the transmission of a message and therefore must be dealt with *before* the message can be accepted and understood.

Nonverbal Variables

Space and Distance

Communication often becomes difficult and may become ineffective if the receiver feels either crowded or isolated, if he feels that his privacy has been violated or his personal territory has been encroached upon. This aspect of communication may be difficult to assess because we seldom think about it unless there is a problem, and therefore may not be accustomed to consciously considering it. It is usually easier for the nurse to discover she is invading a patient's personal space than it is to find out that he feels isolated. You will need to make these assessments early so you can position yourself effectively before any problem arises.

Personal Appearance

Most people dress up for the important events of life, and one indication of the importance of an event may be the personal grooming done in preparation for it. A person's appearance also reflects the importance attached to routine activities, and is frequently noted by the other people in the situation. Patients and families often deduce that, because certain members of the health care team are well groomed, they value both their jobs and the people they care for. Some nurses, however, feel that their grooming and appearance is a personal matter which has no bearing on the quality of their nursing care.

Appearance is indeed a personal matter, but it also affects nursing care. The appearance of the nurse affects the patient's perception of the care he is receiving, and this perception, for the patient, is equal to reality. Each patient has an image of "a nurse" and may find the discrepancy between his expectations and reality unsettling or even frightening. Some patients are disturbed to find the nursing staff without caps and, in some situations, without white uniforms. They feel less safe and secure because it is harder to identify a nurse: "You can't tell what kind of worker is coming into your room."

Nurses who maintain that "the uniform does not make the nurse" have a point to be sure; but the fact that human interaction is influenced by the appearance of each party is an equally valid point for consideration. The degree to which a given patient finds his nurse's uniform and appearance reassuring, confusing, provocative, or pleasing determines the effect that this aspect of nonverbal communication will have on nursing care. Policy decisions in this area should be made in the best interest of patients. Children usually respond favorably to colored uniforms; in some settings, geriatric patients may find comfort and security with nurses in traditional white uniforms. If you are committed to the establishment of a therapeutic relationship with patients, your choice of uniform and grooming becomes important when setting your priorities within the context of nursing. The nonverbal message conveyed by appearance can either add to or detract from subsequent verbal messages.

Facial Expression

You cannot evaluate the impact of your facial expression on communication without feedback from patients, friends, peers, family, or videotapes. This feedback is necessary if you are to determine such things as whether the facial expression which you intend to look accepting and nonjudgmental actually conveys acceptance, or whether it is so blank that it suggests boredom and inattention. Without such feedback, a nurse could not discover, for example, that her habit of frowning when she concentrates or listens attentively makes her appear critical and disapproving. Few people are likely to volunteer this type of information, so you will need to ask for feedback from people whom you respect and trust.

Touch

In a professional context, touch is a potentially powerful means of communication that should be used carefully and selectively. Some people do not like to be touched by a person they do not know well and will recoil at the touch of a person who seems to touch too casually and too frequently. Just as some people talk too much, others seem to touch too much; indiscriminate touching can evoke a negative response that influences all future communication.

On the other hand, the act of touching can convey concern, caring, and empathy and may take such forms as clasping a patient's hand during a difficult conversation or a painful procedure, giving an unhurried backrub, rocking an infant or child, brushing the hair back from a patient's forehead, and holding a patient close during a moment of intense grief or pain.

Verbal Variables

Size and Structure of Message

A person tends to reject a message that is vague, inappropriately long, complex, or disorganized. There is a limit to the amount of information that can be processed by a person at any given time, and humans tend to respond in a manner similar to ways in which a computer reacts to overloaded circuits. A computer blows a fuse, scrambles the messages, or shuts itself off. A person either turns out the message, or selects some portions and ignores the rest.

Vocabulary

A message may be poorly understood because the receiver is unable to translate it into words and phrases that are meaningful to him. This problem is usually obvious when a second language is involved, and as a result, steps are taken to alleviate the situation. Many large agencies have a list of available translators but if translators are not available, the patient's family or friends may take turns serving in this capacity.

The problem of vocabulary is even more serious when professional jargon, slang, or street language is causing the difficulty because the receiver may be unwilling to admit that he is unable to "understand the English language." He finds himself in a situation in which the individual words sound familiar but the combination and usage of these words produce an incomprehensible message.

Pacing

The speed with which the message is delivered plus the presence, absence, and length of pauses help determine whether the overall communication is satisfying, irritating, or frustrating. Feedback from the other person

will help you pace yourself; if such feedback is not given voluntarily or spontaneously, you will need to seek it by asking, "Am I going too fast?" or "Does it bother you when I pause to think about what you have said?"

COMMUNICATION TECHNIQUES

Each person has a pattern and style of communicating with people that has developed over the years and that is probably comfortable and satisfying. *Professional expertise* can be acquired by refining and expanding these existing competencies and by learning additional, rather specialized skills.

Because many nursing interactions are deliberately structured to accomplish some specific purpose, the nurse must be able consciously to select and use the approaches and techniques which she thinks will be most effective. Some people seem to be naturally good communicators; they are open and sensitive and seem to know intuitively what to say and how to say it. The majority of the population is not blessed with this talent. The *ability to communicate effectively can be learned,* however, and although it is not easy for some people, each nurse can acquire an extensive repertoire of important and useful communication skills. The more skills a nurse has at her command, the more selective she can be in choosing approaches that might work in a given situation.

Skills and techniques which are basic to therapeutic communication include:

Attending, Picking up and responding to cues, Listening, Suspending judgment, Responding to content, Responding to feelings, Clarifying the patient's meaning, Validating your own perceptions, Asking questions, Using silence, Confronting, Describing behavior and avoiding labels, Using feedback.

These skills are described in the pages that follow.

Attending

One of the most basic communication skills is that of giving your full attention to another person. This includes making him both *physically and psychologically comfortable* because he cannot benefit fully from an interaction if he is uncomfortable or distressed. Therefore, do whatever needs to be done to make the patient as physically comfortable as possible.

Psychological comfort is the result of your efforts to make the patient feel at ease while talking with him.

First of all, your body posture should convey acceptance, equality, and interest. *Position yourself at the patient's level;* it is not psychologically comfortable to be in an inferior position with someone towering over you. If there is no chair available, sit on the patient's bed rather than stand over him (unless this is contraindicated by some medical precaution or isolation procedure).

Face the patient, lean forward a bit, and maintain eye contact with him, letting him know that, for the moment at least, he is your primary concern. If you have ever talked with someone who had the knack of making you feel special—as if you were the only person in the world who mattered—then you know how much this skill can facilitate effective communication. If the subject under discussion is very personal or potentially embarrassing, it is important to ensure the patient's privacy. Pull the bedside curtains, ask relatives to step outside for a moment, or find a secluded spot down the hall. Do whatever seems necessary to make the patient comfortable.

Finally, never underestimate the value of a cup of tea or coffee. Food and drink are among the most basic human needs. Even though the other person may not be experiencing real hunger or thirst, the symbolic nourishment of a cup of tea or coffee conveys your desire to nurture and heal him as well as your acceptance of him as a person. The old saying "Let us break bread together," refers to this sense of fellowship and caring, and the sharing of a cup of tea may be a significant step in forging the bonds of mutual trust and respect.

Picking Up and Responding to Cues

The word *cue* is used to denote any verbal or nonverbal response from a patient that indicates that some type of intervention is needed from you. A cue serves as a prompt for the next person's actions, much as the prompter in the theater provides a prompt or cue whenever an actor does not know what to do or say next.

Nonverbal Cues

The physical appearance, energy level, and posture of the patient are cues to his level of well-being and the type of intervention needed. Your interaction with a person who is well groomed and who moves with determination will be much different from your interaction with a patient of similar age and diagnosis who looks disheveled, appears apathetic, and moves with reluctance and uncertainty. Each patient needs something from you, and his nonverbal cues will help you begin to assess those needs.

Cues from the environment are important, such as the presence or absence of family photographs, the type of reading materials, and any indications of hobbies or interests. Rooms full of antique furniture or marijuana growing on the window sill each suggest a certain lifestyle and provide cues that may guide your nursing interventions. Verbal cues are certainly important; but a picture is said to be worth a thousand words, and a careful observation is equally valuable.

An observation must be evaluated and put into context because it is a momentary impression and lacks the benefit of time. It captures the moment, like a photograph, but cannot indicate relationships as a movie can. You cannot see what the situation was like before you entered the picture, nor can you know what is likely to occur next. You can respond only to what you see and hear and then try to determine possible relationships. If something seems different or does not quite fit, you may need to pursue that cue more vigorously. If a patient's mother, who has always been carefully groomed and wearing lipstick and perfume, is wearing no makeup and looks as if she had slept in her clothes, her nonverbal cues merit attention.

Verbal Cues

Sometimes, the actual words spoken by a patient are of less consequence than other verbal cues which indicate that communication is difficult or blocked in some way. Such verbal cues include repeatedly changing the subject, answering questions inappropriately, giving only noncommittal or one-word answers, interrupting, asking the same questions over and over, and asking trivial questions when there are important issues at stake. Any of these behaviors, especially when repeated or forming a pattern, are verbal signals that something is wrong and that attention must be paid to the communication process itself.

Responding to Cues

Your response to cues, verbal or nonverbal, will vary from patient to patient and situation to situation. In one instance you may respond quickly and openly. In another situation you will bide your time; you will take a *wait and see* approach and collect more data. In still different circumstances, you will slowly and gently begin to explore the situation.

Occasionally, you will deliberately choose *not* to respond to a cue. This is very different from *missing* or *ignoring* a cue. It could be that the cue represents a behavior that is neither appropriate nor effective for the patient, so you make a conscious decision not to reinforce that behavior with a response. Sometimes it is good not to respond to a cue if responding might hurt the patient. For example, if a child is trying hard not to cry during a procedure and you know it is very important to him not to cry in front of a certain person who is present, it would hurt him if you were to say, "You look about ready to cry. Go ahead; it may make you feel better." At a later time, the child needs an opportunity to cry and may need to be encouraged to do so, but at the moment, such a response is likely to shatter his composure and cause him humiliation and pain. In this situation, as in every other, your action will be influenced both by *your ability to analyze and interpret the cue* and by *the number of responses in your repertoire.*

Listening

To give a patient your full attention, you may need to develop new or additional listening skills. In many social and business interactions, people tend to expend minimal energy on listening. They listen enough to transact some necessary business, to seem interested, or to get the gist of a conversation; but very often their minds are far away. In a therapeutic interaction, this level of listening is inadequate because it does not enable you to respond fully to the patient, and to structure the communication deliberately to meet the patient's needs.

To be effective, you need to tune out all distractions in the environment and to concentrate on three things: what the patient is saying; what you, the nurse, are saying; and the relationship between the two.

Listening to the Patient

In many conversations, a person uses the time when the other person is talking to formulate his own next remark. He never really listens because he is deciding what to say next. In a professional conversation, a skilled therapist or nurse avoids this pitfall through the use of short periods of silence. The helping person first concentrates on what the other person is saying and then waits quietly for a moment or two to formulate her own response. If such a pause seems awkward at first, a helping person may want to say something like "I need a minute to think about what you just said."

A nurse trying to develop her listening skills will find it helpful to note the conditions under which she finds it difficult to listen. It may be that you find it hard to listen when you are pressured for time, when the other person has a marked accent, when there are a number of activities in the same room, or under a variety of other conditions. Once you have identified the conditions that make listening difficult for you, you can set about learning to cope with the problem. It is beneficial to practice listening under problem conditions that gradually *increase in intensity.*

The usefulness of verbal cues is determined to a large extent by your ability to listen to two things at once. You need to be able to *listen to the actual content* of a person's words and, at the same time, *listen for the underlying message.* They may be quite different. For example, a patient may be complaining bitterly about the hospital food, but the nurse may sense that food is not the issue. She may therefore decide not to get involved in a discussion of diets and menus but to respond to what seems to be an underlying anger. In doing so, the nurse may discover that the patient is angry about a number of things but is afraid to complain about them for fear the staff will get angry and not give him safe care. In a case like this, if the nurse had responded to the literal meaning of the patient's words, nothing would have been accomplished because the patient's real concern would have been missed.

In addition to listening for underlying messages, it is important to listen for *recurrent themes.* A patient may return to the same theme or issue again and again, perhaps on different occasions, stating it first one way and then another. A patient might mention that her brother had died with a similar diagnosis; on another occasion she might describe her mother's funeral, then later talk about her increasing tendency to lose things. The next day she might note that she has just read of the deaths of several well-known figures and later talk about her difficulties in trying to keep her plants alive. This patient would seem to be giving her nurse cues to indicate that she needs to talk about some aspect of death or dying. Because she seems unable to address the issue directly, the nurse may need to help by observing, "in the past few days, I've noticed that you have mentioned your brother's death, your mother's funeral, losing things, the deaths of a senator and an entertainer, and your plants dying. I wonder if you are beginning to think about your own death or the death of someone close to you?" It takes practice to be able to identify recurrent or underlying themes because most people do not routinely relate what was just said to what was said an hour ago or yesterday.

It is equally important to *note gaps in a conversation.* If you are listening with a purpose and know what to listen for, you will notice the instances in which the patient does *not* mention something that should be relevant. If he repeatedly omits any reference to a seemingly relevant person, object, or event, you may need to explore the omission.

Listening to Yourself

In some settings, people chatter or ramble on and on, often so unaware of what they are saying that occasionally a person will ask in surprise, "Did I really say that?" As a helping person, you need to be aware at all times of what you say and how you say it. Listen to your choice of words, the organization of your thoughts, the tone of your voice, the enunciation and pronunciation of your words, and the rapidity with which you speak.

Check the number of times you have to say, "No, that's not really what I mean," or "That's not what I meant to say." Such statements are confusing and sometimes upsetting to a patient. Thinking *before* you speak and listening *while* you speak will help you avert some of these difficulties.

Listening to the Interaction

It is important to *examine the relationship* between what the patient said and what you said because the manner in which each affects the other will affect the course of the overall interaction. Questions that might help you examine this relationship include: "Does either of us interrupt frequently, as if we were not even listening?" "Do I find myself getting irritated with the patient if he takes a long time to say something?" "Does my mind wander?" "Do I get defensive or argumentative if the patient disagrees with me or criticizes any aspect of his care?" "Do I change the subject if the topic is embarrassing or the conversation begins to get emotional?"

The basis for this type of evaluation is hard, intense, concentrated listening.

Suspending Judgment

Hasty judgments and unwarranted conclusions are impediments to all communication and are especially detrimental to a professional interaction. The patient-nurse relationship, especially in the early stages, can be marred by jumping to conclusions based on insufficient data. It is necessary to make *tentative* assessments as an interaction progresses, but it is important to substantiate each one before a response is made or any action is taken. It is essential that you examine the patient's behavior in its context and that you verify your interpretation of that behavior in order to avoid misinterpreting either the nature or the intended effect of the behavior.

It is difficult to state accurately the nature of an isolated bit of behavior. For example, it is hard to differentiate quickly between the giggles of a good-natured and "silly" preadolescent and the giggles of an extremely nervous one. A young mother who recently learned she has cancer may have been sobbing all through visiting hours despite her husband's efforts to comfort her. She may be crying, however, not over her diagnosis, but over some tragic news her husband brought from home.

It is also difficult to determine quickly the intended result of a given behavior. A middle-aged patient who seems to be rude, arrogant, and irritating may indeed be rude, arrogant, and irritating. But your interaction with him is likely to be different if you know that his behavior stems from his efforts to test the level of your acceptance of him as a person. Similarly, it makes a difference if a nurse knows that the antisocial behavior of a 9-year-old is directed not toward keeping her *away* but toward getting her attention and drawng her toward him because he gets minimal attention from the staff when he is quiet and good.

By deliberately suspending judgment until a behavior has been more fully examined, you prevent nontherapeutic or even harmful responses on your part. It is difficult if not impossible to undo the damage that premature or unwarranted words and actions can do to a relationship.

Responding to Content

Before you can help another person effectively, you must understand his situation and *he must know that you understand it.* It is not enough to be sensitive and fully aware of a person's situation and what he is experiencing; you must be able to convey that understanding to the person you are trying to help.

This understanding, called *empathy,* is the sharing of another's experience, the understanding that comes from placing yourself in his position, "walking in his shoes," trying to view the situation through his eyes. This is an active process in which you ponder such questions as: "What would it be like to become a widow?" "How would I have felt at fourteen if my father had been an alcoholic?" "If I were the head nurse, how would I cope with that inept staff nurse?"

As you try to identify the reactions you might have if you were you in the other person's situation, it is helpful to recall past situations in your life which were similar in some way to the present one, situations with elements in common with the one you are now considering. You may not have been widowed, but you may have experienced intense loneliness, great loss, or deep feelings of helplessness. You may not have had an alcoholic father, but you may be able to recall the experience of having conflicting feelings of shame and loyalty toward a person close to you.

While trying to analyze how you might feel in the situation, try to understand what the situation may be like for the person already in it. You may not know that person well, but using your knowledge of people you do know well makes it possible to predict with some degree of accuracy what he may be feeling. For example, although you may not yet be well acquainted with a particular 17-year-old male patient, you probably are acquainted with a number of other 17-year-old boys. You are likely to know at least a few teenagers from similar cultural, socioeconomic, and geographical backgrounds; and you have studied the developmental tasks and stages of that age group.

With all these data as a base, it is possible for you to describe several ways in which the situation might affect this patient who is still a stranger to you and to anticipate ways in which he might respond. As you interact with him, your empathy and understanding will become more accurate and sensitive. This understanding must then be put into words because *empathy is not very helpful to the patient unless he is aware of it.* It is true that some understanding can be conveyed nonverbally, but most of the time, it is words that help us gauge the depth of another's concern and caring.

Your verbal response to the patient must be genuine. If, in a rare situation, a patient's situation is beyond your comprehension, it is not helpful for you to pretend you understand. A phony, false response is easily detected by a patient, and will undermine your credibility and hinder the development of a trusting relationship. It is better to say something like "I've never experienced anything like that and it's hard to imagine what it must be like for you. But if you can describe it a little more, I'll try to understand enough to help you."

The response with which you try to convey to the patient your understanding of his message should *rephrase the patient's message precisely but in different words.* Using the very same words sounds parrotlike. An effective response might begin "In other words . . ." or "You are saying that . . ." Finally, the response should be free from unnecessary details so that the message of understanding is clear and easily understood.

Responding to Feelings

As you try to understand what the patient is experiencing and what the experience means to him, you will become increasingly aware of his feelings. This understanding of his feelings must be shared with the patient just as you shared your understanding of what he had told you about the situation or experience (Fig. 9.4). Empathy and understanding of the experience are conveyed by rephrasing what the patient has said; understanding of the patient's feelings is conveyed by using words that are precisely *interchangeable* with the ones the patient used. These words can be likened to very specific synonyms that express not only the same category of feeling but the same intensity of feeling. Skill in selecting and using interchangeable words rather

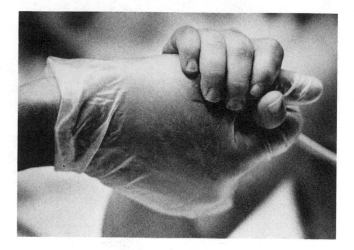

Figure 9.4 *Sharing feelings promotes the understanding which is necessary for effective communication.*

than the patient's own words shows the patient that you listened carefully and understood; he knows you are not merely parroting his words without thinking.

A careful assessment of the patient is needed before the nurse can select a truly interchangeable word that matches both the *category* of feeling and the *intensity* of the feeling. For example, if a patient says he is angry, you need to determine how angry he is before you can select a response that indicates an understanding of his feeling. The words *furious* and *annoyed* are both related to the category of anger, but furious indicates a high intensity of anger, whereas annoyed denotes a relatively mild feeling of anger. Therefore, *furious* and *annoyed* cannot be used interchangeably for angry.

A patient may be unable or unwilling to describe his feelings verbally, making it necessary for you to deduce the nature of his feeling from his nonverbal messages. You can usually relate his nonverbal cues to some major category of feelings, such as anger, fear, confusion, happiness, sorrow, helplessness, and strength. This tentative, initial assessment is shared with the patient, and he is then able to confirm or deny its accuracy. A simple restatement can communicate an understanding of feelings. A more complete statement that puts those feelings into context and states the feeling plus the reason for the feeling conveys a greater understanding.

It sometimes seems *risky* to respond to a patient's feelings because we cannot predict the outcome and tend to fear the worst. Fear of not being able to handle the situation, of the patient losing control and shouting or crying, causes some nurses to retreat to a position of safety in which the patient is encouraged to exercise self-control, restraint, and discipline, to be polite and brave and not give in to his feelings. Such emphasis on suppressing or repressing feelings will result in a *superficial* calmness that is neither helpful nor healthy for the patient.

You cannot help a person unless you understand both his situation and his feelings. It is true that, as you help him explore his feelings, he may express them more fully and may begin to cry or seem to get increasingly angry. With help, however, he will be able to work through these feelings, resolve the situation, and move on to a higher level of well-being.

The helping process can occasionally be demanding and exhausting. Nurses often feel drained and depleted, as if they have nothing left to give. At such times, you will need to seek renewal from whatever source is most helpful to you, whether it be friends, music, art, physical activity, or meditation. This process of restoration is similar to that needed after vigorous physical activity, but the need for it is sometimes less obvious and thus often ignored. You will need to develop support systems and identify sources of renewal early in your career, so you can maintain a high level of psychological health and well-being.

Patients need help coping with their feelings *as quickly as possible* because a person experiencing strong emotion cannot attend to anything else (Fig. 9.5). If he is expending all his energy in dealing with his emotions, he may be unable to comprehend or respond to many of the messages directed at him. A person who is panic stricken, extremely angry, or sobbing with grief, for example, cannot concentrate on things outside himself. Therefore, his feelings must be dealt with *before* he can be expected to attend to business matters, learn about his condition, or plan for the future. The same is true of happy feelings because intense joy, the thrill of achievement, or the excitement of a special event can momentarily block a person's ability to concentrate on anything else.

A person experiencing a strong emotion must be given time to cope with that emotion before he is expected to start another task. The amount of time needed may vary from a few minutes to a few days or weeks or even longer. The amount of help needed will also vary. One patient may need only someone to listen; another may need help in identifying and verbalizing the feeling and even more help in deciding what action, if any, needs to be taken.

Clarifying the Patient's Meaning

As the patient explains his position or makes a point, there will be statements you do not understand or fully comprehend. As future interactions rest on a clear understanding of what the patient has said, the nurse must provide ample opportunity for *clarification*. This is usually not at all difficult if two potential stumbling blocks are recognized and prevented.

The first block is an occasional reluctance on the part of the nurse to admit that she does not understand what the patient has said. This may happen if the patient's occupation or background has led the nurse to feel that she "ought" to be able to understand or that it is her fault if she does not. This might happen if the patient has been stereotyped by a single label, such as lawyer, nursing supervisor, priest, or professor.

The nurse may also be reluctant to admit she does not understand when the patient is using words she fears may have a connotation that might prove embarrassing. The nurse may be reluctant to ask the meaning of some street terms, for example. It may seem risky; but no matter how difficult the task, the patient must be given the opportunity to clarify his meaning because he has a *right to be understood.*

A second block to clarification occurs whenever a patient feels that he is being criticized for not making himself clear. This will happen if your request for clarification is carelessly made or poorly stated. If you phrase a request for clarification in terms of *your own need,* however, there is less chance that the patient will feel criticized. Such phrases are: "I'm not sure I understand. Do you mean that . . . ?" or "It would help me if you could give me an example," or "Would you explain to me the difference between . . . and . . . ?" These accepting, nonjudgmental phrases produce very different results from critical remarks such as "You are not making yourself clear" or "You haven't made much sense so far." Blocks to clarification can be averted if the nurse values an accurate understanding of the patient's meaning enough to verbalize her need for clarification.

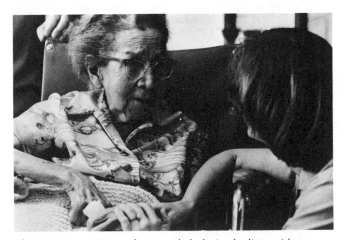

Figure 9.5 *A patient often needs help in dealing with strong emotions which interfere with health and well-being.*

Some of the ways a nurse can ask the patient for clarification include:

- Asking for additional information
- Asking for examples or illustrations
- Asking the patient to identify similarities and differences
- Asking the patient to restate or rephrase what he has said
- Identifying any points that seem incongruent or inconsistent and asking for clarification

When seeking clarification by any of these means, it is important to remember that the patient may be unable or unwilling to use certain words or phrases. For example, a patient might be talking about his forthcoming exploratory surgery and mention the word *tumor*. The nurse, knowing that the physician has talked with the patient about the possibility of cancer, might ask the patient if he is afraid the surgeon might find *cancer*. The patient may act flustered and tonguetied and be unable to say the word even after the nurse has spoken it; but the nurse will have enabled him to nod or otherwise acknowledge his fear and will have opened the way for further discussions.

Some patients are unable to use a word with strong emotional or sexual overtones. In such cases, the nurse will need to say the word and let the patient merely indicate whether or not it is the right one. She may also need to put into words for the patient any negative or angry feelings he may have about the staff, the hospital, or his family. Any nurse can probably remember instances in which she was grateful when someone put into words what she was feeling, enabling her to say, "You said it; I didn't." *Clarification must be done by the patient* because he is the only one who really knows what he means, but *the process is initiated and encouraged by the nurse.*

Validating Your Own Perceptions

Even after the patient has clarified his meaning, it is not safe to assume you completely understand him. You must put into words your understanding of his meaning, must state your perception, so that he can say, "That's right," or "No, that's not what I mean." This process, called *validation,* communicates your present level of understanding to the patient. If your understanding is adequate, the conversation can proceed; if not, the patient has an opportunity to explain further what he means or what he is feeling before a serious misunderstanding arises.

One aspect of validation, called *owning,* refers to the practice of stating that the perceptions to be validated are one's own, that one accepts them or owns them. Therefore, a validation statement often includes an "owning" phrase such as "as *I* see it," "if *I* understand correctly," or "let me see if *I've* got this right." The phrase often used in groups is "I'm only speaking for myself." The advantage of an owning phrase is that it helps to distinguish between a statement of understanding of the patient's feelings or ideas and a premature labeling of the patient. There is a difference between saying, "It seems to me that you are afraid," and saying, "You're afraid," before it is possible to be certain.

Asking Questions

The type of questions asked influences the amount and type of information received. A *narrow* question that focuses the patient's attention on a narrow segment of his life will obtain a specific bit of factual information. Questions such as, "How much do you weigh?" and "Do you know how to test your urine?" elicit one- or two-word answers. A *broad* question, on the other hand, will evoke an idea, a viewpoint, or an explanation. Examples of broad questions are: "What part of weight control is hardest for you?" and "Would you tell me how you test your urine?" Broad questions yield some factual information plus some even more important data about the patient's attitudes, level of understanding, and feelings.

The type of question asked is influenced by the *purpose* of the question. When the question is asked for the purpose of obtaining specific information, such as during an admission interview, a health assessment, or a medical history, narrow questions are appropriate and necessary. During the process of therapeutic communication, broad questions are more effective. A good rule to follow is this: Whenever possible, avoid asking questions that can be answered by a single word, including *yes* and *no.* It takes no longer to ask a broad question, and yet you obtain so much more information. It is worth noting that, once a satisfying communication process has been established, the patient is likely to give a great deal of information, regardless of the type of question asked.

In addition to avoiding yes–no questions whenever possible, the nurse should avoid leading questions. A *leading question* is one that implies the "correct" or acceptable answer. Because the answer is predetermined by the person asking the question, the question is pointless, for most people tend to give the expected answer whether it is true or not. Examples of leading questions are: "You certainly can take your own bath, can't you?" "Now, you surely aren't going to cry and upset your daughter again when she comes this afternoon, are you?" "You really weren't going to eat that candy bar, were you?"

LEADING QUESTIONS SERVE NO USEFUL PURPOSE. The answers obtained are often not true or valid, and the question endangers the patient-nurse relationship by putting the patient in a position in which it may seem preferable to lie. Leading questions reflect the bias of the person asking the question, often contain a veiled threat, and tend to coerce some patients into a specific response or behavior.

Using Silence

Although silence is initially a difficult technique to use, it is so valuable when used with sensitivity that it very quickly becomes worth all the effort required to become proficient in its use. Types of silence range from awkward pauses to thoughtful intervals and long periods of comfortable, companionable silence. The latter types of silence require a relatively relaxed and trusting relationship. Before this has developed, silence may occur because a person cannot think of anything to say, refuses to talk, or is unable to talk because of nervousness or anxiety. Such situations are difficult for the nurse because it is often hard to differentiate between the patient who wants to talk but is unable to, and the patient who can communicate but chooses not to. The latter instance creates a dilemma for the nurse because, while she is trying to develop a therapeutic relationship with the patient, she must at the same time respect his right to remain silent.

Silence, when mutually acceptable to both parties, is valuable because it permits thoughtful analysis of what is being said, gives a person time to collect himself during a stressful interaction, and allows time to think through an important or difficult response rather than blurt out the first thing that comes to mind.

It is hard for many people to learn to use silence consciously and deliberately as a tool. You may find it helpful to pace yourself in the acquisition of this skill by gradually increasing the length of your silences. If you have a tendency to break a silence as quickly as possible, try counting. When the first silence occurs, slowly count to 5 before saying anything. On subsequent occasions, count to 6, then 7, and continue until you can tolerate a silence of 15 seconds. A 15-second silence may seem as long as eternity, but over the years, with continued practice, you will be able to use silences of 30 seconds or more to increase the effectiveness of your nursing interactions.

You need to remember, of course, that, although you may feel comfortable with silence, the patient may be acutely uncomfortable. If so, you will need to mod-ify the use of silence or help the patient learn to be more comfortable with it, because silence is useful only when it is *acceptable to both parties.*

Confronting

In ordinary usage, the word *confrontation* sometimes denotes an angry conflict. It is often used to describe an assertive position in which one faces the reality of a situation. In the context of therapeutic communication, the word is used somewhat differently: *confrontation* is somewhat like holding a mirror up to a patient so he can see himself as you see him. It is the process of helping him see that his verbal and nonverbal messages are not congruent with each other, that they are inconsistent. For example, incongruence would be evident in a patient whose posture, facial expression, and gestures indicate depression and sadness while he brightly says that he feels "just fine."

Whenever there is a discrepancy between a patient's verbal and nonverbal messages, the *nonverbal message is more reliable.* A person has little or no control over nonverbal responses such as blushing, fainting, trembling lips, sweating palms, or shaking hands. Since these responses are not easily manipulated, they are likely to be more accurate than a verbal response. Therefore, whenever you find that verbal and nonverbal messages are not congruent, it is usually safe to *trust the nonverbal ones.* Confrontation is done in a gentle, concerned way, with no hint of criticism or censure. The discrepancy is noted in a matter-of-fact but caring manner that invites the patient to explore the discrepancy with the nurse, such as: "You say you are not nervous, but your hands are trembling and you look ready to cry."

Describing Behavior and Avoiding Labels

The ability to separate the *behavior* from the *person* who exhibits the behavior makes it possible for the nurse to discuss a situation without making value judgments about the person or using labels that may hurt him. It is one thing to say to a child, "Your room needs to be cleaned," and quite another to pass judgment on that child by saying, "You are so sloppy." The latter statement is destructive to the child's self-esteem and is not helpful because it provides no guide for action.

A statement that describes the behavior in question sometimes includes a search for understanding, such as, "It is really important for you to force fluids. Is there a reason why your intake is lower today?" This approach will have a very different effect than a statement such as, "You know you should drink more, so why are you so uncooperative?"

Labeling often takes place in the hospital during a change-of-shift report when nurses tend to take short-cuts in talking about patients. A nurse might carelessly label a patient depressed, uncooperative, or confused without describing the behavior she observed which would have verified and substantiated her one-word description. This label is likely to be remembered and repeated during the next change-of-shift report, with the result that subsequent nursing care may be based in part on someone's preconceived and biased idea about the patient rather than on an assessment of the patient's present behavior.

In addition to the detrimental effect on both communication and nursing care, *labeling is dangerous when charting is being done* because it is hard to substantiate. The patient's chart is a legal document, and every nurse is accountable for what she has written. A statement such as "patient continues to be uncooperative" is open to many interpretations and would be difficult to defend in a law suit. On the other hand, a precise description of the patient's behavior can be factual and defensible if enough detail is provided. Examples of such descriptions, though incomplete when out of context, would be: "Patient ate a candy bar from the vending machine while fasting for a diagnostic test," and "Refused all 10 AM medications on the ground that she 'feels better without them.'"

Labeling is obviously detrimental when the label is negative, but it is equally dangerous to use a positive label indiscriminately. A patient can be deprived of important nursing interventions if he is labeled "very cooperative" rather than being more accurately described as a frightened person who acquiesces with all suggestions, complies without question, and often fails to ask for medication when he needs it. A patient who is labeled "good" may be easy to care for, but his care is not likely to be professional until his responses and behavior have been assessed and interpreted.

Using Feedback

Feedback in therapeutic communication is used in the same way that it is used in any system: to determine the state of the components and relationships within the system and to provide the data that will allow the system to maintain a steady state or to move in a specified direction. For example, feedback may cause you to think: "Everything is going well, so I can keep using this approach awhile longer," or "Something is wrong; I feel as if we are talking *at* each other rather than *with* each other."

Receiving Feedback

The feedback you *receive* may be either solicited or unsolicited. Solicited feedback is obtained when it is ac-tively sought from a patient or a member of his family. You may want to know, for example, whether or not a given nursing interaction was effective. When seeking this kind of information, the questions need to be phrased so that it will elicit specific feedback; otherwise, the feedback may be so general it is meaningless. If you want to examine whether or not you listened and observed effectively, for example, you could ask: "Were there any times when you thought I wasn't listening?" "Did you try to tell me anything you don't think I heard?" "Were there things I failed to observe?" The value of specificity can be illustrated by contrasting the feedback from the above questions with the limited feedback likely from a vague question such as "Were things OK when we were talking today?"

Unsolicited feedback is sometimes nonverbal. Even so, it is usually fairly easy to differentiate between positive and negative feedback, although it may not be possible to identify the cause immediately. You may be able to tell, for example, that something is wrong, but not know whether the cause is boredom, fatigue, bad manners, medication, or a hot, stuffy room. Regardless of the cause, the feedback is valuable because it indicates that a change is necessary.

In addition to feedback from others, the *feedback that comes from within oneself* can be invaluable. Intuition, feelings, and physiological responses can provide strong and accurate information that, if acknowledged, will indicate either that the communication is effective or that some changes should be made.

Giving Feedback

The feedback a nurse gives can be given spontaneously or in response to queries from the patient. In any case, it must be given to let the patient or family member know whether to continue a course of action or change it. The patient or family member may seek feedback from the nurse for a variety of reasons: the nurse may be the only person available; the patient may trust the nurse and value her opinion; or he may be so anxious that he seeks feedback from every person he meets. Regardless of his reason for asking, the feedback given should be sensitive and helpful.

Positive feedback is usually no problem. It is easy and satisfying for the nurse to let a patient know that he is doing well, that she understands and empathizes with him, and that she respects him and feels comfortable with him. Considerable thought must precede negative feedback, however. Negative feedback to the patient is often most effective when it is stated in terms of the nurse's *own reaction* to the patient's behavior. Feedback phrased "I am confused about . . ." "I get nervous when you . . ." or "I feel angry when I see . . ." allows the patient to draw his own conclusions about the effect of his words or behavior and is less threatening than statements such as "You make me nervous" or "You make me angry." Such statements are often referred to as *I statements* and *You statements.*

There are times when a *skilled* therapist or nurse must give frank and honest feedback that may be momentarily hard and hurtful for the patient, but the nurse's interaction with the patient will usually be less intense than that of a therapist, and her feedback will usually help without hurting. Diplomacy, tact, caring, and genuine acceptance help in phrasing negative feedback in a supportive way.

TAKING ACTION

The initial phase of therapeutic communication is directed toward the development of trust, rapport, and understanding. Empathy and acceptance of the patient's feelings and ideas will make him feel better for the moment, but without *action* there is no change in the situation that caused the initial distress or discomfort. Merely sharing feelings is not enough. The first phase of a therapeutic interaction is followed, therefore, by the second phase, the action phase or working phase. (In some instances, this terminology is a bit misleading because, if the patient initially rejects or mistrusts you, you may actually work harder, spend more time, and expend more energy during the first phase than during the second phase.)

The action that is eventually taken should be directed by the needs and desires of the patient, although it is influenced by input from the nurse, the health team, the family, and other relevant people. The nurse's knowledge and expertise are essential in helping the patient to develop and implement a course of action; but if such action is to be meaningful and truly helpful to the patient, it must have its origins *within the patient.* Effective action cannot be imposed on the patient from the outside by another person, no matter how knowledgeable and competent that person may be.

At the onset, and at intervals throughout the action phase, you will need to ask the patient, "What can I do to help?" or "What would be helpful to you right now?" Such questions enable the patient to indicate his perception of his current needs which will help you decide where to start in the situation. The patient may say anything from "Just stay with me" to "Please talk to my mother (husband, physician) for me." The request may be appropriate or unreasonable. In any case, the request gives you additional cues as to how the patient views his situation.

The action phase of therapeutic communication can be encouraged and guided by the nurse, but it is usually not appropriate to give advice or tell the patient what he ought to do. The giving of advice implies that the advice giver has the answer or solution to a problem, and this is not usually true, especially in the early stages of problem solving. There is no single right answer; the patient must select for himself what seems to be the best solution in light of all the circumstances. The nurse should *assist the patient in obtaining the information needed for an informed decision* and help him as necessary with the decision-making process, but must remember at all times that the patient has a fundamental right to the freedom of choice, including the choice of doing *nothing* about an apparently distressing situation.

EVALUATING YOUR VERBAL RESPONSES

Throughout the process of therapeutic communication, you are in a position either to enhance or to interfere with its effectiveness. Your responses, both verbal and nonverbal, are crucial and should be evaluated from time to time.

Evaluating the responses you made during a professional interaction will identify the areas in which you were most effective. You will also be able to examine areas in which you feel you either failed to respond, or responded inappropriately or less effectively than you would have liked. Such an evaluation will give direction to your efforts to increase your expertise in therapeutic communication.

Process Recordings

To evaluate an interaction, you will need a tape recording or written transcript of the conversation. This will enable you to analyze your responses in the context of what the patient said and did. This transcript should be a *verbatim account* of the conversation; if not taped, it must be written as soon after the interaction as possible, while the words are still fresh in your memory. Most people are not accustomed to recalling the exact words of a conversation, and it is difficult to do so at first; therefore, your first process recording should encompass only a 3-to-5-minute segment of a conversation. As your skill increases, you will be able to recall much longer interactions with considerable accuracy.

One format for writing a process recording consists of three columns in which you record what the patient said and did, what you thought and felt at the moment, and what you then said or did. By reading across the columns, you will be able to analyze each of your responses in relation to the events that prompted you to make the response.

```
┌────────────────────────────────────────────────────────┐
│  Process Recording                                      │
│                                                         │
│  What the patient    What I thought    What I said      │
│  said and did        and felt          and did          │
└────────────────────────────────────────────────────────┘
```

Each entry in the *first column* should state precisely what *you saw and heard.* In addition to an accurate recording of the patient's words, notations regarding the patient's facial expression, gestures, tone of voice, sighs, and silences should be included.

The content of the *second column* should indicate *what you thought and felt* and will be influenced not only by the patient's message but also by your reaction to the message. This column should include the thoughts you were thinking as you formulated your response and also mention your feelings of pleasure, anger, panic, curiosity, embarrassment, or whatever influenced the forthcoming response.

The *third column* should record *what you said and did.* In addition to your verbal response, it should include any nonverbal responses such as, "I was too embarrassed to answer, so I just kept on making the bed"; "I put my arms around her shoulders and held her close"; or "I was so nervous I had to leave the room."

Evaluation of the Process

Once the interaction has been recorded, you can examine it for both process and content. With respect to the *process,* you might ask the following questions:

- Were my responses prompted by the patient's words or actions?
- Was I really listening and observing?
- As I reread the process recording, can I identify cues I missed or ignored?
- Did the patient hear me? Were his words and actions based on what I had just said or done?
- In retrospect, were my thoughts and feelings in line with what I had just seen and heard, or were they inappropriate because I failed to pay attention?
- Is there a flow of ideas and feelings between the patient and myself, or is the interaction disjointed and choppy, like a series of unrelated exchanges?

Evaluation of the Content

In addition to examining the relationships within the conversation, the actual *content* of your responses should be analyzed. One way to do this is to evaluate the sensitivity of each response.

- A *sensitive* response is understanding, accepting, and helpful
- A *neutral* response is neither hurtful nor very helpful
- A *nonsensitive* response lacks understanding and is hurtful and rejecting

Sensitive Responses

A response is *sensitive* if it focuses on the patient, promotes understanding of his feelings and ideas, and conveys the nurse's acceptance and understanding. Examples of sensitive responses would be:

- Picking up and following (or at least acknowledging) the patient's cues, both verbal and nonverbal
- Accepting the patient's feelings and ideas as valid and important and using them as a basis for further interaction
- Encouraging the patient to begin or continue to express his feelings and ideas
- Attempting to put into words your own perceptions of what the patient seems to be feeling and saying, and then acknowledging these perceptions as your own
- Waiting for a validation of your understanding before adding your own ideas, feelings, or advice and before proceeding to another point or topic
- Asking questions to better understand what the patient thinks and feels rather than just to get specific factual information

Neutral Responses

A response is *neutral* if it focuses on the routine activities or social niceties of everyday life and results in maintenance of the status quo. Examples of neutral responses are:

- Giving a simple reminder or direction such as "Be sure to drink lots of fluids" and "You can turn over now so I can rub your back"
- Giving a direct answer to the patient's request for information without pursuing the topic
- Referring to policy or rules and giving reasons in a neutral, noncritical way
- Giving an explanation
- Asking a factual question
- Stating what you will do (or try to do) about a problem

Nonsensitive Responses

A response is *nonsensitive* if it focuses on a problem or issue instead of on the patient, denies the importance of the patient's concerns, or conveys rejection of the patient and his feelings and ideas. Examples of non-sensitive responses are:

- Ignoring or missing the patient's cues, verbal or nonverbal
- Responding only to the literal meaning of the patient's words
- Denying the validity and importance of the patient's questions and statements; indicating that the patient's ideas or feelings are wrong, inaccurate, inappropriate, undesirable, or unimportant
- Criticizing; saying, "You shouldn't . . ." "Don't . . ." "You are always . . ." or "You never . . ."
- Giving advice or your own point of view *before* it is asked for
- Assuming that you understand the patient's feelings and ideas and not validating your understanding
- Changing the subject; shifting focus from the patient to other people, things, or events
- Arguing
- Defending behavior of self or staff before focusing on the concerns of the patient
- Rejecting the patient's ideas, actions, or feelings

Checking Your Progress

To evaluate the responses on the process recording, it may be helpful to assign a numerical value to each response: 1 for a hurtful response, 2 for a neutral response, and 3 for a helpful response. To assign a value to a response, it is necessary to *relate that response to the patient's last response*. Unless you know what preceded your response, you cannot evaluate it accurately.

You can total the values you assign to your responses and divide by the number of responses to obtain an overall, or average, score. The score for your first process recording is apt to be a 2 or less because nurses and other helpers who have not had prior training in therapeutic communication tend to make responses that are not helpful. With practice grounded in theory, however, the level of sensitivity rises quite rapidly.

The level reached depends somewhat on the level at which the person started. A person who normally argues, criticizes, or gives advice freely might have an initial score of 1. A subsequent score of 1.8 or better would indicate significant progress because the level of sensitivity has risen from hurtful to nearly neutral. The responses may not be helpful yet, but they are no longer hurtful. Eventually, the scores will move from neutral

into the sensitive range. An initial score between 1 and 2 can be disheartening, but unless you come from an unusually sensitive, expressive, and verbal family, you may have had no opportunity to learn this type of skill. Most people, before training, do not have a repertoire of sensitive responses readily available.

INDIVIDUALIZING THE COMMUNICATION PROCESS

Many aspects of the communication process have been studied and researched, and general principles have been derived that explain, at least partially, the dynamics of effective communication. As a result, *communication skills can be learned, refined, and expanded*. There is, however, no set of rules or techniques which will always yield predictably good results. Each nurse must integrate the principles of effective communication into her own patterns of human interaction and create an effective way of communicating with patients that is natural, genuine, and satisfying for her.

PATIENT TEACHING

The stress felt by many patients and their families is increased by inadequate communication skills. If conversation in the home has usually been casual or superficial, they are likely to be unable to talk with each other about pain, fear, discouragement, or death. If family members are unaccustomed to saying "I love you" to each other, they may need much help in learning to do so during a crisis or terminal illness.

Some families can learn from the nurse as she engages in therapeutic conversation with them, but others will need to be taught consciously and deliberately. It will be necessary to explain the importance and benefits of open, direct, and honest communication, and you will need to give them feedback about their progress.

It is important to note, however, that some patients and families are *unable* to change their long-standing patterns of communication within a short period of time, even though they may want to do so.

RELATED ACTIVITIES

1. The single most common communication problem for most inexperienced nurses is that of giving advice too freely. For at least a week, change your initial response *every time* you are tempted to advise another person. Substitute a comment such as "Tell me a little more about it" or a question such as "What ideas do

you have about things that could be done?'' for the advice you were inclined to offer, and note the effect of such a delay in advice giving on both yourself and the other person.

SUGGESTED READINGS

Almore, Mary G: Dyadic communication. *Am J Nurs* 1979 June; 79(6):1076–1078.

Benderly, Beryl Lieff: Dialogue of the deaf. *Psych Today* 1980 Oct; 14(10):66–77.

Carlson, Robert E: *The Nurse's Guide to Better Communication.* Glenview, IL, Scott, Foresman and Co, 1984.

Christo, Shirley: A nursing approach to adult aphasia. *Can Nurse* 1978 Sept; 74(8):34–39.

Diaz-Duque, Ozzie F: Overcoming the language barrier—advice from an interpreter. *Am J Nurs* 1982 Sept; 82(9):1380–1382.

Duldt, Bonnie Weaver, Kim Giffin, and Bobby R Patton: *Interpersonal Communication in Nursing.* Philadelphia, Davis 1984.

Ekman, Paul, Wallace V Friesen and John Bear: The international language of gestures. *Psych Today* 1984 May; 18(5)64–69.

Ferszt, Ginette G, and Phyllis B Taylor: The patient's right to cry. *Nursing 84* 1984 March; 14(3):65–67.

Forsyth, Diane McNally: Looking good to communicate better with patients. *Nursing 83* 1983 July; 13(7):34–37.

Goleman, Daniel: Can you tell when someone is lying to you? *Psych Today* 1982 Aug; 16(8):14–23.

Grasska, Merry Ann, and Teresa McFarland: Overcoming the language barrier—problems and solutions. *Am J Nurs* 1982 Sept; 82(9):1376–1379.

Hein, Eleanor C, and Maribelle B Leavitt: Providing emotional support to patients. *Nursing 82* 1982 June; 12(6):127–129.

Holderby, Robert A: Conscious suggestion: Using talk to manage pain. *Nursing 81* 1981 May; 11(5):44–46.

Knowles, Ruth Dailey: Building rapport through neuro-linguistic programming. *Am J Nurs* 1983 July; 83(7): 1010–1014.

Mitchell, Ann Chappell: Barriers to therapeutic communication with black clients. *Nurs Outlook* 1978 Feb; 26(2):109.

Morgan, Rosemary Hrubec: Breaking through the sound barrier. *Nursing 83* 1983 Feb; 13(2):112–114.

O'Sullivan, Ann Lawrence: Privileged communication. *Am J Nurse* 1980 May; 80(5):947.

Piotrowski, Marcia M: Aphasia: providing better nursing care. *Nurs Clin North Am* 1978 Sept; 13(3):543–554.

Platt-Koch, Lois M: Soap opera: catalyst to communication. *Am J Nurs* 1984 Oct.; 84(10):1244–1246.

Ramaekers, Sister Mary James: Communication blocks revisited. *Am J Nurs* 1979 June; 79(6):1079–1081.

Richardson, Karolee: Hope and flexibility—your keys to helping OBS patients. *Nursing 82* 1982 June; 12(6):65–69.

Scheideman, Jean M: Problem patients do not exist. *Am J Nurs* 1979 June; 79(6):1082–1083.

Steffee, Donna Rae, Karen A Suty, and Primo V. Delcalzo: More than touch: Communicating with a blind and deaf patient. *Nursing 85* 1985 Aug; 15(8):36–39.

Summers, Ann: Billy was totally unresponsive. *Am J Nurs* 1979 July; 79(8):1262–1263.

10

Teaching and Learning

Prerequisites and/or Suggested Preparation
Suggested preparation for this chapter includes Chapter 1
(Nursing as a Profession) and Chapter 9 (Communication) or the
equivalent content from another source.

TEACHING AND LEARNING

Teaching is the process of facilitating learning. It is a deliberate, intentional action undertaken to help another person learn to do something he presently cannot do.

Learning means that a person becomes capable of doing something he could not do before. Learning results in a wide range of behaviors, from motor skills to intellectual skills. A person is said to have *learned* when he can explain, discuss, demonstrate, make, or prepare something by using some set of ideas, motor skills, or both.

The thing to be learned may be called an objective, a goal, or a purpose. Whatever the term, it indicates the nature and focus of the learning. In most instances of effective learning, the objectives are developed by *patient, family, and nurse working together.*

Teaching as a Process

Teaching is but one aspect of the teaching-learning process, and it is an artificial separation to speak of either teaching or learning in isolation. Teaching is a *two-way interaction;* and in general, any one-way communication is not teaching.

Teaching is a process which is similar in many ways to nursing process, and the teacher may describe the activities in terms of assessment, planning, intervention, and evaluation.

The first step in teaching is the *assessment* of the learner, the teacher, and the teaching situation. Data must be collected about the learner's ability to learn, his physical and psychological readiness to learn, his medical and nursing diagnoses, his physical condition and prognosis, the treatment regimen, his attitude and motivation. This information is all needed to describe or diagnose the specific patient teaching situation accurately.

During the *planning phase,* input from the patient that was obtained during the assessment phase is used in making preliminary plans, which are then discussed with the patient. The patient's input is reflected in the goals and objectives that will direct the teaching. During this phase, outcome criteria are established that will enable the nurse and patient to evaluate the effectiveness of the patient teaching.

The *intervention phase* of teaching includes all the activities of teaching, such as demonstrating, explaining, and using group discussion and printed materials.

The *evaluation phase* of teaching enables the nurse to determine the effectiveness of her teaching as measured in terms of the objectives and criteria. She can evaluate the patient's learning to date and, depending on the outcome, make additional assessments, and provide for additional teaching or remedial teaching as needed.

PURPOSES OF PATIENT TEACHING

In accordance with the Patient's Bill of Rights and recent court decisions, the patient has the right to know enough about his diagnosis, treatment, and prognosis to make informed decisions, to participate effectively in his own care, to protect himself from complications, and to seek a higher level of health for himself and his family.

The purposes or goals of patient teaching may be divided into three major categories: to promote health, to prevent illness, and to cope with illness. These categories often overlap.

To Promote Health

Teaching to promote health includes all teaching that helps to improve the quality of life, furthers optimal physical and psychological growth and development, increases self-esteem, and promotes self-actualization. Examples of such teaching would include teaching a young mother about the importance of sensory stimulation for her infant, teaching a family about the relationship between communication patterns within the family and the mental health of each member, and teaching a group of parents about the significance of each stage of growth and development.

To Prevent Illness

Teaching to prevent illness helps to eliminate or reduce preventable illness, discomfort, and misery. Examples of such teaching include genetic counseling, helping people decrease the possibility of stress-related illnesses, and efforts to prevent obesity, drug abuse, and adolescent pregnancies.

To Cope With Illness

The patient and his family need to learn how to participate in any prescribed nursing and medical regimens and how to live with a condition that cannot be cured or relieved. The patient and family may need to learn how to promote satisfying interactions with a dying person, how to live with the residual paralysis of a stroke, how to prevent complications such as infection or contractures, or how to cope with problems such as mental illness, alcoholism, child abuse, or mental retardation.

AREAS OF PATIENT TEACHING

The patient and his family need and have the right to acquire the *knowledge* and *skills* that will enable them to function at an optimal level despite the limitations or restrictions of their current situation.

Knowledge

The knowledge needed may be divided into three areas: (1) Knowledge of the patient's physical and mental condition (2) Knowledge of the health care delivery system and (3) Knowledge of the patient's immediate environment.

Knowledge of the Patient's Condition

In general, the patient and his family have the right to know as much as desired about the patient's condition. The amount of material presented and the manner of presentation will depend on the age, ability, interest, and condition of the patient and family, and the information must at all times be accurate, honest, and understandable.

With respect to the patient's condition, there are at least six major areas of concern about which most patients seek information and about which they should be knowledgeable: (1) language and terminology, (2) anatomy and physiology, (3) diagnosis, (4) prognosis, (5) therapy, and (6) predictable events.

LANGUAGE AND TERMINOLOGY. The patient needs to understand the words and abbreviations relevant to his situation. This knowledge is necessary for effective communication and for adequate understanding of subsequent teaching.

ANATOMY AND PHYSIOLOGY. The patient can participate more fully in his own treatment regimen, whether it is preventive or therapeutic, if he is knowledgeable about his body and its functioning. The nurse cannot assume that the patient and his family understand basic anatomical and physiological concepts, because many people are woefully ignorant about their own bodies. Sometimes this lack of understanding is apparent even from a casual observation, such as the announcement by a patient in the waiting room of an orthopedic surgeon that she needed to have an operation to "fix the cartridge in my knee." It was evident that the woman knew little or nothing about the structure of her knee in general, or about cartilage in particular. One of the difficult tasks of teaching is to assess how much the patient already knows and to determine what knowledge is necessary for adequate understanding and cooperation on the part of the patient.

Among other things, the patient needs to know the normal values for relevant measurements and laboratory tests, as well as the norm for his own condition, if he is to understand and to some extent interpret the changes in his own condition. For example, he needs to know both the range of normal blood pressures and his own pattern of readings to understand the significance of his latest blood pressure.

DIAGNOSIS. Except under unusual circumstances, the patient needs to know the nature of his illness or condition. If a diagnosis has not yet been made, he needs to know the name and purpose of the diagnostic tests and the outcomes or results as soon as they are available. It is usually the prerogative of the physician to give this information, but you can support the patient and encourage him to seek the information he needs if his physician does not volunteer it.

PROGNOSIS. Once the diagnosis has been made, the patient needs to know what it will mean to him, what the outcome is liable to be, and what is likely to happen to him in the days that lie ahead. The nurse may need to help him put his concerns into words so that he can discuss them with his physician. An open, honest, and frank discussion will relieve the patient of unwarranted worry and will enable him to make realistic plans for the future.

In some situations extensive teaching may be needed by one or more members of the family before they can accept the patient back into the family system, especially when the patient's prognosis necessitates extensive or difficult adjustments in family relationships.

TREATMENT. The patient and his family need to know:

- That they have the right to accept or reject treatment that is offered
- What the alternatives or other options are
- What the outcomes might be, both with and without treatment
- That a second opinion may be desirable (and that it will be paid for by some insurance plans)
- The meaning of informed consent

Before the patient and physician or nurse agree on a treatment regimen, the patient needs to know the anticipated or hoped for results; the nature of any risk, side effects, or adverse reactions; and the cost in terms of time, energy, money, and discomfort. The patient needs to know the name and dose of any drugs prescribed, as well as possible side effects and incompatibility with other drugs, alcohol, or foods.

PREDICTABLE EVENTS. One of your greatest contributions to the patient is your ability to provide anticipatory guidance. "Forewarned is forearmed" is as true in the area of patient teaching as in any other aspect of life. The patient who knows what to expect is better prepared to cope with a given situation than the patient who is taken by surprise by fairly common events or happenings. For example, most patients need to know in advance the nature and probable duration of discomfort after surgery, and that it is important to help a spouse anticipate the changes in behavior that accompany the various stages of dying.

The process of teaching about predictable events varies from patient to patient. Some patients are future oriented and are able to read about or discuss events that may not happen for a number of weeks or months. Other patients learn best at a time closer to the event. They are not as concerned about what *will* happen as they are with what is happening *now*. In either case, the nurse's task is to help the patient and family explore and cope with situations that, although understandable and predictable, are unique and unknown to this particular patient and family.

Knowledge of the Health Care Delivery System

The patient's need for knowledge of the health care delivery system is related to his need for psychological safety, his need to belong, and his need for self-esteem. You can help satisfy these needs by teaching the patient those things that will help him feel confident of his ability to manage himself within a vast and often impersonal system. The nurse's teaching should include material related to four areas of concern to the patient and his family: (1) Personnel (2) Organization and structure (3) Routines and procedures (4) norms and expectations

PERSONNEL. First of all, the patient needs to know the name and the role or position of each person with whom he will be directly involved. The person who is entering a large teaching hospital for the first time needs to learn the difference between an intern, a resident, and an attending physician as well as the difference in role of the medication nurse, the treatment nurse, the floor nurse, and/or the primary nurse.

ORGANIZATION AND STRUCTURE. The patient often needs to learn the relationship of one agency to another or one department to another. He needs to know what resources are available within the community, and what the routes of access are.

The nurse may need to interpret the role of a given member of the health team and clear up any misconceptions before the patient is able or willing to use the service that is available. The patient may not accept the services of the medical social worker, for example, if he believes that social workers are "for poor people who can't pay their bills."

ROUTINES AND PROCEDURES. On occasion, the nurse may be the person who explains complexities of the health care system, interprets or cuts through the red tape and policies of the agency, and assures the patient that certain restrictive requirements are routine and not personal.

NORMS AND EXPECTATIONS. The nurse may need to help the patient learn what he can expect of the staff and what the staff expects of him. There will be less irritation, frustration, and misunderstanding if expectations are openly expressed and discussed as needed. For example, a patient may feel angry or distraught because the clinic physician does not tell him the details of his condition and therapy. The physician's position may be: "I'll tell him anything he wants to know, but he never asks, so I assume he knows as much as he wants to." You may need to teach the patient how to seek the information he desires.

Much knowledge about norms, expectations, and limits can be gained through trial and error or by observation, but in many situations the patient can acquire the needed knowledge more quickly and effectively if you deliberately teach him those things that will enable him to *participate effectively in his own care.* This is especially true of children and adolescents, who tend to be more assertive in their search for norms and limits and who may unintentionally irritate or alienate the staff in their efforts to discover what is expected of them and what they, in turn, can expect of the staff. People who are passive, shy, or unsure of themselves often need extra help in this area.

Knowledge of the Immediate Environment

The security and safety of the patient are closely related to his understanding of his current environment. He needs to know: (1) the nature of any real or potential hazards (2) the name and location of things and places and the time when various events will occur and (3) the details of routines and procedures that involve him

Skills

In addition to *knowledge* about his condition, the health care delivery system, and his immediate environment, the patient needs to learn a number of *skills* to feel

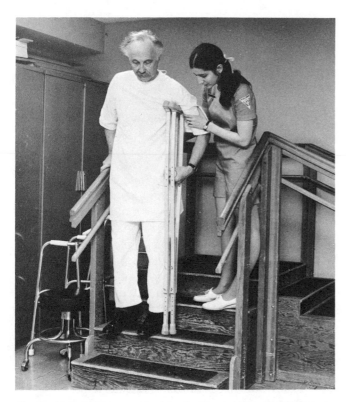

Figure 10.1 *Before a patient is discharged from the hospital, he must be taught the skills necessary to manage at home.*

competent and maintain his self-esteem (Fig. 10.1). He needs to be able to do both those things that are expected of him and those things that he either wants to do or feels compelled to do. These skills include such diverse abilities as being able to read a thermometer, change a dressing, or incorporate a special diet into family meal planning.

TIMES FOR TEACHING

The *activities of teaching* may take place at any time, but *learning* occurs only when the patient is ready to learn. At other times he may listen politely and may even memorize some of the factual material, but he may not learn anything that will help him to improve his health or well-being.

For the hospitalized patient, there tend to be three periods of concentrated teaching: (1) upon admission, (2) at the onset of tests or therapy (including pre- and postoperative teaching), and (3) upon discharge. These are valid times for concern about the patient's needs, but they are *not necessarily* the most appropriate times for effective teaching. The patient's stress level may be so high at these times that he may be unable to do

more than look attentive and listen politely. At such times, patient teaching should be geared toward helping the patient meet his *most basic needs*. He needs to learn those things that will help him cope with his immediate situation, but a time of great stress is *not* an appropriate time for extensive teaching.

The optimal times for more extensive teaching occur when the patient is as physically comfortable and as psychologically relaxed as possible and when he needs to learn how to do something that seems desirable to him. Many nurses use the phrase "the teachable moment." Unfortunately, this sometimes seems to imply that the occasions for teaching are fleeting and spontaneous while in reality, teachable moments can be *created* by the nurse. The skilled teacher recognizes and uses those occasions when the learner is anxious, eager, or "dying to learn," but she is thoroughly capable of creating a situation in which the patient can and will learn those things he deems important for his well-being. The nurse's sense of timing is critical. The mother who is fatigued by the care of a colicky infant or a sick husband may not seem very teachable to a public health nurse who is determined to teach her about immunizations on a given visit. That same mother may be very eager to learn at another time, however, when she is not so tired or distracted.

OTHERS WHO TEACH PATIENTS

The nurse is usually the primary health teacher, but many people contribute to the process of patient teaching. These contributors include physicians and other members of the health care team, friends, families, former patients, and various agencies.

Neighbors, spouses, parents, and grandparents are effective teachers. In fact, the advice and teaching of a respected lay person may at times be heeded more quickly than the teaching of a professional person, especially if ethnic values, folklore, or tradition is involved. These lay people are aware of the patient's value system, lifestyle, and fears and aspirations, so their teaching is likely to be direct and relevant. The nurse must expend considerable effort and energy to teach in a manner which is equally relevant and meaningful.

Former patients are able to teach new patients effectively, partially because of their empathy and understanding, and partly because of their enthusiasm and interest in helping another person learn to live with a given condition or disease. Examples of organized teaching by former patients are the ostomy clubs and the Reach to Recovery programs for women who have had a mastectomy.

ASSESSMENTS RELATED TO PATIENT TEACHING

Effective teaching depends on an accurate assessment of: (1) the learner (2) the learner's readiness to learn (3) the teacher and (4) the teaching situation

Assessment of the Learner

To meet the learning needs of a patient, it is necessary to obtain objective data *about* the patient, and subjective data *from* the patient.

Data About the Patient

Objective data that describe the patient can be obtained from a wide variety of sources. Observation of the patient yields information about sex, race, approximate age, general physical and mental condition, and overall capacity for sight, hearing, and speech. The patient's chart or referral form gives the highlights of the patient's medical history, present condition, prognosis, and current therapy. The records or chart may give family composition, occupation, birthplace, and religion. Information on educational background or intelligence may be deduced from conversation with the patient and occasionally from his choice of reading materials.

Data From the Patient

Some of the material most relevant to patient teaching can be obtained or derived only from the patient. His attitude toward learning, his background and motivation, his interest and readiness to learn, and his needs and abilities can be assessed only in conjunction with the patient himself.

Assessment of Readiness to Learn

There are four conditions to assess in determining readiness to learn that are especially significant in the context of patient teaching: comfort, energy, motivation, and capability.

Comfort

The term *comfort* includes both physical and psychological comfort and is closely related to Maslow's hierarchy of needs. Basic physiological needs must be met in order for the patient to be *physically comfortable,* and his security needs must be met for him to begin to feel *psychologically comfortable.* These lower level needs must be met before higher level needs emerge and he is ready to learn.

PHYSICAL COMFORT. Physical comfort implies the absence of those conditions or symptoms that, if present,

would make a person uncomfortable. Six of the most common sources of discomfort are pain, nausea or dizziness, itching, fatigue or weakness, hunger or thirst, and the need to urinate or defecate. The nurse cannot assume that a recent nursing intervention has eliminated a discomfort or that an absence of complaints indicates comfort. The fact that the patient has received medication for his pain does not guarantee that he is now free from pain.

PSYCHOLOGICAL COMFORT. Psychological comfort implies the absence of those emotions that, if present in more than minimal amounts, would make a person uncomfortable. Some of the most common of these emotions are fear, anxiety, worry, grief, anger, and guilt. The nurse may notice behaviors or nonverbal cues that lead her to suspect the presence of one or more of these emotions; but because they are not directly observable, each must be validated. The nurse may need to say something like: "We had planned to discuss your medications this afternoon, but you look worried to me, and it seems hard for you to lie still. Is this a bad time for you to try to learn about your drugs?"

One attribute of a skillful nurse is her *ability to modify her planned intervention on the basis of new data.* If the nurse discovers that her patient is uncomfortable, either physically or psychologically, her most appropriate intervention would be to relieve the discomfort before proceeding wih the planned instruction. *An uncomfortable person is not ready to learn.*

Energy

Another condition that influences readiness to learn is the amount of energy currently available to the learner. Human energy is finite; it is not unlimited. If large amounts of either physical or psychic energy are currently being expended, there may be none available for learning. The amount of energy available for learning is closely related to the patient's physical condition, his reaction to his stage of illness, and the current number of stressors in his life.

A patient who is literally fighting for his life in a critical care unit has no energy for anything else. A person who is actively denying his illness has little energy for learning about that illness. An elderly person who has just been moved from his home to an extended care facility is likely to have little energy in excess of what is needed for the adjustments to an entirely new lifestyle. In some situations the amount of energy available for learning may increase rapidly, within a few days; in other situations, it may take a few weeks or even months for a noticeable increase in energy to occur.

A person's energy is also affected by his body rhythms.

Some people have dramatic peaks of energy during each day in accordance with their circadian rhythms. The person who "doesn't wake up until noon" does not learn effectively during the early morning hours, making it frustrating and unsatisfying for all concerned when teaching sessions are scheduled at that time.

Motivation

It is not usually possible to deduce a person's motivation from the behavior he exhibits as he proceeds to meet a given need. We can infer, for example, that a patient who is intent on learning all he can about his condition, treatment, and prognosis is probably highly motivated. But we cannot determine the *nature* of his motivation merely by observing his behavior as a learner. The patient may in fact be unaware of his own motivation; and even if he is aware of it, he may be unwilling to disclose it. The patient may be motivated to learn by a need or desire to get well; to retain a label of "good patient"; to be able to return to work; to please others, especially the professional staff; to manage his own care; or any of a variety of other needs or desires. It is important to resist the tendency to *assume* you know why your patient wants to learn. In any group of eager learners, each of whom is exhibiting almost identical behaviors, there may be as many sources of motivation as there are learners.

The behaviors that result from each of these diverse motivations may be identical. The patient may lean forward, ask questions, take notes, ask for a fuller explanation, seek out the nurse, request books and pamphlets, plus any of a variety of other behaviors that might indicate motivation to learn.

The *absence* of any discernible desire to learn is closely related to a patient's perception of his situation and his expectations for the future. If he presumes that his situation or condition cannot be improved, if his past experiences lead him to believe that no amount of energy and effort is likely to help, he is not likely to be motivated to learn or to participate in his own care. The *possibility of attainment* is an important aspect of motivation; people tend to strive for those things that are real possibilities for them. If a patient rejects the nurse's teaching, saying, "I can never do it anyway," or "Nothing can help me," contact with other people who have successfully mastered a similar condition or disability may increase the patient's perception of the possibility of attainment and, consequently, his motivation to learn.

Capability

Assessment of capability must be made concurrently with or subsequent to the formulation of objectives and the identification of prerequisite skills. In other words, the nurse cannot tell whether a person is capable of learning something until she knows what capabilities *are necessary*, what attributes and abilities *are required*.

Capability is influenced or determined by heredity, age, maturation, stage of development, past learning, physical and mental health, and environment. Some limitations of capability can be alleviated or removed. Inability to read can be remedied by education; inadequate strength, by exercise; and poor eyesight, by eyeglasses. Capabilities dependent on maturation or development cannot be altered. An infant cannot be taught to walk until his muscular, skeletal, and nervous systems are sufficiently developed. A child cannot understand abstract concepts until his cognitive abilities are adequately developed.

INTELLECTUAL AND EMOTIONAL CAPABILITY. There are at least five *intellectual skills* to be assessed in determining whether a learner possesses the intellectual ability needed for the competence he seeks:

1. Basic mathematical skills (for calculating dietary requirements, or reading a thermometer, for example)
2. Reading skills, for reading directions and instructions
3. Verbal skills, for communicating with others involved in care of self or family; for expressing self
4. Problem-solving skills, for assessing situations and knowing when and how to seek help and assistance
5. Ability to comprehend and follow instructions, for ensuring safe, effective care at home

In addition to assessing essential intellectual (cognitive) *skills*, the nurse must determine whether the patient knows the *concepts and facts* necessary for him to understand the new material. For example, does the learner have the basic understanding of the anatomy and physiology of his own body needed to comprehend the nurse's explanations?

A person's past experiences tend either to attract him toward a specified goal or to turn him away from it, and a person's *attitudes* and *value system* often exert powerful influences on his readiness to learn. For example, it would be helpful to assess whether a patient with hypertension appreciates and values the importance of keeping his hypertension under control before you try to teach him about the prescribed treatment.

PHYSICAL CAPABILITY. If the patient is to learn or acquire a psychomotor skill, four aspects of physical capability must be assessed:

1. *Size.* Are the patient's height and weight adequate with respect to the task and equipment involved?
2. *Strength.* Does the patient have the strength to follow the prescribed regimen?
3. *Coordination and dexterity.* Can a patient with a pronounced tremor of his hands measure his liquid medication safely, for example?
4. *Senses.* Is the patient able to see, hear, smell, taste, and feel well enough to learn the designated task?

Once you have assessed the various aspects of capability, you will be able to decide whether or not the learner is capable of learning the new material or acquiring the new skill. In some instances the objectives may need to be revised to accommodate some limitation of the learner's ability. In other situations preliminary teaching, treatment, exercise, or other intervention is needed to overcome a learner's limitation or deficit. In rare circumstances you may find that the proposed objectives are completely unrealistic in light of the learner's capability and that entirely different goals must be set. Difficult as this may be, it is better to discover the discrepancy between expectations and capability as the result of careful assessment than to discover it as a result of the learner's failure to reach the stated objectives.

Most assessments of readiness to learn must be done quickly if the nurse is to be able to do any teaching within the limits of a home visit, a clinic appointment, or an 8-hour shift in an acute care setting. Readiness must be assessed before each teaching interaction because the status and condition of the patient or family may change rapidly from one visit to another or from one shift to another. Some assessment data will remain valid from one teaching interaction to the next, while other data will change. The learner's capability will remain fairly constant, and motivation may change very slowly, but his levels of *comfort and available energy* may change dramatically within a very brief period of time.

Style of Learning

In addition to assessing the patient's physical and intellectual capabilities, the nurse needs to explore the ways in which he learns best. He can probably tell the nurse, for example, whether he prefers to have her start at the beginning and *explain everything*, to merely answer his questions, or to provide him with materials to read.

In addition to his style of learning, the patient's memory and ability to concentrate should be assessed.

MEMORY. Patients are often confronted with a number of things to be memorized, ranging from lists of acceptable foods to the names and dosages of current medications. For some people, this is easy; for others, it is well-nigh impossible. A careful assessment is necessary to identify the patient whose memory is faulty and enable you to modify your teaching methods accordingly.

ATTENTION SPAN AND CONCENTRATION. You will need to determine whether a given patient learns best from a long, uninterrupted teaching session or from a series of short ones. It is also important to identify those people who need a quiet place, free from all distractions, in order to concentrate.

Assessment of the Teacher

It is important to assess the attitudes, knowledge, and skill of the teacher.

Attitudes

Your effectiveness as a teacher will be significantly influenced by your attitudes toward the patient and toward the subject matter. You may have very positive feelings toward a given patient and still encounter difficulties in teaching him because of the nature of the content. Every nurse has some topics with which she is less comfortable, and these discomforts can be significant enough to interfere with effective teaching. For example, you may have no difficulty in teaching a patient who had a heart attack the things he needs to know about the physiology of his heart, and yet have trouble teaching that same patient about the sexual aspects of his rehabilitation.

It is important to identify areas of teaching which are stressful to you, to determine the *basis* for any reluctance or problems in teaching, and take appropriate remedial action. Neither nurse nor patient benefits when a nurse refuses to acknowledge strong feelings that create a block or barrier to patient teaching.

Knowledge

Patient teaching is influenced by the nurse's knowledge of relevant content. Whereas knowledge does not *guarantee* that teaching will take place, it *increases the probability*. An intense commitment to patient teaching almost inevitably leads to increased knowledge because the nurse actively seeks the information needed to teach each patient.

Skill

In assessing your ability to teach, you will be concerned with two kinds of skills: those related to the particular condition or illness, and those basic to teaching. Both are essential. You must be *able to do* whatever it is that the patient needs to learn and, in addition, be *able to teach* him how to do it. For example, the nurse who plans to teach a young couple how to care for their premature infant must first of all be skilled in the care of premature infants and, second, be skilled in teaching nervous, apprehensive parents.

Assessment of the Teaching Situation

Once the learner and the teacher have been assessed, the *teaching situation* should be assessed in terms of resources and support.

Resources

People are without doubt the most important teaching resource. Effective teaching can take place in crowded quarters, with few if any teaching materials *if* the people involved are knowledgeable, skillful, and committed to patient teaching. People likely to prove helpful to the nurse are, first of all, consultants and specialists in the field of nursing. The clinical nurse specialist in cancer nursing, the nurse in charge of the pain clinic, or one of the nurses from the orthopedic unit may help a nurse plan to meet the teaching needs of her patient, for example.

Support

Of all the kinds of support relevant to patient teaching, three of the most important are legal, collegial, and familial.

LEGAL SUPPORT. The nurse practice acts in some states include teaching in the legal definition of nursing. In these states, teaching is not only supported, *it is mandated by law*. It is not an optional activity.

COLLEGIAL SUPPORT. Collegial support refers to the value and emphasis placed on patient teaching by other members of the health care team and by their concept of who should do the teaching. In some settings, much of the formal teaching is done by a patient educator while in other institutions, each nurse is expected and encouraged to teach her assigned patients. A few physicians prefer, and insist upon, teaching their own patients, but increasing numbers of doctors acknowledge patient teaching as a significant nursing intervention.

FAMILIAL SUPPORT. Whenever possible, assess the family support system *before* you begin to plan for patient teaching. Assess the possible effect of the patient's condition on the rest of the family and determine the extent to which the patient depends on other people for some aspect of the behavior you hope to teach. It is both nonproductive and frustrating to spend time and energy helping a patient learn something he can never fully use because of some constraint in his family system. For example, the pregnant teenager may become knowledgeable and motivated to seek adequate nutrition for herself and her unborn baby from state or federal food plans, but be prevented from doing so by a father who, angered by her pregnancy, will not permit her to accept welfare to obtain the food supplements he cannot or will not buy.

The nurse will need to assess the relationship of the patient (the expected learner) to others who may in fact be the more significant learners. If, for example, a family is experiencing a great deal of stress in coping with the care of a parent on home dialysis, the anxiety of a school-aged child and his subsequent behavior may prove disruptive to all normal interaction in the family. In such a situation the child is one of the primary learners, so an essential task of the nurse is to teach the child to cope with his own feelings about his parent's illness and pending death.

Ideally, the nurse should actually meet the various members of the family and assess the varying degrees of support. On those occasions when this is not possible, a beginning assessment can be made by asking a variety of questions such as: "How do you expect your (husband, wife, child) will react to (your diet, your need to be on the first floor, etc.)?" "What kind of changes will this . . . make in your day-to-day routines?" "Who is most likely to help you with . . . ?" Of all the initial data to be collected, information related to the patient's family system is among the most important. Without a basic knowledge of the patient's support systems, patient teaching can be based only on assumptions, which can lead to faulty and ineffective teaching.

The *assessment phase* of teaching is the keystone for subsequent success or failure.

OBJECTIVES AND CONTENT

The process of describing what can realistically be accomplished in a given teaching situation follows a careful assessment of the learner, the teacher, and the situation. The expected outcome is called a goal or an objective. Goals are usually broad and general, whereas objectives are narrow and specific. Goals often represent long-range intentions and aspirations, while objectives usually represent immediate or short-range outcomes, outcomes that are related to a specific learning experience.

Educational Objectives

According to Robert Mager (1962), each educational objective has three parts: the *behavior*, the *conditions*, and the *criteria*. An objective attempts to answer three questions:

1. What should the learner be able to do? (the behavior)
2. Under what conditions should he be able to do it? (the conditions)
3. How well should he be able to do it? (the criteria)

Behavior

The behavioral portion of an educational objective is a statement of the learner's ability to do something at the *end* of the learning experience. Some of these abilities are very narrow and specific, such as the ability to walk with crutches. Others are much broader, such as the ability to maintain a prescribed diet while eating in college dining rooms or restaurants.

To be useful, an educational objective must describe a behavior that can be *observed and measured.* Such an objective is called, appropriately enough, a *behavioral objective.* The objective must contain an active verb, a verb that indicates what the learner will do if he successfully meets the objective. He *may* run a mile, *point* to three objects, *draw* a diagram, *recite* a poem, or *do* any one of hundreds of other actions.

These actions are all observable, in contrast to such activities as thinking, understanding, or knowing. An observable behavior is one that can be seen or heard by another person.

Behavioral objectives are important because they permit feedback about learning. If the learner has met the objectives, effective learning has taken place, and feedback about this achievement serves as a necessary reward and reinforcement for teacher and learner. If the objectives were *not* met, such feedback indicates that the teacher must change either her method of teaching, or the objectives themselves. If a nurse does not have objectives for her teaching, she cannot tell if the patient has achieved the desired or expected learning. The learning cannot be evaluated because neither patient nor nurse has stated what was desired or expected.

Conditions

Most learning results in the ability to perform a task under *one rather specific set of circumstances* but not under others. For example, a child might learn how to ride a bicycle *safely* on the streets of his suburban neighborhood, but he would not be expected to be able to do so on a major highway or through the business district of a large city.

An objective for a freshman nursing student might include the behavior "to feed a patient." If no conditions are stated, the natural assumption would be that she was expected to be able to feed *any* patient. This is unrealistic. She might be able to feed a convalescent patient; but until she received further teaching, she could not be expected to feed an infant who had just had surgery for a cleft palate, a patient who was nauseated from chemotherapy, or a patient whose swallowing reflex was impaired.

It is important to determine the *conditions* under which the patient or family will *actually be doing* the desired activity and then teach for performance under those conditions. The objectives for the learning should reflect that situation. For example, if a patient will be caring for his colostomy in the shared bathroom of his rooming house, that situation needs to be simulated as closely as possible in the teaching. He is ill prepared for discharge if he knows how to care for himself only in the privacy of a well-equipped hospital bathroom.

Many times, the conditions are stated as "givens." The objective may read "Given . . . (the conditions), the learner will . . . (the behavior). For example: "Given regular supervision by a private pediatrician, the mother will . . ." or "Given the assistance of a home aide, the patient's wife will be able to . . ."

Criteria

The criteria of an objective answer such questions as: By what standards? By whose authority? To whose satisfaction? In giving range-of-motion exercises, for example, what constitutes full range of motion: the textbook description? the patient's comfort? the physiotherapist's recommendation?

The criteria also indicate *how well the task must be performed* to be considered acceptable. In a mathematics examination, what degree of accuracy is expected: 100%?, 65%? Some behaviors must always be 100% perfect; for example, there can be *no* deviation or error in sterile technique. At the other extreme, some criteria may rest *within the learner.* Such a criterion may be a learner's comfort or satisfaction, as determined by the learner.

The phrase "according to Hoyle" represents an example of criteria or standards. Just as Hoyle can be designated as the authority for rules of card games, so can other authorities or criteria be designated as the standard of desired performance for any behavior. Many objectives state an authority or standard against which the learner's performance can be measured. The criteria portion of an objective often includes a phrase such as: "as listed in the hospital diet sheet," "as described in the agency manual," or "as demonstrated by the physiotherapist." Sometimes the criteria specify that an acceptable performance must be completed in a certain length of time or in a specified number of attempts.

Ideally, criteria should be written and reviewed with the learner *before* the learning experience. In this way he not only knows what behavior is expected of him but knows the quality of the expected behavior. He knows the basis on which he will be judged and has a standard whereby he can evaluate his own performance. Even if the criteria are not available in written form, they can be communicated orally to the patient with similar results. When the learner knows what is expected of him, misunderstandings or disagreements about achievement are minimized.

Ideally, objectives are written out. This helps to ensure *clarity* (so that each objective will be thought through, clearly and logically), *consistency* (so that the nurse can remember and carry out the plans she has made with each patient), and *continuity* (so that other members of the staff can contribute to the patient's learning when the nurse is not present). In day-to-day nursing practice, there may be many times when it is not possible to sit down and write out objectives, but every nurse can think each one through carefully and develop the skill of formulating objectives mentally.

Mutual Development of Objectives

Time is one of the nurse's most important resources; given that it is often in short supply, it behooves her to use it wisely. One way to do so is to make sure that the objectives for patient teaching are acceptable to both nurse and patient. If the patient participates in developing the objectives, there is usually less question of

their acceptability. This premise must be validated, however, because a nurse represents authority to many patients, who will follow her lead in developing objectives as readily as they will follow directions about a treatment.

A patient may try to be a "good patient" by complying in the hospital with a routine or procedure he has neither the intention nor the ability to follow at home. The patient who agreeably participates in a discussion of low-salt diets may be thinking, "Nurse, you're wasting your time. I live with my sister, and she'll fix the meals just the way she has for the past 25 years." The teaching, in this situation, is a waste of the nurse's and patient's time unless it is directed toward *mutually acceptable* and *mutually significant* objectives.

The patient and nurse must assume joint responsibility for the patient's education. The patient must be an active participant in the educational process, make his needs known, give feedback to the teacher, and participate in the evaluation of his progress and performance. The patient is likely to learn more effectively if he also has an opportunity to participate in the planning, implementation, and evaluation of his learning. Participation includes the development of objectives (Fig. 10.2).

It is usually unwise to permit the patient to assume full control of his learning for a variety of reasons. He

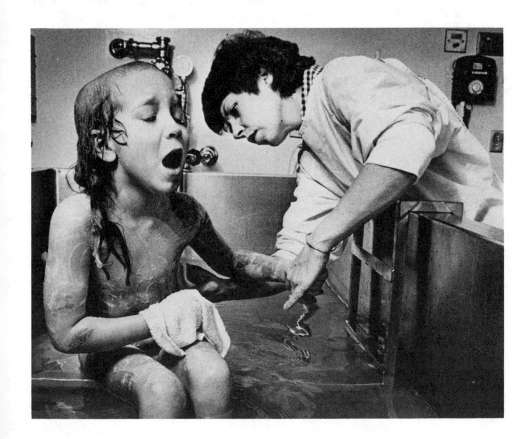

Figure 10.2 Before Renee could go home, her mother had to master her bath procedure. She had to learn how to protect the new grafts, prevent infection, cope with Renee's pain, and manage her own stress.

lacks the knowledge to identify those things about his condition that may be critical or even life-threatening; his psychological status at the moment may interfere with logical thought and planning; or he may lack the energy and motivation to seek learning experiences. In other words, he may be too ill, depressed, upset, tired, or discouraged to try to figure out what he needs to learn to improve his lot. Therefore, it is not fair for the nurse to dismiss her responsibility with the thought, "If he had wanted to know, he would have asked."

The nature of the objectives depends on input from the patient, the physician, the family, the nurse, and any other people who are significant in the health care and family systems. The nurse's input consists of a knowledge of what is *needed* by the patient, and the patient's input consists of what is *wanted* by the patient. Sometimes these overlap; other times, the distance between them is great. Your skill as a teacher will be reflected in your ability to integrate your input and the patient's into a meaningful set of objectives.

You will eventually develop your own approach to this process, but initially you might try the following one: As you conclude the assessment phase, you might say something like this: "You seem to want to learn . . . and . . . From my experience, I can pretty well predict that you will also need to know how to . . . and . . . Given these needs and interests, let's decide where to start. Which ones seem most important to you?"

As you and the patient work to develop a meaningful set of objectives, you may find it helpful to couple the desired behavior with the patient's reason for wanting to learn it. The format "to learn . . . so that . . ." is often useful; for example, "I want *to learn* to use a walker *so that* I can get to the bathroom at home when everyone is at work." If you know the patient's reason for wanting to learn something, you can put that task into a context that may identify a need for more teaching.

Objectives and Continuity of Learning

The fragmentation of our current health care delivery system makes it imperative for the patient to be involved as much as possible in setting goals and objectives for his own learning. He may well be transferred from unit to unit, from facility to facility, and *he may be the only person who is fully aware of his objectives and progress to date.*

A patient may move from an intensive care unit to a progressive care unit, then to a regular medical-surgical unit within the same acute care setting, and then to an extended care facility, and finally home. Despite these moves, the patient and his family may be able to structure for themselves some kind of continuity if they

were involved from the beginning in the setting of objectives. This responsibility for continuity should not be delegated or deliberately shifted onto the patient, however, for it is a *nursing responsibility.* In some places, nurses are actively seeking innovative ways to ensure continuity of teaching as the patient moves from unit to unit and from facility to facility. In situations in which nursing has not yet assumed this responsibility or has not yet implemented an effective plan for doing so, the use of well-stated objectives can help the patient to gain at least minimal control over his own learning.

The opportunities for meeting long-range objectives are severely limited by the shortness of many hospitalizations. To facilitate any long-range teaching, such as teaching the parents of a premature infant, the hospital nurse will need to contact a community health nurse or clinic nurse who may follow the patient. A request for follow-up teaching may be an established part of an agency's referral system and it is important that each referral include the behavioral objectives relevant to the patient's needs and an assessment of his learning to date.

The Domains of Learning

Human behaviors and actions were divided by early Greek philosophers into three domains, and this same threefold division is still evident today. We speak of *knowledge, attitudes, and skills* or of *thinking, feeling, and acting.* With reference to educational objectives, we speak of the *cognitive, affective, and psychomotor* domains or classifications. These domains are significant because the characteristics of learning within each domain influence the selection of teaching methods and the method of evaluation.

A behavioral objective in the *cognitive domain* deals with the recall or recognition of information, and the development of intellectual abilities and skills. Objectives in the *affective domain* describe changes in feeling, tone, emotion, interest, and attitudes and are related to values as well as degrees of acceptance or rejection. The *psychomotor domain* emphasizes muscular or motor skills—tasks that require coordination and dexterity and often some manipulation of materials or objects.

Writing Objectives in Each Domain

PSYCHOMOTOR DOMAIN. Objectives in the psychomotor domain are the easiest to write in behavioral terms because the action is obvious. The verbs are specific, and the behavior is easily observed. Examples of psychomotor objectives are: to give an injection, to walk with crutches, to apply hot packs, to read a thermometer, to bathe a baby.

If a nurse encounters difficulty in teaching or evaluating a psychomotor skill, it may be that the skill she is trying to teach is composed of several component skills, each of which should be taught and evaluated separately. For example, the objective "to breast feed a baby" is composed of at least three subobjectives, each of which needs to be taught, unless it has already been reached. These objectives are: to prepare and keep the nipples in good condition, to handle the baby, and to actually nurse the baby. Each skill is essential. If the mother has never picked up or held an infant, she is likely to need help in doing so before she will be able to position the baby for feeding. Sometimes it is helpful to state a subobjective as follows: "to learn . . . in preparation for . . ." This format indicates clearly that the objective is a contributing objective and makes explicit its relationship to a main objective.

COGNITIVE DOMAIN. Objectives in the cognitive domain are harder to write because you cannot *observe* an intellectual activity or behavior; you can only infer its occurrence from some product that results, such as the answers to a test. You cannot watch a person think or remember or calculate, but you can observe him make a list, take a test, describe an event, or state the facts. Therefore, in writing a cognitive objective, avoid all abstractions such as to know, to realize, and to understand, and use instead a verb that will result in an action or product you can *see* or *hear*. There must be a behavior that can be observed if the objective is to be considered behavioral. Examples of behavioral cognitive objectives might include:

Stating the name and dose of current medications
Describing the characteristics of a 2-year-old child
Listing the seven warning signs of cancer
Describing the safety measures needed for an elderly person who is returning home after fracturing his hip

AFFECTIVE DOMAIN. Objectives in the affective domain are the hardest of all to write in behavioral terms. It is difficult to avoid using abstractions such as to value, to appreciate, and to believe, and to use instead words that indicate a measurable behavior. Mager (1968) uses the concept of *approach* behaviors in writing affective objectives. He uses actions that indicate that the learner is *moving toward* the desired behavior as evidence that the learner is beginning to value it positively, that he sees some worth in it. Examples of behavioral objectives in the affective domain might include:

Verbalizing fears about surgery to parents or nurse
Adhering to prescribed diet

Seeking support from members of a group
Keeping clinic appointments
Complying with medical regimen

As attitudes and feelings are often difficult to change, the learner may seem slow to reach objectives in the affective domain. His progress will be easier to support and evaluate if the behavior in each objective is small enough to accomplish and measure in a relatively short time. An objective that requires a patient to "adopt and sustain a lifestyle compatible with the treatment of high blood pressure" cannot be attained for many months or even years. A more useful objective would be: "to do one thing each day for the next month to minimize the effects of an identified stressor." Both nurse and patient can note progress toward the second objective, and the nurse can modify her teaching as needed to help the patient accomplish it.

Teaching in Each Domain

PSYCHOMOTOR DOMAIN. Teaching in the psychomotor domain usually requires a demonstration plus considerable feedback and opportunities for practice. Elements of the other two domains are usually present in varying degrees, especially in the early phase of learning a psychomotor skill. Initially, the learner needs an explanation—a *cognitive* (theoretical) basis for the motor skill he is to learn. Teaching in the *affective* domain may be needed if he is fearful, apprehensive, or resistant.

Some of the general assessments that must be made were mentioned in the section on assessment of the learner. Specific psychomotor assessments would include an evaluation of strength, dexterity, coordination, and sense of balance. Optimal eyesight must be ensured through good lighting and clean eyeglasses as needed. If equipment is to be used, it should be adjusted whenever possible to the height and size of the patient.

One consideration that is quite specific to the psychomotor domain is that of clothing. In general, the patient should wear comfortable, supportive shoes instead of slippers. Street clothes are preferable to gowns and robes for three reasons: (1) the patient is less likely to become tangled up in folds of a robe or gown, when trying to learn to transfer from wheelchair to toilet, for example; (2) some skills are learned more easily if there are no loose sleeves to contaminate a sterile field or get caught in a mechanical device; and (3) the nurse can more readily evaluate the patient's performance, as during crutch walking, if his movements are not obscured by a robe.

Two more assessments are needed for teaching in

the psychomotor domain: How does the patient feel about learning this skill? and How does he learn best? The way a person feels about learning a motor skill is influenced by his perception of himself as clumsy or adept. The person who views himself as clumsy must worry about the nurse's reaction to his lack of coordination in addition to being concerned about learning the motor skill. Fear of operating mechanical or electrical equipment may range from mild apprehension in some people to near-panic in others, especially if the equipment is attached to a person and there is even the remotest possibility of injuring that person. Some people are very fearful of any procedure involving oxygen. No matter what a nurse thinks of such reactions, she must accept the person's feelings about learning a given motor skill as both valid and significant and provide the support needed as the person tries to learn the task.

The patient's perception of how he learns best is also important in teaching a psychomotor skill. He will probably be able to identify himself as a "tell me" or a "show me" person. A *tell me* person is verbally oriented and often prefers to read a set of instructions for himself and then proceed to follow them. Other people are equally intense *show me* people. Ask your patient how he learns best and how he would like to proceed. His self-knowledge and insights are likely to be most helpful as you prepare to teach a psychomotor skill.

COGNITIVE DOMAIN. Teaching in the cognitive domain usually involves the transmission of information from one person to another person or group of people, commonly through an explanation or lecture, although a variety of media may be used.

The assessments specific to the cognitive domain include an assessment of general intellectual ability plus specific assessments of the abilities needed to reach each objective. For example, an objective that requires an elderly patient to "state the name, dose, and main effects of each drug you are currently taking" might seem reasonable to the nurse but overwhelming to a patient who has not tried to memorize anything in years, especially if he has recently been plagued by a failing memory. He may truly be *unable* to memorize and recite the information. Rather than subject him to the frustration of trying and the humiliation of failing, the nurse may need to teach him to post the information in several places at home and carry it with him at all times.

If a patient seems unable to meet the cognitive objectives, reassess his ability. Confusion or a decrease in level of alertness may be caused by a reaction to drugs or a change in the patient's physical condition. Whatever the cause, the difficulty must be corrected before teaching can proceed; if it cannot be corrected, the objectives should be modified.

AFFECTIVE DOMAIN. Teaching in the affective domain usually seeks to change, or at least modify, an attitude or an emotional response, to create interest, or to develop a tendency to act in a certain way. This kind of change is most likely to be brought about by interaction within a small, supportive group or as a result of an extensive one-to-one interaction with a person who holds the desired attitude or emotional response. Affective learning does *not* usually result from a lecture or an explanation.

Teaching in the affective domain may need to precede teaching in the other two domains, especially in situations in which the learner has strong feelings about the subject or skill to be learned. A person who is in the throes of a strong emotion is unable to attend to anything else until his emotional response has been dealt with.

A change in attitude takes place slowly; it cannot be forced. It is usually futile to try to deal directly with an attitude by confronting the person and asking or demanding that he change his attitude.

Selection of Content

In patient teaching, the content to be learned consists of the knowledge, attitudes, and skills that are needed by the patient to attain the objectives that he and the nurse have established. Content is elusive because it is an abstract concept; strictly speaking, one cannot select content at all. If anyone were to ask a nurse to select the content for teaching a newly diagnosed diabetic, the answer should be, "That's impossible; there is no such thing as the content for a newly diagnosed diabetic!" *Content is derived from objectives,* and objectives are specific to each patient. The needs, and therefore the objectives, are very different for a 7-year-old girl whose care will be managed by her parents, a 16-year-old athlete whose only concern at the moment is the effect that diabetes and "needles" will have on his Olympic aspirations, and a 35-year-old man who is preoccupied with thoughts of complications such as amputation and blindness. There will be some commonalities among the objectives for these three patients, but that does not mean that a nurse could ever arbitrarily select the content for a "newly diagnosed diabetic."

The first step in determining the content for patient teaching is to separate those things that are *necessary* to meet the objectives from those things that are *nice* to know. Professional input can and should be divided into two categories: the content that is *necessary* for the protection, safety, and well-being of the patient and the content that *might be* desirable, informative, and possibly useful. These distinctions often are difficult to make because they change from time to time with a given patient and also from patient to patient. At the onset of an acute illness, the teaching needed may seem very limited in scope and depth, but any more information would be superfluous and unnecessary for the patient's immediate needs. Later on, information that was unnecessary at the onset of the illness becomes very necessary.

For example, the family of a patient admitted to the hospital with a massive stroke does not need to be taught about rehabilitation until it is known that the patient will recover and they are able to look to the future. As the patient and family begin to move toward objectives that are related to physical therapy, speech therapy, and other aspects of rehabilitation, the nurse will need to identify more content, which she again categorizes into what is necessary and what is nice to know. The patient and family need to know how to help prevent contractures of the joints; they do *not* need to know the terms flexion and extension in order to do this (the words bend and straighten will do). Some people will want to know the correct terminology, and they certainly have the right to know, but it not necessary in order to exercise the affected extremities.

Input for the objectives and the resulting content comes from both professional and personal sources. *Professional input* comes from the nurse, the physician, and other members of the health team. *Personal input* comes from the patient and his family.

Professional Input

The nurse's knowledge and expertise, coupled with that of other members of the health team, provide the basis for patient teaching. Without this solid base of accurate, factual knowledge, the content of patient teaching would be flimsy indeed.

The nurse's contribution will be based in part on her own experiences with other patients who have had similar conditions or problems, and in part on the experiences of other nurses, which are available to her through professional journals and textbooks. This information enables the nurse to hypothesize and to predict with a fair degree of accuracy some of the teaching that is likely to be needed by a given patient.

There will be many instances in which neither nurse nor physician will have some of the competencies needed to prepare a teaching plan for a particular patient. In such cases the selection of content for that patient's teaching will be greatly influenced by the contributions of a physical therapist, a nutritionist, a rehabilitation specialist, a psychiatric consultant, or some other member of the health care team.

The phrases *acts of commission* and *acts of omission* might well be applied to the selection and teaching of

essential content. It is easy to see how a nurse could be held liable for an act of *commission* if *inaccurate* information caused a patient to jeopardize his well-being, or if *incorrect* information caused him to do something that had a detrimental effect on his condition. On the other hand, it is equally reasonable that nurse and physician be held accountable for acts of *omission* if they *fail* to give adequate information. Failure to teach a person who is on anticoagulant therapy that he should carry essential information in his wallet could result in grave consequences if he were injured and taken, unconscious, to a nearby hospital for emergency surgery, for example. In some instances the responsibility for failure to teach essential content must be shared by both physician and nurse; in other situations the responsibility must be borne by the nurse alone.

Personal Input

Input from the patient will be based on his desire to know and his fears or concerns, and will indicate what he wants to accomplish and how he expects to cope with his situation or condition. Input from the family will be based on the family's response to the patient's situation or condition and will reveal, either directly or indirectly, some clues to the effect on the family. As members of the family indicate the things they want to know, you will be able to assess the impact of the current situation on the family and discover ways you can teach them to cope more effectively.

Patients differ in their search for knowledge, partly because of their individual reactions to health and illness and partly because of their personal concern or lack of concern for details. The person who never reads the details of a lease, contract, or guarantee may show little concern for the details of a consent-for-treatment form. The person who habitually responds to difficulty or trouble with "I don't want to hear about it" may react in similar manner to information related to his diagnosis, treatment, and prognosis. Other people find considerable comfort and security in the acquisition of knowledge.

The information sought by the patient may be almost identical to the information he needs to know. He may ask, for example, "What are the precautions I must take? What are the possible complications? Are there any side effects to this drug?" In other situations, however, there may seem to be little relation between the information the patient seeks and that which professional people have indicated is necessary. Regardless of similarities and differences, both categories of information are important and must be included. The information the patient *must* know to meet the objectives that have been established plus the information that the patient *wants* to know prescribes the content for patient teaching.

METHODS OF TEACHING

In an ideal situation, the choice of teaching methods would be determined by the objectives and the nature of the material as well as by the number and characteristics of the learners. In real life, the choice of method will also be influenced by the amount of space, time, and other resources available. A large medical center, for example, might have an extensive library of audiovisual materials for patient teaching; but in a small rural setting, a nurse might have to draw her own sketches. Five of the most frequently used teaching methods are: explanation, group discussion, demonstration, role playing, and the use of printed materials. Other methods are discussed in the bibliographic selections.

Explanation

An explanation is perhaps the most frequently used (and abused) method of teaching. *Properly used,* an explanation is given in response to the learner's need, real or potential. When misused, an explanation is likely to be the result of one person telling another person what he must do and why. The content of the explanation may be almost the same in each case, but the approach and results are very different.

An explanation may either be initiated by the teacher in anticipation of the learner's needs or be given in response to a learner's question.

Teacher-Initiated Explanations
The content of a teacher-initiated explanation is selected by the teacher on the basis of:

- Past experience in similar situations
- Observations or assessments made in the present situation
- Agency policy or protocol

When you initiate an explanation, it is important, first of all, to enhance the patient's motivation to learn. This can often be done by establishing a need, or by making an activity seem worthwhile and desirable. It is a mistake, for example, to launch without warning into an explanation of how to cough, turn, and deep breathe after surgery regardless of a patient's interest or to tell him only what will happen if he does not do so. It is more effective to spend a few minutes *describing the advantages* of coughing, turning, and deep breathing, thereby making it a desirable activity: "After surgery, you will be able to . . . and will notice less . . . if you will cough, turn, and deep breathe at frequent intervals."

When you initiate an explanation, assess the following as you proceed:

- The patient's knowledge and past experience—he may, for example, have had three barium enemas before this one, making your explanation unnecessary and repetitious
- His understanding—he may have had three barium enemas before this one but without understanding why they were done or what was indicated by the results
- His reaction—his verbal or nonverbal indications of relief, confusion, interest, and so on will indicate how the explanation should be modified

Explanations in Response to a Patient's Question
The format and wording of the patient's question may give the nurse some clues to the *meaning* of the question to the patient. Questions that ask who, what, where, when, and how are often simple requests for information, although the person may sometimes be expressing his underlying fear, anger, or other emotion through these questions. An explanation is useful if the patient is seeking information; an explanation is of little use if the patient is expressing his feelings.

A question that begins with *why* usually questions the purpose, rationale, reason, or basis for a decision or action. It usually involves values and beliefs and may have a high emotional component. It is important to listen for the underlying concern of questions such as: "Why do I have to. . . ?" "Why does the doctor. . . ?" and "Why do you always. . . ?" The nurse may be tempted to become defensive and offer explanations to justify her behavior or that of the staff when, in reality, the patient may be asking, "Are these things happening because I am critically ill?" or wondering "Are you really competent?" If this is the case, an explanation of nurse or staff behavior is not likely to be as helpful to the patient as an opportunity to discuss his fears would be.

Before giving an explanation, therefore, make sure you understand both the question itself and what the question *means* to the patient. Clarify your understanding of the question, rephrase it, and validate your perception. Sometimes it is advisable to answer the question briefly and then take time to explore the patient's reason for asking it.

In some situations you may choose to end your explanation with a bit of information or a question to stimulate the learner, to whet his curiosity, to give him something to think about and provide the basis for more questions.

It is for some reason you are unable to give an explanation, an honest response such as "I don't know, but I'll find out" or "I'm concentrating on your IV right now—I'll be able to answer in just a moment" conveys interest and encourages future questions.

Before leaving the patient or changing the subject, ask the patient questions such as: "Does that answer your question?" "Does that help to clear it up for you?" "Is there anything else I might be able to explain to you?" This gives you a chance to watch for cues that indicate understanding or the lack of it, such as a gaze of bewilderment or a nod of understanding. You can verbalize these observations to the patient and, based on his response, modify or expand your explanation as needed.

Group Discussion

Group discussion is an excellent method of teaching in the affective domain. In the context of patient teaching, group discussion provides an opportunity for patients and families to share experiences and support each other, and to explore meanings and examine values. Group discussion provides an opportunity for people to learn from each other, to learn from someone "who really knows," from someone with a similar problem, from someone who has found an answer. Groups might be formed of patients who are terminally ill, obese adolescents, parents of handicapped children, or single parents, for example. In group discussion, previously learned material plus some new material is applied and integrated, giving new insights and meanings, and solutions to problems.

Establishing Norms for the Group
It is important to spend a few moments at the beginning of a group session to clarify expectations, describe the schedule, indicate scheduled breaks (have a watch available or designate someone to keep track of time), attend to any cultural or ethnic details, and bring new members up to date. Time spent on introductions is almost always worthwhile in establishing rapport between members, especially if each member describes in a sentence or two his current situation and his reason for being present.

Promoting Discussion
The discussion can be initiated by presenting a predictable problem, something your experience has found to be common to many patients and families. You might present a hypothetical situation for discussion or merely

state, "I have found that many patients experience . . ." This approach may seem safer and less threatening to a new group than exposure of a personal situation or experience. In some situations, you can stimulate discussion with questions such as "What do you expect will happen if. . . ?" and "What do you anticipate will be the hardest part of. . . ?" When the members of the group feel safe and secure enough with each other, individual members will spontaneously bring up for discussion problems they have encountered, or report on developments in their situations since the last meeting of the group.

You can promote discussion by reading the verbal and nonverbal cues as the discussion progresses and by encouraging wide participation while respecting each person's right to remain silent and listen. Use caution in calling on specific people, because a person may be too deeply involved to be able to participate at a given moment. Encourage people to seek clarification and validation from each other and to express their empathy and concern openly. Reinforce desired group behaviors, and refocus attention and discussion as needed.

Evaluating the Discussion
Whenever feasible, it is desirable to have the group spend a few minutes evaluating the outcomes. A few questions such as "What happened in our group today?" "What did you learn today?" or "In your opinion, what was the important thing that we discussed today?" will usually help members of the group to identify the significant aspects of the session. By comparing the responses of the group with your objectives for the discussion, you will be able to estimate the effectiveness of the interactions.

Demonstration

Demonstrations range in complexity and scope along a continuum from a spontaneous "Here, let me show you" through a planned, more formal demonstration. A spontaneous, spur-of-the-moment demonstration is neither better nor worse than a carefully planned and executed one; the choice depends on the situation. You cannot afford to miss an opportunity for teaching by delaying until you have had time to plan a demonstration, but neither can you afford to give a formal demonstration using a casual approach or a spontaneous one.

This method of instruction to help the patient acquire a skill that will enable him to maintain his own health, participate in his own care, and care for himself or others. The skill may be manual or interpersonal. The demonstration of a manual skill, when followed by a practice session, effectively combines the learning

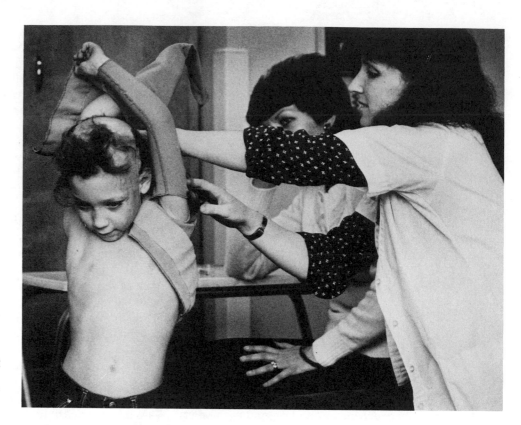

Figure 10.3 *Therapist Gabby Liddard teaches Renee's mother how to help Renee into the jobst which will help minimize scarring by exerting a constant, even pressure on the grafted skin.*

that occurs through hearing, seeing, touching, and manipulating (Figs. 10.3 and 10.4).

A demonstration may also be used to orient a person to a procedure or process. The nurse may demonstrate, in advance, a treatment the patient will soon experience or show him what will happen during a forthcoming procedure. The opportunity for the person to *see* and *handle* any equipment that will be used results in much greater learning than merely being told about it. Such demonstrations may be given to an individual patient or a group of patients.

Spontaneous Demonstrations

A spontaneous demonstration is a nursing intervention that responds to a person's need to learn how to do something *at once*. The nurse may notice a person's frustration at being unable to complete a task, or a person may ask for help in doing something. A new and urgent need may suddenly have arisen as a result of a change in the patient's condition or situation.

If a demonstration is needed, show him what he *currently needs to know* and then plan an appropriate follow-up, rather than overwhelm him with more than he can handle at the moment. A spur-of-the-moment demonstration may involve a sense of urgency that makes it difficult for the learner to absorb as much as he might in a less hurried situation. If you are not able to do the follow-up teaching yourself, you can describe

the need for additional teaching in a referral to another agency.

Planned Demonstrations

PREPARING IN ADVANCE. To prepare for a demonstration in advance, practice both the demonstration and the verbal explanation as needed and decide where you will place equipment, how you will dispose of waste materials, how you will open containers, and so on. It is most disconcerting to find oneself in the middle of an otherwise smooth demonstration with both hands full and the cover not yet unscrewed on the next piece of equipment to be used.

Assemble the equipment and do the demonstration or procedure in the way it will be currently experienced or used by the patient. It may be necessary to delay a demonstration until the actual equipment to be used is available, until you can visit the patient's home, or do whatever must be done to make the demonstration relevant to the people involved.

Decide how to present the rationale and the reason for each action. Depending on the characteristics of the learners, you may teach by rote memorization, by inquiry, or by some approach midway between the two. For example, you might: (1) teach *the* way to do the task (2) teach *one* of many ways, or (3) help the learner devise *a* way to accomplish the task. A child, a very

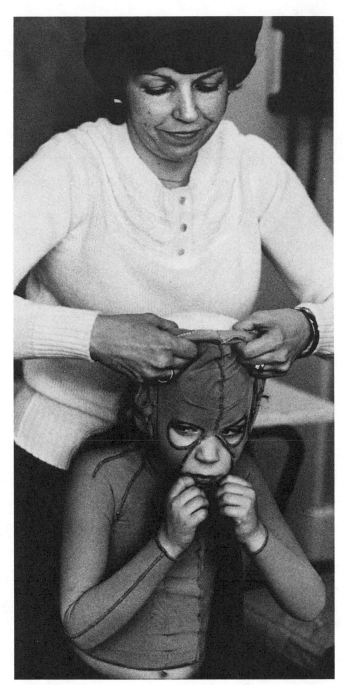

Figure 10.4 Renee's mother demonstrates her ability to apply the jobst because such a return demonstration is an effective method of evaluating the learning which has taken place.

anxious person, or a retarded person will probably learn more effectively from a simple, direct, structured approach that says, "This is the way to do it." With this approach, there is no confusion or ambiguity.

An intelligent adolescent, however, may do better with an introductory demonstration, followed by an exploration: "What would be the best way for you to accomplish the same thing?" When using the latter approach, you will need (1) to be open to a variety of answers from learners, some of which may seem very unorthodox and (2) to thoroughly understand the underlying principles of physics, microbiology, physiology, or whatever is needed to evaluate the safety and effectiveness of the learner's proposed method of doing the task.

Decide in advance how you will manage the transition from your initial demonstration to a satisfactory *return demonstration* by the learner. In some situations it will be feasible for you to demonstrate an activity and for the learner to repeat the demonstration at once. In many other situations the first and last demonstrations will be separated by a number of other sessions that are characterized by a gradual decrease of participation on your part and a gradual increase in learner participation.

The number of demonstrations needed will depend on the capability of the learner, the type or complexity of the skill to be acquired, and the level of learner competency required.

DEMONSTRATING. Whenever possible, it works well to run through the procedure or demonstration rather quickly to give an overview and enable the learners to get a sense of what is to be learned. The nurse should, of course, mention that a slower, more detailed demonstration will follow.

DEMONSTRATING AGAIN. In a more detailed follow-up demonstration, make clear to the learners whether you are showing them *the* way (for example, how to keep an object sterile) or *one* of many ways to do something. The repeat demonstration would also include an expanded explanation giving a more complete rationale for each action than was given the first time.

If the task is complex or anxiety producing, try to repeat the demonstration a third time, this time, directing the learners to interrupt as needed and encouraging them to ask questions.

ARRANGING FOR PRACTICE AS NEEDED. If the task involves sterile technique, it is usually helpful to let the learners handle the unsterile equipment until they are thoroughly familiar with it. For example, the nurse can let a diabetic patient manipulate an unsterile syringe and needle and get the feel of it. The need to be dexterous with sterile equipment from the very beginning places an unnecessary double burden on the learner—that of learning to maintain sterility while learning to manipulate the syringe at the same time.

ARRANGING FOR A RETURN DEMONSTRATION. Having the learner do a return demonstration allows you to assess his performance and evaluate his skill. You can evaluate his understanding by assessing his ability to recognize and correct his own errors, and by his ability to correct errors that you point out.

ENSURING TRANSFER OF LEARNING. Help the learner anticipate possible problems and reasonable solutions. Ask him, "What would you do if. . . ?" and help him work through any problems you can predict he might encounter. If he is in a hospital, ask him to have his own equipment brought in to him so he can practice with it before discharge. As soon as he is thoroughly comfortable with the task, discuss the maintenance of equipment, the purchase of replacement parts, and possible substitutes in an emergency. Give him any available printed materials which he can use to review at a later date or to supplement your teaching.

Occasionally, you may be caring for a patient or family who cannot tolerate extensive preparation or formal instruction. In such a situation, integrate the necessary demonstrations into other nursing interventions, showing in a seemingly casual way how to do one aspect of the necessary skill at a time.

Role Playing

Role playing occupies a unique place among teaching methods and strategies. On one hand, it seems simple and spontaneous, very much like the pretend play of childhood. On the other hand, it is a complex and powerful way to facilitate learning. *Role playing* may be described as a brief, usually spontaneous interaction in which several people play out roles that are assigned but unrehearsed. Both the players and any others in the group usually become deeply involved.

Role playing provides an opportunity for learners to explore alternative ways of acting or responding in a situation to see how others might do something, to hear how various responses sound, and to practice a new behavior in a safe and supportive setting. Role playing also may be used to promote involvement in a situation, to evoke an emotional response, to give a common basis for discussion, or to focus a generalized or diffuse discussion.

The cues and possibilities for using role playing are often subtle and easily missed, but you will find opportunities for role playing with increasing frequency as you become aware of patient comments or statements that suggest a need for working through a situation or a problem. For example, the statements "I don't think I could do that" and "I could never do that" often indicate a *need to test out a new behavior* or *to prepare for a future event*. Role playing gives people an opportunity to act out and cope with the fantasies that will emerge in response to the question "What might possibly happen if you. . . ?" Role playing gives the learner an opportunity to plan ahead and to be prepared with several possible responses to the worst things that could possibly happen in a given situation. It gives a learner a chance to figure out ways to handle a variety of possible responses to possible reactions of others.

Some role-playing situations will involve only you and your patient as you help him practice a new behavior or test a new approach to a difficult situation. Sometimes you will use role playing as you teach the patient's family or a small group of patients and families. When more than two persons are involved, the following steps will usually increase the effectiveness of the role playing.

1. The first step in role playing is to describe the situation briefly. Next, describe the roles, giving age, sex, and relationships of players, and ask for volunteers. In almost every situation, someone will volunteer for each role. It may even be the most unlikely person because there is a certain safety in playing the role of someone else, and it provides a chance to do or say things one never would in real life.

2. Once players have been designated, give any necessary directions. Very few are needed, and they usually are given to all players within earshot of everyone. Have the players move close together. No props are needed, and there is no script, of course. You may want to clarify briefly or review the purpose and intent of the role playing and tell the group what to look for.

3. Stop the action after 5 to 6 minutes, sometimes less, rarely more. Stop the action at a logical pause, at the conclusion of a specific interaction, as soon as any conflict seems to be resolved and while interest is high. Do *not* let the role playing die and the action peter out, because attention and interest will drop and the desired learner involvement will cease.

4. Use the role-playing experience. Much learning occurs immediately after role playing, especially if the teacher follows the suggestions listed below.

   a. Ask each player to describe his feelings; they may or may not have been expressed freely or accurately in words during the role playing. The audience needs to hear such comments as "I was furious, but I didn't feel I had a right to . . ." or "I felt so scared of her that I couldn't think of anything to say."

b. Ask the audience to describe their feelings about the interaction and the feelings the scene evoked. For example, a member of the audience might say, "I felt like I did when I first heard that Carrie had leukemia." It is important not to rush; this period may give a person an opportunity to express feelings that have up until now been difficult to verbalize.

Printed Materials

Depending on the learner, printed materials may be used in three ways: (1) in lieu of other forms of teaching (2) to supplement other media, and (3) to stimulate review at a later time. The usefulness of printed materials depends on the characteristics, condition, and needs of the patient. There are three important guidelines for using printed materials:

1. Do not *assume* that the patient can read. It is tragic, but true that some high school graduates are unable to read above a third or fourth grade level and that there are large numbers of functional illiterates in this country. People are often adept at concealing this deficiency, so careful detective work may be necessary. Watch for behavior such as: the gracious acceptance of a brochure or pamphlet, which is then set aside to be "read later"; rapid or cursory attention to the material; an unusually long time spent "looking" at the material; books and magazines in the room that are apparently never read and may be there for appearance only; and *vague* responses to questions about his reaction to the material you have given him. Granted, these behaviors may be noted in people who are highly literate, but the appearance of several in the same patient might signal an inability to read.

2. Do not *assume* that the patient can see well enough to read. An older person may be literate, but his eyesight may have failed so much that he is now unable to read. He may have left his glasses at home if it was an emergency admission to the hospital. His eyeglasses may need to be changed; or he may need glasses, surgery for cataracts, or treatment for glaucoma. The patient may tell you this, or he may exhibit behaviors similar to those listed for the patient who cannot read.

3. Evaluate the reading level of the proposed materials. A careful assessment of both patient and the available printed material should enable a nurse to match the learner to the appropriate educational matter. During the course of conversation, ask him what he likes to read. The fact that one patient reads *The National Enquirer* while another reads *The New York Times* is more significant than the fact that both are high school graduates.

In addition to readability, the nurse needs to evaluate printed materials for style and format. If the style is dull, the type is small, and the page appears crowded with words, the patient is not likely to read the material.

PATIENT TEACHING

It is important for every person to understand that he is responsible to a large measure for his own health, and that in order to fulfill that responsibility, he must acquire the necessary information and skills. Persons who are eager to learn must know that they have a *legal right* to be taught those things which are significant to the outcome of their condition. Persons who are *passive* recipients of health care need to be encouraged to become active participants in decisions related to their health and well being, and to begin to seek information related to those decisions.

All individuals and their families need to be taught how and where to get information, and ways to evaluate the source and accuracy of the information obtained.

RELATED ACTIVITIES

Scarcely a week will pass that you will not find something in a newspaper or magazine that will help you to teach. A picture or an article may describe a situation that will provoke discussion, give an example of a hard-to-teach concept, or explain an abstract idea in simpler terms than you had thought possible.

These items, saved over the years, are almost useless if dumped in a box or drawer but are invaluable if filed for easy access. No matter how extensive a personal collection of educational materials may become, it will be of little use if you cannot locate the materials easily or, worse yet, do not even know or remember what you have. The following suggestions are helpful in developing a rich and useful file of educational materials.

1. Decide on a filing system. As soon as you begin to collect materials, decide how you will catalog them. You might categorize by disease, by nursing diagnosis, by categories used in various nursing indexes, or by a system of your own devising. The type of system used is less important than the fact that you have one.

2. Clip and collect materials. Keep a pair of scissors handy and cut out pictures and articles from magazines, newspapers, old textbooks, and advertising brochures. Save news of clubs, organizations, and agencies your patients and their families might contact for help.

Make copies of materials you cannot cut out. Save articles related to research on subjects of interest to you. Save pertinent book reviews and selected bibliographies on topics such as explaining death to children. The items you save may be single pictures or printed matter ranging in length from a few sentences to a long article. Send for reprints such as *The Reader's Digest* series on the various organs and systems of "Joe's Body."

3. Sort and file the materials. For an investment of $12 to $15, you can buy approximately 100 manila folders, enough to last for many years. As you file each item, it is important to date it and indicate its source. Such information is necessary when you periodically clean and sort your file and when you want to seek more information on the subject.

4. Use the materials. Refer to the materials for your own information; share them with patients; make copies to use in preparing booklets or pamphlets for your patients; share the items with colleagues as the occasion arises.

5. Sort and discard at intervals. Set aside an evening every month or so to file your most recent acquisitions. It is important to discard materials, as well as to save them. If you spend an afternoon once or twice a year discarding outdated or unwanted materials, your files will always be in usable condition and will be an asset in your professional career.

SUGGESTED READINGS

Billie, Donald A ed.: *Practice Approaches to Patient Teaching.* Boston, Little Brown, 1981.

Byrne, T Jean, and Dorcas Edeani: Knowledge of medical vocabulary among hospitalized patients. *Nurs Res* 1984 May/June; 33(3):178–181.

Claytor, Kaye: If you need a patient-ed booklet. *RN* 1984 July; 47(7):57–61.

Doak, Cecilia Conrath, Leonard G Doak, and Jane H Root: *Teaching Patients With Low Literacy Skills.* Philadelphia, Lippincott, 1985.

Levin, Lowell S: Patient education and self care: How do they differ? *Nurs Outlook* 1978 Mar; 26(3):170.

Loughrey, Linda: Dealing with an illiterate patient . . . you can't read him like a book. *Nursing 83* 1983 Jan; 13(1):65–67.

Mager, Robert F: *Preparing Instructional Objectives.* Belmont, California, Fearon, 1962.

Mager, Robert F: *Developing Attitudes Toward Learning.* Belmont, California, Fearon, 1968.

Murray, Ruth, and Judith Zentner: Guidelines for more effective health teaching. *Nursing 76* 1976 Feb; 6(2):44–53.

Narrow, Barbara W: *Patient Teaching in Nursing Practice.* New York, Wiley, 1979.

Rankin, Sally H, and Karen L Duffy: *Patient Education: Issues, Principles, and Guidelines.* Philadelphia, Lippincott, 1983.

Rankin, Sally H, and Karen L Duffy: 15 problems in patient education and their solutions. *Nursing 84* 1984 April; 4(4):67–81.

Redman, Barbara K: *The Process of Patient Teaching in Nursing.* ed.5. St. Louis, Mosby, 1985.

Schulman, Steven: Facing the invisible handicap (learning disability). *Psych Today* 1986 Feb; 20(2):58–64.

Timely Teaching (continuing education feature): *Am J Nurs* 1985 July; 85(7):797–812.

    McHatton, Maureen: A theory for timely teaching.

    Miller, Eleanor, Barbara B Blumberg, and Blake Brown: What do patients know about clinical trials?

    Waidly, Erika: Show and tell: Preparing children for invasive procedures.

    —————— The SMOG readability formula.

11

Principles of Physics Relevant to Nursing

Prerequisites and/or Suggested Preparation
There are no prerequisites to this chapter.

During the early part of this century, only the physician was expected to take the patient's temperature and blood pressure; nurses were not considered capable of using a thermometer or blood pressure cuff and stethoscope. Today, nurses are involved in the use of complex and sophisticated equipment such as cardiac monitors, kidney dialysis machines, respirators, and pacemakers. Nurses participate in the use of laser beams, radiation therapy, fiber optics, and ultrasound technology.

Nursing has long been recognized as both an art and a science, and rapid advances in medical and non-medical technology now demand an increasing emphasis on science, especially physics. For example, nursing will inevitably be involved in space travel and colonization, and a nurse responsible for the well-being of space travelers and settlers will need to know the effects of weightlessness on circulation and blood pressure, and how to manage IV fluids in the absence of gravity.

Selected principles from physics which are critical to an understanding of many nursing procedures are introduced in this chapter. These principles have been grouped into a single chapter to reduce the need to explain each principle each time it is mentioned in a subsequent chapter. Concepts related to nuclear radiation are included in Chapter 26 and concepts related to osmosis and filtration are included in Chapter 31 (Fluid and Electrolyte Balance).

FLUID FLOW

A critically ill patient is often described as having "tubes coming out in all directions," a description that may be literally true. A patient could, for example, have tubes in his stomach, trachea, urinary bladder, peritoneal cavity, subclavian artery, and a major vein. His nurse must know the purpose of each tube, as well as how to adjust the flow of fluid to or from his body through each tube. The basis for such knowledge is an understanding of the principles of fluid flow.

Since tubes are used to transport fluid from one place to another, their effectiveness depends upon the rate at which fluid flows through the tube. The rate of flow depends upon (1) pressure which forces fluid through the tube, and (2) resistance to that flow.

Pressure and Fluid Flow

The pressure exerted by fluid in a container is called *hydrostatic pressure,* and depends on the *weight* of the liquid and the *height of the column* of liquid. The weight of a liquid is determined by its density (specific gravity). If the weight of one liquid is double that of another liquid, the pressure it exerts will be double.

The *column of fluid* (head of fluid) is the fluid in a container and its tubing, such as IV fluid or the fluid for an enema. The height of the column is measured from the top of the fluid in the container to the level of the bottom end of the tubing. If the height of one column of liquid is double that of another column of liquid of equal density, the pressure exerted will be double.

The pressure exerted by a column of fluid is measured at the base of the column. Hydrostatic pressure is usually measured in grams per square centimeter or pounds per square inch, and the size and shape of the column do not affect the pressure. For example, all 2-feet-high columns of water exert the same *pressure per square inch* whether the bottom surface of the column is 1, 9, or 200 sq inches. If the container is raised to a height of 3 feet, the height of the column is increased, and the hydrostatic pressure is also increased. If the container is lowered, the pressure is decreased.

Pressure in Flowing Fluids

Pressure Gradient

The pressure of a fluid is determined by the weight (density) of the fluid and by the height of the column of fluid. The difference in pressure between the upper and lower levels of a column of fluid is called the *pressure gradient.* Fluid flows from an area of greater pressure toward an area of lower pressure.

Whenever the pressure from a column of fluid is greater than any pressure against the outlet of the tubing, the fluid will flow toward the outlet of the tubing. If pressure encountered at the outlet of the tubing were greater than the pressure in the tubing, the fluid would be forced back toward the container. In order for IV fluids to flow *into* a vein, for example, the pressure of the IV fluid must be *greater* than the pressure of the blood against the outlet of the tubing. If the pressure of the blood were greater than the pressure of the IV fluid, blood would flow out of the vein, and into the IV tubing.

The rate of flow through a straight tube is in proportion to the pressure gradient between the top and the bottom of the column of fluid. Fluid will flow as long as there is a pressure gradient, but when there is no longer a difference in pressures, the fluid stops flowing. The pressure gradient can be increased or decreased by changing the height of the column of fluid (the head of fluid). *Raising* the container of fluid increases the head of fluid which increases the pressure and the pressure gradient, thereby increasing the rate of flow. Conversely, *lowering* a container of fluid decreases the head of fluid, the pressure, and the pressure gradient, and consequently slows the rate of flow.

Increasing Fluid Flow by Increasing Diameter of Tubing

Original diameter = $(1)^4$ = $1 \times 1 \times 1 \times 1$ = 1 unit of flow.

Double diameter = $(2)^4$ = $2 \times 2 \times 2 \times 2$ = 16 times as much flow.

Triple diameter = $(3)^4$ = $3 \times 3 \times 3 \times 3$ = 81 times as much flow.

Quadruple diameter = $(4)^4$ = $4 \times 4 \times 4 \times 4$ = 256 times as much flow.

Resistance

The two factors which determine the rate of fluid flow are the *pressure* exerted by the fluid and the *resistance* encountered by the fluid. The two factors act in opposition. Pressure tries to force fluid to flow *in*, and resistance tries to keep it *out*.

Resistance is determined by (1) the diameter of the tubing (2) the length of the tubing, and (3) the viscosity of the fluid.

Diameter of the Tubing

When the diameter of the tubing is increased, the flow of fluid increases *tremendously*. This increase is proportional to the *fourth power* of the diameter of the tubing. Therefore, all other things being equal, doubling the diameter of a tube increases the rate of flow through the tube *16 times* ($2^4 = 16$), and tripling the diameter of a tube increases the rate of flow 81 times ($3^4 = 81$).

A decrease in the diameter of the tubing causes a corresponding decrease in the rate of fluid flow. It is not necessary to decrease the diameter of the entire tubing in order to slow the rate of fluid flow, because a *narrowing at any point* along the tubing creates the same effect. The rate of fluid flow through IV tubing, or enema tubing, for example, is slowed by tightening the clamp, and increased by opening the clamp.

Viscosity

Viscosity is the tendency of a liquid to resist flow; it is sometimes described as the friction within the fluid.

Decreasing Fluid Flow by Decreasing Diameter of Tubing

One-half diameter = $(\frac{1}{2})^4$ = $\frac{1}{2} \times \frac{1}{2} \times \frac{1}{2} \times \frac{1}{2}$ = $\frac{1}{16}$ as much flow.

One-third diameter = $(\frac{1}{3})^4$ = $\frac{1}{3} \times \frac{1}{3} \times \frac{1}{3} \times \frac{1}{3}$ = $\frac{1}{81}$ as much flow.

One-fourth diameter = $(\frac{1}{4})^4$ = $\frac{1}{4} \times \frac{1}{4} \times \frac{1}{4} \times \frac{1}{4}$ = $\frac{1}{256}$ as much flow.

The viscosity of a fluid is the ratio of its viscosity to that of water and is measured in terms of a unit called a centipoise. A few approximate representative values: water 1.00; ether 0.23; blood 2.5 to 14.0; olive oil 84.0; and castor oil 986.0. The more viscous the fluid, the slower it will flow. Therefore, if a thick fluid is diluted it will be less viscous and will flow faster.

Viscosity is affected by temperature, and viscosity increases as temperature decreases—hence the old-timer's phrase, "slower than molasses in January." Warming a fluid will make it less viscous and will let it flow faster.

The viscosity of blood varies with body temperature and fluid balance. Viscosity decreases with increased muscular activity and increased body temperature. Blood viscosity increases dramatically when the water content of the blood drops during dehydration; the blood becomes "thicker" and flows much more slowly.

Friction

Friction of any kind slows the flow of fluids through a tube; three factors which influence the amount of friction encountered by a fluid are length, diameter, and inner surface of the tube.

The rate of fluid flow varies inversely with the *length* of the tube. The molecules of fluid rub against the wall of the tube; the longer the tube, the more friction there is and the slower the flow of fluid.

The tubing used for patient care should be short enough for adequate fluid flow, but long enough to permit the patient to move around without pulling on it. The tube should not be so long that the patient might get tangled up in it.

The *diameter* of the tube affects the amount of friction encountered. A narrow tube creates greater friction than a wide one because a greater proportion of the fluid is in contact with the walls of the tube.

A tube with a very *smooth* inner surface produces very little friction. The fluid flows along in sheets and is called *laminar* flow. A tube with a rougher inner surface produces slower, irregular, *turbulent* flow. Plastic tubing is likely to have a smoother inner surface than rubber tubing.

Changing the Rate of Fluid Flow

Before taking any action which would alter the rate of fluid flow through a patient's tube, it is essential that you *positively identify* the tube you are concerned about. There may be several tubes which are identical in appearance, and it is essential that you trace the selected tube from its source to its outlet to make sure that you have the right one. In some situations, an error in changing the flow rate can be life threatening or fatal.

The rate of flow of a fluid can be increased by *increasing the pressure* on the fluid and/or by *decreasing the resistance* against the fluid. These changes can be brought about by:

- Raising the container of fluid, thereby increasing the pressure and the pressure gradient
- Decreasing the friction by using a larger tube, shortening the tube, or using tubing with a smoother inner surface
- Decreasing the viscosity, when appropriate, by warming or diluting the fluid

FLUIDS AT REST

Pascal's Law

The pressure at any point within a fluid *at rest* is the same as it is at any other point. If this were not so, the fluid would be moving from points of higher pressure to points of lower pressure, and the fluid would no longer be at rest—it would be flowing. Because the pressure throughout a fluid at rest is constant, *Pascal's law* states that *an increase in the pressure on any part of the fluid is transmitted undiminished to all other parts of the fluid.* This law applies to all fluids within the body, such as spinal fluid, urine, blood, and intraocular fluid. This law is applied in nursing to the operation of a hydraulic patient lifter and to the use of air or water mattresses.

Hydraulic Lifter

The mechanism of the hydraulic patient lifter consists of two connected cylinders filled with oil. One cylinder is much larger than the other; each cylinder contains a piston. When pressure is applied to one piston, the pressure is *transmitted undiminished* through the fluid to the other piston (Fig. 11.1). If, for example, a pressure of 50 lb/sq inch is exerted on the smaller piston, that same pressure of 50 lb/sq inch is relayed to the larger one, and *each square inch* of the larger piston will lift 50 pounds. If the surface area of the larger piston is 10 times that of the smaller piston, the large piston will lift 10 times the weight that can be lifted by the smaller one. If the top surface of the small piston is 1 square inch, and the surface of the large piston is 10 square inches, the pressure or force that can be exerted by the larger piston is 50 lb/sq in × 10, or 500 lb. A pressure of 50 lb on the small piston, therefore, exerts a pressure on the large one that enables it to lift 500 lb. By using a hydraulic lifter, a nurse is able to lift a heavy patient with relatively little effort and very minimal danger of back injury (see Chapter 29).

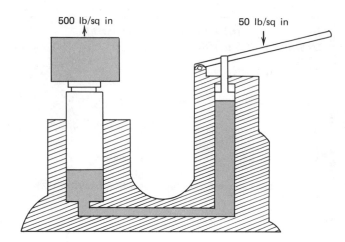

500 lb/sq in   50 lb/sq in

Figure 11.1 Hydraulic jack.

Air and Water Mattresses

Pascal's law explains the effectiveness of air and water mattresses in helping to prevent pressure (decubitus) ulcers (bed sores). When a person lies on an ordinary mattress, there is uneven pressure on the surface of his body.

The soft tissues over bony prominences such as the hips or coccyx are compressed between the bone and the mattress. Circulation through this compressed tissue is slowed drastically, and if the pressure is prolonged, the tissue dies from lack of oxygen and nutrients. The resulting area of dead and injured tissue is called a decubitus or pressure ulcer, and can take months to heal.

Air or water mattresses are used to *prevent* or treat pressure ulcers because, according to Pascal's law, all pressure from the patient's body is *evenly* distributed throughout the mattress by the air or water. As a result, there are no areas of concentrated pressure.

Foam rubber mattresses contain air in each tiny space of the spongy rubber. They are less beneficial than air mattresses but more effective than regular mattresses in preventing pressure ulcers.

ELECTRICITY

Electricity is a form of energy that involves a flow of electrons from one atom to another. Some substances, such as metals and water, transmit electrons freely; they are said to be good *conductors* of electricity. Substances such as dry air, rubber, and glass do not transmit electrons and do not conduct electricity; they are called *insulators* or nonconductors.

There are two types of electricity. *Static electricity* is the accumulation of electrical charges *on the surface* of a nonconductor. *Dynamic electricity* is the **flow** of electrical charges *through* a conductor.

Static Electricity

Friction between two objects which do not conduct electricity causes electrons to accumulate on the surfaces of each nonconductor. This accumulation of electrons creates static electricity, as commonly occurs as a result of friction between rubber soles and a wool rug, between bedding and a rubber sheet, and between tires and the pavement. In each instance, since neither object conducts electricity, electrons accumulate on each nonconductor. This accumulation can be removed by a *spark* or by *conduction.*

A spark from static electricity is small and passes unnoticed in most situations, but a spark in the operating room, for example, is hazardous because certain anesthetics are explosive. In that setting, every effort is made to (1) keep static electricity from accumulating on any surface, and (2) make sure that, if it does accumulate, the electrical charge will be discharged by preplanned conduction rather than by a spark.

To prevent a buildup of static electricity and to decrease the risk of an explosion in the operating room, materials that tend to accumulate charges of electricity are not permitted. Garments of silk, nylon, or dacron, and rubber-soled shoes cannot be worn.

Dry air tends to promote static electricity, so the humidity in the operating room is kept relatively high. Water is a good conductor of electricity, and moist air tends to carry charged particles away and thereby decrease any possible accumulation. Clothing, drapes, and towels in the operating room are made of cotton, linen, or rayon because these fabrics absorb moisture readily and therefore tend to conduct electricity rather than generate sparks. Antistatic sprays are also used to help control static electricity.

Shoes, floors, and equipment must be made *conductive* to permit the discharge of electricity **before** enough accumulates to generate a spark. A conductivity tester is used to determine how well an object can conduct a charge of static electricity; if an object is found to resist conduction, it is either prohibited or modified to make it more conductive. For example, shoes can be fitted with special metal clips or tapes that will conduct any accumulation of static electricity from a person to the floor, where it can be conducted out of the operating room.

The transmission of electricity from an object to the ground is called grounding (the electricity travels through a conductive material to the *ground*). Defective wiring in a piece of equipment can cause a short circuit of electricity through the body of a person using that equipment since the current has no other place to go. In order to prevent such an accident, the wiring in modern buildings is usually grounded for safety with a third wire (ground wire). If the wiring is grounded, the electricity from a short circuit will follow the ground wire because it offers less resistance than a person's body, and a fatal accident may be averted. It is important to note, however, that grounding does not offer protection if the person is in water or on a wet surface. For example, a person in a bath tub will be electrocuted if an electrical appliance such as a radio or a hair dryer falls into the water even though the appliance may be plugged into a grounded outlet.

Dynamic Electricity

Electricity that *flows through* a conductor is *dynamic.* Static electricity can be considered dynamic at the moment of a spark; but when the spark jumps, the electrical charge is discharged, and no electricity remains. Dynamic electricity, on the other hand, continues to flow as long as there is a source such as a generator, a battery, or a power plant.

Dynamic electricity (usually referred to simply as electricity) can be dangerous and often fatal under two conditions: (1) When *large* amounts of current from an external source enter the body through the skin (macroshock) and (2) when *minute* amounts of current enter the heart via electronic equipment implanted in or near the heart (microshock).

Macroshock occurs whenever a person touches a source of electricity while he is grounded. Water conducts electricity, so it is extremely dangerous to touch a frayed cord or faulty light switch with wet hands or while standing on a wet surface. The current will pass *through* the person's body en route to the ground, making him part of the electrical circuit. Safety measures are designed to interrupt this circuit. Such practices include using nonconductive gloves and tools, wearing rubber-soled shoes, and standing on a nonconductive surface such as a thick, dry board while working with electricity. These precautions will break an electrical circuit so the current does not pass through the body.

Blood, urine, and saliva are good conductors. Electrical impulses can flow through the body of the victim of an electrical accident and enter the body of a rescuer. Therefore, a rescuer should not touch a victim until the electrical current has been shut off or until the victim has been separated from the source of electricity. A dry wooden stick, a piece of rubber, dry rope, or some other nonconductive object can be used to separate the victim from the source of electricity.

Cardiopulmonary resuscitation should be started as soon as the victim has been removed from the source of electricity, and emergency medical help should be sought at once. An electrical shock can cause severe burns (either on the skin or deep within the body), severe muscle contractions, and death from cardiac or respiratory arrest.

Microshock can be a hazard whenever a patient is being diagnosed, monitored, or treated with electrical equipment; the risk is even greater when there is a catheter, probe, or wire connecting his heart to a piece of electrical equipment. Minute amounts of current, far too weak to be felt by another person, can cause a fatal ventricular fibrillation if the current is conducted *directly* into a patient's heart.

The staff caring for patients who are at risk for electric shock need intensive training in ways to safeguard the patient. All equipment should be checked regularly by a qualified technician. Two warning signals related to microshock: (1) any evidence of electrical interference or "noise" on monitors or EKG equipment, and (2) a tingling sensation felt when a piece of electrical equipment is touched. Both situations should be reported, investigated, and corrected at once.

HEAT TRANSFER

A nurse uses the principles of heat transfer to maintain the body temperature of a premature infant, treat a victim of hypothermia, reduce a fever, prevent or treat heat stroke, and teach a person to apply hot packs safely. In each instance, the nurse's success or failure is influenced by her understanding of the interaction between heat transfer and the body's physiological processes.

Heat is a form of energy produced by the motion of molecules. The speed with which the molecules move determines the *intensity of heat* (temperature), which is measured in degrees. When the speed of the molecules of a substance is increased, the temperature of that substance is raised. The temperature of an object depends on the speed with which its molecules are moving and is not affected by the volume or size of the object. A large object and a small object will have the same temperature if their molecules are moving at the same speed.

The *quantity of heat,* on the other hand, is determined by the sum total of kinetic energy of all the molecules of an object. A large volume of water at 68 degrees C has a greater *quantity* of heat than a small volume of water at 68 degrees C. The intensity of heat (the temperature) is the same for both, but the large volume can give off more heat than the smaller volume. The quantity of heat is measured in calories or in British thermal units (Btu).

Temperature Gradient

When there is a difference in temperature between two objects or substances, heat is transferred from the warmer to the cooler object. The warmer object loses heat and its temperature drops. The cooler object absorbs heat and its temperature rises. The transfer of heat slows as the temperatures begin to equalize and stops when the temperatures are the same. The speed of heat transfer depends on the difference in temperatures (the temperature gradient); the greater the difference in temperature, the more rapid the transfer of heat. A change in temperature is always caused by the *transfer of heat;* it is not possible to transfer cold. An object becomes cooler when it *loses heat;* it cannot become cooler by receiving cold.

Types of Heat Transfer

The transfer of heat can take place by any one of three processes: conduction, convection, and radiation. In most siuations, however, heat is transferred by a combination of the three.

Conduction

The *conduction* of heat is the passage of heat through an object or a substance, or from one object to another one which is touching it. When one end of a metal rod is heated, the heat travels through the rod by conduction. Substances such as metal, which conduct heat rapidly, are called good thermal conductors. Substances that conduct heat poorly, such as cork, are called insulators and are used to block or prevent the transmission of heat.

Of the three states of matter (solid, liquid, and gas), gases are the poorest conductors. Trapped *air,* therefore, is an effective insulator. Thermal window glass, building insulation, down jackets, and thermal blankets all retain heat in proportion to the amount of air that is trapped between the panes or among the fibers. Moving air, on the other hand, is not an effective insulator.

When various objects of the same temperature are touched, some feel colder than others. For example, a metal doorknob, a wooden table, and a wool blanket, all at room temperature, will feel warmer or colder as a result of differences in conduction. A metal doorknob conducts heat away from the fingers so rapidly that the fingers feel cold, making the doorknob seem colder than room temperature. Wool, because of its trapped air, conducts heat poorly. Since the wool does not conduct heat, little heat is transferred from the fingers, and the blanket feels warmer than room temperature.

A knowledge of conduction is important in nursing

because it provides a basis for guidelines that will protect patients against injury from heat or cold. Prolonged contact with ice or an object at near freezing temperature will injure body tissues by the very rapid loss of heat. It is possible to regulate and slow the transfer of heat *from* the body to an ice pack by insulating the body with a layer of trapped air. This can be done by inserting a layer of fabric such as outing flannel or terry cloth between the skin and the ice-cold surface. A piece of smooth sheet would be unsatisfactory because it would not trap enough air within its fibers to be an effective insulator.

Insulation is also used to prevent too rapid a transfer of heat when heat is applied to the skin. An excessively rapid transfer of heat will burn the patient's skin. This danger is minimized by insulating the skin from the heat with a layer of trapped air or some other poor conductor such as oil or petroleum jelly.

Water conducts heat about 28 times more effectively than air; therefore, the transfer of heat by conduction can be increased or decreased by the use of water. Heat is conducted much more rapidly by a hot, moist compress than by a hot, dry compress, and as a result, the potential for burning a patient's skin is increased.

Convection

Convection is the process by which heat is carried from one place to another by the *movement of a heated gas or liquid.* Hot water running into a container of cool water will eventually warm all the water, and hot air from a fireplace carries heat around the room. Although air at rest (trapped air) is a poor conductor of heat, air *in motion* transfers heat by convection very effectively. Examples of heat transfer by convection include forced air (hot air) heating systems, the cooling produced by currents of air from a fan, and the warming produced by currents of warm water in a whirlpool bath.

Radiation

Heat is transferred by radiation in the form of waves which produce heat when they are absorbed by an object. Dark-colored and rough-textured surfaces absorb heat waves readily, and heat is transferred to such surfaces effectively. Light colors such as white or silver, and smooth, shiny surfaces reflect radiation and shield the underlying object from heat.

The transfer of heat from a radiant object such as the sun *to the body* is affected by the color and texture of a person's clothing. The transfer of heat *from the body* by radiation accounts for about 60 percent of the body's heat loss. It is for this reason that the addition or removal of clothing or bedding is an important factor in the regulation of body temperature.

STABILITY AND BALANCE

The principles of stability and balance form the basis for good body mechanics, and are important to nurses for two reasons. First, the risk of back injury is high in nursing, therefore prevention of injury is the only way a nurse can avoid jeopardizing her career. Second, many families and patients, especially those with muscle weakness or paralysis, need to learn how to prevent injury and increase the patient's ability to move about. In order for the nurse to participate in efforts to teach effective body mechanics, a knowledge of the principles of stability and balance is necessary.

Stability is the ability of an object to resist a force that tries to push or pull it over. An unstable object will topple in response to a very small force. A stable object will remain upright even though considerable force or pressure is applied against it.

It is common knowledge that a tall, thin object is less stable than a short, fat one. The scientific explanation for this phenomenon involves several principles of stability and balance.

Principle No. 1. The stability of an object depends on the relationship between the height of its center of gravity and the size of its base of support.

Although the force of gravity acts on all parts of an object, each object has a center of gravity. *Center of gravity* is defined as the internal point at which all the mass or weight of the object is centered. The center of gravity of a symmetrical object is the same as its geometrical center. If a symmetrical object were suspended from this point, it would remain balanced, without tilting or tipping, no matter what the position of the object.

The center of gravity is much harder to locate in an irregularly shaped object. In an adult human being, the center of gravity is located in the pelvis. The problems of stability become more complex when a person picks up a heavy object and the extra weight is added to his body weight. Because the center of gravity represents the point where the weight of an object is centered, any weight that is added to the object will change the location of the center of gravity. The center of gravity moves in the direction of the additional weight since that weight must be included in the total weight that will be represented by the new center of gravity.

The relation of the height of the center of gravity to stability can be stated as follows: given two objects with identical bases of support, the object with the lower center of gravity is more stable. The relation of base of support to stability can be stated as follows: given two objects with centers of gravity of equal height, the object with the larger base of support will be more stable.

Principle No. 2. The stability of a given object can be increased by lowering the center of gravity, enlarging the base of support, or both.

A low center of gravity contributes to stability, thus one way to increase the stability of an object is to *lower its center of gravity*. The *location* of the center of gravity within an object does not shift when the object is moved about, but the *height* of the center of gravity can be raised or lowered by changing the position of the object.

Any rectangular object, such as a stick of butter, is more stable when placed on its long side than when standing on end. The same is true of human beings. A person is more stable and less likely to tip over when squatting than when standing erect, and is even more stable when lying down.

In many situations it is neither advisable nor possible to increase the stability of an object by lowering its center of gravity. When the center of gravity cannot be lowered, stability can be increased by *enlarging the base of support*. The base of support of an object can be enlarged in three ways: from side to side, from front to back, or in both directions at once.

When the base of support is increased in either direction, an object becomes more stable in that direction but is no more stable in the other direction than it was before. In other words, when a base of support is increased from *side to side*, a force applied to the side of the object will no longer tip it over, but a force applied to the front or back will still tip the object over.

A person enlarges his base of support by placing one foot forward and the other back, by separating his legs, or both. The direction of the enlargement of the base of support depends on the type of activity to be undertaken while in that position.

Principle No. 3. For an object to be balanced, its line of gravity must pass through its base of support.

The *line of gravity* is a vertical line (imaginary) that extends downward from the center of gravity. An object is balanced and stable if its line of gravity passes through its base of support. The line of gravity need not pass through the center of the base of support; it need only pass through some part of it. Therefore, movement of the upper part of the object, which may cause the center of gravity to shift a bit, does not necessarily unbalance the object; it will remain balanced as long as its center of gravity is over some part of its base of support.

PATIENT TEACHING

Increasing numbers of patients are being cared for at home, and home care often involves the use of complex equipment. All persons who will be using such equipment need to understand enough about the relevant concepts of physics to ensure the patient's safety and well-being. The malfunction of equipment such as a hydraulic lifter or electric wheelchair can seriously disrupt the patient's daily routine; in some situations, the patient's very life depends upon the proper functioning of equipment such as a kidney dialysis machine or respirator. Body mechanics will be important as well.

It is not enough for the patient and family to have a general idea of how things work; it is important in every situation that they understand the scientific basis for the functioning of essential equipment.

RELATED ACTIVITIES

1. Visual aids can increase the effectiveness of your patient teaching as well as your own understanding of various concepts of physics which are difficult to explain with words alone. The science editors of magazines such as *Time* and *Newsweek* frequently present remarkably clear and concise explanations of complex phenomena such as the use of laser beams, ultrasound waves, and fiber optics in medicine. Some magazine and newspaper articles include diagrams which illustrate the principles involved. Use a clearly labeled manila envelope or folder to start an ongoing file of materials related to physics which will enhance your nursing effectiveness and patient teaching in the years ahead.

2. As soon as time permits, enroll in a basic physics course through your local community college or high school adult education program. As the age of space travel and advanced technology begins to involve the health of increasing numbers of people, an extensive knowledge of physics will become essential for the professional nurse.

SUGGESTED READINGS

Erickson, Roberta: Tube talk: principles of fluid flow in tubes. *Nursing 82* 1982 July; 12(7):54–62.

Flitter, Hessel Howard, and Harold R Rowe: *An Introduction to Physics in Nursing.* ed.7. St. Louis, Mosby, 1976.

Freeman, David L: Lasers in the O.R. *Am J Nurs* 1986 Mar; 86(3):278–282.

Jensen, J Trygve: *Physics for the Health Professions.* ed.2. Philadelphia, Lippincott, 1979.

Zettel, Estar: Beaming in on the GI tract (with lasers) *Am J Nurs* 1986 March; 86(3):280–282.

12

Concepts from Pathophysiology Relevant to Nursing

Prerequisites and/or Suggested Preparation
A knowledge of human anatomy and physiology is prerequisite
for this chapter.

The television program *Quincy* has done much to emphasize the importance of the pathologist in forensic medicine (medicine in relation to the law), but unfortunately, it does not portray the much greater significance of less dramatic, day-to-day contributions of the pathologist. The program demonstrates the importance in criminal investigations of an autopsy to determine the time and cause of death, but, because of the nature of the plots, there is no mention of three other vital functions of the pathologist. These are (1) to help the physician make a diagnosis, (2) to determine the cause of death in non-criminal cases, and (3) to describe the effect on the body of new drugs and treatments.

The pathologist helps the physician *make a diagnosis* by examining questionable cells and tissue under the microscope. One of the commonest examples is the *biopsy* which indicates to a surgeon whether or not a lump is malignant (cancerous). Such an examination can be done during an operation.

The use of an autopsy to *determine the cause of death* is important if the death was unexpected, cannot be explained on the basis of observable symptoms, or there is more than one possible cause of death.

Perhaps the most significant contribution of the pathologist is his ability to *describe the effect of new treatments and drugs*. For example, information about the size and distribution of clots resulting from the use of the first artificial heart led researchers to both modify the design of the device and evaluate the use of anticoagulant drugs. It will be the findings of the pathologist that will help researchers such as those studying AIDS to know if their discoveries are valid.

PATHOLOGY

Pathology is the study of the nature and cause of disease, and *pathophysiology* is the study of how normal body processes are altered by disease. The pathologist is a specialist in *laboratory medicine*, in contrast to the physician, who is a specialist in *clinical medicine*. The pathologist obtains his data both by the microscopic examination of tissue and by gross examination (observations that can be made by the naked eye and by the sense of touch).

The terminology related to pathology and pathophysiology is extensive and precise, and it is important to nurses for two reasons. First, the *use* of appropriate terminology aids communication among physicians, nurses, and other members of the health care team. Second, an ability to *translate* the language of the medical sciences into lay terms enables the nurse to interpret for the patient and family the information given them by the physician. Each nurse, therefore, must be able to understand the language of pathophysiology in order to read patient charts, laboratory reports, research studies, and professional journals, and to translate relevant medical information into words comprehensible to patient and family.

Terminology

The *etiology* of a disease or condition is its cause. If the cause has not yet been determined, the phrase "of unknown etiology" applies. A condition is said to be *idiopathic* when the cause is not known.

Pathogenesis refers to the development of a disease. The onset is called the *prodromal* stage. There may be a period during which the disease is well established but not yet apparent. This stage, of which the patient is unaware, is the *subclinical stage;* and the term might apply to the early stage of cancer or diabetes, for example. A disease in the subclinical stage could be detected by laboratory tests but not by physical examination of the patient.

The *acute stage* occurs when a disease is fully developed and at its peak. The acute stage is the most severe, and is self-limiting because the patient either recovers, enters a chronic stage, or dies.

Some conditions do not reach an acute stage. Some infections, for example, are mild and are described as *subacute* or *low-grade* infections.

A disease or condition that cannot be cured and that might well be present for the rest of a person's life is said to be *chronic*. Many chronic diseases such as rheumatoid arthritis, multiple sclerosis, ulcerative colitis, and leukemia are characterized by alternating periods of freedom from discomfort (*remissions*) and periods of acute distress (*exacerbations*). During the "good times," which may last from a few weeks to a few years, the disease is said to be in *remission*. The symptoms have disappeared or lessened in severity, and the patient can lead a relatively normal life. When a natural remission coincides with a new form of treatment, the remission may well be attributed to the new treatment, leading patients and families to believe that the new drug or treatment was responsible for the remission, and that a "wonder drug" or "cure" has been found. This phenomenon contributes to the continued acceptance of "quack" treatments by people who are desperate to find the relief which current medical therapy cannot always provide.

Disease is manifested both by subjective data (symptoms) that are known only to the patient and by objective data (signs) that can be observed or detected by another person. *Subjective* data would include a headache, dizziness, blurred vision, pain, or nausea, for example. These symptoms are well known to the patient, but another person can become aware of these symptoms only from the patient's comments or behavior. *Objective* signs, on the other hand, can be observed, heard, measured, or felt by another person. Examples of objective data include body temperature, blood pressure, and a rash or cough.

A specific cluster or combination of signs and symptoms is called a *syndrome* and is sometimes used to identify or describe a specific disease entity. For example, *Reye's syndrome* is an acute and often fatal disease of childhood characterized by acute edema (swelling) of the brain, low blood glucose levels, and infiltration and dysfunction of the liver. This combination of signs may appear after a variety of common viral infections, but the relation between the infection and the brain and liver changes is not known. A syndrome often bears the name of the person who first observed its occurrence. Reye's syndrome was named for an Australian pathologist who first recognized it in 1963.

The outcome or after effect of a disease is the *sequel;* the plural form, *sequelae,* is usually used. A new or different disease condition which is secondary to the initial pathology is called a *complication.* Many complications are caused by incomplete or faulty medical or nursing care, or by failure of a patient to comply with the prescribed therapy, and many complications are therefore preventable.

Lesion is a nonspecific term that refers to an area of abnormal tissue. Examples of lesions include ulcers, boils, pimples, blisters, and bed sores.

CAUSES OF DISEASE

The theory of multiple causation (Chap. 8) indicates that no disease is caused by a single factor. A causative organism or event can often be identified, but an individual's bodily response will be determined by many factors. Of 10 people exposed to a person with tuberculosis, for example, only one or two may actually develop tuberculosis. The development of the disease will depend on the number and virulence of the tubercle bacilli and on such variables as age, health status, nutritional state, history of previous exposure to tuberculosis, lifestyle, and current level of stress. These factors and others determine a patient's resistance or susceptibility to the disease.

The causes of disease include:

- Lack of oxygen and essential nutrients to the cells
- Physical injury (thermal, mechanical, or electrical)
- Chemical injury
- Infectious agents
- Abnormal cell growth
- Degenerative changes

Lack of oxygen and essential nutrients is usually caused by an inadequate blood supply to an area (*ischemia*). This can result from poor peripheral circulation to the hands and feet, for example, or from the *blocking* (occlusion) of an artery by a large blood clot, or by a *narrowing* (stenosis) of the artery which supplies the area.

Physical injury can be thermal, mechanical, or electrical. *Thermal* injuries are caused by excessive heat or cold and include burns, sunstroke, heat exhaustion, frost bite, and freezing. *Mechanical* injuries are caused by pressure, force, or friction. A blow from, or contact with, a blunt object will produce a fracture, bruise, or a concussion; a sharp object produces an injury such as an incision, a cut, a stab wound, or a puncture wound. *Chemical* injury can be caused by poisons or drugs taken into the body as well as by acids or alkalis which are spilled on the skin or splashed in the eyes.

Infectious agents can cause either local or systemic injury and disease. A *local infection* is one which is confined to a well-defined area of the body, such as an infected cut or tonsillitis. A *systemic infection* such as typhoid fever or the "flu" involves the entire body.

Infectious agents include bacteria and viruses, and, in a slightly different context, lice, ticks, hookworms, pinworms, itch mites, and others. A wound or lesion is said to be *secondarily infected* when an infection is superimposed on the original wound or lesion. For example, a child's chicken pox lesions can become secondarily infected if he scratches them with dirty fingernails.

Abnormal cell growth may be the result of (1) a change in the *size* of the existing cells, or (2) an increase in the *number* of cells present (the addition of new cells). A disturbance in the *size of existing cells* results in an increase or decrease in the size of the tissue or organ involved. *Hypertrophy* is an increase in the size of each cell; *atrophy* is a decrease in the size of each cell. Hypertrophy of a muscle often results from extensive exercise of that muscle. This can occur in the skeletal muscles of a body builder, for example, or in the overworked cardiac muscles of a failing heart, which causes an enlarged heart. Atrophy of a muscle occurs when it is not used because of paralysis, pain, or other condition. Lay people refer to atrophy as the process of "wasting away."

The growth of new cells (in contrast to the enlargement and growth of existing cells) produces a *neoplasm,* which means "new growth." A neoplasm (tumor) can be either *benign* (noncancerous) or *malignant* (cancerous). A benign neoplasm remains localized. It does not spread or invade other tissues, but it can injure surrounding cells by creating pressure on them as it grows. A malignant neoplasm does not remain localized; it spreads to other parts of the body. Malignant cells *metastasize* (spread) by direct invasion into adjacent tissue or they can be spread via lymph or blood to distant parts of the body.

DISEASE PROCESSES

There are relatively few ways in which the body can react to injury and disease. Five of the most basic disease processes are inflammation, healing, necrosis, infection, and circulatory responses. Different combinations of these disease processes plus differences in the location, severity, and duration of the injury, as well as specific responses of the individual patient, make possible a wide variety of disease conditions.

Inflammation

The injury or death of body tissue prompts an inflammatory response in the adjacent tissue. The *inflammatory response* is largely vascular, and its effects are caused by an increase in blood flow through the area.

It is important to note that inflammation and infection are *NOT* the same. The inflammatory process is the body's normal response to all cellular injuries and can occur in the *absence* of any bacterial or viral infection. For example, inflammation is present under an unbroken blister, around a surgical incision, and in a sterile urinary bladder that has been irritated by a sterile catheter. On the other hand, inflammation is also present in every infected wound. Although infection is not a necessary part of the inflammatory process, inflammation is an essential part of the body's response to infection.

The inflammatory process is characterized by five signs, which have been known as the *cardinal signs of inflammation* for over 2,000 years. These signs are redness, pain, warmth, swelling, and decreased function and they are sometimes called by their Latin names of *rubor, dolor, calor, tumor,* and *functio laesa.*

Redness (*rubor*) is caused by the rapid dilation and filling of capillaries in the area of the injury. The increased blood flow produces a condition of *hyperemia* (excess blood) or congestion, and the area appears red or inflamed. Pain (*dolor*) occurs when nerve endings are irritated by the release of substances such as histamine from the injured cells and when there is pressure from the swelling that is part of the inflammatory process.

Warmth (*calor*) is produced by an increased flow of blood into an injured area near the surface of the body. Because the temperature of the blood is warmer than the temperature of the surface of the body, the injured and inflamed area soon feels warmer than the surrounding surfaces. There is no noticeable increase in temperature when the injured area is deep within the body because temperature of the internal tissues already equals the temperature of the blood.

Swelling (*tumor*) is caused by an accumulation of fluid and cells in the interstitial spaces of the inflamed tissue. The inflammatory process increases the permeability of the small blood vessels, and fluid escapes into the interstitial spaces. The accumulated fluid and cells are called *exudate.* Exudate may be colorless and clear, and contain few cells or, if the area is infected, it may be thick with leukocytes, dead cells, and microorganisms. Loss of function (*functio laesa*) is caused, at least in part, by the patient's reluctance to move a body part that is swollen and painful.

In the inflammatory process, the increased flow of blood to an area transports extra fluids, nutrients, and leukocytes to the site of the injury. The fluid dilutes and weakens the injurious agent and any toxins that may have been produced. The extra nutrients provide the materials needed for tissue repair and healing. The leukocytes destroy and remove dead cells, debris, and any microorganisms which may be present.

Leukocytosis is an increase in the number of circulating white blood cells. It is present in most bacterial infections; it appears early and is pronounced in patients whose resistance is good.

When the injurious agent and its by-products have been removed, diluted, neutralized, or walled off, the inflammatory process slows and normal cellular activity is resumed. The blood vessels regain their semipermeability, and the flow of exudate ceases. The swelling subsides as excess fluid is removed, the irritation of nerve endings decreases, and pain is diminished. Discoloration fades, and waste products are carried away from the site.

If tissue damage was minor, the area is quickly restored to its previous state, a process referred to as *resolution.* If tissue damage was more extensive, the injured area cannot be restored by resolution, and the damaged tissue must be replaced with new cells by the processes of healing.

Healing

Two types of tissue repair are involved in healing. The first type is called *regeneration* and it is the replacement of injured cells with new cells identical to the ones that were destroyed. The second type of repair involves the growth of connective tissue and the development of

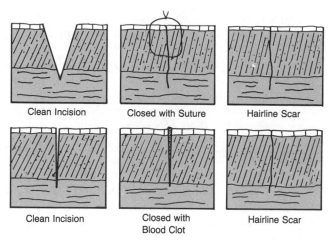

Figure 12.1 *Healing by first intention (primary union).*

scar tissue. Some tissues, such as skin, bone, and the lining of the mouth, regenerate easily and quickly but other tissues, such as nerves and heart muscle, regenerate poorly or not at all.

When tissue cannot regenerate, the wound heals by the development of scar tissue. Newly developed scar tissue is called *granulation tissue*. It is loose, very vascular, pink, and easily injured. Granulation tissue, therefore, must be protected from friction and other damage during this stage of healing.

When the edges of an injury or surgical incision are brought together and kept together, the wound is said to heal by first intention (Fig. 12.1). Blood clots cause the edges of the wound to adhere to each other, and sutures are used as needed to keep the edges together. When the wound edges can be closely approximated and held in place, the wound will often heal without a scar. Healing starts within a few days and is quite complete within a few weeks.

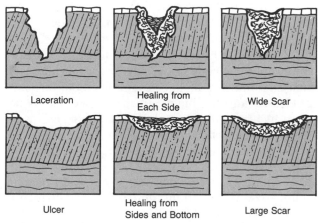

Figure 12.2 *Healing by secondary intention (granulation).*

When the wound edges are not approximated or when they are infected, the wound must heal by second intention, and the space gradually fills with scar tissue (Fig. 12.2). Some wounds are broad and shallow (saucer shaped) so it is not possible for the edges to be brought together. Such a wound must be repaired by growth from the sides and bottom. The process is slow, and the length of time for healing depends on the size and location of the wound, the circulation to the area, and the nutritional status of the patient. A wound heals very slowly if circulation is poor and the patient is undernourished, because cell growth and repair cannot take place without an adequate supply of essential nutrients (Table 12.1).

Several types of problems can result from the healing process, such as the *shortening of scar tissue* or the *overgrowth of new tissue*.

Scar tissue tends to shorten and become more dense as time passes. Extensive shortening and tightening of

TABLE 12.1 FACTORS WHICH AFFECT HEALING

Circulation	Adequate arterial blood is needed to furnish oxygen and nutrients. Adequate venous circulation is necessary to remove waste from area (bacteria, toxins, and cellular debris).
Infection	Both localized and systemic infections slow the healing process. Disturbance of the body's immune system makes any wound susceptible to infection and retards healing.
Nutrition	Adequate intake and utilization of amino acids, vitamins A and C, and zinc are essential. A high protein diet may be required.
Drugs	Adrenal corticosteroids influence the inflammatory process and may delay healing.
Wound edges	Approximation of the wound edges promotes healing and protects the wound from infection.
Immobilization	Restriction of movement is necessary for proper healing of bones, and of tissues near a joint.
Contamination	Wounds contaminated with foreign bodies such as bits of wood, dirt, or glass heal poorly.
Type of tissue	Tissues such as skin, muscle, bone, and endothelium regenerate; nerve fibers do not.
Age	The healing process tends to slow with age, due in part to changes in circulation and nutrition.

scar tissue can result in *contractures* that limit movement and produce extensive disfigurement. Contractures are common after severe burns, and multiple operations may be needed to loosen the tissue over a joint and permit adequate motion of that joint. If a scar encircles a hollow passageway such as the esophagus, the urethra, or a portion of the intestines, the scar may shorten and tighten enough to constrict the passageway and interfere with its function. The narrowed portion is called a *stricture.*

The growth of excess tissue during healing can cause cosmetic problems. A minor problem is created when a small amount of *granulation tissue* protrudes above the surrounding skin. The protruding tissue is sometimes called *proud flesh;* and it can quite easily be removed by electrical cautery or by surgical excision. A more serious problem is created by the growth of excessive *connective* tissue (*keloid tissue*). It is disfiguring if it occurs on the face, neck, or other exposed portion of the body because keloid tissue is hard and irregular, and can be quite large. Removal is not always successful because the overgrowth tends to recur. Black and Asian people are most frequently affected by keloid growths, and there may be a genetic disposition to keloids in some families.

Another problem of healing is the development of *adhesions.* When some types of tissue are injured, the inflamed surfaces sometimes adhere to adjacent surfaces. Occasionally, the two surfaces fuse together as the inflamed surface heals, forming an adhesion. Surfaces which are especially susceptible to the formation of adhesions are the pleural membranes of the chest and the surfaces of the intestines. Some adhesions are of little consequence, but others impair the function of an underlying organ enough to require corrective surgery to separate the adhering surfaces.

Necrosis

As soon as a group of cells or an area of tissue dies, the process of *necrosis* begins. The dead cells release enzymes which, although not harmful to living cells, begin to dissolve the dead cells. The adjacent living tissue also releases enzymes as part of its inflammatory response to cellular death. The dead tissue that is surrounded by living tissue is referred to as *necrotic tissue.* (When the entire body dies, the terms necrotic and necrosis are not generally used.)

There are numerous types of necrosis, and the differences are readily discernible under a microscope. *Liquefactive necrosis* occurs when dead tissue is liquefied by enzymes. This process produces a liquid-filled hole and occurs in necrotic brain tissue. *Caseous necrosis* oc-

curs when necrotic tissue crumbles but does not liquefy. The dead tissue bears a resemblance to cheese, hence the name caseous necrosis. One of the commonest causes of caseation is tuberculosis. *Coagulation necrosis* is a form of necrosis in which the dead tissue does not liquefy or crumble but retains its anatomical structure for some time. This type of necrosis usually occurs in tissue which has died as a result of *ischemia* (inadequate blood supply to the tissue). Gangrene is a form of coagulation necrosis and is caused by the action of saprophytic bacteria, which exist only on dead tissue. The dry, shriveled, black areas of gangrenous tissue on an extremity are called dry gangrene, whereas a gangrenous section of bowel, for example, is called moist gangrene.

Small numbers of dead cells are quickly destroyed by enzymes and carried away by leukocytes, whereas large areas of necrotic tissue over wounds such as extensive burns or a large bedsore are hazardous and must be treated promptly and vigorously. Dead tissue is an excellent culture medium and a focus for infection. Necrotic tissue forms a black crust called a *slough*, which is sometimes cast off (sloughed off) during the inflammatory process.

If the slough is tenacious and remains in place, it must be removed because living tissue cannot heal when it is covered by dead tissue. The removal of necrotic tissue is called *debridement*, and the process, which is similar to the removal of a firmly attached scab, is stressful and painful for the patient.

Debridement can be done surgically, mechanically, or by the use of enzymes. Surgical removal may require the use of an anesthetic. Mechanical debridement is accomplished by the use of wet-to-dry dressings. When wet dressings are allowed to dry, the necrotic tissue sticks to the dressing and is pulled away from the wound when the dried dressing is removed. Another type of mechanical debridement involves the use of continuous wet dressings and soaks or baths which loosen necrotic tissue. Finally, necrotic tissue can be removed by using a proteolytic enzyme solution which digests dead tissue without injuring live tissue.

The presence of necrotic tissue can cause systemic changes in a patient's body, such as a fever and an increased number of leukocytes in the blood. Enzymes are released into the blood stream by necrotic tissue, and an increased blood level of certain enzymes is an important diagnostic indication that there is necrotic tissue somewhere in the body. For example, three enzymes which are released when a person has a myocardial infarction (''heart attack'') are SGOT (serum glutamic-oxaloacetic transaminase), CPK (creatine phosphokinase), and LHD (lactic dehydrogenase). The presence of these enzymes in the blood indicates that the person has probably had a myocardial infarction.

Infection

The presence of infectious organisms within the human body *does NOT* necessarily mean that the person has an infectious disease. The body encounters a wide variety of microorganisms each day, but its defenses effectively destroy or repel most infectious agents before they can multiply enough to cause disease.

The *first line of defense* against infection includes the skin, the lining of the mouth and pharynx, the cilia of the respiratory tract, the acidity of the stomach, and the peristaltic movements that periodically empty the intestinal tract. The *second line of defense* is the inflammatory process. Microorganisms that successfully penetrate the first line of defense are counteracted or attacked by phagocytes, antibodies, or other components of the inflammatory process. The activities of the lymphatic system constitute the *final line of defense*.

If the body's defense system is unable to keep an infection localized, a systemic infection may result. *Bacteremia* refers to the presence of bacteria in the bloodstream. Most microorganisms which enter the bloodstream are quickly destroyed by white blood cells, but if the bacteria are especially virulent or numerous, the body defenses may be inadequate to cope with the overwhelming infection, and a condition called *septicemia* (blood poisoning) results.

The exudate produced by the inflammatory process is often clear with few cells (*serous exudate*), like the fluid in a blister, for example. If an infection is present, the exudate will contain large numbers of leukocytes and bacteria and is known as a *purulent exudate*. Under certain circumstances the enzymes that are released liquefy the surrounding tissue (*liquefaction*), and the combination of liquefied tissue, white blood cells, and bacteria is called *pus*. This process is called *suppuration* and when it is localized, it produces a pus-filled cavity known as an *abscess*.

An abscess can be very difficult to heal because the process of liquefaction tends to steadily enlarge the cavity. Treatment usually involves surgical *incision and drainage* of the abscess (I/D). When an abscess is not drained, it may extend along under the surface, producing a hollow, blind tract called a *sinus*. In other situations, the abscess will eventually create an opening to the surface of the body or into an adjacent hollow organ. This connecting passageway is called a *fistula*. Some infections are not localized but are diffuse, spreading rather rapidly along the loose connective tissue of an area of the body to produce a condition called

cellulitis. In such a situation, the entire area is inflamed and characterized by redness, heat, swelling, and pain.

Circulatory Disturbances

Hyperemia

Hyperemia (congestion) is an excess of blood within the blood vessels. This condition is caused either by an increased flow of blood to the area or by a decreased flow from the area. An *increased arterial flow* to an area is part of the inflammatory process. *Decreased venous flow* from an area can be caused by pressure on, or obstruction of, the veins, or by the heart's inability to efficiently pump blood through the veins (cardiac failure).

Ineffective blood flow *from* an area creates an accumulation of blood and a pressure that dilates the veins in that area. If such venous congestion is longstanding, the veins become permanently dilated, hard-walled, and tortuous, and are called *varicose veins* or *varices*. *Hemorrhoids* are varicose veins around the rectum and anus.

Ischemia

Ischemia is the opposite of hyperemia; it is an *inadequate* blood supply to an area or organ. Ischemia results in a deficit of oxygen (*anoxia*) and nutrients in the cells of that area or organ. There is often a corresponding accumulation of waste products because there is not enough blood flow to carry them away. Ischemia is frequently caused by an obstruction such as a blood clot, or by a narrowing of the arterial blood vessels, which prevents blood from reaching the area.

The symptoms and effects of ischemia depend in part on the area involved. An inadequate blood flow to the brain gives symptoms such as mental confusion, whereas ischemia of muscle tissue produces pain. Prolonged or complete ischemia results in death of the tissue. For example, prolonged ischemia of the foot can lead to gangrene of the toes, and ischemia of heart muscle (*myocardial infarction*) results in death of the involved heart tissue.

Hemorrhage

Hemorrhage is the escape of blood from the confines of the cardiovascular system. A hemorrhage can be massive, rapid, and life threatening as a result of damage to a major artery, or it can be minute and slow from very small blood vessels as the result of a bruise. Even a small hemorrhage, however, can create a potentially fatal pressure if it occurs within a confined space. For example, since the skull is rigid, the accumulation of blood from a cerebral hemorrhage can create a life-threatening pressure on the brain, and a hemorrhage into the nonelastic pericardial sac can produce a potentially fatal pressure on the heart. The significance and effect of a hemorrhage, therefore, depends on the amount of blood lost from the general circulation and on the location of the hemorrhage.

Pinpoint hemorrhages in the skin or mucous membranes are called *petechiae*, whereas larger, blotchy areas of hemorrhage (bruises or black-and-blue spots) are called *ecchymoses*. The swelling caused by an accumulation of blood in body tissue is called a *hematoma*.

Shock

Shock is a circulatory disturbance in which the blood pressure is inadequate to circulate blood to vital tissues and organs. Shock may be caused by a decrease in the volume of blood in the body (*hematogenic shock*), by failure of the heart to pump the blood which is available (*cardiogenic shock*), or by an increase in the size and capacity of the vascular bed (*vasogenic shock*).

HEMATOGENIC SHOCK. The volume of circulating blood can be decreased by the loss of whole blood as a result of hemorrhage, or by the loss of plasma fluids as a result of extensive burns. When the blood *volume* is inadequate, it is impossible for blood to reach all the organs and tissues. This condition is also known as *hypovolemic shock*.

CARDIOGENIC SHOCK. The blood volume may be adequate to sustain life, but unless the heart is capable of pumping the blood through the vascular system, the blood cannot circulate through the tissues and organs. Some of the causes of cardiogenic shock are myocardial infarction, accidental injury to the heart, complications of cardiac surgery, and congestive heart failure.

VASOGENIC SHOCK. Shock can occur despite normal blood volume and heart action if the size of the capillary bed is greatly increased by severe vasodilation. A normal blood volume simply cannot adequately fill the expanded capillary spaces. Such marked vasodilation is usually caused by impaired functioning of the nervous system, and the result is often called *neurogenic shock*.

The status of a patient in shock is extremely unstable; unless treatment is prompt and vigorous, irreversible changes occur and death results.

Edema

Edema is an accumulation of fluid in the interstitial spaces of an area. Factors related to the flow of fluids into and out of the interstitial spaces are described in Chapter 31 (Fluid and Electrolyte Balance).

Effusion

An accumulation of fluid within a body cavity is called an *effusion*. Fluid in the pleural cavity, for example, is pleural effusion. Fluid in the peritoneal cavity (peritoneal effusion) is also referred to as *ascites*. Fluid can also accumulate in a joint or in the pericardial sac.

Arteriosclerosis

Arteriosclerosis (hardening of the arteries) refers to a number of conditions characterized by thickening and hardening of the walls of arterial blood vessels. One of these conditions is *atherosclerosis*; the terms arteriosclerosis and atherosclerosis are often used interchangeably. Atherosclerosis is a condition in which the arterial blood vessels are narrowed or obstructed by irregular, elevated masses of fatty material and connective tissue called *atherosclerotic plaques*. These plaques obstruct the flow of blood through the artery and, in addition, roughen the lining of the blood vessel, thereby promoting clot formation. Atherosclerosis is an example of the multiple causation theory of disease (Chap. 7) because its etiology is so complex that it is not possible to indicate a single cause or even a predominant one.

Thrombosis

Thrombosis is the formation of one or more blood clots within the blood vessels of a living person. Clots form after death, but such a clot is not usually called a thrombus. A thrombus forms because the lining of the blood vessel has become rough or irritated, because the flow of blood has been slowed or otherwise altered, or because the clotting mechanisms of the blood have been changed by disease or drugs. The condition in which there is clot formation plus inflammation of the vein (phlebitis) is called *thrombophlebitis*.

Clot formation in an *artery* results in ischemia in the tissues or organ supplied by that artery. Clot formation in a *small vein* usually results in the development of collateral circulation in that area, whereas clot formation in a *large vein* produces passive congestion.

Both thrombosis and thrombophlebitis are dreaded complications of prolonged bed rest or immobility and are caused, in part, by prolonged pressure on veins and slowed venous circulation.

Embolism

Embolism is the name given to the movement of portions of a substance through the bloodstream from one place to another. This substance might consist of pieces of a blood clot, clumps of cancer cells, air bubbles, or other foreign matter; but unless otherwise specified, the term *embolus* usually refers to a fragment of a blood clot.

TABLE 12.2 CHARACTERISTICS OF BENIGN AND MALIGNANT NEOPLASMS

Characteristic	Benign Neoplasm	Malignant Neoplasm
Growth	Pushes surrounding tissue aside; slow growth; encapsulated	Infiltrates surrounding tissue; rapid growth; nonencapsulated
Recurrence	Does not recur after removal	Tends to recur after removal
Tissue destruction	Little destruction	Extensive destruction
Spread	Does not spread	Spreads to different parts of the body via blood and lymph
Microscopic appearance	Cells tend to look like parent cells	Cells seldom resemble normal parent cells
Systemic effects	Causes pressure on adjacent tissue; seldom fatal	Often causes extensive damage; usually fatal unless growth can be controlled

A large thrombus (*blood clot*) can fill a blood vessel almost completely for a distance of 6 in or more. When a piece of this long clot breaks off, it is an embolus. It is carried by the blood through smaller and smaller blood vessels until it becomes lodged and can travel no farther. The blood supply to that area is cut off by the clot, thus, if a major organ such as the brain, heart, or lungs is involved, the results are serious, and can be fatal.

Abnormal Cell Growth

Neoplasm, meaning "new growth," refers to a wide variety of rapidly proliferating cells. The word tumor, formerly used primarily to refer to one of the cardinal signs of the inflammatory process, is now used as a synonym for neoplasm.

A *benign* (noncancerous) neoplasm is smooth, regular, localized, well differentiated, and often encapsulated. It grows rather slowly and can usually be removed with minimal difficulty.

A *malignant* (cancerous) neoplasm is irregular in shape, grows rapidly, invades adjoining tissue, and often metastasizes to distant parts of the body.

Much of the current research related to the cause and treatment of cancer is focused on questions of cellular growth and replication. In normal cells, mitosis yields two identical cells, each with a normal arrangement of chromosomes. The abnormal mitosis of cancer cells produces changes in the cellular membranes and growth limits of the cells. The subsequent rampant growth of these abnormal cells causes them to invade

and destroy other cells, and to rob them of essential amino acids (Table 12.2).

Neoplasms are classified and named according to their type and the kind of tissue from which they originate. For example, the suffix *-oma* is used to denote a *benign* neoplasm, and the two suffixes *-sarcoma* and *-carcinoma* denote *malignant* neoplasms. For example, the word oste*oma* indicates a benign bone tumor, and the word osteo*sarcoma* indicates a malignant bone tumor. The

TABLE 12.3 SELECTED BENIGN AND MALIGNANT TUMORS

Type of Tissue	Benign Tumor	Malignant Tumor
Epithelial		
Skin	Papilloma	Squamous cell carcinoma
Glandular	Adenoma	Adenocarcinoma
Connective tissue		
Fibrous	Fibroma	Fibrosarcoma
Fat	Lipoma	Liposarcoma
Cartilage	Chondroma	Chondrosarcoma
Bone	Osteoma	Osteosarcoma
Blood vessel	Hemangioma	Hemangiosarcoma
Lymph vessel	Lymphangioma	Lymphangiosarcoma
Muscle		
Smooth	Leiomyoma	Leiomyosarcoma
Striated	Rhabdomyoma	Rhabdomyosarcoma
Nerve cells	Neuroma	Neurogenic sarcoma
	Neurofibroma	Neurofibrosarcoma
Hemopoietic	Lymphoma	Lymphosarcoma

word aden*oma* denotes a benign glandular tumor and the word adeno*carcinoma* denotes a malignant glandular tumor (Table 12.3).

Disease Processes of the Skin

Diseases that involve the skin are many and varied; they include such diverse conditions as acne, measles, hives, syphilis, and cancer. The causes of such disturbances are most commonly bacterial or viral infections, drug reactions, parasites and insects such as lice and fleas, fungus diseases such as ringworm and athlete's foot, contact with irritating chemicals, and injuries such as cuts and burns.

Some disease conditions of the skin are easily diagnosed and treated; others require the specialized knowledge and skill of an allergist or a dermatologist. The skin responds to injury or disease through a variety of lesions which are not specific for any particular disease, but which are common to many. A *vesicle* (blister), for example, may develop in response to friction, heat, chemicals, or a virus.

Common Lesions

The ability to differentiate among the various skin lesions is necessary in order to establish both nursing and medical diagnosis and to prescribe the proper treatment. In addition to proper identification of the type of lesion, the location and distribution of the lesions is often important in making a diagnosis. For example,

---

Types of Mechanical Injury of the Skin

- *Contusion.* Injury to underlying tissue in which the skin is not broken; a bruise.
- *Excoriation.* Any superficial loss of skin.
- *Abrasion.* Loss of outer layers of skin by friction, as in a "skinned" knee.
- *Laceration.* A break in the skin with jagged, irregular edges (in contrast to the straight, regular edges of an incision).
- *Puncture wound.* A stab wound; a wound made by a long, sharp object; a wound that is deeper than it is long.
- *Maceration.* A condition in which the skin becomes spongy, soft, and fragile as a result of soaking or prolonged contact with moisture.

---

the rash of measles appears on the face first and then extends to the trunk and extremities, whereas the rashes of other diseases follow entirely different patterns of appearance.

See box below for descriptions of common lesions of the skin, some of which are shown in Figure 12.3.

Burns

An extensive burn is one of the severest insults (injuries) that the body can experience because the skin is the body's first line of defense against infection. Any break in the skin is a possible portal of entry for micro-

---

Common Lesions of the Skin

- *Macule.* A small, flat, discolored area that cannot be felt with the fingers; a large macule is a *patch*.
- *Papule.* A small, solid, raised, discolored area; a large papule is a *plaque*.
- *Nodule.* A solid, raised lesion that extends deeper into the skin than a papule; a tiny lump.
- *Vesicle.* A small blister.
- *Bulla.* A large blister.
- *Pustule.* A blister filled with pus.
- *Wheal.* An elevated lesion of variable size and color; often part of an allergic response such as hives.
- *Ulcer.* A depression or excavation that follows the sloughing of necrotic tissue; frequently shallow and saucer-shaped.
- *Fissure.* A linear split or crack.
- *Crust.* A layer of solid matter formed by dried exudate or secretions.
- *Comedo.* (pl. comedones) A blackhead; a plug of keratin and sebum within a hair follicle.

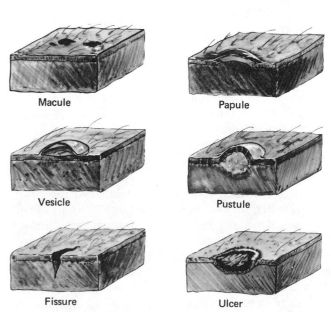

Figure 12.3 Common lesions of the skin.

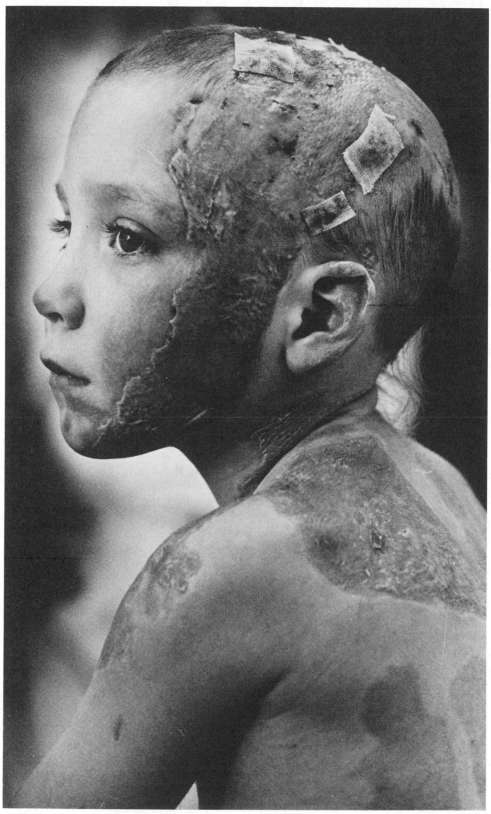

Figure 12.4 *Healing grafts of meshed skin on Renee's head, neck, and shoulder, and healed donor sites across her back. Although most of Renee's face was not burned, these scars may cause stress to Renee and her family for years to come.*

organisms, and the destruction of large areas of skin can render the body nearly defenseless. Intensive care in special burn units has successfully counteracted many systemic responses to the loss of skin, such as excessive loss of fluids and inability to maintain a normal body temperature, but exposure to the environment of large areas of unprotected tissue frequently results in infection despite heroic efforts to prevent it.

One measure of the severity of a burn is the depth to which it penetrates the skin and underlying tissue. *Superficial* (or first-degree) burns are confined to the epidermis (outer layer of skin). Common examples are sunburn or brief contact with a hot cooking utensil. The skin turns pink or red, and *desquamation* (peeling) is common after 3 to 7 days. This type of burn can be extremely painful because of injury to the numerous nerve endings in the skin.

Partial-thickness (or second-degree) burns involve more of the skin than the epidermis. The skin is partially destroyed, and its appearance varies with the depth of the destruction. The skin may still be intact but badly blistered, or the epidermis may be gone and the surface may appear mottled or red, wet and shiny, or swollen. The burn is painful and will take about 1½ to 4 weeks to heal, depending in part on whether or not the area becomes infected.

Full-thickness (third degree) burns result in total destruction of the skin with injury to the subcutaneous tissue and sometimes with injury to the underlying muscle and bone. The burn looks charred and is covered with a thick, dry, tough, dark crust of necrotic tissue called *eschar.* If the burn completely encircles a body part, the eschar must be quickly split or removed because it is tight and nonelastic and will impede circulation when the underlying tissues begin to swell during the inflammatory process. Sensation is diminished or absent in the eschar and the underlying tissue because the nerve endings have been destroyed.

Full-thickness burns do not heal spontaneously; eschar must be removed by debridement, and skin grafting must be done. These treatments may involve numerous operations over a number of months; plastic surgery is often required to repair the scars and deformities incurred during the initial life-saving therapy (Fig. 12.4, see previous page).

Most burns are a combination of all three categories of burns, and the severity of a burn depends not only on the depth of the burn but the extent of the area covered. An initial rough estimate of the percentage of body surface burned can be obtained by the use of the "rule of nines," which divides the body surface into units or multiples of 9 percent. There are three areas that each constitute 9 percent of the body's surface, and four areas that constitute 18 percent each. The three 9

percent areas are the two arms, and the head and neck. The four 18 percent areas are the back of the torso (trunk), the front of the torso, and each leg. The genital area is 1 percent, giving a total of 100 percent. From these allotted percentages, it is possible to calculate the percentage of body surface that has been burned.

The rule of nines provides a rough estimate in an emergency situation but does not take into account the differences caused by age. For example, the leg of an adult constitutes about 40 percent of his body weight, whereas the leg of an infant is only about 28 percent of his body weight. Therefore, more precise formulas must be used to assess the extent of a patient's burns as soon as any necessary life-saving measures have been instituted in the burn unit or emergency room.

The body's response to extensive burns involves every system of the body and nearly every type of pathophysiological response, including changes in respiration, metabolism, and kidney function, inflammation, necrosis, and healing; complications range from contractures to a type of stomach ulcer (Curling's ulcer) that develops in response to the stress of severe burns.

Fractures

Fracture is the term applied to a disruption in the continuity of any bone. Some fractures are life threatening because of damage to other tissue which results in hemorrhage and shock, but many are uncomplicated and heal quickly. Fractures can be caused by a sharp or heavy object, or they can be caused by an unusual or abnormal muscular action or stress. A *pathological fracture* is caused by minor trauma or pressure on a bone which has already been weakened by a disease condition such as cancer or osteoporosis (porous bones). Some of the common types of fractures are described below.

1. *Closed (simple) fracture.* The skin is intact over the fracture, and since the bone does not protrude, infection is not a concern at the time of the injury (Fig. 12.5a).
2. *Open (compound) fracture.* The skin has been broken either by the ends of the bone or by an external object such as a bullet. Since the skin is the body's first line of defense, the fractured bone and the tissues around it are open and susceptible to infection (Fig. 12.5b).
3. *Complete fracture.* The fracture line extends completely through or across the bone (Fig. 12.6a).
4. *Incomplete fracture.* The continuity of the bond is not completely disrupted (Fig. 12.6b). This fracture is often referred to as a *greenstick fracture* be-

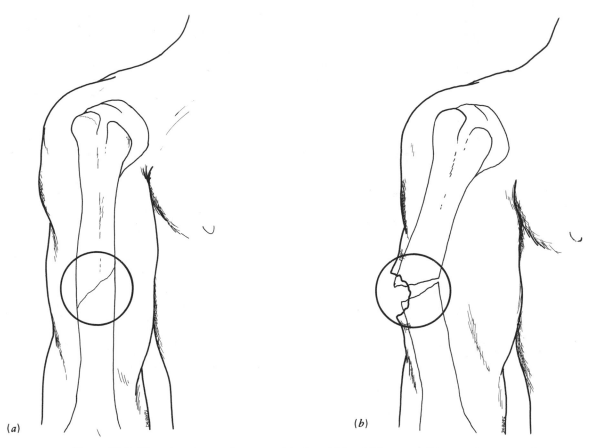

Figure 12.5 Closed and open fractures: (a) closed (simple) fracture; (b) open (compound) fracture.

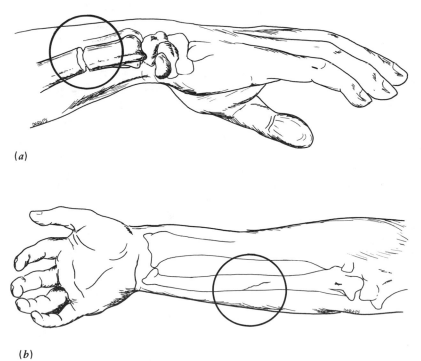

Figure 12.6 Complete and incomplete fractures: (a) complete fracture; (b) incomplete (greenstick fracture).

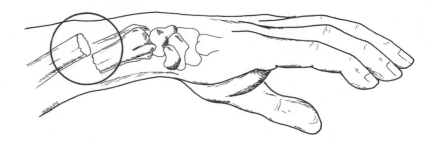

Figure 12.7 Displaced fracture.

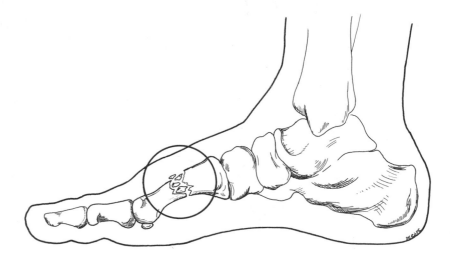

Figure 12.8 Comminuted fracture.

cause it resembles the break in a young sapling in which the wood cracks on one side but does not break all the way through. Such a fracture is more common in children than in older people, whose bones are brittle and snap easily.

5. *Displaced fracture.* The pieces or ends of bone have been displaced away from the fracture line (Fig. 12.7).
6. *Comminuted fracture.* There is more than one fracture line; the broken ends may be crushed and fragmented (Fig. 12.8).
7. *Complicated fracture.* The injury is complicated by damage to adjacent tissue such as nerves, blood vessels, muscles, or underlying organs.

Since bone has the power of regeneration, fractures heal by the growth of new bone cells rather than by the development of scar tissue. Newly created cells of bone and cartilage surround the fracture, forming a soft enlargement called a *callus*. Calcium salts are then deposited throughout the callus and the callus is converted to bone which eventually becomes as strong as it was before.

PATIENT TEACHING

The increasing emphasis on self-care and home care means that lay people need to understand some of the basic concepts of pathophysiology, especially those concepts related to inflammation, infection, and healing. They need to know, for example, that the skin is the body's first line of defense, that it must be kept intact, and therefore, one should never break a blister.

People need to learn to make careful observations of all wounds, and be able to differentiate between a wound which is reddened as a result of the normal inflammatory process and one which may be infected. The ability to make careful observations coupled with an understanding of basic concepts of pathophysiology will make it possible for a person to know when to seek nursing or medical assistance.

RELATED ACTIVITY

1. As part of your efforts to acquire a professional vocabulary, from now on try to recall the medical term for each pathological condition you see. It is difficult

to learn new names for familiar lesions, and therefore, the process must be deliberate and conscious. You will still use a layman's term or slang phrase when it is appropriate to do so, but when communicating with professional colleagues, you need terms which are more precise than pimple, sore, bump, or black and blue spot.

SUGGESTED READINGS

Boyd, William, and Sheldon Huntington: *An Introduction to the Study of Disease*. ed. 8. Philadelphia, Lea & Febiger, 1980.

Bruno, Pauline: The nature of wound healing. *Nurs Clin North Am* 1979 Dec; 14(4):667–682.

Cohen, Stephen, and Geraldine K Glass. Skin rashes in infants and children (programmed instruction). *Am J Nurs* 1978 June; 78(6)1041–1072.

Guyton, Arthur C: *Textbook of Medical Physiology*. ed. 6. Philadelphia, Saunders, 1980.

McConnell, Edwina A: Leukocyte studies: What the counts can tell you. *Nursing 86* 1986 March; 16(3):42–43.

Muir, Bernice: *Pathophysiology: An Introduction to the Mechanisms of Disease*. New York, Wiley, 1980.

Price, Sylvia Anderson, and Lorraine McCarthy Wilson: *Pathophysiology: Clinical Concepts of Disease Processes*. ed. 3. New York, McGraw-Hill, 1986.

Randall, Brenda Joy: Reacting to Anaphylaxis. *Nursing 86* 1986 March; 16(3):34–39.

Siskind, Jill: Handling hemorrhage wisely. *Nursing 84* 1984 Jan; 14(1):34–41.

Part Three

Individuals and Families

13

Human Needs

Prerequisites and/or Suggested Preparation
Chapter 7 (Health and Illness) and Chapter 8 (Stress, Adaptation, and Coping) are suggested as preparation for this chapter.

THEORISTS AND BASIC HUMAN NEEDS

Theories of human growth and development have been described but few of the theorists deal with the *factors which must be present for optimal growth and development*—the basic human needs. Nor do they specifically address the issue of *health*; they do not identify or describe the factors which are necessary for the maintenance of health, the prevention of illness, or the restoration of health.

Nurse theorists, because of the nature of the nursing profession, have recognized for many years the relationship between health and the meeting of human needs, and have explored this relationship as a basis for nursing practice.

Florence Nightingale

In 1859, when she was 39 years old, Florence Nightingale wrote *Notes on Nursing*. This book was intended not to be a training manual for nurses, but rather a guide to help women take care of sick members of their households, and help keep others from becoming sick. It sold 15,000 copies the first month (a goodly number for the year 1859), and was based on 14 years of experience and observation in England and Europe, including two years of service during the Crimean War. Nightingale had spent many years trying to formulate a system for improving the quality of nursing, and about six months after the book was published. She established the Nightingale Training School of Nurses in London.

Notes on Nursing is delightful to read—it is practical, philosophical, witty, and *nearly a hundred years ahead of its time*. The terminology is different from that in use today, but Nightingale addressed the issues of sanitation, environmental pollution, epidemiology, hospital infections, nursing process, and nursing standards. Regardless of the topic, however, her attention was always focused on the *patient and his needs*.

She had accumulated much evidence to support her theory that much misery was caused not by disease but by failure to meet the patient's needs. This viewpoint is evident in the following passages from the second page of her text:

In watching diseases, both in private houses and in public hospitals, the thing which strikes the experienced observer most forcibly is this, that the symptoms or the sufferings generally considered to be inevitable and incidental to the disease are very often not symptoms of the disease at all, but of something quite different—of the want of fresh air, or of light, or of warmth, or of quiet, or of cleanliness, or of punctuality and care in the administration of diet, or all of these. And this quite as much in private as in hospital nursing.

The reparative process which Nature has instituted and which we call disease, has been hindered by some want of knowledge or attention, in one or all of these things, and pain, suffering, or interruption of the whole process sets in.

If a patient is cold, if a patient is feverish, if a patient is faint, if he is sick after taking food, if he has a bed-sore, it is generally the fault not of the disease, but of the nursing.

In modern, air conditioned homes and hospitals some of these problems have been alleviated, such as the need for fresh air and proper sanitation. But in some settings, the problems have merely been transformed— the foul odor from unwashed bedding and infected wounds in 1859 has been replaced by the foul odor (or imperceptible dangers) of industrial fumes and other kinds of air pollution. The cause of the problem may have changed, but the basic human need for fresh air remains.

Florence Nightingale did not categorize patients' needs, nor did she describe them as problems or nursing diagnoses as modern writers might. She did, however, discuss each one in meticulous detail and with a remarkably perceptive concept of holistic nursing. Her appreciation for the relationship between mind and body is indicated by the following passage from p. 59.

The effect in sickness of beautiful objects, of variety of objects, and especially of brilliancy of colour is hardly at all appreciated. . . . People say the effect is only on the mind. It is no such thing. The effect is on the body, too. Little as we know about the way in which we are affected by form, by colour, and light, we do know this, that they have an actual physical effect.

The validity of using the patient's needs as a basis for nursing care is shown by the fact that 125 years after Notes on Nursing, nursing theorists continue to use basic needs as a framework for nursing care:

Basic Needs Identified by Florence Nightingale (1859)

1. Fresh air
2. Light
3. Warmth
4. Cleanliness of environment
5. Personal cleanliness
6. Elimination
7. Positioning
8. Variety
9. Prevention of "hospital diseases"

From Nightingale, F: *Notes on Nursing: What It Is and What It Is Not*, 1859, 1969, Dover Publications, Inc, New York.

Faye Abdellah

In 1960 (101 years after *Notes on Nursing* was written), Faye Abdellah and her colleagues developed a nursing theory which emphasized nursing care which treated the *whole* patient and attempted to meet or resolve his problems, whether they be physical, psychological, social, or spiritual. The nurse was viewed as a problem solver, and the specific needs which were identified are often referred to as "Abdellah's 21 nursing problems."

Abdellah's 21 Nursing Problems (Needs)

1. To maintain good hygiene and physical comfort
2. To achieve optimal activity, exercise, rest, and sleep
3. To prevent accident, injury, or other trauma and prevent the spread of infection
4. To maintain good body mechanics and prevent and correct deformities
5. To facilitate the supply of oxygen to all body cells
6. To facilitate the maintenance of nutrition to all body cells
7. To facilitate the maintenance of elimination
8. To facilitate the maintenance of fluid and electrolyte balance
9. To recognize the physiological responses of the body to disease conditions—pathological, physiological, and compensatory
10. To facilitate the maintenance of regulatory mechanisms and functions
11. To facilitate the maintenance of sensory function
12. To identify and accept positive and negative expressions, feelings, and reactions
13. To identify and accept the interrelatedness of emotions and organic illness
14. To facilitate the maintenance of effective verbal and nonverbal communications
15. To facilitate the development of productive interpersonal relationships
16. To facilitate progress toward achievement of personal spiritual goals
17. To create and/or maintain a therapeutic environment
18. To facilitate awareness of self as an individual with varying physical, emotional, and developmental needs
19. To accept the optimum possible goals in light of limitations—physical and emotional
20. To use community resources as an aid in solving problems arising from illness
21. To understand the role of social problems as influencing factors in the cause of illness

---

From Abdellah, Faye G, et al.: *Patient-centered Approaches to Nursing,* Macmillan, New York, 1960.

Henderson's Basic Needs

1. Breathe normally
2. Eat and drink adequately
3. Eliminate by all avenues of elimination
4. Move and maintain desirable posture (walking, sitting, lying, and changing from one to the other)
5. Sleep and rest
6. Select suitable clothing; dress and undress
7. Maintain body temperature within normal range by adjusting clothing and modifying the environment
8. Keep body clean and well groomed and protect the integument
9. Avoid dangers in the environment and avoid injuring others
10. Communicate with others in expressing emotions, needs, fears, questions, and ideas
11. Worship according to his faith
12. Work at something that provides a sense of accomplishment
13. Play or participate in various forms of recreation
14. Learn, discover, or satisfy the curiosity that leads to "normal" development and health

---

From Henderson, Virginia: *The Nature of Nursing,* Macmillan, 1966, p. 49.

Despite the differences in specificity and terminology, there are significant similarities between the needs identified by Florence Nightingale and the problems (needs) listed by Faye Abdellah.

Virginia Henderson

In 1964, Virginia Henderson defined nursing as the process of:

helping people (sick or well) in the performance of those activities contributing to health or its recovery (or to a peaceful death) that they would perform unaided if they had the necessary strength, will, or knowledge. It is likewise the function of nurses to help people to be independent of such assistance as soon as possible.

In accordance with her definition of nursing, Virginia Henderson listed 14 basic needs of all patients (see above). These needs were stated simply and directly, and encompass virtually all health related aspects of the patient's life.

Abraham Maslow

Abraham Maslow was a psychologist, not a nurse, but his theoretical concept of a *hierarchy of human needs* is an integral part of many nursing theories. It is useful

> ### *Abraham Maslow's Hierarchy of Needs*
>
> 1. Physiologic needs
> 2. Safety and security
> 3. Love and belonging
> 4. Self-esteem
> 5. Self actualization
>
> ―――――――――――――――――――――――――
> Adapted from Maslow, Abraham H: *Motivation and Personality*, 2nd ed.
> Harper and Row, New York, 1970.

because the categories of needs are broad and inclusive, and it is significant because a person's physiological and psychological needs are viewed together within a larger framework related to what Maslow refers to as "the further reaches of human nature."

Maslow's *hierarchy of needs* is used as the framework for the discussion of basic needs and nursing which follows because it is appropriately inclusive and because it is especially applicable to the practice of nursing at every level.

MASLOW'S HIERARCHY OF NEEDS

Abraham Maslow (1908–1970), a distinguished psychologist, believed the best way to understand human motivation was to study the most highly developed, fully human people he could find, people who were exceptionally productive, healthy, creative, happy, and mature. He studied the lives of hundreds of people ranging from presidents and artists to homemakers and scientists. Despite their many differences, these people had one thing in common: they were, according to Maslow, all self-actualized.

Maslow concluded from his research that human beings are dominated by a number of *basic needs* that tend to direct behavior until each need is satisfied. Although these basic needs are interrelated, they tend to be hierarchical. The lower level needs must be satisfied before higher level needs can be met; in fact, higher level needs do not even emerge until lower level needs have been at least minimally satisfied. For example, a person's need for food can, at times, dominate his behavior. His mind will be preoccupied with thoughts of food; he is likely to expend all available physical energy on attempts to get food; and he may even behave in a dangerous and irrational manner. Once his need for food has been met and his hunger has been relieved, higher needs will emerge and motivate him until they in turn are satisfied.

Maslow identified the following five groups of needs

as basic to human motivation: (1) physiological needs, (2) safety and security, (3) love and belongingness, (4) self-esteem, and (5) self-actualization (Fig. 13.1). Of these needs, the physiological ones are the most basic, the most powerful, and the most obvious. They include need for oxygen, fluids, food, shelter, sleep, and sex. If one or more of these needs is not met at least minimally, a person will be unable to meet higher level needs. For example, a person who is suffocating from lack of oxygen may also have unmet self-esteem or security needs, but these he will ignore until he is no longer panicky about his oxygen supply and until he is able to breathe adequately with minimal effort and exertion.

As soon as physiological needs have been adequately met, a group of needs emerges which Maslow describes as safety needs. These needs include both physical and psychological safety and security. When both the physiological needs and the safety needs have been met, the belongingness and love needs emerge, followed in turn by esteem and self-actualization needs. The need to know and to understand and esthetic needs are among the highest level needs.

Although the basic needs usually emerge in an order similar to the one described above, *they do not form an*

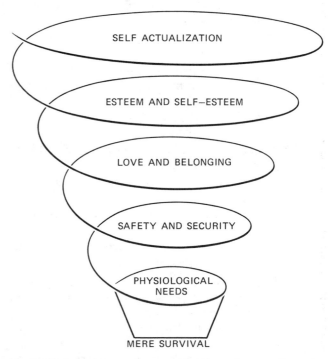

Figure 13.1 *Unmet needs at any level can hamper the satisfaction of higher level needs. The lower the level, the more fully those needs must be met in order for upper level needs to emerge. Extensive interference with physiological needs, for example, can place all higher level need fulfillment in jeopardy.*

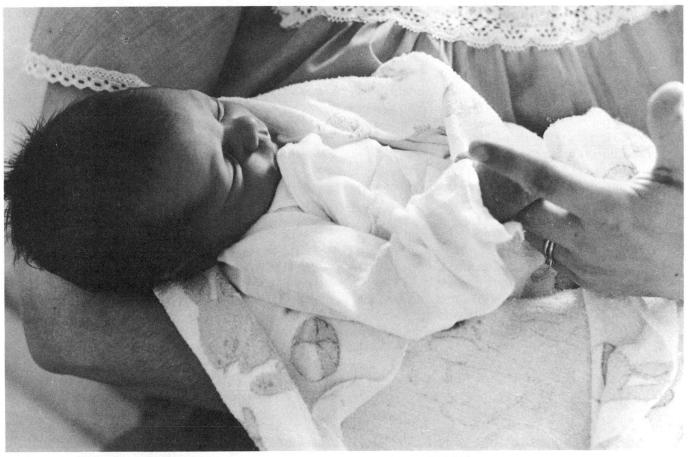

Figure 13.2 The early satisfaction of basic needs provides the foundations for self-actualization.

absolute hierarchy. There are many exceptions. The potential for satisfying higher-level needs may have been dulled in people who have lived at a bare subsistence level for many years. A psychopathic personality may be unable to give and receive love even though his lower level physiological and safety needs may have been adequately met. On the other hand, some outstanding people have devoted their lives to ideas or causes with almost complete disregard for their own lower-level needs. Maslow believed that people born into situations that enable them to satisfy their basic needs very early in life develop such strong, unified characters that they can withstand the loss or frustration of these lower level needs for considerable lengths of time (Fig. 13.2).

Most people manage to satisfy many or most of their lower level needs, but from time to time, a few of these needs may be unmet or only partially satisfied. During an illness or in time of crisis, a person may experience a sudden upsurge of unmet lower level needs. It is these *unmet needs* that have the greatest effect on a person's behavior and that significantly affect the nurse-patient interaction. Once a need has been satisfied, it has little

effect on behavior and motivation, for a need that has been met is no longer a need.

Maslow's hierarchy of needs contributes to the nurse's theoretical basis for assessing patients, anticipating patient needs, planning nursing care, and understanding patient responses or lack of responses to nursing interventions, including patient teaching. There are two essential steps in using Maslow's theory of basic needs. First, the nurse must be able to recognize the signs, symptoms, and behaviors that might indicate an unmet need. Second, the nurse must be able to determine how the unmet need might influence nursing care.

Physiological Needs

Oxygen

Inability to meet the need for oxygen can result in the most urgent of all emergencies. All tissues are susceptible to lack of oxygen, but the brain is permanently damaged within a very few minutes by inadequate oxygenation. Emergency resuscitation measures often restore respiration; and the patient may recover, either partially or fully, from the episode. In an emergency situation there is usually no doubt that a basic need is not being met. In less dramatic situations, however, the patient's unmet need for oxygen may be unnoticed or overlooked.

INDICATORS OF AN UNMET NEED FOR OXYGEN. Information related to the need for oxygen is obtained from assessment of the patient's pulse, respiration, color, alertness, and composure. A pulse that is difficult to palpate, labored or difficult respirations, pallor or cyanosis of the skin, mental confusion, lack of energy, or apprehension may indicate an inadequately met unmet need for oxygen.

IMPLICATIONS FOR NURSING. Because a person's physiological needs are most crucial, his need for oxygen must be granted high priority. Before starting to care for any patient, the nurse must make a quick assessment of the patient's oxygenation and take any action that may be indicated. In addition to assessing his physiological needs, it is important to meet the psychological needs of a patient in respiratory distress because fear, anxiety, or apprehension can increase a person's need for oxygen and at the same time make respirations less effective, more difficult, or more labored.

Fluids

The impact of prolonged or extreme thirst and dehydration on higher level needs is quite obvious. No one would attempt to interest the dehydrated survivor of a desert accident in discussing art or politics; his need for fluids is overwhelming. The more common deprivations of liquid are less obvious, however, and can be overlooked. People with diarrhea or vomiting who are not under medical or nursing supervision often exhibit varying degrees of dehydration as do people who are not fully mobile and therefore not able to obtain liquids as needed.

INDICATORS OF AN UNMET NEED FOR FLUIDS. A careful assessment of a patient's condition may reveal one or more of the following indications of unmet need for fluids: poor turgor (elasticity) of the skin; dryness of the mouth, lips, skin, and hair; constipation; and dark urine with a higher than normal specific gravity. Because fluid and electrolyte imbalances are closely interrelated, the patient with an inadequate fluid intake may also exhibit some degree of mental confusion, irritability, or sluggishness.

IMPLICATIONS FOR NURSING. Although a patient may not complain of discomfort or thirst, the stress of an unmet need for fluid may cause both physical and psychological discomfort, and he may be unable to concentrate

on prescribed exercises and treatments. In addition, a dry or cracked tongue and lips may make it uncomfortable for the patient to speak and therefore hard for him to communicate.

Food

Except in situations involving famine or disaster, the nurse is unlikely to encounter many starving patients. She will, however, need to intervene in situations in which a patient and his family are *malnourished* or *undernourished*. If the nurse suspects that a person's nutrition is inadequate or faulty, many professional skills will be needed in order to help that person because the psychological, social, cultural, and physical aspects of nutrition make it one of the most complex of the basic needs.

INDICATORS OF AN UNMET NEED FOR FOOD. Some of the clues to unmet food needs are unplanned weight loss, failure to grow or gain weight, pallid skin, dull hair, listlessness, and lack of energy. The quantity and quality of food eaten should be taken into consideration before the nurse assumes that these symptoms or conditions are caused by some disease.

The indicators listed above are often the result of an inadequate food intake but similar effects may result from an adequate intake of poor-quality food. If the basic need for food is equated with optimal nutrition, then excessive weight gain and obesity may also be considered indicators of an unmet basic need.

IMPLICATIONS FOR NURSING. Adequate nutrition is essential for physical fitness, a sense of well-being, and the energy needed to meet higher level needs. Therefore, the malnourished or undernourished patient cannot be expected to have much energy available for recovery, growth, and learning. In some situations a person's nutrition must be improved before other therapy can be effective; in other situations, therapy or teaching related to nutrition is required before a person's nutrition can improve. A careful nursing diagnosis is needed to differentiate between the two types of situations.

An elderly widow, living alone, may be undernourished and losing weight because: (1) she cannot afford enough food, (2) she may be too feeble to prepare three meals a day, (3) she may have no appetite because of illness or loneliness, or (4) she may have no way of obtaining groceries regularly. A nurse who scolds the woman for not eating, or merely teaches her about the need for adequate nutrition, will accomplish nothing. The woman's self-esteem (a basic need) will be lowered by the scolding, and the underlying situation will remain unchanged by even the best of teaching.

Unmet nutritional needs cannot always be equated with unavailability of food. Fad diets, preference for junk foods, irregular patterns of eating, ignorance, or psychological quirks can contribute to poor nutrition. Parental neglect and child abuse, illness, pride resulting in rejection of food stamps or welfare, and psychological problems can also block satisfaction of the need for food. Because many influences on food intake have emotional overtones, a gentle and accepting attitude by the nurse is needed to help a person explore the problems related to his unmet nutritional needs.

Shelter and Maintenance of Body Temperature

Except for the increasing numbers of street people (homeless people), relatively few people in this country are without shelter of any kind, although many live in substandard housing. Shelter and protection from extremes of heat and cold are necessary for life and therefore constitute one of the most basic needs in Maslow's hierarchy. Except in an emergency or disaster, the basic need may not be the need for shelter as such but for maintenance of a normal body temperature. Rapid changes or prolonged extremes of environmental temperature are especially difficult for very young, elderly, feeble, or inactive people, and an abnormal body temperature is stressful to any person.

INDICATORS OF AN UNMET NEED FOR PROTECTION FROM EXTREMES OF TEMPERATURE. Some indicators of unmet needs for shelter or temperature control are color and condition of the skin, body temperature, position of body, and level of activity and alertness. Some physiological responses to extremes of heat and cold are dramatic and obvious, such as burns, frostbite, sunstroke, shivering, and sweating. Other responses are less intense but equally significant indicators. Such responses to cold include sluggishness, a huddled posture, a curled position in bed, rubbing of the hands, pulling of clothes around the body more snugly, and low levels of energy and attention. Responses to heat which may be missed or misinterpreted include restlessness, irritability, loosening of clothes, thirst, lethargy, and decreased attention span.

In most instances the physiological response to an extreme of temperature does not vary with the cause. The body's response is the same whether the extreme of temperature is caused by disaster, neglect, or therapy. The body's response to cold, for example, is similar whether the cold is caused by a blizzard, an unheated house, a hypothermia machine, or excessive air conditioning.

IMPLICATIONS FOR NURSING. It may take a very careful assessment and a great deal of perception to discover that a patient's apparent lack of motivation, attention, and general unresponsiveness is due to the discomfort of being too warm or too cold. Either condition detracts from the ability to meet higher level needs.

Sleep

Each person's need for sleep must be adequately met on a fairly regular basis if he is to function at an optimal level. Satisfaction of the need for sleep depends on both the quantity and quality of sleep and is affected by a person's diurnal rhythm. When normal patterns and rhythms of sleep are interrupted by illness, insomnia, work, or the environment, the resulting fatigue and stress limit the probability of meeting higher level needs.

INDICATORS OF AN UNMET NEED FOR SLEEP. Some indicators of unmet sleep are rather obvious, such as dark circles under the eyes and falling asleep during the day. Other signs include a lowered level of energy and motivation, irritability, difficulty in concentration, slowed reactions, and lowered mental acuity. Because some of these indicators are also symptoms of illness, the nurse will need to validate her assessment in order to determine whether the observed behaviors are the result of illness or of inadequate sleep.

IMPLICATIONS FOR NURSING. Whenever possible, noncritical treatments and patient teaching should be scheduled when the patient is as rested and alert as possible. Fatigue makes learning, exercise, and other aspects of therapy much more difficult.

Sex

Maslow included sex as one of the basic needs that must be satisfied for the higher level needs to be met. Although sexual behavior is influenced by many needs, especially by the love and belonging needs, Maslow indicated that sex can be studied as a basic physiological need (1970, p.44).

Because of the cultural, moral, and psychological aspects of sex, this need is perhaps the most difficult of the physiological needs with which the health care worker has to deal, especially when helping a physically handicapped, elderly, retarded, or institutionalized person. With the increasing acceptance of sex and sexuality as integral aspects of human life, people expect to receive knowledgeable and concerned assistance with various physiological problems such as infertility, birth control, venereal disease, and menopause. In addition to the physiological aspects of sex, the nurse may find it necessary to assist families with problems of sexuality that relate to other needs (love and belonging, esteem, and self-actualization needs).

INDICATORS OF UNMET PHYSIOLOGICAL NEEDS RELATED TO SEX. Unmet sexuality needs might be indicated by difficult or painful intercourse, failure to conceive, painful menstruation, unwanted pregnancy, difficult or disturbing menopause, overt or excessive masturbation, and improper sexual advances.

IMPLICATIONS FOR NURSING. To treat the patient as a whole person, the nurse must be prepared to recognize and respond to any clues that might indicate that a patient has unmet needs related to sex. This will require of the nurse a knowledge of human sexuality, the ability to communicate openly with a patient or client, and an awareness of the nurse's own feelings and attitudes toward sex.

Many nurses find it no more stressful to take a sexual history and to discuss a person's sexual needs with him than to take a dietary history and to discuss his nutritional needs. Other nurses, because of their own culture, upbringing, and values, find it difficult to do more than answer a person's questions accurately and factually.

A nurse may find that she needs to spend considerable time and energy working through her own beliefs and values. For example, a nurse who believes that premarital sexual intercourse is a sin is likely to find it difficult to work as a public health nurse in a neighborhood in which many girls are sexually active at age 13 or 14 and where the rates of teenage pregnancy and venereal disease are high. Regardless of personal beliefs and values, the nurse's interactions with the patient and family can be effective if she accepts the fact that she cannot and should not impose her values on other people. A nurse need not approve of the behaviors she encounters in patients; but to function effectively, she must be able to accept each patient as a worthy and valued person. A nonjudgmental attitude, regardless of personal beliefs, will enable a nurse to help each patient.

Safety Needs

Once a person's physiological needs have been met, the safety needs emerge. Until this time, he may have had to take chances with his own safety to meet his basic physiological needs. When they have been adequately satisfied, he then begins to seek a safe, orderly, predictable world. Although Maslow usually referred to safety as a singular need, there are two components to safety in the context of the health care delivery system: psychological safety and physical safety.

Psychological Safety and Security

To *feel safe and secure*, a person needs at least a *minimal understanding of what to expect* in terms of people, interpersonal relationships, routines, procedures, equipment, and other aspects of the environment. He also needs to understand the way in which his body, mind, and emotions function. This need for psychological safety and security becomes more pronounced whenever a person enters a new situation, and becomes even more intense when he is vulnerable and apprehensive because of illness. In some instances the nurse can help to meet the patient's need for psychological safety by including carefully planned explanations and demonstrations throughout all her early contacts with the patient. Some of these explanations will be based on the nurse's past experiences and her knowledge of the types of fears and anxieties which are frequently encountered by patients; other explanations will be based on the individual patient's comments, questions, and other verbal or nonverbal cues.

INDICATORS OF UNMET NEEDS FOR PSYCHOLOGICAL SAFETY AND SECURITY. The needs for psychological safety and security are difficult to assess because the related behaviors are easily misinterpreted. The person who fails to keep clinic appointments because he is awed and frightened by the clinic setting may be thought to be lacking motivation. The patient who refuses to drink the fluids ordered for him because he is afraid of asking for the urinal too often may be labeled "uncooperative." The patient in a research center or teaching center who will follow only those orders issued by his attending physician or a familiar nurse because he is terrified of being experimented on is more likely to be considered obstinate than he is to be assessed as frightened. Much of the behavior labeled uncooperative, difficult, noncompliant, or demanding stems not from malice or ill will on the part of the patient but from unmet safety needs. An assessment of psychological safety needs requires considerable skill and patience because there is no readily identifiable set of indicators. Clues must be sought in such diverse behaviors as: frequent and often repetitious questions, frequent or seemingly unreasonable requests, demands for a ritualized schedule or rigid routine, and the physiological signs of fear or anxiety. The fearful and insecure patient may be either unusually passive and cooperative or may refuse to comply at all without extensive explanations.

IMPLICATIONS FOR NURSING. Much of the initial patient teaching in any setting is planned to relieve the patient's anxiety and help him feel comfortable. Once the initial explanations have been given, however, the focus of the teaching often shifts rather rapidly from helping the patient adapt to a new situation to an emphasis on things he needs to know. If this shift is abrupt or occurs too quickly, the patient's ongoing need for psychological safety will not be met. Unless a situation is relatively stable and unchanging, the patient's needs will change frequently, perhaps from day to day. Preoperative threats to safety and security will be replaced by postoperative threats, which may be followed in turn by apprehension related to discharge and the worries that often accompany convalescence. A worried, anxious patient is unable to concentrate on things to be learned, so the only teaching which is likely to be effective under these situations is that teaching which is designed to reduce anxiety and thereby improve future learning. An ongoing assessment of the need for psychological safety and security is critical throughout all patient-nurse interactions, whether in an acute care setting, a clinic, or the patient's home. Failure to meet the psychological safety needs can seriously impede a patient's progress, whereas adequately met safety needs free a person to move to a higher level of need fulfillment.

Physical Safety

According to Maslow, safety needs do not emerge until physiological needs have been met. Although this may be true with respect to the patient, the *nurse cannot wait to attend to safety needs* until the patient's physiological needs have been met; she will need to meet his safety needs and physiological needs simultaneously. Since the patient or family are often not aware of potential threats or dangers, the staff in a health care delivery system must assume almost total responsibility for meeting many of the patient's physical safety needs.

INDICATORS OF UNMET PHYSICAL SAFETY NEEDS. In some situations there may be no clues or indicators from a patient that a physical safety need was not met until there is tangible bodily evidence that his body has been threatened or injured. Examples of such evidence include nausea from an incorrect dose or overdose of a drug, joint contractures from poor positioning, muscle atrophy (wasting) from inadequate exercise, fever from an infection, bedsores from prolonged pressure over a bony prominence, and a bruise or fracture from falling out of bed. All of these are the *result of unmet safety needs.*

The patient's expression of concern for his physical safety is more frequently related to pain or discomfort and may be indicated by a question such as "Will it hurt?" Questions and comments such as the following are more often an indicator of a safety need than an indication of intellectual curiosity: "How fast is my IV supposed to run?" "What makes that clicking noise in the machine?" "I usually get a large and a small white pill in the morning; why do I now get two small ones?"

IMPLICATIONS FOR NURSING. The patient and family need to be taught to recognize and identify the possible dangers related to a specific age (such as the accidental poisoning of toddlers), a specific situation (such as anticoagulant therapy), or a specific environment (such as highly waxed floors in the home of an aged person). They should be taught how to protect themselves and others from injury, infections, and disease. They also need to be taught basic first aid, including mouth-to-mouth resuscitation and the Heimlich maneuver for choking. The patient must be taught how to protect himself from complications related to his present disease or condition. Although the need for patient teaching related to physical safety may seem less urgent than some other teaching needs, failure to do such teaching may seriously hamper the patient's progress or endanger his life and well-being.

Love and Belonging Needs

When the physiological and safety needs of a person have been met, the need for love, affection, and belonging emerges. Each person yearns for affectionate relationships with people and seeks a place for himself within each group in which he finds himself (Fig. 13.3). If he feels relatively safe and secure, he is able to expend considerable energy to meet this need. Maslow differentiated between these love needs and sex, which he considered a physiological need. His view of love closely parallels that of Carl Rogers, who has defined love as "being deeply understood and deeply accepted." Maslow found that growth and the development of one's potential are inhibited by the absence of love. Clinicians have proved that babies who are not given adequate expressions of love will fail to thrive, will sicken, and may eventually die. The clinical term for this medically recognized condition is the *failure to thrive syndrome.*

Within the health care delivery system, the need of the patient and family for love, understanding, and acceptance is often expressed as a protest against the frequent dehumanization of health care. These expressions of need range from the complaints of individual patients to documentary films about the inhumanity of some medical and nursing care. A patient or family member may comment: "Nobody cares, nobody knows how I really feel; I'm just another number in this hospital"; or "I've been waiting out here for three hours now—I don't think anyone even knows I'm here." Such feelings affect the patient's reaction to therapy, his response to teaching, and his motivation for recovery.

INDICATORS OF UNMET LOVE AND BELONGING NEEDS. In accordance with the flight-or-fight responses to stress, the person with unmet love and belonging needs may either *passively accept* the situation or *actively seek* to be noticed and recognized within the health care delivery

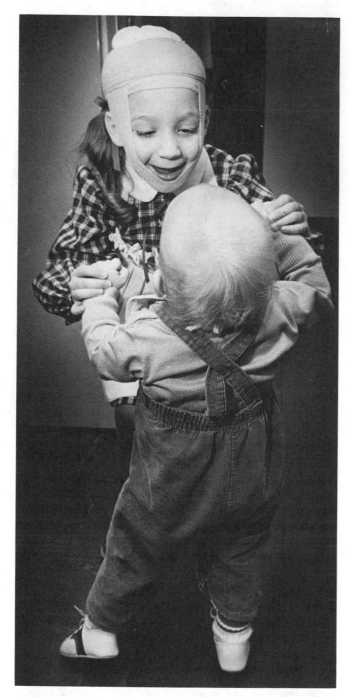

Figure 13.3 *This interaction between Renee and a young cousin illustrates the basic need of all humans, regardless of age, for love and belongingness as described by Maslow. The picture also demonstrates the significance of touch as a form of nonverbal communication.*

system. Unless the nurse is meticulous in her assessment of the patient or family, these responses may be misinterpreted, with little if anything being done to meet the underlying need. The passive patient who is feeling hurt and dehumanized may be described as a good patient and left alone, while the assertive patient who is also feeling hurt is described as a difficult patient and also left alone. In each instance the basic needs continue to be unmet.

Assessment of the quiet, noncomplaining person is difficult. His behavior is not disruptive and may even be satisfying to the staff. He may seek approval and acceptance by being eager to please, agreeable, compliant, and easily satisfied. He may try to be helpful in order to prove that he belongs. As all these behaviors may be misinterpreted or pass unnoticed, a nurse needs to be especially thorough in her assessment of any patient who seems to be almost too good or too quiet or too cooperative.

Identification of the patient who is actively seeking a place in the unit or group is often less difficult. The indicators of his unmet love and belonging needs may include ringing his call bell frequently; complaining about many things, both important and trivial; stopping by the nurses' station a number of times each shift; asking many questions; spending considerable time in the patients' lounge; and other types of attention-seeking behavior. Some of these behaviors tend to alienate the staff; as they withdraw from him, his needs are unmet to an even greater degree.

IMPLICATIONS FOR NURSING. Satisfaction of love and belonging needs should start with the very first contact with a patient and family and may even precede other types of interaction. For example, in a clinic setting, eye contact and a smile in passing will acknowledge the patient as a person even before he is called in for his scheduled appointment. When the nurse introduces herself and calls that patient by name, she again acknowledges him as a person and a member of the unit.

One of the most significant ways in which the nurse helps to meet love and belonging needs is to teach the patient and his family or friends how to grow and develop in their relationships with each other despite a serious illness, poor prognosis, or pending death. In addition, the nurse can do many things to meet the patient's love and belonging needs. In general, any nursing action that decreases a person's feeling of being ignored will help to meet that person's need for acceptance and belonging. When talking with a patient, such fundamental behaviors as fully facing the patient, maintaining eye contact, and sitting down with him whenever possible help him feel that the nurse is reaching out to him in an accepting way.

Whenever a nurse plans her nursing care or patient teaching with little or no input from the patient, she increases his sense of isolation and aloneness, and reinforces his feeling that he does not count for much within the health care delivery system. *Mutual goal setting* assures the patient and family that they are members of the health team, that they are accepted, and that they are understood.

Esteem Needs

Although the esteem needs are sometimes treated as a single need, Maslow identified two sets of esteem needs: (1) self-esteem and self-respect and (2) the respect and esteem of other people (1970, p. 45).

Self-esteem and Self-respect

The esteem needs are critical for the promotion of health, especially mental health, even though health care workers sometimes place a much higher priority on physiological needs and safety needs. If the promotion of mental health is accepted as a goal of nursing practice, attention to the esteem needs must be as carefully planned and as deliberate as the attention to lower level needs.

The self-esteem needs include the need for competence, skill, mastery, independence, and confidence. Although everyone does not enter the clinic or hospital with the same degree of self-esteem and self-respect, it is important that each person leave with his own feelings of self-esteem and self-respect intact or even enhanced.

INDICATORS OF AN UNMET NEED FOR SELF-ESTEEM AND SELF-RESPECT. Unmet self-esteem needs are indicated by feelings of dependence, lack of confidence, lack of competence, and lack of ability. These feelings are likely to be reflected in statements such as: "I just can't get around anymore; I guess I'll have to give up my job"; "Somebody will have to irrigate my colostomy for me—I just can't"; or "I'll never be able to stick to that diet."

Each person has his own way of dealing with unmet esteem needs. A few people will reveal their feelings, but many more will conceal them as best they can. All of the nurse's psychosocial assessment skills will be needed to differentiate between the quietly self-confident person and the person who, though seemingly assured, feels incompetent or inferior. As the nurse makes this assessment, it is necessary to determine which aspects of any unmet self-esteem needs are part of a long-standing pattern of behavioral responses and which ones are health related or illness induced. A successful lawyer who feels confident and respected in a courtroom may feel awkward, awed, and incompetent when confronted with braces and traction or by an authoritarian physician or nurse.

IMPLICATIONS FOR NURSING. The effort to maintain and increase a patient's level of self-esteem and self-respect must start with the first contact between patient and nurse. The initial patient teaching should help the patient to feel competent and to feel that he has retained a fair amount of his independence and autonomy. If a patient does not know how to do what is expected of him, he will feel awkward, helpless, or incompetent; therefore, early patient teaching must make certain he is able to fill out his menu, call for the nurse, and get to the bathroom (or use the bedpan or urinal). It is vital that the patient *be able* to do these things rather than merely know how to do them. A person who has been told what to do but is unable to do it because of arthritis, confusion, pain, anxiety, or some other reason will suffer an increasing loss of self-esteem.

The focus of patient teaching should be directed toward the patient's acquisition of those skills and understanding that will result in increased self-esteem and self-respect. This increased self-esteem may be noted in statements such as: "I *can* get around—today I got on and off the toilet alone"; "I'm learning to be an accountant so I can keep working"; "I did it, and I never thought I'd be able to"; "I guess I really can take care of her at home"; and "I did it all by myself this time!"

Respect From Others

In addition to feeling good about himself, a person needs to know that others share that feeling and opinion. Maslow believed that a stable and healthy self-respect is closely related to deserved respect from others (1970, p. 46). This need for respect and approval of others can be noted in questions such as: "How am I doing, doctor?" and "Am I doing it right, nurse?" The person who is trying to stop smoking, to calculate a diabetic diet, or to walk with an artificial leg needs feedback and reinforcement. Each one needs to know that the people he considers important believe that he is becoming more capable and more competent in the areas with which he has been struggling.

INDICATORS OF AN UNMET NEED FOR RESPECT FROM OTHERS. Indicators of an unmet need for respect from others may include decreased motivation, minimal expenditure of energy, and discouragement. A person, consciously or unconsciously, usually tries to live up to the expectations of those who are significant in his life. If other people seem to be uninterested or seem unimpressed by a patient's efforts, he may well figure, "Why bother? I'm not getting anywhere." If others seem to expect him to fail, he is likely to do so. On the other hand, if the nurse is interested and aware of the patient's progress, a genuinely enthusiastic "You're doing fine" or "That's better than you did yesterday" will tend to raise the person's self-esteem and spur him on to even greater effort (Fig. 13.4).

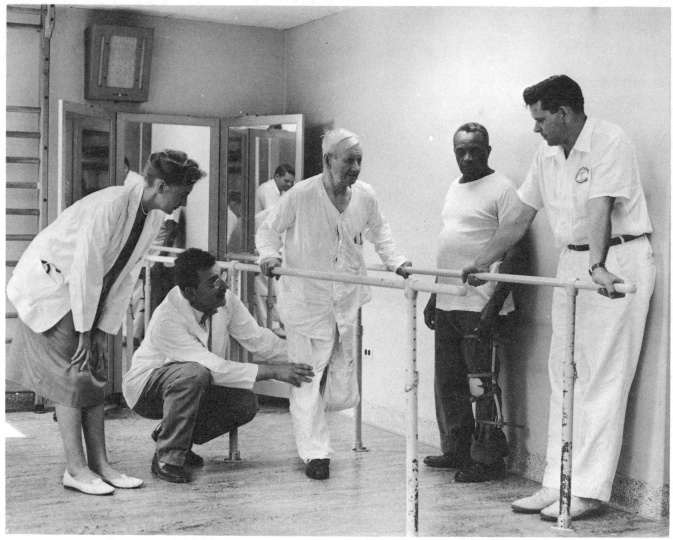

Figure 13.4 *The physical support and encouraging presence of these people combine to help this man adjust to his below-the-knee amputation.*

IMPLICATIONS FOR NURSING. It is not enough merely to teach the patient how to do those things he is expected to be able to do with respect to his health care. Teaching must also include giving encouragement, support, and positive reinforcement as the patient progresses and also during his inevitable periods of discouragement and frustration.

Higher Level Needs

Maslow originally defined the basic needs as *deficiency needs* because each one meets the following conditions:

1. Satisfied needs help prevent illness
2. Unmet or inadequately met needs breed illness
3. The meeting of needs cures illness (1962, p. 20)

For example, pure air, good nutrition, security, and love tend to prevent physical and/or mental illness. Air pollution, malnutrition, fear, and neglect tend to foster illness; whereas the restoration of pure air, good food, security, and love help to cure physical and mental illness.

As a result of his later research, Maslow (1970) developed another list of needs in higher categories, which he calls *growth needs*, as opposed to the basic deficiency needs. All of these higher needs, which include the need for self-actualization and esthetic needs, are related to the delivery of health care; but the application of these needs is beyond the scope of this book. Let it suffice to say that Maslow stated:

living at the higher need level means greater biological efficiency, greater longevity, less disease, better sleep, appetite, etc. The psy-

chosomatic researchers prove again and again that anxiety, fear, lack of love, domination, etc. tend to encourage undesirable physical as well as undesirable psychological responses. Higher need gratifications have survival value and growth value as well. (1970, p. 98)

PATIENT TEACHING

An understanding of Maslow's basic concepts can help people accept and cope with a variety of troublesome or baffling behaviors. A parent who recognizes the implications of *an unmet need* for sleep will be less likely to punish an unruly toddler who is in fact not naughty at all but merely tired and overstimulated. The attention-getting (and sometimes obnoxious) behavior of a child or adult is easier to cope with if it is accepted as indicative of a legitimate and often critical need for belonging and respect rather than as a deliberate attempt to irritate and frustrate other people. Lay people do not need to know the terminology of Maslow's theory of a hierarchy of needs, but they do need to be taught that: (1) human behavior is affected by a number of physiological and psychological needs, (2) human life and well-being can be enhanced to the degree that these basic needs are fulfilled, and (3) exploration and identification of any unmet basic needs is an initial step in the process of helping both children and adults to reach their full potential.

RELATED ACTIVITIES

1. An important step in the process of learning to use Maslow's theory is the examination of your own basic needs and your behavioral responses. During a period of 24 hours, identify six to eight instances in which one of your basic needs was not met to your satisfaction. In each instance, try to determine whether or not failure to meet the need was related to another more pressing need. For example, was failure to meet your need for a good night's sleep caused by *esteem needs* and the resulting pressure for good grades, by *love and belonging needs* which might be met at a certain social event, or by *safety and security needs* created by news of a prowler in the neighborhood? In each instance, briefly analyze your response to the unmet need and try to identify any pattern of responses.

2. Think of four or five recent situations in which your self-esteem has been high, and *identify the ways in which other people contributed to that feeling.* What did they do or say? Using the words or behavior of those people as examples, think of three ways in which you could help to meet the esteem needs of: (1) a new mother who is finding it difficult to breastfeed her baby, (2) an older person who must resort to using a cane, or (3) a child who just failed a spelling test. (Merely *telling* the person that the use of a cane is not very important or that one failure is okay will *NOT* increase his or her self-esteem!) It will be interesting to compare notes with your classmates and discover how similar or different your ways of helping might be. If they are very different, what might account for the differences?

3. Analyze two situations in which you feel that the behavior of one person was misjudged or unfairly criticized by one or more other people who were unaware of the needs which affected the person's behavior. In each situation, how might the situation have been prevented, or what could be done to help prevent similar misunderstandings in the future?

SUGGESTED READINGS

Driscoll, Richard: Their own worst enemies. *Psych Today* 1982 July; 16(7):45–49.

Goble, Frank G: *The Third Force: The Psychology of Abraham Maslow.* New York, Pocket Books, 1970.

Kagan, Jerome, interviewed by Elizabeth Hall: The fearful child's hidden talents. *Psych Today* 1982 July; 16(7):50–59.

Luckmann, Joan, and Karen Sorenson: When patients' actions tell you about their feelings, fears and needs. *Nursing 75* 1975 *Feb*; 5(2):54.

Maslow, Abraham: *The Farther Reaches of Human Nature.* New York, Viking Press, 1972.

——— *Motivation and Personality.* ed. 2. New York, Harper & Row, 1970.

——— *Toward a Psychology of Being*, ed. 2. New York, Van Nostrand Reinhold, 1968.

Nightingale, Florence: *Notes on Nursing: What It Is and What It Is Not,* New York, Dover Publications, Inc., 1859, 1969.

Rogers, Carl: *Freedom to Learn.* Columbus, OH, Merrill Press, 1969.

——— *On Becoming a Person*, ed. Sentury, Boston, Houghton Mifflin, 1961.

Tinelli, Sharon Olson: The relationship of family concept to individual self-esteem. *Issues Ment Health Nurs* 1981.

Yura, Helen, and Mary B. Walsh: *Human Needs 2 and the Nursing Process*, New York, Appleton-Century-Crofts, 1982.

14

Perinatal Development

Pamela Forand Ryan

Prerequisites and/or Suggested Preparation
An understanding of the anatomy and physiology of the male and female reproductive systems is prerequisite to understanding this chapter, and suggested preparation includes Chapter 13 (Human Needs).

Of all the ways in which nurses promote health, none is more significant than the measures undertaken to ensure the healthy prenatal development of a new baby. Even before the moment of conception, nursing interventions are directed toward ensuring an optimal situation for the developing individual.

This broad emphasis on preconceptual and prenatal health is reflected in the terms that apply to an evolving field of nursing practice. In years past, the term *obstetrical nursing* referred to the care of the mother during her pregnancy, labor, and delivery, and for the immediate care of the newborn. A generation or so ago, the importance of the mother-child relationship was recognized, and this area of nursing practice was referred to as *maternal-child nursing*. At present, the significance of the family unit is acknowledged by the term *child-bearing family nursing* which focuses on the interrelated needs of mother, baby, father, and siblings.

The overall health of any nation is related to the physical and psychological status of its infants at birth, and the most effective way to improve the health status of infants is to focus on those defects, deformities, and deficiencies which can be prevented or minimized. Examples of conditions which are either reducible or preventable include: prematurity, low birth weight (baby is not premature but is significantly underweight), infant drug addiction, congenital defects, inherited diseases, and some types of mental retardation.

Since nursing interventions related to these conditions must take place as early as possible, preconceptual teaching must take place during early adolescence, and prenatal care must begin with the onset of pregnancy. Opportunities for early intervention are not always available or utilized, but provision for such care is a top priority for both nursing and society as a whole. Infant mortality rates in the US do not compare favorably with those of other industrialized nations, and nursing is committed to minimizing this unfortunate discrepancy. Some of the ways to accomplish this task are to increase opportunities for adolescent education, provide preconceptual education to prospective parents, offer genetic counseling, give prenatal care, and provide education about childbirth.

The health of the newborn is influenced by genetic, physical, psychosocial, and socioeconomic factors which should be assessed by the nurse and parents together whenever an opportunity for such an interaction can be created. Such assessments and subsequent teaching may take place in the office of a midwife or physician, clinic, high school or adult education program, or hospital outreach program.

THE PRECONCEPTUAL PERIOD

The building blocks for a baby's growth and development begin long before conception, and it is imperative that prospective parents appreciate the value of being physically and psychologically ready to have a baby.

Environmental Factors

The term *environmental factors*, in the context of the preconceptual and prenatal periods, refers to all those factors external to the fetus itself. Such factors include the mother's health, nutrients available for the fetus, and toxic substances.

The Prospective Mother

Ideally, the preconceptual care of the mother begins during her childhood with the early development of good health practices, appropriate immunizations, and proper nutrition which will provide a solid biological foundation for future childbearing. The psychological basis for future parenting begins by experiencing the love and nurturing of attentive parents, and by fantasizing and role playing while "playing house."

Whenever feasible, a thorough health assessment should be done prior to conception, regardless of the age of the prospective mother, to identify and correct

---

Assessments Relevant to Prospective Parents

- Physical Factors
    - Health history of prospective parents and grandparents
    - Current health habits of prospective parents
    - Health status of prospective mother
- Genetic Factors
    - Family history of unusual traits or abnormal conditions
    - Existence of known genetic traits, dominant or recessive
    - Ethnic predisposition to specific disease condition(s)
- Psychosocial Factors
    - Age and *maturational level* of prospective parents
    - Relationship between prospective parents
    - Relationships between prospective parents and grandparents
    - Circumstances surrounding anticipated pregnancy
    - Expectations and attitudes toward pregnancy and parenthood
- Socioeconomic Factors
    - Adequacy of housing, income for prenatal expenses
    - Possible impact of parenthood on education and/or career

any medical problem that might interfere with the normal growth and development of the anticipated baby.

The Prospective Father

Information about the effects of paternal preconceptual conditions is limited and speculative in nature. Some studies have shown a relationship between some chronic diseases such as diabetes and congenital anomalies and low birth weight infants. There is evidence that chronic drug and alcohol abuse by the prospective father results in genetic damage which is, in turn, submitted to the offspring, and new research is beginning to explore the theory that the seminal fluid of drug users may have a harmful effect on the fetus in utero.

The psychological readiness of the prospective father is influenced by the parenting he received as a child, his current attitude toward women, developmental level, willingness to assume the responsibilities of parenthood, and his reasons for wanting to become a father.

Responsibility for Environmental Factors

The responsibility for control over preconceptual environmental factors affecting the growth and development of the fetus does not lie with any one person or group of persons; rather, it is a shared responsibility. Families must assure that their growing children develop good habits of nutrition, exercise, rest, and recreation. Parents and schools must work together to provide adequate family life education programs with access to information related to contraception and sexually transmitted diseases, as well as the use and abuse of drugs and alcohol. Health care providers must increase their efforts to educate the public about the importance of preconceptual care, to provide adequate health care facilities, and to support family planning services.

It is imperative that all family related agencies and institutions redouble their efforts to reduce the numbers of adolescent pregnancies for the good of the nation, the young parents, and the baby itself. Infant mortality is highest in young women under 16; pregnancy poses serious threats to the young mother for three reasons. The pregnancy draws on the nutritional stores needed for the adolescent's own growth, the psychological demands associated with pregnancy can interfere with her own psychological development, and the tendency to drop out of school can place her in economic jeopardy, often for the rest of her life.

Genetic Factors

Genetic Counseling

About 25 percent of birth defects are due to genetic factors, and genetic counseling is the only readily avail-

able strategy for *preventing* such deformities and deaths. Genetic counseling is important when there is a family history of congenital defects, when a previous child has been born with a hereditary disease, or when the mother might be a carrier of a disease which affects males only.

When prospective parents who are at risk for genetic defects are identified in the preconceptual period, they can take advantage of genetic counseling before a pregnancy occurs, when a wider range of options is available to them. These options include childless marriage, adoption, and the possible abortion of an affected fetus.

Genetic factors which place a prospective parent at risk include:

- Maternal age over 35 with an increased chance of a baby with Down's syndrome
- Ethnic background with a high frequency of genetic disorders such as sickle cell anemia
- Family history of genetic disorders such as Huntington's chorea or hemophilia
- A reproductive history of miscarriages and stillbirths
- Presence of maternal diseases related to high incidence of birth defects

If preconceptual counseling is not available, parents who are concerned about genetic defects may choose to take advantage of new techniques of prenatal diagnosis.

AMNIOCENTESIS. Amniocentesis is a test which enables a physician to determine whether a baby will be born with a hereditary defect. It is used to diagnose chromosomal abnormalities. A small amount of amniotic fluid is withdrawn through a needle, which is inserted through the mother's abdomen under local anesthesia and positioned in the amniotic sac. The fluid is submitted to the laboratory, where culture and chromosome analysis are done. The procedure must be done between the fourteenth and sixteenth weeks of gestation, and 2 to 4 weeks are required before the results become available.

CHORIONIC VILLUS SAMPLING. A recent development in prenatal diagnosis is chorionic villus sampling, which can be done at eight to 12 weeks of gestation. The aspiration or biopsy of villi from the developing embryo poses little documented risk to the fetus, and the results are available within 1 to 2 weeks. This earlier diagnosis allows the parents more time for decision making, and also more privacy since the pregnancy is not yet physically obvious to others. If extensive or extreme abnormalities suggest the possibility of an abortion, the risk is reduced because the procedure can be done earlier.

Determination of Sex

The sex of the baby is determined at conception when sperm and ovum unite. Each sperm and each ovum contains 22 autosomes (chromosomes) plus 1 sex chromosome known as the X or Y chromosome. A sperm can contain *either* an X or a Y chromosome; whereas an ovum always contains 2 X chromosomes. If the fertilized ovum contains 2 X chromosomes (one from each parent) the baby will be a girl. If, however, the fertilized ovum contains an X from the mother and a Y from the father, the baby will be a boy. The fact that the father determines the sex of the baby can be very important when counseling a family in which the mother is "blamed" for not producing a male heir.

It would be reasonable to assume that 50 percent of babies would be males and 50 percent would be females; however, there is a higher conception and birth rate among males for some unknown reason. This is offset by a higher infant and childhood mortality rate among boys; thus, there are more women in the world than men.

Nursing Role

The nurse plays a vital role in the hereditary aspects of the preconceptual or prenatal period. She can help to identify clients at risk and assist them in obtaining counseling, and in some settings she can also provide follow-up care by maintaining contact with the family and developing a close relationship with them. This might involve interpreting and reinforcing the advice given, assisting the family in problem solving, supporting them in their decision, and reinforcing their coping skills. Ultimately, the nurse has a tremendous impact on the future growth and development of the planned-for-baby.

Pre-Embryonic Stage

The pre-embryonic phase lasts for 2 weeks, during which the fertilized ovum (zygote) makes its way down the fallopian tube into the uterus where it will become implanted and receive shelter and nourishment for the remainder of the pregnancy.

This mass of cells has all the basic elements to develop into an embryo. It begins to hollow out, expand, and divide into two layers: an inner layer from which the fetus will develop, and an outer layer which will provide nourishment for the fetus.

Embryonic Loss

Approximately 35 percent of pregnancies never progress beyond the pre-embryonic stage, and these pregnancies are usually missed by the parents and perceived as "late" periods. These losses occur because any interference with growth and development during the pre-embryonic stage usually results in failure of the fertilized ovum to progress beyond the initial 2 weeks. A number of factors may interfere, the most common being some type of chromosomal abnormality which is often referred to as a "blighted ovum."

Since human growth is sequential, each stage of a pregnancy depends on the successful completion of the previous stage. The pre-embryonic stage is completed with the implantation of the fertilized ovum into the endometrium (lining) of the uterus, and the next stage is ready to begin.

THE PRENATAL PERIOD

One of life's greatest miracles is the way in which two tiny specks of tissue—an ovum and a sperm—combine, grow, and develop to become a human being. The interval between the moment of conception, when ovum and sperm unite, to the moment of birth, when a fully formed baby joins his waiting mother and father, is the most rapid period of growth and development in a baby's life. During this prenatal period, the developing baby increases in size over two billion times while passing through three stages—pre-embryonic, embryonic, and fetal—each of which has inherent milestones and dangers.

Embryonic Stage

The embryonic stage begins once implantation is completed and lasts for 6 weeks. This phase is characterized by rapid cell division. During this most crucial period of development, essential organs begin to develop, and any *interference* with development during this stage will lead to *major congenital anomalies.*

Development of Support Structures

Once shelter and nourishment have been assured, the embryo, as it is now called, can begin its growth in earnest, a process which is regulated by the genetic structure of the embryo, enzymes, and hormones. Support structures develop from the inner layer of cells which is made up of hairy projections called *chorionic villi.* The villi that are closest to the thickened endometrium of the uterus become the *placenta* by the end of the first month. The placenta serves as the source of nutrients for the baby, oxygen and waste exchange between mother and baby, and hormone production to sustain the pregnancy. The villi farthest from the uterine wall degenerate, leaving the *chorionic membrane* to surround the growing embryo.

Differentiation of Germ Layers

Simultaneously, the embryonic cells differentiate into three distinct layers which are called *primary germ layers:* (1) the endoderm, (2) the ectoderm, and (3) the mesoderm. At this point, the components for organ development are complete. Table 14.1 lists the organs that arise out of each primary germ layer.

Interference with development during this period of time will result in severe abnormalities in the baby. Coexisting congenital defects will appear in organs arising out of the same germ layer, but some factors, such as rubella (German measles), will interfere with the development of all three layers.

By the time the embryonic stage of growth and development is completed at 8 weeks, the embryo resembles a human being with human characteristics, and the basis for the next stage of development has been established.

Fetal Stage

The final stage of prenatal development, the fetal stage, is the longest, lasting from the end of the eighth week of pregnancy until the baby is born. No further germ layers will form, and every organ structure that will be present in the newborn is evident in what is now the *fetus.* This is a period of refinement of structures as well as organization and perfection of the functions of the structures. The pace of growth is very rapid and occurs

TABLE 14.1 ORGAN DEVELOPMENT FROM PRIMARY GERM LAYERS

Ectoderm

Epithelium of skin, hair, nails
Sebaceous glands
Sweat glands
Epithelium of nasal, oral passages
Salivary glands
Mucous membranes of mouth, nose
Tooth enamel
Nervous system

Mesoderm

Muscle
Bone
Cartilage
Dentin of teeth
Ligaments
Tendons
Areolar tissue
Upper urinary tract: kidneys, ureters
Genitals
Cardiovascular system
Lining of pericardial, pleural, peritoneal cavities

Endoderm

Epithelium and glands of digestive tract
Lower urinary tract: bladder, urethra
Thyroid, thymus glands
Epithelium of respiratory tract (except nose)

in three directions: (1) head to toe (cephalocaudal); (2) near to far (proximodistal); and (3) general to specific (differentiation). During this stage, physiological development continues and the psychosocial development of the fetus begins.

Physiological Development

The duration of the pregnancy is calculated in two ways. The parents may think in terms of *9 calendar months* of pregnancy counted from the last menstrual period, while the physician counts in *lunar months* of 28 days each beginning with the time of conception 2 weeks after the last period. The duration of pregnancy, according to the physician, is 10 lunar months or 40 weeks, referred to as *weeks of gestation.* These weeks and months are further divided among three trimesters.

ULTRASOUND. Direct methods are now available that make it possible to more accurately determine fetal age and to detect any interference with growth and development. Ultrasound (sonogram) is a safe diagnostic tool which utilizes sound waves to project intrauterine images onto a screen. It is useful for assessment of gestational age, multiple pregnancy, sex of the fetus, and, more recently, the diagnosis of structural abnormalities.

THE FIRST TRIMESTER. The pre-embryonic and embryonic stages take place during the first 2 lunar months (weeks 1 to 8) of the first trimester. During this 8-week period, the cardiovascular system begins to function while rudimentary body parts, head and facial features, and external genitalia are formed. During the third lunar month (weeks 9 to 12), the kidneys begin to function and nail beds, teeth, and bones appear. The gender is distinguishable and the fetus moves about freely even though the mother is not yet able to feel these movements.

THE SECOND TRIMESTER. The second trimester begins in the fourth lunar month (weeks 13 to 16), which marks rapid skeletal development, uterine development in the female fetus, and the appearance of downy body hair. The fifth lunar month (weeks 17 to 20) is characterized by *quickening* (''feeling life'') and heart sounds which can be heard through a stethoscope. Permanent tooth buds, eyebrows, and head hair appear, while the skeleton begins to harden. By the sixth lunar month (weeks 21 to 24), this ''miniature baby'' might live outside the protection of the uterus, although its chances of survival are small. The fetus may respond to external sounds and shift around as if trying to become comfortable. Its body becomes straighter and the skin has a red, wrinkled appearance.

THE THIRD TRIMESTER. The survival rate of a baby born during the seventh lunar month (weeks 25 to 28), or the beginning of the third trimester, increases to 10 percent. The fetus assumes a head-down position in the uterus, and its eyelids open. During the eighth lunar month (weeks 29 to 32) the testes of a male fetus descend into the scrotum; the fetus begins to store fats and minerals. Its skin begins to lose its reddish color, and fingerprints are set. The mother may feel vigorous movement as the fetus responds to environmental stimuli such as noise or change in the mother's position. Lunar month nine (weeks 33 to 36) is characterized by increased fat and iron stores, development of the lungs, and decreased movement as the uterine space becomes cramped. The final lunar month (weeks 37 to 40) is a time for firming of bones and skull, plumping of the body, and storage of fats and minerals as the fetus prepares for its impending birth.

Length and weight changes that accompany these other physiological developments are shown in Table 14.2.

TABLE 14.2 FETAL GROWTH IN LENGTH AND WEIGHT BY TRIMESTERS, LUNAR MONTHS, AND WEEKS OF GESTATION

Trimester	Lunar Month	Weeks of Gestation	Length (inches)	Weight (oz)
1st	1	4		
	2	8	0.5	1/30
	3	12	2.6	1.75
2nd	4	16	4.4	4.0
	5	20	6.0	8.0
				lb
	6	24	8.0	1.3
3rd	7	28	14.4	2.5
	8	32	17.0	3.5–4.0
	9	36	18.0	5.0–6.0
	10	40	20.0	7.0–7.5

Psychosocial Development

There is little hard evidence to prove that psychosocial development of the fetus begins in utero, but it is accepted that such attributes as intelligence and personality are affected by an interrelationship between heredity and environment both before and after birth. These psychosocial characteristics develop and unfold as the child grows, but there is no objective way to prove that this development began before birth. Most mothers of several children will agree, however, that each baby behaved differently while she was pregnant—one was active *all* the time, another was usually quiet, and yet another seemed to quiet down when she rocked gently for a while.

PATERNAL INTERACTION. Some fathers who had spent a lot of time ''talking to the fetus'' report that their newborns seem to recognize their voices. This is contrary to the more common belief that babies always respond more quickly to the higher-pitched voices of their mothers.

PARENTAL ATTACHMENT. How the parents feel about this baby-to-be certainly is important to the future healthy psychosocial development of the baby. Klaus and Kennell (1982) found that the mother's attachment to her baby begins during the pregnancy as she accepts her pregnancy and begins to see the baby as a separate individual. Fathers, too, begin to attach to the baby during pregnancy, but at a much slower pace than mothers.

The increasing emphasis on the importance of the parents' psychological well-being and interest in the psychosocial development of the fetus during pregnancy has created an expanded role for nurses. It is now appropriate for the nurse to monitor the parents' psychological progression through the pregnancy, to help them identify developmental tasks which should be completed (Chapter 16) and to help them limit the stressors of pregnancy.

Factors Affecting Fetal Development

The mother-to-be and the fetus comprise a complex, interacting system. This system is affected by a number of diverse factors such as nutrition, teratogens, maternal disease, and genetics, any of which can pose a threat to the development of the fetus.

Nutrition

Prenatal nutrition is considered one of the most important factors affecting the health of both mother and baby. Pregnancy is not the time for the overweight mother to go on a diet, and a proper diet with adequate protein intake is essential, as is a prescribed vitamin and mineral supplement. Protein intake is especially important during the last 2 months of pregnancy when growth of the fetal brain is at its peak. Government programs such as WIC (a supplemental feeding program for *w*omen, *i*nfants, and *c*hildren) have been established to assure that mothers of limited financial means receive proper nutrition during pregnancy. Proper nutrition for pregnant teenagers is often difficult to achieve because many of them are weight conscious, have poor eating habits, or lack the money to buy the proper nutrients.

Teratogens

Any chemical or substance which causes abnormal development of the fetus is known as a *teratogen*; even brief exposure of the mother to some teratogens during the prenatal period poses a severe threat to the normal growth and development of the baby-to-be. Commonly encountered teratogens include: x-rays, medications, alcohol, illicit drugs, cigarettes, and caffeine. Less common teratogens include toxic chemicals and waste products.

The extent of damage to the fetus depends on: (1) the strength of the teratogen, (2) the affinity of the teratogen for a specific type of fetal tissue, and (3) the length of exposure to the teratogen. Fetal tissues are most susceptible to damage during their crucial developmental times as shown in Table 14.3. These time periods are significant because many of them start *very early*, often *before* the woman knows she is pregnant.

X-RAYS. Exposure to x-rays poses a high risk for fetal abnormality because rapidly growing tissue is extremely susceptible to radiation. Therefore, it is wise to

TABLE 14.3 CRUCIAL DEVELOPMENTAL PERIODS FOR SELECTED TISSUES

Organ	Gestational Weeks
Brain	2–11
Eyes	3–7
Cardiovascular	3–7
Renal	4–11
Genital	4–14
Lips, palate	7–10

avoid *all* x-ray examinations if pregnancy is possible or known to exist.

MEDICATIONS. A pregnant woman should check with an obstetrician before taking any type of medication, no matter how safe the drug may seem or how infrequently it is to be taken. One or two doses of some drugs such as thalidomide (a tranquilizer) are enough to cause extensive congenital deformity, and a drug which has not received FDA approval should *never* be taken. The antibiotic tetracycline causes brown stains to appear on the child's teeth at about the age of 6 or 7 years, and aspirin taken within a week of delivery increases the bleeding time of both mother and baby. The label of any over-the-counter (nonprescription) drug should be read and followed exactly.

ALCOHOL. Habits of the mother, which may or may not have long-term effects on her own health, can have devastating, irreversible effects on the fetus. Episodes of heavy drinking in the first trimester can cause severe damage to the fetus, but even light drinking throughout the pregnancy can lead to physical and mental retardation. Exposure to alcohol in utero may very well be the most common cause of mental retardation and the number one teratogen in the US.

ILLICIT DRUGS. There is little documented evidence about the effect of all illicit drugs on fetal development because many of these drugs are taken with other teratogenic substances. There is evidence that marijuana and other drugs cause chromosomal and genetic damage, and heroin-addicted mothers routinely give birth to heroin-addicted babies who must suffer withdrawal in the crucial newborn period.

NICOTINE. Smoking affects fetal growth by interfering with the amount of oxygen and nutrients that reach the fetal circulation. Mothers who smoke have constricted blood vessels, including those vessels which supply the placenta. Less blood reaches the placenta which decreases the nutrition of the fetus. Mothers who smoke are more likely to give birth to growth retarded, low birth weight babies and to have a higher incidence of sudden, premature separation of the placenta.

CAFFEINE. It is possible that the use of caffeine by the mother may interfere with fetal development. Caffeine is known to cross the placental barrier, but most studies on its teratogenic potential have been done on animals. Some studies have shown that caffeine is associated with birth defects, while others have not proven such a relationship. Therefore, until the evidence of caffeine's safety is complete, limited use of caffeine is advisable.

INFECTIONS. The fetus is well protected from most maternal infections, but some viruses and bacteria (biological teratogens) do cross the placental barrier and reach the growing fetus. Rubella is probably the most common infection associated with abnormalities, but defects can also be caused by maternal exposure to toxoplasmosis, syphilis, chickenpox, cytomegalovirus, and herpes simplex.

Maternal Disease

Some maternal diseases cause growth retardation and anomalies. The decreased oxygen supply related to maternal heart disease, the constricted vessels in hypertensive mothers, and the vascular changes in diabetic mothers are related to small for gestational age (SGA) infants; on the other hand, large for gestational age (LGA) babies are often the result of high blood glucose in diabetic mothers. Cesarean delivery can protect newborns from sexually transmitted diseases present in the mother.

Genetics

It is not always possible to predict adverse genetic factors in the preconceptual period, and many babies with genetic defects are born to unsuspecting parents. Many of these disorders fall into one of two categories: (1) single mutant genes which follow mendelian laws for inheritance, such as cystic fibrosis and hemophilia, or (2) chromosomal abnormalities with a loss, addition, or alteration of chromosomes, such as Down's syndrome (mongolism).

Nursing Role

Nurses play a vital role throughout pregnancy to assure that the environment of the fetus (the condition of the mother) is an optimal one for adequate fetal growth and development. Ideally, the first prenatal visit includes a thorough examination of the mother plus detailed health histories of both parents which will uncover potential problems and allow early corrective interventions. Monitoring of the mother's health habits and fetal growth during subsequent prenatal visits assures that development is progressing as it should so that mother and baby are ready for the next phase.

LABOR AND DELIVERY

The process of labor and delivery, by which the fetus makes the change from intrauterine life to extrauterine life, is a short but crucial developmental time. For 10 lunar months, the fetus has been nourished and protected within the confines of the mother's uterus, but with the advent of the birth process, the infant faces major stressors. These stressors have the potential for impacting the future growth and development of the soon-to-be newborn.

Process of Birth

The process of childbirth has been called by many terms including accouchement, confinement, parturition, and travail, but labor is probably the most fitting description because it involves a great deal of work. Labor is a time of change—a beginning and an end. The nurse plays an important role in this miracle called childbirth, making sure that the process goes as smoothly as possible. It is the nurse's responsibility to:

1. Assess the physical status of the mother and fetus
2. Ascertain the parents' expectations for the birth
3. Determine significant social, cultural, and psychological factors
4. Intervene to facilitate labor for the mother
5. Protect the mother and fetus from preventable complications and hazards
6. Help the mother cope with her discomfort

Stages of Labor

FIRST STAGE. The first stage of labor, or dilating stage, begins with the first regular contractions and continues until the cervix is completely dilated (opened) and effaced (thinned). This is accomplished when the presenting part of the fetus, usually the head, exerts pressure against the cervix under the force of the uterine contractions. It is the longest of the stages, lasting 10 to 12 hours with a first baby and 6 to 8 hours with subsequent babies.

SECOND STAGE. The second stage of labor, the expulsion stage, begins when the cervix is dilated and effaced and ends with the birth of the baby. During this stage, which lasts 1 to 2 hours for a first baby and ½ to 1 hour for others, the baby makes its way down the pelvic passageway and, with the delivery, one phase of the newborn's life has ended and a new one is beginning.

THIRD STAGE. The remainder of the *products of conception* (the placenta and membranes) is expelled during the third stage of labor, a process which lasts 10 to 20 minutes. During this period, the newborn is given initial care, and breast feeding may be initiated.

The next 1 to 2 hours is truly a transition period for parents and newborn alike. The physiological equilibrium of mother and baby must be restored, and parent-infant interactions need to be initiated.

Initial Care of the Newborn

The most critical period in a newborn's life is the first 24 hours after birth—half of all neonatal deaths occur in this time period. Other events which occur, and the care given during this transition from intrauterine to extrauterine life, can affect the quality of the newborn's life for years to come. The primary concern of those caring for the newborn is its survival, beginning with assuring that the baby's respiratory system has been activated and that he is protected from heat loss and a marked drop in body temperature. The cord is clamped, initial contact with the parents is made, the baby is weighed and identified, and vitamin K is administered by injection to prevent neonatal hemorrhage. Many states require that silver nitrate or erythromycin be instilled in the infant's eyes to protect him against blindness from possible maternal infections such as gonorrhea. This practice is a controversial issue, and parents need to be aware of legal requirements as well as their own rights.

APGAR SCORING. A quick physical assessment of the newborn is made in the delivery room at 1 minute and again at 5 minutes, using the Apgar scoring system developed by Dr. Virginia Apgar in 1953 (Table 14.4).

THE NEONATAL PERIOD

The first 28 days of a baby's life constitute the *neonatal period*, a time when this developing person must make many adjustments to life on his own. Physiological equilibrium must be achieved, while a foundation is being laid for accomplishing all the developmental tasks of the future. On a very basic level, the neonate begins to achieve self-awareness, adjust to other people, express feelings, learn a system of communication, and experience loving. A solid foundation in the neonatal period for all of these developmental tasks, which are described in detail in Chapter 15, is important for the health and well-being of this new life.

Characteristics of the Normal Newborn

A normal part of pregnancy includes fantasizing by the parents-to-be about what the baby will be like. During the early days and weeks after the birth, these prebirth fantasies must be reconciled with the actual characteristics of the newborn if the parents are to properly respond to and care for the infant. Knowing what to expect of a normal newborn is essential to this process.

Physical Characteristics
While each baby is a unique individual, at no other stage in life will the neonate share more common characteristics with other neonates than in the first 28 days.

TABLE 14.4 COMPONENTS OF APGAR SCORING SYSTEM

Sign	0	1	2
Heart rate	Absent	Slow; <100	>100
Respiratory effort	Absent	Slow; weak cry	Good; strong cry
Muscle tone	Limp; flaccid	Some flexion of extremities	Active motion; good flexion
Reflex irritability	No response	Grimace; weak cry	Vigorous cry
Color	Pale; blue	Pink body; blue extremities	All pink

Apgar score = Total of scores for each sign
   Score 7–10 is good
   Score 5–7 is poor—infant may need assistance to maintain life
   Score 0–4 is very poor—infant needs immediate cardiac and respiratory assistance;
                     those who survive have high incidence of neurological
                     deficits

The baby's head appears large in proportion to the rest of the body, accounting for one-quarter of the body weight; the abdomen protrudes due to weak muscles and relatively large size of abdominal organs; and short arms and legs are kept flexed or semiflexed. The rapid physical growth of the fetus continues for 18 months, with gains of 5 to 7 oz weekly, and growth of 1 inch monthly, the norm for the first 6 months.

The baby's face is round and puffy, with a pug nose, receding chin, and fat cheeks, which help him nurse more easily. The eyes are usually a slate blue color, regardless of what they will be in the adult, and they may be closed even when the baby is awake. Swollen eyelids, crossed eyes (strabismus), flickering eye movements (nystagmus), and tearless crying are all normal. The two soft spots on the baby's head are the *fontanelles*, and serve to protect the soft brain tissue while allowing room for rapid growth.

Behavioral Characteristics

The new baby is helpless, with uncoordinated, uncontrolled movements. Long periods of sleep alternate with shorter periods of waking, most of which are spent in feeding during the initial weeks. The newborn frequently coughs, gags, and drools during these early feedings, and bowel movements follow shortly after the feeding, especially in a breast-fed baby. A newborn communicates his discomfort and needs by crying, and in the beginning, new parents find it difficult to determine from the cry whether their infant is cold, hungry, wet, or in pain. Some infants who are tense or restless will often settle down when they are quietly talked to and held.

REFLEXES. Several reflexes are present at birth which allow the baby to grow and develop until the nervous system matures. Rooting, sucking, and swallowing reflexes allow the baby to seek and ingest food, while protective reflexes such as sneezing and turning the head to the side when face down serve to safeguard the baby. Major reflexes are assessed each time the neonate is examined, and any deviation from normal indicates that a more detailed assessment is in order.

SENSES. Babies are born with functioning senses, which are far more subtle than those of the fully developed adult. The baby's eyes are sensitive to bright light but can focus on and track objects that are near. The human face is the most powerful stimulus, but bold patterns and sharply contrasting colors also attract attention. Blinking and jerking in response to loud noises indicate that babies can hear, but they seem to prefer soft, rhythmic sounds that resemble the mother's heartbeat. A preference for a sweet rather than a bitter substance by 3 to 4 days suggests that taste is a functioning sense at birth or shortly thereafter, while the sense of smell is evidenced by the ability of breast-fed babies to distinguish the odor of their own mother's milk, by the age of 10 days. The neonate is sensitive to touch and pressure and needs adequate tactile stimulation for normal development to occur.

TEMPERAMENT. The personality of the newborn evolves over time, but his *temperament* is present at birth. The way in which he characteristically reacts to situations is evidenced by such things as activity level, adaptability, intensity of reaction, and distractability.

Factors Affecting Growth and Development

Once the baby has made it through the crucial prenatal period and the stress of labor and delivery, his growth and development depends as much on complex psychosocial factors as on important physiological factors.

Nutrition

Everyone needs good nutrition for optimal health, but at no time is it more important than during infancy. Because infancy is a time of extremely rapid growth, nutritional deprivation will cause inadequate growth in length, failure to gain weight, and interference with central nervous system development. The infant's rapid rate of growth and immature digestive system create special nutritional needs which are met best by breast feeding or by bottle feeding with a formula that closely resembles breast milk.

Breast feeding has many advantages, not the least of which is the opportunity for deep intimacy and bodily contact between the baby and his mother. Human milk contains the necessary nutrients in proper proportion and easily digested form, and also contains antibodies from the mother which afford the baby an extended period of protection from infection. If the mother needs to stop breast feeding for any reason, she can feel confident that even a brief period of nursing gives her baby the best possible start, both physically and psychologically.

For many mothers, breast feeding has the additional advantage of being both *inexpensive* and *convenient*. On the other hand, certain drugs and foods eaten by the mother are transmitted to the infant through breast milk, and the mother must monitor what she eats while she is nursing.

The *LaLeche League International* is an organization established by mothers to disseminate information on breast feeding to new mothers and also to professional persons. There is a local LaLeche group in nearly every city which will give help and encouragement to any nursing mother who may need it.

Bottle feeding, of course, is not influenced by what the mother eats and, since today's formulas closely resemble the composition of breast milk, bottle feeding can be a suitable substitute for breast feeding. If the baby is *held closely while he is fed,* his psychological need for closeness and intimacy can also be met as adequately with bottle feeding as with breast feeding.

Sensory Stimulation

Stimulation is an important aspect of the infant's care and plays a major role in its psychological development and learning. Jean Piaget, a Swiss psychologist, calls this the *sensory motor period* because the baby learns through sensory stimulation and responds with motor movement and the development of motor skills. Appropriate stimulation of the newborn's senses is necessary for normal patterns of growth, development, and attachment. Early sensory stimulation is provided by colorful mobiles, music, fondling, changes of position, and interactions with parents and siblings. Each infant is unique, and it is important for parents to be in tune to their baby's responses so that he isn't understimulated or consistently overstimulated by noise, movement, or rough handling. Stimulation can be active or passive, purposeful or spontaneous, but it does need to be appropriate to the infant's personality and level of sensory development.

Bonding

Bonding is the term used to describe the psychological affiliation between a child and his parents and siblings. The process begins with a period of acquaintance when parent and infant gain information about each other through sight, touch, voice, hearing, and smell. This is followed by a period of attachment when mutual interaction and interdependence lead to a closer affiliation. Bonding is a close and long-standing affiliation which serves to bring individuals together, to keep them together, and to facilitate interaction. Bonding is the basis for constructive social relationships, including those of the family into which the new infant has been born; therefore, bonds must develop between mother and infant, father and infant, and siblings and infant.

MOTHER AND INFANT. Until recently, most of the literature on bonding addressed only the affiliation between mother and infant and focused heavily on the period immediately following delivery. Some studies have tried to determine if there is a "maternal sensitive period" when optimal affiliation can occur. There does seem to be a time in the first minutes and hours after birth when the mother responds to her infant in a fairly consistent way. These responses include: (1) assuming an en face position in which eye contact with the newborn

is established, and (2) conducting tactile exploration of the baby, first with her fingertips and then with the palms of her hands. While it is ideal to provide time for mother and baby to become acquainted right after birth, it is not always possible. Researchers are beginning to discover that humans are very adaptable and that mothers and infants seem to be able to form a bond even under adverse circumstances such as delayed contact because of prematurity or illness of mother or baby.

The mother brings many things to this first period of acquaintance including her life history, her self-concept and personality, her perception of the birth experience, and her fantasies of what the baby will be like; on the other hand, the baby brings only his actual appearance and his behaviors. It is these behaviors, such as cooing and smiling, which serve as the baby's part of the reciprocal interactions necessary for attachment.

FATHER AND INFANT. Recent changes in childbearing practices have finally begun to incorporate the father in all aspects of perinatal care, including opportunities for father and infant to establish the important psychological affiliation. Involvement in his wife's pregnancy and his presence during delivery have promoted the father's initial bonding and future interaction with his infant. Observations of fathers with their newborns show that they respond in a similar manner to the ways in which mothers respond; however, as babies grow and develop, fathers tend to take on different roles from mothers, spending less time in caregiving and more time in playing. The fathering role, while different from the mothering role, is an important and unique part of a child's development.

SIBLINGS AND INFANT. Few specific data have been reported on the early affiliation of the infant and his siblings, but the relationships are certainly significant. If the older child is helped to hold, rock, amuse, and care for the infant, the relationship is likely to be loving and satisfying. If the older child is continually directed to "stay out of the way" or to "leave the baby alone," lifelong feelings of envy, resentment, or jealousy are likely to arise.

Nursing Interventions

Physical and behavioral assessment of the neonate is important during the neonatal period because the nurse often spends more time with the baby than the physician does, and therefore is often in a better position to note problems and detect deficiencies. Health care of the newborn is affected by the availability of affordable care, by the attitudes and values of the parents, and by the lifestyle of the family. Some newborns receive virtually no medical care or nursing supervision, while others receive regular attention from highly qualified pediatric nurses and doctors.

The nurse must capitalize on each opportunity to observe the parents with the infant, whether in a clinic, pediatrician's office, or home, and to assess for strengths and potential problems in the family relationships. It is imperative that any necessary interventions be initiated early so that both physical and psychological development of the infant can progress in a normal way.

PATIENT TEACHING

In the past, women have made the first prenatal visit to the physician for the purpose of verifying a suspected pregnancy. The current availability of kits for determining whether or not a woman is pregnant may eliminate an early visit to the physician or midwife, and may, in some situations, delay essential prenatal care.

It will be important to teach the general public that although such kits serve a purpose, the need for *early* prenatal care and supervision is as urgent as ever.

RELATED ACTIVITIES

1. Study the relationship between the use of home pregnancy testing kits and the timing of initial prenatal care by asking doctors, midwives, and clinic staff whether or not there is any noticeable trend toward delayed prenatal care in women who use such kits.

If such a relationship is found to exist, or such a trend seems to be developing, write to the manufacturers of such kits and urge that information related to prenatal care be added to the package, or printed more prominently. Consider the possibility of writing a brief item for your local newspaper or one of the magazines for women and/or adolescent girls.

SUGGESTED READINGS

Brooten, Dorothy, and Clara H Jordon: Caffeine and pregnancy. *JOGN Nursing* 1983 May/June; 12(3):190–195.

Buckner, Ellen B: Use of Brazelton Neonatal Behavioral Assessment in planning care for parents and infants. *JOGN Nursing* 1983 Jan/Feb; 12(1):26–30.

Graham, D, S Jacques, and V DeGeorges: The role of ultrasound in the diagnosis and management of the obstetrical patient. *JOGN Nursing* 1983 Sept/Oct; 12(5):307–312.

Hangsleben, Karin Larson: Transition to fatherhood: An exploratory study. *JOGN Nursing* 1983 July/Aug; 12(4):265–270.

Hogge, Joan S, W Allen Hogge, and Mitchell S Golbus: Chorionic villus sampling. *JOGN Nursing* 1986 Jan/Feb; 15(1):24–28.

Jankowski, Carole B: Radiation and pregnancy: Putting the risks in proportion. *Am J Nurs* 1986 March; 86(3):260–265.

Judd, Judy M: Assessing the newborn from head to toe. *Nursing 85* 1985 Dec; 15(12):34–41.

Klaus, Marshall H, and John H Kennell: *Parent-Infant Bonding.* ed. 2. St. Louis, Mosby, 1982.

Marecki, Marcia et al: Early sibling attachment. *JOGN Nursing* 1985 Sept/Oct; 14(5):418–423.

Pillitteri, Adele: *Maternal-Newborn Nursing: Care of the Growing Family.* ed. 2. Boston, Little, Brown & Co, 1981.

Reeder, Sharon J Luigi Mastroianni, and Leonide L Martin: *Maternity Nursing.* ed. 15. Philadelphia, Lippincott, 1983.

Schuster, Clara Shaw, and Shirley Smith Ashburn: *The Process of Human Development: A Holistic Life-Span Approach.* Boston, Little, Brown and Company, 1986.

15

Individual Development

Patricia A. Duncan

Prerequisite and/or Suggested Preparation
The basic concepts of systems theory (Chapter 5 or its equivalent from another source) is suggested as preparation for this chapter.

GROWTH AND DEVELOPMENT

The effectiveness of a health care worker depends in part upon an understanding of the commonalities and differences among the people the worker is trying to help. This understanding comes from knowing how people in general grow and develop, how a specific person became the person that he or she is, and what changes in the person are likely to occur during the next stage of development. For example, the care of a 3-year-old in a pediatric unit will be more effective if the nurse knows what 3-year-olds are like in general, what is unique about this particular 3-year-old, and what changes may accompany his next stage of development.

The terms *growth* and *development* denote both universality (commonality) and individuality (uniqueness). In most instances, the commonalities are greatest at birth, while individuality becomes more pronounced as the person matures. For example, newborn infants around the world are quite similar in size, reflexes, sensory development, and needs. As each baby develops, however, it is influenced by its family and by the culture and society of which it is a part. The inborn personality of the baby and influences from the world around it combine to produce a unique individual.

Commonalities of Growth and Development

From conception to death, an individual is growing and developing—physically, cognitively, emotionally, socially, and spiritually. The changes which result from this process follow *specific* principles and patterns. These changes are sequential and can be identified, observed, and reported.

The principles of *physical growth* are the same for all

1. Try to get child to smile by smiling, talking or waving to him. Do not touch him.
2. When child is playing with toy, pull it away from him. Pass if he resists.
3. Child does not have to be able to tie shoes or button in the back.
4. Move yarn slowly in an arc from one side to the other, about 6" above child's face. Pass if eyes follow 90° to midline. (Past midline; 180°)
5. Pass if child grasps rattle when it is touched to the backs or tips of fingers.
6. Pass if child continues to look where yarn disappeared or tries to see where it went. Yarn should be dropped quickly from sight from tester's hand without arm movement.
7. Pass if child picks up raisin with any part of thumb and a finger.
8. Pass if child picks up raisin with the ends of thumb and index finger using an over hand approach.

9. Pass any enclosed form. Fail continuous round motions.
10. Which line is longer? (Not bigger.) Turn paper upside down and repeat. (3/3 or 5/6)
11. Pass any crossing lines.
12. Have child copy first. If failed, demonstrate

When giving items 9, 11 and 12, do not name the forms. Do not demonstrate 9 and 11.

13. When scoring, each pair (2 arms, 2 legs, etc.) counts as one part.
14. Point to picture and have child name it. (No credit is given for sounds only.)

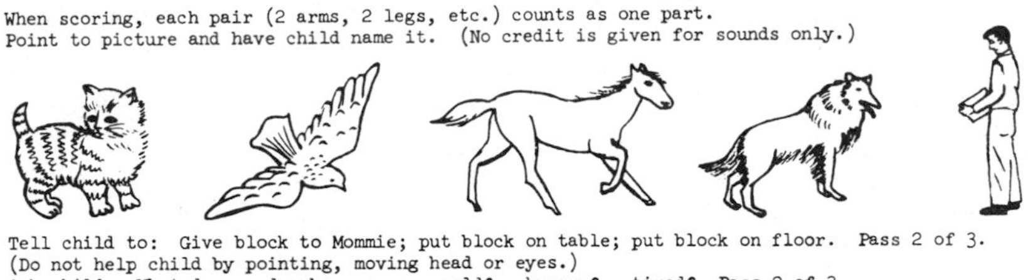

15. Tell child to: Give block to Mommie; put block on table; put block on floor. Pass 2 of 3. (Do not help child by pointing, moving head or eyes.)
16. Ask child: What do you do when you are cold? ..hungry? ..tired? Pass 2 of 3.
17. Tell child to: Put block on table; under table; in front of chair, behind chair. Pass 3 of 4. (Do not help child by pointing, moving head or eyes.)
18. Ask child: If fire is hot, ice is ?; Mother is a woman, Dad is a ?; a horse is big, a mouse is ?. Pass 2 of 3.
19. Ask child: What is a ball? ..lake? ..desk? ..house? ..banana? ..curtain? ..ceiling? ..hedge? ..pavement? Pass if defined in terms of use, shape, what it is made of or general category (such as banana is fruit, not just yellow). Pass 6 of 9.
20. Ask child: What is a spoon made of? ..a shoe made of? ..a door made of? (No other objects may be substituted.) Pass 3 of 3.
21. When placed on stomach, child lifts chest off table with support of forearms and/or hands.
22. When child is on back, grasp his hands and pull him to sitting. Pass if head does not hang back.
23. Child may use wall or rail only, not person. May not crawl.
24. Child must throw ball overhand 3 feet to within arm's reach of tester.
25. Child must perform standing broad jump over width of test sheet. (8-1/2 inches)
26. Tell child to walk forward, ⌒⟳⌒⟳⌒⟳→ heel within 1 inch of toe. Tester may demonstrate. Child must walk 4 consecutive steps, 2 out of 3 trials.
27. Bounce ball to child who should stand 3 feet away from tester. Child must catch ball with hands, not arms, 2 out of 3 trials.
28. Tell child to walk backward, ←⌒⟳⌒⟳⌒⟳ toe within 1 inch of heel. Tester may demonstrate. Child must walk 4 consecutive steps, 2 out of 3 trials.

DATE AND BEHAVIORAL OBSERVATIONS (how child feels at time of test, relation to tester, attention span, verbal behavior, self-confidence, etc,):

Figure 15.1 Denver Developmental Screening Test.

humans and the sequence of *psychosocial development* is similar for persons within a given culture. Every person demonstrates the characteristics of babyhood, childhood, adolescence, and adulthood in sequence, although the length and relative importance of each stage is culturally determined. For example, some cultures foster a long period of adolescence while others use elaborate rituals or rites of passage to mark an abrupt change from childhood to adulthood.

Every person develops through stages devoted to play, preparation for adulthood, doing the work of an adult and raising a family. This sameness of growth and development among individuals comprises the *universality and commonality* of mankind.

Characteristics of the Denver Developmental Screening Test (DDST)

- Areas Tested

    Personal/social skills: relating to people, independence.

    Language skills: use and interpretation of spoken word.

    Fine motor/adaptive skills: eye-hand coordination; problem solving; perception.

    Gross motor skills: coordination, locomotion, posturing.

- Age Range

    Newborn

    Infants and children to age 6

- Use

    An assessment tool, *NOT* intended to be a diagnostic test.

    Screens for developmental delays in infants and children.

    Also identifies children with *potential* developmental problems.

    Positive or suspicious findings require retesting and/ or referral for diagnostic testing.

- Advantages

    Standardized test with proven reliability and validity.

    Takes into consideration whether child was full term or premature.

    Not harmful or frightening to child.

    Minimal cost, testing materials readily available (toys, blocks, raisins, yarn).

    Training of tester requires only a few hours.

- Disadvantages

    Requires 20 minutes for testing.

    Space needed for testing.

    Does require some training of tester.

Individual Differences

At the same time, each person is a highly *unique* individual. Individual differences may be due to genetic factors, environmental factors, or life experiences; these differences require careful attention if the nurse is to give effective, holistic care.

Individual differences are meaningful only in the context of commonalities. A nurse must know what is normal for a given age or stage of development before she can evaluate the status of a specific individual. A knowledge of normal growth and development enables the nurse to recognize deviations from the norm, and to know, for example, when a child is unusually slow to walk, to respond to other children, or to use language effectively. The ability to make such assessments is necessary in order for the nurse to intervene effectively, either directly or indirectly by referring the child and his parents to a specialist for further evaluation and treatment.

One way to evaluate a child's development is to compare his capabilities with an established set of characteristics which have proved to be normal for a given age. One of the best examples of a reliable standardized test is the Denver Developmental Screening Test, shown in Figure 15.1 and described in the boxed material.

A knowledge of what is normal for each stage of development, enables the nurse to provide *anticipatory guidance* to patients and families. For example, the nurse can help the parents of a 1-year-old look ahead to the toddler stage and plan how they can protect him from the hazards which are associated with a toddler's need to climb and explore (Fig. 15.1).

THEORIES OF GROWTH AND DEVELOPMENT

There is no single theory which explains all aspects of growth and development. At present, each researcher studies and investigates the specific aspect of growth and development which concerns him most. These selected aspects are called *domains* and include the biophysical, cognitive, social, emotional, and spiritual domains of growth and development. Each of these approaches contributes to an overall understanding of the growth and development of an individual, and little by little a fairly complete picture of the process emerges.

Domains of Growth and Development

Research related to growth and development is categorized into one of the following domains or spheres of activity as follows:

Biophysical: physical growth and development at all levels; cells, organs, body structure and systems.

Cognitive: intellectual development; the ability to know, perceive, think, reason, understand, interpret, problem-solve.

Social: development of relationships with others, both individuals and groups, within the family and community.

Affective: internal responses to external events; emotions, feelings.

Spiritual: related to one's beliefs about a power or being greater than oneself; usually related to moral and ethical behavior.

The two terms, growth and development, are sometimes used interchangeably but within the context of nursing, the following distinctions between the two terms are usually made:

The term *growth* is used most often to refer to physical changes which are basically *quantitative* and related to what can be measured or weighed such as height, weight, head circumference. There are *limits* and *specific end points* to growth.

The term *development* refers to a lifelong process of growth, maturation, and learning. It is a process of movement toward a more advanced, effective, skillful state. In general, there are no end points to development, and normal individuals are considered to have an almost unlimited potential for ongoing development.

Patterns of Growth and Development

Development of the individual is not random or haphazard; it is *sequential, orderly, and predictable.* Two of the most obvious examples of the orderliness and predictability of the growth process are the cephalocaudal sequence and the proximodistal sequence. The term cephalocaudal sequence refers to a head-to-foot direction. Major growth and development occurs first in the head, then the trunk, then the legs. This begins in utero and continues throughout the life span. At birth, the head is 20 percent of the body mass, and the legs are very small by comparison. In adulthood, the head is only 8 percent of the body mass, and the trunk and legs are large and heavy. Control of the head is achieved by the infant long before he has any control over his legs.

The *proximodistal* sequence refers to development from the midline of the body outward. Muscles and joints closer to the midline of the body are *proximal* to the midline and can be controlled by the individual before those which are *distal* or farther away from the midline of the body. Arm control is achieved before hand control, and hand control is achieved before finger control. This sequence accounts for the fact that large muscle control precedes fine muscle control.

The principle of *differentiation* means that growth and development progresses from the general to the specific, from the simple to the complex. For example, the hand movements of an infant progress from gross, *aimless* movements to purposeful grasping with the whole hand and finally to fine finger coordination. A baby almost literally cries with his whole body, but the body movements of a sobbing child are usually limited to the upper body, and the movements of a crying adult are usually limited to the eyes and face. Infants respond to people in general before they can differentiate and recognize their parents and siblings.

Basic Principles of Growth and Development

1. *Growth and development are continuous processes which follow predetermined patterns.* These patterns are definite, orderly, predictable, and sequential. Individual differences do exist but they do not greatly influence the overall processes.

2. *Development involves both maturation and learning.* Maturation is the process of genetically programmed physiological growth. Examples of maturation include teething and the changes which accompany puberty.

Maturation and learning are interrelated because certain types of learning cannot take place until the individual is mature enough (maturational readiness), and maturation can be slowed if there is no opportunity to learn. For example, a child cannot walk until certain physical changes have occurred to provide the necessary strength and coordination. In other words, he cannot walk until he is mature enough.

On the other hand, if the child is not given the opportunity to learn, development may be retarded. A child who has very limited contact with other people will not learn to talk as readily as the child who is surrounded by people who talk and read to him.

Maturation is related to an overall readiness to learn. When maturational readiness is present in any domain, the individual will learn more readily and effectively. No amount of practice or training will be effective if maturational readiness is not present.

3. *Each individual follows the predetermined patterns of human growth and development in his own way.*

Differences in individual growth and development are due in part to:

- heredity
- the rate of the individual's maturational process

- environmental influences and learning
- health status
- gender
- intellectual development
- parental attitudes and interest
- position in family constellation
- environmental stimulation

The rate of growth is not the same for all children nor is it consistent for the same child. Sudden spurts or surges of growth are common, and are usually followed by periods in which little or no change seems to

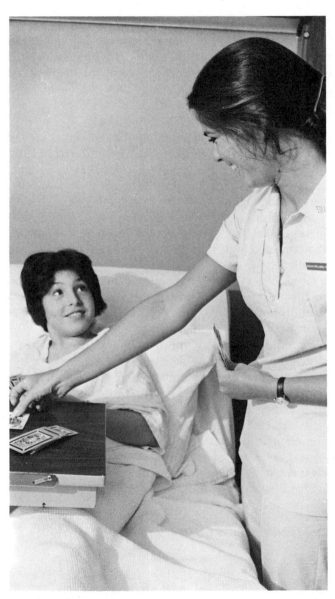

Figure 15.2 *The nurse uses her knowledge of developmental needs to plan activities for this hospitalized adolescent patient.*

occur. Rates of growth and development vary for each individual child in each domain, and parents often need help in understanding and using this concept because they tend to compare aspects of the growth and development of one child with its own siblings or with other children. Knowledge of the normal range of rates and patterns of growth and development will help parents, nurses, teachers, and other professionals to view each child's progress realistically and to intervene more effectively.

4. *Each stage of the life cycle has traits and tasks that are characteristic of that stage.* There are *traits* which are characteristic of each domain of development at each stage, such as the negativism of age 2, and the need to reminisce during late adulthood.

There are *developmental tasks* to be achieved for each stage of the lifespan. These tasks involve specific behaviors and skills that must be learned for successful achievement of that stage and optimal preparation for future stages. Examples of such tasks: infancy, learning to eat solid food; early adulthood, establishing a relationship with a member of the opposite sex; late adulthood, adjusting to retirement (Fig. 15.2).

5. *The basis for the attitudes, traits, behaviors, and lifestyles of the individual is formed during infancy and early childhood.* This early foundation highly influences the development of the individual as he grows older. This is true for all domains of development.

THEORISTS

Freud

Sigmund Freud was an Austrian physician (1865–1939) whose early work involved scientific investigation of the nervous system. In his medical practice, he focused on nervous disorders, and he eventually became interested in working with the psychoanalytic technique of *catharsis* which involved the patient's talking at length about his problem while the physician listened.

Freud's work with patients who had nervous disorders led to his development of the first major theory of personality. Since his theory proposed a concept of childhood sexuality, which was revolutionary, especially during the late Victorian era, it is not surprising that his ideas were unacceptable to many and were widely challenged. Many other theorists were influenced by his research, although some of them later developed their own theories.

Personality Structure

Freud considered the personality to be composed of the *id*, the *ego*, and the *superego*, and believed that the functions of these three aspects of personality were directly related to the three principles of *pleasure, reality*, and the *ideal*.

The *id* includes instincts and reflexes and is the source of psychic energy. The id's function is to reduce tension within the individual. This tension is experienced as discomfort or pain, and Freud believed that a person instinctively acts to reduce or remove tension.

Freud called this process of avoiding pain and seeking pleasure or gratification *the pleasure principle*. It is a process by which an individual tries to minimize discomfort and to maintain a balance or feeling of constancy whenever he is experiencing change. Freud considered the id to be unchanging over time, although he believed that it could be influenced by another part of the personality, the ego. The impulsive, demanding, pleasure-seeking aspects of the id are readily apparent in the infant whose ego and superego are not yet developed. The infant or toddler cries when he is uncomfortable or frustrated, is concerned only with himself, acts on impulse, demands instant gratification of his needs and desires, and pursues those activities which give him pleasure.

Since the reduction of all tensions is not possible through the primitive actions of the id, further personality development is necessary.

The *ego* functions to *govern the id* in order for the individual to interact effectively with the world around him. The ego operates on the reality principle. The *reality principle* causes the ego to mediate the individual's interaction with the external world through the processes of learning, memory, thinking, perception, and problem-solving. The development of these psychological processes enables the individual to control his impulses and instinctive behavior, to behave in socially acceptable ways, and to plan and work or wait for the satisfaction of his needs and desires.

The *superego* is related to the individual's moral development, and guides the person to seek good and avoid wrong in accordance with the *ideal principle*. The lay term for the superego is the *conscience*. The conscience involves that which is good and desirable, and thus encourages the individual to act in ways which are valued as morally right by parents or society at large. The conscience also involves that which is considered *undesirable* by parents or society. The development of both aspects of the superego is influenced first by parental values and moral codes, and then by the society with which the individual has contact.

The concept of what is good and right and "ought to be done" is developed through praise, rewards, and approval; the concept of what is wrong and "ought *not* to be done" is developed through negative feedback, punishment, and deprivation.

The superego integrates the individual's moral code into his personality, and bestows rewards or punishments upon the ego. Rewards may be in the form of a favor to the self (a special treat) or a feeling of pride. Freud believed that the superego's self-punishment for a wrongdoing could be in the form of accidents, illness, losing things, or feelings of guilt and shame.

According to Freud, these three systems—the id, the ego, and the superego, function together to maintain a balanced personality. Harmony and balance between the systems is necessary for mental health and the ability to meet one's own needs. Disharmony among them was believed to indicate imbalance and impede the functioning of the individual.

Stages of Development

Freud believed that an individual experiences tension in first one and then another part of his body from birth through adolescence, especially during the first 5 years. The tension related to each body part is the basis for a specific stage of development, and each successive stage dominates that point in life.

At each stage of development, the individual tries to reduce tension and to gain pleasure and gratification in relation to the body parts involved. Psychosexual energy (libido) supplies the necessary energy and organizes the behaviors of the individual.

Resolution is the term applied to the effective completion of a stage or phase of development. It means that the needs of that stage have been resolved and satisfied.

Resolution of one phase allows the person to go on to the next stage. Incomplete resolution results in a fixation at that stage. This occurs if needs are not met or if they are overindulged.

Freud believed that the major tasks of personality development were complete by age 6. Adolescence initiates a revival of earlier childhood conflicts, but if earlier stages were effectively passed, the adolescent would be expected to continue into adult heterosexual relationships successfully. Development was believed to be complete at the end of adolescence.

ORAL PHASE. During this phase, the infant derives pleasure and gratification from activities involving the mouth

---

Freud's Stages of Development

Oral	Birth to 1 year
Anal	1–3 years
Phallic	4–6 years
Latency	6–12 years
Genital	12 years and older

such as sucking, feeding, vocalization, and exploratory play. Freud identified the five modes of functioning of the mouth as (1) taking in, (2) holding on, (3) biting, (4) spitting out, and (5) closing. He believed that if the child uses one mode predominantly during this phase, it will be also used in later life. Thus, an individual may have traits reflective of early adjustment such as acquisitiveness (taking in), tenacity (holding on), verbal aggression (biting), rejection (spitting out), or negativism (closing). Ideally, the infant will use *all* modes rather than predominantly one, and will not rely on the mouth as the major source of tension reduction and gratification.

Fixation during this stage due to incomplete resolution may be manifested in adult years by alcoholism, smoking, overeating, and excessive talking. Freud believed that incomplete resolution of this stage could be related to poorly timed or unsatisfactory weaning. An infant's survival depends upon the mother's care, and poor resolution of the task of weaning from bottle or breast may lead to problems related to dependence, including either overdependence or an inability to be dependent when necessary and appropriate.

ANAL PHASE. Physiologic changes at this time permit both bowel control and an awareness of sphincter muscles. The toddler becomes aware of body sensations related to elimination and is ready to exert control over these sensations. Tension is experienced by the child as the result of fecal material pressing against the anal sphincter and rectal walls. A bowel movement reduces tension and thereby produces pleasure and gratification.

Freud believes that the pleasure experienced by the child interacts with parental attitudes and behaviors during toilet training to influence the child's personality. The child takes pride in the bowel movement he has brought about, and is likely to be disturbed by negative parental attitudes.

When parents have a calm, easygoing attitude toward toilet training, with appropriate praise for the child's progress toward socially acceptable patterns of elimination, the child is likely to move through this stage without difficulty. On the other hand, when parents display attitudes of disgust or displeasure toward the bowel movement which was satisfying to the child, or when toilet training is too early or rigid with harsh punishment for failures, the resulting conflict between the parent's authority and the child's pleasure may lead to difficulties both now and later. The child may refuse to part with that which has given him satisfaction in the past, and the parents may resort to the use of enemas or suppositories to force the child to have a bowel movement.

Freud believed that conflict during the anal stage of development could lead to retaliation in later life in the form of messiness, extravagance, wastefulness, or the opposite—meticulousness, frugality, and miserliness. He also believed that unwarranted or *extravagant* praise during this phase could lead to an increase or excessive desire to please others in adulthood.

PHALLIC PHASE. During the preschool years, the genital area becomes the source of pleasure and gratification. Small children touch or fondle their genitals because it feels good, and masturbation provides pleasure. This activity is viewed by many parents as abnormal, sinful, sexual, or repulsive, and they may react in an emotional, distraught manner. Harsh scolding or punishment by parents can lead to sexual problems because the child comes to believe that that part of his body is unacceptable or not good. On the other hand, if parents can remain calm and unruffled by the child's masturbation, the child can be taught that although playing with his genitals may feel good, it is not socially acceptable in front of other people. The child then passes through this phase with a positive feeling about his body and an intact self-esteem.

Sexual longing for the parent of the opposite sex is present during this phase, although the process differs for boys and girls. The male loves his mother and wishes to have her to himself. He is in rivalry with his father and wishes him out of the picture. This is known as the *Oedipus complex*, after a Greek mythological figure who killed his father to marry his mother. The boy finds himself in an impossible position, and feels overwhelmed and fearful of the father. Freud believed that the boy fears castration (removal of the testicles) by his father, and used the term *castration anxiety* to describe this tension.

The Oedipus complex is resolved by the child's recognition of the impossibility of the situation. This occurs as the child matures, and a result of lack of encouragement from the mother. With resolution, the boy identifies with the father, and moves on to the next stage of development.

According to Freud, during the phallic stage of development, a girl becomes aware that she doesn't have a penis and she blames her mother. Identification with the mother decreases and love for the father increases. Freud believed that the girl, therefore, experiences a form of castration complex (penis envy) in relation to the father. He named this the Electra complex with reference to a Greek princess who helped to assassinate her mother because of love for her father. Resolution of this conflict and identification with the mother occurs as the girl recognizes the impossibility of possessing the father.

The end result of the phallic stage is identification

with the parent of the *same sex*, although the conflict (Oedipal complex, Electra complex) reemerges to a lesser degree during adolescence. Freud viewed non-resolution of this phase as resulting in homosexuality.

This part of Freud's theory has come under fire by many in today's society. It is hard for many people to accept the concept of penis envy, and the notion that a female is lacking because she doesn't possess a penis is inconsistent with the status of women in today's world. Current studies describing the behavior of girls and boys during the preschool years seems to refute the concept of a castration complex as an aspect of normal development.

LATENCY PHASE. Freud viewed the period between the ages of 6 and 12 years as a quiescent time during which earlier turmoils are not evident. Following the completion of the phallic phase, until the age of adolescence, the child's energies are focused on school skills and the development of peer relationships, particularly with same sex friends. Mostly tranquil in appearance, this phase is a time for integration of all development to date.

GENITAL PHASE. This phase brings back the unresolved conflicts of earlier stages in an attempt to achieve final resolution for the remainder of the person's life. The focus is on other people as objects to love, in contrast to the earlier focus on oneself. Freud believed that the aim or outcome of this stage is the joining with another person in a mature sexual relationship to reproduce and establish a home and a place in the community. This phase lasts the remainder of the individual's life.

Erikson

Erik Erikson was trained in psychoanalysis by Anna Freud, Sigmund Freud's daughter. He began his career in Vienna, and later practiced, taught, and studied in the United States. Although Erikson's theory is based on Freud's theory of personality development, there are significant differences between the two.

Freud believed that the development of an individual's personality was largely complete by the end of adolescence, while Erikson believed that the process continued throughout the entire life span of the person. In addition, Erikson's outlook was more optimistic, and he believed that each stage provided new opportunity for growth, and that resolution of previously unresolved stages may be achieved at a later time given the appropriate conditions. Erikson's theory views the social aspects of the individual as crucial to normal development.

Erikson described eight sequential stages in the development of a strong ego. During each stage, there is

Erikson's Eight Stages of Man	
Age	**Developmental Conflict**
Infant	Basic trust versus mistrust
Toddler	Autonomy versus shame and doubt
Preschool	Initiative versus guilt
Schoolage	Industry versus inferiority
Adolescence	Identity versus role confusion
Young adulthood	Intimacy versus isolation
Middle adulthood	Generativity versus stagnation
Late adulthood	Ego integrity versus despair

a specific attribute or quality to be acquired. Just as Freud talked of conflict and tension within the developing child, so Erikson theorized that there is conflict and struggle within each of his eight stages of man. He believed that each stage represents a developmental crisis which has two possible outcomes. One of these possible outcomes denotes successful resolution of the development conflict while the other possible outcome indicates failure to resolve the conflict. *Successful resolution* of a given stage means that the individual has moved one step closer to a strong ego and well developed sense of identity. Delay or *lack of resolution* of any stage can impede or slow healthy development, although Erikson believed that this might be corrected later in life.

Erikson's Eight Stages of Man

1. *Basic trust versus mistrust.* The development of trust during infancy depends upon the quality of the mothering or parenting relationship. When the infant's needs are fully and consistently met, his discomfort and tension are decreased and the infant experiences comfort, pleasure, and a sense of security. If the infant gets no consistent response to his cries of hunger or discomfort, he has no reason to trust the sensations that he is experiencing or to trust that people are reliable and responsive to him. He learns that he has little or no influence on the people around him. The consistency with which the infant's needs are met when he is cold, wet, hungry, or in pain has ramifications beyond the infant's trust of the parent—it forms the basis for a *general state of trust* which is basic to the development of a healthy personality.

Erikson believed that it is also important for the parent to convey to the child a sense of meaning and trust at a wider societal level. The infant needs to learn that the people around him are sensitive and responsive to his needs, that there is consistency in the way in which they interact with him. If interactions with the infant are inconsistent and unpredictable, the infant does not learn to trust. If, for example, when the infant cries from hunger, he is sometimes fed and sometimes ignored, he learned that his cries have no predictable effect, that his cries are untrustworthy as a means of getting comfort, and that he cannot trust people to respond to him.

Failure to achieve trust results in mistrust, and Erikson cites infantile schizophrenia and adult depressive and schizoid stages as possible outcomes.

2. *Autonomy versus shame and doubt.* A toddler is mobile and physically able to do things to assert his growing sense of autonomy and independence. Cognitive and language skills contribute to his developing sense of self. Given the development of basic trust in the mothering one and in his external environment, the toddler begins to develop self-control and self-esteem. The successful outcome of this stage is characterized by a toddler's proud declaration, "I can do it myself!"

The toddler is a tireless bundle of energy and curiosity with little concept of the potential dangers which surround him. He must be given every opportunity to experiment and test new capabilities and skills while being provided with supervision and protection from emotional and physical harm. Choices should be given to enhance his sense of autonomy and control and opportunities to attempt achievable tasks should be provided.

This is the age of "No," often referred to as the "terrible twos," and the negativism typical of this age is part of the child's move toward autonomy and his need to test the control of others. Parents often need help in understanding and accepting this stage as normal because many tend to view it as an undesirable contest of wills.

Erikson uses the phrase "shame and doubt" to describe failure to achieve autonomy. It refers to the child's feeling of self-consciousness, a feeling of being exposed, and that everyone is looking at him.

Firm and consistent guidance is needed to help the toddler establish boundaries between what is and what is not acceptable behavior. This guidance is crucial in teaching children to deal with frustration, to learn early concepts of compromise, and to realize that there are boundaries to what a child can or should control.

Erikson states that a sense of self-control and self-esteem produces a lasting sense of good will and pride, while an absence of self-control or overcontrol by others creates a lasting propensity for shame and doubt.

3. *Initiative versus guilt.* The term *initiative* means that the preschool child undertakes, plans, and carries out a task for the sake of being active and doing some-

thing, whereas during the previous stage many actions were, more often than not, acts of defiance or attempted independence.

The preschooler is actively involved in learning about himself, and in trying out new skills and behaviors. There is identification with the same-sex parent, but also now an ability to relate to people other than his parents—peers, other adults, and those who live only in his now-active imagination. These others provide the child with a new world of possibilities for what he might become.

The negative aspect of this stage is *guilt*, which is experienced as a result of having gone too far in one's actions. The child's developing superego and conscience can make him try to overcontrol and overrestrict himself and others, and can make him develop deep resentment toward those who do not live up to his new conscience. Failure to achieve a balance between his desire for initiative and his need for self-control can lead to either decreased initiative and a frightened state of inhibition, or an overcompensation in which the child continually "sticks his neck out." The beginnings of psychosomatic illness may form during the conflict between wanting to take the initiative and being scared of doing so. Illness can make it difficult or impossible to do certain things, and thereby, *unconsciously*, the child might begin to use illness as an escape from difficult situations.

Masturbation by the preschooler and talk about toileting and body parts is common, and parents need to set limits on impulsive or socially unacceptable behaviors without imposing guilt.

4. *Industry versus inferiority.* The schoolage child is actively involved in learning the skills necessary to function productively in the world outside the family. The child who has mastered previous developmental tasks and who has achieved an appropriate level of physical, cognitive, and language development will enter school and take on this new learning with zest. This is the time of life when the child is likely to become interested in a hobby. The period is one of building on and enhancing what has come before. It is a time of learning to work with others, to set realistic and achievable goals, to learn the fundamentals of technology and the basic concepts of one's culture.

It is important for the child to find activities that are *meaningful* to him, but this is not always an easy task for a schoolage child in our technological society. In earlier times, each child was responsible for certain tasks and chores, and he knew that the family's comfort and well being depended in part upon how well those chores were done. In some cultures today, many parents find themselves in a difficult situation. There may be few really significant tasks for the child, and the parent must rely on hobbies, sports, or community activities to keep the child busy and out of trouble. Concerned parents sometimes involve the child in much that is not of the child's choice or liking. The parent needs to be available to the child without imposing because too much intrusion from the parent is as much of an impediment as too little at this time.

Successful completion of this stage results in a sense of pride and accomplishment coupled with confidence in one's self and one's abilities. Failure to complete this stage brings a sense of inferiority, a feeling of being unable to do anything right, and an unwillingness to risk trying to do so (Fig. 15.3).

5. *Identity versus role confusion.* During this phase, adolescents seek to find congruence and agreement between how they see themselves and how others perceive them, and they rework earlier conflicts in the process. The choice of an occupation is one of the most crucial decisions and involves an often difficult compromise between the adolescent's dreams of what he would like to become and the reality of his actual abil-

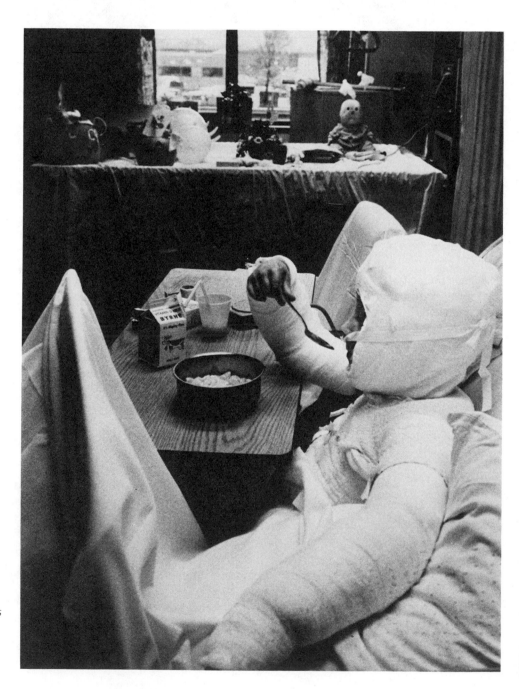

Figure 15.3 *Renee's insistence upon feeding herself despite her bulky dressing indicates that she has successfully progressed through Erikson's stage of* autonomy vs. shame and doubt. *She is now involved in the tasks of middle childhood which Havighurst describes as achieving personal independence.*

ities and talents. In addition, the choice involves a search for connections between past experiences and likes, and possible future career choices.

Questions of sexual identity create a conflict at this time due to bodily changes and impulses. This conflict is resolved through friendships with both sexes, and by talking at great length about a multitude of issues related to identity. Idealism is strongest at this stage. Conformity to the peer group is often a defense against confusion and uncertainty. It is a way of acquiring, at least temporarily, a set of social values which help to determine one's place in the group.

Failure to achieve identity results in role confusion regarding sexual and occupational identity, and tends to leave the adolescent in a state of uncertainty, with no clear sense of direction regarding the person he wants to become as an adult.

6. *Intimacy versus isolation.* Intimacy involves sharing a commitment to a relationship which is mutually self-giving, one which is not self-centered. Young adults are ready to enter intimacy once they have achieved identity in the areas of sexuality and occupation. Intimacy is usually thought of in relation to a person of the opposite sex who is a possible marriage partner, but intimacy also involves friends of the same or opposite sex.

The achievement of intimacy brings with it the capacity to establish a mutually satisfying sexual relationship with another person.

Failure to achieve intimacy results in isolation and the need to keep a distance between oneself and other people, a need to defend one's "territory" of person and space. This results in an inability or unwillingness to develop mutually satisfying relationships, and causes the young adult to interact with others in a competitive or combative manner. The individual is concerned about being victimized or exploited in relationships and thus avoids closeness and maintains a strong sense of territoriality.

7. *Generativity versus stagnation.* During the seventh stage, the adult in midlife shifts the focus from self to future generations and society. Generativity is often viewed narrowly as the raising of one's own children. Erikson goes beyond this to include any form of guidance for the next generation. Community activities, political involvement, volunteer activities with youth groups in the community, and professions such as teaching and nursing are all expressions of generativity. Productivity and creativity are additional aspects of generativity.

Failure to reach the stage of generativity results in stagnation in which concerns about oneself take precedence over concerns about the welfare of others. Stag-

nation results in self-absorption which precludes faith and involvement in the future of the human race.

8. *Ego integrity versus despair.* The task of later adulthood is to come to terms with one's own life and accept what has been and what is. Those who achieve integrity live with a sense of hope for the future and a desire to use their remaining time well. The clarification and acceptance of the life one has lived provides a sense of meaning and purpose.

The person who has achieved integrity has accepted and adjusted to the ups and downs of his life, and to the way in which his life has affected, and has been affected by, the lives of others. Life review or reminiscence is a vital process during this stage. The result is a strong philosophy that anticipates death with dignity.

The individual who does not achieve ego integration experiences despair. There are many regrets and an inability to be enthusiastic or hopeful about the past, present, or future. This state *differs from the temporary despair* which most people experience from time to time, particularly when poor health, loss of loved ones, or financial problems intervene. Those who do not achieve integrity are dissatisfied with their lives, feel disgust and disappointment, and fear death.

It is important to note that Erikson did not see his eight stages as self-contained and mutually exclusive. He believed that

- The eight stages occur in sequence
- The successful accomplishment of one stage is an important foundation for the next
- Failure to accomplish one stage makes the next one more uncertain and difficult
- Unsuccessful resolution of a stage can be corrected in later life given the appropriate conditions
- The basic conflict of any stage does not end with that designated life stage

Erikson believed, for example, that the conflict between trust and mistrust may predominate the conflicts of infancy, but it does not end there—it recurs throughout life. The older individual must learn how to know whom to trust, and under what circumstances. If an individual never learned to trust himself and others as an infant, the task of doing so becomes harder as time passes, and subsequent stages are more difficult to achieve. Erikson believed, however, that such deficits could be overcome.

Piaget

Jean Piaget, a Swiss psychologist, proposed a theory of intellectual development in children characterized by sequential stages, each of which must be mastered before the child can proceed to the next stage. He believed that, from birth on, children are actively involved in learning. They receive information and stimulation from their own bodies, from other people, and from the environment. Piaget's theory provides information about the child's ability to learn at any given stage and the importance of providing appropriate learning opportunities at certain stages.

Piaget believed that the final stage of cognitive (intellectual) development ends around age 14, and that after this there are no further *qualitative* changes in the cognitive structure, but that *quantitative* changes continue throughout life. According to his theory, an individual would not acquire any new or different cognitive skills after age 14; he would merely expand and refine those which had been acquired by midadolescence.

Two of the terms basic to Piaget's theory are assimilation and accommodation. *Assimilation* is the process by which new information is integrated into existing cognitive abilities. It is the process by which the child combines a new situation with his existing intellectual skills to solve a problem or make a decision.

Accommodation is the changing of already established intellectual capabilities, or the development of new ways to adjust to new information. This allows for new and adaptive behavior and new ways of coping when the individual is confronted with new information or circumstances.

Sensorimotor Period

This period extends from birth to 2 years and is divided into six substages.

SUBSTAGE 1: REFLEX REACTIONS. From birth to the age of 1 month, the infant's behavior is based on reflexes related to sucking, hearing, vision, and touch. The infant reacts to stimuli; there is little or no intentional activity as yet.

SUBSTAGE 2: PRIMARY CIRCULAR REACTIONS. The term *circular reaction* refers to behavior that promotes repetition and the infant from 1 to 4 months begins to prolong and repeat behaviors which were initially a reflex action. Whereas the newborn infant sucks as a reflex when something touches his mouth, systematic and repetitive thumb sucking begins when the older infant has acquired hand-to-mouth coordination. The infant becomes aware of novel events and shows early signs of curiosity. He will imitate the actions of others in a primitive way.

SUBSTAGE 3: SECONDARY CIRCULAR REACTIONS. From 4 to 8 months of age, the infant's repetitive responses change

from those concerned with his own body (primary reactions) to those concerned with his environment (secondary reactions). The beginning of intentional movements can be observed as the infant shakes a rattle to make a noise or pushes a mobile to keep it moving. He begins to be aware of his effect on things and acts to make things happen. At this stage, the infant recognizes familiar people and objects, will reach for objects, and will look for an object when it is made to disappear.

SUBSTAGE 4: COORDINATION OF SECONDARY REACTIONS. From 8 to 12 months, *intentionality* is well developed. The infant now uses means to reach ends, e.g., he pulls the string of a toy to bring it closer. He is developing a sense of self, can differentiate between self and other people or objects, and reacts to separation from his mother. *Object permanence* is present. This means that the infant is aware that an object is present even if it is hidden, and he enjoys simple hiding games. Bedtime and bathtime rituals become important at this stage.

SUBSTAGE 5: TERTIARY CIRCULAR REACTIONS. Between the ages of 12 and 18 months, the child repeats those actions which please him, but he does not always repeat them in the same way. His reactions become varied, and indicate the beginning of trial and error experimentation. The child tries to produce effects that are satisfying to him and is incessantly curious and constantly exploring.

SUBSTAGE 6: INVENTION OF NEW MEANS. During the next 6 months, from 18 to 24 months of age, the child begins to use symbols or visual imagining to "figure things out." He is beginning to pretend, and can remember, plan, and solve simple problems which he encounters. He can repeat the acts of another person when that model is no longer present.

Period of Preoperational Thought

Between the ages of 2 and 7 years, sensorimotor experiences continue to be important, but the child begins to function in symbolic and representational realms. He works directly with words and ideas and does not need to have the objects or events present. The child uses toys or objects to represent the real thing. At about age 4, he becomes less egocentric and thinks more complexly. He begins to establish cause and effect relationships as evidenced by frequent use of the word "because."

According to Piaget, the child between 2 and 7 years is not yet able to deal intellectually with *problems* of time, space, causality, measurement, numbers, quantity, and volume; he is certain that everything is just as it appears. He can tell which object is shortest or longest, or which container is fullest, but cannot deal with transformations of shape. He does not realize that the *volume* of one cup of liquid in a tall narrow glass remains the same when it is poured into a short squat glass. During this stage, the child develops a sense of the past, present, and future, but has little idea of the length of time in terms of hours, weeks, or years.

Period of Concrete Operations

During the early and middle school years, ages 7 to 11 years, the child learns to *solve problems* in a concrete manner. He learns to think logically, and can categorize (place related items in groups) and seriate (arrange objects in a special order). He begins to discuss causes, effects, relationships, and hierarchies.

During this period, the child becomes increasingly less egocentric, and is gradually realizing that other people have different points of view and see things differently than he does. Social interaction is a necessary condition for learning the reciprocity of viewpoints and ideas.

Period of Formal Operations

As this period begins, the child has learned to solve concrete problems and is now ready to deal with abstract problems. Between the ages of 11 and 14 years, the child begins to use specific mental operations such

---

An Example of Cognitive Development/ Developmental Concepts of Death

- Infancy to 2 years
    No real concept of death
    Beginning of experiences with separation
- 3 to 5 years
    Death seen as temporary and reversible
    Believes that the deceased is "sleeping"
- 6 to 8 years
    Believes that death comes from without (external sources)
    Death personified as skeleton, ghost, bogeyman
    Beginning awareness of finality
    Associates death with old age
- 9 to 11 years
    Beliefs are more aligned with adult concepts of death
    Interested in cause of death and what happens after death
- Adolescence
    Fears death
    Fascination with phenomenon of death
    Wishes to fulfill ambitions and dreams before dying

---

as logical thinking, scientific reasoning, exploration of both sides of a question, building and testing a hypothesis, reflection, prediction, and evaluation. Piaget asserts that after this stage, the individual refines and expands the use of these operations by means of frequent and repeated practice throughout life.

Havighurst

Robert J. Havighurst, an educator, built his theory from the concepts of Eric Erikson. Havighurst's developmental theory was designed for educators, but it is applicable to nursing practice, especially in the areas of patient and family teaching and anticipatory guidance.

Havighurst's development theory is based on learning "To understand human devclopment, one must understand learning. The human individual learns his way through life" (Havighurst, p. 10). He described a series of *developmental tasks,* each of which needed to be accomplished at the appropriate stage of the life cycle for optimal health and growth.

A developmental task is a task which arises at or about a certain period in the life of the individual, successful achievement of which leads to his happiness and to success with later tasks, while failure leads to unhappiness in the individual, disapproval by the society, and difficulty with later tasks. (Havighurst, 1972, p. 2)

Havighurst described developmental tasks arising from a combination of internal and external forces. The *internal* forces are the result of physical maturation, such as the strength and coordination which are needed to stand erect, the changes associated with puberty, and the physical changes of aging. The *external* forces arise from the demands and expectations of society. Parents, peers, neighbors, and community groups all exert pressure upon the individual to learn to behave in ways that are both expected and acceptable within that culture.

Developmental tasks also result from a third force, namely personal values and aspirations. Based upon his abilities, and his perception of the pressures and opportunities afforded by his culture, the individual develops a set of motives and values which influence the things he chooses to learn and the tasks he is willing and able to accomplish.

Researchers have studied the phenomenon of "critical periods" or "sensitive periods" in the life of an individual during which a given developmental task is accomplished most easily and with optimum results. Such a period is referred to as the *teachable moment* and occurs at the convergence of physical readiness, societal pressure, and personal interest. *Premature* pressure to achieve a certain developmental task is not fruitful; it

Havighurst's Developmental Tasks

INFANCY AND EARLY CHILDHOOD

1. Learning to walk
2. Learning to take solid food
3. Learning to talk
4. Learning to control the elimination of body wastes
5. Learning sex differences and sexual modesty
6. Forming concepts and learning language to describe social and physical reality
7. Getting ready to read
8. Learning to distinguish right from wrong and beginning to develop a conscience

MIDDLE CHILDHOOD

1. Learning physical skills necessary for ordinary games
2. Building wholesome attitudes towards oneself as a growing organism
3. Learning to get along with age mates
4. Learning an appropriate masculine or feminine role
5. Developing fundamental skills in reading, writing and calculating
6. Developing concepts necessary for everyday living
7. Developing conscience, morality, and a scale of values
8. Achieving person independence
9. Developing attitudes towards social groups and institutions

ADOLESCENCE

1. Achieving new and more mature relations with age-mates of both sexes
2. Achieving a masculine or feminine social role
3. Accepting one's physique and using the body effectively
4. Achieving emotional independence of parents and other adults
5. Preparing for marriage and family life

6. Preparing for an economic career
7. Acquiring a set of values and an ethical system as a guide to behavior; developing an ideology
8. Desiring and achieving socially responsible behavior

EARLY ADULTHOOD

1. Selecting a mate
2. Learning to live with a marriage partner
3. Starting a family
4. Rearing children
5. Managing a home
6. Getting started in an occupation
7. Taking on civic responsibility
8. Finding a congenial social group

MIDDLE AGE

1. Assisting teenage children to become responsible and happy adults
2. Achieving adult civic and social responsibility
3. Reaching and maintaining satisfactory performance in one's occupational career
4. Developing adult leisure time activities
5. Relating oneself to one's spouse as a person
6. Accepting and adjusting to the physiological changes of middle age
7. Adjusting to aging parents

LATER MATURITY

1. Adjusting to decreasing physical strength and health
2. Adjusting to retirement and reduced income
3. Adjusting to death of spouse
4. Establishing an explicit affiliation with one's age group
5. Adopting and adapting social roles in a flexible way
6. Establishing satisfactory physical living arrangements

results only in wasted energy, frustration, and possibly a sense of failure. On the other hand, the ability of parents or teachers to predict when an individual is likely to be ready to tackle a given developmental task will facilitate the process with gratifying results.

Havighurst differentiated between recurrent and nonrecurrent tasks. Some tasks, such as learning to walk, talk, and read need to be learned only once. Other tasks tend to recur at various times, even though in slightly different form. Some of these recurrent tasks are learning to get along with one's age mates, participating as a responsible citizen, and learning one's sex role. Recurrent tasks are present in each stage of life, and the process of learning and accomplishing these tasks extends throughout each individual's lifetime.

Researchers have derived the following principles which contribute to our understanding of the significance of developmental tasks:

1. Every person faces certain responsibilities of growing up at every stage of his life.
2. A person must accomplish the developmental tasks of any given period in his development if he is to grow on to the next level of his maturation (Fig. 15.4).
3. Growth responsibilities are so urgent and insistent that they take precedence over outside pressures.
4. No one else can accomplish for the individual the developmental tasks that he faces.

5. Very few developmental tasks can be mastered in isolation.

6. A teacher or parent who encourages and assists a child to accomplish his developmental tasks, helps to promote the child's development. (Adapted from Duvall, 1964, p. 42)

The significance of Havighurst's theory is twofold. First, each individual must take an active role in his own development, and second, appropriate interventions by concerned persons at the sensitive times or teachable moments can facilitate this process. Significant interventions include: anticipatory guidance by which the person is helped to understand and prepare for the tasks which lie ahead, the provision of a supportive environment in which to learn, and reward or recognition for tasks well done.

Kohlberg

In an era when there is much controversy over separation of church and state, and conflict between groups such as the Moral Majority and other segments of the population, the moral development of the individual is of great concern to parents and educators. Lawrence Kohlberg and other researchers are trying to identify the developmental stages of morality, and the degree to which they are successful will affect the ways in which parents, educators, and the clergy can influence the moral standards of our time. (See page 230.)

INTERRELATEDNESS OF THEORIES

Although the attention of a given theorist is focused on a particular and limited aspect of individual growth and development, these specific theoretical concepts can be combined to give a more global understanding of human development. Each theory contributes different insights which, when taken together, provide a holistic view of a person at a specific stage of development.

Most of the concepts complement each other; they are usually not contradictory, and therefore, it is not necessary to choose one or the other. For example, with respect to development during the first year of life, the following concepts are interrelated and can be used to provide a basis for understanding *one* aspect of infant behavior:

Freud—oral phase focuses on satisfaction associated with the mouth

Erikson—the development of trust when the infant's need for food is met

Piaget—the repetitive behavior of intentional and purposeful sucking

Havighurst—developmental task of learning to take solid food

When these concepts are synthesized, a nurse could derive guidelines such as the following:

- The *manner* in which an infant is fed affects his psychosocial development (the infant should be fed in response to his cries of hunger and the feeding should be a loving social interaction between infant and caregiver).

- The *process of feeding* is as significant as the kind and amount of food given (the infant needs an

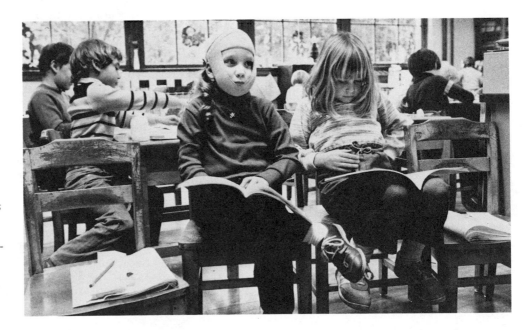

Figure 15.4 The intent expressions on the faces of Renee and her classmates illustrate Erikson's fourth stage of development industry vs. inferiority. It is during this stage that children are receptive to the systematic instruction which will prepare them for the demands of their culture and society. (See Havighurst's tasks of middle childhood in text.)

Kohlberg's Stages of Moral Development

PRECONVENTIONAL LEVEL OF MORALITY

Stage 0	Age: 0–2 yr	Egocentric judgments on basis of what child likes (helps) him, or doesn't like (hurts) him; reacts to hurt with anger and to pleasure with love
Stage 1	Age: 2–3 yr	Fear of hurt or punishment is dominant factor in determining right or wrong
Stage 2	Age: 4–7 yr	Conforms to rules out of self-interest or in relation to what others will do in return for good behavior

CONVENTIONAL LEVEL OF MORALITY

Stage 3	Age: 8–9 yr	Seeks and gains approval; good relationships = right; broken or bad relationships = wrong
Stage 4	Age: 10–12 yr	Age of accountability; personal concern for doing duty, showing respect for authority and maintaining social order; rigid adherence to law and order

POSTCONVENTIONAL LEVEL OF MORALITY

Stage 5	Adolescence	Rights and responsibility balanced in social context; rational thinking; values will of majority; doesn't expect to get something for nothing, to take and not give, to belong without producing
Stage 6	Age: Adult	Mature, moral, self-motivated individual; self-evaluating; self-actualizing; internalized standards; places integrity before expediency.

Life Spans and Contributions of Selected Development Theorists

Theorist	Born	Died	Primary Contribution
Sigmund Freud	1856	1939	Personality development
Jean Piaget	1896	1980	Cognitive development of children
Robert Havighurst	1900		Development tasks throughout life
Erik Erikson	1902		Levels of psychosocial development
Evelyn M. Duvall	1906		Stages of family development
Lawrence Kohlberg	1927		Stages of moral development

New parents need to learn what to expect from a child during a given developmental period so that their expectations can be realistic and appropriate. Many parents need considerable support during a phase or stage which is difficult for a given child; they need to know that "this too shall pass" and that the troublesome behaviors are not a permanent part of the child's personality.

Many adults find it helpful to learn that researchers are exploring the phases and stages of adult life, and that adults can pass through difficult phases without permanently damaging important relationships.

RELATED ACTIVITIES

1. Analyze your own developmental level in terms of Erikson's eight stages, Havighurst's developmental tasks and Kohlberg's stages of moral development. Identify those stages or tasks which you have completed, and use those tasks which lie ahead as one basis for making decisions about your immediate future.

adequate amount of sucking, and weaning should be carefully planned).

No single theory of human development is comprehensive enough to account for all the variables which contribute to the uniqueness of each individual, and it is the task of nursing to combine the information which is currently available into useful guidelines for nursing interventions.

PATIENT TEACHING

It is important for patients and families to learn that: (1) human development is sequential and predictable, (2) each phase and stage provides an essential foundation for the next period of development, and (3) each phase can be facilitated by family support, understanding, and encouragement.

SUGGESTED READINGS

Assessing the Elderly (continuing education feature). *Am J Nurs* 1985 September and October. Part 1: Burggraf, Virginia and Barbara Donlon: Assessing the elderly—system by system. *Am J Nurs* 1985 Sept; 85(9):974–984. Part 2: Henderson, Martha L, Antoinette M. Hays, and Frances Borger: Assessment of mental status. *Am J Nurs* 1985 Oct; 85(10):1103–1111.

Barry, Patricia D: *Psychosocial Nursing Assessment and Intervention* (chaps. 2 & 3). Philadelphia, Lippincott, 1984.

Coles, Robert: *The Moral Life of Children*, Boston, Atlantic Monthly (distrib. by Little, Brown and Co.), 1985.

Coles, Robert: *The Political Life of Children*, Boston, Atlantic Monthly (distrib. by Little, Brown and Co.), 1985.

Dennis, Lorraine Bradt, and Joan Hassal: *Introduction to Human Development and Health Issues*. Philadelphia, Saunders, 1983.

Erikson, Erik: *The Life Cycle Completed*. New York, Norton, 1982.

Flavell, John H: Really and truly (appearance vs. reality for children). *Psych Today* 1986 Jan; 20(1):38–44.

Gardner, Howard: The seven frames of mind (measurement of human potential). *Psych Today* 1984 June; 18(6):20–26.

LeShan, Eda J: *The Wonderful Crisis of Middle Age*. New York, Warner Paperback Library, 1973.

Long, Kathleen Anne: Are children too young for mental disorders? *Am J Nurs* 1985 Nov; 85(11):1254–1257.

Murray, Ruth Beckman, and Judith Proctor Zentner: *Nursing Assessment and Health Promotion Through the Life Span*. ed. 3. Englewood Cliffs, NJ, Prentice-Hall, 1985.

Nissenson, Marilyn: Therapy after sixty. *Psych Today* 1984 Jan; 18(1):22–26.

Pines, Maya: Can a rock walk? (cause and effect for children). *Psych Today* 1983 Nov; 17(11):46–54.

Schuster, Clara Shaw, and Shirley Smith Ashburn: *The Process of Human Development: A Holistic Life-Span Approach*. Boston, Little, Brown and Company, 1986.

REFERENCES

Erikson, Erik H: *Identity, Youth and Crisis*. New York, W. W. Norton and Company, 1968.

Erikson, Erik H: *Childhood and Society*. ed. 2. New York, W. W. Norton, 1963.

Freud, Sigmund: *A General Introduction to Psychoanalysis*. New York, Simon-Schuster, 1969 (Pocket Book ed.).

Ginsberg, Herbert, and Sylvia Opper: *Piaget's Theory of Intellectual Development: An Introduction*. Englewood Cliffs, NJ, Prentice-Hall, 1969.

Havighurst, Robert J: *Developmental Tasks and Education*. ed. 3. New York, David McKay, 1972.

Piaget, Jean: *The Psychology of Intelligence*. Totowa, NJ, Littlefield, Adams and Company, 1969.

Piaget, Jean: *The Language and Thought of the Child*, Cleveland, Meridian Books, World Publishing Company, 1967.

16

Family Development

Prerequisites and/or Suggested Preparation
Knowledge of the basic concepts of systems theory (Chapter 5)
and of the stages of individual development (Chapter 15) is
necessary for understanding this chapter.

There is a complex relationship between every individual and his or her family, and few nursing interventions can be fully effective unless these relationships are taken into account. The nurse must know enough about the family to be able to place the patient in some sort of context—from what kind of setting did he come and to what situation will he return?

Consider the case of two young lawyers, both hospitalized for relatively minor injuries received while skiing. The background information is almost identical for each of them. Each lawyer was born near Boston, attended Harvard law school, is married with two preschool age children, and drives a luxury car. Each lawyer is a Democrat, Catholic, and physically fit except for the current problem. Given these data, it would seem logical to use similar approaches to each lawyer's nursing care and patient teaching, and it would probably be appropriate to do so whenever the illness is a minor one.

If, on the other hand, each lawyer had suffered a catastrophic illness such as cancer, AIDS, or quadriplegia following an automobile accident, a single or common approach to the two situations could not be used. The effects of any major illness are not confined to the patient, and members of his family will be affected in one way or another whether they want to be or not. An acutely ill person is not self-sufficient, and his health care will be influenced by the help and support he receives (or does not receive) from his family. Therefore, a nurse will need to understand the general nature of important patient-family relationships before she can help the patient cope effectively with his situation.

Patient-family relationships will influence the outcome for each of the two seriously ill young lawyers as they try to find answers to questions such as the following:

- Who will help my wife to cope with my condition?
- Where should I go when I leave the hospital? Could I be cared for at home?
- If I can't work, how will we manage financially? Should we sell our expensive house and car?
- How will all this affect my parents? and my children?
- Holidays and vacations are very important to my whole family? What will happen now? Can I still participate?

Neither lawyer can find answers to such questions without interacting with a variety of other people, and the nurse must understand the basis for such interactions before she can help either patient cope with his stress and anxiety.

Keeping in mind the *similarities* between the two patients, great *differences* in their situations emerge when their families are taken into account. For example:

Lawyer #1: Descended from long line of lawyers, judges, and politicians; parents wealthy, accustomed to keeping servants and receiving services of all kinds; acquainted with many important people in the health care field; family interested and concerned but very busy with professional careers.

Lawyer #2: Oldest of eight children; two others also attended college (all on scholarships); parents immigrated to this country in 1935; father is successful shopkeeper; family maintains close ties with ethnic neighbors (mother still speaks very little English); both parents in poor health and have a general mistrust of "modern medicine"; family is close knit, very proud of lawyer.

The above information is certainly *not* complete enough to be adequate for decision making and planning, but it serves to show the intricacies of the situations, and to emphasize the need for understanding *each family* before patient care is planned. Each patient will be affected by his family's reaction to his illness, by the relationships between himself and his family, and by the interactions between the nurses, doctors, and his family. For example, it is possible that health care workers will treat the two sets of parents differently. Attitudes toward a wealthy professional couple may be quite different from attitudes toward parents who are less confident and who don't trust the health care delivery system, especially when one of them speaks little English. Each patient will be sensitive to the ways in which his parents are treated, and will respond accordingly.

THE STUDY OF FAMILIES

Each family is a *unit* with a unique personality, structure, and attributes. In addition to its uniqueness, however, each family exhibits certain characteristics which are common to all families and it is these commonalities which form the basis for the study of family life. Some of these aspects of family life are: communication patterns, power structure, roles within the family, values, patterns of coping, culture, emotional relationships, economic considerations, and health practices.

Concepts and Definitions

For the purposes of this text, the term *family* is used to designate any unit of two or more people who are emotionally involved with each other and living together as a result of birth, marriage, or choice. This definition is more inclusive than the older, more traditional concept of a family as a husband, wife, and their children. It is broad enough to include a wide variety of families, including an unmarried couple, single or unmarried parent and child, commune family, homosexual couple, childless couple, or elderly siblings living together. It also includes a single adult living alone with strong family ties, such as a young woman with a new job and her first apartment. In each of these families there is involvement, mutual commitment and obligation, and a sense of unity based on marriage vows, birth, or mutual consent.

The preceding definition of a family states that the members are involved with each other, but does not specify the nature of the involvement. Ideally, the involvement would be one of love, caring, concern, mutual respect, and support. Unfortunately, family involvement often includes anger, bitterness, lack of respect, jealousy, submission, and even abuse of vulnerable members. Given this range of possible attitudes and behaviors, it is important to assess a given family systematically, in terms of those aspects of family life which are common to all families. If the focus of study is not directed toward specific interactions within the family, it is very easy to become judgmental and ascribe negative values to a family which is markedly different from our personal concept of what a "good" family should be like.

Every family manages its money, communicates, and recognizes authority figures within the family, and these things can be studied without labeling the family good or bad, normal or deviant, functional or dysfunctional. It is possible for a family to be strong, healthy, supportive, and effective and still seem very strange indeed to a nurse who knows little about subcultures and value systems which are different from her own. (See box.)

Some of the terms used by theorists when studying and describing a family include: *nuclear family, family of origin,* and *extended family* plus the newer term *blended family.*

- Nuclear family—refers to a husband, wife, and their children
- Family of origin—the family into which a person is born
- Extended family—consists of the nuclear family plus persons who are related by blood such as grandparents, cousins, aunts, and uncles, and usually refers to those relatives who are actively involved in some way with the nuclear family
- Blended family—consists of husband, wife, children of previous marriages of one or both partners, and possibly children from the present union

---

Traditional and Evolving Family Forms

TRADITIONAL FAMILY STRUCTURES

Nuclear family. Husband, wife, and children living in common household; single or dual careers.

Nuclear dyad. Husband and wife living alone (childless or children have left home); single, or dual careers.

Single-parent family. One head of household with preschool or school age children; results from separation, divorce, abandonment, or death; parent may or may not have career depending upon financial aid from absent parent or other sources.

Three-generation or extended family. Any of above families plus one or more grandparents living in common household.

Single adult living alone.

EVOLVING FAMILY STRUCTURES

Commune family. Either a household of monogamous couples with shared facilities, resources, and rearing of children, or a household of adults and children (a group marriage). The latter usually has a charismatic leader, sometimes involves cultism, all are "married" to each other, and all participate in raising the children.

Unmarried parent and child family. Marriage either not desired or not possible; child is natural offspring or adopted; usually mother and child.

Unmarried couple and child family. Either a common-law marriage with natural or adopted children, or a social contract marriage involving an ideological commitment to a relationship not recognized by law.

Co-habiting couple. Couple living together without marriage.

Homosexual union. Same sex couple living together as marriage partners.

KIN NETWORK

Any combination of the above families plus other relatives living geographically close and sharing goods and services.

Approaches to the Study of Families

Just as the theorists who study individual growth and development approach the topic from a variety of directions, so do those who study the family. These approaches to the study of family life include: family interaction, the family as a social institution, the structure and function of the family, the developmental stages of the family, and the family as a system. Of all these approaches, the systems approach and the developmental approach are currently used most frequently in day-to-day nursing practice. These two approaches are not contradictory, and it is useful to use both perspectives when studying a given family.

Some of the other approaches are used by nurses with special training who are engaged in family counseling and therapy.

Systems Approach

This approach is based on general systems theory (Chapter 5) and the family is viewed as a single system which interacts with many other systems. The terminology of systems theory is used to describe both the family system and its subsystems (the individual members of the family). Terms commonly used include the following: system, component, input, feedback, boundaries, output, and equilibrium.

BOUNDARIES. The size of any system is determined by the placement of its boundaries, and the boundaries of the family may be set around the nuclear family alone, or may be expanded to include all or part of the extended family. According to systems theory, the boundaries of a system are set arbitrarily at any given point in time, and can be changed as needed to permit the continued study of the system as it expands or contracts. This concept is important because it permits the boundaries of a family system to expand to include the addition of children or the spouses of grown children, and it also permits boundaries to contract as children grow up and leave home, or family members die.

COMPONENTS. Members of the family are called either *subsystems* or *components* of the family system. All components of a system are interrelated, and in accordance with systems theory, whatever happens to one member of a family affects all other members, and whatever happens to the family as a whole affects each individual member. Within the family there are a number of naturally occurring groups (subsystems) such as husband and wife, siblings, parent and child, husband and his parents, wife and her parents, and grandparents and grandchildren. The relationships within each subsystem are unique, and the interests and needs of one subsystem may conflict with those of another. For example, the needs of husband and wife for adult recreation may conflict with the children's expectation to be included in all activities. Each family member belongs to several subsystems, and the individual's relationship with one subsystem affects his relationships with other subsystems of the family.

The family is a component or subsystem of many larger systems such as their extended family, church, neighborhood, village, political party, and nation. Whatever happens within their church, neighborhood, or other larger system will affect the family as a whole, and each member of it.

INPUT. The family is an open system which interacts with other systems, and whose subsystems interact with each other. Input into the family takes the form of information, energy, or materials just as for any other system. Family input includes everything from money and bills to visits with friends, parent-teacher conferences, and health care. Some families are less open than others, and tend to be aloof, suspicious, or unfriendly, and to isolate themselves from the majority of other systems. Such families have a very limited and restricted input.

OUTPUT. The output of a family is the sum total of actions of the members of that family. A family's output includes the money it pays for food, clothing, and shelter; the work done by its members; prayers for other people; volunteer work; mischief done by the children; letters and telephone calls; criminal or antisocial acts; discoveries and inventions; political and all other activities. The output of some families is minimal and seems to exert little influence on other systems. The output of other families is detrimental to society, and the output from some families is beneficial almost beyond measure.

FEEDBACK. According to systems theory, feedback is a portion of the output of a system which is fed back into the system for the purpose of self-regulation of the system. In a family, feedback is obtained through communication and the observation of the ways in which certain behaviors affect other people. Each family member can determine whether or not he or she was understood, and whether or not a certain set of actions achieved the desired results.

Feedback becomes input when it is received by an individual; it provides the information which lets that person decide whether to continue his course of action or make some changes. Negative feedback indicates the need for a change, and positive feedback indicates that the individual is on the right track. Even small children use feedback from parents or siblings to decide whether or not a certain behavior is acceptable or desirable.

The family system as a whole uses feedback from neighbors, relatives, teachers, professional people, police, and others to evaluate themselves as a family. The acceptance or rejection of the family by other systems provides the positive or negative feedback which is needed for the self-regulation of family functioning.

EQUILIBRIUM. Equilibrium is usually referred to as *stability* in the context of a family system. Each family experiences its ups and downs, periods of tension and disruption, and crises from time to time, but a *healthy family is essentially stable* in the long run. Each time the family or one of its members experiences a noticeable change, feedback mechanisms provide the information needed to evaluate the change and take any action necessary to restore a stable situation.

Stability in a family means that people and activities are dependable and quite predictable, and that no matter what happens, things get back to normal fairly quickly. Some families are very unsettled and seem to go from one upheaval or crisis to another. This may be due to dysfunctional patterns of interaction, lack of accurate and complete information for decision making, or lack of energy or resources to take appropriate and effective action.

Developmental Approach

Theorists who use a developmental approach to study the family view the family as a *unit which has a life cycle* with predictable, orderly *stages of development*. In addition to the developmental tasks of each individual, as described by Havighurst and others (Chapter 15), there are developmental tasks *for the whole family* which must be accomplished at each stage of family development.

Theorists who use this approach believe that the developmental tasks for each stage of family life must be met before the family can move on to the next stage of family development. The tasks are derived from biological requirements, social imperatives, and individual goals and values.

Successful achievement of these family tasks provides for optimal development of the family as a unit as well as for the development of each individual member.

There is some variation within these tasks depending on the life cycle stage of the family at any given point in time, and they are influenced by factors such as culture and socioeconomic status, but there are eight tasks which are essential for the survival and development of all families. These tasks are related to the following*:

1. *Physical maintenance*—providing shelter, food, clothing, health care.
2. *Allocation of resources*—meeting family needs and costs, apportioning material goods, facilities, space, authority, respect, affection.
3. *Division of labor*—deciding who does what, assigning responsibility for procuring income, managing the household, caring for family members, and other specific tasks.
4. *Socialization of family members*—guiding the development of each member toward socially ac-

ceptable patterns of controlling elimination, food intake, sexual drives, sleep, aggression.

5. *Reproduction, recruitment, and release of family members*—bearing or adopting children and rearing them for release at maturity, incorporating new members by marriage, and establishing policies for the inclusion of others: in-laws, relatives, step-parents, guests, family friends.
6. *Maintenance of order*—providing means of communication, establishing types and intensity of interaction, patterns of affection, and sexual expression by ensuring conformity to family norms.
7. *Placement of members in the larger society*—fitting into the community, relating to church, school, organizational life, political and economic systems, and protecting family members from undesirable outside influences.
8. *Maintenance of motivation and morale*—rewarding members for achievements, satisfying individual needs for acceptance, giving encouragement and affection, meeting personal and family crises, refining a philosophy of life and a sense of family loyalty through rituals, family traditions, festivals.

Duvall's Theory of Family Development

Evelyn Duvall studied with Robert Havighurst, and in 1942 they collaborated on the first published work related to the concept of family developmental tasks. Over the years, she refined her family life cycle approach and described eight successive stages and the tasks for each stage throughout the life cycle (Table 16.1).

TABLE 16.1 DUVALL'S EIGHT STAGES OF FAMILY LIFE

Stage I	Beginning family (married couple without children)
Stage II	Early childbearing family (oldest child is an infant up to age 2½ years)
Stage III	Family with preschool children (oldest child is 2½ to 5 years old)
Stage IV	Family with school children (oldest child is 6 to 13 years old)
Stage V	Family with teenagers (oldest child is 13 to 20 years old)
Stage VI	Launching center family (from the time the first child leaves until the last is gone)
Stage VII	Family in the middle years (empty nest to retirement)
Stage VIII	Family in retirement and old age (from retirement to death of spouses)

*Adapted from Duvall, pp. 27–28.

Families in the first five stages, from marriage until the first child is ready to leave, are referred to as *expanding* families. Families in the last three stages are referred to as *contracting* families.

When Duvall did her major research on family development, the nuclear family was the basic family structure in the U.S. and she used the age and school placement of the oldest child to determine a family's life cycle stage. Since that time, many different patterns of family life have evolved, and her classic stages must be modified for those families who by choice or circumstance do not fit the nuclear family structure. For example, the couple without children would go through stages I, VII, and VIII of the stages in Table 16.1. Blended families or families whose children are widely spaced may have an overlap of stages.

Other changes in family life have altered the timing of different stages for many families. For example, the empty nest may be delayed because more adult children are living at home now as a result of divorce or separation, unemployment, or the high cost of separate housing. In such situations, the transition between stages VI and VII is prolonged and the developmental tasks of each stage are modified.

Duvall's theory of family development is still widely used because the majority of the developmental tasks *need to be done* whether or not they are actually done, and regardless of how they are done (Table 16.2). For example, before a baby is born, the tasks of the "family" are similar whether the mother is the wife in a traditional nuclear family, an unwed teenager, or a career woman who is unmarried and pregnant by choice. The task of getting and spending income must be accomplished whether it be by pursuing a professional career or applying for welfare benefits.

Current research will eventually explain and describe many of the new and evolving forms of family life and Duvall's theory will be modified or replaced.

Duvall's Family Developmental Tasks

I. DEVELOPMENTAL TASKS OF THE BEGINNING FAMILY. The first stage of the family without children is divided into two phases, each with its own developmental tasks. These phases are the *establishment phase*, and the *expectant phase*.

Establishment Phase: (1) Establishing a home base in a place to call their own. (2) Establishing mutually satisfactory systems for getting and spending money. (3) Establishing mutually acceptable patterns of who does what and who is accountable to whom. (4) Establishing a continuity of mutually satisfying sex relationships. (5) Establishing systems of intellectual and emo-

tional communication. (6) Establishing workable relationships with relatives. (7) Establishing ways of interacting with friends, associates, and community organizations. (8) Facing the possibility of children and planning for their coming. (9) Establishing a workable philosophy of life as a couple.

Expectant Phase: (1) Arranging for the physical care of the expected baby. (2) Developing new patterns for getting and spending income. (3) Reevaluating procedures for determining who does what and where authority rests. (4) Adapting patterns of sexual relationships to pregnancy. (5) Expanding communication systems for present and anticipated emotional needs. (6) Reorienting relationships with relatives. (7) Adapting relationships with friends, associates, and community activities to the realities of pregnancy. (8) Acquiring knowledge about, and planning for the specifics of pregnancy, childbirth, and parenthood. (9) Maintaining morale and a workable philosophy of life.

II. DEVELOPMENTAL TASKS OF THE CHILDBEARING FAMILY (oldest child newborn to 30 months). (1) Establishment of the family as a stable unit. (2) Reconciliation of conflicting developmental tasks of family members. (3) Mutual support of developmental needs of each member to strengthen each individual and the family unit. Also: (1) Adapting housing arrangements for the life of the little child. (2) Meeting the costs of family living at the childbearing stage. (3) Reworking patterns of mutual responsibility and accountability. (4) Reestablishing mutually satisfying sexual relationships. (5) Refining intellectual and emotional communication systems for childbearing and rearing. (6) Reestablishing working relationships with parents. (7) Fitting into community life as a young family. (8) Planning for further children in the family. (9) Reworking a suitable philosophy of life as a family.

III. DEVELOPMENTAL TASKS OF THE FAMILY WITH PRESCHOOL CHILDREN (oldest child 2½ to 6 years). (1) Supplying adequate space, facilities, and equipment for the expanding family. (2) Meeting predictable and unexpected costs of family life with small children. (3) Sharing responsibilities within the expanded family and among members of the growing family. (4) Maintaining mutually satisfying sexual relationships and planning for future children. (5) Creating and maintaining effective communication systems within the family. (6) Cultivating the full potential of relationships with relatives within the extended family. (7) Tapping resources, serving needs and enjoying contacts outside the family. (8) Facing dilemmas and reworking philosophies of life in ever changing challenges.

IV. DEVELOPMENTAL TASKS OF THE FAMILY WITH SCHOOLAGE CHILDREN *(oldest child 6–13 years)*. (1) Providing for children's activity and parent's privacy. (2) Staying financially solvent. (3) Cooperating to get things done. (4) Continuing to satisfy each other as marriage partners. (5) Effectively utilizing family communication systems. (6) Feeling close to relatives in the larger family. (7) Tying in with life outside the family. (8) Testing and retesting family philosophies of life.

V. DEVELOPMENTAL TASKS OF THE FAMILY WITH TEENAGERS *(oldest child 13–20 years)*. (1) Providing facilities for widely different needs. (2) Working out money matters in the family with teenagers. (3) Sharing the tasks and responsibilities of family living. (4) Putting the marriage relationship into focus. (5) Keeping communication systems open. (6) Maintaining contact with the extended family. (7) Growing into the world as a family and as persons. (8) Reworking and maintaining a philosophy of life.

VI. DEVELOPMENTAL TASKS OF THE LAUNCHING CENTER FAMILY *(first child gone to last child's leaving home)*. (1) Rearranging physical facilities and resources. (2) Meeting costs as a launching center family. (3) Reallocating responsibilities among grown and growing children. (4) Coming to terms with themselves as husband and wife. (5) Maintaining open communication within the family, and between the family and others. (6) Widening the family circle through release of young adult children and recruitment of new members by marriage. (7) Reconciling conflicting loyalties and philosophies of life.

VII. DEVELOPMENTAL TASKS OF A FAMILY IN THE MIDDLE YEARS *(empty nest to retirement)*. (1) Maintaining a pleasant and comfortable home. (2) Assuring security for the later years. (3) Carrying household responsibilities. (4) Drawing closer together as a couple. (5) Maintaining contact with grown children's families. (6) Keeping in touch with brothers' and sisters' families and with aging parents. (7) Participating in community life beyond the family. (8) Reaffirming the values of life that have real meaning.

VIII. DEVELOPMENTAL TASKS OF THE AGING FAMILY *(retirement to death of one or both spouses)*. (1) Finding a satisfying home for the later years. (2) Adjusting to retirement income. (3) Establishing comfortable household routines. (4) Nurturing each other as husband and wife. (5) Facing bereavement and widowhood. (6) Maintaining contact with children and grandchildren. (7) Caring for elderly relatives. (8) Keeping an interest in people outside the family. (9) Finding meaning in life.

Factors Which Influence Family Development

Every family on the face of the earth is influenced by a wide variety of forces outside the family. These forces provide input into each family system and affect family development to a greater or lesser degree. They cannot be avoided, although some isolated, relatively closed family systems do manage to exclude some of the effects of such factors.

Family size and composition are two of the most significant determinants of family development because a family consisting of two parents and one child is obviously going to function differently than a family with nine children, for example. But given any group of families of equal size, it is differences in the following factors that will make each family unique:

- *Geography:* Small town, rural, or inner city? Industrialized or developing nation? Warm, tropical, temperate, or frigid climate?
- *Political situation:* Democratic, repressive, or revolutionary? Militaristic, corrupt, or constitutional?
- *Family economics:* Affluent, welfare, or borderline? Upwardly mobile, unemployed, or destitute?
- *Living conditions:* Spacious home, crowded flat, public shelter? Refugee center, longtime family home, or trailer park?
- *Ethnic background:* Part of the predominant culture or member of minority group? Isolated or surrounded by others of similar culture background? Political refugee or family of a foreign ambassador?
- *Generation:* New immigrant, or long-established descendent of an 18th century immigrant?
- *Language:* Fluent in local language, unable to communicate, or multilingual?
- *Education:* Literate or illiterate? Professional, semi-skilled, or untrained?
- *Religion:* Important, peripheral, or absent? Members of emerging church, cult, or mainstream traditional church?
- *Family health:* Optimal, borderline, or ravished by diseases prevalent in the area?
- *Value system:* Conservative and traditional, liberal and evolving, rebellious, or avant-garde?

Each of the above factors exerts an influence on a family's growth and development as well as on the development of each member of the family. The amount of influence exerted by each factor will vary from family to family, but all of the factors are interrelated—

Brief Summary of Population Trends in the U.S. (Based on 1980 Census)

- It is very unlikely that we will ever again grow as rapidly as during the 20 years following World War II.
- We are moving south and west, out of large cities, and to suburbs and the countryside.
- Our minority populations are growing much faster than the rest of the population.
- Our population is aging and will continue to grow older.
- More of us are living alone and our families are smaller.
- We're better educated.
- We're getting married later.
- Slightly over half of all women now are in the work force, and many hold jobs previously monopolized by men.
- Our incomes continued to grow in the 1970s but the gains were largely offset by increases in the cost of living.
- The poverty rate dropped slightly during the 1970s for the total population, but it dropped substantially for senior citizens.
- More of us are buying our own homes, despite higher costs.

Source: U.S. Department of Commerce, Bureau of the Census, *We, The Americans,* 1984, p.15.

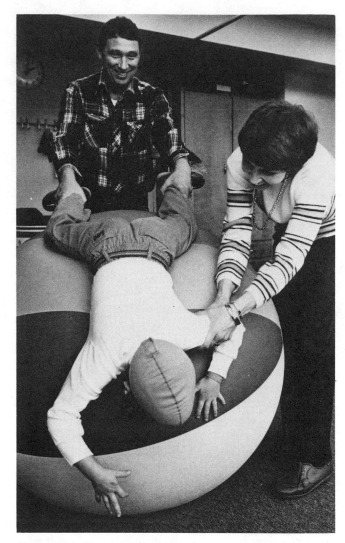

Figure 16.1 *The enthusiastic involvement of Renee's parents in her physical therapy illustrates one of the primary functions of a family—that of helping each other cope with the demands of stressful situations.*

none of them can operate in isolation. Each factor represents an interaction between the family system and several other systems within the community. For example, the educational status of the family is influenced by the family's value system, the geographic availability of schools and colleges, the status of men and women, financial resources, and the political climate of the country.

Interaction among all the forces which affect family development results in a set of attitudes which tend to direct the life of the family (Fig. 16.1). These attitudes are culturally derived, and develop over a number of years, involving several generations of the family. Significant attitudes are related to vital topics and issues such as:

- *Marriage* (divorce, racial intermarriage, living together)
- *Status of children* (an economic necessity, something to be endured, a blessing, the "property" of the parents)
- *Status of women* (equality, women's work versus men's work within the family, handling of money, decision making)
- *Work* ("being on welfare is an acceptable way of life," "anyone can get ahead if he works hard," "material things are not important so take time to smell the roses")
- *Health* (go to the doctor if you don't feel well versus if you can get out of bed you can go to work)

It is highly impractical and unrealistic for a nurse to try to assess all these aspects of family life in detail for every family she cares for, but it is *possible and essential* for each nurse to *take them into consideration* when she is planning nursing care.

NURSING AND THE FAMILY

The nurse is one of the health care workers most likely to avoid stereotyping and jumping to conclusions such as "Mr. Brown has a good job, he lives in a nice section of the city, and his family visits him quite frequently; *therefore,* he probably has an O.K. family situation and won't have any problems when he goes home."

The professional nurse avoids such pitfalls of over-generalization and the stereotyping of families by fostering her innate qualities of curiosity and wonderment. As she cares for each patient and interacts with members of his family, she thinks:

"I wonder why John acts so irritable and depressed just before visiting hours each day. His family is so pleasant."

"The Smith baby is almost 6 weeks old, and his grandmother has still not picked him up or looked directly at his hare-lip and cleft palate. I wonder what I can do to help her?"

"I wonder what is making it so difficult for Mr. Thompson's children to make plans about his care after his stroke? Is it finances, family tradition, sibling rivalries, geographical distances, or what?"

Preparation for Nurse-Family Interactions

Schools of nursing approach the study of families in a variety of ways. Some programs focus on the individual patient first and focus on the family unit at a later time. Other schools progress from studying the family as a unit to studying various age groups within the family. Some programs incorporate a focus on the family throughout the entire curriculum while others concentrate on family life during a unit on public health or community health.

Regardless of the formal placement of such studies, it is extremely important for even the beginning student to include the concept of family into *every nursing experience*. It is only by consistent, regular, and conscious attention to patients' families that you will automatically include significant family relationships in each of your nursing care plans.

In some instances, involvement with the family will be joyous such as helping a mother breastfeed her first-born or monitoring the successful correction of a baby's deformity. In other situations, involvement will be difficult and frustrating such as helping a family cope with attempts at suicide, dealing with abusive parents, or helping a patient and his family plan for the patient's impending death.

Nursing involvement with the family ranges from a simple awareness and concern for the family, through

> ### Examples of Nurse-Family Interactions
>
> - Counseling families about family planning, prenatal care, mental health, hereditary problems, or plans for retirement.
> - Teaching families more effective ways of parenting; accident prevention, normal growth and development, anticipatory guidance, discipline, immunization, and nutrition.
> - Motivating families to assume responsibility for their own health through self-care and attention to nutrition, recreation, exercise, and the environment.
> - Helping families balance the needs and demands of a chronically or terminally ill member against the needs of the rest of the family.
> - Strengthening and supporting vulnerable families who are confronted with actual or potential problems of alcoholism, child abuse, mental illness, violence, incest, drug abuse, or depression.
> - Helping families cope with the complexities of various health care delivery systems with respect to their rights and options, available resources, procedures and policies.
> - Teaching families how to care for a patient at home, including care during minor illnesses, convalescence, chronic conditions, and terminal illnesses.

direct teaching and emotional support of the family, to family therapy for disturbed, multiproblem families. The latter type of nursing involvement is a nursing specialty called family therapy or family nursing and requires advanced preparation, usually at the graduate level.

The techniques and skills which are required for both assessment of the family and effective intervention are based on therapeutic communication (Chapter 9). The interaction starts with the very first meeting with the family, and continues for the duration of the nurse's contact with the patient and family.

There are a number of things which affect the nurse's contact with the family. These include fatigue, lack of energy, pressures of time, personal attitudes toward the family, any apparent disinterest or rejection on the part of the family, and concern about the outcome if the problem is a sensitive or difficult one. Despite these very real concerns, the effective professional nurse is the one who does whatever she can with whatever skill she has to include the family in planning nursing and health care.

FAMILY HEALTH CARE

The nurse is often the only professional health care worker who works with the family as a whole, who has an awareness of the overall needs of the family, and who is able to help the family develop a unified approach to the family's health. Except for the fortunate families who have access to a "family doctor," health care is fragmented for the average family. For example, within the space of a few months, a family could be involved with the following health care resources:

- Obstetrician or obstetrics care—for pregnant mother
- Pediatrician or well baby clinic—toddler's immunizations
- Surgeon and hospital staff—10-year-old's appendectomy
- Home health aides—care of grandfather after a stroke
- General practitioner—treatment of mother's "flu"
- Industrial nurse—regarding father's weight at yearly physical

In each of the above contacts, it is likely that the health care given was focused almost *exclusively* upon the problem or condition of the one person who was perceived to be the patient, with little or no attention paid to the family. In some instances, such an approach might be appropriate, but *only* if the nurse has assessed the situation and made a conscious decision that such a narrow focus is appropriate. In each of the contacts mentioned above, a nurse could assess the level of stress and coping by asking a few strategic questions and engaging the family members in a meaningful conversation, no matter how brief. Such a conversation might reveal the existence of any urgent needs or problems which would otherwise be missed as a result of the unfortunate fragmentation of care currently imposed upon most families.

The need for attention to the overall needs of the family is especially acute when cultural differences are involved. For example, the rural family who has just moved to the city, the political refugee family who has been given sanctuary by a church, or the newly retired couple who has just arrived in Arizona after leaving their home of 60 years in Maine—all these families are likely to have needs and concerns which transcend the immediate health problem of a given family member. In many situations, cultural differences are not readily apparent but are nevertheless significant. For example, the cultural differences between living in a small town in Maine and a retirement community in Arizona could be as great as or greater than those on either side of the border between France and Holland.

Many of the problems which beset families from a given culture are not nursing problems, cannot be solved by the nurse, and should not be tackled by the nurse,

but the *impact of these problems* on the mental and physical health of the family *cannot be dismissed.*

Examples of such problems are:

Inner city families—air pollution, noise; lack of space and privacy; feelings of alienation; fear of violence; exposure to drug abuse and crime.

Rural families—sanitation and water (dependence upon wells and septic systems); lack of access to cultural and civic resources; limited health care facilities; limited transportation for poor and elderly.

Families with working mothers—management of housekeeping; affordable and acceptable substitute child care; decreased time for involvement in school, church, and civil activities; decreased time and energy for attention to family's growth and development.

Foreign families—limited ability to express needs; loneliness; anxiety; difficulty in meeting spiritual, social, and nutritional needs; difficulty in reconciling old and new cultures and maintaining self-esteem; reconciling differences within the family arising from the different rates at which various age groups accept the new culture and/or reject the old.

CULTURE AND ETHNICITY

Increased tourism, immigration, business relocations, and political activities have increased the contacts between people of different cultures. Cultural diversity used to be centered in large cities or selected areas of the country but today it is manifest throughout the land, and in no aspect of human life is the impact greater than upon the health of those involved.

Culture can be defined as the combined manifestation of the beliefs, behavior, social forms, traditions, and taboos of a racial, religious, or social group. The term *ethnicity* refers to the culture of a specific racial or national group, and recently, to the culture of a minority group.

Some cultures are well defined, well known and well accepted by large segments of the population. Examples include such diverse groups as orthodox Jews, Jehovah's Witnesses, British royalty, and Swedish communities in Minnesota. Other cultures, or subcultures, are not well accepted and may be rejected, avoided, or even harassed. Examples of the latter include some religious cults, homosexuals, illegal Mexican aliens, and street people. Each of these diverse cultural groups has its own code of behavior, social norms, patterns of trust, and channels of communication which must be taken into account before their health care needs can be met.

When you are in a situation in which you have frequent contact with members of a specific cultural group, it will be important for you to study in detail the background of that culture and learn as much as you can about the people with whom you are working. But, until then, your energies should be directed toward understanding the relationship between nursing and culture *in general* rather than trying to learn the specifics of selected cultures.

Memorization of a few facts about a given culture is a dangerous practice. At best, it leads to superficiality and ineffective nursing interventions and at worst, it leads to stereotyping and labeling of individuals with potentially harmful results. For example, it is not possible for any author to "describe briefly" the care of native Americans. The needs of an Indian woman who has never been off her reservation on the plains of Dakota bear little resemblance to the needs of a prominent Indian leader who has met with the President of the United States, and served on a number of national committees. It is not possible to generalize the "care of the black patient": the nursing care and health needs of the Rev. Jesse Jackson (recent candidate for president, world traveler, and diplomat) following minor surgery are far different from the care needed by a frightened black refugee from Haiti following identical surgery.

It is important to avoid at all cost any tendency to believe and perpetuate statements such as "Black people enjoy eating collard greens and chitlins," "Orientals are stoic with respect to pain but Italians are emotional about it," or "Homeless street people *prefer* to live on the streets."

Guidelines for Transcultural Nursing

- Acknowledge your own cultural background and heritage
- Avoid stereotypes; identify your cultural biases and prejudices
- Prevent or minimize any language barriers
- Learn as much as you can about the patient's culture
- Explore the patient's view of the situation
- Involve family members; consider family role changes
- Identify other persons who are significant in patient's situation
- Take cultural food preferences and practices into account
- Evaluate nursing effectiveness frequently; take appropriate action

---

Most health care workers in the United States would agree that it is impossible to describe a "typical" American patient but they often fail to realize that it is equally impossible to describe the reactions and needs of a "typical" Catholic, Italian, or Vietnamese patient.

Assessment of Cultural Differences

In some instances it is relatively easy to spot a person of a different culture. In the United States for example, a different culture might be signified by an Oriental facial structure, the inability to speak or understand English, the wearing of an Indian sari, or the horse-drawn transportation and distinctive clothing of an Amish farmer.

But a far greater number of cultures and subcultures in the United States are not readily identifiable and in many instances, members of those groups receive less than optimal health care because their needs are either not recognized or not acknowledged. Some of these subcultures are:

- Migrant workers
- The very rich
- Runaways
- Persons from remote areas of the Appalachian mountains
- Prostitutes working in a given section of a city
- "Pro-natural" advocates of communal living
- Teenage drug abusers in a given high school
- Recovering alcoholics who belong to Alcoholics Anonymous
- Health "addicts" who frantically pursue health to excess

These groups represent only a few of the many hundreds of cultures and subcultures which have special health needs. In each instance, the group tends to have a code of behavior, a certain form of language or jargon, prescribed areas or territories, strong feelings about authority figures or professional people, and a set of beliefs about health and their own bodies.

A nurse may be involved with an entire family, all of whose members belong to a given cultural group, such as the family of a multi-millionaire tycoon or a transient family of fruit pickers. On the other hand, the nurse may be dealing with a family in which only one member belongs to a certain subculture, and where health needs are not being met because of alienation, misunderstanding, or rejection.

It is often not possible to identify an individual as a member of one cultural group or another by appearance (blue jeans, designer jeans, and dungarees look very similar to an untrained eye) or by demographic data such as name, age, and address. The nurse, therefore, must be on the lookout for clues and cues which would indicate that an individual's family relationships and health needs are significantly influenced by his cultural group. The only way to obtain the data which will be needed in order to understand the patient's situation is to use the techniques of therapeutic communication (Chapter 9) and to explore each verbal or behavioral cue with sensitivity and skill.

Aspects of Culture To Be Assessed

There are at least 10 areas of culture which should be assessed in order to give the most effective nursing care possible. These are: (1) language, (2) space and territoriality, (3) time orientation, (4) gender roles, (5) nutrition, (6) disease risks, (7) health beliefs and practices, (8) responses to birth and death, (9) family relationships, and (10) acceptance by the community.

1. Language and Patterns of Communication

When a patient or his family does not speak or understand English, an interpreter must be used, and communication is difficult for all concerned. An even more serious situation may exist when the patient speaks English but both patient and nurse have different meanings for the words that are being used. The nurse *assumes* that the patient understands what she is saying,

---

Guidelines for Using an Interpreter

- Select an interpreter who is suitable. Consider the cultural attitudes of patient toward age, sex, and social class of interpreter (some material will be private and personal).
- Do not assume that every bilingual person is qualified to interpret. Try to find a trained medical interpreter.
- Allow plenty of time for the interview. Everything must be said twice. (Simultaneous translation is not effective.)
- Speak in short sentences to enhance accuracy of interpretation.
- Verify that both interpreter and patient understand your meaning.
- Be attentive to patient's nonverbal responses.
- Build rapport with the interpreter and maintain open communication.
- Ask for interpreter's impression of overall situation but do not permit interpreter to interject personal opinions or beliefs into the translated message.
- Be sure interpreter understands the ethical aspects of working in a health care setting.

---

and the patient *assumes* that his interpretation of the nurse's meaning is correct. Even if he suspects that there is a communication gap or barrier, he may be too embarrassed to mention it. The commonest examples of such problems involve "street language," current slang, and professional or occupational jargon. A similar problem occurs when a person's second language is perfect textbook English which does not include current cliches, catch-words, slogans, "in" jokes, and abbreviations.

2. Space and Territoriality

A person's concept of his own personal space is influenced by his culture, and it is extremely important to take these differences into account when you plan nursing care. The care of his personal belongings and the respect with which his possessions are handled are of vital concern to some people and of little concern to others.

Cultural differences determine the distance which must be maintained between two people, and whether or not casual touching is permitted. Some cultures place significance on the heights of the positions of the persons involved. A sitting or lying position may seem to indicate dependency, or seem inferior to a standing one, for example.

Eye contact is related both to communication and to territoriality, and is often misinterpreted. Some nurses feel that a person who will not look them in the eye is sneaky or evasive, when in reality, that person may feel that he is showing respect by not presuming to establish eye contact with an authority figure or an important person like a nurse.

3. Time Orientation

Since many aspects of nursing care involve the setting of short range and long range goals, it is important to know how the patient and family view the dimension of time. Some cultures value punctuality while others take a leisurely, almost careless approach to schedules. Members of some cultures are future oriented, including a strong belief in life after death, while others do not plan ahead and purposely live one day at a time.

4. Gender Role

Nursing involves close physical and psychological relationships between men and women, and it is important to know when these interactions might be a problem for a patient and his family. Some cultures have rigid codes of behavior regarding exposure of the body, especially in the presence of a member of the opposite sex, and failure to take these restrictions into account could cause tremendous stress and anxiety. Examples of such restrictions include the role of women in countries of the Middle East, and the church laws of some fundamental sects.

Another potential problem related to gender is that of the reluctance of some males to accept guidance, suggestions, or orders from a female nurse.

5. Nutrition

Cultural beliefs about nutrition are important for both physiological and psychological reasons. Each person should have access to food which will meet his nutritional needs and at the same time not violate any of his religious requirements or ethnic preferences. It is imperative, for example, that kosher food be available for an orthodox Jew, and that appropriate and nutritionally balanced foods be available for the person who is a strict vegetarian. Meals should be psychologically satisfying as well as nutritious, and efforts should be made to provide foods that are *familiar* and enjoyable. Rice and pasta may provide similar nutrients, but they are not interchangeable for ethnic groups which normally eat one or the other.

6. Disease Risks

Community health nurses must be knowledgeable about the health problems and diseases which are likely to beset the cultural groups with which they are working. For example, people in some rural areas of the south are more likely to be infested with hookworms than are people in cities. Venereal diseases are a hazard for prostitutes and many runaways, the incidence of Tay-Sachs disease is highest among Jewish babies, and foot problems are extremely common among street people. It is not realistic to try to learn the specific risks for all cultures, but each nurse must know the hazards for the cultural groups *with whom she is working* in order to do an effective job of case finding, patient teaching, and prevention.

7. Health Beliefs and Practices

One of the most significant effects of culture on family life and the welfare of the individual involves beliefs regarding the causes of illness. These beliefs are deeply ingrained within the individual, and will influence his response to health care. For example, the patient teaching and nursing care of a patient with kidney failure will depend upon which of the following is believed to have caused his illness:

- A pathophysiologic process
- Failure to follow the laws of nature
- The malicious behavior of other people; voodoo; hexes
- Punishment for sin

- The logical result of not taking care of oneself
- Witchcraft
- Evil forces; the evil eye
- Failure of society to provide affordable health care
- Being out of harmony with the environment

Nurses believe that disease and illness are caused by a combination of bacterial or viral infection, failure of the body's immune system, stress, and environmental factors, and they tend to find many of the causes listed above unlikely or unbelievable. This gap between the beliefs of some nurses and patients creates a barrier which is often difficult to overcome.

Many patients and families never express their true beliefs about the cause of a given illness because of fear of ridicule or rejection. For example, a nurse who does not understand the basic concept of voodoo can never expect to get a complete and honest nursing history from some patients.

In addition to knowing what members of a given cultural group believe about the *causes* of illness, it is important to understand their beliefs about the *treatment* of illness. When the patient and family do not have access to their preferred mode of treatment, or when that method has failed, they may submit reluctantly to scientific or modern treatment. The success of the new treatment will depend in part upon the manner in which the patient and his family are helped to bridge the gap between their feelings about the two modes of treatment.

Examples of treatments which are familiar to some cultures are: the wearing of protective amulets, incantations, herbal teas and ointments, exorcism of evil spirits, the laying on of hands by the elder members of the group, removal of the hex or spell, fasting, and the ministrations of a healer. Some health care workers become frustrated and intolerant when a patient is re-

---

Hexes and the Hospitalized Patient

- *What is a hex?* The spell of an ill-wisher or malicious person which is believed to have caused the present illness.
- What is the impact on the patient? The associated anxiety and despair can be fatal. Confidence and hope that the spell can be removed is life-giving. The patient will not recover until the hex is removed.
- How can the hex be removed? The family may hire an appropriate specialist to remove the spell. An anthropologist may be able to remove the spell or recommend an appropriate practitioner. Contact the nearest university for the names of such persons.

luctant to seek the benefits of modern health care and they fail to realize that great patience and sensitivity are needed in order to help a patient and his family to abandon, even temporarily, the beliefs and practices of their culture.

8. Responses to Birth and Death

Cultural differences in the way families react to the processes of birth and death are based on many other aspects of family life. These include beliefs about life after death, gender roles, family relationships, attitudes toward children and the elderly, the continuity of generations, the value of human life, and the laws of nature (Fig. 16.2). Birth and death situations tend to be dramatic events, and cultural influences are more apparent at such times than they are in less stressful happenings.

9. Family Relationships

Before a nurse can effectively help a family plan for the health care of one of its members, it is important to understand the structure and functioning of the family and to get at least tentative answers to questions such as the following: Who is the head of the family: mother? father? grandmother? Who makes the final decisions? Are elderly parents revered, considered a burden, or simply tolerated? Are feelings expressed openly or kept hidden? How do members of this culture treat people

who are too ill or too old to work? Answers to these and similar questions will help the nurse to set realistic and appropriate goals for patient teaching and the care of a given patient.

10. Acceptance by the Community

Health care workers matter of factly counsel patients and families to make use of community services and resources but such advice is not helpful to a family

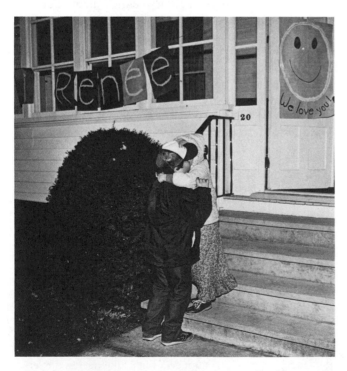

Figure 16.2 Getting re-acquainted with one's brother is one of the best parts of going home.

Suggestions for Working With a Patient of a Different Culture

- If a patient is unwilling or unable to do as he is directed or requested, find out why. Assess his personality, past behavior, and present condition. If no explanation is found, assess his cultural background.

- Accept the patient as he is! Actually put into practice some of the cliches of nursing, such as "Respect the dignity of man" and "Every individual is unique."

- Make sure that all communication, both verbal and nonverbal, is sensitive and appropriate. Do not respond to the patient or family with amazement, surprise, or disbelief. Use the term "different" when referring to the patient's beliefs and practices rather than words such as strange, peculiar, or funny.

- Avoid making superficial generalizations. Do not make casual statements or feign understanding. Saying to a Jehovah's Witness "I knew a Jehovah's Witness once and he _____" is not sensitive or helpful. It implies that all members of the group are alike, and that their culture is not very complex and is easy to understand.

- Read and study about the culture. Observe, watch, and experience everything you can. If it is feasible, learn the language and taste the food.

- Minimize the patient's feelings of alienation. Avoid the use of alienating pronouns such as the use of "we" (the majority culture) versus "they" (members of the different culture). Avoid stereotyping by saying "Mr. Amoli believes _____" and not "They all believe that _____." Do not contribute to any insensitive behavior by the rest of the staff (no flippant remarks or "innocent" ethnic jokes).

- Respect the patient's value system. Refrain from giving advice, making judgments, or giving your opinion about his values and beliefs. A nurse can *respect and accept* a patient's behavior and beliefs without approving of them!

- Follow acceptance with action. Acceptance of the patient's cultural background should be followed by whatever patient teaching may be necessary in order for him to: (1) choose from the health care options that are available to him, (2) give informed consent for treatment, and (3) participate knowledgeably in his own care.

whose culture is not well accepted by neighbors and service agencies. In such situations, alternative sources of assistance must be sought. A similar situation can occur within a hospital or other health care facility if the patient's culture is rejected by one or more members of the staff.

PATIENT TEACHING

Many families seem to drift along from year to year, responding as best they can to whatever comes their way. They seem unable to anticipate the changes that are likely to take place, and are, therefore, often unprepared for the situations they must face.

It is important to help such families gain greater control over their lives in order to reduce stress and enhance family functioning. This can be done by 1) providing information about some of the predictable events of family life and their possible effects, and 2) teaching the family how to plan ahead.

Information related to predictable events will include the stages and phases of both individual and family development as well as the implications of specific milestones such as graduation, promotion, moving, and retirement. Families can be helped to plan ahead by encouraging them to *ask questions well in advance* of forthcoming changes. Examples of such questions include:

"What will it be like to leave home and have my own apartment?"

"Grandpa can't live alone much longer—what are some possible ways of taking care of him when that time comes?"

"A lot of people at work are being transferred to other plants—if that happens to me, what can we do to make the move as easy as possible for all of us?"

Some families will need considerable support and encouragement in order to ask such questions if their usual responses in the past have been "I don't even want to think about it" or "There's no point in worrying about it, so let's drop it." Attitudes are hard to change, and it will take such families a long time to fully appreciate the benefits of becoming knowledgeable about family development, and actively influencing one's family life.

RELATED ACTIVITIES

Before you begin to assess the families with whom you are working, it will be helpful to study your own family. The following questions will help you examine your family in a new light, especially if the questions are used as a basis for a general family discussion.

1. How does your family define itself? Who is 'in' and who is 'out'? Which relatives are always invited to family dinners?

2. Are the boundaries of your family system rigid or flexible? How easy or difficult is it for a person to enter your family by marriage, adoption, or other relationship? What happens to relationships within your family when a member is lost by death, going to college, moving away, or any other reason, good or bad?

A discussion of these questions with other family members is likely to reveal a variety of different perceptions of family relationships which will be helpful to all concerned.

SUGGESTED READINGS

The Family

Barry, Patricia D: The family as a system (chap. 8) in *Psychosocial Assessment and Intervention*. Philadelphia, Lippincott, 1984.

Carley, Lori: Helping the helpless: The abused child. *Nursing 85* 1985 Nov; 15(11):34–38.

Coakley, T Anne, Paul R Ehrilich, and Elaine Hurd: Health screening in a family clinic. *Am J Nurs* 1980 Nov; 80(11):2032–2035.

Dowling, Claudia: The relative explosion: America's new kissin' kin. *Psych Today* 1983 April; 17(4):54–59.

Duvall, Evelyn: *Family Development*. ed.4. Philadelphia, Lippincott, 1971.

Friedman, Marilyn: *Family Nursing: Theory and Assessment*. New York, Appleton-Century-Crofts, 1981.

Hymovich, Debra P, and Martha Underwood Barnard (eds): *Family Health Care* (Vols. I & II) ed.2. New York, McGraw-Hill, 1979 Vol I: General Perspectives; Vol II: Developmental and Situational Crises.

Meredith, Dennis: Mom, dad and the kids. *Psych Today* 1985 June; 19(6):62–68.

Murray, Ruth Beckman, and Judith Proctor Zentner: *Nursing Concepts for Health Promotion*. ed.3. Englewood Cliffs, New Jersey, Prentice Hall, 1985.

Sanders, Frances V, and Elizabeth M Plummer: Assault on the aged: Is your patient a secret victim?. *RN* 1983 July; 46(7):21–25.

Smitherman, Colleen: Parenthood (chap. 14) in *Nursing Actions for Health Promotions*. Philadelphia, Davis, 1981.

Welch-McCaffrey, Deborah: When it comes to cancer, THINK FAMILY. *Nursing 83* 1983 Dec; 13(12):32–35.

Culture and Ethnicity

Brown, Helen Byers: Won't or can't? (effect of cultural background). *Am J Nurs* 1980 July; 80(7):1296–1299.

Davis, Ruth W, and James E Hooker; If the patient is a suspected criminal. *Nurs Outlook* 1979 July; 27(7):1250–1252.

DeGracia, Rosario T: Cultural influences on Filipino patients. *Am J Nurs* 1979 Aug; 79(8):1412–1414.

Floriani, Carol Milardo: Southeast Asian refugees: Life in a camp. *Am J Nurs* 1980 Nov; 80(11):2028–2030.

Fustero, Steven: Home on the street. *Psych Today* 1984 Feb; 18(2):56–63.

Gordon, Verona C, Irene M Matousek, and Theresa A Lang: Southeast Asian refugees; life in America. *Am J Nurs* 1980 Nov; 80(11):2031–2036.

Henry, Beverly Marie, and Elizabeth DiGiacomo-Geffers: The hospitalized rich and famous. *Am J Nurs* 1980 Aug; 80(8):1426–1429.

Kimball, Kathryn A: Caring for a special patient (mental retardation). *Nursing 83* 1983 Oct; 13(10):74–75.

Kubricht, Dottie W, and Joe Ann Clark: Foreign patients: a system for providing care. *Nurs Outlook* 1982 Jan; 30(1):55–57.

Meleis, Afaf I: The Arab American in the health care system. *Am J Nurs* 1981 June; 81(6):1180–1183.

Rosenblum, Estelle H: Conversation with a Navajo nurse. *Am J Nurs* 1980 Aug; 80(8):1459–1461.

Part Four

Nursing Process

17

Overview of Nursing Process

Prerequisites and/or Suggested Preparation
Chapter 1 (Nursing as a Profession) is prerequisite to understanding this chapter, and Chapter 4 (Conceptual Frameworks and Nursing) is suggested as additional preparation.

NURSING PROCESS

Nursing process is the term currently applied to a systematic and logical approach to nursing practice. It is an orderly sequence of steps that organizes the separate activities of nursing into an effective and unified whole.

Nurses have always maintained that nursing is both an art and a science, and nursing process combines the most desirable elements of the *art of nursing* with the most relevant elements of the *scientific method*. This combination is important because reliance on the *art* of nursing alone could give gentle, concerned care that might at the same time be haphazard, inconsistent, or only minimally effective. On the other hand, nursing care based on the scientific method alone could be efficient and effective, but impersonal and dehumanized. The use of nursing process helps the nurse to combine expert knowledge with intuition, art with science, and spontaneity with systematic action.

Nursing process is a series of activities by which the nurse collects the information she needs, uses that information to identify patient needs, makes a nursing care plan, implements the plan, and evaluates the effectiveness of her nursing care. These activities are not new; they have been carried out by skilled and scholarly nurses for many, many years, even though the activities were not called nursing process. These activities are similar to the steps of logical thinking or the scientific method; they are *not* unique to nursing.

It is agreed that nursing process consists of a number of steps or phases, but there is no consensus about the number of phases because the activities are not mutually exclusive, and often overlap. Different terms are used by different authorities to identify these steps, but differences in terminology are relatively unimportant *if the basic process is well understood,* and if nurses who are working together use mutually acceptable terminology to communicate effectively with one another.

This substitution of terms for well-understood concepts is similar to the quick mental translations we all make every day. For example, most adults are able to recognize the common meaning of such diverse statements as: "The old man died and was taken to the burying ground." "The elderly gentleman passed on and was taken to the graveyard." "The patriarch drew his last breath and was carried to the cemetery." These statements are admittedly simpler and more concrete than the phrases used in nursing process, but the principle is the same. With the possible exception of a few scientific principles, *any idea can be expressed in more than one way.* The words used may differ from time to time, from place to place, and from theory to theory, but the underlying truths remain constant. In this book, five phases or steps are identified and are termed assessment, diagnosis, planning, intervention, and evaluation.

Nursing process is used in all settings with individuals, families, or community groups. It is a thought process that can be done with incredible speed by an experienced nurse in an emergency situation, or it may be done slowly over a long period of time by a community health nurse dealing with the nursing needs of a school system or community. Each phase of this process is described in this chapter; the *skills* basic to each phase are taught in separate chapters (Chaps.18–22).

ASSESSMENT PHASE OF NURSING PROCESS

Assessment is the term applied to all the activities by which the nurse gathers necessary information about a patient or a client. Areas to be assessed include the patient's condition, family, culture, environment, diagnosis, and treatment.

Assessment can be considered the foundation or keystone of nursing process because the effectiveness of the total process depends on it. A precise nursing diagnosis or effective nursing action cannot result from an incomplete or inaccurate assessment; therefore the quality of nursing care can be no better than the quality of the nurse's assessment.

Purposes

The overall purpose of assessment is to provide a basis for planning effective nursing care, but there are a number of contributory purposes. Assessment is undertaken to:

- Provide the basis for accurate nursing diagnoses
- Provide a basis for informed and effective decision making
- Promote a holistic rather than fragmented approach to patient care
- Collect data for people conducting nursing research
- Facilitate the evaluation of nursing care

Areas to Be Assessed

Most professional nurse practice acts state that the nurse is expected to diagnose and treat human responses to illness and disease. Because the patient's perception of his condition influences his psychological and physiological responses to it, nursing assessments must describe both the condition and the patient's responses to it (Table 17.1).

TABLE 17.1 SIGNIFICANT AREAS OF NURSING ASSESSMENT

1. *The patient's perception of his current health status* (how he feels, what symptoms he is experiencing, and why he is seeking medical or nursing care)

2. *Health-related stressors in his life and his strategies for coping with them*

3. *Lifestyle* (his daily routines and his ability to perform the activities of daily living)

4. *Developmental level*

5. *Basic physiological needs* (his ability to carry out basic body functions related to breathing and circulation, elimination, nutrition, rest and sleep, hygiene and grooming, sexuality, and mobility and exercise)

6. *Other basic needs* (as described by Maslow and others)

7. *Sensory status* (his vision; hearing; taste; ability to speak; ability to experience pressure, heat, and cold)

8. *Resources* (his abilities, strengths, assets, and sources of support such as friends and family)

9. *Deficits* (his limitations, weaknesses, liabilities, financial problems, loneliness, fear, and so on)

10. *Goals* (what the patient expects to gain or how he expects to benefit from medical and nursing interventions)

11. *Help needed to achieve goals* (what assistance the patient needs and is willing to accept)

Nursing assessments frequently obtain valuable information that also contributes to the physician's data base, but this is an added benefit. The purpose of a *nursing assessment* is to obtain information that will enhance the quality of *nursing care* although that same information may contribute indirectly to the physician's goal of treating a specific disease.

Sources of Data

Sources of information about the patient are many and varied. These sources include: the patient, persons who know the patient well, members of the health care team, the patient's chart and records, reference materials, and the nurse herself. In many situations the use of these sources is limited only by the time and energy of the nurse and by a need for practicality and reasonableness.

The worth of any source of information can be partially measured by the following criteria:

- A source of data is *valuable* if the information can be obtained with economy of time and energy, and if the information is accurate, current, and understandable

- A source of data is *poor* if finding it requires considerable time and energy, or if it yields information that is old, inaccurate, or hard to understand

Patient

The prime source of information about a patient is the patient himself. Some data from the patient can be verified by data from other sources; if a patient says he has a fever, the use of a clinical thermometer will confirm or reject this statement. Much of the data given by the patient cannot be verified by an outside source, however. There is no objective means for verifying the patient's statement that he is dizzy, weak, or in pain.

Data on the patient may, therefore, be either subjective or objective. *Subjective data* include information which can be provided only by the patient (the subject), such as his perception of what he is experiencing or his attitudes, desires, feelings, and needs. *Objective data* can be determined by a person other than the patient through observation or measurement of the patient, by physical examination, or by laboratory tests. A patient's height, weight, temperature, and blood pressure are all *objective data*, for they can be measured by another person; nausea, dizziness, or the nature and extent of a patient's pain are *subjective data*, for they cannot be measured or described by anyone but the patient.

Data may also be categorized as either constant or variable. A person's birth date, place of birth, sex, and color of eyes remain constant; but his weight, blood pressure, and body temperature will vary from day to day and sometimes from hour to hour. Variable data must be frequently updated.

Significant Others

People who know the patient well are able to contribute useful data. Family, neighbors, and friends are important sources of information, especially if the patient is unconscious, confused, or a child. Teachers, scout leaders, and baby-sitters can be significant sources of information.

In certain situations, some information must be kept confidential. Occasionally, important information must be shared, but the name of the informant need not be revealed. For example, a neighbor's information about an abused child can be directed toward the proper authorities without identifying the neighbor.

Members of the Health Care Team

Doctors, social workers, respiratory therapists, fellow nurses, and members of other disciplines who have worked with the patient are invaluable sources of information. Anyone who has been in contact with him, from the candy striper who visits each afternoon to the maid who says that she "jollies him along a bit" as she cleans his unit each morning, is likely to have bits of information that may be useful.

Patient's Chart and Records

The patient's chart contains much information on the patient's past medical history, family medical history, symptoms, course of disease or illness, treatment, and progress. It includes observations made by the nurse during her assessment of the patient; findings obtained during the physician's physical examination; measurements of weight, height, blood pressure, temperature, and pulse; and the results of laboratory tests, x-ray films, and biopsies. Information obtained by the clerk in the admitting office such as age, birthplace, occupation, address, marital status, and religious preference offers clues that are helpful in understanding the patient and his concerns.

Reference Materials

Textbooks, journals, slides, tapes, and other resources are invaluable aids to understanding the theoretical basis for the patient's condition and treatment as well as his nursing care. Nursing journals enable the nurse to learn from researchers and practitioners who have cared for patients with problems similar to the ones with which she is now concerned.

Nurse

The knowledge the nurse has acquired and her past experiences are valuable resources on which to draw for information relative to the patient's care. It is not always easy to make a deliberate and conscious effort to recall some half-remembered fact, principle, or personal experience, but the effort is worth it because the process of recalling information strengthens the memory and increases the likelihood of recall the next time that information is needed.

Selectivity in Assessment

The nature and extent of assessments in a given nursing situation depend on the condition and needs of the patient. For example, the assessments made in an emergency situation must focus almost exclusively on basic physiological functions; it would be most inappropriate in an emergency to try to do an extensive assessment of the patient's cultural background, developmental level, or lifestyle.

The information needed to plan care for a toddler who fell from his high chair is different from that needed to plan care for an elderly woman who fell and broke her hip. In addition to obtaining data necessary for both, the nurse caring for the toddler needs to find out how he tells his parents that he is hungry or thirsty, whether or not he is toilet trained, and if so, what words or signs he uses to indicate a need to use the toilet. Information about favorite toys or a security blanket, and

Guidelines for Selective Nursing Assessments

- Seek only that information which is likely to be useful in planning nursing care for a specific patient. Your knowledge of developmental stages, disease processes, and potential problems will make it possible to predict which areas are likely to be of concern, and to seek the data needed for intelligent and effective action.
- Do not seek information already available from another source. It is a duplication of effort to gather information already obtained by the physician or the admitting office. It is annoying to the patient to have a number of people ask him for the same bits of information. His trust in the health care team can be undermined if he senses a lack of communication among its members, which causes him to wonder, "Don't those people ever talk to each other? I've answered the same questions about four times now."
- Be *non-selective* in the receipt of data from the patient and family. Information offered by the patient and family must be accepted as representing a valid concern *at that moment*. The information may be distorted by fear, worry, or despair, and subsequent information may reveal more significant concerns, but at the moment, all statements must be accepted in good faith until they are disclaimed or discredited.

about his usual reaction to separation from his family is essential in planning to meet the needs of a child. On the other hand, assessment of religious preference, hobbies, educational background, and ways of coping with stress have little relevance for nursing care of the toddler, although these same items of data are likely to be significant in planning to meet the needs of the elderly woman who will have limited mobility for some time.

Selectivity is an important aspect of nursing assessment because it is wasteful to expend time and energy seeking information that is unnecessary or already available from another source.

Even though selectivity is important, it is essential for the nurse to know the full range and scope of assessments that can be made. Knowledge of important areas of assessment serves as a guide during the assessment process and helps to prevent omissions that might otherwise occur.

Methods of Collecting Data

The methods used to collect data during the assessment phase of nursing process are extensions of those the nurse has used all her life: observing, listening, questioning, reading, and sensing. These methods, described briefly below, are applied to nursing in greater detail in Chapter 18.

Reading Includes searching and reviewing the literature as well as selecting from the patient's chart and other records the information which will be useful in planning that patient's care.

Interviewing Includes listening and questioning as well as other basic communication skills needed to take a nursing history.

Observation Includes the use of all one's senses (tasting, touching, smelling, hearing, and seeing) to obtain information. People who have paid little conscious attention to these senses will find it necessary to do so in nursing because a skilled nurse is able to detect a significant change in a patient's condition through her senses, often before that change is identifiable through other means. The nurse whose fingertips can detect an elevated temperature, whose nose detects the fruity, sweet breath of a patient in a state of diabetic acidosis, or who realizes from a kiss that the salty taste of a infant's cheek may indicate cystic fibrosis is a nurse who can recognize and respond to early changes in a patient's condition.

Physical Assessment. Physical assessment includes four essential techniques: auscultation (listening), palpation (feeling), inspection (looking), and percussion (tapping). These techniques are taught in Chapter 18.

Preparing Data for Use

Information collected from many sources and at different times must be examined and organized before it can be used.

First of all, the data must be sorted and categorized. As this is done, gaps and overlaps will become evident, and relationships will be suggested. The nurse may notice that isolated comments that seemed of minor importance at the time assume a new significance when grouped together. For example, she might have noted three things: (1) the patient asked her doctor for a laxative; (2) the patient's daughter asked the nurse if her mother had wanted an enema that morning; and (3) the patient commented, as the nurse helped her fill out her menu slip, "I don't like salads of any kind—or any fresh fruits or vegetables, for that matter." Each of these three bits of information, when considered separately, might be insignificant. All three items considered together, however, suggest the possibility of a bowel problem despite the fact that, when the nurse took a nursing history, the patient stated she had no problems with elimination.

Second, after the information has been sorted and categorized, some of it must be verified or validated. Some bits of information will seem to contradict other bits; some data will seem inconsistent; other information just will not fit in at all. It is not possible or practical to verify every bit of information, but top priority should be given to verifying any questionable data related to patient safety.

Third, as data begin to accumulate, it will be necessary to retain only the most useful information and discard the rest. Some patients give far more information than the nurse needs or can use, so that, despite her efforts to be selective, extraneous and unnecessary material is collected. This material merely clutters the nurse's head and, if written down, clutters charts and records, thereby hindering the effective use of nursing process.

Last, it is important to share data with other people working with the patient, either orally or in writing. Unless the material is privileged information, it should be shared so that all staff caring for the patient work from a common base of knowledge which will facilitate continuity of care and a consistent approach to the patient's problems.

Attitudes Basic to Assessment

Activities related to assessment have been referred to as "getting one's facts straight," "sizing up the situation," "collecting information," and "obtaining a data base." These activities depend, in part, on the development or maintenance of essential scientific attitudes. Four attitudes basic to effective assessment are curiosity, openness, persistence, and skepticism. These attributes, coupled with clinical assessment skills, will produce assessments which can provide a sound basis for nursing actions and indicate directions for needed research and study.

Curiosity

Nursing assessments carried out in routine fashion yield a certain amount of useful information, but the results are meager indeed compared with the data collected by a *curious* nurse. Such a nurse wonders: "Why is this patient still vomiting?" "Why does this patient seem so different from the textbook description?" "Could there be a connection between that patient's confusion and the new medication she is taking?" "Is there a better way to turn this patient who screams every time she has to be moved?" Questions such as these are likely to yield new insights and information that will enhance and expand nursing knowledge.

For example, changes in hospital policies about the separation of small children from their parents were initiated by pediatric nurses who were curious about the behavior of small children both during and after hospitalization. These nurses discovered that *separation from parents* could be more traumatic to a sick child than the hospitalization itself. As a result, hospital policies were changed to permit and encourage parents to stay in the hospital with their children and to participate in their care. Curiosity, therefore, is an attribute to be cultivated and fostered among nurses because the questions and assessments that result often provide the impetus for studies and research that improve patient care.

Openness

Many important advances in nursing have been made by nurses who were not actively pursuing an idea or seeking an answer but who were open and receptive to the world around them. Nurses who are attentive to cues and stimuli from the patient, his family, and his environment and who follow up these observations with relevant assessments are likely to make discoveries that, when coupled with data from other observations, may lead to improved patient care.

Some nurses have an unfortunate and restricting tendency to block out or shut out everything that seems unusual, unsettling, or at odds with the expectations of the nursing staff. In such instances, opportunities for exploration and study are missed, and nursing care becomes increasingly routine and progressively less effective.

Persistence

Another attribute which is necessary for making adequate assessments is persistence. It is frustrating to seek certain data only to find that the laboratory report is not back yet, the night nurse's charting is vague and ambiguous, or the patient refuses to talk to you. When essential data are not available, it may take considerable ingenuity to think of alternative sources of information, or to think of different ways of getting the information from the sources at hand.

Skepticism

Nursing assessments are more accurate when the nurse pays attention to her feelings of skepticism about what she has seen or heard. These feelings will range from vague doubts and little nagging suspicions to downright disbelief, and it is the nurse's responsibility to respond to feelings of uncertainty by validating the source and credibility of things she sees and hears. The patient, his physician, or a nursing colleague may misspeak themselves or make an error in judgment. Laboratory results can be erroneous; equipment gauges can malfunction; and orders can be inaccurately transcribed.

Even observed patient behavior may be atypical of that patient.

A nurse is accountable for her actions, including her nursing assessments, and *any tendency to accept unsubstantiated data must be rigorously counteracted.* Clues to such tendencies can be detected through a nurse's use of phrases such as: "I guess . . . ," "I suppose . . . ," "They say . . . ," and "I assumed . . ." A nurse who accepts and believes everything without question risks injury to the patient and her own career. A nurse cannot make assumptions such as "The doctor wouldn't have ordered that medication if it wasn't right," nor can she fail to take action when she has doubts such as "I didn't think that special diet looked quite right, but I figured the diet kitchen ought to know."

Use of Assessment Forms

Almost every agency and institution has developed one or more forms for use in making nursing assessments. These are often referred to as nursing history forms; they range from complex checklists to simple outlines. Checklists sometimes include the majority of all possible areas of assessment, including such things as the composition of the family unit, the presence or absence of dentures, eyesight and hearing, bowel habits, sexuality, and the number of pillows used at night.

Other forms simply list the major categories of assessment. This list serves as a guide for the nurse, who then asks broad, open-ended questions, listens carefully, and selectively records the information that seems significant. The quality of nursing assessment depends on the *expertise of the nurse* rather than on the type of forms used, and a skillful nurse can make a complete and accurate nursing assessment without using any type of printed form or outline.

DIAGNOSTIC PHASE OF NURSING PROCESS

Nurses must assume increasing responsibility for managing those areas of health care which are unique to nursing. Such aspects of care are separate and distinct from those areas of care included in medical management, and are being described by nurses with increasing specificity. In order for nurses to manage those areas of care which they are licensed to treat, nurses must be able to diagnose the patient's responses to his condition, and then plan the appropriate nursing care.

Traditionally, much of nursing practice has been based on orders written by a physician. The implementation of orders written by a physician is still an important aspect of nursing practice, but in addition, the nurse is now obligated to diagnose and plan within the limits of the state in which she is practicing. A given patient may have one or more medical diagnoses plus one or more nursing diagnoses, and his care will be directed by both medical orders and nursing orders. These diagnoses and orders are complementary; they cannot be contradictory.

In the context of both medicine and nursing, a diagnosis is derived from currently available data and identifies one aspect of a patient's condition. One essential purpose of a diagnosis is to facilitate communication between members of a given profession. The physician, for example, uses terminology that has been classified and accepted by physicians around the world to communicate a great deal of information in a few words. The use of a diagnosis such as peptic ulcer, mumps, or cystitis conveys considerable information about a patient from one physician to another because both understand the usual symptoms, cause, underlying pathology, and therapy for that diagnosis.

Medical Diagnosis

A medical diagnosis is concise, often only two or three words, and indicates a specific *disease* or *illness*. The physician makes his diagnosis by organizing and interpreting relevant facts obtained from the patient, from a physical examination of the patient, and from diagnostic tests. Because a disease or illness is the focus of a medical diagnosis, the same diagnosis may be used throughout the duration of the illness, regardless of the patient's condition. A diagnosis of appendicitis is appropriate whether the patient is experiencing early symptoms, awaiting surgery, or recovering from surgery.

Nursing Diagnosis

A nursing diagnosis is very different from a medical diagnosis. It is a concise statement of a patient's *response* to his illness, disease, or condition, and the *nursing diagnosis will change whenever the patient's response changes.* A nursing diagnosis denotes a physical or psychological response of a patient to his condition and describes a nursing problem, one that nurses are licensed to diagnose and treat.

A nursing diagnosis may be related to the medical diagnosis, but it is separate and distinct. It is concerned with those areas of health care that are exclusively within the sphere of nursing. Nursing diagnosis and nursing orders relate to the *independent* functions of the nurse, whereas the implementation of orders based on the medical diagnosis represents the *dependent* function of the nurse.

The making of a nursing diagnosis is a relatively recent activity, and as yet, there is no generally accepted format or terminology for nursing diagnoses. As a result there is much variation in the phrasing of diagnoses, and some of them are long and complex. Progress toward greater precision is being made by both clinicians and researchers, but it is not likely that nursing diagnoses will ever be reduced to the brevity and specificity of a medical diagnosis. A medical diagnosis indicates a single, well-defined condition or disease process, such as appendicitis, which is remarkably constant from one body to another. There can be no *single* nursing diagnosis related to appendicitis, however, because no two persons respond to appendicitis and its related problems in the same way.

Given three patients who are scheduled for an appendectomy, the pathology of the disease process is quite uniform from one patient to another, but the human responses may be very different. There is little similarity between the responses of a 6-year-old patient who has never been away from his home and his parents before, a 17-year-old football player at the beginning of the football season, and a 40-year-old patient who had a "very bad time" after a previous operation. Although all three patients have a medical diagnosis of appendicitis, each will have a *different nursing diagnosis*. The 6-year old, for example, might have a nursing diagnosis related to fear of being left alone, while the 17-year old might be beset by anger and hostility be-

TABLE 17.2 COMPARISON OF MEDICAL AND NURSING DIAGNOSES

Nursing Diagnosis	Medical Diagnosis
Identifies a human response to a disease, illness, condition or situation	Identifies a specific disease or illness
Derived from patient's physical and psychological reactions	Derived from patient's symptoms, physical examination, and diagnostic tests
Changes whenever patient's responses change	Usually remains constant throughout course of illness; additional diagnoses added as needed
No consistent classification or terminology	Terminology classified and accepted by medical profession
Serves as guide for nursing care; leads to nursing plans and nursing orders	Serves as guide for medical management, parts of which may be implemented by nurse; leads to medical prescription and doctor's orders

cause of missing the most important game of the season. The 40-year-old patient may be upset by fear of prolonged vomiting after surgery plus fear of complications, such as an infection in the incision. The nurse may implement similar medical orders for each patient, such as medication for pain, ambulation, and diet; but the patient's *personalized, individualized care will be based on the nursing diagnosis*, not on the medical diagnosis.

Process of Diagnosing

Data collected during the assessment phase of nursing process have little value until they are analyzed and interpreted. A patient's weight and blood pressure, the specific gravity of his urine, and the level of his blood cholesterol, for example, have little meaning until these measurements are compared either with previous measurements for that same patient or with values considered normal for patients of similar age, size, and condition. As data are being collected, therefore, the nurse needs to know the standard against which the data will be compared. Possible standards include laboratory values, standard charts of height and weight, textbook descriptions, generally accepted concepts (such as Erikson's developmental stages and Maslow's hierarchy of needs), standardized tests (such as the Denver Developmental Test and the Apgar Rating Scale for newborn infants), plus previously collected data about the patient.

The use of collected data enables the nurse to determine whether or not a patient's condition or responses have changed since the last time they were assessed. The use of standards enables her to determine whether the condition or behavior she has observed is within the range considered normal. In many instances data must be compared both with previous measurements and with established standards. For example, the fact that a community health nurse finds a patient's blood pressure to be unchanged on three successive weekly visits has little meaning unless it is known whether or not the blood pressure is normal. Three unchanged readings that are elevated indicate that the patient's hypertension is not controlled and that a change in therapy is needed. Three unchanged readings that are normal indicate that the present therapy is effective.

In addition to comparing data with previous measurements and observations, and with established standards, the nurse must look for relationships between the various bits and pieces of information. Some information that seems unimportant or trivial when viewed in isolation becomes significant when considered in context with other data. For example, the fact that a child is not hungry, *or* seems tired, *or* failed two tests in school may be unimportant. But if the child has a poor appetite *and* is listless, *and* is failing in school, the combination of symptoms may indicate a serious problem.

Ruling Out Problems

Making a definitive nursing diagnosis includes the process of ruling out other possible diagnoses. The physician often makes one or more definite diagnoses plus one or more tentative diagnoses, which he shows to be tentative by the abbreviation R/O (rule out). This means that the physician must collect additional data that will either support or rule out the tentative diagnosis.

During the process of making a nursing diagnosis, the nurse may hypothesize several diagnoses that seem likely on the basis of data already collected. Each possible diagnosis must then be substantiated or rejected (ruled out) on the basis of additional data from the patient or other sources. A tentative nursing diagnosis is ruled out if it becomes evident that the patient is coping well and has no problem in that area. It is trite but true that what is a problem for one patient may be no problem at all for another. Going up and down stairs on crutches, for example, is no problem for a paraplegic patient who has been using crutches for many years, but it may seem like an insurmountable problem for a new amputee.

Three criteria for ruling out a problem or diagnosis are described by Little and Carnevali (1976, p. 147). They believe a problem should be *ruled out* if the nurse finds that:

1. No unusual stress is present (there is no problem).
2. Unusual stress is present, but the patient's way of coping and his resources are adequate (the patient can manage without nursing assistance).
3. Any unusual stress that can be anticipated probably will not exceed the patient's resources and ways of coping (no problems are expected).

When a problem or diagnosis has been ruled out, a notation to that effect is usually made on the patient's chart or record. For example, in some households, a sick infant could quickly fatigue the mother and upset the household. A community health nurse might expect this to be the case with a family she is visiting, but find that there is no such problem. She might note, "Baby is still irritable and fussy during night and often cries for several hours. Father cares for infant on alternate nights, and grandmother baby-sits for several hours during afternoon so mother can rest when she has been up during night. Family coping well." Such a statement is referred to as a diagnostic statement, which in this case is a positive one. It is also referred to as a *positive diagnosis* or a *healthy diagnosis.*

If, however, a patient is unable to cope with the demands of his condition or situation because of health-related concerns, a problem either exists or is likely to exist in the future. Any discrepancy between the demands of daily living and the patient's ability to meet those demands constitutes a problem. When either the demand or the ability to meet the demand is related to health, the problem may be a nursing problem. If so, a nursing diagnosis is needed to indicate the type of nursing care needed.

Ruling In Problems

A nursing problem is *ruled in* if the nurse's assessment indicates that one or more of the following conditions are present:

1. Health-related stressors have reduced the patient's normal abilities, resources, or ways of coping.

Examples of Problems Caused by Disturbed Ability To Cope With Demands of Daily Living	
Condition	**Examples**
Patient's ability to cope with normal demands of daily living is *reduced* by health-related factors.	Unable to do grocery shopping because of weakness and pain in legs
	Unable to tolerate regular diet because of missing teeth and painful gums
	Reluctant to leave house because of frequent "accidents" caused by loss of bladder control
Changes in health status or situation demand new or additional coping abilities.	Learning to give insulin to 10-year-old son
	Learning to walk after an above-the-knee amputation
	Discovering that a teenage daughter is pregnant
Increased demands of daily living are likely to exceed patient's ability and resources at some point in the future.	Mother caring for son with steadily deteriorating condition
	Parents confused about care of 15-year-old retarded boy who has become very interested in girls
	Elderly woman caring for spouse and tiring as help from neighbors starts to taper off

2. Changes in the patient's situation or health status demand new or additional abilities, resources, or ways of coping.
3. Health-related stressors eventually are likely to exceed the patient's resources and ability to cope (Little and Carnevali, 1976, p. 154).

If the demands placed on a patient or family, whether they be *physical, psychological, intellectual,* or *social,* are equaled or exceeded by the ability to meet those demands, the patient or family will be able to manage.

- If usual coping ability equals usual demands, the patient can manage
- If extra coping ability equals extra demands, the patient can manage
- If reserve coping ability equals future demands, the patient can manage

If the demands placed on the patient or family are greater than the ability to meet those demands, a problem exists. The relation between ability to cope and demands or stress can be described in terms of balance and imbalance. When stress and coping are balanced, there is no problem; but when stress of any kind outweighs a person's coping ability, a problem exists.

The Nursing Diagnostic Statement

The relation between any kind of demand on the patient and his resources and deficits must be organized into a diagnostic statement that will indicate the type of nursing care or assistance the patient needs. A diagnostic statement may be termed a problem statement, a patient problem, or a nursing diagnosis. When the term diagnosis is used, it is imperative that the full term *nursing diagnosis* be used to prevent any possible confusion with the medical diagnosis.

A nursing diagnosis should be concise yet complete enough to communicate the nursing needs of the patient to all who read it. In general, a nursing diagnosis that includes a statement of the patient's problem and its cause will give an indication of the nursing care needed. Neither a statement of the problem nor the cause alone is adequate for planning care. For example, the notation of a specific behavior without a cause, such as "crying and unable to sleep," is not very helpful. The next nurse who cares for that patient has little indication of the nursing needs of that patient because she does not know whether the patient is crying and unable to sleep because of pain, loneliness, or the sound of ambulances beneath the hospital window.

On the other hand, a nonspecific behavior with a cause is no more helpful than a specific behavior without a cause. A nurse cannot tell from a notation that a patient is *"upset* by activity in the unit" whether he is angry, confused, or frightened. The combination of a specific problem and its cause, however, when stated as a diagnosis such as "crying and unable to sleep because of activity around him in unit" gives direction for nursing intervention. This nursing diagnosis indicates that the patient needs assistance in meeting his need for sleep and that the cause is not physiological but related to the environment. Further assessment will be needed to determine whether it is more feasible to reduce the activity around the patient, move the patient to another room, or teach him new ways to cope with the excessive stimuli.

Many patients have multiple problems and therefore require more than one nursing diagnosis. Priorities are then set among the diagnoses, so that the most urgent ones can be dealt with first.

In summary, a nursing diagnosis is a concise description of a patient's *response* to his situation, illness, or condition. A nursing diagnosis provides direction for nursing care by indicating both the problem and its probable cause, and must be precise enough and complete enough to facilitate communication among nurses. The specific skills basic to the formulation of a nursing diagnosis are taught in Chapter 19.

PLANNING PHASE OF NURSING PROCESS

When a nursing diagnosis has been made or a problem has been identified and stated, it is often advisable for the nurse to validate the diagnosis or problem before proceeding to the planning phase. If the patient was involved in making the diagnosis, validation may not be needed. If, however, the nurse hypothesized the diagnosis from the data available to her without direct input from the patient, her diagnosis must be validated with the patient if he is capable of responding. Some validation is as simple as saying to the patient, "On the basis of . . . and . . . , it seems that you are having trouble with . . . Is that the way it seems to you?" Or, "I've noticed that . . . and I read in your chart that . . . It seems as if . . . is a problem for you. Am I right in thinking so?" If the assessments were accurate and the diagnosis is precise, the patient will most likely agree with the diagnosis. If not, he will disagree, and the nurse can proceed to revise the diagnosis until it is deemed accurate by the patient.

If the patient is unable to participate in the validation of the diagnosis, the nurse may need to seek the assistance of the family or another member of the nursing staff. Such validation is important because it is wasteful to spend time and energy making plans on the basis of an inaccurate or inappropriate diagnosis.

Occasionally, a diagnosis is based entirely on objective data and need not be validated if the nurse is certain that her observations and measurements were accurate. For example, if the patient's skin is flushed and feels hot and dry to the nurse's touch, and he has a rectal temperature of 40 degrees C (104 degrees F), it is not necessary or even reasonable to ask the patient to validate a diagnosis related to elevated body temperature.

Once the nurse has validated the accuracy of her diagnosis, she can proceed with the planning phase of nursing process. The five major activities essential to this phase are described briefly here and explained in greater detail in Chapter 19.

The activities of planning are:

1. Developing objectives (what needs to be done?)
2. Selecting nursing interventions (how can it be done?)
3. Writing nursing orders (who will do it? where? when?)
4. Organizing and planning nursing care (how can it all get done?)
5. Establishing criteria for evaluation (how can success be measured?)

Developing Objectives

An objective is a statement that gives direction to a person's efforts and activities. An objective has often been likened to a road map: it helps one choose a destination, find the best way to get there, and know when the destination has been reached. Without a map, a person might eventually reach his destination through trial and error, but such a journey would be wasteful of time, energy, and money. It might take years of wandering to reach a destination less than 1,000 miles away.

In nursing, there is no time, money, or energy to waste. Time with patients is limited; the cost of health care is very high; and nurses cannot afford to squander energies on haphazard actions. Therefore, objectives must be set before each nursing interaction. These objectives may be termed goals, purposes, or expected outcomes. Regardless of the name used, an objective describes the end result which is sought and hoped for by patient and nurse. In this text, the words goals and objectives are used interchangeably.

Throughout this book, it is always assumed that the patient will participate in setting the objectives for his care whenever he is able to do so. If patients are unable to participate, as are infants and patients who are confused, comatose, critically ill, or simply too sick to care, the nurse must set the objectives for nursing care. In a majority of instances, however, the patient is both willing and able to help set the goals for his care, and the nurse works *with* him in doing so; she does not set goals for him.

A useful and effective objective is one which is:

- Mutually acceptable to nurse, patient, and family
- Appropriate in terms of the medical and nursing diagnoses, and treatment plans
- Realistic in terms of the patient's capabilities, time, energy, and resources
- Specific enough to be understood clearly by the patient, family and other nurses
- Measurable enough to facilitate evaluation

An objective is *mutually acceptable* to patient, family, and nurse when all relevant people agree that the goal is important, reasonable, and worth working for. The goal must be compatible with the lifestyle of both the patient and his family if it is to be achieved and maintained.

An objective is *appropriate* if it is consistent with both medical and nursing diagnoses and plans for therapy. An objective that involves taking a lonely patient to the lounge to play cards is *not* appropriate for a patient who is on bed rest following a massive heart attack.

An objective is *realistic* if a patient's resources and abilities are adequate. It is not realistic to expect an elderly woman with painful, crippling arthritis to be able to use crutches soon after breaking her ankle, nor is it realistic to expect a young couple whose infant just died to consider planning for another child before they have had time to grieve fully.

An objective is *specific* when the desired behavior is clear cut and not open to interpretation. A specific objective usually contains an active verb, which denotes an action or response that can be *seen* or *heard*. For example, a goal of "getting around more easily" is general and not very helpful. A goal of "walking to the bathroom and back without help" or "being able to move self from bed to chair and back again" is specific enough to be understood by all concerned.

An objective is *measurable* enough to permit evaluation when the patient's actions and responses can be seen, heard, felt, or measured by another person. An objective of "feeling comfortable" cannot be evaluated directly, but behaviors which are related to comfort, such as moving about in bed, putting on makeup, asking for reading materials, and discussing discharge plans can be observed directly.

When the objectives for nursing care have been formulated, they are ranked in order of priority. Urgent goals related to the relief of severe pain or acute discomfort, life-saving measures, or intervention in an emotional crisis must take top priority while less urgent or long-range goals are held in abeyance.

Selecting Nursing Interventions

When the objectives for care have been established, the nurse selects one or more nursing interventions which are likely to be effective in that situation. The beginning practitioner may have only a few interventions to choose from, but an experienced nurse will know of, and be able to use, a large number of appropriate measures. In fact, one of the hallmarks of an expert practitioner is her extensive repertoire of possible interventions. A beginning student may be able to think of only two things to do for a patient in pain: to give the medication ordered by the physician or to change the patient's position. An experienced and skillful nurse may, in addition to these two interventions, choose to apply heat or cold, rub or massage certain body parts, use distraction and diversion techniques, initiate some type of behavior modification, use imagery, administer a placebo, apply a local analgesic, or, after proper training, use hypnosis or relaxation therapy.

To avoid the noncreative and repetitious use of only one or two interventions, it is helpful to do a bit of private brainstorming with questions such as "What are the possibilities?" and "What sorts of interventions can I choose from to reach this particular objective?" When a nurse consistently tries to extend her repertoire of possible nursing interventions, the breadth and depth of her expertise will expand and the likelihood of her being able to help in a wide range of patient situations increases.

The nurse can learn new interventions, approaches, and techniques from many sources, including:

- Other nurses, aides, orderlies, specialists, and consultants (most colleagues are willing to teach those who are willing to ask for help)
- Family and friends of the patient (never underestimate the usefulness of tried and true home remedies)
- Journals, books, charts, records, and films
- Trial and error (test your hunches and see if they work)
- Workshops, teaching days, and staff development programs
- Personal research (systematically test several approaches and compare the results)
- Application of scientific theory and principles

From all nursing interventions relevant to a given situation, the nurse selects a few that seem likely to be effective. For each of these, she postulates the probable results and the likelihood of success. For any possible intervention, some results will be desirable; others, undesirable. For example, a different position might ease the discomfort of a patient in pain, but the process of moving him might interfere with an ongoing treatment or procedure. Each patient situation is different, and each patient is unique so there can be no automatic choices or selections. The nurse is obligated to select the intervention most acceptable to both the patient and herself, based on the data she has at the moment.

Before making a final selection of a nursing intervention, the nurse must assess the resources available and the strengths and deficits of those involved.

Nurse: Can she carry out the desired action? Does she have the necessary skill? Could she do it with help? Should someone else do it?

Patient and family: What can they contribute? What are their strengths, weaknesses, and attitudes about the proposed action?

Staff and other members of the health team: Are they likely to support or reject the proposed approach?

Equipment: Is everything that might be needed available? If not, can it be obtained?

Time and energy: Does the nurse have the time and energy for this action? Is her assignment or case load such that this action is feasible?

It is pointless to select a nursing intervention that might be ideal in many ways but that is in reality out of the question because of missing equipment, nonacceptance by other staff, lack of time, or inadequate skill on the nurse's part.

Writing Nursing Orders

A nursing order* is not the same as a physician's order that is carried out by a nurse. Even though a physician's order is transcribed and written down by a nurse, carried out by a nurse, and the results noted and charted by a nurse, it is *not* a nursing order.

Doctors' orders direct the *dependent* functions of the nurse; nursing orders direct the *independent* functions of the nurse. The scope of possible nursing orders will vary from state to state in accordance with the nurse practice acts of each state. The legal definition of nursing practice in each state determines the nature of those activities judged to be distinct, separate from, and independent of medical practice.

Many nurses are unaccustomed to the concept of nursing orders, and there are many areas of concern

*There seems to be no rational explanation for why a parallel grammatical construction is not used for nursing orders and physician's orders. The term physician's or doctor's orders is traditional, but the corresponding term nurse's orders is seldom used.

and unanswered questions such as: Who should write nursing orders? The head nurse? The team leader? The individual staff nurse? The clinical nurse specialist? Where does the power lie with respect to nursing orders? By what authority can one nurse write orders for another nurse to carry out in her absence? These and other questions are both practical and philosophical in nature, and there will be no easy answers. One thing is certain, however, and that is a need for nurses to make nursing diagnoses and write nursing orders which will direct those aspects of patient care that are unique to nursing practice.

The characteristics and attributes of nursing orders are described in Chapter 20.

Planning and Organizing Nursing Care

The process of planning nursing care involves deciding how to organize an assignment or case load in order to complete all required activities and to include as many optional ones as possible. This process ranges in scope from merely pausing for a moment to figure out how to get everything done, to writing detailed nursing care plans that become part of the patient's chart or record.

When organizing the nursing care for assigned patients, the nurse must take into account the time at which different required activities have been scheduled and also the desired sequence of activities. If a treatment or diagnostic test is scheduled for a specific hour, for example, other activities must be scheduled either before or after that event. If there is a conflict, or if that schedule is not a good one for the patient, it may be possible to reschedule the test or treatment. Until this is done, however, that event must be accommodated in the nurse's planning, for it cannot be ignored or delayed.

The sequence of activities may be very important. For example, if a patient has been ordered to get out of bed for a prescribed period of time each day but finds it too painful to do so, it may be desirable to administer his pain medication about 20 to 30 minutes before he must move about so that his pain will not rob him of the benefits of the prescribed activity. It is sensible to do all treatments potentially involving soiling, such as giving an enema, *before* clean linen is put on the bed. Toenails should be cut *after* they have been softened by soaking.

It is helpful to estimate the length of time it will take to complete all required care—all the things that must be done. This time can be called "must do" time. When this time is subtracted from the total time available, the difference equals the amount of time available for desired activities. Total time less "must do" time equals "can do" time. As a nurse becomes proficient, she finds she can combine activities and do two or three things at once: she can soak a patient's feet, for example, while brushing the patient's hair and helping her to cope with the anxiety created by her pending transfer to a nursing home.

Finally, a nurse can save time and energy if she "uses her head to save her heels," as the old saying goes. Learning to think ahead means that *one* planned trip down a long hospital corridor can replace many unnecessary trips to the kitchen, linen supply cart, utility room, and nurses' station later on. It is both frustrating and inefficient for a nurse to reach a patient's room, only to discover that she needs to go back down the hall to get a piece of equipment or to report an observation to the head nurse.

Establishing Criteria for Evaluation

It is difficult to assign the activity of *establishing criteria for evaluation* to a specific phase of nursing process because it can be done quite effectively at different times. The purpose of establishing evaluation criteria is to provide a basis for determining whether or not a given nursing action was effective. The criteria or standards for measuring success are derived from answers to the questions "How will the patient look or act if the intervention is effective?" and "What are the desired outcomes of this intervention?" Some nurses find it helpful to include the criteria for evaluation in the objectives for nursing care, such as "to walk the length of the hall and back without having to stop and rest, without shortness of breath, and with no increase in pulse rate." Other nurses find such a statement cumbersome and prefer to write an objective, select a nursing action likely to meet that objective, and finally, establish outcome criteria.

The criteria for evaluation (outcome criteria) must be closely related to the nursing diagnosis because the diagnosis dictates the purpose, direction, and desired outcome of nursing interventions. For example, in some situations, one standard for judging the effectiveness of nursing actions taken to relieve pain might be that the *patient will fall asleep.* In another situation, it might be important for a patient in pain to move about in bed to stimulate his circulation after surgery, and for him, an increased *willingness to move* is a more appropriate measure of successful pain relief than falling asleep would be.

Outcome criteria *must* be established *before* the evaluation phase of nursing process can be entered, and they *should* be established before or during the implementation phase to provide a basis for feedback during the giving of nursing care. If a nurse knows the type of patient response that will indicate that her nursing care is effective, and if her patient shows no sign of responding in that way, she can modify her approach or switch to another intervention that might prove more successful.

IMPLEMENTATION PHASE OF NURSING PROCESS

The nursing care planned for a patient may be implemented by the nurse directly or indirectly. The nurse may actually give the care herself, or she may delegate that responsibility to another member of the nursing staff or to a member of the family. Care by others can be effective if the nursing orders are detailed enough to ensure that the type of care she has planned will actually be given.

In addition to complete and detailed nursing orders, two other factors affect the quality of care given, namely the *attitudes* and the *competency* of the person giving care. A concerned, caring attitude is fundamental to effective nursing care, and each nurse must develop the interpersonal skills which will permit her to share that concern with the patient and his family. Some nurses seem to work equally well with patients of any age or sex and with any type of illness, but a majority of nurses develop rather specialized concerns that draw them toward a specific group of patients, such as critically ill infants, adult surgical patients, adolescents, terminally ill patients, or drug abusers. It is the *art of nursing* that is revealed in the relationships which are basic to the implementation phase of nursing process.

Second, a concerned and caring attitude must be coupled with a high degree of *skill and competency* if the planned nursing care is to be effective (Fig. 17.1). Schools of nursing and the in-service education departments of agencies and institutions have a degree of responsibility for helping each nurse become skillful and competent, but it is the *responsibility of the individual nurse* to evaluate her own performance at regular intervals. She must seek assistance, instruction, or advanced training as needed whenever new equipment and techniques are introduced into nursing practice. Each nurse is accountable for maintaining a high level of expertise throughout her nursing career, and this responsibility cannot be shifted to other people or to a department or institution. *Continuing education is a personal responsibility.*

Criteria for Nursing Actions

There are six criteria used for evaluating the excellence of any nursing action: safety, effectiveness, efficiency, economy, comfort, and legality.

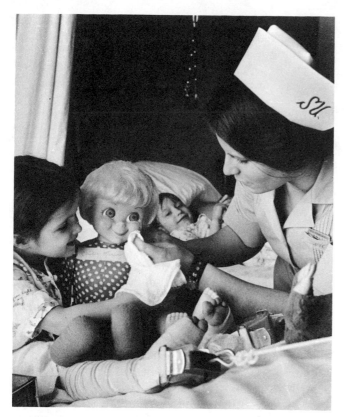

Figure 17.1 Attention to things that are significant to the patient conveys concern and caring.

Safety

Safety is the most significant of the criteria because, unless a patient is safe, the other criteria count for naught. A person is more vulnerable to both physical and psychological trauma when he is ill, and a nursing action that endangers him in any way cannot be considered effective.

Effectiveness

A nursing action is effective if it is safe, first of all, and, second, if it achieves the desired outcome. To judge the effectiveness of any nursing action, the nurse needs to know the anticipated or expected outcome. She needs to know, for example, the desired effect of each medication she gives, the expected physiological reaction to hot packs, and the desired effect of an ear irrigation. Effectiveness is evaluated by asking whether the intervention did what it was supposed to do.

Efficiency

A nursing action may be safe and may eventually achieve the desired effect, but it may be done in such an inefficient manner that much time and energy are wasted, leaving the patient (and possibly the nurse) unduly tired

and dissatisfied. Good body mechanics, careful organization of activities, and the prevention of wasted motion, plus the skill and competence that permit adequate speed, will ensure appropriate efficiency.

Economy

Nurses have an obligation, as do all citizens, to do everything possible to help control the ever-increasing cost of health care, and one of the most significant ways to do this is by not wasting either time or materials. Before the advent of disposable equipment and the practice of charging patients for the supplies used in their care, each ward or unit was issued the supplies and equipment needed for the day or week. After being used, most of these items were washed and returned to a central supply service, where they were repackaged and sterilized for future use. Nurses, of necessity, tended to be careful of equipment and supplies because any waste or extravagance might mean a shortage, either on one's own shift or on succeeding shifts.

In recent years, however, disposable items are ordered as needed for each patient, and he is billed accordingly. This creates the illusion of a never-ending supply of each item, and because the price of an item is not apparent, it is easy to be unintentionally extravagant. It is easier to wipe up spilled liquids with one of the patient's absorbent pads than it is to go and get some paper towels or find a mop, for instance. Each unnecessary use of disposable materials increases the patient's bill, which in turn increases the cost of his health care, the cost of insurance premiums, and the cost of taxes if the health care is state or federally funded.

Comfort

Excellence in nursing care requires that the patient be physically and psychologically comfortable (except in those instances when the patient must experience something that is momentarily uncomfortable, such as an important exercise or change of position).

Attention to seemingly small details, such as giving adequate explanations, being gentle in moving the patient, pulling the curtains to ensure privacy, and introducing patients to each other helps to provide the comfort and security that characterize excellence in nursing practice.

Legality

Every nursing action must come within the limits of nursing practice established by law in a given state or district. Every nurse is responsible for learning about her legal obligations and limitations whenever she moves to a new agency or geographical area.

Nursing Care Plans

Nursing process contributes to the development of a *nursing care plan*, but the two are *not* equal or even similar. Many people use the phrases "using nursing process" and "using nursing care plans" interchangeably, but this is inaccurate and misleading. Nursing process is, by definition, a *process*, a series of actions. A nursing care plan is a *product*, something that is made, created, or developed. The relationship between the two is similar to the relationship between the process of building a house and the blueprint for that house. The blueprint is a tangible end product of one step in the process. Just so, a nursing care plan is a tangible end product of one phase of nursing process.

The steps of nursing process involve mental activities, the results of which can be verbalized and described in writing if desired. Nursing students are often required to fill out a nursing process form for each assigned patient so that instructors can evaluate their progress in learning to use nursing process. This form usually includes space for a written nursing care plan for the patient. The completed forms demonstrate to the instructor the student's ability to use nursing process. Once a student has learned to use nursing process, practice in using it allows nursing process to become an integral part of her overall thought processes. When this has occurred, it is no longer necessary for her to focus consciously on the various steps and phases, nor to write out her plans for every patient; nursing process has become for her the framework within which the activities of nursing are organized.

Written nursing care plans help to ensure continuity and quality of care and provide one basis for the evaluation of patient care. Written care plans, therefore, are often required by institutions as well as by insurance groups such as Medicare.

EVALUATION PHASE OF NURSING PROCESS

Evaluation is the process of comparing something with a standard to determine its worth, merit, success, or value. Standards are absolutely essential for the judging of any product or performance, for judging everything from lemon pies or roses to ballet or wrestling. It is impossible to evaluate a product or performance unless the judge knows the characteristics that distinguish excellence from mediocrity. The judge must know exactly what to look for. In nursing, the standards used are often referred to as *outcome criteria* or *criteria for evaluation.*

Evaluation is an ongoing process throughout all phases of nursing process. The nurse must compare the feedback she receives during each phase with certain standards for that phase in order to know whether she should continue or change her course of action. In addition to this ongoing evaluation of the progress being made, a more extensive evaluation is made at the end of a given patient's care, or at the end of a shift or assignment.

Evaluation focuses, first of all, on the implementation of nursing care. If the outcome criteria have been met, if the objectives have been attained, and if both patient and nurse are satisfied with the outcome, nursing care was appropriate and effective. If, however, the objectives have not been met, and if either nurse or patient feels uneasy or dissatisfied with the nursing care and its results, a more extensive evaluation must be done to determine whether the problem stems from poor implementation, from faulty planning, from an inaccurate diagnosis, or from an incomplete assessment.

Although it is not possible to rank the phases of nursing process by importance, evaluation is one of the most critical phases because it provides a basis for the improvement of patient care, which is an ultimate goal of both medicine and nursing. The skills needed for the evaluation process are presented in Chapter 22.

In summary, nursing process is a systematic way of organizing the activities of nursing practice to ensure the highest possible quality of patient care. Although in this text, nursing process is applied most frequently to the care of sick people, it is equally useful in meeting the nursing needs of families and communities; it is used in the promotion of health and the prevention of illness as well as in the treatment of illness.

RELATED ACTIVITIES

The steps or phases of nursing process are not unique to nursing. They were derived from the steps of scientific methodology and can be applied to almost any undertaking. In order for these steps to become an integral part of your approach to both nursing and everyday situations, it is helpful to experiment with their application.

During the coming week, select at least one situation in which you will be required to take some action. Examples of such an activity include: conducting a meeting, taking a trip, knitting a sweater, cleaning your room, entertaining guests.

Use the steps of nursing process or logical thinking throughout the activity as follows:

1. *Assessment.* What data would be helpful *before you start?* What should you know about the situation, your own knowledge or ability, the equipment to be used, and so on?
2. *Diagnosis* (analysis of the situation). Based on the information available to you, how would you describe the situation?
3. *Planning.* Based on your analysis of the situation, what *might* you do? How might you do it? What preparation do you need? What help might you need?
4. *Implementation.* What did you actually do?
5. *Evaluation.* How did it turn out? How do you know? What criteria did you use for evaluation?

- If the activity was successful, which step was most significant?
- If the outcome was not as successful as you would have liked, work *backward* through the steps of the process until you can identify the step which was different.

Examine your approach to other types of activities in order to find out whether or not you *frequently* omit or neglect the step that was inadequate, or any other

phase of the process. If so, make a concentrated effort to focus on that step in the future as preparation for the use of nursing process.

SUGGESTED READINGS

Atkinson, Leslie D, and Mary Ellen Murray: *Understanding the Nursing Process,* ed. 3. New York, MacMillan, 1986.

Lamonica, Elaine: *The Nursing Process: A Humanistic Approach.* Menlo Park, CA, Addison Wesley, 1979.

Marram, Gwen, Margaret W Barrett, and E M Olivia Benis: *Primary Nursing: A Model for Individualized Care.* ed.2. St. Louis, Mosby, 1979.

Marriner, Ann: *The Nursing Process: A Scientific Approach to Nursing Care,* ed.3. St. Louis, Mosby, 1985.

Murray, Ruth, Marilyn M Huelskoetter, and Dorothy Lueckepath O'Driscoll: *The Nursing Process in Later Maturity.* Englewood Cliffs, NJ, Prentice-Hall, 1980.

Yura, Helen, and Mary B Walsh: *The Nursing Process: Assessing, Planning, Implementing and Evaluation.* New York, Appleton-Century-Crofts, 1983.

Yura, Helen, and Mary B Walsh: *Human Needs and the Nursing Process.* New York, Appleton-Century-Crofts, 1978.

Yurick, Ann Gere: *The Aged Person and the Nursing Process.* New York, Appleton-Century-Crofts, 1980.

18

The Assessment Phase of Nursing Process

Prerequisites and/or Suggested Preparation
Chapter 17 (Overview of Nursing Process) and Chapter 12 (Concepts from Pathophysiology Relevant to Nursing) are prerequisite to understanding this chapter. In addition, Chapter 9 (Communication) is prerequisite to Section 2 of this chapter (Interviewing).

Section One

The Assessment Process

Assessment

Areas to Be Assessed

Phases of the Assessment Process
Instantaneous Appraisal
First Impressions
Detailed Assessment

ASSESSMENT

Assessment is the process of obtaining essential information about a patient, and the quality of any nursing assessment depends on the *skill* and *selectivity* of the nurse. Skill in collecting data is absolutely essential; but unless the skill is used selectively, the assessment process is likely to be ineffective.

Failure to be selective and to focus the assessment process on those areas which are essential in a given patient situation results in a shotgun approach. This means that large amounts of information are collected in the hope that some of the information will be useful. The phrase *shotgun approach* reflects the difference between using a rifle and using a shotgun for hunting. A shotgun fires many lightweight pellets over a large area and is used to hunt small, rapidly moving objects such as ducks. A rifle fires a single, heavy bullet toward a large, slower moving target such as an elephant or a deer. Each gun has its use, and they are not interchangeable. Marksmanship is critical when a rifle is used, and if a person's aim is poor, he must improve it because he cannot use a shotgun instead. Pellets would be ineffective against the tough hide of an elephant or the thick fur of a bear. The same is true with nursing assessments. A nurse cannot afford to use a shotgun approach because her aim is poor; she must not collect data at random simply because she cannot decide what information is essential. She must improve her marksmanship and collect information with skill, precision, and accuracy. Focusing the assessment process on relevant and important areas decreases the amount of time and energy spent on needless assessments. There is usually, for example, no need to do as complete an assessment on a patient scheduled for corrective surgery on a toe, as on a patient scheduled for open heart surgery. Selectivity in assessment is especially important in the emergency room, at the scene of an accident, or during a disaster.

AREAS TO BE ASSESSED

In general, there are three areas to be assessed: the patient's past health history, his current health status, and the care and assistance that is needed or anticipated. These three areas encompass what has happened to the patient in the *past*, what is happening to him *now*, and what is likely to happen to him in *the future*. These areas of assessment are inseparable and must be included in every assessment because the patient's present situation is based on his past experiences and, to a large extent, influences what he will experience in the future.

Figure 18.1 shows the interrelatedness of these three areas of assessment and indicates that nursing diagnoses are derived from the central core of this interrelatedness. An example of this interrelatedness is: "Shortness of breath (present) as a result of emphysema (past) now necessitates the occasional use of oxygen at home (assistance needed)." Another example might read: "Weakness and low back pain (present) resulting from recent injury (past) necessitates accepting help with household chores and learning how to lift properly (assistance needed)."

In addition to the importance of the central overlapping areas, the overlap between adjoining assessment areas is important in planning nursing care. A patient's past health history affects both his present health status and the type and extent of care needed. The continuing effect of former conditions, such as scars, handicaps, limitations, and residual disease processes can affect a patient's present health status in the form of chronic illness or persistent health problems. There is no way a patient can ever "start fresh" or "start with a clean slate" with respect to his health; his *current health status is always affected in some way by his past*. Even if there is no physical trace of some earlier problems or illnesses, a patient's recollection of his experiences will affect his perception of the care he now needs and the assistance he is willing to accept for his current problem. He may seem to need a specific type of therapy and assistance but be unable to acknowledge that need or accept the therapy and assistance. Or, past experiences may cause him to feel that he needs far more care and assistance than his condition seems to warrant.

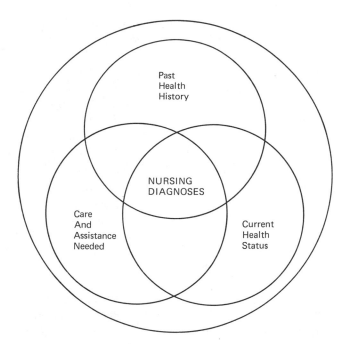

Figure 18.1 Interrelatedness of areas of assessment.

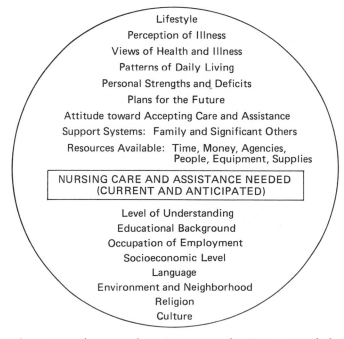

Figure 18.3 Elements of current health history to be assessed.

Some of the major elements to be assessed with respect to past health history, current health status, and nursing care and assistance needed are shown in Figures 18.2–18.4. In every patient situation, the elements to be assessed should be chosen for their relevance to that particular patient's situation.

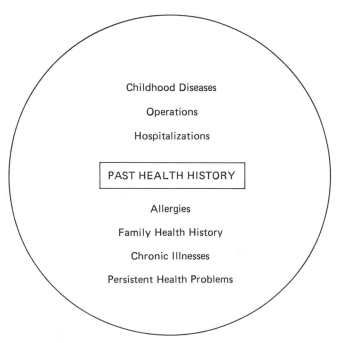

Figure 18.2 Elements of past health history to be assessed.

Figure 18.4 Elements of nursing care and assistance needed to be assessed.

PHASES OF THE ASSESSMENT PROCESS

The assessment process can be divided into three phases: instantaneous appraisal, first impressions, and detailed assessment.

Instantaneous Appraisal

An instantaneous appraisal, which takes only a few seconds, is done on the nurse's first contact (or each new contact) with every patient and is designed to answer only one question: Is this person in acute distress? The answer to this question determines the nurse's subsequent course of action. If the patient is found to be in acute distress, the nurse will take *immediate appropriate action* while continuing to make additional assessments relevant to the distress. Examples of appropriate action might be calling for help, applying pressure to control bleeding, or using the Heimlich maneuver if a person is choking.

The clues that indicate acute distress are *readily observable*. If a patient is having difficulty breathing, is in severe pain, or is vomiting, choking, or bleeding profusely, he is in acute distress. If he is pale, agitated, perspiring profusely, crying, incoherent, hysterical, trembling, or violent, he is in acute distress. Any of these conditions or a combination of them demands a nurse's immediate attention. Acute distress takes precedence over everything except an even more critical life-and-death situation. All routines and procedures are postponed until a patient's obvious distress has been alleviated to a tolerable degree. It is poor nursing practice to disregard a patient's distress and proceed as if he were calm and comfortable.

During this instantaneous appraisal, four bits of data can be obtained. A patient's *sex, color,* and approximate *age* can be assessed with a glance. In addition, the patient's *name* can be obtained from the patient if he is able to talk, from his identification bracelet, from family or friends, or from identification found in a wallet or purse. It is important to get and *use* the patient's name as quickly as possible because use of his name contributes to the patient's sense of security and helps to ensure safety through proper identification of the patient.

First Impressions

If the initial appraisal indicates that a patient is not in any sort of acute distress, the nurse can proceed to obtain and examine data from her first impressions of the patient. First impressions give minimal baseline data on a patient's physical, emotional, sensory, and interactive states and indicate obvious areas for subsequent assessment. The process of using first impressions requires that the nurse mentally place the patient on each of four continuums according to his physical, emotional, sensory, and interactive status:

Status	Positive	Negative
Physical	Comfortable	Uncomfortable, in some distress
Emotional	Confident	Scared, nervous
	Calm	Distraught
Sensory	Oriented	Confused
	Alert	Not alert
Interactive	Active	Passive, withdrawn
	Cooperative	Not cooperative

Other adjectives can be substituted for the ones in each continuum because it is not the terminology that is important, but rather the conscious and deliberate process of using your first impressions.

First impressions are involuntary; they occur whenever two people meet, and normally each person mentally applies certain descriptive adjectives to the other. In a professional context, the adjectives are used somewhat differently. A professional health care worker does *not* label a patient with the adjectives that come to mind. A nurse does not, for example, label a patient "confused" on the basis of her first impression of that patient, but that impression does provide a *starting point* and can indicate a need for detailed assessment. Adjectives serve only as a kind of shorthand a nurse can use as she proceeds to watch for behaviors that will clarify her first impressions. With respect to a patient who seems confused, a nurse might notice that he asked three times where he was, cannot remember how he got to the hospital, and lost his way to the bathroom twice in 1 hour. These *behaviors* can be reported and charted, thereby providing other staff with data that are accurate and precise rather than general and abstract. A phrase, such as "patient is confused," is subject to many interpretations and should *not* appear on the patient's chart, which is a *legal document*.

Using first impressions of a patient does not mean jumping to conclusions. Using first impressions does not in any way reduce the need for a detailed assessment, nor does it reduce the extent of that assessment. First impressions do provide useful data that give direction to a nurse's initial interactions with a patient.

The accuracy of a nurse's first impression of a patient depends on her ability to read the patient's verbal and nonverbal cues. *Nonverbal* cues can be derived from the patient's activity (ex., pacing, constantly moving about in bed, picking at the bedclothes, lying quietly), posture (ex., slumping, erect, slouching), grooming (ex., neat, disheveled, clean), and facial expression (ex., appearing angry, worried, happy, calm). *Verbal cues* are picked up by using basic communication skills (Chapter 13).

Finally, each aspect of a nurse's first impressions should give rise to the questions: What is the basis for this impression? What makes me think that this may be true? Why do I feel this way? The process of searching for the cause or basis of an initial impression leads to the next phase of the assessment process.

Detailed Assessment

The third phase of the assessment process is much longer than the others and results in the collection of specific and detailed data. Because the psychosocial and physical aspects of a patient are interrelated and interdependent, it is not appropriate during initial assessments to focus exclusively on either one except in some special areas such as psychiatric nursing. An apparent problem, such as an abnormal gait, may have a physiological basis, but it could also have a psychological cause or even a financial one related to ill-fitting shoes.

An altered psychological state, such as extreme irritability, can have physiological causes, such as drug toxicity, systemic illness, or brain damage. Data from initial, general assessments must be analyzed and interpreted to determine what kinds of specific assessments are needed. Subsequent assessments may focus heavily on either the psychosocial or the physiological aspect, but never to the complete exclusion of the other.

There are six categories of assessment activities: (1) interviewing, (2) observing, (3) measuring, (4) physical examination, (5) assisting with diagnostic tests, and (6) using charts and records.

Each of the six categories is explained in the following sections, and the basic skills related to each are described. The emphasis in each instance is on methods of assessment and data collection, not on the data per se. The technique of percussion is taught in this chapter, for example, but a description of the data obtained by percussion of the chest is deferred to Chapter 32 (Respiration).

Section Two

Interviewing

Interviewing

Use of Questions

Informal Interview
  Questions About Past Health History
  Questions About Current Health Status
  Questions About Care and Assistance Needed

Formal Interview

Interview Guides
  Topical Outline
  Question Format

Patient Interview Guide
  Rationale for Questions

INTERVIEWING

The process of interviewing a patient differs from therapeutic communication in that it *seeks information;* it is not intended to resolve problems, find solutions, explore feelings, or prompt decisions. The nursing interview, often called taking a nursing history, is part of the assessment process, and its purpose is to collect data that will help provide a sound basis for nursing care.

A nurse sometimes interviews a patient to obtain specific data related to his admission to the health care system or to obtain data needed for a research study, but most nursing interviews are conducted to obtain a nursing history.

A nursing history differs from a medical history in both purpose and format. The *medical history* seeks specific, factual information about a disease, an illness, or a condition. The *nursing history* seeks information about a patient's physical and psychological responses to his disease, illness, or condition. The medical history usually follows a traditional, standardized format, but there is no such standardized format for a nursing history. Nursing interviews can be organized around nursing problems, basic needs, body systems, or any other approach to nursing practice, and the interview can be formal or informal.

USE OF QUESTIONS

Both formal and informal interviews depend on a nurse's ability to formulate questions that will elicit relevant and essential information. The types of questions which are needed are determined by the type of information sought. A narrow, sharply focused question is used to seek specific, detailed, factual information. A broad, open question is used to obtain data about a patient's feelings, perceptions, attitudes, and beliefs. Each has its uses and purpose, and they cannot be used interchangeably.

Since the purpose of an assessment interview is to collect data, many of the questions must be specific and narrow, such as: "How long have you had this pain?" "Do you give yourself an enema very often?" and "Under what circumstances do you get short of breath?" These narrow, direct questions seek a specific factual answer and are of necessity quite different from the broad, open questions which are essential to therapeutic communication (Chapter 9).

It is advisable, whenever possible, to avoid asking Why questions. Why questions often evoke memories of childhood criticism, of bombardments of queries beginning "Why did you. . . ?" or "Why didn't you. . . ?" A patient may not know why he said or did what he did, and yet he may feel pressured to come up with a reason. On the other hand, he may know full well the reason for his behavior or beliefs but be unwilling to share that reason with anyone for fear it is not an acceptable one.

INFORMAL INTERVIEW

Much attention has been paid to descriptions of a formal interview, and it is an increasingly common sight to see a nurse sitting at a patient's bedside or in a clinic with clipboard and pen. By comparison, the informal interview has been underrated and underestimated. This

---

Comparison Between Therapeutic Communication and Interviewing

- Similarities
  Both are purposeful and deliberative
  Both keep social interaction to a minimum
  Both are basic to effective nursing care
- Differences
  The purposes of *therapeutic communication* are to: explore feelings, teach, give psychological support, facilitate decision making; set objectives, and solve problems. The purposes of an *interview* are assessment and the collection of data.

---

is unfortunate because it has the greater potential for increasing the effectiveness of nursing care simply because it can be done in a greater number and variety of situations: when entering a patient's home, while admitting a patient to a health care facility, or while talking with a patient in a waiting room.

Both the formal and the informal nursing interview seek information about (1) a patient's past health history, (2) his current health status, and (3) the care and assistance needed, but the informal interview is usually more direct and seeks to obtain the most urgent data very quickly.

Questions About Past Health History

It is possible to obtain the information necessary to initiate immediate nursing care by asking only a few questions such as "What brings you to the hospital (or clinic)?" or "Tell me a bit about your problem." The answers to these questions will indicate some of a patient's expectations regarding health care and will also give some clues to the patient's perception of his illness and its possible outcome. Answers may range from "to get my hernia fixed so I can pass the physical for a new job" and "to find some way to cope with the pain—it's getting worse every day" to "I don't know—my doctor just said he was sending me to the hospital." These answers may indicate whether a patient is discouraged, anxious, or optimistic about his forthcoming experiences.

Questions About Current Health Status

Simple, straightforward questions such as "How do you feel now?" or "You look upset and ready to cry. Are you frightened?" will help you assess the urgency with which you must approach a patient's care. Possible answers might include: "I'm feeling just fine—no problems at all"; "The pain is so bad I don't think I can stand it much longer"; or "I'm afraid I'm going to faint."

Questions About Care and Assistance Needed

"What can I do right now to help you?" "What might make things better for you?" "What kind of help will you need in caring for yourself?" These questions may seem basic and obvious, but improbable as it may seem, many patients enter and leave a hospital or clinic without anyone ever asking *directly,* "What can I do to help you?" or "What do you need?"

Answers to a nurse's questions about the care and assistance needed by the patient will include such widely diverse responses as: "Could I have a drink of water, please?" "Would you tell me again how you work this thing to call the nurse?" "Would you call my sister? She doesn't know where I am"; and "Sometimes I wet the bed when I get scared at night." A patient's statements about his reason for seeking care, the description of his problem, and the care and assistance he needs will help the nurse to individualize her nursing care even before she is able to do a complete nursing history. For example, only a few questions were needed to elicit the following information which illustrates the difference in needs of two patients, each with a diagnosis of low back pain.

Patient 1. 22-year-old native American; looks apprehensive and tense; states he injured his back earlier in the week. Indicates that the pain is worse than it has ever been, but states angrily that he doesn't need anything except to get back to work.

Patient 2. 45-year-old owner of popular Italian restaurant. Dozing at intervals; looks relaxed. Says he has had a nagging backache for several months and that it has not improved with rest at home. States that his back feels fine while he is in bed and that all he needs at the moment is for the television set and telephone to be connected.

In these two situations, the answers to the nurse's question, "What do you need?" indicated that the needs of the two patients are very different, and that the focus of her nursing interventions must be different in order to be effective.

To summarize briefly, the short, informal interview yields information which is helpful in meeting a patient's *immediate* needs. It gives direction to a more extensive, ongoing assessment, and it identifies the nurse as a caring person with skill in getting right to the heart of the matter. The informal interview is usually integrated into other, ongoing nursing activities and is likely to be viewed by a patient as an expression of interest and concern, whereas a formal interview can seem rather cold and impersonal.

FORMAL INTERVIEW

A *formal assessment interview* is a nursing action that is not usually combined with another activity. The nurse usually works from a printed form, a checklist, or an outline which may consist of topic headings or ques-

tions. The use of a predetermined format helps to guarantee a nursing history that is complete and comprehensive. It also helps to avoid digression, thereby minimizing wasted time.

Guidelines for Taking a Nursing History

1. *Introduce yourself* if the patient does not know you, giving your title, role, or position. Sit down so that you are at the patient's level.

2. *Explain the purpose of the interview.* Indicate the likely length of the interview. If you will be making notes, explain what you are writing and why.

3. *Make the patient as comfortable as possible.* Attend to his physical needs before expecting him to focus his attention on the interview.

4. *Vary your format and process to accommodate the needs of the patient.* Problems such as deafness, a language barrier, aphasia (inability to talk), or a critical illness require some modification of approach. Be ready to postpone parts of the interview if the patient shows signs of fatigue or distress. Other adaptations may be needed if the patient is a child or if the setting is unusual, such as a prison, store-front clinic, or refugee camp.

5. *Do not collect information which is available elsewhere.* It is frustrating for the patient and a waste of time and energy for several people to ask him for identical information.

6. *Collect only data that will be useful and usable.* Unless the information will make a difference in the patient's care, the process of collecting it is little more than professional busy work.

7. *Adhere to your time limit as closely as possible.* Stick to your purpose and avoid digression. If some point under discussion seems especially significant, make a mental or written note of it and make plans with the patient to discuss it later. If some point elicits a strong emotional response, a sense of urgency, or a crisis, *stop the interview* and deal with the immediate situation. Make plans to resume the interview at a later time or else to deal with the patient's reactions more fully at a later time.

8. *Respect the patient's right to privacy and his right to refrain from answering your questions.* Many things inhibit self-disclosure and keep a patient from sharing information about himself. If a patient chooses not to answer some or all questions, either forego that portion of the interview, or explore with him the reasons for his discomfort with the assessment interview.

9. *Remember that the purpose of an assessment interview is to collect data; it is not to solve problems or make decisions.*

Reasons Why a Patient May Be Unwilling to Answer Interview Questions

- Past experiences may have led him to mistrust nursing personnel.
- He may not be convinced that the assessment has value; it may seem repetitious if other staff have already asked similar questions.
- He may be denying the reality of his illness and be unable to talk about it.
- It may seem to him that the priorities of the nursing staff are inappropriate if, for example, he is still waiting for his pain medication while you have time to sit and ask questions.
- He may fear criticism and be afraid that you will not approve of his answers.
- He may be a member of a religious, ethnic, or other minority group who have experienced discrimination or disdain in the past, and may be reluctant to reveal his affiliation with that group even though his beliefs significantly affect his responses to health and illness.
- You and the patient have not yet established a professional relationship based upon mutual trust and respect.

INTERVIEW GUIDES

The nurse may use either a printed form or an interview guide for a formal assessment interview. A *printed form,* when properly filled out, guarantees that the information deemed necessary by the staff will be obtained. It does not, however, foster creativity in assessing patient needs, nor does it fully use a nurse's skill in interviewing. An *interview guide* places greater responsibility on the nurse and changes her task from one of filling out a required form to one of interviewing the patient. In some situations the outcome will be similar, but in many instances an interview is considered complete when the form has been filled out rather than when the data necessary to plan the patient's care have been collected.

Minimal structure produces the greatest amount of useful material in the shortest time possible provided the nurse: (1) is firmly convinced that the data she seeks are essential for planning nursing care, (2) accepts the need for selectivity in collecting data, and (3) is skillful and competent in interviewing patients. Otherwise, a structured, printed form may be more productive.

The information obtained from a nursing history should be shared with colleagues to ensure continuity of care for the patient, and therefore it is necessary to make this information accessible and easy to locate in the patient's chart or record. Some people find it easier to obtain information from a completed interview form because the same data always appear in the same place on the form. Others prefer notes from a topical outline because all extraneous material is omitted, only relevant information is included, and the resulting history is shorter. If notations are both concise and precise, if the data are categorized and headings are underlined, and if only relevant material is included, a nursing history from an outline will be brief enough and clear enough for the staff to read and use without difficulty.

Topical Outline

Interview guides may be in the form of a topical outline or a series of broad questions. An outline developed by Little and Carnevali (1976) includes a list of areas for possible assessment which serves as a reminder for the nurse (Figure 18.5). The flexibility of this format is demonstrated in Figures 18.6 and 18.7; note that each history omits three or four categories, adds one or two additional categories, and does not follow the order of the lefthand column exactly. Note the precision with which the nurse separates objective data from subjective data in Figure 18.7. Notice that the heading does not ask for information available elsewhere (such as street address, name of physician, or medical diagnosis) but that it does ask by what name the patient prefers to be called.

Question Format

The interview guide that follows is an example of a guide based on questions rather than a topical outline. It consists of 20 questions, each of which deals with an area of concern rather than a specific detail or fact. With slight modification in wording, these questions can be used with people of all ages and in all settings. There are innumerable ways to phrase each of these questions, but a nursing student usually memorizes these or similar questions for her first interviews. It is easier to conduct an interview when one does not have to think about what question should be asked next. As your skill in interviewing increases, you will develop a set of questions of your own that are relevant to the setting in which you are working and with which you feel comfortable.

PATIENT INTERVIEW GUIDE

I. PAST HEALTH HISTORY
   1. Would you tell me a little about yourself, your family, your way of life?

2. What sort of things do you do or try to do to keep healthy?
3. What things in your life seem to make it hard to keep healthy?
4. How do you usually react to being ill?
5. How do you like other people to treat you when you are ill? What kind of assistance or care has been helpful when you were sick in the past?

II. CURRENT HEALTH STATUS
6. What were the symptoms of this problem or condition?
7. What did you do when you noticed these symptoms?
8. Does anything seem to relieve these symptoms, even temporarily?
9. How do you feel now?
10. What do you know about your illness or condition?
11. What have you been told about the treatment or tests that have been planned for you?
12. What have you heard about the likely outcome of all this?

13. Who or what has been your chief source of information?

III. NURSING CARE AND ASSISTANCE NEEDED
14. What, if anything, don't you understand as well as you'd like to?
15. What do you think will be the hardest part of this situation (illness, hospitalization)?
16. Many aspects of your life will be disrupted, at least temporarily, by treatments, or by hospital rules and regulations. Which of these disruptions may be hard for you to deal with?
17. What do you think may be the major effect of this illness or condition on your family and yourself?
18. What would you like to be able to do to help yourself get better or be more comfortable?
19. What kinds of help are you going to need in order to manage?
20. Who might be able to provide this help (care, assistance)?

Each of these questions was designed to assess an aspect of a patient's strengths and needs; the questions

SAMPLE NURSING ASSESSMENT FORM

Name _____ Age _____ Date _____

Prefers to be called _____ Assessment made by _____ RN

Areas	Subjective/Objective Data
Client perceptions of: Current health status Goals Needed/usable services	
Functional abilities: Breathing/circulation Elimination Emotional/cognitive Mobility/safety Nutrition Hygiene/grooming Sensory input Sexuality Sleep/rest	
Resources & support systems: Environmental Personal/social Other	

Figure 18.5 *A nursing assessment form. (Reproduced with permission from D. Little and D. Carnevali: Nursing Care Planning, 2nd ed. Philadelphia: JB Lippincott Company, 1976, p. 143)*

SAMPLE NURSING ASSESSMENT FORM

Name __Miss Rose Stevens__ Age __48__ Date __7/7__

Prefers to be called __Miss Stevens__ Assessment made by __Mary White__ RN

Areas	Subjective/Objective Data
Client perceptions of: Current health status Goals Needed/usable services *Functional abilities:* Breathing/circulation Elimination Emotional/cognitive Mobility/safety Nutrition Hygiene/grooming Sensory input Sexuality Sleep/rest *Resources & support systems:* Environmental Personal/social Other	*Current Health Status:* Having severe back pain that responds to moist heat, pain medication, and muscle relaxants at home. A diabetic since 1957—tends to run trace or neg on urinalyses. On lente insulin. Has schedule of rotating sites—some atrophy of upper arm sites. *Goals:* Get pain under control so she can go on planned vacation trip 8/1 to France. *Needed Services:* Prefers to continue to give own insulin. *Breathing/Circulation:* R-20 (uncomfortable, medication wearing off). Pulse, 88 reg. Color of feet and legs good/warm, pedal pulses present. Knows importance of foot care to a diabetic. *Mobility/Safety:* Does not want to move because of spasms. Wants help turning. No pain in using arms, hands. *Nutrition:* Diabetic exchange diet. Eats 7:30/12/5:30. Snack (protein) at bedtime. Knows food composition. Weight seems normal for height. No food dislikes or allergies. *Sensory:* Wears contacts. Slight hearing loss—right side. Lives alone in rural area. Teaches French in high school Sept.-June. *Sleep/Rest:* Prior to back pain slept 8 hours uninterrupted. For past week has slept no longer than 1-2 hours at a time and only 4 hours in a 24-hour period. Most comfortable on back, uses no pillow. *Hygiene/grooming:* Grooming seems important. Hair coiffed, nails manicured. Extensive toiletries. Gowns and robe well cared for, neatly packed. Showers daily at bedtime. *Emotional/Cognitive:* Despite reportedly severe pain speaks quietly with restraint. Describes diabetic management and experiences of back pain with precise terminology. *Personal/Social:* Sister and her family live 20 minutes from hospital. Are available to help. Ph: 273-6410. Prefers visitor restriction if in pain (except for sister). *Diversion:* Has FM radio with her and some nonfiction books.

Figure 18.6 *Nursing assessment form, completed sample. (Reproduced with permission from D. Little and D. Carnevali: Nursing Care Planning, 2nd ed. Philadelphia: JB Lippincott Company, 1976, p. 144.)*

Name	Arthur Longbranch		Age	47	Date	6/22/75

Prefers to be called __"Art"__   Assessment made by __Jill Sutter__   RN

Areas	Subjective/Objective Data
Client perceptions of: Current health status Goals Needed/usable services *Functional abilities:* Breathing/circulation Elimination Emotional/cognitive Mobility/safety Nutrition Hygiene/grooming Sensory input Sexuality Sleep/rest *Resources & support systems:* Environmental Personal/social Other	*Perceived health status:* (subjective) Right inguinal hernia repair in A.M. Hospital stay expected: 3–4 days. Older brother had same surgery 6 months ago, no problems; no previous hospital admissions. Expects spinal anesthesia—some concern re aftereffects. Doctor told him he was in good condition. No other medical problems. (objective) Uses medical terminology. *Goals:* (subjective) To be out of hospital in 3–5 days, up day of surgery. To return to job as accountant in 2 weeks and to his golf game in 6 weeks. *Expected care:* (subjective) Doctor will order medications to control pain and sleep as needed. Brother said backrubs at bedtime promote relaxation. No limitations on visitors. *Hygiene/grooming:* (subjective) Usually showers at breakfast every day. Shaves two times daily, at breakfast and after supper. (objective) Trimmed moustache, long sideburns, toupee. *Sensory input:* (subjective) Glasses for close work, none for distance, checked 6 months ago. No difficulty hearing. *Sleep/rest:* (subjective) Usual sleep pattern, 10:30 P.M. to 6:30 A.M. without waking. Usual treatment for sleeplessness: reading and hot cocoa; sleep not often a problem unless worrying. *Nutrition:* (subjective) Three meals, 7:30 A.M., 12 noon, 6 P.M., no snacks except coffee. Drinks 10–12 cups/day. Dislikes: strong vegetables, mayonnaise, casserole dishes. No food allergies. (objective) Height, 6 ft; weight, 180 lb. Looks well nourished. *Elimination:* (subjective) Bowel movement after breakfast every day. Treatment for constipation: 1 cup prune juice in the morning. No nocturia, frequency, or burning. *Social/recreation:* (subjective) Plays bridge once a week with fellows in office. Plays golf two times a week. Enjoys lake fishing, boating, reading (mysteries), gardening—roses, orchids. (objective) Has *Sports Illustrated, U.S. News and World Report, Newsweek* at bedside. *Support systems:* (subjective) Wife, employed school teacher. Married 20 years 2 daughters. 16-year-old at home, 18-year-old away at Univ. Family will visit evenings. Hospital insurance and sick leave. (objective) Picture of wife and daughters outside their home on bedside stand. *Breathing:* (subjective) Does not smoke. No history of chronic respiratory disease. (objective) Respirations 14, No symptoms of resp. infection.

Figure 18.7 Nursing assessment form, completed sample. (Reproduced with permission from D. Little and D. Carnevali: Nursing Care Planning, 2nd ed. Philadelphia: JB Lippincott Company, 1976, pp. 145–146.)

were not designed to obtain large amounts of specific, factual information. As each question, or a similar one, is asked, it is important to keep in mind the purpose or intent of that question. The nurse should assume, until she has reason to believe otherwise, that whatever a patient chooses to tell her is important to him and is uppermost in his mind. The information he selects from all possible information he might give in answer to her question will indicate his areas of concern. The specifics of his answers may be less significant than the underlying themes. For example, the specific sex and ages of a patient's children are usually less important than the recurrent themes of frustration, isolation, and despair as he talks of lack of respect, lack of family unity, lack of concern for one another, and that "we scarcely even talk to each other anymore."

None of these questions was designed to elicit data specific to culture or ethnicity, but an astute interviewer will recognize cues from the patient which may suggest a need for further exploration of these areas, often at a later time.

Rationale for Questions

I. PAST HEALTH HISTORY

1. Would you tell me a little about yourself, your family, your way of life?

    This question is asked in order to elicit data relevant about a patient's developmental stage, self-esteem, work, hobbies, family composition, and so on. The nurse needs to read between the lines to determine whether a patient considers his life satisfying and meaningful and whether he feels worthy and respected. A patient's selection of content and his facial expression, tone of voice, and gestures will provide additional data about his situation. The needs and nursing care of a patient who enthusiastically describes his family and job are likely to be different from those of a patient who says, "There isn't anything of importance to tell—I just do the best I can and hope things will get better."

    The patient is free to select what he wants the nurse to know, and this may vary from his marital status, to his upcoming retirement, the high cost of living, worry over a child, or loneliness since the death of his wife. Careful analysis of the data at a later time may indicate a need to assess a given area further or to begin to assess an area the patient omitted or avoided, but at the time of the interview, the patient's *self-selection* of areas of concern enables the nurse to start her nursing interac-

tions from the patient's own perception of his needs.

2. What sorts of things do you do, or try to do, to keep healthy?

    The nurse uses this question to elicit attitudes about health and the prevention of disease. Does the patient seem to pursue health actively, or is he passive, merely hoping that he does not get sick? Do his answers indicate a sense of autonomy or a sense of being powerless to control or influence his own health?

3. What things in your life seem to make it hard to keep healthy?

    This question is asked in order to determine a patient's perceptions of stressors, such as the high cost of food, irregular time schedules of the family, easy fatigue, inadequate recreation, and cultural conflicts about the promotion of health. It would be impossible to discuss or even identify all such stressors, so it is necessary to accept a patient's comments as a valid assessment of his perceptions at the moment.

4. How do you usually react to being ill?

    This question may reveal attitudes of fear, denial, fatalism, or an overly rational approach. It may give clues to other types of responses to illness, such as worrying about money, changing physicians at frequent intervals, or becoming very nervous and irritable.

5. What kind of care or assistance has been helpful when you were sick in the past? How do you like people to treat you?

    This question helps identify possible approaches to the nursing care of the particular patient. For example, does the patient indicate a preference for being left alone when he does not feel well, a need to be pampered, or a need to assume a dependent role? Is it helpful to him for someone to take charge of things, or does he struggle to stay in control of his own situation?

II. CURRENT HEALTH STATUS

6. What were the symptoms of this problem or condition?

    Answers to this question will indicate a patient's awareness of his own body. Were the symptoms rather advanced before he even noticed or acknowledged them? If the situation involves a psychosocial problem, the patient's answer will indicate his awareness and perception of difficulties within his individual or family system. The nurse should listen carefully to the patient's choice of words and to his ability to express himself, and note any embarrassment he seems to feel in talking about certain symptoms.

7. What did you do when you noticed these symptoms?

   This question may reveal attitudes toward self-treatment versus medical care, attention to early symptoms, denial or rejection of illness, and patterns of a patient's response to stress (the fight-or-flight response).

8. Does anything seem to relieve these symptoms, even temporarily?

   This question helps assess a patient's reliance on or faith in drugs, prayer, home remedies, and other ways of coping.

9. How do you feel now?

   This seems like a simple question, but it allows a patient to expand on the description of his symptoms that he gave to the physician and to explain, perhaps for the first time, his psychological reactions to his situation or condition. He is able to say, "I feel hot (dizzy, nauseated, short of breath)"; "I feel scared (discouraged, exhausted, depressed, resigned)." The answers to this question will give direction to the nurse's initial interventions.

10. What do you know about your illness or condition?

    The nurse should use this question to listen for accuracy and adequacy of knowledge, vocabulary, and understanding of medical terms and also for a patient's perception of whether physicians and nurses tend to give information or withhold information.

11. What have you been told about the treatment and tests that have been planned for you?

    The rationale for this question is similar to that for question 10. The answers to questions 10 and 11 both give direction to patient teaching.

12. What have you heard about the likely outcome of all this?

    The nurse should note that this question does not ask, "What has your physician told you?" It leaves the patient free to quote friends, the newspaper, his doctor, or any other source that seems significant to him. This question may elicit specific factual information, or it may elicit cues to attitudes of fear, optimism, resignation, desperation, or anxiety. This is one of the most important of all the questions because of the insights it may provide into patient motivation and behavior.

13. Who or what has been your chief source of information?

This question may already have been answered, at least in part. An absence of professional sources may indicate poor communication with physicians and nurses. Sources such as neighbors or friends have implications for patient teaching. Questionable sources, such as tabloid newspapers, must be *accepted without comment* at the time of the interview because rejection or criticism of such sources may be taken personally by the patient, and any feeling of rejection by the patient will undermine the trust the nurse is trying to foster during the early phases of their relationship.

III. NURSING CARE AND ASSISTANCE NEEDED

14. What, if anything, don't you understand as well as you'd like to?

    A patient's answers indicate his priorities and provide a valid starting point for patient teaching. His answers may also indicate whether or not he feels that he "ought" to understand the things that have been explained to him, and yet he is free to reveal any lack of understanding without fear of being considered dumb or inattentive.

15. What do you think will be the hardest part of this illness (situation, hospitalization)?

    The answer to this question will indicate some of the current major stressors for the patient. Possible stressors include pain, lack of privacy, loss of independence, financial insecurity, separation from spouse, family, or lover, fear of mutilation or disfigurement, embarrassment, and so on. It is impossible to predict what the stressors may be for any given patient without input from the patient. For example, the major stressor for each of three women of the same age who are scheduled for a mastectomy might be, respectively, the resulting disfigurement, dread of being "out of control" while anesthetized, and fear of being unable to cope with pain.

16. Many aspects of your life will be disrupted, at least temporarily, by treatments, or by hospital rules and regulations. Which of these disruptions may be hard for you to deal with?

    The answer to this question may be related to the previous answer, or it may be very different. A patient may answer in terms of sleeping patterns, eating habits, sex, social activities, limited communication, and so on. The answers will help the nurse plan nursing interventions that will foster effective adaptation by the patient to his stressors.

17. What do you think may be the major effect

of this illness or condition on you and your family?

This question may yield clues to patient-family relationships and to the nature and extent of a family's concern, understanding, willingness, and ability to be involved in the patient's situation. It may also indicate a patient's ability to plan for the future, and the degree to which his appraisal of his situation is realistic or accurate.

18. What would you like to be able to do to help yourself get better or be more comfortable?

This question is likely to reveal information about a patient's personal goals and aspirations. The answer may indicate dissatisfaction (such as a lack of self-discipline in adhering to prescribed treatment) or a feeling of inadequacy. It may reveal things a patient believes he could probably do for himself if he had the necessary encouragement, equipment, permission, or whatever. A patient's answer may indicate his attitudes toward his prognosis, recovery, and the reality of his situation.

19. What kinds of help are you going to need in order to manage?

Answers to this question constitute an initial assessment of a patient's strengths and deficits as the patient begins to identify the type of care and assistance he will need to cope with his current health problems. In certain situations some of a patient's needs are obvious, such as the physical needs of a dying patient; but other needs can be identified *only by the patient*. He may say, "I'll be okay if I know someone will come in every half hour without fail during the night so I'll know I'm not alone"; or "Please let me keep my radio on low through the night."

One patient may need help in interpreting his needs to his family. Another may need help in adapting a procedure so that it will be compatible with his life as a forest ranger. Still another patient could be discharged and go to his daughter's home if he could find some way to get his twice-weekly injections.

20. Who might be able to provide this help (or care or assistance)?

Answers to this question provide a beginning assessment of a patient's attitude toward asking for and accepting help from others as well as an assessment of the patient's sources of help and support, and his knowledge of community agencies and services. For some patients, a major nursing intervention may be assistance in identifying and contacting sources of help. For others, an important need is assistance in learning how to ask for and accept help of any kind.

Section Three

Observation

The Process of Observation

Things to Be Observed
   Signs of Distress
   Real or Potential Hazards
   Condition or Status of the Patient
   Patient's Immediate Environment
     Patient's Reaction to His Immediate Environment
   People Significant to the Patient
     Patient's Reaction to People Significant to Him
   Patient's Larger Environment

THE PROCESS OF OBSERVATION

In nursing, observation is the intentional and purposeful use of *all five senses* to gather information about a patient and his situation. A nursing observation yields direct, first-hand bits of information that are obtained through the faculties of hearing, sight, taste, touch, and smell. Three of these faculties are used in a *specialized, intensive* manner during the physical examination of the patient; these are referred to as inspection (looking), auscultation (listening), and palpation (touching) and are described in detail in Section 5 of this chapter.

Observation in nursing is deliberate and conscious; it is not a casual or an incidental activity. It is a continuous process; a skillful, professional nurse is, of necessity, always observant. She can no more be observant only in isolated instances than an honest nurse can be honest just in selected situations. The intensity and focus of the observations will vary from one situation to another, but a nurse must always be alert, observant, and ready to respond in appropriate fashion.

A nurse would be overwhelmed by the multiplicity of stimuli from her observations if she were not able to screen and filter out the unimportant ones. This screening is done on the basis of her knowledge in three areas:

- What *should* be observed in a given situation
- Which norms are relevant to a given situation
- The patient's previous condition or status

The process of identifying significant observations requires the nurse to make a quick mental comparison between what she has observed and what she would expect to find in that situation. For example, in a well-baby clinic, the nurse's knowledge of normal patterns of growth and development would indicate that a 6-month-old infant who weighed 10 lb was not developing properly. Even before she weighed the baby, her initial observation would indicate the need for an extensive assessment.

A nurse working nights will be able to tune out all the normal nighttime sounds. She will not need to investigate every sound she hears, but she will respond to a patient whose cough sounds different and to a patient whose suction machine is making a different sound. An experienced nurse in the newborn nursery, in the midst of many crying babies, will notice the high-pitched cry characteristic of some brain-injured infants, sometimes even before a medical diagnosis has been made.

If a nurse's observations are to be useful in planning nursing care, she must be able to describe what she has seen, heard, felt, smelled, or tasted so she can share her observations with others. Each description must be *precise, accurate, complete,* and *phrased in accepted terminology.* Whereas a lay person might report that a bed-ridden patient has a "small red spot on his back," a nurse would be more precise and specific in her description. The lay person's report fails to answer questions such as: Where is the spot—over the sacrum or the scapula? What size is a "small spot?" The size of a pimple? Of a half-dollar? What kind of spot is it? Is it draining? Is it healing? Is it covered with a scab? A nurse describing the same area might report: "a reddened area the size of a quarter over the sacrum; not tender; skin intact; redness disappears with massage."

The ability to describe and share observations is important for three reasons. A precise, accurate description makes it possible to: (1) plan effective nursing care, (2) evaluate the outcome of nursing care, and (3) collect information that could be used to study patient responses to various nursing actions and that might

result in the discovery of new techniques and approaches in nursing.

THINGS TO BE OBSERVED

Nursing observations should be systematic and organized so that observations are made in sequence without gaps and omissions. Each nurse eventually develops a personal pattern or system for making observations, and it may be similar to or markedly different from the pattern shown in Figure 18.8. In this illustration, the observational process is viewed as if it progressed through a series of concentric circles or waves that move outward from the patient to his immediate environment and on to the people who are significant in his life and then to his larger environment.

Since the first phase of every patient assessment is an appraisal of possible distress or danger, the first observations are directed at that concern. The sequence of observations might then proceed as follows:

1. Signs of patient distress
2. Hazards or dangers, real or potential
3. The condition or status of the patient and the functioning of his equipment
4. The patient's immediate environment
5. The patient's reaction or response to his immediate environment
6. The people who are significant to the patient (family, friends, staff)
7. The patient's response to significant people
8. The larger environment (neighborhood, community)

Signs of Distress

The first observation in any situation is made to seek signs of physical or psychological distress. These observations include any *sounds* of distress heard when a patient is out of sight, such as a patient sobbing in the next unit or unusual sounds from the bathroom.

Real or Potential Hazards

Observations of real or potential hazards can usually be made rather quickly as the nurse enters a patient's home or walks into his hospital unit. Once a nurse has developed a *habit* of checking for hazards whenever she enters a patient's room or home, the process can be speeded up by recalling the hazards that might be *specific to a given age or condition.* The things that might be dangerous for a toddler are quite different from those

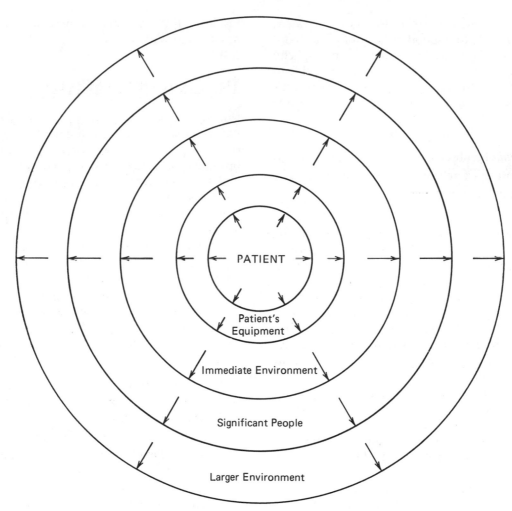

Figure 18.8 A pattern of systematic observation.

that are hazardous for an elderly person, and the related observations are thus somewhat different.

Examples of real or potential patient hazards include:

- A crib side left down
- Liquids spilled on the floor
- An untied shoelace
- A reddened pressure area over the sacrum
- The absence of a hospital identification bracelet
- Scatter rugs in the home of an elderly patient
- A salt shaker on a salt-restricted dinner tray
- Peeling paint on or near an infant's crib

Observation of such hazards, followed by prompt action, can avert danger and discomfort for a patient or his family.

Condition or Status of the Patient

Regardless of the age or condition of a patient, there are a number of observations that should be made. The items that follow illustrate the range and scope of data that can be obtained by observation:

- Sex
- Race
- Approximate age
- Size (approximate height and weight)
- Level of consciousness
- Affect (facial expression)
- Posture and symmetry of sides of body
- Movement and activity (balance, strength, endurance)
- Grooming (hair, skin, clothes, cleanliness)

- Condition of skin (wounds, lesions, bruises, texture)
- Color (nailbeds, mucous membranes, conjunctivae, skin)
- Respiration (rate, depth, sounds)
- Temperature of skin
- Drainage, discharge, exudates (blood, urine, feces, vomitus, sputum, drainage from wounds or from a suction machine)
- Prostheses (artificial eye, limb, dentures, wig)
- Odors (breath, drainage, discharge, perspiration, feces, urine)

In addition to the general observations she makes on every patient, the nurse must observe those things that are *specific* to a particular patient's condition. For example, she would examine the pupils of a patient with a head injury, and she would check the circulation in the toes of a patient with a newly applied long leg cast. For each patient, the nurse needs to ask: "What observations are important to the care of this patient?" and "What information do I need to plan his care or to evaluate the effectiveness of care already given?"

In addition to observing the condition of a patient, she must observe the functioning of his equipment. In some institutions this responsibility is shared with specialists, such as an IV team or the respiratory therapist. An IV therapist may be responsible for starting an IV, and for changing the needle and tubing at prescribed intervals, but the nurse may be responsible for checking the IV frequently enough to be able to alert the therapist to any difficulty that should arise.

A patient's equipment should be checked frequently enough to ensure proper functioning so that the patient will receive optimal benefit and will be spared any possible discomfort or injury. Questions to be asked include: Are all fluids flowing properly? Are drainage tubes open and draining well? Do the gauges indicate the prescribed amount of suction or pressure? Are hot packs still hot or ice bags still cold?

Patient's Immediate Environment

On entering a patient's home or hospital room, a nurse should assess its safety, cleanliness, temperature, light, convenience, comfort, and esthetic qualities. The influence of the environment on a person's physical and mental health has been acknowledged for centuries, and formed the basis for many of the teachings of Florence Nightingale. Since that time, management of a patient's environment has become an increasingly important nursing responsibility.

In some situations the nurse will be able to alter a deficient or disturbing environment by adjusting the lighting or temperature, removing supplies and equipment that are no longer needed, removing soiled dressings or body wastes, or arranging furniture for the convenience of the patient. In other situations the nurse cannot remedy the situation herself but must work with the landlord, homeowner, department of health, or hospital administrator. But regardless of who finally assumes responsibility for the problem, the nurse is responsible for observing the patient's immediate environment and initiating any remedial action that may prove necessary.

Patient's Reaction to His Immediate Environment

Environmental conditions that could result in an accident, an infection, or a disease must be corrected as soon as possible, but a decision to modify any other aspects of the environment depends on the patient's *reaction* to them. A patient whose eyes are sensitive to light may want to keep his shades down and his room quite dark. The dim light may seem oppressive to his nurse but not to him. A person with limited mobility may keep everything within his reach and, as a result, may seem to be surrounded by clutter. A person with few friends or a limited income may tend to treasure and seemingly hoard his possessions and may be unwilling to part with such things as nearly dead plants, overripe fruit, or empty candy boxes.

Careful observation is needed to determine the *meaning of the environment* to the patient and whether or not any nursing intervention is warranted. Every person values his personal space and his territorial rights and it is therefore inappropriate for a nurse to rearrange, clean up, or alter any aspect of a patient's environment that is nonhazardous unless the patient requests it or concurs that it should be done.

People Significant to the Patient

Because a patient's health and well-being are influenced by the people around him, it is important to observe those who seem to be significant in his life. This may be done directly, through contact during visiting hours, or during the home visits of a community health nurse, for example, or it may be done indirectly through telephone conversations, photographs, or letters. Such contact with people who are significant to the patient will enable the nurse to make a tentative assessment of such factors as their health, attitudes toward the patient, ability to communicate, and their outlook on life. The mere fact that a patient has a married son is of little use in planning for the patient's discharge; what matters is whether the son is outgoing, healthy, financially secure, and concerned, or whether, for example, he is chronically ill, poor, alcoholic, and alienated from his father. The mere existence of a relative, friend, neighbor, or pastor has little relevance for nursing care until the nurse has been able to observe and learn something about that person.

Patient's Reaction to People Significant to Him

It is necessary for the nurse to remember that her own reaction to people of importance to a patient is relatively insignificant compared to the *patient's reactions* to them. A son who is perceived by the staff to be arrogant and condescending may be perceived as confident and successful by his mother. A sister who seems thoughtful, interested, and concerned to the staff may be deemed a meddling nuisance by her brother.

Observation of a patient before, during, and after contact with his friends and relatives will help the nurse assess the nature of his relationships and the amount of support he receives from them. Headaches, nervousness, anxiety, and other indications of stress and tension suggest a difficult or negative relationship. In some situations the identification of a difficult relationship, followed by help in improving that relationship, may be one of the most significant nursing interventions.

It is equally important to observe the reactions of a patient to significant members of the health team. You may observe that a patient is fearful, apologetic, or assertive toward the staff in general or that he reacts in an atypical fashion to a single member of the staff. If your observations suggest that the patient's relationship to one or more staff members might interfere with his health care, further assessment is needed to explore the nature and scope of the problem and to determine what, if anything, should be done about it.

Patient's Larger Environment

The community health nurse, school nurse, industrial nurse, and others have an opportunity to observe a patient's home, neighborhood, and/or his community. These nurses can assess such factors as sanitation, employment, crime, transportation, recreation, medical care, and other resources, some of which may be critical for everyone in that area. Other factors are critical for certain groups, such as the elderly or the handicapped, or for people in special situations, such as those in a migrant camp, an Indian reservation, or a children's summer camp. Nursing observations of a patient's larger environment often form the basis for significant changes or reforms that enhance the health and welfare of all who live or work in that environment.

Section Four

Measurement

MEASUREMENT*

Measurement is a form of assessment that determines the dimensions, capacity, quantity, or degree of something. Some of the things commonly measured in nursing are height, weight, temperature, pulse, respiration, blood pressure, and the volume of fluids such as urine. A single measurement is rarely significant or useful; it must be used in conjunction with other data. A weight of 120 lb, for example, is meaningless without height and age. A 4-foot-tall, 10-year-old girl who weighs 120 lb is obese, but a 6-foot-tall adult weighing 120 lb is not. A temperature of 39 degrees C (102.2 degrees F) will be interpreted differently if the patient's temperature has been 39 degrees C for 2 weeks, has been normal until today, or has suddenly dropped from much higher readings.

Data obtained by measurement must be accurate and precise. A patient's weight is not "about 160 lb." Either it is 160 lb or it is not. If the weight is 159 or 161 lb, it should be reported as such. For each type of measurement, the degree of precision is determined by the equipment used. For example, bathroom scales are calibrated in pounds, and the accepted degree of precision would be 1 lb. Baby scales are calibrated in ounces, and the accepted degree of precision would be 1 oz. An infant's weight, therefore, should be precise to the nearest ounce and should be stated as 6 lb, 2 oz, for example.

Accuracy depends on: (1) the vision and hearing of the nurse, (2) the precision of the instrument or tool used, and (3) the conditions under which the measurements are taken.

Systems of Measurement

Many hospitals use the metric system of measurement exclusively, while some use both the metric and the apothecary systems. Most hospitals measure fluid volume in the metric system, and equipment is calibrated accordingly. Length is consistently measured in centimeters by the physician, so nurses find it useful to carry a small centimeter ruler for measuring scars, bruises, or other surface areas. A few basic equivalents are given below; extensive conversion tables are included in the appendices.

---

*The taking of necessary measurement is an essential part of the assessment phase, but the *interpretation* of the data obtained is a *different activity* and part of the next phase of nursing process. This section, therefore, explains how to take correct and accurate measurements but does not describe the physiological significance of various measurements.

APPROXIMATE EQUIVALENTS

1 in = 2.5 cm	1 cm = 0.4 inch
1 ft = 0.3 m	1 m = 39.4 inches
1 lb = 0.45 kg	1 kg = 2.2 lb
1 qt = 1.0 liter	1 liter = 1.0 qt

HEIGHT

One of the commonest measurements is height. It is important in assessing a child's rate of growth, and it is used in conjunction with age in assessing a patient's weight. An infant is measured while lying on its back with knees extended, and feet at right angles to the table. Accuracy of measurement is increased by placing one flat object against the infant's feet and another against the top of his head and measuring the distance between the two surfaces.

Height is measured in feet or meters; 1 foot = 0.3 meter.

WEIGHT

A change in body weight may be a symptom of disease, a manifestation of inadequate or faulty nutrition, an indication of altered fluid balance, or a reaction to therapy. Some patients are weighed daily, and because a change in body weight may be a basis for alterations in diet or medication, these patients must be weighed with great accuracy.

The patient on daily weights should be weighed at the *same time* each day, on the *same scales*, wearing the *same amount of clothing*. Patients are usually weighed before breakfast and after the bladder or catheter bag has been emptied. A fresh paper towel should be placed on the platform of the scale under the patient's bare feet because the scale is not usually washed between patients.

If a patient is unable to stand, he is transferred to a stretcher scale and weighed. The weight of any sheets, pads, blankets, or pillows must be subtracted from the overall weight.

Infants are weighed without clothing, before feeding, at the same time each day. The tray or platform on which the baby is laid will feel cold to the infant, so a diaper is placed under him. The weight of the diaper is then subtracted from the overall weight. If for some reason an infant is weighed with clothes on, an identical set of clothes must be weighed and that weight subtracted from the overall weight of baby and clothes. Some breastfed infants are weighed before and after feeding if there is concern about the amount of milk the baby is getting.

Weight is measured in pounds or kilograms; 1 kg equals 2.2 lb.

CIRCUMFERENCE

Changes in the circumference (girth) of a patient's chest, abdomen, or extremity can be a significant symptom. An enlarged abdomen, for example, may indicate an accumulation of fluid within the peritoneal cavity (ascites). A decrease in the circumference of a patient's calf or thigh could indicate atrophy (wasting away) of the muscles. It is important to measure the circumference of a baby's head at regular intervals until age 2 because changes in the circumference of the skull indicate the rate of growth of skull and brain. The skull is measured along an imaginary line above the eyebrows in front of and over the occipital protuberance in back.

You measure circumference by wrapping a tape measure around a body part. The tape should be snug enough to stay in place without slipping, but not tight enough to depress the underlying tissue. Subsequent measurements of the same body part should be made at the same point; and if frequent measurements are to be made, accuracy is increased by marking the patient's skin above and below the tape to indicate the exact point of measurement. A cloth, flexible steel, or paper tapemeasure may be used. A cloth tapemeasure should be checked for accuracy periodically because cloth has a tendency to stretch with age.

Circumference is measured in inches or centimeters; 1 inch equals 2.5 cm.

DIAMETER AND AREA

Any description of a lesion, bruise, wound, scar, or lump must include its size, and a small pocket ruler enables a nurse to measure accurately the area to be described. When it is not feasible to use a ruler, it is helpful to compare the area to that of a familiar object such as a coin; with practice, a nurse learns to describe a lesion with accuracy as being the size of a half dollar, for example (Fig. 18.9). Lumps and masses can be described in terms of a pea, a cherry, a walnut, or an egg until they can be measured accurately.

FLUID VOLUME

Body fluids which are commonly measured include urine, blood, vomitus, drainage from chest tubes, liquid fecal matter, gastric drainage, and fluid withdrawn from any body cavity. Large amounts of fluid can be measured with reasonable accuracy by using a container calibrated in increments of 10 to 20 cc, but small amounts of fluid must be measured more precisely by use of a measure calibrated in increments of 1 to 2 cc. For example, the urine of a patient whose daily output of urine is 2,000 cc or more could be measured with reasonable accuracy to the nearest 10 to 20 cc each time he urinates, but the urine of a patient in kidney failure whose total daily output of urine is less than 100 cc must be measured accurately to the nearest cubic centimeter.

To measure small amounts of fluid accurately, a clear plastic or glass measure must be used so that measurement can be made at eye level. It is *not* accurate to look down into a nontransparent container and try to read the calibrations.

All discharge, drainage, and fluid excreta should be measured and recorded except for the urine of people who have no urinary or fluid balance problems and whose urine, therefore, need not be measured. Fluid spilled or excreted onto bedding, clothing, or a rug cannot be measured, so the amount must be estimated. This is difficult to do because the fluid is soaked up and spread by capillary action. It may be helpful to practice estimating fluid volume by spilling a measured amount

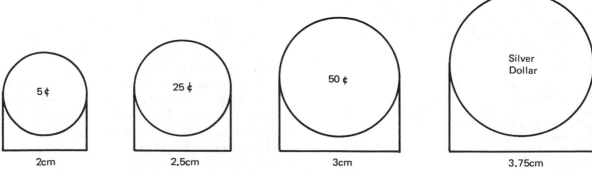

Figure 18.9 *Approximate equivalent surface areas (actual size).*

of colored water or juice onto a towel or piece of sheeting and noting the size of the spot made by each amount of fluid.

TEMPERATURE

Body temperature is one of the most sensitive and reliable indicators of physical health and illness. In health, body temperature remains surprisingly constant despite environmental and physiological influences; therefore, any noticeable change in temperature signals some physiological disruption. Parents as well as nurses are able to detect the presence of a fever from a variety of clues, such as a hot forehead, flushed face, and increased thirst. In addition, a person often exhibits an individual, characteristic appearance and behavior each time he has a fever. A parent may state, for example, "I always know when my child has a fever—his palms feel hot, his eyes are bright, and he seems especially animated." Such indications of fever should be validated with a thermometer, and the temperature should be recorded for comparison with later measurements.

Body temperature is one of the four indicators traditionally referred to as *vital signs* (temperature, pulse, respiration, and blood pressure). Vital signs are taken to obtain baseline data about a patient or to monitor the progress of a patient's disease or condition. *Baseline data* is a term that refers to the normal or usual state of a person, which provides the basis for interpreting other data in the future. These data reveal the pattern of minor fluctuations which is normal for a given patient, a pattern that must be known so that subsequent changes can be recognized.

Body temperature is also measured to monitor changes in a patient's condition. Changes in temperature are important in detecting and diagnosing an illness or disease, in gauging the progress of a patient's condition, in serving as an early warning of complications, and in evaluating the effectiveness of therapy. Frequency of temperature measurement ranges from a few times per year for a healthy adult to every 15 to 20 minutes for a patient whose temperature is extremely high or low. A commonly used routine interval is every 4 hours (q 4h), often around the clock. Some agencies, however, now take each patient's temperature only once a day, with additional measurements taken *as indicated.* It is important to distinguish between measurements that are necessary and justified and those that are taken because of policy or routine. A patient who is afebrile (without a fever) should *not* be awakened during the night for a routine temperature check, but it is important to awaken a patient for an unscheduled temperature check if a nurse suspects his body temperature has changed. If, while a nurse is checking a patient's IV at 3 am, his skin feels hot to the touch, she should check his temperature then, not at 8 am when it is scheduled to be taken.

"Taking his temperature" is one of the immediate responses of a parent to a sick child. The phrase "he has a temperature" is often used to indicate the presence of a fever; and while the phrase may be appropriate for use by lay people, it is inadequate for professional use. It is not accurate because every person has a temperature. Correct usage is, "He has an elevated temperature," or "He has a fever."

Sites

Body temperature is measured most frequently at four sites: mouth, rectum, axilla, and esophagus. The selection of a site depends on the age and condition of the patient and on the degree of precision required.

Mouth

Taking an oral temperature is less intrusive and more acceptable to most people than taking a rectal temperature. Two drawbacks to its use are: (1) the measurement may be inaccurate if the patient cannot or will not keep his mouth closed, and (2) a glass thermometer can be broken if the patient bites it. An oral temperature, therefore, should *not* be taken on any of the following patients:

- Infant or small child
- Unconscious patient
- Confused or irrational patient
- Patient who must breathe with mouth open
- Patient who has had oral surgery
- Patient with an oral infection
- Patient with a history of convulsions

Rectum

A rectal temperature has long been considered more reliable than an oral temperature, but recent research is challenging the validity of that position. A rectal temperature is taken whenever an oral temperature is likely to be unsafe or inaccurate. A rectal temperature should not be taken on a patient who has a rectal disorder or who has had rectal surgery. A rectal temperature should not be taken on a patient who is in a cast or in traction unless he can be turned enough for the nurse to see the anus and be able to insert the thermometer safely.

Axilla

An axillary temperature is taken when neither a rectal nor an oral temperature is possible. The disadvantages of an axillary temperature are: (1) the reading is lower than for all the other sites and (2) it takes the longest time to get an accurate temperature. The thermometer is held in place by pressing the patient's arm against his chest to ensure as much contact and accuracy as possible.

Esophagus

An esophageal temperature measures a patient's internal, or *core temperature*. The procedure is more complex than for the other temperature measurements, so it is done most frequently in an intensive care unit when precise information is needed about a patient's temperature. A temperature-sensitive device, usually electronic, is passed down the patient's esophagus, often in conjunction with a nasogastric tube. It is left in place for as long as measurement of the patient's core temperature is essential.

Types of Thermometers

Glass and Mercury

There are three common types or shapes of glass and mercury thermometers: oral, stubby, and rectal. The *oral* thermometer has a long, slender bulb, which supposedly increases its accuracy by allowing more mercury to come in contact with the blood vessels under the tongue. The *stubby* type has a shorter, rounder bulb and can be used to obtain either oral or rectal temperatures. The bulb end of a *rectal* thermometer is blunt so that it is less likely to injure the rectal mucosa when it is inserted.

Heat from a patient's body causes the mercury to expand along a scale that may be either centigrade or Fahrenheit. There is a slight constriction in the glass which keeps the expanded column of mercury from dropping back toward the bulb end. After the thermometer has been read, the column of mercury is moved back toward the bulb end by shaking the thermometer briskly, either by hand or by a centrifuge. The mercury should be below the 35.5 degrees C (or 96 degrees F) mark before the thermometer is used again.

A glass thermometer is relatively cheap because it will last indefinitely if handled with care. Unfortunately, the expense from breakage is high in some institutions, and other types of thermometers are being used. A glass thermometer must be disinfected between patients, unless each patient has his own thermometer. A glass and mercury thermometer is fairly slow compared with an electronic thermometer. A glass rectal thermometer must be left in place for at least 3 minutes; and an oral one, for approximately 8 minutes. More research is needed because there is no consensus on optimal times; recommended times for an oral temperature, for example, range from 5 to 11 minutes.

Electronic

An electronic thermometer consists of a temperature-sensitive probe, or sensor, attached by a wire to a digital display unit (Fig. 18.10). The probe is covered with a disposable cover, then positioned in a patient's mouth or rectum, and left in place for 20 to 30 seconds. The temperature is read from the digital display unit. The electronic thermometer is fast, accurate, and easy to read. Disposable probe covers eliminate the need for disinfection. The initial cost is high.

Tape or Patch

A small strip or patch of temperature-sensitive tape serves as a thermometer when applied to a patient's abdomen or forehead. The tape changes color at different temperatures. If a precise measurement is important, a temperature outside the normal range should be checked with a glass or an electronic thermometer.

Taking a Temperature

There are so many types of thermometers and patient situations that it is not feasible to outline a detailed procedure for each. It is possible, however, to sum-

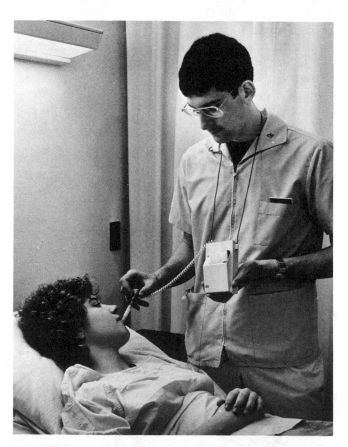

Figure 18.10 *Electronic thermometer equipment can be worn around the neck to leave both hands free to work with the patient.*

marize the *essential* elements of taking rectal and oral temperatures. An essential element of a procedure is one that *must* be present for the procedure to be considered well done and effective.

Taking a Rectal Temperature

A rectal temperature is usually taken with the patient lying on his side. The buttocks are separated enough to make the anus clearly visible, and the lubricated end of the thermometer is inserted about 1½ in (less for a child). It may be necessary to hold the thermometer in place if the sphincter muscles of the rectum tend to force the thermometer out. If a patient has large or painful hemorrhoids, it is usually difficult to insert a thermometer without causing considerable discomfort. The rectal area must be exposed with good light so that the nurse can try to separate the hemorrhoids (bulging grapelike protrusions of vein), and try to find an opening through which she can insert the thermometer. *Never try to force a thermometer into place or try to insert it blindly.* Sometimes the patient is able to insert the thermometer with minimal discomfort, or you may be able to obtain an order for oral temperatures.

For both esthetic and sanitary reasons, the cover of the probe of an electronic thermometer should be wrapped in tissue before it is discarded if it is soiled. A glass and mercury thermometer must be wiped clean so that the numbers are clearly visible to ensure an accurate reading.

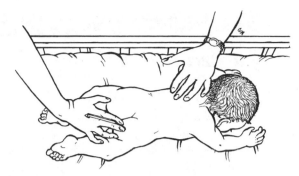

Figure 18.11 *When taking an infant's temperature, the hand holding the thermometer must also hold the baby's buttocks to prevent injury in case he moves.*

Taking a Baby's Temperature

When taking the temperature of an infant or a toddler, it is necessary to hold the thermometer in place. The child is placed in a prone position across the nurse's lap or on his stomach on a bed or table. A child is likely to move suddenly, so he must be protected from sudden penetration of his rectum by the thermometer. *The hand that holds the thermometer should hold the child's buttocks* so that, should he move, the nurse's hand and the thermometer would move with him as a unit (Fig. 18.11). When the thermometer moves with the child's body, there is little danger of injury.

PROCEDURE 18.1

Taking an Oral Temperature*

SUMMARY OF ESSENTIAL NURSING ACTIONS

1. Make sure that an oral temperature is safe and appropriate for the patient.
2. Maintain medical asepsis throughout the procedure.
   - Use patient's own or a clean thermometer, or use a disposable probe cover on an electronic thermometer.
   - Put used thermometer or probe cover in proper place at end of procedure.
3. Make sure that the thermometer is ready for use.
   - Mercury in glass thermometer should be below 35.5 degrees C or 96 degrees F.
   - Signal on electronic thermometer should indicate readiness for use.

4. Prepare patient as indicated by age, condition, and situation.
   - Direct patient to keep thermometer under tongue with lips closed.
   - Remind patient not to bite thermometer.
5. Leave thermometer in place for length of time specified by school or agency policy.
6. Make good use of time needed for glass thermometer to register (take pulse and respiration, straighten unit)
7. Read thermometer, and record or report temperature accurately.

*See inside front cover.

Taking a Rectal Temperature*

SUMMARY OF ESSENTIAL NURSING ACTIONS

1. Make sure that a rectal temperature is necessary.
2. Maintain medical asepsis throughout the procedure.
   - Use the patient's own or a clean thermometer, or a fresh disposable cover for probe of electronic thermometer.
   - Do not place used (soiled) thermometer or probe cover directly on patient's bedside stand or other equipment. If you must lay it down, place it on a tissue or paper towel.
3. Make sure that the thermometer is ready for use.
   - Mercury in glass thermometer should be below 35.5 degrees C or 96 degrees F.
   - Signal on electronic thermometer should indicate readiness for use.
   - End of glass thermometer or probe cover should be lubricated with a substance such as vaseline.
4. Prepare patient as indicated by age, condition, and situation.

   - Assist or move patient into a safe, comfortable position.
   - Restrict movement of infant or child gently but securely.
   - Separate buttocks until anus is *clearly visible*.
5. Insert lubricated end of thermometer the appropriate distance for age and size of patient.
6. Hold thermometer in place as indicated by patient's age and condition.
7. Keep thermometer in place for length of time specified by school or agency.
8. Make good use of the time needed for glass thermometer to register (talk with patient, take pulse and respiration)
9. Read thermometer accurately.
   - Wipe soiled end of glass thermometer as needed to permit accurate reading.
10. Record or report temperature accurately.

*See inside front cover.

Reading and Recording a Temperature

A glass thermometer must be wiped clear of mucus or feces so that the column of mercury will be clearly visible. To read the thermometer, hold it parallel to the floor, at eye level, and slowly rotate it back and forth until you can see the mercury. The patient's temperature is indicated by the line opposite the end of the column of mercury.

On a centigrade scale, there are 10 divisions for each degree, so the temperature is read to the nearest 0.1 degree C.

On a Fahrenheit scale, there are five divisions for each degree, so each line represents ⅕, or 0.2 degree

F, and the temperature is read to the nearest 0.2 degree (Fig. 18.12).

Figure 18.13 shows two thermometers that you can read for practice. Write down your answers and check them against the figure caption.

An electronic thermometer is read directly from the digital display unit. You read a tape or patch thermometer by comparing the color of the tape with a color key.

In most institutions the vital signs of all patients are recorded in a vital signs notebook or on a work sheet by the person taking them. Later they are transferred to the permanent graphic sheet in each patient's chart. The graphing of vital signs is often done by the ward clerk or secretary.

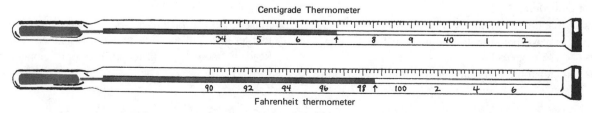

Figure 18.12 *Normal centigrade and Fahrenheit readings are 37°C and 98.6°F.*

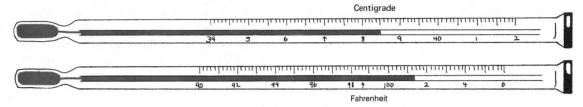

Figure 18.13 *Centigrade reading, 38.5°; Fahrenheit reading, 101.3°.*

Conversion Between Systems of Measurement

Many hospitals have adopted the metric system of measurement, and use centigrade thermometers exclusively. Other agencies and most lay people use Fahrenheit thermometers. Therefore, nurses must be able, for the foreseeable future, to use both systems of measurement. Conversion tables (see Table 18.1) are convenient, but a nurse should be able to use a formula to convert from one system to another in the event that a conversion table is not available.

To convert from degrees C to degrees F, multiply by $\frac{9}{5}$ and add 32.

Example: $(100 \text{ degrees C} \times \frac{9}{5}) + 32 = 180 + 32$
$= 212 \text{ degrees F}$

to convert from degrees F to degrees C, subtract 32 and multiply by $\frac{5}{9}$.

Example: $(212 \text{ degrees F} - 32) \times \frac{5}{9} = 180 \times \frac{5}{9}$
$= 100 \text{ degrees C}$

TABLE 18.1 TEMPERATURE CONVERSION SCALE

Degree Centigrade	Degree Fahrenheit
35.5	95.9
36.0	96.8
36.5	97.7
37.0	98.6
37.5	99.5
38.0	100.4
38.5	101.3
39.0	102.2
39.5	103.1
40.0	104.0
40.5	104.9
41.0	105.8
41.5	106.7
42.0	107.6

Note: Each 0.5 degree C = 0.9 degree F. Therefore, a change of 0.5 degree C = a change of 0.9 degree F.

If you are uncertain about which formula to use, or whether you remember it correctly, you can check the formula you have in mind by changing the temperature of boiling water from one scale to the other, as in the examples above. If the formula is incorrect, it will be immediately apparent because you will get an incorrect boiling temperature.

RESPIRATION

The general term *respiration* encompasses both external and internal respiration. External respiration is the process of breathing and is assessed, in part, by describing the rate, depth, and other characteristics of inspiration and expiration. The term respiration, when used in the context of vital signs (temperature, pulse, respiration, and blood pressure), refers to external respiration and is used in that context throughout this chapter. Internal respiration refers to the cellular exchange of carbon dioxide CO_2 and oxygen O_2 and is assessed through data obtained from laboratory analysis of a patient's blood. Internal respiration is not considered part of a patient's vital signs.

Assessment

Respiration is assessed by describing its rate, depth, rhythm, and the ease of breathing.

Rate
The normal respiratory rate of adults ranges from 16 to 20 breaths per minute. Infants, children, and elderly people have a faster rate. Respiratory rate is affected by emotions, physical activity, disease conditions, drugs, pain, and fever. For example, an increase in body temperature of 1 degree F results in an increase in respirations of approximately 4 breaths per minute. Increased intracranial pressure depresses the respiratory center in the brain, as do a number of drugs, thereby causing decreased respiration.

A respiratory rate over 24 is called *tachypnea*. A respiratory rate under 10 is called *bradypnea*. *Apnea* is the temporary absence of respiration. Episodes of apnea are timed and reported in number of seconds' duration. Prolonged apnea results in death.

Depth

The volume of air in each breath is about 500 cc for a healthy adult but may be greatly increased or decreased by physical activity, disease conditions, and drugs. The depth of respirations is described as *shallow, normal,* or *deep.* A patient is said to be short of breath (SOB) when his respirations are shallow and rapid. Shallow, rapid respirations are termed *hypoventilation,* whereas deep, rapid respirations are termed *hyperventilation.*

Rhythm

Respirations arc normally *regular* and *even* as well as *noiseless* and *effortless.* The most common disturbance of rhythm is called *Cheyne-Stokes respiration,* and is caused by damage to the respiratory center of the brain. These respirations, which are often seen just before death, gradually increase in rate and depth, then decrease, and finally cease for a brief period of 20 or 30 seconds. These gradual increases and decreases in rate and depth, separated by periods of apnea, are repeated in a regular pattern. Cheyne-Stokes respiration may persist for a long period of time and may be either effortless or difficult.

Difficult Respiration

Dyspnea is a condition in which respirations are difficult, labored, or painful. The patient is in obvious distress and is fighting for breath. Dyspnea may be caused by such conditions as the narrowing of air passages from asthma or a severe allergic reaction, increased secretions in the lungs, an acute airway obstruction, or an inability to inspire effectively.

Orthopnea is a condition in which a patient's dyspnea can be relieved by placing the patient in an upright position. The patient usually sleeps sitting up or propped up on pillows. Orthopnea is frequently measured in terms of the number of pillows needed for him to breathe at night, such as one-, two-, or three-pillow orthopnea.

Measurement

Respirations are measured by watching and counting the rise and fall of the patient's chest. This must be done unobtrusively because a person tends to alter his breathing if he is aware that he is being watched. An effective way to count respirations is to place the patient's arm across his chest while his pulse is taken and keep it there for the respiration count which is done while you are holding the patient's wrist as if still taking his pulse. If the respirations are shallow and hard

to see, it is possible to feel the patient's chest rise and fall.

An infant's respirations must be counted before his temperature or pulse is taken, because either of these activities might startle him and cause him to cry, thereby altering his respiratory rate.

PULSE

When the heart contracts during systole, about 70 cc of blood is forced into the aorta by the left ventricle. This blood increases the volume of blood already in the aorta and thus exerts additional pressure against its walls. These surges of increased pressure are transmitted as waves throughout the arterial blood vessels of the body. These waves, or pulses, can be felt, or palpated, wherever a peripheral artery can be compressed against an underlying bone. The commonest sites for palpating a pulse are the carotid, temporal, brachial, radial, popliteal, femoral, dorsalis pedis, and posterior tibial arteries (Fig. 18.14). The pulse rate can also be determined by auscultation (listening) with a stethoscope over the apex of the heart (apical pulse).

An apical pulse is taken on infants and small children; a radial pulse is most common for adults. The radial site is readily accessible, and the pulse is usually strong and easily located. The femoral, popliteal, and pedal (dorsalis pedis) pulses are used to assess circulation in the legs. The carotid pulse is used in many emergencies because it is accessible, is conveniently located near the site of resuscitation efforts, and is often palpable when the peripheral pulses can no longer be detected. The carotid, temporal, or apical pulse is used when the radial site is covered with a cast or dressing or is otherwise inaccessible.

A pulse is palpated with the second, third, and fourth fingers. The thumb is not used because it has a pulse of its own, which might be confused with the patient's pulse. A pulse is usually counted for 15 seconds, and the rate is multiplied by 4 to give the number of heartbeats per minute. Some schools and agencies require pulses to be counted for longer than 15 seconds, but others believe errors in counting might make the longer time less accurate. If any irregularity, change, or abnormality is noted during a 15-second count, the pulse should be counted for a full 30 or 60 seconds.

Assessment

The pulse is taken to assess heart function and to assess the adequacy of blood flow to an area of the body. The characteristics of a pulse that contribute to such as-

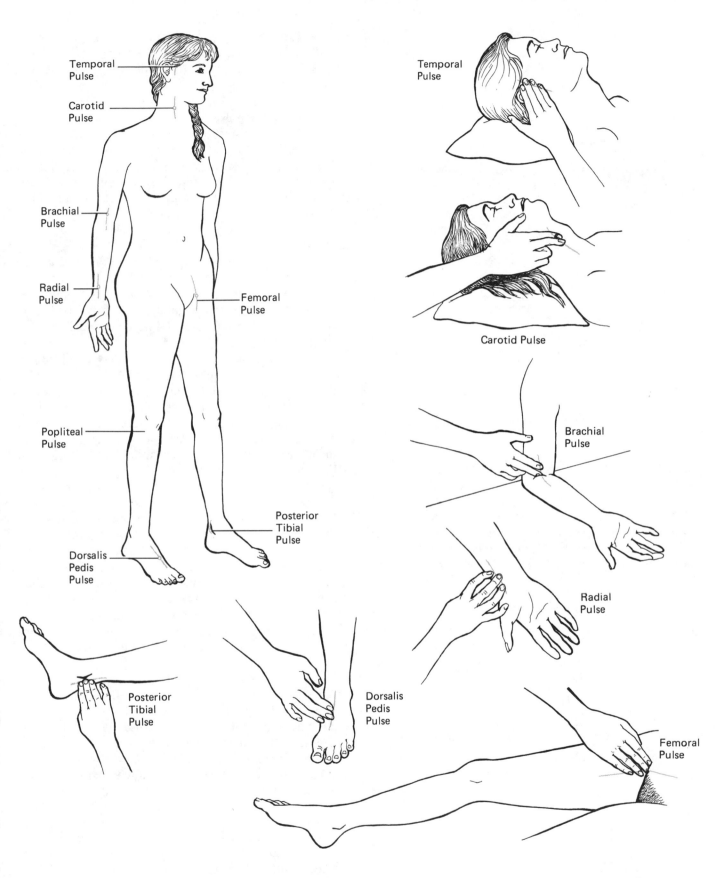

Figure 18.14 *Pulse sites and techniques for palpation.*

293

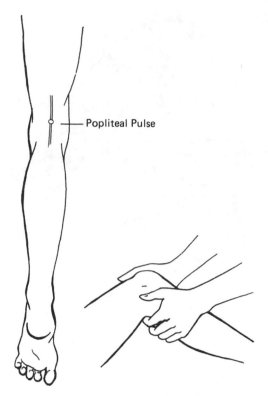

Popliteal Pulse

Figure 18.14 *(Continued)*

sessments are (1) rate, (2) rhythm, (3) tension, and (4) volume.

Rate

The pulse rate indicates the number of heartbeats per minute. The normal range for adults is 60 to 80 beats per minute, although athletes often have a much slower rate because of a well-conditioned, efficient heart action.

The pulse rate is affected by age, sex, physical or emotional activity, and illness (see Table 18.2). Anything that stimulates the sympathetic nervous system, such as heat and pain, will increase the pulse rate. An

TABLE 18.2 PULSE RATE ALTERATIONS THROUGHOUT LIFE

Age	Pulse Rate/Minute
Birth	120
1 year	110
5 years	95
10 years	85
Adolescent	80
Adult	75
Athlete	60

increase in body temperature of approximately 0.5 degree C will increase the pulse rate by 7 to 10 beats per minute. The pulse rate is affected by drugs such as digitalis, and the pulse rate can thus be used to monitor the effect of the drug. For example, digitalis is often withheld if the pulse rate drops below 60.

An adult pulse rate over 100 beats per minute is called *tachycardia,* and a rate under 50 beats per minute is called *bradycardia.* An increased rate is more common than a decreased rate during illness, so it is important to report a decreasing pulse rate promptly because it may be especially significant.

Rhythm

The rhythm of a pulse is either *regular* or *irregular.* An irregular pulse indicates an irregular heartbeat (arrhythmia). The irregularity may occur in a pattern at predictable intervals (a regular irregularity), or it may occur in random fashion at unpredictable times (an irregular irregularity).

An *intermittent* pulse rhythm includes periods of regular pulse rhythm alternating with periods of irregular rhythm. A *bigeminal* pulse consists of a pause after every two beats. A *dicrotic* pulse feels double to the touch.

A *premature beat* is a weak contraction that precedes a normal one, and the heart may seem to be skipping or fluttering. When a patient is conscious of his own heartbeats, the sensation is called *palpitation.*

Tension

Tension and *compressibility* are terms used to describe the contour of the artery, and the characteristics of the artery *between pulses.* In health, an artery feels firm, straight, smooth, and round. With a condition such as arteriosclerosis, the artery feels hard, tortuous, cordlike, irregular, and twisted. It tends to roll about under the fingers. When a patient's blood volume is low, as during a severe hemorrhage, the artery feels very soft, and minimal pressure is enough to obliterate it.

Volume, Strength, or Force

The strength or volume of a pulse reflects the volume of blood ejected with each beat of the heart. A *normal* pulse feels full and has a strong pulsation. A *weak* pulse is described as feeble or thready, and may be imperceptible at some peripheral sites. A weak pulse is usually rapid because the body tries to compensate for the decreased volume of each beat by beating faster. The heart tries to maintain a constant cardiac output; if the stroke volume decreases, the rate must therefore increase to maintain a uniform output. A *bounding* pulse is strong and difficult to obliterate by compression. It is the result of an increased stroke volume of the heart.

PROCEDURE 18.3

Counting the Patient's Radial Pulse and Respirations*

SUMMARY OF ESSENTIAL NURSING ACTIONS

1. If this is feasible, position patient's arm across his chest.
2. Use your first three fingers to palpate patient's radial artery (inner aspect of wrist just above his thumb).
3. Count pulse rate accurately for length of time specified by school or agency.
4. Note rate, rhythm, tension, and volume (strength) of pulse.

*See inside front cover.

5. *Without moving your hand or the patient's arm,* count his respirations unobtrusively and accurately for the length of time specified by school or agency.
6. Note rhythm (regularity), depth, and ease of respirations.
7. Count the pulse and respirations of an infant or small child when it is as calm as possible, usually *before* the temperature is taken.

Apical Pulse

The apical pulse is not palpated as other pulses are. The apical pulse is taken by auscultation over the apex of the heart. The apex of an adult's heart is located about 7.5 cm (3 inches) to the left of the sternum, slightly below the left nipple.

Apical pulse sounds are fairly high pitched, so the diaphragm head of the stethoscope is used, rather than the bell. (See Section 6 of this chapter for more detailed information on auscultation and the use of a stethoscope.) The diaphragm should be placed directly against a patient's skin, *not* over his clothing. If a female patient has pendulous breasts, it will be necessary to lift the left breast in order to place the stethoscope on the chest wall as close to the level of a nonpendulous nipple as possible.

Each heartbeat consists of two sounds, which are counted as one beat, and which are heard as *lub-dub.*

The first sound is the closure of the atrioventricular valves (primarily the mitral valve), and it signals the start of the period of systole. The second sound is the closure of the semilunar valves (pulmonic and aortic), and signals the start of the period of diastole.

An apical pulse is taken on infants and children because it is more accurate than trying to palpate a radial pulse. An apical pulse is taken on adults whenever the radial pulse cannot be palpated accurately either because it is weak or imperceptible or because it is irregular.

Apical-Radial Pulse

An apical-radial pulse is taken whenever there is reason to believe that the apical and radial pulses might be different. Some cardiac arrhythmias include irregular beats that are too weak to be transmitted to the peripheral arteries and therefore cannot be felt as part

PROCEDURE 18.4

Taking an Apical Pulse*

SUMMARY OF ESSENTIAL NURSING ACTIONS

1. Try to relieve the patient's anxiety or apprehension if this procedure is unfamiliar to him or if his cardiac condition is unstable.
2. Maintain privacy by pulling curtains around the bed of hospitalized patient before exposing chest.
3. Properly position the earpieces of your stethoscope.
4. Position diaphragm head of stethoscope over apex of heart.

*See inside front cover.

- Place diaphragm directly on skin (not over clothing).
- Position it about 7.5 cm (3 inches) to left of sternum and slightly below left nipple.
- Lift the breast if it is pendulous and position the head of the stethoscope beneath it.

5. Count the heart rate accurately for the length of time specified by school or agency.
- Count the two heart sounds (lub-dub) as one beat.

of the radial pulse. The difference between the apical and radial pulse rates is called the *pulse deficit*. The size of the pulse deficit is one measure of the severity of the arrhythmia. The more serious the arrhythmia, the greater the number of beats too weak to reach the radial pulse, and the greater the difference between the apical and radial pulse rates (the pulse deficit). A newly detected pulse deficit should be reported to the physician at once.

An apical-radial pulse is taken by two nurses using the same watch or wall clock (Fig. 18.15). When both pulses have been located, both nurses start counting at an agreed-upon point, such as when the second hand reaches a particular number or when one nurse gives a prearranged signal to start counting. The pulse rates are counted simultaneously for an agreed-upon length of time, usually 30 or 60 seconds. *Both* rates are recorded in the appropriate place on the patient's chart.

It is possible for one nurse to obtain an *approximate* apical-radial pulse by taking first one and then the other, but this is *not* precise and should be done only when a second nurse is not available, such as during a home visit.

BLOOD PRESSURE

Blood pressure is the force exerted by the blood against the walls of a blood vessel. The *diastolic blood pressure* is the pressure of the blood during cardiac diastole, the period when the ventricles are relaxed and filling. It is the minimal, constant pressure against the vessel walls. The *systolic blood pressure* is the maximum pressure of the blood during cardiac systole, when the left ventricle contracts and forces additional blood into the aorta, thereby increasing the pressure against the vessel walls.

Blood pressure is measured in millimeters of mercury (mm Hg), and the measurement equals the height to which the blood pressure can raise a column of mercury against the force of gravity. An average systolic

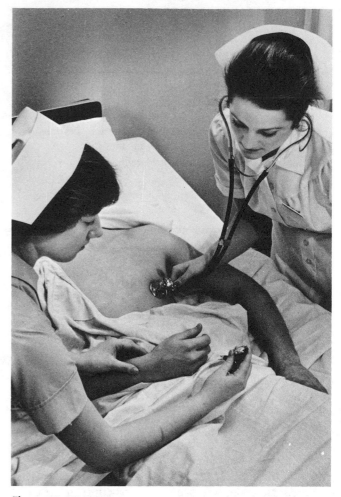

Figure 18.15 *Two nurses must count an apical-radial pulse simultaneously.*

pressure for a young adult is 120 mm Hg, and the average diastolic pressure is 80 mm Hg. This blood pressure (BP) is written 120/80, and the form of the notation is the basis for the common practice of reporting a BP as "120 over 80."

PROCEDURE 18.5

*Taking an Apical-Radial Pulse**

SUMMARY OF ESSENTIAL NURSING ACTIONS

1. Explain your actions if this procedure is new to the patient or he is concerned about the status of his heart.
2. Secure the assistance of another nurse.
3. Decide who will count the apical pulse and who will count the radial pulse.

4. Agree upon the point at which you will both start counting, using the *same watch or clock*.
5. Silently count the pulse rates for the length of time specified by school or agency.
6. Record both rates as indicated by agency policy.

*See inside front cover.

Blood pressure varies with age and is affected by stress, anger, pain, physical exercise, position, disease, and drugs. There is a range of normal BP for every age; it is important to know a patient's usual BP because a change of 20 to 30 mm Hg could be very significant for that patient even though the changed BP is well within the normal range for his age. Blood pressure increases slowly from infancy through middle age, when it begins to increase more rapidly (Table 18.3).

A person is said to be *hyper*tensive if his BP is persistently elevated beyond 140/90. *Hypo*tension is a condition in which the BP is persistently below average for a given age. *Orthostatic hypotension* is a form of low BP that occurs when a person suddenly assumes an erect position.

It is as important for a person to know his normal BP as it is for him to know his weight or blood type. Hypertension is a major health problem, and an awareness of one's blood pressure is an important aspect of prevention and early diagnosis and treatment. Except in situations in which specific information might increase a patient's anxiety and worry to an intolerable level, a patient should be told his blood pressure.

Equipment

The blood pressure of a critically ill patient in an intensive care unit can be measured *directly* by means of a catheter inserted into a major artery and attached to electronic equipment. Such measurement is potentially hazardous and is used only in special situations.

Blood pressure is measured *indirectly* with a stethoscope and a sphygmomanometer (sfig'mo-mah-nom'e-ter). The sphygmomanometer is an inflatable cuff attached by tubing to either a mercury or an aneroid manometer. A mercury manometer contains an upright column of mercury and a scale calibrated in millimeters. An aneroid manometer contains a spring and a round dial with a needle that points to the pressure. Its dials are calibrated from a mercury manometer. The aneroid manometer is compact and portable and easy for a person such as a community health nurse to carry; but unless it is well cared for and recalibrated at intervals, it may be less accurate than a mercury manometer.

Size of Cuff

The cuff of the sphygmomanometer should be an appropriate size for the patient. The standard sizes are newborn, infant, child, adult, large adult, and thigh. The choice of a cuff depends on the circumference of a patient's arm or leg. The inflatable bladder inside the cuff should extend at least halfway around the limb.

The width of the cuff is also important, and it is generally accepted that the width of the cuff should be 20 percent wider than the diameter of the arm or leg. This guideline, however, is one of those rules that are widely accepted and quoted but rarely used because there is no practical way to do so. In this case, there is no practical way to determine the diameter of an arm or leg quickly. To do so would require either calipers or a ruler, tape measure, and a knowledge of algebra. It is important to use *your best judgment and common sense* when trying to find an appropriate size of cuff, especially if a patient is short and fat, or tall and thin. A cuff that is *long* enough to encircle the plump arm of a short fat person may be too wide, and a small cuff *short* enough to fit the thin arm of a very slim tall person is likely to be too narrow.

A cuff that is *too narrow* will give a falsely high reading because it does not cover enough of the artery and excessive pressure is needed to compress the artery. A cuff that is *too wide* will give a low reading.

Application of Cuff

The cuff consists of an inflatable bladder with a larger fabric covering. It should be wrapped *smoothly, evenly,* and *snugly* around the arm or leg because a cuff that is wrapped too loosely or unevenly will give a distorted reading. On an arm, the cuff is placed so that the lower edge of the bladder is centered about 2.5 to 5 cm (1 to 2 inches) above the inner aspect of the elbow (the antecubital space).

When a leg is used to measure BP, the popliteal artery behind the knee is used. If this is possible, the patient is helped into a prone position (on his abdomen). If not, he is positioned on his side with the knee slightly flexed. The cuff is wrapped snugly, smoothly, and evenly around the thigh, just above the knee, and the stethoscope is placed over the popliteal artery behind the knee.

TABLE 18.3 BLOOD PRESSURE ALTERATIONS THROUGHOUT LIFE

Age (yr)	Blood Pressure (mm Hg)
Infant	90/60
3–6	110/70
7–10	120/80
11–15	130/80
15–20	130/85
20–40	140/90
40–60	160/95
60–75	170/95
75 and older	180/100

Adapted from The American Heart Association.

Measurement

Because the sphygmomanometer is not in contact with the blood, it does not measure BP directly. It measures the *amount of external pressure* needed to offset the blood pressure and to stop the flow of blood through the arteries.

Measurement by Auscultation

Auscultation of the brachial artery with a stethoscope just below the blood pressure cuff reveals characteristic sounds when the cuff pressure is increased or decreased. These sounds were first described in the early 1900s by a Russian physician named Korotkoff and are known as Korotkoff sounds. Before the cuff is inflated, no sounds are heard because the artery is not compressed and it can pulsate freely. Characteristic sounds are heard when the cuff is partially inflated and the artery is slightly compressed. When the pressure of the cuff *exceeds the systolic pressure,* the brachial artery is fully compressed; blood cannot flow through the artery and there is no pulsation. When the artery is not pulsating, there are no sounds.

When the cuff is partially deflated and the pressure in the cuff *equals the systolic pressure* of the heart, the blood begins to flow through the partially compressed artery and it pulsates with each beat of the heart. This blood flow produces a clear, sharp, distinct tapping sound, and the reading at which it is first heard is the patient's systolic blood pressure. When the cuff is further deflated and the pressure in the cuff *equals the diastolic blood pressure,* the blood flows freely and sounds are no longer heard. The point at which the sound disappears is accepted in some agencies as the diastolic blood pressure, although other agencies use the change of sound that precedes the cessation of sound as the diastolic pressure. The American Heart Association accepts as the diastolic pressure the point at which the quality of sound *changes* from a clear, distinct tapping sound to a soft, muffled sound or murmur. Some hospitals and agencies use all three measurements: the *clear tapping sound* (the systolic pressure), *muffled sound or murmur* (the first diastolic sound), and the *cessation of sound* (the second diastolic sound). These measurements are recorded as 130/86/82

$$\text{or } \frac{130}{86/82} \text{ for example.}$$

If only one diastolic pressure is being used in an agency, the nurse needs to ask whether it indicates the change of sound or the cessation of sound so that her method of measurement will be consistent with the one used by the rest of the staff. Even with a consistent method of measurement, there is likely to be some variation between readings because diastolic readings especially tend to vary with the quality and placement of the stethoscope, and the hearing of the nurse.

Measurement by Palpation

In addition to auscultation of the brachial artery, blood pressure can be determined by *palpation of the radial artery.* The radial pulse disappears and reappears as the cuff pressure is increased and then decreased. The point at which the radial pulse reappears is the systolic blood pressure. The diastolic pressure is difficult to determine by palpation, but an experienced practitioner can detect a quick whipping or snapping sensation at that point.

The palpatory method of taking a BP is used in emergency situations when the patient is in shock and his cardiac output is too low to produce a pulsation strong enough to be auscultated. It is also used during the initial physical assessment of an adult patient in order to prevent an error that can be caused by a phenomenon known as an *auscultatory gap,* which occurs in patients with hypertension. In such cases, the first Korotkoff sounds may be heard at a high pressure and then disappear, only to reappear at a lower pressure. If, initially, the cuff is not inflated enough, the silence of the auscultatory gap may be mistaken for the silence that precedes the first Korotkoff sounds. If the top sounds are missed, the sounds that *follow* the auscultatory gap will be mistaken for the first Korotkoff sounds, making the systolic pressure seem much lower than it actually is.

This error can be prevented by palpating the radial pulse and then inflating the cuff until the pulse can no longer be felt. *The radial pulse is palpable during an auscultatory gap,* so if the cuff is inflated *until the pulse is obliterated,* the gap will have been passed. Upon deflation, the point at which the pulse returns will be the systolic pressure. This palpated systolic measurement indicates the mm Hg which will be needed for accurate measurements using the auscultatory method, and the BP cuff is then inflated above that point when the BP is taken.

Guidelines for Taking Blood Pressure

Important points related to taking a BP include the following:

- Take a patient's BP *whenever his condition warrants it* as well as at the time scheduled. Routinely scheduled BP's should be taken at the same time each day with the patient in the same position

PROCEDURE 18.6

Taking a Blood Pressure*

SUMMARY OF ESSENTIAL NURSING ACTIONS

1. Prepare the patient's arm.
   - Expose the arm from axilla to elbow.
   - Place it in a relaxed supported position about heart level
2. Position the blood pressure cuff properly.
   - Make sure the cuff size is appropriate.
   - Center the lower edge of the inflatable bladder about 1 in above the bend of the elbow (the antecubital space).
3. Make sure the gauge is easily visible and registers zero.
4. Position the stethoscope correctly over the brachial artery.
5. Inflate the cuff about 30 mm Hg above the likely systolic pressure.

6. Deflate the cuff slowly enough to obtain an accurate reading.
7. Note the reading at which the Korotkoff sounds specified by the agency are heard (first sound plus change of sounds and/or last sound).
8. If necessary to recheck your reading, wait 1–2 minutes before doing so.
9. If an auscultatory gap is suspected, or if the blood pressure is too low to be auscultated, use palpation of the radial artery and the blood pressure cuff to determine the systolic pressure.

*See inside front cover.

each time (sitting, standing, lying down). Consistency of measurement is important in obtaining accurate data.

- Position the arm so it is relaxed and supported at heart level with the elbow slightly flexed.

- Inflate the cuff about 30 mm Hg *above the likely systolic pressure* as determined previously by the palpatory method or indicated by previous readings. *Inflating the cuff any higher than necessary produces unnecessary pain and discomfort.*

- Decrease the cuff pressure at a rate of *2 to 4 mm Hg/per second.* Decreasing the pressure too slowly prolongs the patient's discomfort; decreasing the pressure too rapidly makes an accurate reading unlikely.

- If you are not sure that your reading was accurate, *wait a full minute* and then retake it. The pressure of the cuff causes a temporary venous congestion in the arm which must be relieved before the second measurement can be accurate.

- Blood pressure is affected by stress, illness, emotions, and physical activity and it must be taken at regular times for several days to determine the normal BP for a given person; a single measurement can be misleading.

- BP should *not* be taken on an arm that has been injured or diseased, that has an IV running, or that is on the side of a patient's radical mastectomy. An unimpaired arm should be used for BP measurement.

Section Five

Physical Examination

PHYSICAL EXAMINATION

In a literal sense, the terms *physical examination* and *physical assessment* are interchangeable, but in practice, the terms are used differently. *Physical examination* usually refers to a comprehensive evaluation of a patient's overall physical condition; *physical assessment* commonly refers to the evaluation of a specific body part or system, such as an assessment of a patient's respiratory status. This chapter generally reflects that distinction.

A physical examination is done:

- As part of regular, preventive health care
- To detect any problems that might affect performance in college, military service, summer camp, police work, a new job, or other new situation
- As part of the admission procedure in a hospital
- To make a diagnosis
- To determine the extent of a disease or condition

Relevant portions of the physical examination are done to:

- Determine the progress of a disease condition
- Evaluate a patient's physical response to therapy

- Obtain data as a basis for making decisions about care and treatment.

Nurses in screening centers, neighborhood health centers, private practice, and primary care often give complete physical examinations; but more frequently, a nurse does that part of a physical examination which will provide the information she needs for planning and evaluating nursing care. For example, before chemotherapy for cancer, a thorough assessment of the patient's mouth is needed to plan care that will prevent or minimize some of the devastating side effects of the drug on the mouth. A community health nurse will assess the heart and lungs of a patient with a history of congestive heart failure who is finding it difficult to breathe, and the school nurse will assess the muscles and nerves of a child who has begun to fall frequently.

After each assessment or examination, the nurse will *treat* those conditions that are *within the province of nursing,* such as the need for intensive mouth care. She will report to the physician those conditions that need medical diagnosis and treatment, such as pleural fluid or a suspected neurological disturbance.

PSYCHOLOGICAL PREPARATION OF THE PATIENT

Many people experience considerable stress during a physical examination, either because of embarrassment or because of anxiety about the outcome. *Embarrassment* may result from one or more of the following:

- Exposure of body parts
- Manipulation of the body, such as examination of the breasts
- Being questioned about intimate body functions
- Examination of rectal and genital areas

Embarrassment may be intensified by age or by lack of previous experience with physical examinations. Students from grade school through high school seem consistent in their dread and dislike of "school physicals." A person who states, "I've never been sick a day in my life," often finds the first complete physical examination very stressful, especially if she is an older woman who must undergo a pelvic examination.

Careful draping, a chance to undress and dress in private, thoughtful attention to verbal and nonverbal cues, and a thorough explanation of what the patient is to do and to expect will help to minimize embarrassment. When the patient and the examiner are of the opposite sex, it may help to have a third person of the same sex as the patient in the room during potentially embarrassing parts of the examination. It is important to remember that the examination of an adolescent boy by a female nurse or physician may be just as embarrassing for him as the examination of an adolescent girl by a male nurse or physician.

A second source of stress during a physical examinatin is *anxiety about the outcome*. The outcome is almost always significant because of its impact on the person's life. The person who is having a physical examination because of illness or disease is apprehensive—the examination will either help to make a diagnosis or it will fail to yield a diagnosis, thereby prolonging the indecision of not knowing what is the matter. Even a healthy person is beset by thoughts and questions such as: "I won't get the job if I fail the physical—What will I do then?" or "Suppose he finds something wrong that I don't even know I have?"

Measures to relieve anxiety related to a physical examination are similar to those used in conjunction with diagnostic tests and are described in detail in the next section. Briefly, the patient should receive an explanation about the examination, and any questions should be fully answered. He should know the sequence of events, what to expect, and what he will be expected to do. Neither the embarrassment nor the anxiety can be relieved completely, but both can be minimized by adequate preparation and by support during the examination.

PHYSICAL PREPARATION OF THE PATIENT

Physical preparation of the patient includes advance preparation, general comfort measures, and positioning of the patient for the examination.

Advance Preparation

The advance preparation needed is determined either by orders that are specific for a given patient or by accepted protocol. *Protocol* is a term for a set of orders, policies, or treatments that constitutes the standard operating procedure for a designated set of circumstances. An established protocol obviates the necessity for writing the same plans or orders every time a commonly encountered situation arises. These orders or guidelines are sometimes called *standing orders*.

Protocol may cover almost any aspect of health care, from the routine admission of a patient to a hospital, to the patient teaching done after certain kinds of surgery. Protocol for preparation of a patient for a physical examination means that, unless something else is specifically ordered, each patient is to be prepared in accordance with predetermined orders. Examples of such orders are:

- No douching for 24 hours before a pelvic exam and Pap test
- Enemas until clear before a proctoscopic examination

General Comfort Measures

Comfort during the physical examination promotes relaxation, which in turn contributes to the accuracy of the examination. Nervousness, feeling cold, and a full bladder, for example, may cause a patient to tense his abdomen enough to make palpation very difficult. Anxiety and discomfort can elevate the patient's BP as well as his respiratory and pulse rates.

Physical comfort and subsequent relaxation can be increased by attending to a patient's basic needs through such measures as making sure that he is warm enough and telling him where the toilet is. Many patients are reluctant to ask for anything that might be considered unimportant, so the nurse should ask if the patient needs anything, such as a tissue, a drink of water, or a place to put his glasses.

In addition to general comfort measures, patient safety must be ensured. A frail patient may need assistance in getting on and off a high examining table or in maintaining a difficult position during the examination. An agitated, distraught child may need to be held by one of his parents or by a nurse throughout the examination.

Positioning

During a physical examination, the patient is asked to assume one or more of the following positions: erect or standing, dorsal recumbent, lithotomy, Sims, or knee chest.

The *erect or standing position* is used to assess posture, balance, gait, and symmetry of body contours. In the *dorsal recumbent* position, the patient lies on his back with a small pillow under his head (Fig. 18.16). This position is used for examination of the anterior chest,

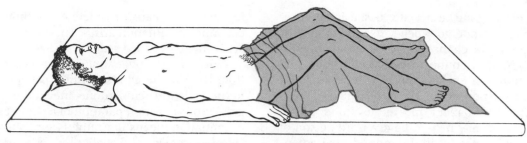

Figure 18.16 *Dorsal recumbent position.*

breasts, abdomen, and legs. The patient's knees are flexed or extended as directed by the examiner.

The *lithotomy* position is used for examination of the vagina, cervix, and rectum. In this position, the patient lies on her back with her knees sharply flexed. Her hips are slid toward the end of the examining table, and metal stirrups are used to elevate and support his feet and legs (Fig. 18.17).

In the *Sims* position, the patient lies on one side with the lower arm behind the back and the upper hip and knee sharply flexed (Fig. 18.18). This position is used for examination of the rectum or vagina.

The *knee-chest* position is embarrassing, difficult to assume, and uncomfortable to maintain. To assume this position, the patient turns onto his abdomen, flexes his knees, and elevates his hips until his body weight rests on his chest and knees (Fig. 18.19). The *hips should be directly over the knees.* Whenever possible, the patient's elbows are flexed and his arms are over his head. A patient may not be able to tolerate this and may have to place his arms at his sides or under his abdomen.

The knee-chest position is used for instrumental examination of the rectum (proctoscopy) or sigmoid colon (sigmoidoscopy). Both physical and psychological support will be needed for a person who is stiff, feeble, or in pain to assume and maintain this position. It can be both painful and exhausting, and such a patient should not be expected to maintain it for more than a moment or two.

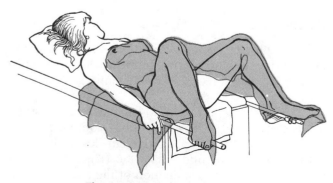

Figure 18.17 *Lithotomy position.*

PREPARATION OF ROOM AND EQUIPMENT

The room should be neat, clean, and as attractive as possible, with all equipment and supplies in good working order and arranged for efficient use by the examiner. Adequate overall lighting is essential, plus extra spot lighting as needed for special examinations, and a provision for darkening the room for eye examinations. If any specimens, cultures, or tissue samples are to be taken, the properly labeled containers should be ready for use.

The basic equipment for a complete physical examination includes:

Stethoscope
Sphygmomanometer
Otoscope
Ophthalmoscope
Tonometer
Tape measure
Reflex hammer
Tuning fork
Vaginal speculum
Watch or clock with second hand
Scale with height measuring rod
Container for soiled instruments
Specimen containers (labeled)
Drapes for covering patient
Penlight
Eye chart
Thermometer
Tongue blades
Head mirror
Adjustable light
Lubricant
Gloves
Alcohol

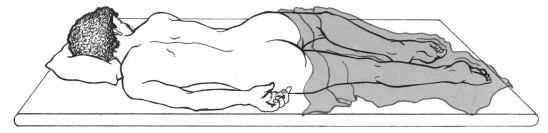

Figure 18.18 *Sim's position.*

Waste container
Skin pen or pencil
Pin
Paper towels or tissues

CONDUCT OF THE EXAMINATION

The purpose of a physical examination determines its thoroughness and extent. A *diagnostic examination,* for example, is likely to be more extensive and comprehensive than a *follow-up examination* after surgery; and the President's yearly physical is more complete than a child's physical for Scout camp.

The examiner's initial contact with the patient provides an opportunity to assess approximate age, sex, any signs of distress, stature, mood, alertness and orientation, speech, grooming, posture, gait, and overall physical condition. The examiner then proceeds to take the patient's medical or nursing history. The patient's height, weight, TPR, and BP are measured and recorded, and the actual physical examination is started.

A physical examination usually follows whatever pattern has proved useful to the examiner. There is no right or wrong sequence, but the examination should be structured and organized in such a way that no parts of it are forgotten or unintentionally omitted. Some parts of the examination are often *deliberately deferred* during an emergency or if a patient is in pain or discomfort, but this is a conscious decision.

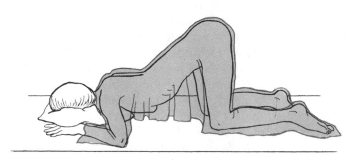

Figure 18.19 *Knee-chest position.*

A commonly used sequence is head to toe. After an initial overall assessment of the patient as a whole, the examiner proceeds to examine the patient's head and neck, anterior chest, posterior chest, abdomen, extremities, genitals, and rectum. This examination may be followed by a neurological examination and a more extensive musculoskeletal examination.

AFTERCARE OF THE PATIENT

If the physical examination has been long and tiring for a patient, the nurse may need to help him dress. A patient may need tissues to wipe away any lubricant from a rectal or pelvic examination and may want to use the bathroom. It may be necessary for the nurse to anticipate a patient's need for certain information. If the examiner gave any explanations at all, the patient may not ask questions because he may think, "The doctor (or nurse) explained it—I ought to be able to remember it for 15 minutes, at least." In reality, the patient may not remember or understand because the explanation may have been unclear, incomplete, or poorly timed. The patient's stress level may have been so high that it was impossible for him even to hear the examiner's explanations or directions.

Spoken or unspoken questions that need answers include: "What do those words mean?" "What does that diagnosis mean?" "What do I do now?" "When is my next appointment?" "Where is that place where I am supposed to go?" "What is that test going to be like?" "What is going to happen now?" Careful answers to such questions coupled with a discussion of the patient's concerns and reactions will relieve anxiety and help ensure the patient's ability to follow any directions given, and to participate in any forthcoming diagnostic activities or treatment.

METHODS OF PHYSICAL ASSESSMENT

Data are obtained during a physical examination through the activities of inspection, auscultation, palpation, and percussion. Each of these techniques enables a nurse or physician to assess a different aspect of an organ or body part and, by combining the data, to describe the size, location, condition, and functioning of a given organ or structure.

Inspection

Inspection is the visual scrutiny of a body part or cavity. The examiner's attention is focused sharply on a specific area and when s(he) has thoroughly inspected that area, the examiner is able to describe its size, shape, color, symmetry, position, and normalcy. Inspection of the patient's skin and mouth can be done with the unaided eye, but a lighted instrument called an *endoscope* must be used to visualize the *interior* of a body cavity, such as the esophagus, larynx, or urinary bladder. The use of this instrument is described in detail in the next section.

Auscultation

Auscultation is the act of listening to sounds produced by body organs and blood vessels. Auscultation is used to assess heart, lung, and bowel function, and it is also used to monitor the fetal heart during labor and delivery. Some auscultation can be done directly by placing an ear against the patient's chest or abdomen, but most sounds are too diffuse or too soft to be heard without a stethoscope.

Equipment

Toy stethoscopes can transmit some heart sounds, and the stethoscopes sold to lay people are sometimes adequate for taking routine blood pressures. *Clinical auscultation,* however, requires a stethoscope of excellent quality which fits the examiner properly. The plastic tips of the earpieces must fit securely and comfortably, and it may be necessary to replace one or both of them if they do not fit the nurse's ear canals properly. The long metal earpieces should be properly angled and strong enough to hold the plastic tips firmly in the ears without discomfort. The rubber tubing should be 12 to 18 in long and appropriate for the examiner's height. The tubing should be thick-walled enough to exclude extraneous sounds but not stiff or inflexible.

The chest piece should include both a diaphragm and a bell. The bell transmits low-pitched sounds best; the diaphragm amplifies and transmits higher-pitched sounds. (A memory device for this relationship is: *bell* and *low* both include the letter l, whereas *diaphragm* and *high* both contain the letter h.)

The stethoscope is one of the nurse's most important pieces of professional equipment; upon purchase, it should be altered as necessary to ensure a perfect fit. The plastic earpieces, the angle of the metal earpieces, and the length of the tubing can be altered or replaced as needed. Because a good stethoscope is expensive, common sense dictates that it be permanently identified with the nurse's name.

A nurse who does not own a stethoscope and shares one which is used by other staff, should first of all clean the plastic earpieces before placing them in her ears. Some nurses carry a few foil-wrapped alcohol wipes in their pockets for this purpose. It is a good technique (and common courtesy) also to cleanse the earpieces after using them.

The earpieces should follow the contour of the ear canal; therefore, the ends of the metal earpieces should point toward the face, not toward the back of the head. Nothing should be allowed to rub against the tubing while you are using the stethoscope because the resulting sounds will distort or mask the body sounds you are listening for.

The position of the chest piece can be changed to accommodate either the bell or the diaphragm. Before you try to use either one, tap the diaphragm lightly with your finger. If the tap is greatly amplified, the diaphragm is in position for use. If the tap on the diaphragm is barely audible, the bell is in position for use.

The diaphragm should be pressed *firmly* against the patient's skin to get the maximum benefit of its potential for amplifying sound. The bell, on the other hand, should be pressed *lightly* because, when pressed too tightly, the skin is stretched across the bell, causing it to resemble a diaphragm.

Auscultatory Sounds

The sounds heard by auscultation are described in terms of four characteristics: pitch, loudness, duration, and quality.

Pitch ranges from high to low and is related to the number of vibrations (frequency) per unit of time. The fewer the number of vibrations, the lower the pitch. In the context of auscultation, the word *frequency* refers to the *pitch* of the sound; it does not refer to the number of times the sound occurs. *Loudness* refers to the intensity of the sound and is described simply as loud or soft. *Duration* refers to the length of the sound and is described as short, medium, or long.

The *quality* of a sound refers to those characteristics that distinguish sounds of equal pitch and intensity, such as some heart sounds and bowel sounds. Some differentiations are quite obvious and easily learned; others are subtle and are learned only by the auscultation of hundreds of patients. These sounds are described by a wide variety of descriptive terms, such as blowing, swishing, gurgling, and crackling. Many sounds have a specific name, such as rale, rhonchus, and bruit. It is important to know and be able to use these terms in order to communicate your findings to others without having to describe each sound. The assessment and interpretation of commonly heard lung, heart, and bowel sounds are described in Chapters 32 and 34.

Any nurse for whom auscultation is difficult or who has a hearing problem (or suspects that she might) is obligated to seek help at once. A nurse has a *moral and legal responsibility* to auscultate with accuracy. Failure to do so because of an uncorrected hearing problem could be a basis for charges of negligence or malpractice.

Palpation

The sense of touch is highly developed in the human hand, and it is possible to make delicate and sensitive assessments on the basis of tactile sensations. These sensations enable the nurse to differentiate between tissues on the basis of the following characteristics:

- Firmness and flaccidness (good and poor muscle tone)
- Hardness and softness (lumps or swelling and normal tissue)
- Roughness and smoothness (rough, scaly skin and normal, smooth skin)
- Hotness and coldness (inflamed tissue and areas of poor circulation)
- Stillness and movement or vibration (presence or absence of a pulse)

Palpation involves the use of the fingers of one or both hands, and it may be superficial or deep. It is done to assess an organ, area of the body, or mass of tissue. The characteristics which can be assessed by palpation are shape, size, location, consistency, tenderness, and mobility. Areas that are examined by palpation include:

Axilla: to detect enlarged lymph nodes

Breast: to locate any lumps or masses

Skin: to assess turgor, temperature, and moisture

Neck: to detect nodules or irregularity of the thyroid gland or lymph nodes

Vagina: to assess shape and consistency of the cervix

Chest: to discern vibrations (tactile fremitus)

Ankles: to evaluate the extent of any edema

Abdomen: to assess size, shape, and location of organs and to detect any lumps or masses

Eyes: to assess intraocular tension

Rectum: to assess cervix or prostate gland through the rectal wall; to detect any masses or irregularity of rectal wall

Effective palpation requires skill, gentleness, warm hands, and short fingernails. The part of the hand to be used depends in part on the type of assessment to be made. The pads of the fingertips are the most sensitive to touch and are used to assess shape, size, consistency, and texture. The palm and the ulnar surface (the outer side) of the hand are most sensitive to vibration and are used to assess the degree of tactile fremitus in the chest. Either the back of the hand or the ulnar surface is used to assess skin temperature.

Sensitivity to touch is *decreased* by heavy pressure and by prolonged pressure, so when you palpate, your *pressure should be light and intermittent*. When deep, firm pressure is needed for a specific assessment, sensitivity of touch can be retained by using two hands, one on top of the other. The lower hand is relaxed and rests *lightly* on the patient's skin. The upper hand presses down on the under hand and provides the pressure necessary for deep palpation (Fig. 18.20). This technique protects the sensitivity of the under hand because all pressure is exerted by the upper hand.

Palpation is difficult when a patient is obese, tense, ticklish, or in pain. It is important to watch for and respond to any verbal or nonverbal expression of discomfort. If the nurse has reason to believe that palpation of an area will be uncomfortable or painful, she should ask the patient to point to the sensitive spots so she can leave the examination of those areas until last. She then proceeds slowly, helping him to relax with all the techniques at her command.

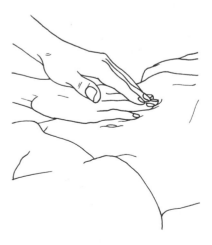

Figure 18.20 *Position of the hands for deep palpation.*

Percussion

Percussion is the act of striking a blow to create a series of vibrations, as with the percussion instruments in an orchestra. In nursing, both direct and indirect percussion are used during physical assessment.

Direct percussion with a percussion hammer is done to test body reflexes. Percussion with the side of the hand produces pain if the underlying tissue is inflamed or infected, and is done to assess the kidneys or sinuses.

Indirect percussion occurs when the examiner inserts something between the object to be percussed and the hammer that strikes the blow. This technique amplifies or clarifies the sound. In nursing, the middle finger of the examiner's hand is placed between the patient and the hammer (the middle finger of the other hand).

Indirect percussion produces both an audible sound and vibrations that are transmitted through the nurse's hands, permitting the use of both hearing and touch. Indirect percussion is sensitive enough to enable the nurse to differentiate between solid and air-filled areas of the body. Differences between the percussion sounds of the abdomen and the chest enable the nurse to locate the level of the diaphragm, for example. Specific assessments of the chest and abdomen that can be made by percussion are described in Chapters 32 and 34. To percuss an area effectively, a nurse must be able to use both hands correctly and to differentiate between the sounds that result from percussion.

Use of Hands for Percussion

1. Hyperextend the middle finger of your nondominant hand and press its distal phalanx and joint on the body part to be percussed (Fig. 18.21). *Make sure that no other part of that hand touches the patient* because such contact will dampen or suppress vibrations just as putting your hand on a drumhead as it is being struck distorts the sound. The finger that is touching the patient and that receives the blow during percussion is called the *pleximeter finger*.

2. Position the middle finger of your dominant hand so that it can strike the pleximeter finger of the other hand. The finger that strikes the blow is called the *plexor finger*. The *tip*, not the pad, of the plexor finger is used, and the nail must be very short to prevent injury to the other hand (Figure 18.21).

3. Hold the plexor finger in a flexed position and aim each blow at the base of the nail of the pleximeter finger. The plexor finger does not move; *all movement comes from the wrist*. Make each blow sharp and quick; the plexor finger should bounce off the pleximeter finger rather than poke or push it. A slow, poorly controlled blow will produce muffled or damped vibrations.

A verbal description of percussion makes the movements sound easy enough. In reality, considerable practice may be needed before *every* blow of the plexor finger strikes between the distal joint and the nail of the pleximeter finger; 50, 75, or even 90 percent accuracy is not good enough for effective percussion. Practice does not require the presence of a patient; it can be done on one's own body, on a desk, or against a wall.

Differentiation of Sounds

There are five categories of percussion notes that can be distinguished by a nurse skilled in percussion. The ability to differentiate between these sounds must be acquired through practice because verbal descriptions are inadequate.

The two most frequently encountered normal sounds are *resonance* and *dullness* (nonresonance). Resonant means resounding, ringing, or echoing, and resonance denotes the presence of these characteristics. Resonance is the low-pitched sound that is heard over normal lung tissue.

Tissue that is more solid than lung tissue does not resonate and therefore sounds dull and flat. Dullness describes the sound produced by percussion over the heart or liver. The resonance of normal lung tissue is replaced by dullness if the lungs become filled with fluid or replaced by the solid tissue of a tumor.

A hollow, air-filled organ is more resonant than lung tissue, and the percussed sound is called *tympany*. Tym-

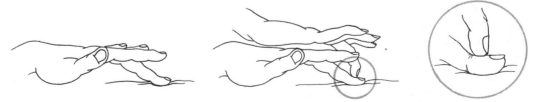

Figure 18.21 *Position of the hands for percussion. Note that only one finger of the lower hand touches the patient and that the plexor finger strikes at a right angle.*

panic means drumlike. Tympany is heard when a puffed-out cheek or an abdomen distended with gas is percussed.

Flatness is an extreme form of dullness that can be heard when a completely solid area, such as a thigh, is percussed. (Some experts use the terms flatness and dullness interchangeably to indicate the absence of resonance.)

Hyperresonance is an ab 'ormal sound that can be heard when a structure contains more air than normal, as when a lung has distended alveoli as the result of emphysema. Since the lung is not a hollow organ, this sound is less resonant than tympany.

The terms used to indicate normal percussion sound can be summarized as follows:

Sound	Intensity	Pitch	Duration
Flatness	Soft	High	Brief
Dullness	Medium	Medium	Medium
Resonance	Loud	Low	Long
Tympany	Louder	Lower	Longer

Some nurses learn to differentiate between percussed sounds very quickly, but others find at first that they simply cannot hear the differences. If you are in the latter group, you will need extensive practice in listening to percussed sounds before you become skillful enough to percuss a patient's chest or abdomen *effectively.* Some students find it helpful to practice on a wall and to listen for a change in resonance which a carpenter hears when he is trying to locate a stud in the wall. The solid wood of the stud will sound dull, whereas the air spaces between studs will sound hollow and resonant. Additional daily practice on yourself, and on family and friends whenever possible, will develop your percussion skills.

Four sites are useful in training the ear to differentiate between percussed sounds. These sites and the sounds produced by each are:

Thigh: flatness
Liver: dullness
Lungs: resonance
Puffed-out cheek: tympany

In addition, an assigned patient will often permit you to percuss his chest and abdomen as part of your clinical activities, thereby expanding the scope of your practice and skill.

PROCEDURE 18.7

*Percussion**

SUMMARY OF ESSENTIAL NURSING ACTIONS

1. Position your *nondominant* hand over the area to be percussed
   - Place hyperextended middle finger on skin.
   - Do not let any other part of that hand touch the area to be percussed.
2. Position your *dominant* hand so that the middle finger of that hand (the plexor finger) can strike the middle finger of the lower hand (the pleximeter finger).
3. Make sure that each blow is effective and precise.
   - Keep plexor finger flexed while percussing.
   - Aim each blow at the base of the nail of the hyperextended lower finger.
   - Strike with the *tip*, not the pad, of the plexor finger.
   - Use *wrist movement* to supply the force for each blow; do *not* move the flexed plexor finger.
   - Make each blow sharp and quick enough to make the plexor finger bounce back.
4. Move hands about over surface being percussed until all areas of dullness and resonance have been accurately identified.

*See inside front cover.

Section Six

Diagnostic Tests

DIAGNOSTIC TESTS

Diagnostic tests are done to obtain objective data that will enable a physician or nurse practitioner to confirm a tentative diagnosis, rule out a possible diagnosis, or differentiate between two or more diagnoses. Diagnostic tests are relevant to the practice of nursing for three reasons. First, the success of a test often depends upon the proper preparation of the patient by the nurse. Second, skillful nursing care following some diagnostic tests is often essential for the patient's safety and well-being. Third, a knowledge of the testing procedure and the results of the test will influence the nursing care that is planned for that patient.

Diagnostic tests are likely to be stressful for the patient because they reflect the uncertainty and ambiguity of the period when nobody knows what is wrong. Each diagnostic test has the potential for confirming a patient's worst fears or for relieving a particular worry. Therefore, the patient approaches any test with mixed emotions. He needs much support and understanding at this time because a test that is routine for the staff may seem to the patient to be almost a life-or-death matter.

The patient and his family need an opportunity to discuss their feelings of apprehension and anxiety both before the test and during the period of waiting for the results. During this waiting period, members of the health team are busy (and accustomed to waiting for test results), but a patient may have little else to think about at this time. He needs to be told whether it will take a few hours or a few days to learn the results, and he needs to be told the reason for any real or seeming delays. The patient's need for emotional support at this time is often overlooked simply because it may not be apparent. Nurses, family, and friends often respond quickly to the needs of a newly diagnosed patient but may be less helpful during the uncertain and anxious period *before* a diagnosis is made.

The patient and family may also need help in coping with the impact of the results. The test results may indicate that the condition is one that cannot be cured but which will be chronic, that surgery is needed, or that more tests will be needed before a diagnosis can be made. The nurse will need to assess each patient's response to test results because any given result can elicit a different response from each patient. One patient's response to a newly diagnosed gastric ulcer might be "Oh no! How can I ever manage?" while another's response might be "That's great! I was so afraid it was cancer!" Responses to a diagnosis will range from hope and relief to despair or deep concern over finances, pain, or family disruption.

PREPARATION OF THE PATIENT

Preparation of the patient for a diagnostic test must include a complete and accurate explanation that answers the traditional who, what, where, when, why, and how questions.

  Why has the test been ordered? (What does the physician expect to find?)
  What will be done? (Will it hurt?)

Who will do the test? (Nurse, physician, or technician?)

When and where will it be done? (In the patient's room? In the x-ray department?)

How will it be done? (In what position? With what kind of equipment?)

There should be no surprises for the patient. He should know in advance, for example, if the test will be done in a dark room or if the head of the examining table will be tilted down during the test. After a diagnostic test, if you encourage each patient to talk about his experience, you will gradually accumulate from your patients a number of significant hints, tips, and ideas that will help future patients cope with the discomfort or stress of a diagnostic test.

When a diagnostic test is done by a technician, as in the x-ray department, a nurse is not usually present. The patient is taken to that department, sometimes by a volunteer worker, and left in the corridor or waiting area. He is tested by the technician, who probably has never seen him before, and returned to the corridor or waiting area to await transfer back to his room. Because the technician has little opportunity to assess the patient as a person, it is vital that the nurse *share pertinent information* about the patient with the technician. Such information might be:

Deafness and inability to hear directions

Dizziness when coming to an erect position

Severe diarrhea all morning

Extreme anxiety, fear, or apprehension

Inability to comprehend and follow more than one direction at a time

Persistent vomiting requiring an emesis basin and tissues to be available at all times

Some patients can and will inform the technician of any difficulty or anticipated problem but others seem unable to do so because of uncertainty, modesty, confusion, or high stress. If a patient is in distress, either physical or psychological, every effort should be made for a nurse, aide, or member of the family to be with the patient during the test. Excuses such as "No one does that" or "It has never been done" are no reason for a vulnerable patient to be left alone at this time. If necessary, the nurse should get a written order from the physician to make sure that the patient will be accompanied.

Regardless of whether a test is done in the patient's unit, a treatment room, or another department, and whether it is done by a nurse, physician, or technician, the attending nurse is responsible for adequate physical preparation of the patient and careful observation of the patient's physical condition after the test.

Adequate physical preparation of the patient helps to ensure that the test can be done as scheduled and that the results will be usable. Faulty preparation often means that the test must be postponed or that the results will be unusable. For example, if a patient mistakenly eats breakfast before an upper GI series, the stomach will contain food, which will distort the x-ray image. The stomach cannot be completely filled with barium and as a result an ulcer, which should show up on the x-ray film as a crater or depression, may not be visible at all. Inadequate preparation or errors in preparation of the patient are costly in time, money, stress, and delayed treatment.

Careful observation of the patient after the test is important because many diagnostic tests are followed by a period of real or potential discomfort. Attentive nursing care is needed to prevent or treat these aftereffects, which will be identified throughout this chapter as each test is described.

TESTS THAT WITHDRAW BODY FLUID OR TISSUE

With the exception of gastric analysis, which may be done by a nurse, tests involving withdrawal of body fluid or tissue are done by a physician. Each test requires penetration of a body cavity and must be done under strict surgical asepsis (sterile technique) to protect the patient against possible infection.

Bone Marrow Biopsy

Analysis of bone marrow is important in the diagnosis of such blood dyscrasias as anemia and leukemia. The most commonly used sites for obtaining bone marrow are the sternum and the iliac crest. Under local anesthesia, the physician inserts a short, thick needle through the bone into the bone marrow cavity. Considerable pressure is needed to force the needle through the bone, and the patient should be prepared for pressure, discomfort, or even pain for a moment. A syringe is then attached to the needle, and 1 to 2 cc of bone marrow is withdrawn. The withdrawal of the marrow produces another instance of momentary pain, for which the patient should also have been prepared. The bone marrow is ejected into a labeled container of preservative and sent to the laboratory.

This test usually evokes considerable anxiety, and the nurse may need to obtain an order for a sedative if the patient is extremely apprehensive.

Preparation of the Patient

To prepare the patient for a sternal biopsy, position him on his back with a folded towel or small pillow between his shoulder blades to elevate the sternum. Shave the area, cleanse the site with an antiseptic solution, and drape the area with sterile towels. Assist the physician as needed, but focus your attention on the patient and his needs.

Aftercare

After the test, apply a small, dry sterile dressing and tell the patient that it is normal for his sternum to be sore for several days.

Gastric Analysis

Gastric analysis is an unpleasant but not painful procedure. A tube is passed through the patient's nose, down his esophagus, and into his stomach for the removal of gastric contents. The volume, composition, and acidity of the contents are analyzed for the diagnosis of conditions such as pernicious anemia and gastric ulcers.

The tube should be large enough to permit aspiration of stomach contents but small enough to avoid major discomfort, and it must be measured and marked so the nurse will know how far to insert it. This is done by measuring the distance from the lower tip of the sternum to the front of the earlobe and on to the bridge

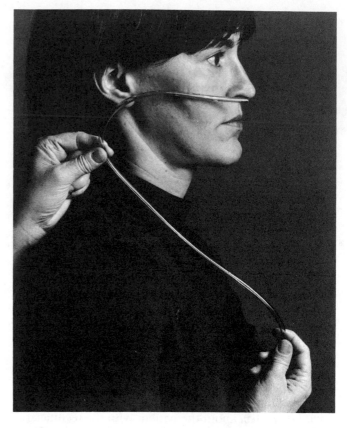

Figure 18.22 *Nasogastric tube measurement is estimated by holding the tube from the nose to the front of the earlobe to the tip of the sternum.*

PROCEDURE 18.8

*Passing a Nasogastric Tube**

SUMMARY OF ESSENTIAL NURSING ACTIONS

1. Mark the distance the nasogastric tube is to be inserted.
2. Position the patient in an upright sitting position.
3. Lubricate the end of the tube with a water soluble substance.
4. Tip the patient's head back and insert the lubricated tip of the tube into a nostril.
5. When the tube reaches the back of the patient's throat, have the patient tilt his head forward and swallow repeatedly.
6. Pass the tube 5–10 cm (2–4 inches) with each swallow.

7. Have the patient take sips of water to promote swallowing.
8. Pause and allow the patient to rest whenever he gags.
9. When the tube has been passed, aspirate to check its position. If no stomach contents are withdrawn, advance the tube another 2 inches, and aspirate again. If the results are still negative, the tube is not in the stomach, and must be withdrawn.
10. Secure the tube to the patient's nose and fasten the end to his gown.
11. Clamp the end if it is to be used for tube feedings, or attach it to suction equipment.

*See inside front cover.

of the nose, and marking that distance on the tube (Fig. 18.22).

If the tube is rubber, it is coiled in a basin of ice to chill it, thereby making it stiffer and easier to insert. The tube is lubricated with a small amount of water-soluble lubricant and inserted into one of the patient's nostrils. When it reaches the back of the patient's throat, he will probably gag, but this sensation will disappear as the tube enters the esophagus. If it persists, you may be passing the tube too slowly or possibly too rapidly. The patient is asked to swallow repeatedly until the mark on the tube reaches his nose. He may be allowed to swallow sips of water during this process unless he has been ordered NPO (nothing by mouth).

Once the tube has been passed, its position in the stomach *must be verified*. The *only positive proof* that the tube is in the stomach is the ability to aspirate gastric contents. If bubbles of air escape from the free end of the tube when it is placed in a glass of water, the tube is probably in the lungs. If the patient coughs, has difficulty breathing, or cannot hum, the tube is in the bronchi or lungs and must be removed and reinserted.

During the test, all or part of the gastric contents are removed with a large syringe. The patient may have been fasting before the test, or he may have been given something to stimulate gastric activity, such as alcohol, caffeine, an injection of histamine, or a test meal of crackers.

The tube is left in place if additional samples are to be taken at a later time. If so, the tube should be taped in place so that a sudden cough or sneeze will not displace it. Subsequent care of the patient depends on the number and intervals of samples to be taken and whether they are to be fasting samples or to follow a test meal.

Lumbar Puncture

A lumbar puncture, or spinal tap, is done for the following *diagnostic* purposes:

- To obtain a specimen of spinal fluid for analysis
- To measure the pressure of the spinal fluid
- To inject air or dye into the spinal canal for x-ray examination

A lumbar puncture is done for the following *therapeutic* reasons:

- To inject medication into the spinal canal
- To remove spinal fluid and reduce the pressure in the spinal canal
- To administer spinal anesthesia

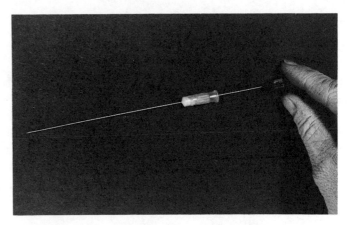

Figure 18.23 *A lumbar puncture needle and stylet, with stylet partially withdrawn.*

After a local anesthetic, a needle is inserted by the physician through the fourth or fifth lumbar space. This is below the level of the spinal cord. A spinal manometer is attached to the needle to measure the pressure of the spinal fluid. The manometer is then removed and a syringe is attached to the needle. The syringe will be empty if spinal fluid is to be removed, or it may contain a dye or medication.

Accidental or unintentional loss of spinal fluid during insertion of the needle is prevented by using a *stylet* to block the lumen (opening) of the needle (Fig. 18.23). A *stopcock* is used to block the flow of fluid while removing the manometer and attaching the syringe. (A stopcock is similar to the three-way spigot on a thermos jug or coffee urn.)

Preparation of the Patient

The patient is positioned on his side with his back at the edge of the bed or table. His spine is flexed with his knees drawn up toward his abdomen, his neck is flexed, and his head is down toward his chest (Fig. 18.24). This position enlarges the intervertebral spaces and facilitates insertion of the needle.

A pillow is placed under the patient's head to keep his head and neck level with his spine, thereby reduc-

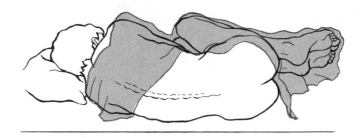

Figure 18.24 *The fetal position with the patient close to the edge of the bed offers the best access for the lumbar puncture procedure.*

ing muscle strain and tension. Another pillow may be placed under the upper arm and leg to keep the upper side of the trunk directly over the lower side. The patient's bowels and bladder should have been emptied to reduce abdominal pressure and subsequent discomfort during the procedure.

The puncture site is shaved if indicated and cleansed with an antiseptic. Strict *surgical asepsis* (sterile technique) is necessary because the procedure invades the spinal canal, thereby exposing its contents to the risk of infection.

The patient should be given a complete explanation that includes being told that:

- He must lie without moving and that the nurse will help him maintain the required position as needed
- He will feel pressure as the needle is inserted but should feel no pain
- He may feel a tingling sensation or momentary pain in his legs or hips if the needle touches any of the nerves that supply that area

Role of the Nurse

In addition to giving emotional support to the patient by talking to him and reassuring him, you will need to attend to his *physical needs*. Observe him carefully for any changes in color, pulse, and respiration that might result from altered spinal fluid pressure. You may need to help the patient maintain the required position. Some patients are too weak, tired, or ill to maintain the position without assistance. Others are physically able to maintain it but, for one reason or another, are unable to remember to do so. You can help by placing one arm behind the patient's knees and the other behind his neck.

Assist the physician as needed. This often involves holding the manometer upright and taking tubes of fluid as they are filled and handed to you. Caution: Because this is a sterile procedure, take great care not to touch the physician's gloved hand or any piece of sterile equipment. If you expect the patient to require your undivided attention, arrange to have a second nurse assist the physician. Finally, make sure that all specimens of spinal fluid are labeled correctly and sent to the laboratory promptly.

Aftercare

After the procedure, apply a small, dry sterile dressing to the puncture site unless the physician has already done so, and help the patient into a comfortable position. If the lumbar puncture was done for *therapy* rather than diagnosis, the nurse should ask the physician about the desired effect of the procedure. Knowledge of the

desired effect will direct your observations toward the important areas of assessment. If, for example, the lumbar puncture was done to reduce an elevated cerebrospinal pressure, your observations would be directed toward watching for indications of a reduced cerebrospinal pressure.

One common complication of a lumbar puncture is a rather severe spinal headache. This may occur after a few hours and sometimes lasts 1 to 2 days. It is eased by lying down and worsened by sitting up and by any sudden movement of the head. The exact cause is not known. Some physicians try to prevent a headache by keeping the patient flat in bed for 12 to 24 hours and forcing fluids to promote replacement of any lost cerebrospinal fluid as quickly as possible. Other physicians believe bed rest is inconsequential, and many lumbar punctures are done on an outpatient basis. If a headache occurs, an ice bag plus bed rest in a quiet, dark room may help, and analgesic medications are usually ordered.

Cisternal Puncture

Cisternal puncture is a procedure similar to a lumbar puncture except that the needle is inserted at the base of the skull, just above the first cervical vertebra. The procedure is done to inject air or dye into the subarachnoid space for x-ray examination of the ventricles of the brain. There are few complications and the test can be done in an outpatient clinic, but many patients are frightened by the prospect of having a needle inserted so close to the brain. Such patients may need sedation in addition to psychological support.

Abdominal Paracentesis

Abdominal paracentesis is the withdrawal of peritoneal fluid from the abdomen. When the procedure is done as a *diagnostic test*, a small amount of peritoneal fluid is withdrawn and examined for the presence of abnormal cells and organisms. When it is done as a *treatment*, a large amount of fluid is withdrawn as part of the treatment for a condition known as ascites (an accumulation of peritoneal fluid).

When a small amount of fluid is to be withdrawn for laboratory analysis, a syringe and long needle are used to aspirate the fluid. If a large amount of fluid is to be removed (up to 2,000 to 3,000 cc), a small incision or stab wound is made between the symphysis pubis and the umbilicus. A trocar and cannula are then inserted. The *cannula* is a rigid, blunt tube through which fluid is drained from a body cavity. The *trochar* is a sharp, pointed instrument that fits inside the cannula and that provides the necessary point for the cannula

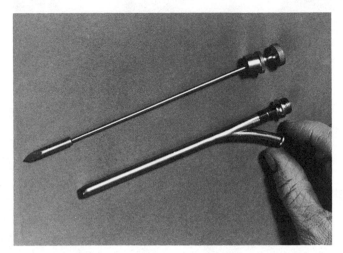

Figure 18.25 Trochar and cannula for abdominal paracentesis. Top: the trochar, a sharp, pointed instrument needed for insertion; bottom: the cannula, for withdrawal of fluid.

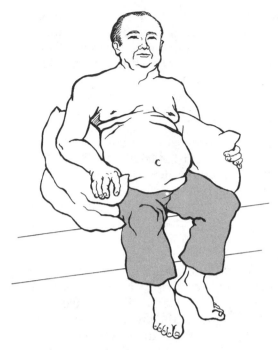

Figure 18.26 Position for abdominal paracentesis.

during its insertion into the body (Fig. 18.25). After insertion, the trocar is withdrawn, leaving the hollow, blunt cannula in place. Flexible tubing can be inserted into or attached to the cannula to carry fluid from the patient to a receptacle. The tubing has a smaller diameter than the cannula, which slows the fluid flow and reduces the intra-abdominal pressure more gradually.

Preparation of the Patient

In addition to basic explanations and psychological support, there are two specific preparations for this procedure. First, the patient must empty his bladder because a distended, full bladder could be punctured by the sharp trochar. If the patient is unable to void, the physician should be notified, as catheterization may be necessary.

Second, the patient must be supported in the designated position because the procedure is likely to be a lengthy one if there is considerable fluid to be withdrawn. Gravity aids the drainage of the peritoneal fluid, so the patient should be in an upright position with feet, arms, and back supported to prevent fatigue. He may sit at the edge of the bed with his feet on a chair and his arms and back supported with pillows. He could sit in a chair with his feet on the floor, and the chair placed beside the bed or a table upon which he can lean. An acutely ill, weak patient may sit in bed with the head of the bed elevated for support, but this position is more awkward for the physician, who must then work from the side of the patient. When the patient is sitting at the edge of the bed or in a chair, his knees should be separated to let the physician position himself as close to the abdomen as possible. The patient should wear pajama pants that can be lowered to his

hips, or else be well draped to prevent embarrassment and possible chilling (Fig. 18.26).

When the patient has been positioned, the abdomen is cleansed with an antiseptic solution. A local anesthetic is injected into the site, the incision is made, and the trocar and cannula are inserted.

Role of the Nurse

The patient's color, respirations, pulse, and blood pressure must be carefully monitored because removal of accumulated peritoneal fluid reduces the intra-abdominal pressure. As a result, an increased amount of circulating blood shifts into the abdominal vessels to compensate for the decreasing pressure. The peripheral circulation will be affected by this shift, and the patient may feel faint or demonstrate early signs of shock, such as pallor, decreased blood pressure, and increased pulse rate. Any changes in the patient's vital signs should be brought to the physician's attention *at once* so that he can interrupt, slow, or stop the procedure.

If the accumulated peritoneal fluid has been exerting pressure against the diaphragm and making it hard for the patient to breathe, he will probably experience considerable relief as the fluid is withdrawn and the pressure is removed.

Aftercare

A few sutures may be needed to close the incision. A heavy sterile dressing is placed over the incision because there is likely to be some leakage of peritoneal fluid for a short while. The dressing should be checked frequently and changed as needed. If considerable fluid was removed, the patient may welcome the support of an abdominal binder. The patient's vital signs should be checked frequently for a few hours.

Thoracentesis

A *diagnostic* thoracentesis is the withdrawal of a specimen of pleural fluid for laboratory analysis. A *therapeutic* thoracentesis is the withdrawal of excess fluid from the pleural space to relieve respiratory distress. The upper level of the fluid is located by percussion and auscultation or by x-ray image, and a needle is inserted into the pleural cavity below that level.

When the site has been anesthetized, the physician inserts a needle through an intercostal space. Because the pressure in the pleural cavity is less than atmospheric pressure, air will enter the pleural cavity through the needle to equalize the pressure, and it must be prevented from doing so. A three-way stopcock attached to the needle enables the physician to open and close the entrance to the needle and also to divert the fluid into tubing that leads to a drainage bottle.

The fact that pressure in the pleural cavity is *less* than atmospheric pressure means that pleural fluid or air does not unintentionally escape from the chest; it must be removed deliberately. Fluid flows from an area of greater pressure to an area of lesser pressure. Therefore, fluid does not leave the chest unless the pleural pressure is greater than the pressure in a syringe or drainage bottle attached to the needle. This difference in pressure is accomplished through the use of suction, and a large syringe can create enough suction to aspirate pleural fluid. A drainage bottle in which a partial vacuum has been created by a suction pump will also pull fluid from the pleural cavity. Thick, viscous material, such as pus, will require greater suction than will a thin, clear fluid.

Preparation of the Patient
The patient's position is intended to enlarge the intercostal space that is to be used for insertion of the needle. This enlargement occurs when: (1) the patient sits with the arm on the side of the thoracentesis site raised over his head or held across his chest, or (2) the patient leans forward on pillows and an overbed table with his arms folded in front of him (Fig. 18.27).

A weak or acutely ill patient who is unable to assume a sitting position *lies on his affected side* with the arm on that side over his head. In this position, the fluid collects at the side of the affected pleural cavity rather than at its base. The needle is inserted close to the outer aspect of the affected side, down toward the mattress or treatment table.

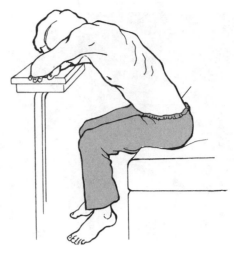

Figure 18.27 Position for thoracentesis.

The patient should be instructed not to cough or move suddenly because such movement might cause the needle to injure the lung, blood vessels, or surrounding tissue. If the patient has to cough, the physician will close the stopcock and withdraw the needle a bit to prevent injury to the underlying tissue.

Role of the Nurse
In addition to providing the patient with physical and emotional support and assisting the physician as needed, the nurse must observe the patient's color, pulse, and respiratory rate at frequent intervals. If a large amount of fluid is withdrawn too suddenly, the abrupt decrease in pleural pressure may cause serious circulatory and respiratory problems. If the patient has been dyspneic, his breathing may become easier as fluid is withdrawn and the pleural pressure is reduced.

Aftercare
A small sterile pressure dressing is applied to the site of the thoracentesis. A chest x-ray film may be ordered for comparison with x-ray films taken before the thoracentesis.

TESTS USING X-RAYS AND CONTRAST MEDIA

An x-ray examination involves the passage of x-rays (roentgen rays) through the body to expose a piece of x-ray film placed under or behind the body. Since dense structures such as bone block the passage of x-rays, the portion of the film behind dense structures is only lightly exposed, and it remains light or white. Hollow and less dense organs permit the passage of x-rays, so the film behind them is heavily exposed and looks very dark.

To visualize and examine a *hollow organ*, a radiopaque substance is used to fill that organ or body cavity and block the passage of x-rays. The radiopaque substance causes the filled organ to appear white on the exposed film, in *contrast* to unfilled organs and cavities; hence the term *contrast medium.*

The radiopaque contrast medium increases the density of the filled organ and creates a contrast between the organ to be studied and the surrounding tissue, which is normally of equal density. A tumor or abnormal structure of the filled organ being studied produces an unfilled area that is dark—a filling *defect.* Any abnormality of the wall of the filled organ, such as an ulcer, creates an irregular line of contrast between the lightness of the filled organ and the darkness of the surrounding tissues.

Proper preparation for these x-ray examinations is essential because the x-ray film is useless unless the organ was *completely emptied* of its normal contents and then *completely filled* with the contrast medium. For example, in a film of the lower colon, a large piece of hard fecal matter and a small tumor could produce a *similar* filling defect—an area that appears dark because more x-rays passed through it than could pass through the radiopaque substance which fills the rest of the colon. Failure to completely empty the lower colon in this case either would result in an inaccurate diagnosis or would necessitate the additional expenditure of time, energy, and money for another test plus a potentially hazardous delay in starting treatments.

These tests are done by specially trained technicians, although a physician may be present to watch and interpret a fluoroscopic examination and to direct the positioning of the patient during some types of tests. The nurse usually has no contact with the patient from the time he leaves the unit until he returns. Her responsibility, therefore, is focused on preparation and aftercare.

Upper GI Series

An *upper GI series*, called a *barium swallow*, permits x-ray examination of the upper portion of the gastrointestinal tract: esophagus, stomach, duodenum, and small intestine. In the x-ray department, the patient is asked to drink a large glassful of thick, chalky barium sulfate, which is usually flavored to make it a bit more palatable. The physician may use a fluoroscope to watch the movements of the esophagus and stomach as the barium is swallowed. The fluoroscope shows motion but does not produce a permanent record.

X-ray study of the stomach is then done, and if the duodenum and small intestine are to be studied, additional films are taken at intervals which coincide with the passage of the barium and the filling of subsequent portions of the intestinal tract.

Some upper GI series also incude the use of an effervescent substance that distends the stomach with gas. The patient is asked to toss about a tablespoon of crystals into his mouth and then swallow about the same amount of water. The crystals dissolve and release bubbles of gas almost immediately. The patient is asked not to burp, and the physician observes the distention of the stomach on the fluoroscope.

Preparation of the Patient

Since the stomach must be empty for an upper GI series, the patient is required to fast, usually from midnight until the time of the test. The test is done with the patient lying on the x-ray table, and if this is the patient's first x-ray examination of this type, he should be warned that the table is hard and cold. He should know that, for this test, the table will be tilted from end to end, and that he will be asked to turn from side to side as the physician and technician seek to find an angle that will show the organ most clearly.

Aftercare

When the patient returns to the unit, he should be given mouth care as desired, and his breakfast. Barium becomes solid as water is absorbed from it, so a laxative is often prescribed to prevent an obstruction of hardened barium in the colon.

Lower GI Series

A *lower GI series*, called a *barium enema*, permits x-ray examination of the colon and rectum. An enema of barium is given to the patient in the x-ray department, and he is expected to retain it until the films have been taken. If the patient thinks he may be unable to retain the barium, he should be instructed to inform the technician, who will use a special rectal tip with a baffle or seal as the enema is administered.

The procedure is uncomfortable, tiring, and embarrassing. A weak, frail, or acutely ill patient may need the support and assistance of a nurse or aide in addition to the help of the x-ray technician. After the test, the barium is expelled into a nearby toilet.

Preparation of the Patient

The lower colon must be empty and completely free of fecal matter, so cleansing enemas are usually given both the night before and the morning of the test. In addition, a strong laxative is usually ordered to clear the lower part of the small intestine because otherwise fecal matter continues to move from the small intestine to the large intestine, and would descend into the colon and ruin the test.

Aftercare

The patient should have an opportunity to wash himself or be washed after the test and to change any clothing that may have been soiled with barium. A cleansing enema is often ordered to remove any remaining barium before it becomes solid. This is especially important for patients with a history of constipation or bowel pathology.

Gallbladder Series

A *gallbladder series* is done to diagnose cholelithiasis (gallstones) or cholecystitis (inflammation of the gallbladder). A radiopaque substance in tablet form is swallowed the evening before the test. It is absorbed by the liver and concentrated in the gallbladder. This concentration of a radiopaque substance will reveal the presence of any stones or any irregularities in the wall of the gallbladder that might indicate inflammation or infection.

Preparation of the patient usually includes a fat-free or low-fat supper the evening before the test plus the correct number of tablets as determined by the patient's weight. The patient should be told that the test is not uncomfortable and takes only a few minutes but that the tablets may cause a temporary side effect such as diarrhea.

Myelogram

A *myelogram* is an x-ray examination of the spinal canal and is done when compression of the spinal cord by a tumor or herniated intervertebral disc is suspected.

A lumbar puncture is done, and a small amount of spinal fluid is withdrawn and replaced with a radiopaque substance. This contrast medium is heavy and does *not* disperse throughout the spinal fluid. The x-ray table is tilted to allow the material to flow toward the suspected area of compression. The needle is left in place throughout the procedure, and at the conclusion of the test the physician withdraws as much of the radiopaque dye as possible. A myelogram can also be done by injecting air into the cisternal subarachnoid space following a cisternal puncture.

Preparation of the patient and aftercare are the same as for a lumbar puncture.

Intravenous Pyelogram

The radiopaque dye used for an *intravenous pyelogram* (IVP) is given intravenously and is concentrated and excreted by the kidneys. The presence of the radi-

opaque dye in the kidney as the dye is being filtered and excreted reveals the size and shape of the kidney, the kidney pelvis, and the ureters. X-ray films are taken at short, carefully timed intervals. The urine is analyzed to determine the amount and rate of dye excretion, which indicates the adequacy of kidney function.

Because concentrated dye produces a clearer image on the x-ray film than does diluted dye, the patient is usually required to fast for 8 to 10 hours before the test so that a mild dehydration will produce a more concentrated urine and dye. In addition, a laxative and enemas are given to clear the intestinal tract of gas and feces, which might obscure the kidneys on the films. If a patient has had an upper or lower GI series recently, any remaining barium must be removed before the pyelogram so that confusing traces of barium do not appear on the films.

The combination of fasting, a laxative, and enemas may prove tiring or even exhausting to a weak, elderly, or debilitated patient, and preparations may need to be modified. It is the responsibility of the nurse to monitor each patient's condition and to *take the initiative* in suggesting that a modification in preparation might be necessary, because neither the physician nor the x-ray technician is likely to be aware of the problem.

Some patients are sensitive to the dye. If the medical or nursing history reveals an adverse reaction to a previous IVP, the physician will probably substitute a retrograde pyelogram (see below) for an IVP which could be hazardous because of the possibility of a severe reaction to the dye.

Retrograde Pyelogram

Retrograde means backward, and a *retrograde pyelogram* differs from an intravenous pyelogram in that the dye passes from the ureters back up to the kidney pelvis rather than moving from the kidney pelvis down to the ureters.

This test is done after examination of the bladder with a cystoscope (see end of section) under local or general anesthesia. The cystoscope permits passage of a catheter up through each ureter, and a radiopaque liquid is instilled in the pelvis of each kidney. X-ray films, which are taken immediately, show the shape and size of the kidney pelvis; subsequent films show the size, shape, and structure of the ureters and bladder as the dye passes out of the body.

The dye for a retrograde pyelogram is different from that used for an IVP; and because it is not given intravenously, the risk of a dangerous reaction is removed.

Preparation of the patient is similar to the preparation for an IVP, and aftercare is the same as care after cystoscopy.

TESTS THAT MEASURE ELECTRICAL IMPULSES

Electrocardiogram

An electrocardiogram (EKG, or ECG) measures and records the electrical activity of the heart. Electrodes (leads) are attached to the patient's body with a special adhesive. These leads conduct the electrical impulses to a recording device that produces a permanent graph of cardiac activity.

The patient should be told that there is no discomfort during the test (except from the adhesive or paste which is usually cold), and that there is no danger of electrical shock. The test measures electrical impulses *leaving* the heart; no electricity enters the body. Female patients are likely to be embarrassed during this test because a technician frequently exposes the entire torso as the leads are applied and leaves it exposed throughout the test. The patient is asked to lie quietly because body movements affect cardiac activity. The test takes only 5 to 10 min. All paste should be removed to avoid any skin reaction.

Electroencephalogram

For an electroencephalogram (EEG), electrodes, or leads, are attached to the patient's scalp with paste, or collodion. The leads may also be attached to the scalp with very tiny needles because the scalp has few nerve endings. The patient is expected to relax in a quiet, dark room, but he is not expected to sleep unless an EEG while sleeping has been specifically ordered by the physician. The test takes about an hour.

Because hypoglycemia (low blood sugar) affects brain waves, the patient is asked not to skip meals or fast before the test. Drugs that affect brain waves, such as anticonvulsants and tranquilizers, as well as stimulants, such as coffee, cola drinks, and tea, are omitted for 24 to 48 hours before the test. Additional preparation, such as washing the patient's hair, depends on the preference of the physician and technician.

TESTS INVOLVING DIRECT INSPECTION OF A BODY CAVITY

Endoscopy is the visual examination of the interior surfaces of a hollow organ or body cavity by means of an *endoscope,* or scope. Each scope is designed for use in a specific body part and is named in accordance with that body part. Examples include: otoscope, bronchoscope, gastroscope, laryngoscope, and sigmoidoscope.

Although endoscopes differ in design, they all include a viewing system and lenses, a light source, a handle, and a power source. Accessories include a suction tip, an electrode tip for cauterization, and forceps for the removal of biopsy tissue or a foreign object. Some endoscopes are equipped with a miniature camera capable of taking color photographs for future study.

A standard endoscope uses a system of lenses and a rigid viewing tube, which is usually metal. A fiberoptic endoscope transmits images and light along flexible bundles of glass or plastic fibers that have special optical properties. The flexibility of a fiberoptic scope makes it both safer and more comfortable for the patient.

Endoscopy is not usually painful, but it is difficult, tiring, and unpleasant. The insertion of a foreign object into a body cavity is an intrusive procedure that is often frightening and embarrassing. The required positions are difficult to achieve and to maintain. For these reasons, the patient needs careful preparation including an explanation and possibly a demonstration of the position and equipment to be used. He will also need psychological and physical support throughout some of the more difficult tests.

Bronchoscopy and Laryngoscopy

Bronchoscopy and *laryngoscopy* are difficult when done with a standard scope because the patient's neck must be hyperextended so that the pharynx and trachea are in a straight line for the passage of the rigid metal tube. The tests are safer, easier, and more comfortable when a flexible fiberoptic scope is used.

Preparation of the Patient
The patient should fast for several hours before the test to decrease the possibility of vomiting and aspirating vomitus into the lungs. Dentures are removed, and a sedative is given. A topical anesthetic is used to decrease the gag reflex, and a general anesthetic is administered to some patients. The patient should be told that the aftereffects, such as a sore throat, difficulty in swallowing, hoarseness, and loss of voice, may be distressing, but that they will be temporary.

Aftercare
Accidental injury to the larynx can cause laryngeal spasms or swelling, so the patient should be observed carefully for any indication of respiratory distress. Swallowing will be impaired, so the patient should be *NPO (nothing by mouth) until his gag reflex returns* after 2 to 8 hours. Advise the patient not to talk, clear his throat, cough, or smoke immediately after the test. An ice collar and lozenges will relieve the sore throat. If a biopsy was done, watch for indications of hidden bleeding, such as coughing or blood-tinged sputum.

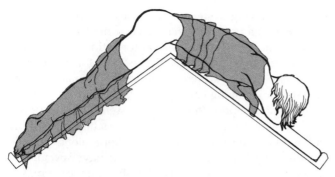

Figure 18.28 Jackknife position for sigmoidoscopy.

Esophagoscopy and Gastroscopy

The patient must fast before either an *esophagoscopy* or *gastroscopy* so that the stomach and esophagus are empty for the clearest possible visualization. An empty stomach also reduces the danger of vomiting and aspiration. Preparation of the patient, passage of the tube, and aftercare of the patient are the same as for bronchoscopy.

Proctoscopy and Sigmoidoscopy

Proctoscopy and *sigmoidoscopy* are difficult and embarrassing for the patient because they are done with the patient in either a knee-chest or a jackknife position (Fig. 18.28). The position, coupled with the nature of the test, make it an unpleasant experience.

The success of the test depends on the quality of the physical preparation of the patient. The rectum and sigmoid colon must be free of fecal matter before the mucosal lining of the walls can be inspected. A cathartic and enemas are usually given during the evening preceding the test, with additional enemas in the morning. Because enemas may irritate and alter the appearance of the rectal mucosa, they are usually *concluded at least 2 hours before the test is scheduled,* to give the mucosal lining a chance to rest and regain its usual appearance. Occasionally, the physician may choose to do the test without preparation of any kind, especially if extreme irritation of the bowel is already a problem.

Because cancer of the rectum is the second most frequent cause of death from cancer in both men and women, many physicians believe that every patient over 40 should have a protoscopic examination each year. When the examination is done in the physician's office, preparation for the test is done at home and the patient must be taught how to give himself an enema if he does not already know how. A proctoscopic examination takes only a minute or two if the rectum is *thoroughly clean,* but it takes longer and is more uncomfortable if preparation is inadequate. Depending on his age and condition, the patient may need to rest before leaving the treatment room or physician's office.

Cystoscopy

For *cystoscopy,* the patient is placed in lithotomy position; and after a local or general anesthetic has been given, the cystoscope is passed through the urethra into the patient's bladder. The walls of the bladder are examined, and if needed, tissue can be taken for biopsy. Therapy can be carried out if indicated.

If a *retrograde pyelogram* is to be done, two catheters are passed through the cystoscope, and one is directed into each ureter. Radiopaque dye is injected through each catheter into the kidney pelvis. If the physician wants to continue to study the functioning of each kidney, the catheters are left in place when the cystoscope is removed. The catheters are carefully labeled (right and left), and each is attached to a separate drainage bottle so that the urine from each kidney can be identified and analyzed separately.

There may be some tissue damage from this procedure and as a result, swelling, difficult urination, and hematuria may occur. The patient's urinary output should be measured for at least 24 hours. The patient should be told that his urine is likely to be tinged with pink but that *any bright red bleeding should be reported at once.* He should also know that the radiopaque dyes may temporarily alter the color of his urine. Fluids, a warm bath, and mild analgesics will relieve discomfort.

Section Seven

The Use of Records and Reports

SOURCES OF INFORMATION ABOUT THE PATIENT

The methods of assessment described in the preceding sections of this chapter have focused on methods of obtaining information directly *from* the patient. In contrast, this section explains the use of records and reports as sources of information *about* the patient.

The major sources of such information are the change-of-shift report, the Kardex, and the patient's chart or record.

Change-of-Shift Reports

At the end of each 8-hour shift, one nurse gives a report to all staff on the next shift. This report helps to ensure continuity of care for patients by making sure that everyone is aware of the current status of each patient. The change-of-shift report may be taped or live, but the format is fairly consistent in either case.

The report on each patient includes the following information: room number, name, age, sex, physician's name, major medical and nursing diagnoses or problems, overall psychological and physiological status, tests scheduled for the day, new treatments ordered, the time non-routine medications were given and their effect, and any new developments or changes in the patient's condition or situation.

Much of the report is factual, but because the psychological responses of the patient affect the patient-nurse relationships, part of any report is likely to be concerned with interpersonal relations. A good report is *nonjudgmental*, and no patient is labeled "good," "difficult," "uncooperative," or any other value-laden term. Instead, the patient's behavior is described in enough detail to allow the staff to understand the situation. A good report is *concise and complete*; all information given is accurate, pertinent, and relevant. The nurse who is reporting is careful to ensure the privacy of each patient by keeping her voice low so that patients in nearby rooms cannot overhear her report.

The following is an example of a typical 8 am change-of-shift report on one patient: "Room 710, Jenny Ward, 85-year-old patient of Dr. Grunder; diagnosis: vulvar pruritus; says she is discouraged over her slow progress and the continued, severe itching, and was crying during the evening; was awakened about 2 am by intense itching of labia and perineum. Calamine lotion with phenol applied; Empirin compound given for pain at 3:15 am; slept remainder of night; scheduled for biopsy of labia this morning—on call to OR at 11 am."

Kardex

The Kardex is a flip-over card file that contains the current data needed for planning basic care for each patient on the unit. The file consists of a double card for each patient (Fig. 18.29), which usually contains the following information:

Demographic data obtained by the admitting office
Current nursing orders
Current physician's orders to be carried out by nurses
Current medications
Scheduled tests or treatments
Safety precautions (including patient's abilities, weaknesses, and deficits)
Factors related to self-care and activities of daily living
Brief record of diagnostic tests or treatments

The back of the Kardex often contains a *patient profile*. This is a brief summary of patient likes and dislikes,

Medications in Pharmacy _____	Blood on Call Date _____	PT OT AM _____	ALLERGIES _____
	No of units _____	PM _____	_____
Valuables in Business Office _____			_____

DIETARY ASSISTANCE

Feed Patient _____

Prepare Food _____

Feed Self _____

ORAL FLUIDS

0700-1500 _____

1500-2300 _____

2300-0700 _____

DIET _____

_____

_____

_____

NOURISHMENT _____

_____

_____

URINE	PROTECTIVE MEASURES	
Partition _____	Side Rails Cont. _____	TPR _____
PH _____	Side Rails HS _____	BP & P _____
	Restrain and _____	Weight _____
Sp G _____	Type _____	I & O _____

MEASURE DRAINAGE	ACTIVITIES	BATH
Urine _____	Bed Rest _____	Complete _____
Hemovac _____	Dangle _____	Partial _____
Wang. _____	BRP _____	Tub _____
Other _____	Commode _____	with assistance _____
_____	Chair _____	without assistance _____
_____	OOB _____	Shower _____
_____		with assistance _____
		without assistance _____

DATE	TREATMENTS AND NURSING ORDERS	TIME	DATE	TREATMENTS AND NURSING ORDERS	TIME

DIAGNOSIS _____	OPERATIONS _____	Religion _____
_____	_____	Last Rites _____
_____	_____	DI _____

ROOM	PATIENT	PHYSICIAN	SERVICE	AGE	Marital Stat	ADM

Figure 18.29 *A sample kardex form.*

family matters, and other data about the patient as a person.

Much of the Kardex is written in pencil so that it can be erased easily and kept current. The Kardex is a method of communication among nurses and is a quick source of information when you are assigned to a newly admitted or unfamiliar patient. It enables you to plan initial care, and will usually suffice as a source of information about the patient until you are able to use the patient's record to obtain more extensive information.

Patient's Record

The patient's record, or chart, is a legal document that includes all information relevant to his diagnosis, care, and treatment. All records contain essentially the same information, although it may be organized in a variety of ways. This information includes:

Demographic data
Consent forms
Patient history
Reports of physical examinations
Reports of diagnostic tests
Nursing diagnoses
Medical diagnosis
Therapeutic orders
Observations of the patient
Record of care and treatment
Progress notes
Summary or discharge notes

In order to use the patient's record to obtain information about him, you must, first of all, be familiar with the organization of the record and know where to find various types of data, such as the patient's past medical history, name of next of kin, consent for surgery or treatment, and religious affiliation. Unless you can quickly locate the information you need, you may be tempted to try to do without it. Second, you must know the terminology, abbreviations, and symbols used in the patient's record. It is impossible to read and comprehend its contents without this knowledge. The process of acquiring an adequate professional vocabulary can be speeded up if you memorize the common prefixes and suffixes that make it possible to analyze an unfamiliar word and figure out its meaning. It is helpful to jot down each unfamiliar word you encounter and to look it up as soon as possible.

An extensive list of abbreviations can be found in Appendix C, and a list of prefixes and suffixes is given in Appendix F. Shorter lists of abbreviations (such as Table 18.2, p. 326) and symbols are interspersed throughout the text as needed.

USES OF THE PATIENT'S RECORD

The patient's record is used for five major purposes: communication, education, research, audit, and patient assessment.

Communication

The patient's record facilitates communication among members of the health care team. All members have access to the record, and all members are able to contribute to it. Communication is thus enhanced within nursing, from nurse to nurse and from shift to shift, and among nurses, physicians, physical therapists, nutritionists, social workers, and others.

Since each chart is stored or microfilmed, the health care team is able to retrieve and use data from the record of a previous hospitalization or visit. Such information may be significant and, in some instances, life-saving.

Education

Access to patients' charts enables medical and nursing students, as well as students from other disciplines, to study the symptoms, diagnosis, and treatment of patients in their care, as well as patients who have been discharged, and patients who have died.

Patients' charts contribute to the ongoing education of physicians by enabling them to study the diagnosis and treatment of difficult cases. The use of computerized records makes it possible for physicians around the world to study the medical management of rare diseases and conditions.

Research

Patient records provide data that enable researchers to compare various medical and nursing treatments, to evaluate the effectiveness of a drug or treatment, to determine the etiology of a new or rare condition, and to gather statistical data related to infections, complications, deaths, and cures from a variety of treatments.

Audit

A regular, systematic review of patient records permits the evaluation of health care given and is the basis for a variety of quality assurance programs. Nursing eval-

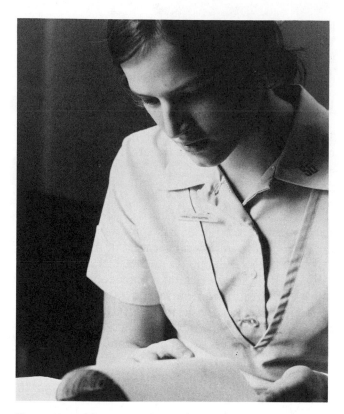

Figure 18.30 *The patient's record provides information for the assessment phase of nursing process.*

uations are usually based on the examination of the recorded nursing history, nursing care plans, nursing interventions, and the subsequent patient responses, both physiological and psychological (Fig. 18.30).

Nurses are developing innovative ways to use the data from patient records as a basis for evaluating the effectiveness of nursing care rather than relying on the opinions of patients, physicians, and peers, or on financial data from agency administrators and insurance representatives.

Assessment of an Assigned Patient

Extensive information must be obtained before nursing or medical care can be planned. Unless the health care worker knows, for example, the psychological and physiological status of the patient, appropriate plans cannot be made. Blood test results must be known before chemotherapy can be started. X-ray results are often needed before surgery can be considered, and physical capability must be known before discharge plans can be completed. The patient's record is the primary source of such information.

Some of the specific ways of using the patient's record are:

1. *To update knowledge and understanding of the situation.* The patient's record enables you to discover quickly what changes have occurred in the patient or in his condition while you were away from him.

2. *To help identify norms for that patient.* Information in the chart gives you a basis for assessing the patient's current status in relation to his previous or usual condition. The chart provides answers to questions, such as: What has the patient's BP been? Is his weight increasing or decreasing? How does he usually react to pain? What is his usual pattern of elimination? How much activity has he been able to tolerate? Some of this information can be obtained from the patient, but it is often neither efficient nor effective to ask the patient for information which is readily available in usable form in his record.

3. *To supplement your own assessments.* Knowledge of the information in the patient's record reduces the time and energy needed for subsequent assessments. There is no need, for example, to ask a patient where he was born because his birthplace is listed with other data obtained by the clerk in the admitting office. In general, a nurse should not collect information already available unless she specifically wants to assess a patient's reaction to her questions.

4. *To explain, confirm, or refute your observations.* If, for example, your detailed and specific observations of a patient's behavior indicated he was confused, his chart might provide initial or tentative answers to questions, such as: When did this behavior start? Has it been noticed by anyone else? Could a medication be responsible for the behavior? Is his cerebral circulation adequate? Could his blood chemistry provide a clue? It is important to *seek an explanation* for any changed behavior or altered physiological response; it is not enough to merely observe and report it.

ORGANIZATION OF THE PATIENT'S RECORD

The organization of the patient's record determines where information is to be entered and is one indication of the manner in which the health care team views patient problems. A patient record can be organized in any way that meets the needs of the people who use it, but most records are organized in one of two formats, either a traditional or problem-oriented format.

The *traditional* patient record is organized according to *the source of the information* contained in the record, and there are usually sections for entries made by physicians, nurses, and special departments, such as x-ray and physiotherapy, and the diet kitchen. The *problem-*

oriented record, on the other hand, is an integrated record in which all information, regardless of source, is organized according to patient problems.

Traditional Records

Although the sequence may vary from hospital to hospital, the information in a traditional patient record is usually organized and categorized as follows:

Patient portrait

Demographic data obtained upon admission

Physician's orders (which may be filed in a separate notebook)

Graphic sheets (showing TPR, BP, weight, intake, output, others)

Report of physician's history and physical examination

Laboratory reports and results of diagnostic tests

Reports from special departments (anesthesia, radiation therapy, social service, vocational rehabilitation)

Nurse's notes (including nursing care plans, nursing history, reports of physical assessments, observations made, and care given)

Discharge notes (patient's condition, progress, and effectiveness of therapy; plans for future care, teaching, or rehabilitation)

A traditional record is functional and efficient, but it does not foster a unified approach to patient care. Each member of the health care team attends to his area of concern, and may be unaware of problems or successes in other areas. The use of a traditional record does not rule out the possibility of a holistic, integrated team approach to patient care, but it does not promote such an approach. In some settings, team conferences or staff meetings promote a unified approach to patient care despite the fragmentation of information in the patient records.

Problem-Oriented Records

The problem-oriented record (POR) is based on a system developed by Dr. Lawrence Weed in the 1960s. This system is patient centered and fosters a collaborative problem-solving approach by all members of the health care team. All health care workers are aware of the existence and impact of all the patient's problems even though each worker's major contribution remains within that worker's area of expertise. The POR aids audit, research, and education because it is possible to trace the identification and management of each problem.

Although the system was designed for use by the entire health care team, it can be modified for use by nurses within the context of a traditional patient record; and many institutions have adapted the system to meet their own preferences and needs. In some settings, the system is focused on the concerns of the medical profession, and the record is named the problem-oriented *medical* record (POMR). In other settings, the system is attentive to the overall health needs of the patient and uses a problem-oriented *health* record (POHR). Regardless of the specific focus, there are four main sections of the record: (1) data base, (2) problem list, (3) initial plan, and (4) progress notes.

Data Base

All members of the health care team contribute to the data base, which includes the medical history and report of the physician's physical examination; the nursing history and assessments; laboratory reports; and the results of diagnostic tests, interviews, and observations. Many agencies use standardized forms to help ensure a complete data base.

Problem List

Analysis of the data which has been collected yields a set of problems, which are *numbered in chronological order* according to the date each was identified (not in order of severity or priority). These problems may be psychological, physiological, cultural, developmental, or socioeconomic. This list of problems is filed in the front of the patient's record and serves as a table of contents for that record. The problem list indicates the date each problem was identified, and the date each was resolved. Input from the patient and family is sought, and new problems are added as they are identified. Only active problems are entered in the problem list; potential problems are considered in the progress notes. Once the initial list has been compiled, each entry in the patient's record is coded by the number of the problem to which it refers.

Initial Plan

The person who has primary responsibility for the patient, usually the physician or primary care nurse, prepares the initial plan of care and outlines an approach to be used for each identified problem. The plan includes the diagnostic work-up or assessment, proposed treatment, and patient education.

Progress Notes

The progress section of the patient's record includes narrative notes, flow sheets, and discharge notes.

NARRATIVE NOTES. Narrative notes are written in a format called SOAP, an acronym for *Subjective* data, *Objective* data, *Analysis*, and *Plan*. Each narrative entry includes the number and name of the problem to which it refers.

Subjective data consist of input from the patient and helps to ensure the participation of the patient in the management of his own care. *Objective* data include observations, measurements, and assessments that describe the patient's response to his disease, care, or therapy.

Analysis refers to interpretation of the data. The person making a narrative entry in the patient's record must analyze the subjective and objective data being entered and attempt to answer questions such as: What do these data mean? What is happening? What caused this phenomenon? This step is critical in the process of resolving patient problems and must precede the formulation of a plan.

The last part of a narrative note is the *plan* or approach that the health care worker believes will help to resolve the problem. Problems vary, of course, in intensity and urgency, and narrative notes need not be made on every problem every day.

FLOW SHEETS. Flow sheets are used to eliminate the inefficient and redundant narrative recording of observations or measurements that must be made at regular intervals. There is no need, for example, to use a SOAP format to record vital signs being taken every hour or to record in narrative form the activity of repositioning a patient every 2 hours, day and night.

A flow sheet permits regularly scheduled activities to be checked off as they are done; these sheets are usually developed for events that take place every few minutes or hours. A flow sheet can also be prepared for events or changes that occur less frequently, such as those that might take place at weekly or monthly intervals in a long-term rehabilitation hospital.

DISCHARGE NOTES. A SOAP format is used to summarize each problem before the patient's discharge and to describe the basis and rationale for each aspect of the discharge plans.

CONTRIBUTING TO THE PATIENT'S RECORD

In addition to *using* the patient's record, the nurse is responsible for *contributing* to it. This activity, called charting, is important because the patient's record is considered a legal document that should contain a complete and accurate account of the care and treatment provided by members of the health care team. Nurses are responsible for recording all essential information related to nursing assessments and nursing care, including treatments that were ordered by the physician and carried out by nurses. The patient's psychological and physiological responses to illness, care, and treatment must be described in appropriate detail. In addition, in some settings, the nurse is responsible for recording the visits or treatments of other members of the health care team, such as physicians, consultants, the nutritionist, a social worker, or a physical therapist. This information must be (1) accurate, (2) legible, (3) concise, (4) clear, (5) current, and (6) technically correct.

Accuracy

The recorded material must be factual and specific so that the information is not subject to a variety of interpretations. Whenever possible, precise measurements should be given rather than vague expressions such as "quite a bit," "a significant amount," "scanty," or "excessive." *Any comments by the patient should be quoted verbatim.*

When information about the patient's behavior is charted, the behavior must be carefully described without labeling the patient. It is not legally acceptable to label a patient "uncooperative," for example, but statements such as, "Refused to change position or to allow nurse to reposition him"; "Refused to talk to nutritionist"; and "Persists in playing radio so loud that other patients complain" are valid and useful. Such statements can be substantiated or verified by other people and, therefore, minimize the possibility of charges of libel by the patient.

The nurse must be careful to differentiate between her observations and her interpretations of those observations. Interpretations of a patient's behavior or response are significant only if they are identified as the nurse's interpretations; they must not be presented as facts.

Correct spelling is necessary to differentiate between drugs with similar names, such as prednisone and prednisolone, and between conditions that are very different, such as apnea and eupnea. A nurse with a severe spelling disability may find it necessary to carry a small pocket dictionary or a list of words that are commonly misspelled.

Accurate charting requires that medications and treatments be charted *after* they have been administered. They should not be charged in advance even though the nurse fully intends to give them. Any number of things might prevent her from actually giving the treatment or medication, and a false entry not only renders the information useless for research, education, or audit but casts a doubt on the accuracy and legality of the nurse's other charting.

The time charted for the administration of medications and treatments should be the actual time, not the scheduled time. Accuracy in charting is increased by the use of military time, which is a 24-hour system. A four-digit number indicates the hours and minutes and makes it impossible to misinterpret am and pm times, such as confusing 12 am with 12 pm (Table 18.1).

Legibility

Charting may be done in either print or script, whichever is more legible. Black ink is preferred because it reproduces better than some types of blue ink when parts of the chart are reproduced for legal or research purposes.

Conciseness

Concise entries make it possible for busy physicians, nurses, students, auditors, and researchers to obtain specific information from a patient's chart quickly and efficiently. Each entry must be complete and accurate, but all unnecessary words should be omitted. The entry should be almost telegraphic in style. The word *patient* or the patient's name need not be included because it is assumed that all entries in a patient's record refer to that patient. Most pronouns can be omitted, as can routine aspects of care. There is no need to chart that the patient's bed was made, for example, or that his tray was served as usual.

TABLE 18.1

Civilian Tme	Military Time
12-hour System	*24-hour System*
1:00 AM	0100
2:00 AM	0200
3:00 AM	0300
11:00 AM	1100
12:00 noon	1200
1:00 PM	1300
2:00 PM	1400
3:00 PM	1500
11:00 PM	2300
12:00 PM	2400[1]

Note: Minutes are written as the last two digits:

0001	1 minute after midnight
0002	2 minutes after midnight
0915	9:15 AM
2115	9:15 PM
2359	1 minute before midnight

Clarity

Words and symbols used by the nurse should convey the same meanings to everyone who reads them. Ambiguous terms or words with a variety of meanings should not be used. Inappropriate abbreviations probably account for more misinterpretations than any other factor. Certain abbreviations and symbols have been accepted and used in medicine and nursing for decades and are well understood by knowledgeable practitioners (Table 18.2).

Other abbreviations emerge from local use and should not be used in another setting where the meanings ascribed to them will be unclear or inaccurate. You are legally responsible for each entry you make in a patient's record, and the abbreviations you use will affect the way in which other people interpret your charting. Whenever you move to a different institution, you should ask for a list of the abbreviations accepted by that agency.

Currentness

Some charting can be delayed until there is an opportune time to do it. Other entries, however, must be made *as soon as the event takes place* because that information may be needed by other members of the health care team. Such events include the admission of a patient to the unit, preparation of a patient for treatment of tests in another department, and preparation of a patient for surgery.

Any treatment or medication that could conceivably be repeated by a second nurse should be charted immediately. Examples of such situations include a *stat order* (a one-time order for a drug to be given at once) or a *prn order* (an order that permits a drug to be given when the patient needs and asks for it). Your charting must be current before you leave the unit for class, coffee break, or lunch so that data relevant to the patient are available to whoever is caring for the patient in your absence.

Technical Correctness

The patient's name and hospital number should appear on each page of the chart. Entries should be in chronological order with the date and time clearly indicated. Each entry must be signed with the nurse's full name and status (RN, LPN, student, other).

Because the patient's record is a legal document, there can be *no blank spaces, ditto marks, erasures, or words deleted.* A line should be drawn through any blank spaces to prevent the insertion of additional data. Reread each entry to make sure that it is correct and that you have omitted nothing. An omission would make that entry inaccurate.

TABLE 18.2 SELECTED ABBREVIATIONS AND SYMBOLS

abd	abdomen	od	once daily
ac	before meals	OD	right eye
ad lib	as desired	OOB	out of bed
adm	admission	OPD	outpatient department
bid	twice a day	OR	operating room
BMR	basal metabolic rate	OS	left eye
BP	blood pressure	OU	both eyes
BM	bowel movement	p̄	after
BRP	bathroom privileges	pc	after meals
c̄	with	PE	physical examination
C & S	culture and sensitivity	PI	present illness
CC	chief complaint	po	by mouth
CTDB	cough, turn, deep breathe	post-op	after operation
D/C or DC	discontinue	pre-op	before operation
DOA	dead on arrival	prn	whenever necessary
DOE	dyspnea on exertion	PT	physiotherapy
DSD	dry sterile dressing	PTA	prior to admission
Dx	diagnosis	qd	every day
EEG	electroencephalogram	qh	every hour
EENT	eye, ear, nose, and throat	q 2h (etc)	every 2 (etc) hours
EKG	electrocardiogram	qid	four times a day
FH	family history	qn	every night
FUO	fever of unknown origin	qod	every other day
fx	fracture	qs	sufficient quantity
Gyn	gynecology	R/O	rule out
H & P	history and physical	ROS	review of systems
HNV	has not voided	Rx	prescription
HS	at bedtime (hour of sleep)	s̄	without
ia	if awake	sc	subcutaneous
I & D	incision and drainage	SOB	short of breath
I & O	intake and output	sp gr or SG	specific gravity
IM	intramuscular	stat	immediately
inc	incontinent	Sx	symptom
IV	intravenous	tid	three times a day
LMD	local medical doctor	TPR	temperature, pulse, and respiration
LMP or LNMP	last (normal) menstrual period	Trach	tracheostomy
LP	lumbar puncture	TWE	tap-water enema
mod	moderate	UCHD	usual childhood diseases
noc	night	VS	vital signs
NPO	nothing by mouth	WBC	white blood cell (count)
O_2	oxygen	WNWD	well nourished, well developed
OB	obstetrics	wt	weight

An error should be crossed out (not blocked out). The word *error* is written across the entry, and the cross-out is dated and signed. Brief corrections can be inserted above the error, dated, and signed. A lengthy correction requires a new entry, complete with date and signature.

PATIENT TEACHING

In order to participate effectively in one's own health care, a person must learn to assess his or her own physical and mental health with reasonable accuracy and attention to detail. The information obtained from such assessments, coupled with information from professional sources, will form the basis for informed and intelligent decision making.

Each person should be taught to:

- *Ask questions.* He should express his concerns and worries, and ask questions of a nurse, physician, pharmacist, informed lay people, and any other knowledgeable persons.
- *Collect data.* He should observe and examine his own body in appropriate detail. He should be able to take his temperature, know what his blood pressure is, be aware of his reaction to various foods, medications, and activities, and be able to describe his feelings and energy level.
- *Keep records.* The human memory is sometimes unreliable, so an individual should be encouraged to keep a written record of relevant data such as immunizations, dates and descriptions of major illnesses and injuries, and changes in body appearance or function which have developed recently or over a period of time.
- *Hypothesize about possible causes of his present condition.* Given the assessment data which he has collected, a person is often able to identify possible cause and effect relationships related to his health. These findings should be explored and validated, and used as a basis for deciding upon a course of action, such as changing one's health habits, consulting a nurse or physician, or arranging for appropriate screening tests.

The process of self-awareness and assessment should begin in childhood and should increase in scope and precision throughout life.

RELATED ACTIVITIES

Nurses and other health care workers have a tendency to make professional judgements which are not fully supported by their assessment data, especially in the realm of psychosocial assessments. It is very easy to go beyond your findings and assume that what you have seen, felt, and heard was accurate and complete.

One way to minimize this tendency is to use a 'soap opera approach.' When you approach your patient, imagine that he is a character in a relatively new television series, and that you have just tuned in for the first time. You know nothing about the character—you don't know anything about his lifestyle, morals, or motives, you don't know anything about his relationships to other characters who are not on the screen, and you know nothing about things that have happened to him in previous episodes. Such uncertainty is unsettling, and if other viewers are present, you will probably ask a number of questions to try to understand the nature of the character and the plot. You would not presume to make any definitive judgements about the character you have started to observe.

The psychosocial assessment of a patient is very similar. You are coming into 'the middle' of a situation possessing *minimal* information about the patient and what has happened before you arrived. If you can remind yourself in each new situation that it will take time to collect enough data to understand both the patient and his situation, you may be able to avoid any tendency toward drawing premature conclusions about the 'character,' the rest of the 'cast,' and the 'plot.'

SUGGESTED READINGS

The Assessment Process

Malasanos, Lois, et al: *Health Assessment.* St. Louis, Mosby, 1981.

Mallick, M Joan: Patient assessment—based on data, not intuition. *Nurs Outlook* 1981 Oct; 29(10):600–605.

Murray, Ruth B, and Judith P Zentner: *Nursing Assessment and Health Promotion Through the Life Span.* ed.3. Englewood Cliffs, NJ, Prentice-Hall, 1985.

Schrock, Miriam Martin: *Holistic Assessment of the Healthy Aged.* New York, Wiley, 1980.

Interviewing

Bernstein, Lewis, and Rosalyn Bernstein: *Interviewing: A Guide for Health Professionals.* ed.3. New York, Appleton-Century-Crofts, 1980.

Duldt, Bonnie Weaver, Kim Griffin, and Bobby R Patton: Interviewing: pulling it all together (chap. 11) in *Interpersonal Communication in Nursing.* Philadelphia, Davis, 1984.

Enelow, Allen J, and SN Swisher: *Interviewing and Patient Care.* New York, Oxford University Press, 1979.

Little, Dolores, and Doris Carnevali: The client, the nurse, and the nursing assessment transaction (chap. 6) in *Nursing Care Planning.* ed.2. Philadelphia, Lippincott, 1976.

Mengel, Andrea: Getting the most from patient interviews. *Nursing 82* 1982 Nov; 12(11):46–49.

Observation

Byers, Virginia: *Nursing Observation.* ed.2. Dubuque, Brown, 1973.

Keeling, Betty L: Making the most of the first home visit. *Nursing 78* 1978 March; 8(3):24–29.

Little, Dolores, and Doris Carnevali: *Nursing Care Planning.* ed.2. Philadelphia, Lippincott, 1976.

Measurement

Adler, Jack, and Nina T Argondizzo: Patient assessment: pulses (programmed instruction). *Am J Nurs* 1979 Jan; 79(1):115–132.

Cudworth-Bergin, Kendell L: Detecting arterial problems with a doppler probe. *RN* 1984 Jan; 47(1):38–41.

Eoff, Mary Jo, and Betsey Joyce: Temperature measurements in children. *Am J Nurs* 1981 May; 81(5):1010–1011.

Erickson, Roberta: Oral temperature differences in relation to thermometer and technique. *Nurs Res* 1980 May/June; 29(3):157–164.

Flynn, Janice Bridges, and Pamela Vickers Moore: Coin-operated sphygmomanometers. *Am J Nurs* 1981 March; 81(3):533–535.

Hill, Martha N: Hypertension: what can go wrong when you measure blood pressure. *Am J Nurs* 1980 May; 80(5):942–946.

Hudson, Barbara: Sharpen your vascular assessment skills with the doppler ultrasound stethoscope. *Nursing 83* 1983 May; 13(5):55–54–57.

Jacobs, Maeona K: Sources of measurement—error in noninvasive electronic instrumentation. *Nurs Clin North Am* 1978 Dec; 13(4):573–587.

Lim-Levy, Fidelita: The effect of oxygen inhalation on oral temperature. *Nurs Res* 1982 May/June; 31(3):150–152.

Physical Exam

Bates, Barbara: *A Guide to Physical Assessment* ed.2. Philadelphia, Lippincott, 1979.

Beaumont, Estelle: Listen here: for the latest word on stethoscopes. (Product Survey) *Nursing 78* 1978 Nov; 8(11):32–37.

Cannon, Christine: Hands on guide to palpation and auscultation. *RN* 1980 March; 43(3):20–27.

Hudson, Margaret F: Safeguard your elderly patient's health through accurate physical assessment. *Nursing 83* 1983 Nov; 13(11):58–64.

King, R Carole: Refining your assessment techniques. *RN* 1983 Feb; 46(2):43–47.

Malasanos, Lois, et al: *Health Assessment.* ed.3. St. Louis, Mosby, 1985.

Diagnostic Tests

Cameron, Terrie J: Fiberoptic bronchoscopy. *Am J Nurs* 1981 Aug; 81(8):1462–1464.

Farrell, Jane: Arthroscopy. *Nursing 82* 1982 May; 12(5):73–75.

Finesilver, Cynthia: Reducing stress in patients having cardiac catheterization. *Am J Nurs* 1980 Oct; 80(10):1805–1807.

Fishbach, Frances: *A Manual of Laboratory Diagnostic Tests.* ed.2. Philadelphia, Lippincott, 1985.

Hanson, Robert L: New approach to measuring adult nasogastric tubes for insertion. *Am J Nurs* 1980 July; 80(7):1334.

Hilton, B Ann: Diabetic monitoring measures: does practice make perfect?: *Can Nurse* 1982 May; 78(5):26–32.

Hollen, Sr. Eileen Marie, Irene Vernaglia Toomey, and Shirley Given: Bronchoscopy. *Nursing 82* 1982 June; 12 (6):120–122.

McManus, Joan C, and Hausman, Kathy A: Cerebrospinal fluid analysis. *Nursing 82* 1982 Aug; 12(8):43–47.

Ordronneau, Noreen D: Helping patients in the radiology department. *Am J Nurs* 1980 July; 80(7):1312.

Rogers, Regina Rae: Your patient is scheduled for electrophysiology studies. *Am J Nurs* 1986 May; 86(5):873–875.

Shaefer, Donald, Betty Collin, and Donald Crell: Preparing a patient for an EEG. *Am J Nurs* 1975 Jan; 75(1):63–65.

Surr, Claire White: Teaching patients to use the new blood-glucose monitoring products—part I. *Nursing 83* 1983 Jan; 13(1):42–45.

——— Teaching patients to use the new blood-glucose monitoring products—part II. *Nursing 83* 1983 Feb; 13(2):58–62.

Widmann, Frances H: *Clinical Interpretation of Laboratory Tests.* ed.8. Philadelphia, Davis, 1979.

Charts and Records

Allison, Shiela, and Kathy Kinloch: Problem-oriented recording. *Can Nurse* 1981 Dec; 77(11):39–40.

Laing, Mary: Flow sheets—meeting the charting challenge. *Can Nurse* 1981 Dec; 77(11):40–42.

Merryman, Pricilla: The incident report: If in doubt, fill it out. *Nursing 85* 1985 May; 15(5):57–59.

Rutkowski, Barbara: How D.R.G.s are changing your charting. *Nursing 85* Oct; 15(10):49–51.

Sklar, Corinne: You and the law: problem-oriented recording—could there be a problem? *Can Nurse* 1982 May; 78(5):47–51.

Ulisse, Gael Calabia: *POMR: Application to Nursing Records.* Menlo Park, CA, Addison-Wesley, 1978.

19

The Diagnosis Phase of Nursing Process

Prerequisites and/or Suggested Preparation

A basic knowledge of the scope of nursing practice (Chapter 1) and an overview of nursing process (Chapter 17) are essential for understanding this chapter.

Nurses have long been accustomed to collecting data that will assist the physician in the development or substantiation of a *medical* diagnosis, but the process of forming a *nursing* diagnosis from available data is still evolving. It took over 300 years for an internationally accepted classification of medical diagnoses to be developed; in contrast, the development of a system of nursing diagnoses has been underway for less than 25 years.

NURSING DIAGNOSIS

The term *diagnosis* can be defined as "the analysis of a condition, situation or problem," and the term is used by workers in a wide range of occupations and professions, from auto mechanics to psychiatrists. A *medical diagnosis* identifies a well-defined disease condition, while a *nursing diagnosis* describes a patient's response to some aspect of such a condition. The significant differences between a medical diagnosis and a nursing diagnosis are related to the *focus* of the diagnosis and the action which follows. A medical diagnosis identifies a pathological condition which will be treated by the physician, whereas a nursing diagnosis describes a patient response which nurses are prepared and licensed to treat. If a diagnosis requires medical intervention, that diagnosis is a medical one: it is not a nursing diagnosis. A nursing diagnosis, therefore, is a clear statement of an existing or potential problem which can be prevented or alleviated by some type of *nursing* intervention.

A well-written nursing diagnosis provides a kind of professional shorthand which facilitates communication between nurses by transmitting a great deal of information in a few words. An effective classification of nursing diagnoses could improve communication between nurses by providing a format for stating a patient's problem so that it is clearly understood by all who read it or hear of it. An agreed-upon terminology could reduce the confusion and misunderstanding which is often dismissed with the phrase "It's all a question of semantics."

The First National Conference on the Classification of Nursing Diagnoses was held at St. Louis University in 1973. Enthusiasm and acceptance of the concept has increased steadily, and the 7th conference was held in 1986.

The North American Nursing Diagnosis Association was established in 1982; by 1984, it had accepted 51 nursing diagnoses (Table 19.1), and is now considering a number of other possible diagnoses which need further study and clarification before they can be accepted. This is an exciting new aspect of nursing with its own

---

> ### The Meaning of "Accepted Nursing Diagnosis"
>
> The term *accepted nursing diagnosis* refers to those diagnoses which, in the opinion of the National Conference Group, identify health problems that can be diagnosed and treated by nurses. At National Conferences, nurses in education, research, and practice review the diagnoses which have been submitted, and then by majority vote, decide which diagnoses are "accepted" and thereby recommended for clinical testing in nursing practice.
>
> At each conference, the terminology and categories of accepted diagnoses may be re-examined and modified as indicated.

emerging field of pioneers and leaders, and the next decade or two will bring forth an abundance of workshops, books, and journals as nursing attempts to further define and describe its unique role within the field of health care.

Components of Nursing Diagnoses

At present, members of the National Conference Group include three components in each diagnostic statement: the problem, its etiology, and the resulting signs and symptoms. Collectively, these three aspects of nursing diagnoses are referred to as PES which is an acronym for *P*roblem, *E*tiology, and *S*igns and *S*ymptoms.

Problem

The *problem* is a clear, concise statement of an existing or potential problem with which the patient must cope. The problem may have been observed (an existing problem), or it may be anticipated on the basis of the patient's condition, or the nurse's experience with other patients (a potential problem).

The term *problem* can be defined as an inability or difficulty in attaining a goal or desired state of being. The patient's problem may be that he is uncomfortable, sick, or in pain. It may be that he feels ineffective because he cannot reach the goals he has set. His life may seem frustrating and unsatisfying because of discrepancies between:

What is and what could be

What is and what should be

What is and what would be if only . . .

WHAT THE PROBLEM IS NOT. The patient's problem is *not* the same as an unmet need. A healthy person needs food and oxygen, but these needs do not usually con-

TABLE 19.1 CATEGORIES OF ACCEPTED NURSING DIAGNOSES

Activity/Rest

Activity intolerance
Activity intolerance, potential
Diversional activity, deficit
Sleep pattern disturbance.

Circulation

Cardiac output, alteration in: decreased
Tissue perfusion, alteration in

Elimination

Bowel elimination, alteration in: constipation
Bowel elimination, alteration in: diarrhea
Bowel elimination, alteration in: incontinence
Urinary elimination, alteration in

Emotional Reactions

Anxiety
Coping, ineffective individual
Fear
Grieving, anticipatory
Grieving, dysfunctional
Powerlessness
Rape trauma syndrome
Self-concept, disturbance in: body image; self-esteem; role performance; personal identity
Social isolation
Spiritual distress (distress of the human spirit)
Violence, potential for

Family Pattern Alterations

Coping, family: potential for growth
Coping, ineffective family: compromised
Coping, ineffective family: disabled
Family process, alteration in
Parenting, alteration in: actual or potential

Food/Fluid

Fluid volume, alteration in: excess
Fluid volume, deficit, actual 1,
Fluid volume, deficit, actual 2,
Fluid volume, deficit, potential,
Nutrition, alteration in: less than body requirements
Nutrition, alteration in: more than body requirements
Nutrition, alteration in: potential for more than body requirements
Oral mucous membranes, alteration in

Hygiene

Self-care deficit (specify level: feeding, bathing/hygiene, dressing/grooming, toileting)

Neurologic

Communication, impaired verbal
Sensory-perceptual alteration
Thought processes, alteration in

Pain

Comfort, alteration in: pain (Acute and chronic)

Safety

Injury, potential for,
Mobility, impaired physical
Skin integrity, impairment of: actual
Skin integrity, impairment of: potential

Sex

Sexual dysfunction

Teaching/Learning

Health maintenance, alteration in
Home maintenance management, impaired
Knowledge deficit (specify) [Learning need (specify)]
Noncompliance (specify) [Compliance (specify)]

Ventilation

Airway clearance, ineffective
Breathing pattern, ineffective
Gas exchange, impaired

*Excerpted from Doenges and Moorhouse: Nurse's Pocket Guide: Nursing Diagnoses with Interventions © 1985 F.A. Davis Company.

stitute a problem because a person simply eats and breathes until the needs are met. If, however, a person is too sick to eat or breathe effectively, or if food and oxygen are not available, a problem exists because the person's normal means of meeting these needs is not adequate.

The problem is *not* a sign or symptom. It is *not* the medical diagnosis. The problem is a statement of the patient's physical or psychological response to his current condition which is, at the moment, unrelieved.

Etiology

The second aspect of a nursing diagnosis is its etiology. The *etiology* is the cause of a problem, which may be physiological, psychological, environmental, sociological, spiritual, or any other set of factors responsible for creating the patient's problem. For example, a patient's failure to follow his physician's orders may be caused by a lack of knowledge and understanding, a denial of his illness, financial problems, lack of family support, an absence of hope, or any of a number of other reasons. It is imperative that the nurse know the etiology of the problem because such knowledge gives direction for nursing intervention. A patient's failure to follow his doctor's orders because of lack of understanding is a much different problem than failure to follow the doctor's order because of financial difficulties, and the interventions must be different for each one.

Signs and Symptoms

The third aspect of nursing diagnosis is the group of signs and symptoms which identify the problem. These are the characteristics of the patient's response, the clues which indicate that the problem exists. Without the identification and validation of the signs and symptoms, the presence of the problem might merely be an assumption, and not a reality.

MAKING A NURSING DIAGNOSIS

The process of making a nursing diagnosis can be divided into four major activities: (1) verifying the data, (2) interpreting the data, (3) identifying the problem, and (4) stating the diagnosis. These activities, though described sequentially, may occur almost simultaneously. None of them is unique to the process of making a nursing diagnosis; they are basic steps in logical thinking and problem solving in general.

Verifying the Data

First of all, the data must be complete if they are to be useful; thus, an ongoing activity is that of looking for gaps or omissions. It is important to study the information available, but it is equally important to be aware of the information that is *not* available. The vague questions that come to mind throughout the day must be transformed into specific questions such as: "There is no report of the patient being catheterized yesterday, and yet the order was written. Does that mean that it wasn't done?" "What happened to the patient last night? He seems much different this morning." "What did the x-rays show?" "Where are the most recent lab reports?"

Reports are sometimes lost, misfiled, or mislaid. Charting is sometimes incomplete. It is your responsibility to seek out the information you need or, in the case of reports from other departments, to initiate a search for missing data. At your request, such a search is often done by the ward secretaries of the units involved.

In addition to noticing gaps and omissions in data, the nurse needs to note any discrepancies that may be present such as a discrepancy between the amount of drug ordered and the amount of drug charted, between the diet ordered and the food the patient is eating, or between the perceptions of the patient and nurse regarding the amount of activity permitted. These discrepancies may be the result of errors in transcribing the original order, in executing the order, or in charting the care given. Such errors render the data useless for planning future care and must be clarified before the data can be used.

An ability essential throughout all phases of nursing process but especially important during the diagnostic phase is the ability to differentiate between facts and assumptions. Assumptions are a necessary part of our everyday activities; it would be impossible to validate and verify the truth and accuracy of everything we see and hear. We must assume, for example, that a 12-inch ruler is 12 inches long, that the person taking x-ray studies is a qualified x-ray technician, and that the milk in an unopened carton is safe to drink. These assumptions are valid because of the checks and balances in our society. The National Bureau of Standards regulates the manufacture of measuring devices; the personnel department of the hospital checks the credentials of its employees; and the state Department of Health oversees the processing and packaging of milk. These assumptions, therefore, are reasonable and warranted.

Other assumptions are neither reasonable nor warranted. Some assumptions are unwarranted because they are based on inaccurate or incomplete data. Other assumptions are unwarranted because of illogical thinking, even though in some cases the basic information was accurate and complete.

Examples of Unwarranted Assumptions Based on Faulty Data

Observation	Unwarranted Assumption	Reality of the Situation
The patient is not complaining of pain.	The patient is not in pain.	The patient may be in considerable pain but does not like to "complain." He does not like to take drugs, fears addiction, and would rather endure the pain.
The patient's daughter visits her elderly father every day.	The daughter is concerned about her father and would like him home with her for awhile when he is discharged.	The daughter has four small children in a tiny three-bedroom house, and thinks her older brother is best able to take care of their father.
The nurse says, "Mr. Jones?" and the patient turns over in bed and gets ready to take his medication.	Patient is Mr. Jones	Patients *usually* respond when spoken to. A patient in bed assumes that the nurse at his bedside came to see him and that she merely used the wrong name. The patient is *not* Mr. Jones.
The patient has tarry black stools. Tarry stools are a symptom of GI bleeding.	The patient has been bleeding, either from his stomach or intestinal tract.	Bismuth preparations turn normal stools black, and the patient has been taking Pepto-Bismol each day for several weeks. The patient is *not* bleeding.

It is obvious that these assumptions were unwarranted, but many similar instances of faulty thinking pass undetected every day. The resulting assumptions are invalid and cannot be used as the basis for a valid nursing diagnosis.

Interpreting the Data

Among the many skills involved in the interpretation and use of assessment data, three skills are especially important. These skills are the ability to: (1) find relationships within the data, (2) use norms and standards, and (3) detect similarities and differences.

Finding Relationships

A mass of unrelated data is of little use as a basis for planning patient care. Such data must be sorted, and classified or categorized to be usable. Some categories are obvious, such as the systems of the body. All physiological data associated with the gastrointestinal tract and the results of related diagnostic tests should be grouped together, for example. Some information may have been collected over a period of time and must be arranged in chronological order before the sequence and progression of events is clear.

Some relationships may be obscure, and their discovery requires expert sleuthing. It may take considerable thought to connect a patient's weakness and easy fatigue with a new medication; to discover that a patient's incapacitating headaches often start about 8 to 10 hours after certain cleaning products have been used; or to see a relationship between a child's loss of appetite, vomiting, and weight loss with the death of his grandmother. An isolated bit of information is seldom useful, and a knowledge of its relationship to other phenomena is necessary before meaning can be ascribed to it.

Using Norms and Standards

To select from all the available data everything that is likely to be significant, two types of norms or standards must be used. First, the data must be compared with the standards accepted as the normal range for the population as a whole, such as height and weight, vision, and red blood cell count. Knowing whether the results of a given nursing assessment are normal or abnormal is prerequisite to using those results.

Second, the data must be compared with the *norms for that particular patient;* the nurse must know what is normal for that person. A BP of 110/80 would be considered normal for a hypothetical average person, but that same BP could represent a state of near shock for a person with hypertension whose BP had not been less than 150/100 in the past 20 years. Similarly, a nurse's concern for a given patient's need for a daily bowel movement is unwarranted if that patient's normal pattern of elimination is a bowel movement every third day. Information is less likely to be misinterpreted when you consistently ask the patient "Is this normal for you?" and "Does this represent a change for you?"

Detecting Similarities and Differences

It has been said that the ability to detect *differences* in things that are similar, and *similarities* in things that are different, is a mark of an educated person. This ability is the result of a person's efforts to find systematic and orderly relationships within his world, and is developed by extensive training and experience. For example, when asked the question "What do irises, roses, peonies, sweet peas, and daisies have in common?" a botanist can describe the structures common to this group of unrelated plants. He is able to see the *similarities in things that are different.* On the other hand, a person who raises prize-winning roses can differentiate among 15 or more varieties of yellow roses that look identical to an untrained eye and can identify each by its botanical name. He can see the *differences in things that are similar.*

In similar fashion, an experienced nurse recognizes the *differences* among patients who share a common diagnosis or condition. A group of premature infants in an intensive care nursery may seem very much alike to an untrained person, but not to the specialist. It is important to be aware of the differences among a group of 80-year-old women in a nursing home, for example, and the ability to see the differences will enable you to care for each as an individual.

It is equally important to be able to recognize *similarities* in the responses of patients with different conditions and diagnoses, such as the responses to pain which are common to many patients regardless of the cause of the pain, which might be caused by cancer, infection, or trauma. The ability to note similarities within differences enables you to use theoretical concepts as a basis for nursing care. It means that it is not necessary for you to start from scratch with each new patient, as if every aspect of the situation were new and different from anything you had ever experienced. You are able to analyze the similarities and differences between patients, and between your patient's condition and the textbook description of a similar patient condition.

Identifying the Problem

Once the available data have been verified and interpreted, the next step in making a nursing diagnosis is identifying the problem. It is necessary to identify the *general* problem area before trying to describe the *specific* problem. Before the nurse can help a crying patient, for example, she must learn whether he is crying because of pain, his forthcoming surgery, finances, or in-law problems. Once the general problem area has been identified, *increasingly specific assessments* must be made until the problem is described in enough detail for a nursing diagnosis to be established.

An early step in forming a nursing diagnosis is assigning the patient's situation, condition, or event to one of the following categories:

> It is not a problem for the patient
> It is a problem, but not a nursing problem
> It is a nursing problem

Since a nursing diagnosis describes a problem amenable to nursing intervention, it follows that problems not amenable to nursing intervention are not an appropriate basis for a nursing diagnosis. Limitations of time, energy, competency, and professional standards make it inappropriate for any nurse to try to solve all of a patient's identified problems. Some problems, such as unemployment, inadequate housing, poverty, and crime are outside the realm of nursing, but the patient's *responses* to such problems may pose a threat to the health or well-being of himself or his family. His response thereby becomes a nursing concern and it is important for the nurse to intervene by referring the situation to a social worker or an appropriate service agency.

A careful distinction should be made between a patient's problem and the nurse's problem. The phrase "difficulty in turning," for example, is vague and does not indicate who is having difficulty, the patient or the nurse. Stated more precisely, the phrase "hard for patient to turn" clearly refers to a patient problem while the phrase "hard to turn patient" refers to the nurse's problem. If a person unfamiliar with the situation can misinterpret a problem statement in any way, the problem should be restated until it is no longer ambiguous.

Stating the Diagnosis

Many patients could, and would if they were asked, diagnose their own nursing needs. The patient may state his perception of the problem (the patient's diagnosis) in a single sentence, or he may intersperse parts of it throughout several sentences or paragraphs; but he will usually include the problem, the cause, and his response or reaction.

The patient is not concerned about the format of a diagnosis and may present the component parts of his diagnosis in any sequence. For example, the following sentences are all constructed differently, but the messages are essentially the same.

> I drink liquor at night because I'm worried and can't sleep.
> I'm worried about my son and I can't sleep, so I drink to feel better.

If I was't worried, I could sleep at night and I wouldn't drink so much.

I can't stop drinking because I'm awake all night worrying about my son.

Any diagnostic statement that fails to include the signs and symptoms (response of the patient to the problem) hampers the nurse because she must know the effect of the condition or situation before she can be sure that a problem exists and that she needs to intervene. In addition to the statement "I can't sleep nights because of worry," the nurse must know how the patient responds to the situation: Does it make him drink excessively, pace the floor, read his Bible, eat compulsively, catch up on reading, or meditate? In short, the response of the patient or family must be known before a problem can be presumed to exist. A situation that might be a major problem for one patient could be of little concern to another. The response of the patient is perhaps the most important aspect of a nursing diagnosis because a nurse treats the patient's response, not the situation.

Although many patients are able to participate in the development of nursing diagnoses, others are not. The nurse must diagnose the nursing needs of infants and toddlers and people who are comatose, confused, or too ill to participate.

Once a patient's problem has been identified and described, it may be necessary to restate it in an accepted format. Some informal diagnoses can be used as stated by the patient to direct and guide the nursing care that will be given in the immediate future. If it seems, for example, that a particular problem can be resolved within your time with the patient, it is not necessary to spend time trying to phrase a formal nursing diagnosis. It need not even be written down. On the other hand, a nursing diagnosis that will be used for a number of days, or even weeks, should be refined and phrased with such clarity that all members of the health care team can understand it easily. It is not enough for a nursing diagnosis to be meaningful to the nurse who writes it; it must communicate her perception of the situation to all who read it.

As yet, there is no universally accepted format for stating a nursing diagnosis. Most schools of nursing have chosen, or are in the process of choosing, a format which all students are expected to use. This format will undoubtedly be modified from time to time as leaders in the development of nursing diagnoses set forth new and more explicit guidelines.

Some hospitals and other health care agencies, especially those who use computers extensively, are seeking standardized formats and a generally accepted classification system.

A Nursing Diagnosis Should Be

- Based on nursing assessments, including both objective and subjective data
- Factual, nonjudgmental, and neutral
- Specific and individualized, based on firsthand knowledge of the patient
- Focused on the patient's response to a disease or condition, not on the disease itself
- Written in clear, simple language
- Based on the problem, etiology, and signs and symptoms

In other situations, nurses are free to use any format that conforms to generally accepted standards for nursing diagnoses.

PATIENT TEACHING

Every person should learn how to present his problem to the nurse or physician in an effective manner in order to avoid wasted time and energy, and to obtain optimal health care. The individual should be able to make a diagnostic statement *using lay language* which expresses his perception of his situation. To help him learn to do so, you will need to ask him three questions related to the three components of a diagnostic statement: the problem, etiology, and signs and symptoms.

1. What seems to be the problem?
2. What do you think caused it? (or might be causing it?)
3. What signs or symptoms have you noticed? What are the characteristics of this condition?

Of these three questions, the second is the one most likely to be especially significant, and yet most often unasked. The patient often has a "good hunch," suspicion, or intuitive guess about the cause (etiology) of his present condition but, for one reason or another, may not tell the nurse or physician. Much valuable time and energy can be lost if the patient lacks the confidence to share his ideas about the etiology because of embarrassment, guilt, fear, or feeling of unworthiness. Examples of causes which may not be reported are: an unhealthy lifestyle, personal stress such as marital problems or large debts, misuse of alcohol or drugs, or a hereditary health problem.

Each person should learn how to participate in the process of diagnosing his own health problems as a step toward achieving more effective health care.

RELATED ACTIVITIES

Select at least five health-related problems which you (or a member of your family) have experienced recently. For each problem write a nursing diagnosis using the PES components (problem, etiology, and signs and symptoms).

1. Categorize the problem by selecting one of the nursing diagnoses from Table 19.1.
2. Identify the cause of the problem.
3. State the signs and symptoms (defining characteristics).

Evaluate each of the diagnostic statements you have written by answering the following questions:

"If this situation were to recur, would this diagnostic statement be clear to all nurses involved in my care?"

"Would this nursing diagnosis give guidance and direction for effective nursing intervention?"

If necessary, rework the diagnosis until you feel that it presents a clear and accurate picture of your state or condition and that it would help to ensure effective nursing care.

SUGGESTED READINGS

Bruce, Joan A, and Marie E Snyder: The right and responsibility to diagnose: The legal side. *Am J Nurs* 1982 April; 82(4):645–646.

Campbell, Clarie: *Nursing Diagnosis and Intervention in Nursing Practice.* ed.2. New York, Wiley, 1984.

Carnevali, Doris L, et al: *Diagnostic Reasoning in Nursing.* Philadelphia, Lippincott, 1984.

Carpenito, Lynda J: *Nursing Diagnosis: Applications to Clinical Practice.* Philadelphia, Lippincott, 1983.

Gettrust, Kathy V, Susan C Ryan, and Diane S Engelman (eds.): *Applied Nursing Diagnosis,* New York, Wiley, 1985.

Gordon, Marjory: *Nursing Diagnosis: Process and Application.* New York, McGraw-Hill, 1982.

Kim, Mi Ja, Gertrude K McFarland, and Audrey M McLane (eds.): *Classification of Nursing Diagnoses: Proceedings of the Fifth National Conference.* St. Louis, Mosby, 1984.

Kim, Mi Ja, et al: *Pocket Guide for Nursing Diagnoses.* St. Louis, Mosby, 1984.

Leslie, Flora M: Nursing diagnosis: use in long-term care. *Am J Nurs* 1981 May; 81(5):1012–1014.

Lunney, Margaret: Nursing diagnosis: refining the system. *Am J Nurs* 1982 March; 82(3):456–459.

Martens, Karen: Let's diagnose strengths, not just problems. *Am J Nurs* 1986 Feb; 86(2):192–193.

Martin, Karen: A client classification system adaptable for computerization. *Nurs Outlook* 1982 Nov/Dec; 30(9):515–517.

Neel, Carol J: Making nursing diagnoses work for you . . . every day. *Nursing 86* 1986 May; 16(5):56–57.

Price, Mary Radatovich: Nursing diagnosis: making a concept come alive. *Am J Nurs* 1980 April; 80(4):668–671.

Tartaglia, Michael J: Nursing diagnosis: Keystone of your care plan. *Nursing 85* 1985 March; 15(3):34–37.

20

The Planning Phase
of Nursing Process

Prerequisites and/or Suggested Preparation
Chapter 1 (Nursing as a Profession), Chapter 17 (Overview of Nursing Process), and Chapter 19 (Diagnostic Phase) are prerequisite to this chapter. The section on the use of objectives in Chapter 10 (Teaching and Learning) is suggested as additional preparation.

The third phase of nursing process is the planning phase. The initial nursing assessments have been completed, the nursing diagnoses have been made, and now the question is: "What is to be done?" The planning phase culminates in a nursing care plan that will answer not only that question, but the questions of How? and When?

The activities of this phase correspond to those by which a physician outlines a plan of treatment for a patient once the diagnosis has been made. These planning activities are extremely important because they make the difference between a haphazard, trial-and-error approach, and a systematic, purposeful approach to both nursing care and medical care.

THE PLANNING PROCESS

There are at least six activities that occur during the planning phase of nursing process. These activities cannot be considered steps because they are not necessarily sequential. Some of the activities can be done concurrently, and others may occur at any time during the phase. These activities are:

1. Setting priorities
2. Setting goals and objectives
3. Stating conditions and criteria
4. Selecting nursing interventions
5. Developing nursing orders
6. Developing a nursing care plan

SETTING PRIORITIES

In any given nursing situation, it is necessary to set priorities among the nursing diagnoses or problem statements so that the most urgent problems can be resolved first. Priority is determined by an analysis of several considerations, among them, the patient's condition, the patient's preferences, the overall plan of therapy, nursing resources, and agency policy.

Factors Influencing Priorities

Patient's Condition
In general, Maslow's hierarchy of needs reflects many of the priorities in patient care. Urgent physiological needs must be granted top priority, followed by safety and psychological security, love and belongingness, and self-esteem. For example, a burned patient's condition must be stabilized and his survival assured before certain psychological aspects of treatment and care can be given a high priority.

Patient's Preference and Sense of Urgency
A patient may be acutely upset or distressed by a problem that seems relatively unimportant or of secondary importance to other people. Problems that seem urgent to the patient and/or the family must be resolved as quickly as possible in order to reduce anxiety and allow the patient's energy and resources to be focused on the next set of problems.

Overall Treatment Plan
Nursing care must be congruent with other aspects of health care, and the priorities of the *overall* treatment plan must be considered when nursing care is being planned. For example, the medical and nursing plans must be consistent with respect to their emphasis on physical activity; one plan cannot promote increased activity while the other is promoting increased rest.

Schedules of various departments must be coordinated so that patient teaching is not planned at a time when the patient is apt to be exhausted from a tiring session in physical therapy, nor a visit from the speech therapist scheduled before the patient has had an opportunity to shave and feel presentable.

Nursing Resources
The time and energy available to the nurse who is assigned to a given patient will affect the setting of priorities. If the nurse's case load or assignment is heavy, or in an emergency situation, she may be unable to attend to anything more than the most basic needs of each assigned patient. Unexpected events and unanticipated changes do happen, but every effort should be made to make sure that each nursing care plan is reasonable, realistic, and practical. A steady succession of unmet goals and objectives is usually a result of poor planning.

Agency Policy
Agency policy may dictate that certain goals be reached before discharge, or that certain skills be attained by the patient before other activities are permitted. In such situations, those goals or skills must be given a high priority, and nursing care must be planned to make sure the goals are reached. If, for example, a developmentally disabled child must be toilet trained before he will be accepted into a day-care program, toilet training then becomes a high priority in the care of that child.

Problem-Oriented Records
If the hospital or health care facility uses a problem-oriented approach, patient problems ae numbered in chronological order, but within the limits of that numbering system, the other considerations for setting priorities for action still apply. The number assigned to a problem does not necessarily indicate its priority.

SETTING GOALS AND OBJECTIVES

There are many synonyms for a goal, including outcome, purpose, aim, intent, and objective, each of which may have several meanings. In this chapter, a *goal* is defined as a desired outcome, an outcome that is both hoped for and worked for. The terms *goal* and *objectives* are often used interchangeably although an objective is often more specific than a goal.

In nursing, goals and objectives are derived from one or more nursing diagnoses which describe the existence of a problem. If the patient were not confronted with a problem or barrier, he would not be in need of nursing care in the form of teaching, psychological support, or physical care and comfort.

The uses and values of goals in nursing are the same as for goals in any situation. Goals give a sense of direction and perspective; their attainment gives satisfaction and a sense of accomplishment; and they provide a basis for evaluating the activities undertaken.

Assessment of the Patient's Problems

The first step in establishing a goal is an adequate assessment of the problem underlying the patient's nursing diagnosis. If a patient's diagnosed problem is caused by lack of direction, by not knowing what to do, or by wanting to pursue several objectives that seem to be in conflict with each other, the nursing goal will be related to clarification of the patient's situation and his attainment of a clear sense of direction.

If a client's problem is related to his indecision over how to achieve a desired objective, such as trying to decide between alternative types of care for an elderly parent, the nursing goal will be related to an exploration of the possible courses of action and the selection of one that is acceptable to those involved.

If a patient's problem is related to barriers that stand between him and his objectives, the nursing goal will be related either to the removal of the barriers, to increasing the patient's ability to surmount the barriers, or to changing the objective. When a patient's problem involves a barrier, it is often helpful initially to assign the problem to one of the following categories:

Nothing can be done about it.
Something can be done about it, and nursing can do it.
Something can be done, but someone else should do it.

It is very difficult for most people to admit and accept the fact that *sometimes nothing can be done about the cause* of a problem; and as a result, considerable energy is expended in irritation, frustration, desperation, or rage over things that cannot be changed. Neither nurse nor patient can change a diagnosis of cancer, or the fact that a baby is deformed. Each person can, however, *modify or change his reaction* to the situation once he has accepted it. The family of an alcoholic cannot change him, for he must do that himself; but family members can learn functional and effective ways of coping with something they have accepted.

The Serenity Prayer, which is basic to the programs of both Alcoholics Anonymous and Overeaters Anonymous, is equally applicable to difficult situations in nursing.

God grant me the serenity to accept the things I cannot change, the courage to change the things I can, and the wisdom to know the difference.

Types of Goals

Goals may be classified as short term, intermediate, or long range. Long-range goals are used in rehabilitation centers, nursing homes, outpatient clinics, and extended care facilities. They are used by community health nurses who work with families over a period of years, and school nurses have long-range goals for children with chronic health problems.

A situation involving long-range goals will usually require intermediate goals as well. The achievement of each intermediate goal tends to encourage the patient to keep on working and tends to decrease the frustration and discouragement that often accompany the seemingly endless struggle to reach long-term goals.

The timing of intermediate goals depends on the timing of long-range goals. If, for example, the long-range goals are expected to be met in 1 month, the intermediate goals would probably be met in 2 or 2½ weeks. On the other hand, if long range means 5 to 10 years for a given patient, the intermediate goals might be set for intervals of 1 or 2 years.

Short-Term Goals

Short-term goals are used under any of three conditions. First, they are used for people who become discouraged or frustrated by any goal that seem remote or difficult to reach. Short-term goals enable these people to experience the success and satisfaction of reaching each of a *series of goals*, the end result of which is the equivalent of an intermediate or long-range goal. The following example illustrates the use of a series of short-term goals for a patient who is frightened and reluctant to move because of severe pain.

Day 1. Dangle feet on edge of bed, with support, for 10 minutes, t.i.d. (3 × daily).

Day 2. Walk from bed to chair, and sit in chair t.i.d. Start with 10 minutes; increase by 10 minutes each time.

Day 3. Walk from bed to door and back. Walk this distance once in AM, 2× in PM. and 3× times in evening.

Day 4. Etc.

Second, short-term goals are used when a patient needs health care only for a short period of time. The nursing goals for a new mother who will be discharged on the second or third day after delivery must, of necessity, be short term. (Long-range goals would have been used during the 9 months of her pregnancy.) The short-term goals might include bathing, diapering, holding, and feeding the infant effectively. If the mother was unable to learn to do this within the time allotted and therefore could not reach the short-term goals, or if other problems arose that could not be resolved within 2 or 3 days, a referral would be made to the appropriate community health agency for ongoing teaching and supervision.

Third, short-term goals are used by nurses whose contact with a patient will be brief even though that patient will need nursing care over an extended period of time. Such nurses would include part-time workers, nurses who float (assigned to a different unit each day), and students who may be assigned to a patient for only a day or two. Each of these nurses is obligated to do what she can to help the patient progress toward goals that have already been established; but in addition, each nurse usually develops additional short-term goals for the time she will be with the patient.

Setting Short-Term Goals

Ideally, patients participate actively in the formation of goals, which are called, logically enough, patient goals. When the nurse's contact with a patient will be brief, her opportunity to include him in setting goals will be very limited. In such circumstances, she must assess the situation and quickly develop a few short-term goals which can be achieved during her time with the patient. Based on information obtained from the patient's chart, the Kardex, and the change-of-shift report plus initial contact with the patient, the nurse can formulate a few nursing goals that, if met, will contribute to his well-being.

Students are often expected to visit their assigned patients during the evening before each clinical experience and then to *write out* their plan of care. Nurses assigned to a unit for a single shift are expected to listen to a report on a patient, skim the chart, read the Kardex

carefully, and mentally establish specific goals for the day. There is usually no time to write a set of goals, but since attention to goals is an integral part of the nurse's thought processes, whenever she approaches a patient's room, she thinks, "What do I want to accomplish while I am with this patient?" The following examples show how a nurse uses basic information about a patient to form short-term goals.

- "The night nurse said that Mr. Jones didn't sleep well. I'll try to find out why, and then see if Mr. Jones and I together can figure out a way to cope with his sleeplessness."
- "When I took Mrs. Baldwin's breakfast tray to her, she looked apathetic and depressed. She isn't wearing any makeup, and her hair looks stringy and dirty. I'll see if she would like a quick shampoo; and while I'm doing that, I'll try to evaluate her emotional status and find out what's going on with her."
- "Mrs. Robinson is only 19, and this is her first hospitalization. I'll see if she knows how to do a breast self-examination, and if not, I'll teach her during her bath."

Short-term goals like these, because they are developed in response to cues from the patient, data from the patient's chart, and the report of the night nurse, are patient centered and valid.

STATING CONDITIONS AND CRITERIA

In nursing, a goal can be defined as a behavior, a change, or a state of being that is sought by, or for, a patient. A goal usually represents potential progress toward greater health or maintenance of an individual's present level of health. The following are examples of patient goals: "to breathe easier," "to be able to manage my own diet," "to get to the bathroom," "to feel less scared about my baby's cleft palate."

These goals, as stated, identify the behavior or ability that is desired; but they are not very useful because they give no guidance to either patient or nurse. There is no description of the conditions under which the behavior will occur, nor of the criteria for knowing when the goal has been reached.

A useful objective has three components: the *behavior*, the *conditions*, and the *criteria*. All three are needed to make a goal specific and realistic, and to provide a basis for measuring success. In other words, any statement that is to give direction to the activities of patient and nurse must include: (1) the desired behavior, (2) the conditions under which the behavior will occur, and (3) the criteria for recognizing satisfactory attainment of the behavior.

The process of describing the conditions and criteria for a given behavior starts with two questions:

Under what circumstances will the desired behavior occur?

How will the patient look or act when this event occurs?

Brainstorming is a valuable technique for answering these questions. The process of listing as many tentative answers as possible increases the possibility of identifying appropriate conditions and criteria, and decreases the likelihood of narrow and restrictive thinking. The following example illustrates a few of the possible conditions and criteria which brainstorming can produce.

Desired behavior: To be able to breathe more easily. Possible *conditions* under which the patient might want to breathe more easily:

- When trying to turn over in bed
- When doing the housework
- When lying down, especially at night
- While jogging
- When dusting and sweeping

Possible *criteria* for measuring success (how will the patient look or act if he is able to breathe more easily?):

- Does not pant or gasp when turning over in bed
- States: "I don't feel short of breath"
- Lips and nail beds are less blue
- Can lie flat; no longer needs three pillows for sleep
- Respirations are slower and less labored
- Less concerned about having portable O_2 tank nearby
- States, "I don't get tired as quickly"

From such a list of possible conditions and criteria, the nurse can select a few that seem relevant to her patient and that are likely to be useful in planning and evaluating his care.

Conditions

Careful identification of the circumstances under which the desired behavior should take place will reduce an idealistic and impractical goal to a manageable, realistic one. For example, the vague goal "to walk again" for a patient with a spinal cord injury could convey the expectation that he will someday be able to walk every-

where, on any surface, under all conditions. A person who writes such a goal probably knows that in all likelihood the patient can never regain such comprehensive walking ability, but the carelessly written goal implies this. Although the patient may never walk easily or rapidly and may never be able to take a back-packing trip over rough terrain, he *will be able to experience success and satisfaction* through a series of specific, realistic goals. His goals can be made realistic by carefully specifying the conditions under which he will eventually be able to walk: to the bathroom without the help of a nurse, from the front door of the house to the car, or in semi-darkness down a theater aisle, for example.

The conditions of a goal may be written as part of the behavior or as a separate phrase. The format is immaterial, but the content must be clear and specific. Even though the words *behavior* and *conditions* may be omitted or unused, the patient, family, and nurse must be in agreement about the behavior that is sought and the conditions under which it will occur. Unless all parties understand and accept the conditions of the goal toward which everyone is working, frustration and disillusionment can be expected because each person will interpret the goal differently. Vague goals such as "to walk again," "to achieve his maximum potential," or "to achieve greater independence" are not helpful to anyone because they are not specific enough to motivate a patient, to guide his efforts, or to evaluate any progress he might make.

Outcome Criteria

In addition to specifying the behavior and conditions of a given goal, it is necessary to describe the ways in which successful attainment of the goal can be recognized. Since a goal is often defined as a desired outcome, the criteria for judging success are called *outcome criteria*, and they are used to indicate how well something has been done.

In most situations, it is not enough to simply *do* something—a poor performance does not constitute successful goal attainment. The minimal acceptable standard of performance must be described. The performance of the patient with a spinal cord injury whose goal was to walk from the front door to the car would probably not be considered successful if it took him 30 minutes, if he fell three times, was extremely short of breath when he got there, and was so exhausted that he had to be lifted into the car. (Of course there are exceptional people for whom getting there at all, in whatever way, would constitute success and whose drive and determination will keep them struggling until it gets easier and easier.) For most patients, reasonable outcome criteria might be being able to walk from the front door to the car without falling, without undue fatigue, without becoming short of breath, and with normal, erect posture.

Outcome criteria may seem elusive and hard to identify at first, but the process becomes natural and relatively easy if, for every goal the nurse sets, she asks herself questions such as:

- How will the patient look if the desired change occurs?
- How will the patient behave if the goal is reached?
- What must he do in order for people to agree that he is successful?
- How well must he do it?

Such questions usually lead to specific, concrete criteria. For example, the following outcome criteria would be useful for a person who is paralyzed on one side following a stroke and whose goal is to use the toilet without assistance:

- Patient's clothing is still clean and dry (does not get wet or soiled in the process)
- Bathroom is as clean after use as it was when patient entered it
- Patient is able to wash his hands after using toilet
- Patient does not slip or fall

Some goals require outcome criteria that are specific and precise and that are based on accuracy, speed, frequency, or amounts. Examples of such criteria are:

- Measures insulin accurately
- Drinks at least 2,000 cc/day
- Walks a mile in 30 minutes (2 times a day)

Characteristics of Outcome Criteria

It is important to separate outcome criteria from closely related aspects of nursing process such as goals and nursing actions, and to be able to identify some of the factors which influence outcome criteria.

OUTCOME CRITERIA DO NOT DEPEND UPON THE WAY THE GOAL IS STATED. The purpose of a goal is to provide direction for nursing care and to facilitate communication of that direction among patient, family, nurse, and other members of the health care team. The *format* of the goal is less important than the clarity of the message, and in many situations the nurse will be free to express the goal as she chooses. In other settings great emphasis will be placed on the difference between *patient goals* and *nurse's goals*. Yet, if the patient has been actively involved in setting a goal, the *intension* of that goal is the same regardless of the way it is stated. In the illustration that follows, the intention of each goal is the same and the end results will be alike regardless of format.

Goal	Patient's Goal	Nurse's Goal
The relief of pain	To experience relief of pain	To relieve patient's pain
The relief of insomnia	To be free of insomnia; to sleep well	To relieve patient's insomnia
Self-administration of insulin	To give my own insulin	To teach patient to give own insulin
Independence in use of toilet	To use toilet without help	To help patient achieve independence in using toilet

In each instance, the *criteria for success will be the same*, regardless of the way the goal is stated.

OUTCOME CRITERIA ARE DIFFERENT FROM A GOAL. A statement of a goal does not indicate how a person can tell if that goal has been reached. A goal of lowered body temperature does not explain what is meant by "lowered body temperature," for example.

The patient's responses to some goals, such as the relief of pain, are basically subjective; and specific outcome criteria are needed to answer the question "How will I know if his pain has been relieved?" Some criteria related to the relief of pain are:

He falls asleep

He states, "I feel better," or "The pain is gone now"

He is willing to move about

He no longer immobilizes the body part, grimaces, or winces

His pulse and respiration, if elevated by pain, have returned to normal

He does whatever the pain was keeping him from doing

None of these *criteria* are the same as the *goal* of pain relief.

OUTCOME CRITERIA ARE INDEPENDENT OF THE NURSING INTERVENTION USED. The criteria listed above for the relief of pain are valid *regardless of the method used to relieve it*. The same outcome criteria are useful whether the method of pain relief is distraction, medication, therapeutic touch, hypnosis, or a hot water bottle. The patient's response to the relief of pain will be similar regardless of the kind of nursing intervention.

OUTCOME CRITERIA DEPEND ON THE PATIENT'S CURRENT HEALTH STATUS AND PREVIOUS LEVEL OF FUNCTIONING. Some criteria can be established only after the patient's normal habits and patterns are known. Outcome criteria for the relief of temporary insomnia, for example, are useless unless they are based on the patient's usual or desired sleeping habits. At first glance, a seemingly valid criteria might be "sleeps 7 or 8 hours without awakening"; but such an outcome criterion is inappropriate for an older person who *normally* sleeps only 5 or 6 hours and who usually gets up at least twice to go to the bathroom. For this person, successful relief of insomnia would be indicated by "sleeps a total of 5 or 6 hours and goes back to sleep within 5 or 10 minues after getting up to go to the bathroom."

Failure to take a patient's previous level of functioning into account is not uncommon. One not-so-funny true story describes a nurse talking with the son of a recently hospitalized elderly patient:

Nurse: "Your father is doing quite well, but we are having trouble getting him to walk more than a few feet.

Son: "Trouble walking! He hasn't been out of bed in the last five years!!"

SELECTING NURSING INTERVENTIONS

In nursing, as in all other endeavors, there are many ways to reach a goal. Several ways may seem equally attractive and equally likely to be effective, so the selection of an intervention to reach a nursing goal requires considerable knowledge and professional judgment.

The first step in the selection of a nursing action is to list as many nursing interventions as possible. This step is crucial because it frees you from a standardized, stimulus-response approach to nursing care. Unless you have deliberately trained yourself to always consider a variety of ways to reach any goal, it is easy to slip into a regrettable pattern of taking routine, unimaginative actions such as:

Stimulus	Response
Patient has a headache?	Give aspirin.
Patient has a poor appetite?	Tell the dietician.
Patient is unsteady on his feet?	Order a walker.
Patient seems lonely?	Inform the family.

For each of the above problems, there are at least five or 10 individualized actions that could be taken

and that would be likely to alleviate the problem rather than simply addressing the symptom of the problem. Some people who are committed to creative problem solving never take action on a problem until at least three possible solutions have been identified.

When a list of feasible nursing actions has been compiled, one is selected. In the end, this selection may or may not prove to be an ideal choice, or even a good choice; but it is selected because *at the time* it seems to be the best one in terms of the preferences of the patient and the nurse, the ability of the nurse, and the resources available to the patient and the nurse. In addition, an action is selected because the nurse expects it to be effective, realistic, and acceptable to all concerned.

DEVELOPING NURSE ORDERS

A nursing order is an order *written by a nurse* that directs the independent activities of nurses toward the attainment of patient goals. Nursing orders are usually written by the nurse who has primary responsibility for the patient, using input from those who share in his care. *Nursing orders increase the effectiveness of patient care* because they increase the probability that care will be implemented as planned, and decrease the likelihood that any aspect of the planned care will be omitted.

A nursing order differs from a medical order in that nursing orders describe an activity and stipulate how it should be carried out, whereas medical orders simply indicate what should be done, with no mention of how. Some examples of medical orders are:

Intake and output for 24 hours
Low salt diet
Out of bed this afternoon
Upper GI series

Medical orders assume that the nurse who transcribes the order will schedule the event as soon as possible and that those who carry out the order know how to do so. The medical order "Out of bed (OOB) this afternoon" does not differentiate among patients with varying capabilities, such as the patient who is eager and able to get out of bed without assistance, the patient who is feeble and needs much assistance, or the patient who is paralyzed and must be lifted OOB. A nursing order, on the other hand, usually specifies *how* the task is to be accomplished, at what time, and for how long.

Nurses write two types of nursing orders, orders which provide a nursing protocol for an identified group of patients and orders for an individual patient.

Nursing Protocol

A well-run household or office functions on the basis of certain routines, expectations, and policies that may be negotiated or modified to meet the demands of specific situations. These guidelines enable members of the household to accomplish certain routine activities with a minimal amount of decision making while devoting more of their available time and energy to especially demanding problems and projects.

In nursing, the ways in which patients progress through some events can be predicted with considerable accuracy, and standardized nursing routines (nursing protocols) can be both effective and efficient. Such events include progression through a sequence of diets followiong noncomplicated abdominal surgery, progressive activity and ambulation after the surgical repair of a fractured hip, and the teaching needed by parents of a premature infant.

Nursing protocols are carefully thought-out guidelines, often developed by a committee, which describe a minimal plan of care for a given condition. These basic orders form the skeleton of the overall nursing care plan and are supplemented by additional, individualized nursing orders. In this text the term *nursing orders* refers to those orders written for an individual patient to ensure personalized, quality care that extends *beyond* the basic care indicated by protocol.

Nursing Orders

Nursing orders, in contrast to nursing protocol, are derived from the nursing diagnosis and from the goals set for an individual patient, and are therefore specific to a given patient. Table 20.1 gives examples of a medical

TABLE 20.1 FACTORS WHICH INFLUENCE A PATIENT'S CARE PLAN

Present situation: Patient, age 67, had surgery 2 days ago for repair of fractured hip.

Medical order: OOB Wednesday; ambulate Friday.

Nursing protocol for all patients with a fractured hip: Prepare patient for ambulation. Teach exercises to strengthen quadriceps and biceps. Schedule and supervise exercises qid (four times daily).

Patient's assessment: "I can't get any rest because they are constantly coming in, and I'm getting worn out and sort of mad."

Nursing diagnosis: Patient irritable and tired because of lack of rest secondary to frequent interruptions.

Nursing order: Incorporate exercises into ADL. Leave patient undisturbed between 10:30 and 11:30 am and 3:00 and 4:00 pm.

order, a nursing protocol, the patient's assessment, nursing diagnosis, and the resulting nursing order in a given situation.

In Table 20.1, the nursing protocol had been developed previously, and the guidelines for preparation for ambulation had evolved as nurses sought ways to help the patient strengthen his arms and legs in preparation for using a walker. The physician made the decision as to when the patient could get OOB and start to walk, but the preparation of the patient for ambulation is a nursing responsibility. The nursing diagnosis describes the patient's response to the exercises prescribed by the nursing protocol, and the nursing order indicates the proposed solution to the problem. The patient was included in planning this approach, and therefore he will not think he is being ignored during the times specified for rest periods.

A nursing order must be congruent with all other orders because the actions that result will be part of the overall therapy. If there should be a discrepancy or conflict between a medical order and a nursing order, it must be resolved at once. Resolution can usually be facilitated by a collegial discussion between nurse and physician about the intent and purpose of each order and of the needs of the patient.

Nursing orders are effective only if the health care delivery system has accepted the concept of nursing orders. Nurses are accustomed to carrying out medical orders, but they are not accustomed to implementing orders by other nurses. An order, in any situation, must reflect both the authority that has been delegated to the person writing the order and the accountability of the person who is to carry out the order. Unless authority has been delegated and accountability has been accepted, any order is meaningless.

The interpersonal aspects of authority and accountability are difficult, but they must be faced or nursing orders will, by default, become merely another euphemism for nursing suggestion, nursing direction, or nursing approach. The staff must recognize that a nursing order is similar to any other order in that a nurse has only three options: carry it out as ordered; negotiate a change in the order; or accept the consequences of not carrying it out (Little and Carnevali, 1976). The last two options require interpersonal skills that may be new and risky for some nurses.

Spontaneous nursing interventions are often effective and significant; but if the effectiveness of a nursing action depends on a *sustained approach over a period of time*, a nursing order must be written so that plans will be made to make sure that the activity is continued for as long as it is needed.

Writing a nursing order is somewhat risky because there are no right orders, no specific, correct orders.

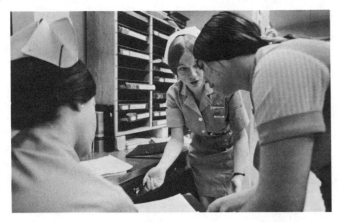

Figure 20.1 *Nursing care plans must be updated frequently to ensure optimal patient care.*

Each order represents a nurse's best judgment at the moment, and an order may or may not achieve the desired results. You will probably not be in a position to write nursing orders for some time, but you can give input to the person who is writing them. You can also hypothesize, "If I were in a position to do so, what would I order?" and thus begin to learn to formulate a nursing order.

DEVELOPING A NURSING CARE PLAN

A nursing care plan organizes the goals, orders, and information about a patient into a meaningful whole. It helps to ensure that needs will be met, treatments will be done as ordered, and progress toward goals will be likely. It serves as a guide to what needs to be done, when, and how (Fig. 20.1).

A nursing care plan usually includes, or refers to, the nursing and medical diagnoses, the goals, the specific nursing measures derived from nursing and medical orders, the times at which nursing actions have been scheduled, deadlines for goals, and outcome criteria. The nursing care plan is revised frequently in response to changes in the patient's condition and needs, and to changes in the involvement of patient and family. Input from the family is especially important in planning for the patient's discharge because a plan that is presented to, or imposed upon, a patient and his family without adequate input is likely to fail.

Standardized plans are devised to provide basic, minimal nursing care to specified groups of patients. These plans are usually noncontroversial because they are often developed through committee or team effort and have been accepted by the staff.

An *individualized nursing care plan* is usually written soon after the patient's admission by the nurse who has primary responsibility for him. A nursing care plan gives you a basis for organizing your clinical assignment. Knowledge of the time and frequency of treatments, tests, or other ordered activities enables you to organize these activities into a realistic sequence. This is especially important if you are assigned to two or more patients. The nursing care plan helps you to assign priorities and to arrange your schedule so that all required activities are done on time.

Student nursing care plans are usually written before care is given to an assigned patient. They are based on data obtained from studying textbooks and the patient's record, and from meeting or interviewing the patient and his family. A student nursing care plan includes the rationale or scientific basis for each nursing intervention as well as detailed data on anatomy, physiology, pathology, pharmacology, and so on. The format for a student nursing care plan is designed to help students learn to prescribe, plan, and implement nursing care. The process is valuable in that it provides a learning experience that will enable the student to prepare the less detailed plans she will use after graduation.

PATIENT TEACHING

It is important that patients and their families be taught three things related to the planning phase of nursing process. First, they need to know that they have a *right* to participate in decisions related to their care, and that they should insist upon being included in planning whenever it is appropriate. Second, they need to know that they have a responsibility to participate in goal setting and planning because their input into this process is essential for its success. Third, patients and families should be helped to set realistic and attainable goals for various levels of both health and illness.

RELATED ACTIVITIES

One way to increase your creativity and your potential for innovative nursing action is to practice the technique of brainstorming. During the next few weeks, think of at least *five* possible solutions to *every* problem, or *five* courses of action for *every* significant decision you must make. For example, instead of thinking "I'm tired of studying, *therefore* I will . . .," say "I am tired of studying and I *could:*

1. _____ , 2. _____ ,
3. _____ , 4. _____ , or
5. _____ .''

Include any remote, far-fetched, improbable, or unrealistic possibility that pops into your mind. Then select the one that is most likely to be satisfying and effective, and do it.

This kind of activity will assist you to establish a pattern of *imaginative, creative thinking* which will help avoid the pitfall of routine solutions and pat answers to complex nursing situations.

SUGGESTED READINGS

Bille, Donald A: Tailoring your diabetic patient's care plan to fit his life-style. *Nursing 86* 1986 Feb; 16(2):55–57.

Bower, Faye: *The Process of Planning Nursing Care.* ed.3. St. Louis, Mosby, 1982.

Forman, Mary: Building a better nursing care plan. *Am J Nurs* 1979 June; 79(6):1086–1087.

Little, Dolores, and Doris Carnevali: *Nursing Care Planning.* ed.2. Philadelphia, Lippincott, 1976.

Sloan, Margaret R, and Barbara Thune Schommer: Want to get your patient involved in his care? Use a contract. *Nursing 82* 1982 Dec; 12(12):48–49.

Vandenbosch, Terry M, et al: Tailoring care plans to nursing diagnoses. *Am J Nurs* 1986 March; 86(3):313–314.

Wells, Marcia: Discharge planning: Closing the gaps in continuity of care. *Nursing 83* 1983 Nov; 13(11):45.

Zangari, Mary-Eve, and Patricia Duffy: Contracting with patients in day-to-day practice. *Am J Nurs* 1980 March; 80(3):451–455.

21

The Implementation Phase of Nursing Process

Prerequisites and/or Suggested Preparation
Chapter 1 (Nursing as a Profession) and Chapter 17 (Overview of Nursing Process) are prerequisite to this chapter. Chapters 18–20 (assessment, diagnosis, and planning phases of nursing process) are recommended.

IMPLEMENTATION

The implementation phase of nursing process logically follows the planning phase, but it frequently begins before all planning has been completed. On paper, the phases appear to be sequential, but in reality, all phases are concurrent to some degree. Nursing process begins with the assessment phase, but it is not possible for the nurse to complete all assessments before she moves on to the next phases. Because the nurse is continually receiving data *from* the patient and *about* the patient, her assessment must be ongoing; it can never be considered complete.

All phases of nursing process overlap, and any discussion of them as separate entities can be misleading. *All* phases are going on to some extent within the implementation phase, and it is wrong to conclude that the nurse ceases to assess, diagnose, and plan simply because her activities at the moment are categorized as implementation.

The duration of the implementation phase ranges from a few minutes or hours to a year or more for some long-range plans or projects. In this chapter, the implementation phase is discussed within the context of a single clinical experience in a hospital or extended care facility. This time span would range from a few hours for a student to a full 8-hour shift for a graduate nurse. Although the *underlying processes are the same,* implementation in other settings, such as a school, clinic, or factory, is somewhat different and is not included here.

The implementation phase of nursing process includes an almost infinite number of activities that are usually termed *nursing actions* or *nursing interventions.* Most of these activities fall into one of three categories: (1) health education and patient teaching, (2) psychological support, and (3) physical care and comfort.

Implementation is based on goals set with or for the patient. Intermediate and long-range goals are usually developed in conjunction with the patient and family, but short-term goals are often developed by the nurse when a patient is too sick or too upset to participate in goal setting. The nurse must set goals for small children and for patients who are comatose, confused, or otherwise incapable of setting them. Patient participation is desirable, but there are many times when the nurse must assume full responsibility for setting the goals that form the basis for the implementation phase.

THE PROCESS OF IMPLEMENTATION

You will develop your own approach and method of implementing a nursing care plan, but there are at least eight basic steps common to every method of implementation:

1. Updating the data base
2. Establishing or reviewing the contract with the patient
3. Modifying the nursing care plan as needed
4. Ensuring the patient's safety
5. Assessing your need for assistance
6. Intervening as planned
7. Analyzing feedback from the patient
8. Communicating findings

Updating the Data Base

Whenever possible, check the patient assignment sheet immediately on reaching the unit so that, as you listen to the change-of-shift report, you can pay special attention to the information about the patients to whom you have been assigned. You should have with you a pen and paper or a pocket-size notebook in which to write down specific details such as the current status of your assigned patient's IV fluids or the time when his last analgesic was given.

Check the Kardex and note any new or changed information, such as a new nursing diagnosis or nursing order or changes in treatment, tests, or medications. Check the TPR book unless the ward secretary has already charted the patient's vital signs on his individual graphic sheet.

Finally, skim your assigned patient's chart and read the physician's latest progress notes, the most recent nursing notes, reports of recent diagnostic or laboratory tests, and any other data that might have been entered since you last studied the chart.

Establishing or Reviewing the Contract With the Patient

Unless you cared for an assigned patient within the preceding day or so, you will need to establish or re-establish your relationship with him. After you have greeted him and introduced yourself describe the extent of your involvement with him. You might say, for example: "Good morning, I'm Susan Jones, and I'll be your nurse until I have to leave for class at 11:30. You are my only patient this morning, so I'll have plenty of time to do things for you. I know that you can't get out of bed, that you need help with your bath, and that your dressing needs to be changed. I read in your chart that you are concerned that you will be weak when you are finally allowed out of bed, so I have planned to teach you some exercises to help restore your strength.

Is there anything else I can do for you this morning? Something which no one else has had time to do yet?"

A brief introduction such as this establishes an informal *contract* or working arrangement. The patient knows your name, the amount of time you can spend with him, your perception of his needs, what you are prepared to do, and that he is free to ask for or suggest additional assistance. Such an introduction sets the tone for the morning and establishes you as a concerned, informed professional person.

Modifying the Nursing Care Plan

The nursing care plan is based on the nursing diagnosis and the goals that have been set for the patient. Since these are likely to be changed whenever the patient's psychological or physical condition changes, it is important to check the Kardex before starting any assignment to validate the nursing diagnosis. It should be both *current* and *accurate*. Note any new or changed orders and revise your plan accordingly.

It is usually helpful to prepare a checklist or flow sheet on which to keep track of the times at which treatments and medications are scheduled and when they are actually given. Such a sheet will help you remember the things you must do and will help you remember the information that you will need when charting and reporting off duty.

If you find that a number of changes have recently been made in the nursing care plan, examine the overall revisions carefully to see if the current schedule is conducive to the patient's well-being. Activities should be grouped and coordinated so that there are periods for rest and relaxation. A schedule that subjects the patient to some type of treatment or activity every half hour all day long is not conducive to his recovery. Try to cluster events in the early morning and before and after mealtimes in order to provide rest periods for a patient who is weak and tires easily. It is also helpful to do several things at once. For example, do range-of-motion exercises while bathing the patient, or teach him while making the bed.

Ensuring the Patient's Safety

Before starting your assignment, review or identify specific precautions to be taken and special observations to be made for that patient. *You should be able to list, without hesitation or uncertainty, the three or four most significant precautions to be taken,* such as keeping the side rails up at all times, or checking the patient's swallowing reflex before offering him fluids by mouth. Make sure you know the *specific observations* that should be made, such as: "Note level of consciousness every hour,"

"Watch for any involuntary, random movements of left arm or leg," "Assess patient's orientation," and "Note any slurring of speech." These specific observations and precautions can be deduced from the Kardex and chart; from a textbook; or from an instructor, a team leader, or an experienced staff nurse. This information will provide direction for an ongoing assessment, and will help you decide which observations must be reported as soon as they are noted and which ones can be reported when you go off duty.

Assessing Your Need for Assistance·

In the majority of nursing situations, you will find that you need assistance of some kind, whether it be help in turning a heavy patient or a consultation about a suicidal patient. The appropriate use of assistance is so important that it is usually included on both student and staff evaluation records. Instructors and supervisors may use complex terminology such as "uses appropriate resources" or "accepts the interdependent nature of nursing"—but the basic concept is simple: there are some things you can't do alone!

Examples of Situations That Create a Need for Help

- Inadequate Strength or Dexterity

  Transferring a helpless, heavy patient from bed to stretcher

  Restraining a struggling infant during a treatment

  Needing an extra pair of hands to manage a complicated piece of equipment

- Lack of Knowledge or Skill

  Trying to understand the physiological basis of hyperalimentation therapy

  Wanting to motivate an apathetic, paraplegic patient

  Having to change the dressing on a badly infected stump following an amputation

- Insufficient Inner Resources

  Feeling very angry over problems created by hospital bureaucracy

  Feeling depressed after prolonged assignment to a group of patients with severe neurological problems

  Trying to cope with sadness and grief over the pending death of a favorite patient

- Lack of Time

  Being unable to complete an assignment within the allotted time

  Having a patient who will need continued care after discharge

Whenever possible, it is good practice to anticipate your need for assistance and plan ahead so that it is available when needed. A need for assistance is usually created by a lack or deficiency in one of four categories: strength and dexterity, knowledge and skill, inner resources, or time.

People vary in their willingness to ask for help, but in nursing, assistance *must* be sought whenever it is indicated in order to:

Ensure patient safety, both physical and psychological

Facilitate the best possible care for the patient

Increase the nurse's knowledge and skill

It is extremely important that assistance be sought from an *appropriate* and *qualified* person (Fig. 21.1). While a nurse's aide or another student could help you do certain tasks, neither of them would be qualified to assist you in a situation which required expert professional judgment and skill. Failure to *seek* and *use* appropriate help could be grounds for negligence or malpractice.

Intervening as Planned

The actual implementation of the nursing care plan, whether it be written or unwritten, is exemplified by Virginia Henderson's definition of nursing:

"The unique function of the nurse is to assist the individual, sick or well, in the performance of those activities contributing to health or its recovery (or to peaceful death) that he would perform unaided if he had the necessary strength, will or knowledge. And to do this

---

Assessment of Your Need for Assistance

1. What kind of help is needed? (Be specific)
2. When is the help needed, and for how long? (At 10 AM for a few minutes? Sometime before you meet with the family? Within the next week or so?)
3. What kinds of help are available to you? (Additional equipment? Your instructor? The hospital chaplain? An experienced staff nurse? A consultant?)
4. How should you ask for help? (Ask another nurse directly? Ask the team leader to assign someone to help you? Make a request in writing, perhaps for a consultant or a follow-up visit by a visiting nurse after discharge?)
5. How should you use the help? (To work with both you and the patient? To work with you behind the scenes and help the patient indirectly? To interact with the patient in your stead?)

---

in such a way as to help him gain independence as rapidly as possible. This aspect of her work, this part of her function, she initiates and controls; of this she is master" (Henderson, 1964, p. 63).

The patient's ability to perform these activities will vary from day to day and, in some instances, from hour to hour as his psychological and physiological condition changes. Great sensitivity is needed to balance the need to have the nurse do things for him against the value of his doing things for himself. An emphasis on patient involvement and responsibility will be effective *only* when the time is right; it cannot be rushed. A premature emphasis on independence is frustrating for all concerned and can only lead to misunderstanding or a battle of wills. For the majority of patients, satisfaction of Maslow's lower level needs for autonomy, independence, knowledge, and competence; and the nurse who recognizes the cues from the patient has an opportunity to teach him those things he is ready and willing to learn.

Using Feedback From the Patient

Data are collected during the implementation phase for two reasons. First, data are collected to assess the effectiveness of the planned nursing care. Verbal and nonverbal feedback from the patient indicates whether or not his elevated temperature is dropping, his pain is relieved, or his hope and his strength are increased. Based on this feedback, the nurse can tell, almost from moment to moment, whether to continue, discontinue, or modify any given nursing action.

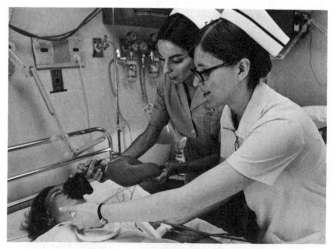

Figure 21.1 Student and instructor work together to adjust a patient's oxygen equipment.

Second, data are collected to generate hypotheses for research and study. Feedback from the patient can stimulate significant questions which have the potential for influencing the nature or quality of nursing care. If, for example, your present patient is the fourth patient in a month to respond in a particular way to a drug or treatment, your curiosity and inquiries could lead you to a study that might benefit many future patients.

Communicating Actions and Findings

The implementation phase is concluded with an oral report to the person who will care for the patient when you leave, plus a written record of your interaction with the patient. (See Chapter 18, Section 7, The Use of Records and Reports.)

An oral report is usually given to one or more of the following people: the head nurse, the team leader, or the nurse to whom the patient is assigned for the next period of time. A useful report is both brief and relevant. It is well-thought-out and often based on a few written notes. The report includes significant events or changes in the patient's condition, the present patient situation, and things to be accomplished or done during the next shift. The person reporting must avoid rambling and including extraneous detail. There is no need, for example, to report that Mr. Jones ate all his breakfast unless he usually does not do so, nor to report bathing him and making his bed, which would be assumed unless the nurse purposely omitted these activities.

An example of a useful report might be: "I was assigned to Mr. Jones in room 410. He received Demerol 50 mg at 10:15 and then was able to sit in a chair for 15 minutes. Dr. Green was in and told Mr. Jones that yesterday's x-rays showed a slight improvement and that he could go home when the present course of chemotherapy is finished on Thursday. Mr. Jones seemed very subdued by the news and says that he's worried about his wife's ability to care for him at home. I arranged for the social worker to come and talk to them during visiting hours this afternoon. Mr. Jones's intake is down—he knows that he is 200 cc behind schedule but thinks he can catch up this afternoon."

FACTORS THAT AFFECT THE IMPLEMENTATION PHASE

Many factors affect the implementation of nursing care, including orientation to the unit, organization, changes, knowledge, nurse's skill, patient's reactions, and the nurse's self-concept.

Orientation to the Nursing Unit

The quality of your Nursing care depends, in part, on how comfortable you feel in the clinical situation. This comfort, in turn, depends on your orientation to the unit. Some agencies have an extensive orientation program, to both the physical and interpersonal aspects of the setting. Other agencies have a minimal orientation, which of course does not preclude a nurse from orienting herself to the unit or agency. A nurse in uniform or a lab coat and wearing an appropriate name tag can gain access to most areas of the hospital or agency by introducing herself to the person in charge and giving the reason for her interest.

A thorough orientation to the nursing unit should include:

- Location of departments and equipment. Where is the admitting office, the chapel, and the x-ray department? Where are wheelchairs, towels, and fruit juice kept?
- Emergency procedures. What are the codes or pages which signify an emergency? What is your responsibility in case of fire? Cardiac arrest? Power failure?
- Policies and rules. When are visiting hours? Does the patient have the right to read his chart? Can patients go home over the weekend?
- Group norms and interpersonal relations. What things must be done and what things are never done on a given unit?
- Assignments. On what basis are patient assignments made? Is the unit organized around functional roles? Primary nursing? Team nursing?
- Hospital system. How is the hospital or agency organized? How are the departments related? Who is your immediate supervisor? Who makes what kinds of decisions?

The answers to these and a multitude of other questions will enhance your ability to implement a nursing care plan because you can do so most effectively when you are familiar with and comfortable in the clinical setting.

Organization

The implementation of a nursing care plan often depends on the ability of the nurse to *organize* the available time, space, and resources. The organization of time involves setting priorities and deciding which things *must be done without fail*, which ones *should* be done, and which ones would be nice to do if there is time. It is helpful to arrange the required activities into a reasonable sequence based on the times the activities are scheduled, and the approximate amount of time each activity will take.

Check on the leeway allowable for each scheduled activity. A medication or treatment scheduled for every 4 hours can probably be given safely within 10 to 15 minutes of the scheduled time. A check on a patient's vital signs, scheduled for every half hour, should occur within 2 or 3 minutes of the designated times because the interval between the checks is so short (10 percent of a 30-minute interval is only 3 minutes, whereas 10 percent of a 2-hour interval is 12 minutes).

A written schedule allows you to pace yourself and to know whether or not your schedule needs to be altered. Whenever possible, your schedule should be loose enough to permit you to cope with unexpected delays and interruptions without panic or undue frustration.

In addition to organizing your time, it is important to organize your work space. Time spent organizing work space in the patient's unit will be saved through increased efficiency and convenience. Excess linen, old newspapers, extra supplies, and waste materials should be removed from the patient's unit. With the patient's permission, personal belongings should be stacked, folded, or put away. Do whatever is necessary to obtain an adequate, usable work space.

Changes

It is unlikely that you will encounter a nursing situation in which the nursing care can be implemented exactly as planned. Almost every situation entails changes in the patient's physical or psychological status, changes in nursing orders or physician's orders, or changes in the times of scheduled treatments or tests. Linen, equipment, or supplies may be unavailable. Patient assignments may be changed.

In each instance, you will need to assess the situation promptly and reestablish priorities for the remainder of the time available to you. An important skill in such situations is the *ability to pause and collect your thoughts before taking any action*. When confronted with potentially upsetting changes, some nurses take several deep breaths; some count to 50 or 100; still others find a quiet place such as a closet or stairway and relax for a moment or two. The choice of technique is unimportant; what matters is the reduction of stress, and the avoidance of hasty, flustered actions in response to the unexpected.

Knowledge

Much of the creativity in nursing depends on a nurse's ability to improvise, adapt, and modify procedures to meet the needs of individual patients. This ability depends, in turn, on your knowledge of the scientific principles which will enable you to decide whether proposed innovations or modifications might lessen in any way the safety and effectiveness of the intervention.

Skill

Excellence during the implementation phase is possible when the nurse is able to execute each activity with exceptional skill and competence. Not all nurses are equally skilled in all facets of nursing, but each nurse can be expected to demonstrate adequate competence in all basic activities, plus a high level of skill in a few areas. Areas in which a given nurse may excel include patient teaching, intensive care, family therapy, geriatric nursing, or adolescent counseling. Within your area of expertise, it is reasonable to expect that your implementation of nursing will be creative, individualized, and highly skilled.

Reaction of Patient and Family

The praise or complaints of the patient and his family will influence your implementation of any nursing care plan. Nursing is an interpersonal process, and both patient and nurse are affected by the attitudes and reactions of the other. Expectations or misconceptions about the roles of patient and nurse will influence the interaction, as will tone of voice, phrasing, nonverbal cues, and timing. A *request* by either party is likely to be respected, whereas an order or demand for the same thing may be rejected. Even though you try to be understanding and accepting of all patients, there is bound to be a subtle difference in your responses to a patient who reacts in a positive way to your nursing care.

Nurse's Self-Concept

The transition from lay person to nurse is often a lengthy and somewhat difficult one, and the implementation of nursing care is affected by the degree to which you feel comfortable and confident in the role of nurse. This confidence is enhanced by behaviors such as:

- Establishing a professional rather than a social relationship with the patient
- Placing your emphasis on helping the patient to meet his needs rather than on pleasing him
- Explaining and giving directions in a positive, assertive way rather than in an uncertain or indecisive manner.

- Answering questions and requests to which the answers are not known with, "I don't know, but I'll find out," rather than with glib generalities or vague references to policies or rules

These and other indications of professional confidence will enhance your implementation of a nursing care plan by fostering the patient's respect and confidence in your nursing expertise.

RELATED ACTIVITIES

Before you start your clinical experiences, evaluate your current organizational skills. If you have reason to believe that you are not an organized person, that you tend to waste time and energy, take the following steps to develop the skills which are basic to the implementation phase of nursing process.

1. Select one of your routine everyday activities, analyze it, and write out an organized set of steps which, if followed, would improve your efficiency. Practice until you notice a distinct improvement.

2. When listing your personal objectives for your clinical experiences, be honest and include the improvement of organizational skills.

3. *Consciously and deliberately* attend to this aspect of implementation during each clinical assignment. Set a reasonable goal for each new experience.

4. Seek help from your instructor or a staff nurse.

5. Routinely evaluate your progress at the end of each clinical experience.

SUGGESTED READINGS

Huttman, Barbara: Quit wasting time with "nursing rituals". *Nursing 85* 1985 Oct; 15(10):34–39.

Huttman, Barbara: All about hectic situations. *Nursing 84* 1984 July; 14(7):34–35.

King, Eunice M, Lynn Wieck, and Marilyn Dyer: *Illustrated Manual of Nursing Techniques.* Philadelphia, Lippincott, 1981.

Lewis, LuVerne Wolff: *Fundamental Skills in Patient Care.* ed.2. Philadelphia, Lippincott, 1980.

Saxton, Dolores F, and Patricia A. Hyland: *Planning and Implementing Nursing Intervention.* ed.2. St. Louis, Mosby, 1979.

Snyder, Mariah: *Independent Nursing Interventions.* New York, Wiley, 1985.

22

The Evaluation Phase of Nursing Process

Prerequisites and/or Suggested Preparation
Chapter 1 (Nursing as a Profession) and Chapter 17 (Overview of Nursing Process) are prerequisite for understanding this chapter. Chapters 17–21 (the first four phases of nursing process) are suggested preparation for this chapter.

Evaluation is an onging process by which the nurse monitors the effectiveness of her nursing care in order to know whether to continue, modify, or abandon a given course of action. Evaluation is often described as the last phase of nursing process, but in reality, it is also an integral part of each of the other phases.

Nursing care is evaluated at both an individual patient level and at institutional levels for a variety of reasons. At an institutional level, nursing care is often evaluated for the following reasons: to assess the satisfaction of the general public with the care provided, to obtain data relevant to the improvement of patient care, to provide a basis for the evaluation of staff performance, and to evaluate compliance with professional standards, insurance requirements, and government regulations.

Evaluation of public reaction to the nursing care of a given hospital or other institution is based on information obtained from patients, families, and visitors. The methods used to gather this information include informal conversations, interviews, and questionnaires given to patients upon discharge. This information about the quality of nursing care is useful but subjective because it is based on attitudes and opinions rather than facts.

Objective and precise information is required to evaluate patients' physical and psychological responses to nursing care. This information is obtained from careful analysis of relevant patient charts by agency personnel or teams of researchers. The results of such analysis provide a basis for decisions related to changes in nursing care.

A similar analysis of patient records by nurses is part of an evaluation process called *peer review*, by which nurses evaluate the performance of fellow nurses.

One method of obtaining information from charts and records is the *nursing audit* which is the systematic examination of patient records by an *audit committee*. Members of the audit committee compare selected records with written insurance requirements, government regulations, and professional standards of care. The committee might audit, for example, the records of all patients who were cared for on a given unit during a certain period of time, or the records of all patients who had suffered a stroke or heart attack. The results of an audit will reveal any irregularities or unacceptable practices related to the length of hospitalization, type of treatment given, and the amount and timing of patient teaching, for example.

At an individual level, each nurse conducts an ongoing evaluation of the care she gives each patient plus a final evaluation at the end of her time with each patient. For example, a nurse would evaluate the care given a certain patient at intervals throughout an 8-hour shift and at the end of the shift would review the goals she had set and the effectiveness of what had been accomplished. When the patient was discharged from her care, the nurse would evauate the patient's overall psychological and physiological responses to her nursing actions, especially those that had been innovative or experimental.

This chapter is primarily concerned with such individual evaluation, but the concepts presented are applicable to nursing audits and other types of evaluation at an institutional level.

THE EVALUATION PROCESS

Some evaluations are complex and highly structured while others are simple and spontaneous, but all evaluations include at least four basic steps:

1. Identification of the standard to be used
2. Collection of data
3. Comparison of data with the standard or criterion
4. Statement of conclusions

Identifying Standards

Standards of care and outcome criteria serve similar functions in the evaluation of nursing care; but, as a rule, *standards of care* are used as the basis for evaluating broad areas of nursing practice, whereas *outcome criteria* are used in evaluating specific activities, such as those associated with the relief of pain. Standards of care may include relevant outcome criteria.

Standards of care should be *based on research findings, theoretical concepts, and currently accepted nursing practice.* For example, standards of care for children who are terminally ill with leukemia might include a goal of *coping with increasing family tension.* If family discussions about death and dying are recommended as one method of coping with such tension, there must be an *identifiable and valid rationale* for that recommendation. Vague reasoning that such family discussions "seem like a good idea" or that they "sound reasonable" is not a sufficient basis for such a standard of nursing care.

Standards of care may be selected or adapted from existing standards and criteria, or they may be developed from a theoretical or experimental base. Any set of standards must be valid and appropriate for the activity to be evaluated, and must be well stated and understandable. Unfortunately, some standards seem to have been hastily prepared. They are poorly written and are either general and superficial, or too detailed and restrictive. It is appropriate, therefore, for any nurse to ask, "Where did these standards come from? Who

ANA Standards of Nursing Practice

1. The collection of data about the health status of the client/patient is systematic and continuous. The data are accessible, communicated, and recorded.

2. Nursing diagnoses are derived from health status data.

3. The plan of nursing care includes goals derived from the nursing diagnoses.

4. The plan of nursing care includes priorities and pre-scribed nursing approaches or measures to achieve the goals derived from the nursing diagnoses.

5. Nursing actions provide for client/patient participation in health promotion, maintenance, and restoration.

6. Nursing actions assist the client/patient to maximize his health capabiities.

7. The client/patient's progress or lack of progress toward goal achievement is determined by the client/patient and the nurse.

8. The client/patient's progress or lack of progress toward goal achievement directs reassessment, reordering of priorities, new goal setting, and revision of the plan of nursing care.

(ANA, 1973, p. 9)

wrote them? Are they based on sound theory and good nursing practice?'' No material (including the material in this text) should be accepted as true or worthy simply because it is in print.

The ANA Standards of Nursing Practice are exam-ples of broad standards for nursing care. These standards can be used in the evaluation of nursing care and the use of nursing process in any setting and for any group of patients or type of patient situation. The seventh and eighth standards refer specifically to the evaluation of the patient's response to nursing care. The ANA has developed additional and more specific standards and criteria for use in evaluating the care of an individual patient.

Collecting Data

The outcome criteria or standards of care to be used for evaluation determine, to a large extent, the amount and type of data to be collected. If, for example, the nurse expects a patient to become more active when his pain is controlled, she will need to collect data on his physical activity. Such information can be obtained by observing or questioning the patient, and from the observations recorded in his chart by others who have cared for him.

The nurse can either collect and use the information that *happens* to be available to her or she can *make*

certain that the information she needs is available. The latter approach is essential if she is conducting a study of patient response to a certain pain-relief measure, for example. For such a study, the nurse would need to tell the staff what data are needed and why, and also how to collect, record, and report them. If the evalu-ation of a phenomenon is important, *data collection can-not be left to chance;* the information must be made avail-able. A special nursing audit will not be valid, for example, if it is based in part on the presence or ab-sence of information that nurses are not, and never have been, expected to record.

In some evaluation situations, questions require only a simple yes or no answer: Did I involve the patient in goal setting? Did the patient learn to use his crutches before discharge? Did the patient's temperature return to normal? In other situations, detailed information is needed. To evaluate the effectiveness of a new ap-proach for increasing the oral fluid intake of toddlers, for example, accurate records of what each child con-sumed are required in order to say with certainty that unlimited Popsicles promote greater fluid intake than the use of straws and Kool-aid.

Comparing Data With Standards or Criteria

The ways in which standards or criteria are used in evaluation range from a simple comparison such as, ''Does this result correspond to this standard?'' to a detailed, point-by-point examination of a patient's record. Regardless of the extent, comparison with a standard is essential; an evaluation is not valid without it. For example, if a nurse states that a certain nursing action was successful, she must be able to indicate the basis for her statement. The nursing action was suc-cessful in *terms of what?*

The patient's response to a nursing action can be compared to outcome criteria which the nurse has de-veloped, wih the responses reported by other nurses in similar situations, or with the responses hypothesized for a research study, but the patient's response *must be compared with some standard* before it can be evaluated.

Stating Conclusions

The end product of the evaluation process is a conclu-sion or judgment about the effectiveness of a nursing intervention. This may be a quick mental note (''It worked!'') or an extensive written summary with rec-ommendations for future nursing action. Such conclu-sions have the potential for influencing subsequent nursing practice by providing a basis for deciding whether to continue, discontinue, or modify a given approach or course of action.

Evaluation of a given situation might indicate that all goals were reached, that the nursing actions were effective and should be tried with other patients. Evaluation in another situation might indicate that some goals were not reached. Failure to reach a goal could be caused by faulty implementation; the evaluator must try to identify any problems of time, organization, skill, energy, or personnel which could have contributed to the failure. If the failure did *not* stem from the implementation phase, the nurse must work backward through the other phases of nursing process until the reasons for failure are identified.

EVALUATING SKILL AND COMPETENCY

In addition to evaluating the effectiveness of her nursing care, a nurse needs to evaluate her competency and skill. Her nursing care may have been effective, but was her performance as good as it could be? You can use the following questions to evaluate your own performance:

- With what are you comparing your performance? You own past performance? Criteria established by your school or agency? The performance of a respected staff member or instructor?
- If you had it to do over, what would you change, and why?

Frequent analysis of your performance will enable you to increase your skill and competency deliberately and consciously.

EVALUATING A PROCEDURE

The implementation of a nursing care plan is affected by the way in which procedures and treatments are done. Nearly every procedure has some unique aspects that require specific criteria for evaluation, but there are six basic criteria common to the evaluation of all procedures: (1) safety, (2) effectiveness, (3) comfort, (4) efficiency, (5) economy, and (6) legality.

Safety

If the safety of the patient is jeopardized in any way at any time, the procedure cannot be considered well done or effective. Regardless of the quality of other aspects of the performance, a procedure is deemed unsatisfactory if the physical or psychological safety of the patient was threatened at any point.

Examples of *safety* criteria are:

- The patient was identified correctly
- Medical and surgical asepsis was maintained
- Any use of restraints was physiologically and psychologically safe
- All equipment was in good working order
- Relevant techniques of alignment, positioning, and body mechanics were used

Effectiveness

A procedure must be effective as well as safe; it must accomplish whatever it is supposed to accomplish.
Examples of criteria for *effectiveness* include:

- The purpose and intent of the procedure were known to all
- The outcome criteria were specific and precise
- The procedure was consistent with the overall plan of therapy
- Modifications were made as needed in response to feedback from the patient
- The procedure was based on scientific principles and theory

Comfort

The physical and psychological comfort of the patient during a procedure is especially important in situations in which fear, anxiety, or muscle tension could block the procedure or distort the results.
Examples of criteria for *psychological comfort* are:

- The patient knew what to expect because the procedure had been explained or the approach used was consistent with the way the procedure had been done in the past
- The patient's privacy was maintained
- The procedure was individualized to meet the needs of the patient
- The patient and family were appropriately involved in the procedure
- The nurse was responsive to feedback from the patient throughout the procedure

Examples of criteria for *physical comfort* include:

- The patient was not in distress of any kind
- The patient was in a comfortable and safe position
- Temperature and ventilation in the room were adequate and comfortable

- The procedure was done with skill and gentleness
- Attention was paid to both the physiological and psychological aspects of an intrusive procedure (a procedure that involves penetration or invasion of a body orifice)

Efficiency

Efficiency is determined by the amount of time and energy used to accomplish a given task. Some levels of efficiency can be determined by time-and-motion studies, but others are less specific and must be evaluated by more general, less rigorous methods.

Some criteria for *efficiency* are:

- The procedure was done quickly, without wasted motion or effort
- No time or energy was lost because of missing or forgotten equipment
- Performance was enhanced by prior organization and planning

Economy

Rapidly increasing health care costs make it necessary for nurses and other health care workers to be more attentive than ever to the conservation of resources and the prevention of waste.

Examples of criteria for *economy* include:

- Neither time, money, resources nor energy was wasted
- When there was a choice, the least expensive yet effective materials were used
- Whenever possible, the patient was taught to use household mateials rather than more expensive, commercially prepared supplies
- The helper or assistant was not kept standing around, wasting time while waiting to help
- Skill and meticulous technique decreased the probability of contamination of equipment and supplies and subsequent waste

Legality

The greatest number of questions on the legality of nursing interventions probably stem from the implementation phase of nursing process, when the nurse is viewed as doing things to and for the patient. Her behavior is no less significant during the other phases, but the potential for error or harm is likely to be greater during implementation of the nursing care plan.

Examples of criteria for *legality* include:

- All nursing orders were within the legal practice of nursing
- There was a valid, signed physician's order for each dependent nursing action
- The nurse was knowledgeable and skillful; there was no possible basis for an accusation of negligence or malpractice

PATIENT TEACHING

Teaching related to the evaluation phase of nursing process is directed toward making the patient aware of his rights, and of his role as a good consumer of health care. Each person needs to know that he has the right and the responsibility to give feedback to members of the health team regarding the quality of his nursing care.

RELATED ACTIVITIES

1. In order for evaluation to be useful as a basis for improving the quality of nursing care, the nurse must be able to analyze all information received carefully and objectively. This is not possible if the nurse has a tendency to become defensive whenever any of the data seem negative or critical. If, in the past, you have tended to become irritated or upset over suggestions that your performance could, or should, be improved, it will be helpful to learn to minimize the stress of such situations and learn to profit from them.

Whenever such a situation presents itself, try doing two things. First, listen carefully (and calmly) to the observer's comments, and then *ask enough questions* to make sure that you understand the *other person's point of view* and the basis for the comments. Second, *before you respond,* ask yourself whether or not the comments are valid and accurate, and plan your response accordingly. This process will slow down or avoid a hasty, ill-considered reaction, and will enable you to decide how you can make the best use of the evaluation you have received.

2. Self-evaluation is an integral part of most evaluation conferences, whether the conference be with an instructor, supervisor, or employer. Explore your current approach toward self-evaluation by analyzing your evaluation of at least one of your activities each day for a week.

Do you tend to be overly critical and seldom satisfied with your performance, or do you find it difficult to see any way to improve what you have done? If you have a *pattern* of responding in either of these two extremes, seek help from an instructor, a classmate or other person in order to learn ways to evaluate your own performance in an objective, analytical way. Aim for self-evaluations which identify and accept both your accomplishments and your present limitations. With practice and assistance, you can learn to objectively compare your performance with what you were trying to accomplish, and thereby obtain a sense of direction for achieving the professional competence you seek.

SUGGESTED READINGS

American Nurses' Association: *Standards of Nursing Practice.* Kansas City, American Nurses' Association, 1973.

Byrne, Karin M, Susan M Lattanzi and Maryellen Morrissey: "Don't let me fall" *Am J Nurs* 1982 Aug; 82(8):1242–1245.

Hurt, Ruth Ann: More than skin deep: Guidelines on caring for the burn patient (outcome criteria). *Nursing 85* 1985 June; 15(6):52–57.

Inzer, Frances, and Mary Jo Aspinall: Evaluating patient outcomes. *Nurs Outlook* 1981 March; 29(3):178–181.

Joint Commission on Accreditation of Hospitals: *Accreditation Manuals for Hospitals* (pp. 37–39). Chicago, The Commission, 1985.

Rice, Berkeley: Performance review: The job nobody likes. *Psych Today* 1985 Sept; 19(9):30–36.

Taylor, Judy A: Are you missing what your patients can teach you? *RN* 1984 June; 47(6):63–69.

Part Five

Nursing Interventions Related to Psychosocial Needs

23

Psychological Support

Prerequisites and/or Suggested Preparation
Communicatin (Chapter 9) and Nursing Process (Chapter 17) are prerequisite to this chapter. Suggested preparation includes an introductory psychology course plus the following chapters in this text or their equivalent: Chapter 5 (Systems Theory) and Chapter 8 (Stress, Adaptation, and Coping).

Section 1

Crisis

Psychological support is the term applied to the nursing interventions used to meet the patient's emotional needs when he is confronted with a crisis, loss, grief, depression, anxiety, or an altered body image.

A person's emotional response to an upsetting or overwhelming situations can be so strong that he is unable to attend to other aspects of his life. He may be unable to think clearly, to interact with other people, or even to attend to his physical needs. In such a situation, the emotional problem must be resolved as quickly as possible in order to reduce the person's stress and enable him to focus his attention on other urgent needs.

CRISIS INTERVENTION

The process by which a trained person helps another person through a crisis is often referred to as *crisis intervention*. The process is not specific to nursing; it is common to all helping professions and can be taught to lay persons. The basic concepts of crisis intervention are relevant to nursing because the very nature of nursing makes it likely that nurses will encounter people in crisis more frequently and with greater regularity than the members of many other professions. The following vignettes depict two of the innumerable types of crises encountered in everyday life.

Mr. Coleman, a businessman, has just been promoted and is finding it increasingly difficult to get his work done. He is irritable and finds it hard to concentrate. He had been hoping for this promotion for over a year and cannot understand his present feelings. His wife has told him that she is quite concerned about the recent changes in his behavior.

Ms. Smith's patient is dying of cancer. She suddenly walks into the nurse's station and bursts into tears. She grabs her purse and coat, says, "I'm leaving," and walks out of the unit, making no provision for the care of her patients for the rest of the day. This behavior is totally atypical, and the staff is dumbfounded.

Both Ms. Smith and Mr. Coleman are in crisis. In this context, the word *crisis* refers to the *reaction* of a person to a given event; the *event* is NOT the crisis. For example, taking care of a dying patient is not, in and of itself, a crisis. Being promoted is not a crisis. But both the nurse and Mr. Coleman have found themselves in situations that seem hazardous to them and are therefore in a state of crisis.

Crisis is a condition, or state of being and the term *in crisis* is similar to the terms in pain, in trouble, and in sorrow. The word crisis is also used to denote the phenomenon that produces that condition or state of being. Just as a pain is responsible for the condition of being in pain, a crisis is responsible for the condition of being in crisis. In this text, therefore, as in much of the nursing literature, the word crisis refers both to the phenomenon and to the person's reaction to it. A crisis is present when a person or family believes itself to be in a hazardous situation. A situation is perceived as hazardous whenever the demands of the situation exceed the ability of the person or family to cope. A very small promotion, for example, might be pleasurable and satisfying, but a large promotion involving new responsibilities, additional skills, and a different lifestyle could result in a crisis. A crisis implies at least a temporary *inability to meet the demands of a situation*. A crisis can be defined as a functionally debilitating mental state resulting from a person's reaction to an event perceived to be so dangerous that it leaves him helpless and unable to cope effectively by usual methods (Dixon, 1979). This condition is a *normal response to a perceived danger*. It is not abnormal and is not a form of mental illness.

A crisis is self-limiting and usually lasts no longer than 6 weeks. Therefore, if a person has been depressed for several years, the depression is likely to be the result of circumstances other than a crisis.

TYPES OF CRISES

There are at least three circumstances likely to make a person perceive a situation as hazardous: threat, loss, and challenge.

Threat

Anything that poses an immediate danger (real or potential) to the psychological or biological well-being of a person or family will be perceived as a *threat*. A snarling dog, an allergic reaction, insufficient food, an angry outburst, or a house fire can threaten the well-being of a person or family and result in a crisis. Whether or not an event is perceived as hazardous depends in part on the person's personality, competency, and need for structure. For example, a snarling dog is a threat to a person who is afraid of all dogs, but that same dog does not necessarily threaten an experienced dog trainer.

A safe situation that is *perceived* as threatening can produce a crisis. A very large barking dog can elicit a crisis reaction in certain people despite the fact that the dog is wagging his tail, is of a gentle breed, and has never made an aggressive move toward anyone. Just so, a certain treatment or illness can be a crisis for a given person even though there is virtually no potential for danger.

Loss

The loss that precipitates a crisis can be either *tangible* or *intangible*. Examples of a *tangible loss* include death, bankruptcy, destruction of property by fire or flood, and loss of friends by moving. To outside observers, the significance of a crisis often seems disproportionate to the size or apparent value of the tangible loss. For example, the disappearance of a beloved mongrel dog can create a crisis for an entire family.

Intangible losses include the loss of prestige or honor, the loss of motivation and a goal (e.g., after completion of a project), loss of self-esteem (e.g., upon failure to win an election), or loss of freedom (e.g., after the birth of a baby). The situation responsible for an intangible loss may have been desired, worked for, and sought after, such as having a new baby or being transferred to a new job. The concomitant losses suffered after achievement can still place those involved in crisis.

Challenge

Any endeavor that involves a conscious mobilization of energy to solve a significant problem or to reach an important goal, such as to climb Mt. Everest or get a doctoral degree, has the potential for engendering a crisis if the person is unprepared or unable to cope with his reaction to the outcome. Coping with success can seem as risky and dangerous to some people as coping with failure does to others.

A current crisis can trigger a reaction to a previously unresolved crisis that places a double burden on the person or family. For example, the sudden death of a young friend can trigger a crisis reaction to the as-yet-ungrieved death of a sibling many years ago.

STAGES OF CRISIS

A crisis is characterized by typical, identifiable stages that are sequential up to the point of reorganization, which can be either successful or unsuccessful.

Denial

During the *denial stage*, the person's verbal and non-verbal behavior indicates a rejection of the event, and he makes statements such as "I can't believe it happened!" "I still don't believe it! or "There must be a mistake!" Denial is influenced by many variables, such as a person's mental health or a lack of evidence to support reality, such as failure to find the body of a person presumed to have drowned.

Increased Tension

During the second stage, one of *increased tension*, the person is still able to function but is becoming agitated. He is irritable and emotionally labile (unstable). He is not yet fully conscious of the nature, extent, or implications of the crisis. He does not yet feel himself to be in crisis.

Disorganization

In the third stage, *disorganization*, the person has become nonfunctioning and may be hysterical. He is unable to carry out his normal activities of daily living because he is totally preoccupied with the event and with his reaction to it. This stage is conscious, and it is the stage in which he is likely to seek help or to accept help that is offered because he is dysfunctional and feels so terrible.

Reorganization

In the fourth stage, *reorganization*, the person in crisis attempts to reorganize his situation and himself, to become a functioning person, to clean up his environment, to continue his activities of daily living, and so on. He tries to get rid of both the crisis and his feelings in one way or another. Either he may try a healthy problem-solving approach, or he may repress the incident and bury it in his unconscious self. The latter is not done consciously. If his attempts are *successful*, a general reorganization is accomplished and the crisis is past.

Attempted Escape

If, however, the person's attempts at reorganization are *not* successful, he will make a conscious effort to escape from the problem. This may involve a physical escape such as moving, taking a trip, or destroying all evidence of the event. He may also consciously try to suppress the problem and get away from it psychologically. *Any attempt to resolve a crisis by escaping will fail* because escape requires a conscious effort to suppress thoughts and feelings. Suppression will alleviate the tension and pain for the moment, but they will still be there tomorrow.

Efforts to escape are followed by local or minimal reorganization rather than general reorganization. This enables the person at least to pull himself together enough to survive as a functioning person, to get to work, and, in general, to carry on as best he can.

NURSING INTERVENTIONS

A person who is upset, agitated, emotionally out of control, or unable to function can be tentatively diagnosed as being in crisis; and it is both appropriate and necessary for someone to intervene at once. It may be determined at a later time that the person's behavior was due to a pathological condition such as some form of mental illness, an electrolyte imbalance, or a drug reaction rather than to a crisis, but *crisis intervention will not hurt the person in any way*, provided the intervener continues to assess and respond to all new data from and about him (Fig. 23.1).

Crisis intervention is a structured process that is easy to learn. As a result, lay people can be quickly trained to become excellent interveners; and each helping person, lay or professional, uses the same interventions in a crisis.

Because many crisis interventions involve people we do not know, such as a person crying in the hospital waiting room or a distraught person at an airport, your first step is to *introduce yourself* and possibly explain your presence there. The second step is to *ask the person's name*, so that you can use it to personalize the

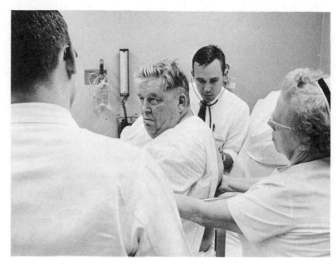

Figure 23.1 *Crisis intervention is an essential part of emergency-room nursing.*

intervention and, if he is confused, to keep him in touch with reality.

If the person seems dazed, bewildered, or immobilized, at the site of a car accident, for example, orient him to time and place, saying something like "Mr. Jones, this is Tuesday afternoon, and you are a few miles from Binghamton. You have been in a car accident. Do you remember it?" After introductions and any necessary orienting, you would:

1. Confront the crisis
   a. Find out if the person feels he is or has been in a difficult or hazardous position.
   b. Be active and direct! Reflection and other nondirective communication techniques will *not* work.
   c. Say something like "It seems that something is very wrong with you," then, "Tell me about it."
   d. The person may not know what is causing his reaction, so ask him how long he has been feeling bad and then get him to describe, in detail, the events of that period of time. Ask what things have changed in his life. There is always a precipitating event, but the person may not be able to make the connection between that event and his present feelings without help.
2. *Help the person to keep his reaction on a conscious level* by saying, "Let's talk about this some more. I think the fact that . . . is upsetting you." Be

careful not to soothe the person and thereby permit him to stop dealing with his crisis.

3. *Help the person learn the facts about the situation.* For example, has a definite diagnosis or prognosis actually been made? Is it true that there is no other flight until tomorrow? Was the driver of the other car really dead or merely unconscious when they carried him away?

4. *Give no false reassurances.* You cannot guarantee anything, and the situation may actually get much worse before the crisis is over.

5. *Discourage any displacement of anger and the blaming of others.* It may have been "the other driver's fault," but that does not change the fact that the person in crisis still has to deal with the consequences of the accident. An angry outburst such as "If that doctor had diagnosed my kidney problem sooner, I wouldn't be in this mess!" does not change the fact that the patient has to deal with his kidney problem. This step is very different from interventions with a depressed person, in which the expression of anger is encouraged (see Section 4 of this chapter).

6. *Help the person to locate and use available support and resources.* Be direct. Point out what these resources can do to help, and describe ways to use that help.

7. *Help with everyday tasks as needed.* Make sure that the person has food or a cup of coffee, a way to get home, a babysitter during hospital visits, and so on. Do not assume that he is "going to be okay," that he will pull himself together and be able to carry on as usual.

Criteria for Evaluation

Crisis intervention is effective when the following conditions prevail:

- The person in crisis has acquired a correct cognitive perception of the event. He knows what actually happened and the cause of the event or the nature of the occurrences that preceded the event. His information about the event is as factual and accurate as possible.

- The person in crisis is able to deal with feelings and thoughts about the event on a conscious level. He is able to recognize and accept his anger, grief, or despair, for example.

- The person in crisis becomes able to manage his feelings through appropriate verbalization, which leads to decreased tension and, ultimately, to emotional stability and control.

- The person in crisis resumes or develops effective patterns of seeking and using help, both with his feelings and with tasks to be done. He uses both interpersonal and institutional resources.

Importance of Nursing Interventions

Crisis intervention is important in nursing because crises are encountered frequently and the ways in which they are handled (or ignored) can profoundly affect a person's life. A person or family in crisis is in a state of disequilibrium, which means that change can be brought about more easily and more quickly than usual. A crisis often provides an opportunity to promote healthy responses, to correct faulty patterns of problem solving, and to resolve old crises that have been reactivated by the present crisis.

When a crisis has passed, it is *possible* for the person or family to be *functioning at a higher level than before.* They will, however, be functioning at the same level or on a lower level if they have *not* been helped through the crisis by the use of crisis intervention. The effectiveness of such interventions is indicated when people who have been in crisis remark at a later date, "It hurt so bad, but I grew so much."

SPECIAL INTERVENTIONS

In addition to the basic skills of crisis intervention, advanced training and specialized skills are needed in some types of crises. This training is usually designed to promote a greater understanding of one's own response to a particular situation or to teach additional techniques of intervention. For example, a community health nurse who has been assigned to provide follow-up care and support to rape victims will need advanced knowledge of the psychological manifestations of a woman's reactions to rape; but in addition, she must have explored her own responses and attitudes toward the act of rape, the victim, and the rapist. In similar fashion, most nurses need help and support as they begin to interact with people who are contemplating suicide or have attempted it, and with the families of such people.

Special techniques must be learned before crisis intervention via a telephone hot line can be done effectively. The absence of all visual information and nonverbal cues make it necessary to have highly developed verbal skills. Telephone contact with a runaway child, potential child abuser, or pregnant adolescent is fragile; and special techniques are needed to keep an unknown and upset person on the phone long enough to be helped.

Section 2

Loss and Grief

Grief, which is a *normal* and *predictable* response to loss, takes many forms, and it may not be recognized if the loss occurred sometime ago or was never identified. In the following vignettes, for example, Mrs. Harper does not connect her present condition (grieving) with the absence of her daughter, possibly because she believes she "ought" to be happy and glad for Jane. Mr. Clark has not resolved the loss of his wife; he has not yet completed the grieving process. Both Mrs. Harper and Mr. Clark need help to avoid the consequences of inadequate grieving.

Mrs. Harper has looked forward to the time when her daughter Jane would be in college and she would have more time for herself. She is disappointed to find that she is accomplishing few of the things she had planned to do. Her friends say, "You seem so irritable lately!" and "You are so emotional—what's wrong with you?" Mrs. Harper doesn't know what's wrong and fears that she has a serious illness, as she is often nauseated.

Mr. Clark has been acting strangely. He refuses to go out of the house and has given up his previous friendships. When friends or neighbors drop in to see him, he seems uninterested in them and occasionally says, "I'm fine." Mr. Clark's wife died abut 9 mo ago, but he still talks about her as if she were alive. His appetite is poor and he is having trouble sleeping.

To help a person cope with loss and grieve effectively, it is necessary to understand the various types of loss, to know the ways people react to loss, and to understand the interventions that are helpful during each phase of the grieving process.

LOSS

Loss is experienced throughout the entire life continuum, from earliest infancy until death. Some losses, such as amputation, robbery, divorce, or death, are obvious and easily identified. Other losses are less tangible and can easily be overlooked or misinterpreted. Examples of such losses include the loss of confidence or prestige, the loss of ability to bear children, and the loss of independence when one grows old and feeble.

Loss occurs whenever something can no longer be seen, heard, felt, known, or experienced. Loss results when something is not to be found and is now missing. There are three major types of losses: loss of a significant person; loss of some aspect of one's physical, psychological, or social well-being; and loss of one's personal possessions.

Loss of a Significant Person

A significant person can be one's parent, sibling, spouse, teacher, playmate, or neighbor. The list is virtually endless, and the commonly used term *significant other* could even include a pet. Significant people can be lost in a variety of ways, including death, moving away, being promoted to a higher grade, having an argument, or running away.

Loss of Part of One's Well-being

Loss of one's well-being includes any loss that damages, lessens, or detracts from one's physical, psychological, or social integrity and health (Lambert and Lambert, 1979):

PHYSICAL WELL-BEING. Loss of limb, eyesight, hearing, hair, strength, mobility, teeth, balance, or normal body function.

PSYCHOLOGICAL WELL-BEING. Loss of confidence, self-control, patience, self-esteem, memory, humor, serenity.

SOCIAL WELL-BEING. Loss of love, support, status, respect, power, or authority.

Loss of a Personal Possession

The loss of personal possessions is often more sudden than the loss of a significant other or the loss of one's health or well-being. Personal possessions may be lost by theft, fire, flood, being misplaced, or wearing out.

SIGNIFICANCE OF THE LOSS

The significance of any loss depends on its meaning for the person involved. The impact of the death of a parent, for example, will vary according to the age of the parent, the age of the child, and the nature of their relationship. The death of a beloved, respected, elderly parent will have a different effect on a person than will the death of an abusive, alcoholic, absentee parent. Similarly, the loss of a home by fire has a different meaning for a well-insured middle-aged couple than for a young couple who built their home all by themselves.

The significance of a loss depends on the amount of change it will inflict on those involved, the meaning of the loss to the person, and the resources and support available to the person as well as his own inner strength. The effect of a loss is also influenced by the amount of preparation or anticipation and the circumstances that surround the event. The effect of losing the family silver, for example, would be different if it were stolen; sold to enable the person to pay medical bills; sold to enable the person to take a trip abroad; or given, as planned, to a granddaughter as a wedding present.

Given the infinite combination of variables that affect a person's reaction to a loss, it is evident that the significance of a loss to a person must be assessed and validated before he can be helped to grieve. A loss that is devastating to one person can be a welcome relief to another, and no one can know for sure which is which without having input from the person.

LOSS, GRIEF, AND NURSING

Grief is a normal response to loss, but it does not come easily. The emotional suffering is sometimes more than a person can bear, and he may try a variety of ineffective strategies in an attempt to avoid the pain of grief. *Effective grieving* in response to loss *is essential for mental health,* and helping a patient or family to grieve is an important nursing intervention (Fig. 23.2).

Nurses need to understand the nature of loss and

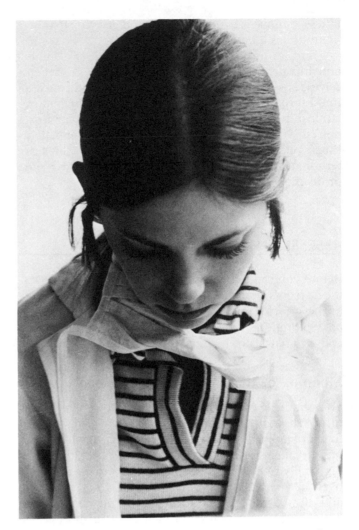

Figure 23.2 *Grief is a normal and essential response to loss.*

grief for three reasons. First, unresolved loss and inadequate grieving lead to depression. In the context of health, depression is *not* a synonym for sadness. Severe depression is pathological and is a form of mental illness (see Section 4 of this chapter for an explanation of depression). As the prevention of mental illness and the promotion of health are integral aspects of nursing, interventions related to loss and grief are essential nursing actions.

Second, loss and grief are important in nursing because they are encountered so frequently. People who are ill usually, if not always, experience one or more losses during the illness. Examples of such losses include loss of a body part or body function, and loss of independence, control, and autonomy. Loss of health and changes in body image bring a loss of what was and "the way I used to be." Because nearly every patient and family suffer losses of some type during an illness, a nurse is exposed to loss and grieving in others many times a day.

Third, an understanding of loss and grief is important in nursing because nurses experience loss themselves. Loss is an inevitable part of life, and because of the interpersonal involvements basic to a helping relationship, a nurse is likely to experience many losses herself. Such losses are encountered whenever patient-nurse relationships or family-nurse relationships are terminated, whether by discharge, transfer, recovery, or death.

ASSESSMENTS

Before you can help a grieving person, you must assess the person's behavior and identify the probable stage of the grieving process. This assessment must include an exploration of the meaning of the loss to the person and an analysis of his reaction to date.

Meaning of the Loss

You should never *assume* that you know what a loss means to another person. For example, the loss of two fingers may be an inconvenience but come as no surprise to a laborer in a hazardous occupation if many of his family and friends have suffered similar accidents over the years. The loss of two fingers would signal the end of a career for a concert pianist, however. If two fingers were lost by a child as a result of his playing with a forbidden tool, he might view the accident as a punishment, while the loss could result in overwhelming guilt for parents who felt that the accident could have been prevented.

The meaning of the loss for the person can usually be determined, little by little, if you do not stifle communication, first, by assuming that you know what the loss means to the person and, second, by acting as if your assumptions are facts. It is appropriate and expedient to hypothesize about possible earnings, but such hypotheses, or tentative nursing diagnoses, must be validated with the patient before they can be used as a basis for nursing intervention.

Reactions to Loss

The process of grieving involves a number of sequential stages: denial, recognition, and reconciliation. Each nursing intervention must be appropriate for the patient's current stage of grieving, so a knowledge of these stages is necessary for an accurate analysis of any given set of behaviors.

Stage Of Denial

Denial is the term used to describe a person's initial reaction to a loss. The person is not yet conscious of any specific emotional reaction. Familiar descriptions of this phase include: "It hasn't hit him yet"; "He's still in a daze"; "He's in a state of shock"; and "He doesn't know what hit him." Typical behaviors of denial include sitting motionless or wandering aimlessly about. Some people respond on an intellectual level and calmly proceed to do all the necessary things with no emotional acknowledgment of the loss. Initial physical reactions include fainting, perspiring, increased heart rate, nausea, diarrhea, crying, confusion, and restlessness.

The duration of the period of denial is affected by the size of enormity of the loss, the expectedness of the loss, the amount of tangible evidence that the loss has occurred, and the ego strength of the person suffering the loss. The stage of denial can range in length from a few hours to a number of weeks. In some situations, the loss overwhelms the person, either because the loss is enormous or because the person has little ego strength and coping ability. In such a case the denial can become pathological and permanent unless the person is helped to grieve *fully* and *effectively*.

Stage of Recognition

Following the period of denial, a person begins to feel his loss and to recognize and become conscious of his emotional reactions. Some responses in this stage are anger, depression, preoccupation, and attempts to deal with guilt. These responses do not all occur in every case, and they are not sequential (Lambert and Lambert, 1979).

Anger following a loss can be directed toward oneself or toward others. A person may express his anger by acts that are harmful or destructive to himself, such as refusing to eat, rest, take prescribed medicine, or meet other basic needs. Anger directed toward others is often expressed by blaming the physician, the nurse, the police, bystanders, or anyone else who could conceivably have prevented or minimized the loss by taking a different course of action.

The *depression* that follows a loss is characterized by insomnia, decreased appetite, decreased energy, and withdrawal from contact with other people. The person's feelings of self-worth and self-esteem may diminish, and he may say, "Don't bother with me," or "Don't waste your time with me."

Preoccupation is evidenced by a constant talking about either the loss or the object that was lost. A person may continually seek more and more information and constantly review the details of the loss. This intense focus on the loss is often an attempt to establish the reality of the loss and to convince oneself that the situation was properly handled. In some instances, preoccupation may idealize the lost person or object, emphasizing the good qualities while unconsciously repressing all negative thoughts and feelings.

Attempts to deal with guilt can usually be recognized by the person's use of 'if' statements, such as: "If only I had told him I loved him"; "If only I had gone back to check the fireplace"; or "If only I had locked the house."

The behaviors that characterize the recognition phase vary according to culture. For example, at one end of a continuum, some societies encourage the free and overt expression of grief, which might include weeping, wailing, preoccupation of the whole tribe or village with the loss for an extended period of time, or the expression of anger through a variety of destructive acts.

Other societies, at the opposite extreme, have developed rituals and procedures for coping with loss in a covert or discreet manner. These include lawsuits, insurance claims, divorces, and memorial services. The proceedings are handled by a specialist, such as a lawyer, a judge, or a funeral director in a socially acceptable manner that often limits the amount of anger and grief that can be overtly expressed.

Stage of Reconciliation

When a person's feelings about his loss have been recognized, accepted, and expressed, that person enters a stage of *reconciliation*. He has become reconciled to his loss, and there is no longer a need for anger or depression. He begins to reorganize those parts of his life that have been affected by the loss. He is less preoccupied with his loss, and the lost person or object becomes a memory. Interest in a possible replacement gradually develops, such as interest in wearing a prosthesis after an amputation.

Reconciliation has been accomplished when *the person accepts the loss and can, without hesitation, express and deal with his feelings about it.* He is reconciled to the loss and is making plans for the future.

NURSING INTERVENTIONS

When your nursing assessment of a person or family who has suffered a loss has established the significance and meaning of the loss and has determined the current stage of grieving, plans can be made for appropriate intervention.

First-Stage Intervention

1. Allow the person the right to deny his loss. Denial is essential when the loss is too painful for the person to face at the moment; the mind is protecting the person. Do *not* destroy or disrupt the person's defenses by forcing him to face reality prematurely.

2. Encourage expression of feelings about the loss. If the person refuses to eat, sleep, or take his medication, do not resort to arguing about it. Instead, help him to put into words his depression, anger, guilt, or other feelings.

3. Help with the activities of daily living as needed or find someone else to do so. In this stage of denial, some people cannot take care of themselves, their families, or their homes.

Second-Stage Intervention

1. It is important to remember that each member of a family will have a different reaction to a loss and may reach the recognition stage at different times. Therefore, when you are helping a family, a variety of interventions may be needed at one time.

2. Help each person to talk about the loss. When feelings begin to be expressed, *do not take the anger personally.* It is very hard to watch and listen to people in this stage because we unconsciously tend to avoid people who are angry, depressed, preoccupied with a single event, or trying to deal with guilt. Such behavior tends to trigger a negative response toward the person, and it may take considerable conscious effort for you to remain involved and effective.

3. Do *not* urge the person to replace the lost object or establish new relationships *at this time.* He is not ready yet.

4. *Do* encourage participation in relevant rituals and ceremonies that help the person acknowledge the separation or loss. Events as diverse as funerals, weddings, graduations, and retirement parties formalize the end of one era or relationship and the beginning of another. The reality of the event is validated by the presence of family and friends, who are then able to support the person or family as needed. *An absence of traditional rituals is a loss in itself* and can leave those involved with an uneasy sense that things are incomplete. This lack of closure makes it easy for susceptible people to deny the reality of the loss and to postpone the later stages of grieving indefinitely.

Third-Stage Intervention

1. Encourage the person to put into words his current perception of himself, how the loss has affected him, and how he has incorporated the loss into his life. Encourage him to describe his current situation and his feelings abut it.

2. Encourage the person to plan for the future, to try new ways of doing things, to establish new relationships, and to test out new responses.

The entire process of grieving can take from 6 months to 2 years. It cannot be hurried or speeded up, but it can be assisted and made more effective. Most people try for about 6 weeks to be helpful to a person experiencing loss, and then they forget. The immediate crisis of loss has passed, and the need for help and support has become less obvious. Unfortunately, intervention and assistance are likely to be needed at intervals throughout the *entire* grieving process, not just during the first 6 weeks or so.

The grieving person or family should be appraised of this fact and should be taught when the initial assistance has decreased or stopped. All members of a family should understand the grief process; they should know the appropriate interventions for each stage, and they should be taught how to help each other as they grieve a common loss.

CRITERIA FOR EVALUATION

A person has grieved successfully when he has completed the stage of reconciliation, when he is able to express and deal with his feelings about the loss, and when he is proceeding to make plans for the future.

If a person has not resolved his loss by the end of 2 years, he should be referred to a mental health specialist for therapy to prevent a serious depression or other mental illness. If at any time a person who has suffered a loss attempts or shows signs of considering suicide, he should be referred at once to a mental health practitioner. He should not be left alone until the suicidal crisis is over.

TERMINATION

Termination is the process of concluding a significant relationship with another person or group of people. Because the process evokes feelings of loss, termination is difficult and often painful, even though it may be part of a desirable event, like graduation or marriage. Termination constitutes the loss of the relationship for both parties, and in addition, the person who is leaving suffers the loss of a familiar situation.

People terminate relationships in many ways and with varying degrees of effectiveness. Some people strive for a well-defined ending, taking a "go, and don't come back" approach. They believe that, once good-byes have been said and there is nothing more to be done, ties should be severed quickly and cleanly. Other people

are unable to acknowledge that a relationship is ending, and they either *prolong* the termination or try to *avoid* it altogether. The *prolongation* of termination is evidenced when fellow employees or vacationers go through the motions of termination, but act as if they are unaffected by either the separation or the leave-taking. They promise to keep in touch and get together soon, even though there is little likelihood of their ever doing so.

The *avoidance* of termination is seen whenever either party busies himself elsewhere at the time of departure. For example, one young woman had invited her neighbors who were moving to come for supper after the moving van left, before they went to a motel to spend the night. One of the neighbors called late in the afternoon to say that the family would not be coming for supper and offered a highly improbable excuse. When the frustrated hostess expressed her dismay and annoyance, the neighbor blurted out, "I always act like this the last few days before we move—I get everyone mad at me, and then I don't have to say good-by." Such behavior does not reduce the stress of a separation; it merely substitutes one emotion for another—a feeling of anger or guilt for grief or sadness. People who avoid termination carry an ever-increasing burden of loose ends, unfinished business, and unended relationships.

Some families tend to manage termination well, and many or all members are present at each leave-taking, regardless of whether the departure is occasioned by a trip, death, or a new job. In other families the adults neither terminate effectively themselves nor teach their children to do so. The family of one man often stated, "Dad never said good-bye to anyone in his whole life." The statement was probably true, and unfortunately neither the man nor his family was able to change their behavior at the time of the man's long dying, which was awkward and empty for all because "Dad didn't like good-byes."

Effective and appropriate termination should be encouraged during childhood because the process is as critical for children as it is for adults and because it is more easily learned as a child than as an adult. Little children should be permitted to cry when they are separated from a trusted adult, and feelings of sadness and grief should be expressed as spontaneously as feelings of joy and happiness. Children should be helped to acknowledge their feelings when a best friend moves away or when they have to leave a favorite teacher, and to recognize the source of such feelings. A child whose cousins must return home after a long summer visit may need help to realize that his feelings of irritability or anger may be related to being left behind by the departing cousins.

Termination is usually easier when a definite date and time can be established and when that time is adhered to and specific plans are made and implemented. References should be made from time to time to the forthcoming termination to minimize any tendency of those involved to avoid the issue. For example, "Tomorrow at this time, you'll be . . ." and "Tuesday will be my last day to take care of you" are matter of fact acknowledgments that the termination is forthcoming. Such statements should be coupled with a brief indication of the speaker's feelings or reaction, such as, "I'll miss you," "I'll be glad for you but sad for me," or "It sure won't be the same without you." No one likes to be ignored or made to feel inconsequential, and it is disconcerting either to leave or to be left when no one acknowledges that the end of the relationship is worthy of notice or mention.

Certain rituals such as a retirement dinner or a going-away party encourage the expression of feelings for many people and enable them to respond when they could not do so on an individual basis. Such events are not common in professional relationships, and terminations in nursing must be accomplished without their benefit.

Some people who are unable to accept and discuss the reality of a forthcoming termination seem instead to test and try the allegiance, love, or caring of the other person. This behavior may be recognized and given labels like "senior stress" or "wedding jitters," but the situation is not relieved until those involved are able to acknowledge, no matter how briefly, their awareness of what is happening.

Termination occurs with increasing frequency in a mobile society. Because successful termination tends to favor the development of new and satisfying relationships, it is important for nurses both to practice and to teach it.

Section 3

Depression

Role of Nursing

Dynamics of Depression

Assessments
Behavior Patterns
Coping Patterns
Responses of the Nurse
Potential for Suicide

Depression and Nursing
Therapeutic Communciation
Physical Care
Establishment of Routines
Referrals

Criteria for Evaluation

Depression is a condition that must be differentiated from "the blues" and from the second stage of the grieving process. Although these conditions bear a superficial resemblance to each other, the causes, manifestations, and nursing interventions are different.

The blues is a term used to describe a *transient* period of lowered spirits in which the person is usually *aware* of the event or conditions that caused his depressed mood. The person feels blue, down, or sad, and may cry easily and unexpectedly. The blues can be caused by such things as the departure of a significant person, failing an exam, or experiencing a disappointment; postpartum blues often occur 2 or 3 days after the birth of a baby. A distinguishing characteristic of the blues is that the sadness lifts when the person becomes caught up again in his usual routines and when he resumes his customary activities. Although lay people use the terms depressed and sad interchangeably, being sad or down is a *normal* condition, whereas true *depression is a pathological condition* that must be diagnosed and treated.

Grief is a normal response to loss; and when sadness (which is a normal part of grief) has been effectively expressed, the person's suffering ends. If, on the other hand, sadness is not expressed and the sense of loss is not resolved, a person may become truly depressed. In a state of depression, a person is not merely sad; he is ill and needs treatment. A grieving person may feel a sense of remorse or guilt for things he wishes he had or had not done, but he rarely sees himself as a worthless person, as a depressed person is likely to do.

The following vignettes give a glimpse of two of the many facets of depression and may help to show that depression is very different from a temporary feeling of sadness or the blues.

Mr. Cunningham moves very slowly and hesitantly as he walks about his living room. He says his whole body aches but that his doctor has told him that there is nothing physically wrong with him. It takes him a good deal of time to complete his sentences, and his listener starts to feel uneasy around him.

Miss Barry has become reluctant to take her medications. She assumes a helpless stance toward her care and passively rejects all attempts to get her involved in her treatment plan. The night nurse reports that Miss Barry rarely sleeps through the night even with the help of sleeping pills. Her appetite is extremely poor, and she seems to be going downhill even though her physical signs indicate that her surgery was successful.

Depression can be defined as an affective (emotional) response involving sadness, hopelessness, dejection, emptiness, and low self-esteem, often accompanied by physical symptoms such as insomnia, anorexia, and psychomotor retardation (Swanson, 1975). In addition, depression:

- Usually involves some type of loss
- Can be a component of physical illness and can complicate or retard recovery
- Is dysfunctional
- Can be caused, precipitated, or worsened in some instances by chemical or hormonal imbalances, such as hypothyroidism

When coupled with *normal* self-esteem, depression is often part of the grieving process, but when coupled with *low* self-esteem, depression is a form of mental illness, such as manic-depressive illness or endogenous depression.

DEPRESSION AND NURSING

The promotion of mental and physical health is a primary goal of nursing, and nurses need to understand the nature of depression in order to prevent it whenever possible. Depression can sometimes be prevented by such nursing actions as crisis intervention and by helping a person to grieve effectively. An awareness of situations or events that can render a person susceptible to depression will enable the patient and nurse to work together to avert it. Examples of possible causes of depression include such things as a change in body image, a threat to self-esteem, a significant loss, and disruption in the family system. A person who has

undergone surgery that seemed to mutilate his body, or a person whose illness has caused him to relinquish his primary role in the family, would be susceptible to depression. Financial worries, a poor prognosis, or changes in treatment, such as the cessation of steroid therapy, have the potential for creating a state of depression.

It is beyond the scope of this chapter to include those forms of depression that constitute forms of mental illness; the material that follows is limited to those aspects of depression that are characterized by behavior patterns related to dejection and low self-esteem.

DYNAMICS OF DEPRESSION

A central aspect of depression is low self-esteem, which prevents a person from dealing with a loss and which can result in unexpressed or unresolved anger. The dynamics of depression usually involve a *series of interrelated events and actions*. An example of such a series of events is:

1. A person fails to develop an adequate sense of self-esteem and feelings of self-worth during childhood and is afflicted by persistent feelings of inadequacy.
2. There is a loss of a valued object, person, or situation. The loss may be real or imagined.
3. At the time of the loss, the person experiences ambivalent (simultaneously positive and negative) feelings toward the object or person. He may love the person but be furious with that person for leaving him.
4. He feels guilty about the anger he harbors and says to himself, "I shouldn't feel this way." He then tries to hide or bury his feelings of guilt.
5. The person cannot tolerate any conscious, uncomfortable feelings such as anger toward the valued object or person. He believes that it is not appropriate for him to feel that way, that he is not worthy enough to criticize, blame, or otherwise reject any part of the valued person, object, or situation.
6. Because he is unable to express his anger, he turns the anger inward on himself and enters a state of depression.

In summary, because of low self-esteem, a person cannot deal with his loss and may experience the effects of unresolved anger. In many instances he is *not aware* of this anger, for it is unacceptable to him and is unconsciously repressed. He is unaware of any feelings of anger and, before treatment, would truthfully deny the existence of anger about the valued object, person, or situation.

ASSESSMENTS

Most of the individual symptoms of depression are not unusual or dramatic, and the occurrence of a small number of them does not warrant even a tentative diagnosis of depression. There are, for example, many causes of insomnia or poor appetite, and there are many reasons why a person might feel pessimistic or might cut down on his social activities. If it only when individual symptoms become part of an *overall pattern* that the possibility or likelihood of depression will become apparent.

Early diagnosis is important, though difficult; and the nurse is obligated to view each patient in a holistic manner that will enable her to see relationships among all aspects of his behavior and to share her observations with other members of the health care team. Case finding is an important nursing responsibility, and if the nurse can recognize the early symptoms of depression, she can refer that person to the appropriate medical or psychiatric resources if her interventions are not sufficient.

Behavior Patterns

In addition to the feelings of sadness, dejection, and downheartedness that persist and often intensify throughout the period of depression, the following behavior patterns are characteristic:

- Changes in body sensation. *Somatization* will occur; that is, unexpressed feelings will find expression in bodily aches and pains. The person may become preoccupied with his body, and he is likely to suffer from insomnia and decreased appetite. His psychomotor movements will be slowed or disrupted.
- Changes in thought patterns. The person becomes pessimistic, sees no possibility of solving his problems, and tends to view things as hopeless.
- Changes in socialization. The person decreases his social participation. He withdraws and decreases his verbal communication (Lancaster, 1980).

Coping Patterns

It is important to assess the strengths of the person, to learn how he has dealt with similar situations in the past, and to discover previously used sources of com-

fort. Depending on the depth of his depression, a patient may or may not be able to give the nurse the information she seeks. If he is not able, the nurse can obtain valuable clues and suggestions from family, friends, or other significant people.

Responses of the Nurse

It is neither easy nor comfortable to be around a depressed person, and it is essential that you monitor your behavior carefully when you interact with a depressed patient. Feelings of depression are *catching*; and a person's feelings of dejection, despair, and hopelessness tend to trigger similar, though less intense, feelings in others. The seeds of depression are part of the human condition, and most people try to protect themselves by staying away from people who are depressed.

The care of a depressed patient can be so depressing that the staff avoids contact with him whenever possible. Therefore, you need to be on guard against any tendency to avoid a depressed patient whose unattractive and uncomfortable behavior tends to repel the very people who could help him.

Potential for Suicide

Many depressed people contemplate, at one time or another, the possibility of suicide as a way to end their mental and emotional suffering, so it is important to assess each patient for suicidal ideation (ideas of suicide). Some of the cues that indicate a person is considering suicide are:

He talks about death.

He talks about the uselessness of life.

He obtains and conceals equipment that might be used to commit suicide, including medications.

He exhibits a sudden change for the better in his mood ("smiling depression").

He talks openly of suicide. People who *talk* about suicide *do* commit suicide!

If you suspect that your patient is suicidal, you should ask him directly if he has thought of killing himself and if he has a plan for doing so. Raising the issue of suicide will *not* make a person consider suicide if he has not already done so. It will only convey your concern for his life and well-being.

If a person is suicidal, a climate of safety and protection should be created. Outside resources—family, friends, clergy—should be encouraged to help support the patient. He should have a responsible person with him at all times until the suicidal crisis is past.

NURSING INTERVENTIONS

Four major aspects of the care of a depressed patient include communication, physical care, routines, and referrals.

Therapeutic Communication

Six guidelines for applying basic communication skills to the care of a depressed patient are:

1. Establish a therapeutic nurse-patient relationship in which the patient feels accepted. Remember that low self-esteem is one cause of his depression.
2. It is *not* helpful to try to cheer the patient. Such attempts cause guilt over not feeling cheerful and increase his sense of unworthiness.
3. It is helpful to accept any expression of negative feelings and to sit quietly with him and not expect him to carry on a conversation with you.
4. Avoid asking the patient to make a decision. This is extremely difficult for a depressed person to do. Do not ask, "Do you want to take your bath now?" but instead make a statement such as "Your bath is ready now. I will help you with it."
5. Any expression of anger will be helpful to the patient, so try to allow him to express anger and avoid taking it personally.
6. The focus of the nurse's role with a depressed person is to help him deal with his feelings.

Physical Care

A depressed person may be virtually immobilized by his depression and unable to assume responsibility for some of his most basic needs. He may sit, unmoving, for hours and fail to eat or drink. His inactivity, poor nutrition, and lack of sleep will lead to physical complications such as constipation and fecal impactions, poor circulation, susceptibility to infection like pneumonia, and malnutrition.

Establishment of Routines

It is helpful and often necessary to set up a structured routine for the patient in an effort to decrease the necessity for decision making and to provide as much stability and consistency in his life as possible. A depressed patient will often sit and stare at his shoes for 15 or 20 minutes, seemingly unable to decide which one to put on first. Larger decisions require even more psychic energy; and during the acute phase of a patient's depression, decisions should be made by someone else whenever feasible.

Referrals

Assistance should be sought from a psychiatric mental health specialist whenever a patient's depression does not respond to the nursing interventions described above or if a suicidal crisis occurs. The psychiatric mental health specialist—a psychiatric nurse, a psychologist, or a psychiatrist—may work directly with the patient or may work indirectly through the referring nurse.

CRITERIA FOR EVALUATION

Nursing interventions have been effective and the patient's depression has been relieved when:

- The patient begins to verbalize feelings of anger as well as sadness
- The patient begins to assume responsibility for his activities of daily living and for meeting his basic needs
- The patient shows increasing interest in participating in plans for his own treatment and care
- The patient views life as having choice, meaning, and hope

Section 4

Anxiety

ANXIETY AND FEAR

It is necessary to understand the differece beween anxiety and fear in order to help an anxious person. *Anxiety* is the mental distress that accompanies the anticipation of some *future* threat or danger. *Fear* is an emotional response to a *present* danger. The source of anxiety may or may not be known. Anxiety is always *vage and ill-defined*, like the anxiety about possible failure on a new job. Fear is caused by a *specific* object or phenomenon perceived as dangerous, like a fire, a snake, or a snarling dog. Anxiety often extends over a number of days, whereas fear is concentrated in the present time.

Both anxiety and fear are emotional responses to some stimulus. Thus, both stimulate the sympathetic nervous system and tend to produce similar physical responses: dilated pupils, increased heart rate, sweating palms, diarrhea.

	Anxiety	**Fear**
Time	Future oriented	In the present
Source	Often unknown, vague, ill defined	Known, specific
Duration	Extended over time	Concentrated in present

Most people do not regularly encounter frightening objects or events, but anxiety is experienced in varying degrees many times each day. Synonyms for anxiety include fretting, apprehension, and nervousness. A knowledge of anxiety is necessary for understanding human behavior because it is a powerful force that can either be directed toward learning and growth or lead to illness and dysfunctional behavior.

SOURCES OF ANXIETY

There are some objects or phenomena, such as an earthquake, assault, or explosion, that almost always generate fear. The same is not true for anxiety because there are few events that are likely to produce anxiety for everyone. For example, an airplane trip can be boring, pleasurable, or anxiety producing, depending on a person's response.

Anxiety is an individual response to an occurrence or event that seems to threaten or affect one's security, either physical or psychological. A few physical conditions such as shock and hemorrhage elicit anxiety in almost every patient. The patient feels anxious and apprehensive, and often describes a vague sense of impending doom. The source of anxiety is usually unknown. The patient may not even know that he is in shock or that he is hemorrhaging internally; he just knows that something is terribly wrong and feels that something awful is going to happen.

Psychological sources of anxiety are intensely personal because people react differently to any given situation. Future events such as an evaluation conference, starting a new job, or entertaining one's in-laws for the first time will produce varying levels of anxiety in different people.

Levels of anxiety occur along a continuum from an *absence of anxiety* that may be either unnatural (ataraxy) or unhealthy (apathy) to states of *severe anxiety or panic* that are equally unhealthy. These levels are described in Figure 23.3, which should be studied carefully. *Middle* levels of anxiety can produce behavior which is directed either toward active efforts to relieve and reduce anxiety, or toward escape and avoidance.

High levels of anxiety produce disorganized or chaotic responses that preclude any rational or effective behavior. The levels of anxiety are sometimes indicated by +'s, as follows: mild anxiety (+), moderate anxiety (+ +), severe anxiety (+ + +), and panic (+ + + +) (Peplau, 1962).

DEVELOPMENT OF ANXIETY

May (1953) has described the *development* of anxiety as follows:

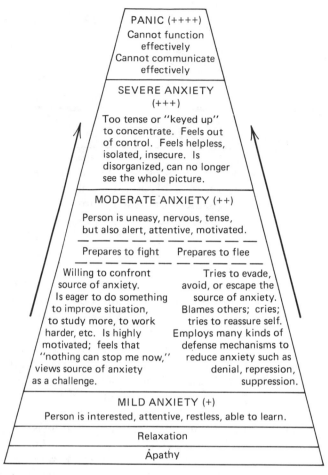

PANIC (++++)
Cannot function effectively
Cannot communicate effectively

SEVERE ANXIETY (+++)
Too tense or "keyed up" to concentrate. Feels out of control. Feels helpless, isolated, insecure. Is disorganized, can no longer see the whole picture.

MODERATE ANXIETY (++)
Person is uneasy, nervous, tense, but also alert, attentive, motivated.

Prepares to fight | Prepares to flee

Willing to confront source of anxiety. Is eager to do something to improve situation, to study more, to work harder, etc. Is highly motivated; feels that "nothing can stop me now," views source of anxiety as a challenge.

Tries to evade, avoid, or escape the source of anxiety. Blames others; cries; tries to reassure self. Employs many kinds of defense mechanisms to reduce anxiety such as denial, repression, suppression.

MILD ANXIETY (+)
Person is interested, attentive, restless, able to learn.

Relaxation

Apathy

Figure 23.3 Behavioral characteristics of various levels of anxiety.

1. Each person holds certain expectations in the form of wishes, wants, desires, or drives. Such an expectation might be: having a happy marriage, being a champion swimmer, losing weight. The expectation may be conscious or unconscious (such as proving oneself superior to a sibling).

2. The possibility or expectation of things working out right is threatened in some way. A few minor arguments with a new spouse can create anxiety for some people about the future of the marriage, for example, and information about the qualifications of other swimmers can create anxiety about winning a swimming meet. Lack of self-confidence or self-discipline can create anxiety about losing weight.

3. Anxiety occurs and the person begins to feel that he or she has lost, or is losing, control over the situation and that the outcome depends on the reactions of the spouse or the qualifications of other swimmers, for ex-

ample. Three major responses to such anxiety are feelings of *helplessness, isolation, and insecurity.* These feelings are present in varying degrees whenever a person is anxious.

4. The early phases of anxiety are largely internal and may not yet have been evident to another person, but, at this point, the anxious person begins to display *relief behaviors.* These are the actions by which he attempts to relieve the distress of anxiety. The anxiety itself (the nervousness, dread, or apprehension) cannot be observed, only the behavior that relieves the anxiety, such as crying, anger, displacement (ritualistic behavior that attempts to retain control), or somatization (expression via bodily aches and pains).

Some relief behaviors such as crying, withdrawal, and somatization are not helpful. Other relief behaviors channel the person's available energy into productive ways to counteract the anxiety, such as learning new ways to communicate with one's spouse, training harder for a forthcoming swimming meet, or trying a new approach to the problem of obesity.

ROLE OF NURSING

It has been said that anxiety is the most unpleasant and, except for loneliness, the most universal of all experiences (Fromm-Reichman, 1960). It is experienced many times a day in response to a wide range of thoughts about various stimuli, such as: "What if my child-support check doesn't come?" "What if this traffic makes me late again?" "I'm not even sure that nursing is the career for me." As an example of the pervasiveness of anxiety, there is a simple sentence of only 10 words that, when spoken by a parent or a person in authority, provokes a degree of anxiety in many people: "I'd like to speak to you for a few minutes."

In addition to the anxieties that accompany the routines of everyday life, anxiety is intensified in any health care delivery system. Most hospitalized patients are made anxious by loss of well-being; loss of autonomy, control, and freedom; loss of familiar routines; and separation from family and friends. Each patient must surrender his role in his family, business, and social worlds and must assume a new role: the "sick role." He must tolerate invasion of his body and his personal space by procedures that are painful, unfamiliar, or embarrassing.

By virtue of their frequent or prolonged contact with patients, nurses are in a position to assess and intervene with those who are highly anxious. Depending on its severity, anxiety can be a motivating or an inhibiting force. It can make a person amenable to taking action that will relieve his anxiety, or it can lead to dysfunctional behavior. The role of the nurse is to reduce anxiety to a manageable level and then help the person deal with it constructively.

ASSESSMENTS

Anxiety is assessed by means of both subjective data furnished by the patient and the observation of certain physiological and behavioral manifestations. When a person is anxious, you will be able to observe some of the typical signs of sympathetic stimulation, such as dilated pupils, a red flush on face or neck, increased perspiration (a cold sweat or sweaty palms), and shaking or tremors plus restless, fidgety movements. In addition to the visible signs of increased activity of the sympathetic nervous system, you will be able to observe other indications of anxiety such as biting nails, talking fast, tics or blinking, hand wringing, and other "nervous" behaviors. Some symptoms cannot be observed and must be reported by the patient; only he can tell you that his heart is "fluttering," his mouth is dry, and he has "butterflies in his stomach" and a lump in his throat. Only he can identify or describe his feelings of dread or apprehension.

As you observe and talk with the patient, try to assess the level of anxiety and communicate your findings by describing both the objective and subjective signs and symptoms. Your observations will help provide a basis for planning appropriate interventions, and are much more helpful than a notation that merely indicates that the patient has 3 + anxiety. Such a notation is easily misinterpreted and is likely to be construed as a diagnosis that is beyond the scope of nursing diagnoses.

NURSING INTERVENTIONS

The type of intervention needed depends on the patient's level of anxiety. Mild-to-moderate anxiety can serve as motivation to acquire the knowledge and skills that will reduce the anxiety. Severe, high-level anxiety, on the other hand, must be reduced to a manageable level before the patient can begin to consider what to do about his situation.

Some of the ways to reduce anxiety are to help the person:

- Become aware of his anxiety by exploring his feelings. Some people deny their distress by stating that they are feeling fine. It may then be necessary for you to confront the person gently with the discrepancy between his verbal statement and his nonverbal cues, saying, for example, "You say you feel fine, but I can see that your forehead is covered with perspiration, your hands are shaking, and you can't sit still." The patient may acknowledge that he *is* feeling a bit nervous, and through the effective use of communication skills, you are likely to be able to help him describe his feelings.

- Focus on, recognize, and name the source of his anxiety. Some reasons for anxiety may seem more acceptable to the patient than others, and care must be taken to identify the *basic, underlying concern* whenever possible. For example, a woman who is scheduled for a mastectomy may blame her nervous mannerisms on a fear of surgery, whereas the unidentified source of her anxiety is the almost unspeakable (for her) thought that after the surgery her husband might find her repulsive, and leave her. In such a case, no amount of preoperative teaching about the surgery wil relieve the patient's anxiety. She must explore her feelings until she can recognize and name the source of her anxiety before it can be relieved.

- Gain insight into his anxiety by exploring the nature and meaning of the perceived threat to his physical or psychological well-being. This can be done by helping him to examine the realities of the situation and to estimate the likelihood that the perceived threat might actually occur. Additional information may be needed to determine whether the threat is based on fact or fantasy.

- Explore ways of coping with anxiety. The person may need to seek additional information or skills with which to counteract the perceived threat. He may need to learn new ways to approach anxiety-producing situations, such as using support groups within his family or community, learning to communicate *directly* with others who are involved, or seeking assistance in raising his self-esteem. It is often necessary to teach the basic steps of problem solving because many people have little or no knowledge and skill in this area.

- Regain a sense of control and security by providing increased structure and routine for a time. This will temporarily relieve some of the ambiguity and uncertainty in his life and will provide a measure of stability during a period of high anxiety.

CRITERIA FOR EVALUATION

Nursing interventions to reduce anxiety will be deemed successful when:

- The signs and symptoms of anxiety are decreased or absent
- The patient is able to focus his attention and concentrate on things that must be done, decided, or attended to at the moment
- He is able to identify and discuss with minimal anxiety the threats he feels might endanger his well-being
- He is able to use problem solving as a method of reducing anxiety

Section 5

Altered Body Image

BODY IMAGE

Body image is a term that indicates the way people think and feel about their bodies. A person is said to have a *healthy* body image when he accepts his body as it is, when he feels that his body is acceptable to other people, and when he is not preoccupied with bodily functions.

A person's body image is basic to his identity and exerts a profound effect on behavior, including social interaction, choice of a career, and sexual behavior. A person who feels attractive, well-coordinated, and strong is likely to feel that he has more options and possible courses of action than does a person who feels ugly, awkward, or weak. Two persons may be equal in height and weight and similar in appearance but present entirely different images to others because of differences in the way they feel about themselves.

Body image is an important aspect of health care because it affects a person's motivation toward the care of his body. As health care moves from mere survival and the conquest of disease toward the promotion of high-level wellness, it becomes apparent that much of the responsibility for the state of a person's health must be shifted from the physician to the individual patient. Improved sanitation, advances in medicine, and new techniques of surgery can reduce deaths from specific illnesses, but wellness cannot be given or bestowed on a person. Each person must assume responsibility from childhood on for engaging in practices that are likely to maintain or improve his health, and the person who values and enjoys his body is more likely to do so than is the person who finds his body unattractive or of little worth.

DEVELOPMENT OF BODY IMAGE

Body image begins to develop immediately after birth and continues to evolve as life progresses. It develops in part from a person's comparisons of himself with the characteristics that are valued by those around him. In a society that values youth, for instance, the wrinkles of impending old age can be a cause for concern or worry, whereas in a culture that reveres its elderly members wrinkles can be a symbol of attainment. Each person tends to comapre his body with others and to wonder whether or not his body is attractive to others. He seeks answers to questions such as: Am I too tall? Too thin? Too pale? Too well-developed? Too clumsy?

It is beyond the scope of this book to trace the develoment of body image through the life cycle, but it is important for the nurse to be aware of opportunities to promote the development of a positive body image.

A person's body is the visible manifestation of his self; and because it can be scrutinized by others, a person's body image is vulnerable to assault, which may be intentional or unintentional, visual, verbal, or physical.

Protection of the patient's body image is a nursing responsibility that is accomplished in diverse ways, such as teaching a person how to cope with the stare of others or helping adults to temper their remarks to children. Parents and teachers can be taught, for example, to refrain from making derogatory remarks such as: ''Pick up your feet—you're clumsy!'' ''I don't know what to do with your hair—it's so thin and unmanageable'' or ''If you'd stop eating chocolate, maybe your complexion wouldn't be so bad.'' Such remarks, made in exasperation by a concerned person, do not help the underlying problem and can be detrimental to the body image of the person to whom the remarks are directed.

The development of body image will warrant increased attention from the school nurse as more handicapped or disabled children are mainstreamed through the public schools as mandated by law. The way in which these children view themselves will be influenced by the verbal messages they receive from teachers, staff, and other children. Studies have shown that the quantity and quality of teacher attention is different for attractive, appealing children than it is for unattractive children, and it is likely that many teachers who intellectually favor the concept of mainstreaming may need help and support in establishing positive relationships with children whose disabilities seem disturbing or even frightening.

ALTERATIONS IN BODY IMAGE

A person's body image is affected by changes in society and by changes in the body itself. A familiar, comfortable body image can be shattered by illness or an accident, or it can be transformed gradually in response to messages from innumerable sources such as women's magazines, television, health clubs, clothing designers, and sex therapists (Figs. 23.4–23.7).

Changes in Society

A person's body image reflects that person's perception of fads, trends, and current values. Some of these influences seem minor and transitory but may be influential at certain stages of body image development. For example, many a girl born with tightly curling hair felt unattractive and out of fashion during the '60s when the vast majority of young girls wore their hair long and very straight, whereas a decade later tight curls were fashionable.

The women's lberation movement has encouraged women to reject the concept of a weaker sex and to view their bodies as strong and capable of performing many tasks and jobs that were formerly deemed unsuitable or inappropriate. Women are being encouraged to value their bodies and to find pleasure and enjoyment in them. Self-care programs are teaching people to become increasingly aware of bodily responses to stress and to know how to prevent and treat a number of body discomforts in a natural, nonmedical manner.

Current emphasis on physical fitness makes it seem desirable to have a body that is capable of participating in a sport, jogging, or even running a marathon race. Many people who have heretofore been complacent abut the bodily effects of a sedentary lifestyle now find themselves uneasy with their body image.

Changes in Body Structure or Function

Alterations in body image occur as the result of both natural and induced changes, which may be either purposeful or accidental. The cause of such changes can usually be identified, but it is not possible to hypothesize whether a given change will enhance or damage a person's body image until one knows how the person perceives the change. Some women feel radiant, beautiful, and fulfilled throughout the bodily changes of pregnancy; others feel awkward, unattractive, and embarrassed. An aging person who feels respected by family and friends may be able to accept the need for a cane or a hearing aid with less negative impact on his body image than can a person who feels that his weaknesses makes him a burden and a nuisance to his family.

Alterations in body image occur following normal developmental processes such as the loss of baby teeth, the physical changes of puberty, pregnancy, menopause, balding, and growing old. Other major causes of altered body image are accidents, disease, and surgery (Figs. 23.5 and 23.6).

The effect of the loss of a body part as the result of an accident differs from a loss by surgery because a person has little or no time to prepare himself for any alteration in body image resulting from an accident. The loss of a leg because of slowly progressive gangrene is likely to have a different impact on body image than the sudden loss of a leg in an industrial accident or war. The impact is not less; it is different.

Alterations in body image will follow surgery of any kind, whether or not the results are visible. A hysterectomy (removal of uterus), for example, produces no visible body change, but its impact on the patient's concept of herself as a woman can be exceedingly great.

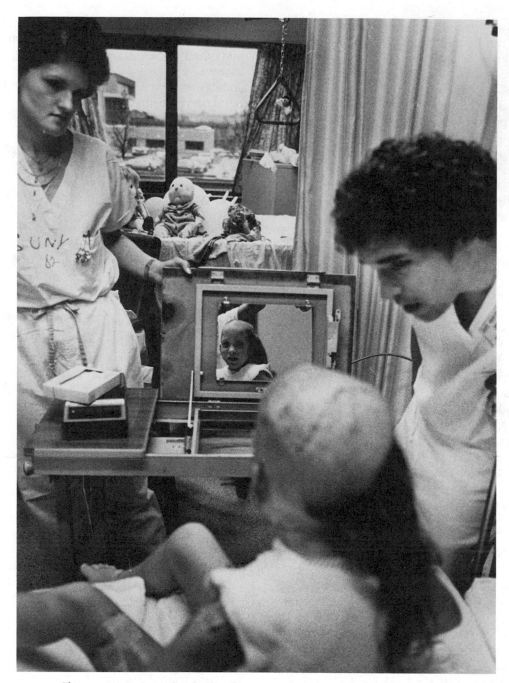

Figure 23.4 Renee's first look at her scars is a tense time for all concerned.

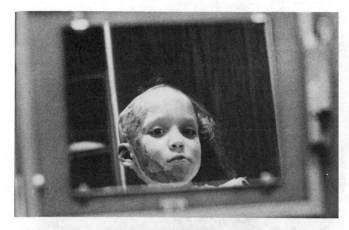

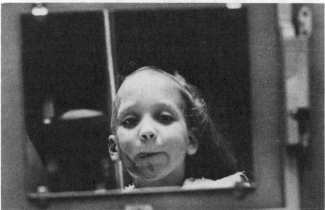

Figures 23.5 and 23.6 *Renee's thoughtful response to the sight of her scars, and her acceptance of them demonstrates a healthy, positive body image. This has been fostered throughout her young life by her parents, and maintained throughout her ordeal by her parents and the hospital staff.*

Many life-saving procedures made possible by medical and technological advances have created major alterations in body image. For example, an organ transplant often leaves the recipient feeling that he is no longer whole or that he is no longer a single complete person. Problems related to an altered body image are often compounded if the donor of the transplanted organ was of a different sex or race. The living donor of a kidney may have perplexing reactions to having part of himself in another person's body.

One of the most complex of all body image alterations follows sexual reassignment. Transsexual patients are usually people who have felt for years that they were trapped in bodies of the wrong gender. After undergoing extensive psychotherapy and hormonal treatment, they have presented themselves for surgery to correct what they consider a mistake of nature. The treatment of a transsexual patient involves major body image adjustments, not only for the patient but for the

nurse as well, and most nurses need support as they learn to interact effectively with a patient who has undergone sexual reassignment.

ASSESSMENTS

Assessment data are often collected over an extended period because changes in body image may evolve slowly, perhaps being delayed by periods of denial, anger, or grief. Some of the assessments to be made include the meaning and nature of the bodily change, the patient's level of self-esteem and security, the patient's pattern of coping, and the nurse's own concepts of body image.

Meaning and Nature of Body Changes

The meaning that body changes have for a patient will be influenced by the speed with which the change occurred, the extent or amount of change, and the patient's perception of how much his life will be disrupted or enhanced. No assumptions can be made. A mastectomy has often been portrayed as one of the ultimate alterations of body image, but for some women the removal of a breast can be *less* traumatic than the complete loss of hair and eyebrows as a side effect of chemotherapy to check the spread of cancer. A mastectomy could also be less damaging to the body image of a famous ballet dancer than the development of a deforming bunion or crippling arthritis.

Age can be a significant determinant of the nature of a change in body image. *Disfigurement* can be less significant to a young child than an accident that limits his mobility and his ability to attain independence and mastery over his environment. An adolescent, on the other hand, is likely to find disfigurement one of the most formidable threats to the development of a positive body image.

Only the patient can say how much and in what ways his life may be changed by his altered body image, and this information can be obtained only through sensitive, skilled communication *over a period of time*. Difficult as it is to obtain the information, it is essential to do so because nursing interventions will differ according to whether the patient feels embarrassed, helpless, stigmatized, useless, ashamed, or angry.

Level of Self-esteem and Security

Although they are difficult to assess, self-esteem and security influence the nature of alterations in body image. A person who feels good about his body may be temporarily devastated by a change in its structure or

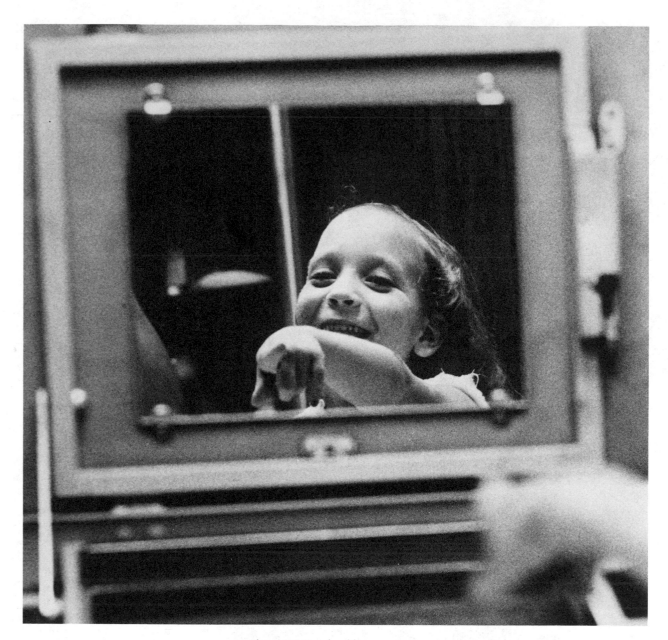

Figure 23.7 A healthy response!

function but is more likely to restructure a positive body image than is a person whose self-concept and body image have always been consistently negative. Several small alterations in body image, with *time for acceptance and integration after each one,* are usually less threatening to a person's security than one very large change.

Patterns of Adaptation and Coping

The nurse needs to assess how the patient usually responds to change or threats to his well-being. Patients who usually deny their feelings will tend to deny the significance of the bodily change and will try to assure themselves that everything will be fine, that things will not be different. Other patients express their feelings freely, and although the process is not easy for anyone involved, the end result is likely to be a healthy adaptation to a changed body image. Interactions within the family are important in assessing the support available to the patient or, on the other hand, what the patient will have to contend with.

Nurse's Own Body Image

It is important to assess your feelings about your own body because, until you understand your own responses, you cannot fully appreciate either a patient's preoccupation with or seeming lack of concern for certain alterations in his body image. It is often useful to consider questions such as: "Do I view my body as a source of pleasure and pride, as a vehicle for accomplishing my daily activities, or as a source of embarrassment or discomfort?" "What aspects of my body and body functioning please me most?" "Would I suffer more from facial disfigurement; the loss of sight, hearing, or speech; paralysis and loss of mobility; or the loss of reproductive ability?" "What alteration in body image would cause me the greatest shame or embarrassment? The greatest anger and frustration?" An honest search for answers to these and similar questions will contribute to your empathy for a patient who is struggling to sort out his feelings and responses.

You must also assess your reactions to bodily changes in your patients, because awareness that certain alterations in body structure or function disturb you will enable you to take steps to keep these feelings from interfering with the patient-nurse relationship. You need to ask yourself questions like: "Do I feel irritated or impatient, for example, with a person whose strength is failing and whose movements are slow or uncertain?" "Am I likely to be unable to cope with a foul body odor, disfigurement, missing body parts, uncontrolled body functions, or wounds that do not heal?" An awareness and acceptance of your feelings will enable you to *seek help* in dealing with them; failure to acknowledge your feelings can interfere with your ability to help your patients.

NURSING INTERVENTIONS

Interventions related to an altered body image include helping the patient to verbalize his feelings, promoting intellectual understanding, helping the patient integrate his feelings and his intellectual understanding, and supporting the family. First, you can help your patient by encouraging him to *verbalize his feelings* about an altered body image, keeping in mind that it is not realistic to expect a person who has never discussed his body image suddenly to begin doing so. Your encouragement of such patients will have to be gentle and without pressure.

You can also encourage a *correct intellectual understanding* of the body change and how it might realistically affect the person's life. A patient may lack knowledge or have distorted views about the probable effects of the body change, and remedying this intellectual gap should enhance positive adjustment. Whenever possible, it is advisable to start the process of adaptation well in advance of probable bodily changes. Examples of

such intervention include early discussion of changes related to puberty, exploration of the probable effects of progressive arthritis, and a full explanation of the possible side effects of chemotherapy before the therapy takes place.

Helping the person *integrate his feelings with his intellectual understanding* is another nursing task. Encourage him to express his feelings as he hypothesizes about the probable impact of the change on his life. He may need help in doing the things that he knows are important but that seem too difficult. He might, for example, know that he must eventually look at and accept his disfigurement, incision, or stump, but be afraid to do so. Just talking about the affected area and asking you how it looks may be an important first step for the patient which indicates the subject is no longer too difficult for him to mention. Your comments such as "It's not quite as red and swollen today" or "There is still a bit of drainage" help to prepare him for what he will see, while supportive remarks such as "It's really hard to get ready to look at the incision, isn't it?" acknowledge the difficulty he is having. Some patients need to cast sidewise glances at a burn or wound before they can bring themselves to really look at it.

Some patients go through a period of testing during which they show the disfigurement or incision to family, friends, and staff to gauge the reactions of others to the bodily change. Opportunities for the expression of anger or grief must often precede nursing efforts to promote acceptance of the change. For some people, denial seems to be the only defense against the seeming stigma or shame of what they perceive to be an unbearable condition, such as persistent urinary incontinence (lack of bladder control).

Finally, the nurse should *support the family* and help them acquire the knowledge and develop the skills and strength to cope with problems related to the patient's altered body image. The family needs an adequate understanding of what is happening and what is likely to occur in both the immediate and distant future, and they often need to be taught how to help. For example, some elderly people feel repulsive and untouchable as they begin to develop tremors, wrinkles, and "age spots" and to acquire spots on clothing from spilled food, or a persistent odor of dribbled urine. The family or attendants may simply not realize the importance of touch in helping such a person feel acceptable and accepted. When they have become aware of the importance of touch as an indicator of acceptance, they may willingly make a conscious effort to grasp the person's hand or touch his shoulder at frequent intervals throughout the day.

Members of a family may need much help in learning to talk to each other about the impact of the patient's bodily changes on him and on themselves. The entire family system is affected, for example, by the mother's loss of a breast, by a grandfather's paralyzed side, or by a father who is unemployed because of a worsening muscle disease.

Timing is important throughout these interventions. Some of them cannot be rushed, and yet they cannot be delayed, because the combination of high anxiety and inadequate support and assistance can lead to ineffective or pathological coping patterns.

CRITERIA FOR EVALUATION

Nursing interventions undertaken to help a person cope with an altered body image can be deemed successful when the patient:

- Is able to express both his feelings and his intellectual understanding of his bodily changes with minimal anxiety
- Is able to consider options and alternatives when trying to solve problems related to his altered body image, such as the use of a prosthesis following a mastectomy
- Incorporates the altered body image into his normal pattern of living

PATIENT TEACHING

Many people are reluctant to seek psychological support or treatment even though their lives are seriously disrupted. In many instances, the nurse must take the initiative to confront a patient and his family with her assessment data, and teach them the importance of seeking and accepting psychological help from a trusted and competent person. The type of help needed will be determined by the nature of the problem, and the helper

---

> ### A Message About Psychologists
>
> Unless specifically exempted by law, psychologists must be licensed and currently registered by the Board of Regents of the University of the State of New York to practice in this state.
>
> If you have a question regarding the status of a psychologist, call the New York State Education Department, Division of Professional Licensing Services.
>
> Toll Free
Dial 1-800-342-3729

---

may be a pastor, neighbor, counselor, physician or other competent and caring person.

It is not safe to undergo treatment with an unknown therapist, and it is essential that you teach the patient the importance of checking the credentials of a psychologist or other therapist. This is such a critical issue that some telephone companies insert a warning such as at the beginning of the list of psychologists in the yellow pages (see box below "A Message About Psychologists").

RELATED ACTIVITIES

Prior to teaching patients about the importance of psychological support, it will be helpful for you to analyze your own attitude toward personally seeking and accepting psychological assistance. You will encounter many difficult and stressful situations in nursing involving patients, families, and professional colleagues, and your career will be influenced by the assistance you receive in coping with your reactions to these situations.

The following questions deserve serious consideration as you prepare to meet the psychological challenges of your profession.

- How difficult is it for you to acknowledge to yourself that you need psychological support?
- How do you communicate this need to others?
- When you need help, do you actively seek assistance or do you wait and hope that someone will notice and offer to help?

If you believe that the process of seeking and using psychological support will be very difficult for you, it is advisable to discuss your situation with your instructor or other knowledgeable person before the need for help arises. This preventive action will help you avoid 'burn out' and other psychological crises common to nursing.

SUGGESTED READINGS

Crisis

Dixon, Samuel L: *Working with People in Crisis: Theory and Practice.* St. Louis, Mosby, 1979.

Hall, Jeanne, and Barbara Weaver: *Nursing of Families in Crisis.* ed.2. Philadelphia, Lippincott, 1979.

Hargreaves, Anne G: Coping with disaster. *Am J Nurs* 1980 April; 80(4):683.

Harrison, DF: Nurses and disasters. *JPN and Mental Health Services* 1981 Dec; 19(12):33–36.

Hoff, Lee Ann: *People in Crisis: Understanding and Helping.* ed.2. Menlo Park, CA, Addison Wesley, 1984.

Janosik, Ellen H: *Crisis Counseling: A Contemporary Approach.* Monterey, CA, Wadsworth Health Sciences Division, 1984.

Krouse, Helene J, and John H Krouse: Cancer as crisis: the critical elements of adjustment. *Nurs Res* 1982 March/April; 31(2):96–101.

Nettler, Gwynne: The quality of crisis. *Psych Today* 1985 April; 19(4):54–55.

Smitherman, Colleen: Crisis (Chap.11) in *Nursing Actions for Health Promotion.* Philadelphia, Davis, 1981.

Loss and Grief

Bower Faye L (ed): *Nursing and the Concept of Loss.* New York, Wiley, 1980.

Campaniello, Jean A: The process of termination. *JPN and Mental Health Services* 1980 Feb; 18(2):29–32.

Carter, Carol: Fear of loss and attachment. *J Gerontal Nurs* 1981 June; 7(6):342–349.

Dimond, Margaret: Bereavement and the elderly: a critical review with implications for nursing practice and research. *J Adv Nurs* 1981 Nov; 6(6):461–470.

Flood, Dianne Milledge, and Sherry Peltz. Helping children and their families grieve. *Can Nurse* 1982 Jan; 78(1):34–36.

Forsyth, Diane McNally: The hardest job of all. *Nursing 82* 1982 April; 12(4):86–91.

Grove, Sheryl, et al.: Encounters with grief (7 articles). *Am J Nurs* 1978 March; 78(3):414–425.

Joyce, Christopher: A time for grieving. *Psych Today* 1984 Nov; 18(11):42–43, 46.

Kuntz, Barbara B: "I didn't think his death would hit me so hard". *RN* 1984 Feb; 47(2):30.

Scheideberg, Donna: "How can you be so sure my baby's dead?" *RN* 1984 Feb; 47(2):29.

Schultz, Clarice A: Sudden death crisis: pre-hospital and in the emergency department. *JEN* 1980 May/June: 46–50.

Sene, Barbara Stankiliweiz S: Termination in the student-patient relationship. In *Psychiatric/Mental Health Nursing, Contemporary Readings.* (pp 181–189), New York, Van Nostrand, 1978.

Sharer, Patricia S: Helping survivors cope with the shock of sudden death. *Nursing 79* 1979 Jan; 19(1):20–23.

Smitherman, Colleen: Grief (Chap. 9) in *Nursing Actions for Health Promotion.* Philadelphia, Davis, 1981.

Stickney, Sandra K: Companions in Suffering. *Am J Nurs* 1984 Dec; 84(12):1491–1493.

Toth, Susan B, and Andre' Toth: Empathetic intervention with the widow. *Am J Nurs* 1980 Sept; 80(9):1652–1654.

Whitaker, Connie M: Death before birth. *Am J Nurs* 1986 Feb; 86(2):157–158.

Depression

Archibald, Joan W, and Marcia A Ullman. Is it really senility—or just depression? *RN* 1983 Nov; 46(11):49–51.

Barry, Patricia D: The depressed patient. In *Psychosocial Nursing Assessment and Intervention* (pp. 201–203). Philadelphia, Lippincott, 1984.

Carmack, Betty J: Suspect a suicide? Don't be afraid to act. *RN* 1983 April; 46(4):43–46.

Depression (continuing education features). *Am J Nurs* 1986 Mar; 86(3):283–298.

————Minot, S. Reid: What does it mean?

————Campbell, Laura: Acute care in the hospital.

————Harris, Beth: Drugs and depression.

————Crockett, Mary Swanson: A case of anger and alienation.

Hart, Nancy A: The suicidal adolescent. *Am J Nurs* 1979 Jan; 79(1):80–84.

Hafen, Brent Q, and Brenda Patterson: Preventing adolescent suicide. *Nursing 83* 1983 Oct; 13(10):47–48.

Hoff, Lee Ann, and Marcia Resing: Was this suicide preventable? *Am J Nurs* 1982 July; 82(7):1106–1111.

Lake, Alice: Childhood depression—The "killer" blues. *Woman's Day* June 7, 1983 66–74.

Rosenfeld, Anne H: Depression: Dispelling despair. *Psych Today* 1985 June; 19(6):28–34.

Smith, Mary L: Depression: you see it—but what do you do about it? *Nursing 78* 1978 Sept; 8(9):42–45.

Smitherman, Colleen: Depression (Chap.10) in *Nursing Actions for Health Promotion.* Philadelphia, Davis, 1981.

Valente, Sharon: The suicidal teenager. *Nursing 85* 1985 Dec; 15(12):47–49.

Valente, Sharon: Stalking patient depression. *Nursing 84* 1984 Aug; 14(8):62–64.

Anxiety

Barry, Patricia D: The anxious patient. In *Psychosocial Nursing Assessment and Intervention* (pp. 198–201). Philadelphia, Lippincott, 1984.

Knowles, Ruth Dailey: Dealing with feelings: Managing anxiety. *Am J Nurs* 1981 Jan; 81(1):110–112.

Smitherman, Colleen: Anxiety (Chap. 6) in *Nursing Actions for Health Promotion.* Philadelphia, Davis, 1981.

Altered Body Image

Barry, Patricia D: Body image. In *Psychosocial Nursing Assessment and Intervention* (pp. 64–66). Philadelphia, Lippincott, 1984.

Blaesing, Sandra, and Joyce Brockhaus: The development of body image in the child. *Nurs Clin North Am* 1972; 7(4):597–608.

Bourne, Barbara A, and Joyce L Kutcher: Amputation: helping a patient face loss of limb. *RN* 1985 Feb; 48(2):39–44.

Dempsey, Mary O: The development of body image in the adolescent. *Nurs Clin North Am* 1972; 7(4):609–616.

Lasoff, Elaine M: When a teenager faces amputation. *RN* 1985 Feb; 48(2):44–45.

Lewis, Carol West: Body image and obesity. *J Psych Nurs* 1978 Jan; 16(1):22–24.

McCloskey, Joanne: How to make the most of body image theory in nursing practice. *Nursing 76* 1976 May; 68–72.

Murray, Ruth L: Body image development in adulthood. *Nurs Clin North Am* 1972; 7(4):617–630.

Norris, Catherine: Body image: Its relevance to professional nursing. In Carlson, CE and B. Blackwell (eds) *Behavioral Concepts and Nursing Intervention*. Philadelphia, Lippincott, 1978.

Smitherman, Colleen: Change in self-concept (Chap. 12) in *Nursing Actions for Health Promotion*. Philadelphia, Davis, 1981.

Stanley, Linda: Does your own body image hurt patient care? *RN* 1977 Dec; 50–53.

Walters, Jean: Coping with a leg amputation. *Am J Nurs* 1981 July; 81(7):1349–1352.

Warlick, Sharon: Sam; the patient nobody wanted to visit. *Nursing 78* 1978 July; 8(7):56–58.

General

Brill, Colleen, and Lyda Hill: Giving the help that goes on giving (self-help). *Nursing 85* 1985 May; 15(5):44–47.

Dewis, Marilyn E, and Joanne Chekryn: The "invisible" spouse. *Nursing 86* 1986 March; 16(3):104.

Fromm-Reichmann, F: Psychiatric Aspects of Anxiety, in Stein M, Vidich AJ, White DM (eds): *Identity and Anxiety*. Glencoe, IL, Free Press, 1960.

Gedan, Sharon: Say good-bye to guilt. *Nursing 85* 1985 July; 15(7):30–31.

Hyland, Patricia A: Time to say good-bye. *Nursing 86* 1986 May; 16(4):128.

Johnson, Suzanne Hall: 10 ways to help the family of a critically ill patient. *Nursing 86* 1986 Jan; 16(1):50–53.

Jones, Marilee K: Caring for the patient who makes caring difficult. *Nursing 86* 1986 May; 16(5):44–46.

Kushner, Harold S: *When Bad Things Happen to Good People*. New York: Scocken Books, 1981.

Lambert, Vicki A, and Clinton E Lambert: *Psychosocial Care for the Physically Ill.* ed.2. Englewood Cliffs, Prentice-Hall, 1985.

May, Rollo: *Man's Search for Himself*. New York, Norton, 1953.

Meer, Jeff: Loneliness. *Psych Today* 1985 July; 19(7):28–33.

Mereness, Dorothy A, and Cecelia M Taylor: *Essentials of Psychiatric Nursing*. ed.11. St. Louis, Mosby, 1986.

24

Sexuality

Prerequisites and/or Suggested Preparation
Suggested preparation for this chapter includes concepts related to values, individual development, therapeutic communication, and body image (Chapters 6, 9, 15, and 23 in this book or equivalent content from another source).

ASPECTS OF SEXUALITY

Sexuality is, in its broadest sense, a composite of the qualities that make a person male or female. It is a combination of the attributes that determine how a person views and uses his physical self, how he reacts to the bodies of other people, and how he perceives the ways in which others respond to him. Sexuality is multifaceted and complex. It is physical, psychological, emotional, personal, interpersonal, cultural, ethical, and spiritual.

Sexuality is *physical* because it involves organs, nerves, hormones and muscles, and because all five senses are involved whenever a person is fully aware of his body, its rhythms and its functions. Sexuality is affected by all basic physiological needs and by good health as well as by disease, injury, and drugs.

Sexuality is *psychological* and reflects a person's sexual self-image and his perception of his gender identity. Each person has a self-concept that is constantly changing and revising itself and that mirrors his view of himself as lovable, fat, unattractive, sexy, or any one of innumerable other adjectives. Sexuality involves the use of each person's defense and coping mechanisms as he deals with his perception of himself.

Sexuality is *emotional.* It can involve feelings of tenderness, anger, love, joy, hate, guilt, desire, or revulsion, among others.

Sexuality is *personal.* Each person has a sexual nature that is uniquely his own. He is what and who he is; there can be no question of rightness and wrongness. His physical self and his perceptions of it belong to him; they are unlike anyone else's.

Sexuality is *interpersonal.* Satisfaction of the need to love and be loved involves an ongoing relationship with at least one other person, although sometimes this "other person" may be a beloved and adoring pet. The need to touch and be touched, and to enjoy a comfortable, sharing relationship with another person requires the ability to establish a meaningful relationship.

Sexuality is *cultural.* It is determined in part by each person's family beliefs and ethnic background, by the attitudes of society, by peer pressure, and by neighborhood norms.

Sexuality is *ethical.* Each person must, sooner or later, confront related ethical issues, such as the legality or morality of women's rights, homosexuality, and sperm banks, for example.

Finally, sexuality is *spiritual.* Many religious teaching include concepts related to reverence and care of the body, the qualities of being male or female, love, and responsiveness. Much of the solace of many religions is derived from the concepts of being held, comforted, cradled, touched, and loved. There are many experiences and aspects of sexuality that transcend human understanding.

Expressions of sexuality vary from era to era, culture to culture, and person to person, but the basic tenets are unchanging. Every person needs a close and satisfying relationship with at least one other person, and he needs to love and be loved, to touch and be touched by that other person.

SEXUALITY AND NURSING

An evolving awareness and acceptance of human sexuality throughout all segments of society have created a corresponding awareness in nursing of the relationship between sexuality and health care. Sexuality is an integral aspect of holistic care, and at present it is not unusual for a nurse's overall plan of care to include nursing interventions related to the sexual needs of her patient. It is not reasonable to expect any nurse to be knowledgeable in all aspects of sexuality, but she should be aware of scope and extent of this topic. In addition to acquiring an overview and a general understanding of sexuality, you will need to obtain the specific knowledge and skills that will enable you to help the patients with whom you choose to work. The material that follows lists some of the aspects of sexuality that are likely to be of concern to your patients and about which you should acquire a beginning level of knowledge and understanding. These aspects can be categorized in numerous ways; in this chapter they are listed as indicators of the education needed by different age groups. In many instances, of course, the assignment of a topic to an age group is purely arbitrary because many topics are relevant to several groups. Areas of sex education that are important to children, for example, are equally important to their parents.

Aspects of Sexuality Relevant to Different Age Groups

Childhood

Gender identification, masculine and feminine roles

Anatomy and physiology of conception, birth, menstruation, nocturnal emission, and masturbation

Potential problems such as molestation, child abuse, incest, rape, sexual experimentation, child pornography

Adolescence

Sexual activity, contraception, venereal disease

Pregnancy, abortion, adoption, teenage parenting

Homosexuality

Runaways, prostitution, pornography

Breast self-examination and testicular examination

Young Adulthood

Marriage, divorce

Family planning, genetic counseling, infertility, adoption

Pregnancy, labor and delivery, lactation, mother and infant bonding

Parenting, single-parent families

Wife abuse, women's self-help groups

Sexual preference and life style

Sexual function and dysfunction

Meeting the needs of the physically and mentally disabled

Middle Adulthood

Menopause and corresponding changes in male sexuality

Cancer of the uterus, cervix, breast, prostate, testicles

Effects of acute or chronic ilness on sexuality

Retirement and sexuality

Late Adulthood

Loss of spouse, loneliness

Sexual needs of the elderly and implications for nursing homes and extended care facilities

Physiological changes, myths and fallacies

Reasons for Not Dealing With Sexuality

Despite an increasing intellectual awareness that a person's sexuality is an integral part of his being, minimal attention is paid to the sexuality of patients in day-to-day nursing practice. At least five reasons can be offered to explain this gap between what could be done and what is actually done in this area.

First, pressures of time and energy create situations in which nursing priorities do not include sexuality. Within the context of traditional nursing practice, sexuality is often viewed as nonessential in comparison to medications, nutrition, or physical therapy. If patients could choose, however, it is entirely possible that some of them would grant sexuality a higher priority than nutrition or exercise.

Second, many hospitalizations are short, and as a result, patient-nurse contacts are often brief. This may negate the likelihood of effective intervention related to sexuality because it takes time to establish the degree of trust and rapport that must be present before a nurse tries to help with any aspect of sexuality.

Third, lack of information or conflicting information handicaps many nurses who would like to be effective in the area of sexuality. Inadequate information about topics such as menopause, sexual activity after a heart attack, or sexuality in childhood, for example, tends to limit the types of patients with whom a nurse feels she can intervene successfully.

Fourth, personal discomfort because of lack of experience, a limited vocabulary, conflicting cultural and moral values, and lack of privacy can make the task of dealing with sexuality seem too risky and not worth the expenditure of psychic energy. For example, merely reading about masturbation is enough to make some nurses anxious. Talking about it is even more stressful, and the care of a patient who masturbates, be he adult or child, may be so disturbing that some nurses must ignore the patient's sexuality in order to continue to help him meet his other needs.

Fifth, a nurse may be knowledgeable and willing to intervene as needed in the area of sexuality, but may lack the necessary skills to do so. Such skills include the ability to note and interpret both subtle and overt cues that a problem exists, to introduce the subject and start the intervention, to take a sexual history, to do appropriate teaching, and to make referrals as needed. These skills can be learned, but their absence can be frustrating in the beginning.

Preparation for Dealing With Sexuality

The areas of preparation needed by the nurse are derived from the reasons why some nurses do not deal with the sexuality of patients. One of the most obvious areas of preparation is the acquisition of knowledge of the subject. The amount and type of knowledge needed will be determined in part by the level at which you plan to intervene. Some nurses merely hope to be able to answer questions without blushing; others expect to make interventions related to sexuality a large component of their nursing practice.

Knowledge can be acquired by taking some of the many available courses on human sexuality, by reading and then discussing the topic with people of different age groups, and by watching the excellent movies and documentaries that have recently been produced. Both knowledge and experience can be gained by doing volunteer work at Planned Parenthood centers, with women's self-help groups, and at adolescent counseling centers, for example. Part of the knowledge you will need includes an extensive vocabulary, which enables you to understand the words and terms used by children, researchers, adolescents, street people, social workers, and other groups.

Another significant area of preparation is related to attitudes and values. It sounds trite and obvious to mention that you will be working with people of different generations, different lifestyles, and different value systems, but these differences are sometimes more significant in the context of sexuality than in other contexts. For example, it is relatively easy to discuss a person's nutrition or exercise needs in terms of his values and lifestyle, but it is not always easy to discuss sexuality with a person whose beliefs and values you find unfamiliar or unacceptable.

The acquisition and development of communication skills, including interviewing and counseling skills, is prerequisite for effective intervention in sexual matters.

The amount of preparation needed depends in part on the goals you have set for yourself, but should in any case be sufficient to enable you to meet three basic goals related to sexuality:

- To begin to understand the scope and ramifications of sexuality
- To accept sexuality as a legitimate and significant aspect of nursing
- To be able to use a few basic nursing interventions that will help a patient meet his needs related to sexuality

SEXUALITY AND ILLNESS

A person's sexuality can be affected by the *outcome* of an illness such as a heart attack or quadriplegia, or can be directly related to the *cause* of the illness, as in repeated attacks of venereal disease. Some problems of sexuality are the result of hospitalization, acute illness, chronic illness, and disturbances of sexuality.

Hospitalization

Any type of institutionalization, whether it be in a hospital, a nursing home, or a prison, can create problems of sexual deprivation. Some of these problems are expressed, overt, or easily hypothesized, such as those of a sexually active young adult who suddenly finds himself confined to a hospital for an extended time and isolated from all significant social contact. Other problems are less obvious, such as those of an elderly woman separated from her husband after 50 years of marriage, or those of an adolescent who fears that the separation brought about by a period of hospitalization will destroy a rather fragile relationship with a new friend.

In addition to the interruption of significant relationships, many hospital practices and policies assault the sexuality of most patients. Some such practices include:

Unflattering, uncomfortable, unisex gowns

Sexually related procedures such as genital care, catheterization, massage, and bathing

Lack of privacy for attention to physiological needs such as bathing and elimination

Lack of opportunity for intimate contact and private communication wth others

Acute Illness

An acute illness such as a heart attack or an accident can suddenly threaten a patient's normal roles and functions, giving him little or no time to prepare for the changes that will occur. Some of these changes are obvious, but less obvious ones may be even more significant. A middle-aged man who suffers a heart attack will undoubtedly be concerned about returning to work, but he may be more deeply concerned about retaining the strong, indomitable male image he has always presented to his adolescent children.

Some types of surgery pose serious threats to the sexuality of some patients. Such surgery includes removal of the uterus, breast, ovary, prostate, or testicle and also the creation of an artificial opening for the excretion of body wastes such as urine or feces.

Chronic Illness

Some chronic or permanent disabilities such as disfiguring burns, an amputation, or a spinal cord injury have a direct and obvious impact on the sexuality of the patient. Other long-term conditions and illnesses exert an indirect influence on sexuality via the side effects of therapy. For example, some drugs, such as those used to treat hypertension, can cause impotence and decreased libido (sexual desire).

Disturbances of Sexuality

Problems of sexuality that are not caused by accident or illness include those related to:

- Sexual preference and sexual behavior patterns
- Gender identity and gender reassignment (sexual transformation)
- Sexual dysfunction or perceived inadequacies such as infertility, impotence, premature ejaculation, and painful or difficult intercourse for a woman (dyspareunia)

ASSESSMENTS

Current nursing literature reflects an emerging interest in sexuality that is consistent with the holistic nature of humans. Unfortunately, however, some authorities urge the nurse to "take a sex history" on each patient. Such advice is ill-founded for two reasons. First, the phrase "sex history" too often refers only to sexual dysfunction, and the format is specifically designed to elicit the information needed to improve sexual relationships. Current use of a sex history as the major tool for the assessment of a person's sexuality tends to overlook the needs of the child, the adolescent, some single adults, and many elderly people.

Second, it is neither advisable nor appropriate to include a sexual history as a routine part of *every* health history. Some people, especially those who have never discussed sex with anyone, will be understandably offended or upset at being asked to discuss sexual matters when hospitalized for a condition such as pneumonia or a fractured ankle that has no obvious relationship to sexuality.

Indications of a Need for Assessment

Assessments related to sexuality should be made whenever you receive verbal or nonverbal cues that a need or a problem exists or is likely to develop and whenever you know from experience or study that a need or problem is likely to arise.

Verbal Cues

Verbal cues can be obvious or subtle, innocent or suggestive, direct or indirect, and can come from persons of any age. The following are a few of the almost infinite number of verbal cues which are likely to be given:

"Where do babies come from?"
"I sure don't think I'll let my husband see this awful scar."
"How soon can we have intercourse after the baby is born?"
"I guess an old codger like me isn't supposed to have feelings."

Each of these statements provides an opening that enables a sensitive nurse to help the patient explore an area of concern. Most verbal cues do not express a need for extensive information but rather indicate a need to explore a troubling issue.

Nonverbal Cues

It is generally agreed that when there is a discrepancy between a person's verbal and nonverbal messages, the nonverbal message is more likely to be accurate. A person may *say* nothing about his sexual needs but may indicate the presence of a concern or need by his nonverbal behavior. Such nonverbal cues are likely to be accurate indicators that a need or problem exists, but they must be explored and interpreted in the context of the person's situation and developmental stage. A few of the many possible nonverbal cues are:

Extreme modesty
Giggling and stealing sidewise glances at other children in the ward
Excessive or overt masturbation (in both children and adults)
Intense interest or embarrassment in response to televised commercials for sanitary napkins, tampons, and douches
Exposure of breasts or genitals that appears to be accidental but is suspected of being intentional
Kissing, touching, or trying to fondle a female nurse's breasts or buttocks

All nonverbal behavior must be put into context, interpreted, and validated by the patient. For example, the significance of dirty jokes depends in part whether they are the "bathroom humor" which is characteristic of certain developmental stages of middle childhood, or the crude jokes and off-color remarks of an adult.

Indicators from Personal Experience or Study

The nurse will discover through reading, study, and talking with colleagues, patients, and families that certain illnesses and conditions frequently create or intensify sexual problems. The relative predictability of such problems is sufficient reason to initiate a rather detailed sexual assessment.

Any condition that makes the patient feel unattractive or undesirable or that might be distressing to other people or make them feel uneasy can create or magnify sexual problems. Some such conditions are:

Severe weight loss or weight gain
Surgery on, or deseases of, the reproductive organs
Pain, either chronic or acute
Altered control of elimination (dribbling of urine, incontinence, presence of an indwelling catheter, colostomy, others)
Disfigurement from severe burns, amputation, or radical head and neck surgery, for example

Paralysis after a stroke or spinal cord injury

Loss of hair after chemotherapy

Side effects of drugs or disease, such as drooling or tremors

Sexual Assessment

When your professional knowledge, cues from the patient, or both indicate the likelihood of a sexual problem or need, a sexual assessment is done. This assessment may range from asking a few questions to a detailed analysis of the patient's sexual attitudes and behavior, past sex history, and current status. The extent of the assessment is determined both by its purpose and by the competence of the nurse.

A detailed assessment is appropriate and necessary, for example, when a patient is being treated for some sexual dysfunction, but it is not always necessary in order to help a patient deal with certain other aspects of sexuality. A specially trained therapist who is helping a paralyzed patient regain the ability to have sexual intercourse will understandably need to ask about the patterns, type, and frequency of sexual activities both before and after the accident. Such information provides a basis for helping the patient devise ways to meet the sexual needs of himself and his partner.

A detailed assessment is not needed, however, to help a patient and his wife discuss the ways in which their fear of future heart attacks might affect their resumption of sexual activity.

NURSING INTERVENTIONS

Your interest in the patient's sexual needs and your desire to help him meet them will be evidenced by a sensitive and considerate approach to every aspect of care. It is important to respect modesty and a need for privacy at all times and to respond to each patient as a sexual being who is either male or female, not an asexual being in a unisex gown and environment.

Most nursing interventions related to sexuality fall into one of four categories: teaching, support, referral, and working for changes in the institution's policies and practices.

Teaching

Teaching the patient and family includes teaching which is specific to a given disease, condition, or therapy; general education about sexuality; anticipatory guidance about forthcoming stages or expected developments; and the dispelling of myths and fallacies.

Guidelines for Sexual Assessments

1. Structure the setting carefully. Ensure as much privacy as possible. Select a time when you are not likely to be disturbed or interrupted, and when the patient is as comfortable as possible.

2. Be matter of fact, serious, and professional. Do not try to cope with your own discomfort or embarrassment by acting cute, cool, flippant, funny, or sophisticated or by adopting any other artificial pose.

3. Introduce the topic by giving the rationale for your concern, based on verbal or nonverbal cues from the patient or your own knowledge and experience. This can be done by making a statement such as "I have been noticing that you . . .", "You have made several remarks lately that make me wonder if . . .", "Many people who have had an operation like yours dread the thought of . . .", or "I have read that after an attack of . . . , people tend to worry about . . ." Allow the patient plenty of time to think abut and respond to your opening and to bring up his own concerns and problems.

4. Whenever possible, start your assessment with areas that seem least likely to be stressful and gradually move to those that could be more stressful.

5. Allow the patient or family member the right to refuse to discuss the matter. Do not take a refusal personally. If you have evidence that your patient might talk with a nurse who is older, more experienced, or of a different sex, ask the patient if this is so and then refer this aspect of his care to someone else.

6. Ask only those questions that you can and will follow up on. Do not seek material you do not need or cannot use.

7. Observe and listen for feedback from the patient related to his understanding of your phrases and terminology. If you do not understand the patient, say, matter-of-factly, "I'm not sure I understand. Does . . . mean the same as . . . ?"

8. Be especially supportive and therapeutic if the patient seems very anxious or uncomfortable. Permit him to digress a bit, to hesitate, to search for words, and so on. He may need tme to get up enough courage to discuss the topic.

9. If there seems to be a problem, ask the patient's perception of it. Do not merely assume that a problem exists.

Support

Support may be expressed through acceptance of the patient, recognition of his concerns and feelings, and willingness to discuss potentially difficult or embarrassing topics. It is helpful to anticipate the patient's concerns and feelings (such as a fear of discomfort during intercourse after childbirth) and to verbalize the possible feelings, thereby giving overt permission to talk about them.

Encourage touching and other expressions of affection during hospitalization. When talking with a patient about sexual activity, such as intercourse after a heart attack, it is good to include the sexual partner whenever possible. Failure to do so can foster suspicion and curiosity about what has been discussed and taught and is likely to decrease cooperation.

Referral

Some patients will be ready to discuss a variety of sexual concerns once they perceive you as a concerned, knowledgeable, and accepting person. Some of their problems may be beyond your current level of competence; in that case, patients should be referred to a person with specialized training. An example of the relation between professional preparation and levels of competence is shown in Table 24.1

You will eventually be able to help those patients who need information, support, and an opportunity to explore feelings; but you should refer patients with sexual problems to a qualified person. Your local Planned Parenthood center has resources for helping with a wide range of problems related to many aspects of sexuality and will be able to facilitate referrals to other agencies or therapists as needed.

TABLE 24.1

	Professional Preparation	Appropriate Level of Therapeutic Intervention
Level 1	Professional nurse	Limited sex education: limited information about sexual feelings, behaviors, fallacies, and myths.
Level 2	Professional nurse with training in sex education and counseling	Specific information about sex and sexuality. Concise suggestions regarding sexual fears, adaptations to illness, and anticipatory guidance.
Level 3	Professional nurse qualified as trained sex therapist	Sex therapy with individual and couples.
Level 4	Psychiatric nurse clinician with master's degree who is a trained sex therapist	Intensive individual psychotherapy, sex therapy, and marital therapy.

Working Toward Institutional Change

Many institutions adhere to practices and policies that are either actually detrimental to the patient's well-being or do nothing to permit him to maintain his sexual identity. There are, for example, restrictions, either verbal or nonverbal, against any attempt by the patient to achieve a degree of privacy by closing his door or pulling the curtains around his bed. Sitting on the bed by a visitor and physical contact such as hugging and kissing are frowned upon if not forbidden.

Nurses may need to take the lead in gradually establishing policies that make it possible for a patient who will be in a hospital, nursing home, or extended care facility for a long time to meet his sexual needs at least minimally. Permission to have the door closed for a little while, an overnight pass to go home, meticulous attention to a patient's need for privacy while bathing or eliminating and during treatments, and the withholding of censure of the patient who masturbates are among the changes that might be made in institutional policy. One nurse reportedly has plans to manage a long-term care facility in which resident couples are permitted to bring their double bed from home. Attempts to make any such changes will be controversial and are likely to elicit a wide range of emotional responses from all concerned, but complete, holistic care is impossible if the patient's sexuality is ignored or blocked.

PATIENT TEACHING

Patient teaching in the area of human sexualiy encompasses an almost limitless range of topics and concerns. Depending upon the age, sex, situation, and needs of the individual, topics for teaching might include: the questionable value of routine circumcision, the relative merits of various methods of birth control, the psychological aspects of a herpes infection, sex education for small children, and the impact of sexually transmitted diseases such as AIDS.

Given the extensive nature of likely topics for teaching, it is impossible for a particular nurse to be knowledgeable and skilled in all areas. It is possible, however, for each nurse to develop three essential competencies as follows:

1. To create a climate or environment in which a person of any age is able to verbalize and discuss concerns about his or her own sexuality.
2. To obtain the needed information promptly and share it with the individual or family as quickly as possible.
3. To make appropriate referrals when the person's needs exceed the nurse's ability to help.

Only two of the many important areas of patient teaching are detailed in this chapter. It is expected that you will acquire the knowledge needed to teach on other topics as you progress through more specialized upper level nursing courses. The two areas included in this chapter are: (1) the individual's responsibility for early cancer detection and (2) the administration of a vaginal irrigation.

Personal Responsibility for Early Cancer Detection

The presence of some forms of cancer cannot be detected by either patient or physician until the disease is well advanced and symptoms appear, but cancer of the breast, cervix, and testicles can be easily detected during its early stages. Cancer of the breast and testicles can be detected through palpation and observation by the patient. Cancer of the cervix is detected through laboratory analysis of vaginal secretions (a Papanicolaou test, usually called Pap test). This test is usually done by the physician, although some women's self-help groups are beginning to advocate self-examinatin of the vagina with subsequent analysis of a Pap smear by a laboratory.

Breast Self-examination

Breast cancer is a leading cause of death from cancer among women, and approximately eight out of every 100 women will develop it. Fortunately, breast cancer can be detected very early through self-examination of the breast, and early detection dramatically increases the chances of a complete cure. About 90 percent of all diagnosed breast cancers are discovered by patients but, if the patient has not done regular self-examinations, the discovery is often accidental after the cancer is well advanced.

When a woman does breast self-examination on a regular monthly basis, she knows the normal texture and contours of each breast and is able to detect very slight and subtle differences. Each woman should report any lump, no matter how small, to her physician at once because prompt diagnosis of a malignancy can often give a complete cure and save her life.

Before teaching a patient how to do a breast self-examination (BSE), it is extremely important to talk with her about what BSE means to her. It is not enough for her to know how to do the examination; most women fail to examine their breasts for psychological, not intellectual, reasons. Some of the reasons and excuses offered for not doing breast self-examinations are: "If I did have cancer, I wouldn't want to know about it," or as stated by one nursing student, "My mother and grandmother both died of cancer of the breast, and I'm too scared to examine mine." The patient who says, "I just don't have the time," may need help in exploring her self-esteem and her priorities in order to discover that time spent on herself is time well spent.

A powerful but usually unexpressed reason among older age groups and some cultural and religious groups is that handling one's breasts is similar to fondling them and thereby somewhat akin to masturbation. Because the risk of breast cancer is very great for women over 50 years of age, it is imperative that the nurse, with great sensitivity and understanding, help such patients deal with their natural reluctance to examine their breasts.

Every female patient with whom you come in contact should be assessed to determine her knowledge of and attitude toward BSE. If she knows how and does it faithfully each month, nothing more need be done. If, however, the patient either lacks knowledge or is unwilling to examine her breasts, teaching is needed. It is indeed tragic for a woman to be hospitalized, in daily contact with many nurses, and then be discharged without having learned to examine her breasts. The illness that brought her to the hospital may have been relatively minor, but failure to learn BSE could jeopardize her life.

BSE involves acknowledgement of its emotional component, use of a mirror, and use of the hands. The patient should be taught to use a mirror to observe her breasts for shape and symmetry. This is done both with her arms overhead and at her sides. Any changes in the nipple or in the size or shape of the breast should be reported to the physician (Fig. 24.1).

She should use her hands to search for any changes in breast tissue and to look for any enlarged lymph nodes in the axilla. Palpation is usually done with the person lying down, though some authorities recommend that palpation be done when the person is in the tub or shower and the skin is wet, on the ground that the fingers will slide over wet skin more easily.

It is important to make certain that the patient understands the reason for each action. If she is taught to examine her breasts using a series of concentric circles, for example, she should understand that this ensures a systematic way of making sure that all breast tissue is examined, but that there is nothing inherently valuable about the use of a circular pattern. Lack of understanding by the patient can negate much of the nurse's teaching, as evidenced by a telephone call received by an office of the American Cancer Society. One woman, who had been taught to examine her breasts while wet, telephoned in great distress to explain that she could not do BSE anymore because she had moved and no longer had a shower!

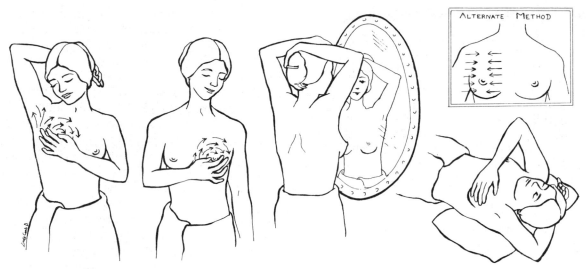

Figure 24.1 *Breast self-examination. Insert shows alternate method of systematic self-examination.*

The most important aspects of BSE are regularity and a systematic pattern of palpation which ensures that every square inch of breast tissue is examined every month. The recommended time is 1 week after the onset of each menstrual period, because the breasts are least likely to be engorged and tender at that time. Postmenopausal women should pick an easily remembered date and do BSE on that date each month.

Although breast cancer is not common among young women, it does occur, and adolescent girls should be taught BSE both for their immediate protection and to establish a lifelong pattern of monthly self-examination. Breast cancer in men is rare, but men should be taught to palpate their breasts occasionally and to immediately inform their physician of the presence of any lumps or other changes.

Testicular Self-examination

Cancer of the testicles can be detected in the early stages by routine self-examination of the testicles. Bimanual palpation of the scrotum will reveal the presence of a lump or a difference in weight between the two testicles. The early stage of cancer is usually painless, and therefore a lump will not be noticed unless the patient examines his testicles regularly.

Testicular self-examination is best done while the man is standing (Fig. 24.2). The man must learn to differentiate the texture and contour of the testicles from that of the scrotum and then check for any difference in weight between the two testes. The early symptoms of cancer are a painless lump and a heavy feeling or sensation of discomfort in the scrotum.

Testicular cancer is not common, but when it occurs, the results are often tragic. The surgery is frequently extensive and destructive if the cancer is far advanced. The situation is doubly tragic because the cancer is curable if detected early enough. The incidence is highest in men 20 to 40 years of age, and the risk is greatest for men who have had, or have, an undescended testicle (cryptorchidism). Testicular cancer is rarely found among blacks or Asians.

Information about educational materials and films is available from your local chapter of the American Cancer Society.

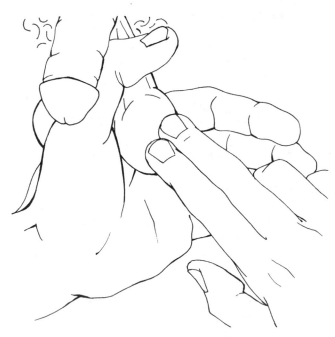

Figure 24.2 *Testicular self-examination.*

Teaching Related to Vaginal Irrigation

Inflammation of the lining of the vagina can result from a wide variety of causes, ranging from simple irritation to a sexually transmitted disease. Regardless of the cause, early symptoms include a vaginal discharge, itching, and often pain. The discharge may be thick or watery, scant or profuse, almost odorless or foul smelling, and white or greenish. The discomfort may be mild or severe, and the itching can be annoying or almost unbearable. It is important for every woman and girl to know that any persistent discharge, pain, or itching should be investigated by a physician. Only the physician can differentiate between a normal, harmless discharge, and the onset of a virulent infection.

Because of the widespread publicity related to sexually transmitted diseases such as herpes, AIDS, and gonorrhea, it is imporant to reassure women that the symptoms of vaginitis do not automatically indicate venereal disease. Young girls who are sexually active are prone to panic over the possibility of a sexually transmitted disease, and postpone or avoid prompt medical attention. They must be taught that vaginitis may be caused by or associated with a disturbance in the pH of the vagina, a yeast or fungus infection, hormonal changes, or an allergic reaction to commercial deodorant sprays and douches.

Vaginal Irrigation

Vaginal irrigations (called douches) are considered necessary for cleanliness by many women, and some believe that a douche can be effective as a contraceptive. Most physicians, however, agree that routine douching not only is unnecessary but may in fact be harmful if the solution used disturbs the normal pH of the vagina, making is suspectible to infection. Douching after in-

tercourse is not an effective contraceptive because sperm may have entered the cervix before the douche could be administered, and too much pressure from a douche may actually force bits of mucus and sperm into the cervix.

The woman who douches routinely in order to feel clean should be taught that daily douches are potentially dangerous except when ordered by her physician for therapeutic reasons. Any douche that removes or alters the pH of normal vaginal secretions renders the vagina susceptible to bacterial, viral, fungus, and yeast infections. Douching for hygienic reasons, in the absence of an abnormal condition, is not necessary; but if a woman does so, douching should be limited in frequency. A warm (never hot) vinegar solution will suffice without disturbing the normal pH of the vagina unduly; 1 or 2 T of white vinegar per quart of water is usually recommended.

Many women who douche for hygienic reasons do so while sitting on the toilet. If, however, the douche is given for therapeutic reasons, the solution may not adequately medicate or remove discharges from all surfaces of the vagina when the woman is in an upright position. Therefore, in the hospital, a douche is usually given on the bedpan or—in the home—with the woman lying in the bathtub.

A douche differs from an enema in that the solution cannot be retained because the vagina has no sphincter. The douche tip or nozzle has multiple openings so the solution sprays against the sides of the vagina as it flows in and out again. Because the vagina is elastic, the douche tip can be rotated without discomfort to wash away a thick or purulent discharge more effectively. The douche container should be held from 1 to 2 ft above the vagina. It is dangerous to hold it higher because the increased pressure could force microorga-

---

PROCEDURE 24.1

*Giving a Vaginal Irrigation**

SUMMARY OF ESSENTIAL NURSING ACTIONS

1. If the vagina is to be irrigated to treat an infection, determine the nature of the infection.
   - If the patient has a sexually transmitted disease, wear gloves.
   - If the patient has diagnosed or suspected gonorrhea, make certain that no solution splashes into your eyes.
2. Position the patient on her back on the bedpan.

3. Lubricate the douche tip with the irrigating solution and insert it 3–4 inches.
4. Hold or hang the container of fluid about 12 inches above the vagina.
5. Rotate the tip back and forth slowly to direct the solution to all sides of the vagina.
6. When all the solution has been used, help the patient to dry her perineal area.
7. Inspect the returned fluid and chart your findings.

*See inside front cover and pages 398–399.

nisms thorugh the cervix; and because the lining of the cervix is continuous with that of the uterus and the open-ended fallopian tubes, microorganisms could eventually infect the abdominal cavity.

Because a douche washes away vaginal secretions and discharges, it should not be administered before a pelvic examination is done unless specifically ordered. The douche would remove specimens needed for examination, thereby depriving the physician of data needed for diagnosis. Douching should not be done for at least 24 h before a Pap test for cancer.

If you give a vaginal irrigation to a patient who has a positive or even a tentative diagnosis of gonorrhea, you must be careful to prevent any of the contaminated solution from splashing into your eyes, which are susceptible to the gonococcus organism. It is also important for you to wear gloves if the patient has a suspected or diagnosed sexually transmitted infection, especially if there is a break in the skin of your hands.

RELATED ACTIVITIES

1. The prevention of teenage pregnancy is a major concern in our society today. The role of sex education is a central issue, with influential groups claiming that it either increases or decreases sexual activity and the probability of pregnancy. Start now to prepare yourself to take an informed and intelligent position, both as a professional and as a citizen, by objectively studying both sides of the question. Read widely and listen to and talk with people of all ages and opinions in order to obtain the data you need for intelligent professional action.

2. Nurses are required by law to report suspected incidents of child abuse, and it is likely that new legislation will soon require the reporting of suspected abuse of elderly people. Familiarize yourself with the phone numbers, process, and legal requirements of the area in which you are now living, and do so each time you move to a different state in the future.

SUGGESTED READINGS

Anderson, Mary Lynn: Talking about sex—with less anxiety. *JPN and Mental Health Services* 1980 June; 18(6):10–15.

Assey, Jane L, and Joan Moore Herbert: Who is the seductive patient? *Am J Nurs* 1983 April; 83(4):531–532.

Baxter, Robert T with Alan Linn: Sex counseling and the SCI patient. *Nursing 78* 1978 Sept; 8(9):46–52.

Brown, Barbara, Barbara Carpio, and Debbie Sue Martin: Wife abuse: an old family problem, a new health problem *Can Nurse* 1982 June; 78(6):23–28.

Carley, Lori: Helping the helpless: The abused child. *Nursing 85* 1985 Nov; 15(11):34–38.

Cohen, Stephen, and Rita RS Gittes: Patient assessment: examination of the male genitalia. *Am J Nurs* 1979 April; 79(4):689–712.

Cohen, Stephen, Joyce E Beebe, and Martina Deyserret: Patient assessment: examination of the female pelvis, Part I. *Am J Nurs* 1978 Oct; 78(10):1717+ (26 pp). Part II *Am J Nurs* 1978 Nov; 78(11):1912+ (28 pp).

Davis, Suzanne Rotz: The breast lumps that *aren't* cancer. *RN* 1983 Aug; 46(8):30–33.

Frank, Ellen Perley: What are nurses doing to help PMS patients? *Am J Nurs* 1986 Feb; 86(2):137–140.

Googe, Mary Catherine Short, and TM Mook: The inflatable penile prosthesis: new developments. *Am J Nurs* 1983 July; 83(7):1044–1047.

Gorline, Lynne L, and Cheryl C Stegbauer. What every nurse should know about vaginitis. *Am J Nurs* 1982 Dec; 82(12):1851–1855.

Greany, Geraldine D: Is she a battered woman? *Am J Nurs* 1984 June; 84(6):725–727.

Griggs, Winona: Sex and the elderly. *Am J Nurs* 1978 Aug; 78(8):1352–1355.

Grimes, David A: Routine circumcision reconsidered. *Am J Nurs* 1980 Jan; 80(1):108–109.

Hanlon, Kathryn: Maintaining sexuality after spinal cord injury. *Nursing 75* 1975 May; 58–62.

Irish, Andrew C: Straight talk about gay patients. *Am J Nurs* 1983 Aug; 83(8):1168–1170.

Koeckeritz, Jane Large: Assessing the genitalia. *RN* 1983 Jan; 46(1):53–59.

Krozy, Ronna: Becoming comfortable with sexual assessment. *Am J Nurs* 1978 June; 78(6):1036–1038.

Lutz, Ronald: Stopping the spread of sexually transmitted diseases. *Nursing 86* 1986 March; 16(3):47–50.

Malinowski, Janet S: Answering a child's questions about sex and a new baby. *Am J Nurs* 1979 Nov; 79(11):1965–1968.

Moore, Karen, Marie Folk-Lighty, and Mary Jane Nolen: The joy of sex after a heart attack: counseling the cardiac patient. *Nursing 84* 1984 April; 14(4):104–113.

Murray, Barbara L, and Linda J Wilcox: Testicular self-examination. *Am J Nurs* 1978 Dec; 78(12):2075–2076.

Pearson, Linda: Climacteric. *Am J Nurs* 1982 July; 82(7):1098–1102.

Poole, Carol Jean: Principles and practice: Neonatal circumcision. *JOGN Nurs* 1979 July/Aug; 8(4):207–210.

Rodgers, Janet A: Women and the fear of being envied. *Nurs Outlook* 1982 June; 30(6):344–347.

Siemens, Sydney, and Rose C Brandzel: *Sexuality*. Philadelphia, Lippincott, 1982.

Stromborg, Marilyn: Screening for early detection. *Am J Nurs* 1981 Sept; 81(9):1652–1657.

Warmbrodt, Lynn: Herpes: The shock, the stigma, the ways you can ease the emotional pain. *RN* 1983 May; 46(5):47–49.

Watts, Rosalyn Jones: Dimensions of sexual health. *Am J Nurs* 1979 Sept; 79(9):1568–1572.

Woods, Nancy Fugate: *Human Sexuality in Health and Illness.* ed.2. St. Louis, Mosby, 1985.

Prevention of sexual abuse of children

Adams, Caren, and Jennifer Fay: *No More Secrets.* San Luis Obispo, CA, Impact Publishers, 1981 (for parents).

Dayee, Frances S: *Private Zone.* New York, Warner Books, 1982 (to be read with children).

Vogel, Carole, and Kathryn Goldner: *The Dangers of Strangers.* Minneapolis, Dillon Press, 1983 (for children).

Wachter, Oralee: *No More Secrets for Me.* Boston, Little, Brown and Company, 1983 (4 short stories for children).

25

Spiritual Needs

Prerequisites and/or Suggested Preparation
Suggested preparation for this chapter includes Chapter 6
(Values) and Chapter 9 (Communication) or their equivalents
from another source.

The nature of the relationship between a person's spirituality and his physical and mental health is not fully understood, but the strength and significance of the relationship has been well documented. Faith and hope have sustained many people during periods of intense physical and psychological suffering, and helping a person to meet his spiritual needs is often one of the most basic and essential nursing interventions.

SPIRITUAL BELIEFS AND RELIGIOUS AFFILIATION

The information which an interviewer obtains about a patient's religion can be misleading unless a distinction is made between *spiritual beliefs* and *religious affiliation.* A patient can be very spiritual even though he states that he does not believe in any religion and belongs to no church or religious organization. Another person may be an active and enthusiastic church member but have little or no interest in spiritual matters.

Some patients do not know that answering questions about their religious preference is optional, and think they must respond to an interviewer. A patient might indicate that he is a Roman Catholic because his parents are, because he was baptized in that faith as an infant, and because he attended a Catholic church as a child. In reality, it may be that he has no *significant* religious affiliation inasmuch as he has not been to church in over 40 years, and his spiritual beliefs may be limited to a few vague concepts from childhood.

A *spiritual belief* refers to belief in a creative force, a higher power, an infinite source of energy, or a divine being. A spiritual belief is based on a person's conviction that there is a power greater than himself that gives order and meaning to life. Some people believe that this power is manifested through nature or supernatural forces; others believe it can appear in human form. A person may believe in one God, or in many gods, which he either fears or worships. Spiritual beliefs may or may not be associated with some form of organized religion.

A *religion* is an organized system of worship. A religion has central beliefs, rituals, and practices that are closely related to birth, marriage, death, and salvation. In some religions the beliefs and practices are complex and sometimes difficult to follow, and there is a rigorous path to membership. In other religions the beliefs and practices may be open to individual interpretation, and membership requirements are less stringent. A small sect may have only a few hundred members; larger religions involve many millions of followers.

There are many reasons, in addition to spiritual ones, for joining a religious group. Some people use their church as an avenue for social action, as an established way to help the poor, the elderly, the hungry, and the homeless. Other people use their church as a source of friends, a place for wholesome recreation, or as a church family when they are separated from their biological families. Still others select their church on the basis of its location, prestige, and membership, as a place to meet the "right" people, and as a place for the important ceremonies of life such as weddings and funerals. Because of the diverse reasons, both spiritual and nonspiritual, why people seek information beyond the name of a patient's religion before she can begin to assess his spiritual needs and beliefs.

Members of a given religious group may agree upon and accept certain beliefs, for example, about the nature of God and the forgiveness of sin, but they may have irreconcilable differences on other points, such as their church's position on birth control, women priests, and homosexuality. There can be a greater difference between the spiritual beliefs of two members of a given church, therefore, than there is between like-minded members of different churches.

Current trends toward an open, questioning approach to all aspects of life encourage the exploration of one's spiritual beliefs. As a result, a patient may be questioning some aspects of his religion just at a time when he desperately wants and needs to rely on that religion for strength and solace as he tries to cope with his illness or suffering. Faith in a higher power or divine being, coupled with a belief that there is a reason or plan for each person's existence, can sustain and support a patient and give meaning to his life. For many patients, their spiritual beliefs and convictions constitute hope, which, though it is elusive and intangible, is often the most critical element of therapy and recovery.

Within the context of nursing, a *spiritual need* is defined as anything which is needed by a patient for him to maintain or increase his faith and fulfill his religious obligations. If, for example, his regular patterns of worship have been disrupted, he will need help in reestablishing a satisfying routine within the hospital or nursing home setting. If his faith has been tested or shattered by recent events, he will need support and understanding as he tries to reconcile his spiritual beliefs with the things that are happening to him. If his illness has created, perhaps for the first time, a growing urge to explore the meaning of pain and suffering and to ponder the eternal question *why,* he may need help in locating and using essential resources.

A patient's spiritual needs are derived both from the requirements or prohibitions of his religion, and from an inner drive to sustain his faith. The former include such things as dietary restrictions, prescribed rituals, or forbidden medical practices; the latter include prayers, celebration of holy days, and visits by spiritual leaders.

ASSESSMENTS

Two types of assessments must be made before a nurse can begin to help a patient meet his spiritual needs. These two areas of assessment are the nurse's own spiritual beliefs, and the nature of the patient's spiritual needs.

Assessment of Nurse's Own Beliefs

An ongoing exploration of the nurse's own spiritual beliefs and attitudes is prerequisite to an assessment of her patient's spiritual needs. Virtually every type of religious affiliation has a strong emotional component that affects a person's relationship with people of other religions as well as with people of the same religion. Your own religious convictions and beliefs will affect your interactions with many patients. In careers such as plumbing, engineering, or music, a person may be able to separate his spiritual beliefs from his work, but such a separation is rarely possible in nursing.

It is true that some nurses, consciously or unconsciously, refuse to become involved in spiritual matters and that others are simply unaware of that aspect of patient care, but in both cases the resulting nursing care is likely to be inadequate and incomplete. The spiritual needs of some patients are as important as their physical needs. For many patients, provision for evening devotions should merit attention equal to that afforded to meals and medications. In fact, if more attention were paid to spiritual needs in some instances, less attention could be paid to medication for problems such as headache, nervousness, and insomnia.

Nurse's Spiritual Beliefs

Any aspects of your religious and spiritual beliefs that are likely to affect your nursing practice should be examined and clarified. Examples of questions to be asked are:

Do you believe that all religions and spiritual beliefs are equally valid, or do you believe that there is only one true religion?

What do you believe about life after death?

How are you likely to respond to a patient or any other person who tries to persuade you or convert you to his way of thinking?

What do you see as the relationships, if any, between sin, punishment, and illness or suffering?

When there is a conflict between religious doctrine and medical practice, which should take preference? Do you believe this to be true for adults, children, or both?

In what ways might it be difficult for you to meet the spiritual needs of a patient whose religious practices are the antithesis of your own, and possibly unacceptable to you?

There are no quick or easy answers to such questions, and your consideration of them at the beginning of your career is just the start of a lifelong endeavor to increase your ability to meet the spiritual needs of your patients.

Assessment of Patient's Spiritual Needs

There are three rules for determining the presence of spiritual needs: (1) make no assumptions; (2) respond to all cues; and (3) respond to your own feelings.

Make No Assumptions About Spiritual Needs

- Do not assume that each person in crisis has a spiritual need.
- Do not assume that an absence of data about religion on a patient's record means that he has no religious affiliation. It may simply mean that he chose not to answer the question.
- Do not assume that a professed atheist or agnostic who is seriously ill does not want, or may not in the future want, spiritual help or guidance. His spiritual needs may change during the course of a long or difficult illness.
- Do not assume that the spiritual needs of a patient have been met just because he has been visited by his rabbi, priest, or minister.
- Do not assume that you can deduce the extent (if any) of a hospitalized patient's interest or involvement in religion solely on the basis of data obtained by the admitting office.
- Do not assume that you can deduce the nature of the patient's spiritual beliefs from the fact that he is an active member of his church or temple. The fact that a patient is of the Jewish religion and participates regularly in temple activities does not indicate whether he considers himself to be a Reform, Conservative, or Orthodox Jew, for example.

Respond to All Cues

NONVERBAL CUES. Examples of nonverbal cues include:

- Devotional materials such as a Bible, pamphlets, and books
- Religious articles such as a rosary, a crucifix, a statue, or an icon

- Visits from a priest, rabbi, or minister
- Posture or position of prayer

The nurse's response to nonverbal cues can be a simple interested comment, a sincere question, or any other sensitive acknowledgement. The *kind* of response is less important than the *act* of a response. When you fail to acknowledge the presence of visible objects or physical positions, your message is: "I choose to ignore these objects or indications of a religious concern."

VERBAL CUES. A patient's verbal cues may include direct questions, indirect inquiries, casual comments, and even hints. These verbal cues are likely to be related to religion, suffering, guilt, fate, dying, and life after death. Examples of such cues are:

"Is there a chaplain here? What's he like?"

"Were you ever taking care of a person when he died?"

"What do you think of all the recent articles about life after death?"

"Do you go to church?"

Many of these questions require a brief, specific, and sometimes factual answer, but as with other areas of professional communication, the underlying message is far more important than the actual words. When a patient asks, "Do you go to church?" he may not be very interested in whether you go to church; he wants to know whether or not it is okay to talk to you about religion. As in all therapeutic communication, it will take considerable skill and concentration to answer such questions briefly and then proceed to discover and respond to the underlying message.

Respond to Your Own Feelings

If your intuition makes you feel that your patient has unmet spiritual needs, you should validate that feeling with him, even in the absence of overt cues of any sort. The approach you use depends on your comfort in raising the subject, but the approach must be clear enough to be understood by the patient. Examples of clear, direct invitations to discuss religion include:

"We have a very nice chaplain here at the hospital. I usually ask my patients if they would like him to stop by and visit."

"I can't explain why, but I somehow feel that you are concerned about religion. Would you like to talk about it?"

The patient may indicate that you are wrong (and he may do so emphatically!), or he may refuse to respond at all, but he will know that the spiritual and religious aspects of his life are of concern to you insofar as they affect his health and well-being and that you are willing to discuss spiritual matters with him if he so desires.

PREPARATION OF THE NURSE

It is neither necessary nor feasible to attempt to learn the details of even the major religions of the world in order to be prepared to meet the spiritual needs of patients. Of course, the nurse should know the basic concepts of the religions she is most likely to encounter in her professional practice, but it is more important to focus attention on the *patient and his perception of his spiritual needs* than on the details of his specific religious affiliation. You need to know the relationships between spiritual beliefs, religious obligations, and health care in general and the meanings these have for a specific patient. In short, you must understand the role of religion in the prevention and treatment of illness.

One of the best ways to acquire such understanding is not by reading or by talking with members of the clergy, but by discussing religion with patients whenever it is appropriate. You will find that many people are willing to share their ideas and beliefs with you when you ask a question like "I don't know very much about your religion. Would you tell me how it helps you when you are sick?" There is no better way to learn, for example, how a Jehovah's Witness who is scheduled for surgery feels about the conflict between his church and the medical profession over the use of blood transfusions during surgery than to ask him directly. Some patients will have had minimal experience in verbalizing their beliefs; others will be very articulate and knowledgeable. Regardless of their ability to express themselves, most patients are willing to explain their religious views and to share their beliefs or disbeliefs with you.

If you are an atheist or an agnostic, or if religion is not important in your life at the moment, the enthusiasm of a devout patient may make you uncomfortable. If so, it might be advisable to acknowledge this discomfort to the patient while continuing to work to meet his spiritual needs.

If you belong to an evangelical religion, you will have to reconcile your zeal and enthusiasm with the need for restraint in professional situations. It is appropriate for you to respond to a *patient's request* for information about your religion; but it is not appropriate for you to try to persuade, convince, convert, or evangelize the patient, no matter how serious his condition or how much you believe he needs it. It may be difficult for you to refrain from such activities; but *you are the patient's nurse,* not his spiritual advisor. Your task is to meet his spiritual needs *as he perceives them,* regardless of how you view his spiritual status.

NURSING RESPONSIBILITIES FOR SPIRITUAL NEEDS

A patient's faith can sustain and support him during difficult times and give meaning to his illness and suffering. The meaning a patient attributes to his condition may be "It's fate"; "That's life"; "It's God's punishment"; "It's a test of my faith"; or any of a number of other beliefs. Such meanings affect the patient's response to his illness or condition. Some beliefs seem counterproductive and seem to work against the efforts of nursing and medicine. If, for example, a patient believes that all humankind is basically evil, that sickness is God's punishment, and therefore that sickness is inevitable, he may feel powerless and thus display little or no interest in trying to prevent illness. It may seem futile to him. If a patient believes that the course or outcome of an illness is determined by fate and that "whatever will be, will be," then decisions related to treatment may have little significance for him.

Although some beliefs may seem to hinder or impede nursing intervention and medical practice, other beliefs, such as the power of prayer and the existence of miracles, are a source of hope, courage, and strength for the patient. Such beliefs enhance the efforts of nursing and medicine and are in many instances an integral part of therapy.

The meaning and significance of a patient's faith in many instances cannot be determined by direct questions. Meaning is assessed through sensitive discussions of matters which concern the patient at the moment. A patient's spiritual life is usually personal and private, and he is not likely to disclose and discuss it until he feels he is in a psychologically comfortable setting with a like-minded and trusted person.

Such conditions are present in some *long-term* health care settings but may be absent in an acute care setting. Large numbers of staff are in contact with the patient each day, but each one may spend relatively short periods of time with him. When the staff seems rushed or primarily task oriented, a patient may find it difficult to initiate or participate in a discussion of spiritual matters.

A patient's spiritual needs are a bit more likely to be met if the agency has a religious affiliation or if the patient has a primary nurse, but in most settings, spiritual needs will not be met until they are granted an *importance equal to that accorded other needs,* such as hy-

giene, nutrition, and exercise. In an acute care center, where nurse-patient contact is often brief or transitory, the nurse must assign a high priority to spiritual needs if they are to be met even at a minimal level. A deliberate and conscious effort will be needed to assess and meet any spiritual needs that are found to exist.

Some nurses are reluctant at first to become involved in the spiritual and religious aspects of a patient's life. Possible reasons include prejudice against people of another religion, stereotyping, and preconceived notions. Some nurses worry about the expectations of the patient's clergy, or fear involvement in an unknown ritual or sacrament.

For some nurses, an even greater concern is that their nursing interventions will somehow cause them to be untrue or false to their own religion. Helping a patient to meet his spiritual needs is *not* the same as practicing that patient's religion. For example, responding to a request from a nearly blind patient to read a letter from his brother who is a Communist party leader does not affect a nurse's patriotism and loyalty to her country, nor does reading, as *a nursing intervention,* a passage from a book that is sacred to the patient in any way indicate that the nurse is practicing that religion or that she is unfaithful to her own religion. Reading to a patient, praying for him, or assisting the clergy merely indicates that, within her professional role, the nurse is helping her patient to meet a basic spiritual need which he is at the moment unable to meet without assistance.

Any conflict, real or potential, between the demands of your profession and your religion can often be resolved by talking with your own clergy or a hospital chaplain. If, however, you should find that you are psychologically, morally, or spiritually unable to do whatever a patient asks of you with respect to his spiritual needs, *you must find another person to help him.* It is poor nursing practice to leave an identified, health-related spiritual need unmet just because you are personally unable to make the necessary interventions.

Types of Nursing Responsibilities

There are seven major nursing responsibilities that help to meet a patient's spiritual needs:

1. Determining the existence and nature of a spiritual need.
2. Helping the patient fulfill his religious obligations.
3. Helping the patient sustain his faith.
4. Supporting the patient when his faith or beliefs are challenged.

5. Considering the impact of religious affiliation on decision making.
6. Including members of the clergy* in health care planning.
7. Developing an open-minded, nonjudgmental attitude toward nonmedical modes of healing.

Determining the Existence and Nature of a Spiritual Need

Once you have reason to believe that a patient will need help in meeting his spiritual needs or religious obligations, you will need considerable skill and sensitivity to assess the *nature* and *meaning* of his needs. It is very easy to misinterpret his behavior and responses. For example, a patient who is comforted by familiar Bible passages, prayers, and hymns may be responding less to the actual words and messages than to the feelings the passages evoke. They may bring back memories of happier days when he felt secure and well cared for. His present interest in a family passage such as the Twenty-third Psalm may be as closely related to his safety and security needs as to his spiritual needs. Although both needs are significant, it is important to know which one might be predominant. Therefore, as you work with your patient, try to understand the meaning various activities have for him.

Such understanding may come slowly because the patient may find his situation painful or too sensitive to discuss. One patient, who lived alone, seemed torn between a desire to talk with a clergyman about her serious medical problem and a tendency to avoid any discussion of religion. Little by little, as the days passed, she disclosed that she had been asked to move out of her daughter's home when the daughter and her husband joined a pentecostal, fundamentalist sect. The patient was considered evil because she watched television and read wordly magazines like *Good Housekeeping*. She was not permitted to see her grandchildren unless the parents were present. The hurt was too deep to permit a quick and open discussion of the problem; but with the support of her nurse, she slowly regained some of her self-esteem, was able to put the situation into perspective, and was able to find solace and comfort in her own faith through discussions with her clergyman.

TWELVE-STEP PROGRAMS. You may have patients who are members of various twelve-step programs, such as Al-

coholics Anonymous (AA) and Overeaters Anonymous (OA), which are spiritual in nature but not affiliated with any religion. Members of these groups have admitted that they are unable to control their compulsive behavior and that their lives have become unmanageable, and hence each member acknowledges a dependence on a higher power—which may be God, the support of the group, or whatever other source of power he may choose. Each member has come to realize that his health, sanity, or very life depends on being sober or abstinent for the rest of his life and that this can only be managed one day at a time with the constant help of his higher power.

Members of OA and AA rely heavily on daily reading for support and strength. The Serenity Prayer is used by both groups and may be repeated many, many times a day, whenever the compulsion to eat or drink becomes obsessive. An alcoholic or compulsive overeater knows that he has a disease that can never be cured, only controlled, and that a single drink or illegal bite will trigger a prolonged binge of weeks or months of drinking or overeating. A member of AA will, therefore, refuse any medication that contains alcohol, such as tincture of paregoric and certain cough medicines. An active member of OA who is tempted to eat between meals will make every effort to contact another OA member by phone. The need to make such as phone call is as much of a spiritual need as reading the Bible, because the OA member has surrendered himself to the higher power of God or the group and his very life may depend on the maintenance of his abstinence.

Other Twelve-Step Programs are springing up across the country in response to the needs of child or spouse abusers, drug addicts, gamblers, compulsive spenders, and other people tormented by compulsive behavior. These programs are based on the principles of anonymity, reliance on a higher power, group support, and a commitment to help others who are still suffering.

NEED FOR VERIFICATION OF SPIRITUAL NEEDS. The spiritual needs of a patient may be closely or remotely related to his present condition, and *he may or may not need help to satisfy those needs.* The behavior demonstrated by the patient and the kind of assistance sought can be easily misinterpreted, and it is therefore important for you to *validate your perception* of the situation with the patient, even though you may be unable, at the moment, to comprehend the scope, significance, or intensity of the situation. You should contact the patient's clergyman, the hospital chaplain, or the clergyman on call *only as requested or agreed to by the patient,* however. Do not take it upon yourself to call a clergyman simply because you presume that such contact is needed or would be helpful.

---

*For the remainder of this chapter, the term *clergy* is used to denote priests, rabbis, deacons, ministes, elders, and all other spiritual advisors inclusively. The term *member of the clergy* or *clergyman* refers to a spiritual advisor, regardless of sex, race, or creed.

Helping the Patient Fulfill His Religious Obligations

Religious obligations that must be met are commonly connected with rituals, sacraments, and ceremonies related to certain milestones of life, such as birth, marriage, and death. These obligations are usually fulfilled by interactions between the patient and his clergyman, and nursing interventions are designed to facilitate that process.

ASSISTING A MEMBER OF THE CLERGY. To prepare the patient and his environment for a clergyman's visit, the patient should be clean, well groomed, attractively attired, and physically comfortable. His unit should be neat and esthetically acceptable. It should reflect the atmosphere that would prevail if the visit were taking place in the living room or parlor of the patient's home. Remove any dead flowers, discard soiled dressings, and empty the emesis basin, urinal, and commode or bedpan as needed. Make sure the bed is neat and tidy and that there is an empty chair at the bedside for the clergyman's use.

To ensure privacy, you may have to reschedule or delay treatments and medications to avoid interrupting the visit. Whenever possible, you should also determine the purpose of the visit in case additional preparation of the patient or unit may be needed. If the priest is to hear the patient's confession, for instance, additional privacy is needed and could be provided by asking an ambulatory roommate and his visitors to sit in the lounge for a few minutes or by taking the patient to an empty room or secluded corner somewhere. Finally, before the clergyman's arrival, ask the patient whether everything is in readiness for the visit and if not, do whatever is possible to make things ready.

Greeting each clergyman as he enters the ward, whether he is there to visit your patient or someone else, is a gracious gesture because he may or may not be familiar with the hospital. If you have never before had an opportunity to talk with the spiritual leader of a religion other than you own, you may feel a bit uneasy at first, but it is neither awesome nor difficult to talk with a priest, rabbi, or other member of the clergy. The nurse could simply say, "I'm Miss Smith; may I help you?" to which the clergyman might respond, "I'm Father Duncan and I'm looking for Mr. Jones in room 317." If it seems advisable, escort him to the patient's unit and ask if there is anything he needs. If the patient is to receive Holy Communion, for example, the clergyman may have brought the necessary articles with him, or he may have planned to use the communion box which is available in most hospitals.

You may need to assist the clergyman. If you know, or discover, that someone will be needed to hold or support a feeble patient, you should offer your assistance or find someone else to do so. If a patient vomits frequently, is likely to faint, or is crying with pain, you should not leave the clergyman alone to cope with the situation unless he verbally indicates that he is capable and willing to do so.

You may feel inept or uneasy in assisting a clergyman of a religion other than you own, but your role, *as a nurse*, is to facilitate the interaction between the patient and his clergyman; it is not your role to enter into that interaction. Your task is to support and care for the patient in such a way that it is physically and psychologically possible for the planned religious activity to take place.

You can also help by arranging for the patient to attend religious services as he wishes and is able. Many hospitals have chapel services at intervals during the week to which patients can be taken by wheelchair or stretcher. In addition, it is often possible to secure a pass for a patient to *leave the hospital* long enough to attend a religious service, especially on an important holy day. Such passes are usually not routine, and therefore the first one may involve considerable negotiation among patient, family, physician, and nursing staff. Depending on the complexity of the necessary arrangements, preparations should be started well in advance of the occasion.

DIETARY OBLIGATIONS. Helping the patient fulfill the dietary obligations of his religion is another nursing responsibility. Although many religions exempt a sick person from rigorous dietary restrictions, a patient may feel uneasy about modifying any long-standing dietary patterns. If he is willing to accept such modifications but is uncertain about their validity, specific verbal assurance by his clergyman may be needed. If, however, a patient wants to maintain his traditional dietary patterns, he should be graciously helped to do so.

Most hospitals are able to provide kosher food for their Orthodox Jewish patients and are able to meet the basic requirements of other religions. Ask your patient, upon admission, if he has any dietary restrictions related to his religion. If these obligations seem to be more rigorous or extensive than usual, arrange for a conference between the patient and the hospital dietitian as quickly as possible.

NEEDS RELATED TO DEATH. Arranging for appropriate care of the body after death is also a nursing responsibility. *Before* an anticipated death, ask the patient or his family if there are religious practices that need to be followed at the time of death regarding sacraments, rituals, and the physical care of the body. Any specific details should be noted on the Kardex for the information of all staff.

In the event of a sudden or unexpected death, you will have to talk with the family as soon as they are able to do so or with an appropriate clergyman about the care of the body.

If the religious and cultural practices of a deceased patient's family involve overt manifestations of grief, such as wailing, moaning, and chanting, it may be necessary to minimize the impact of such responses on other patients. You may be able to move roommates from the room temporarily and close the door, or you may need to take the body and the grieving family to a private place for a short while. It is important for relatives to grieve in their own way, but it is also important to protect other patients from activities and sounds that are easily misinterpreted and therefore distressing or frightening.

Helping the Patient Sustain His Faith

A person's faith must be sustained and nourished, especially under difficult or desperate circumstances. Unless a patient's faith is periodically restored and renewed, it may not be strong enough to support him when he needs it most. There are at least five ways to help a patient manage the devotional practices that will sustain his faith.

FACILITATE PRAYER AND MEDITATION. This can be done by ensuring the privacy that is needed and desired by the patient. If the medical and nursing staff on the ward tend to ignore drawn curtains and closed doors, hang a "No Admittance" sign at the entrance to the patient's unit for a brief period each morning and night. (Be sure to remove it promptly each time or the staff will soon ignore it.) Try to ensure a reasonable degree of quiet and to help the patient to schedule his devotions in accordance with his treatments, medication, and other required activities.

PROTECT RELIGIOUS OBJECTS FROM LOSS OR DAMAGE. Place each statue, icon, or picture in a safe place and tape it in place if necessary. Check all used linen before it is sent to the laundry to prevent the loss of a rosary, crucifix, medal, or other small object. It is helpful, too, to teach the patient that the safety of such objects is a joint responsibility and to help him assume partial responsibility for their protection.

FACILITATE GRACE BEFORE MEALS. A patient who is able to feed himself can delay his eating long enough to say grace if he wants to do so, but the patient who must be fed may not have a chance to say grace in the brief interval between the time when his tray is placed in front of him and the first forkful of food is placed in his mouth. Therefore, before you start to feed a patient,

ask him if he normally says grace before meals and, if so, allow a moment or so for either a silent or a spoken grace. If the patient is aphasic or confused, the nurse may need to say grace. For this reason, a nurse should learn a grace which is commonly used by each of the major religions or a universal one.

When a child is admitted to the hospital, ask him or his parents what table grace, if any, is used at home. If the saying of grace is significant to the child and his parents, place a copy of the grace on the child's chart, in the Kardex, and at his bedside so that it can be said each mealtime. The saying of the family grace can be a significant tie to home and normalcy, but the child may need support in doing so in a strange environment.

READ TO THE PATIENT UPON REQUEST. The patient may ask for a reading from his daily devotional material, from the Bible, or from another sacred book. There will usually be time to honor this request because many commonly used daily devotional materials and familiar passages, such as the Twenty-third Psalm, can be read aloud, thoughtfully and effectively, in 3 or 4 minutes. If you are frequently unable to read to your patient, be sure to find someone who can.

PRAY WITH OR FOR THE PATIENT. If a patient asks you to pray for him, you can do so in a variety of ways. You can offer a silent prayer, read a prayer the patient has chosen, or recite one of your own favorite prayers. You can also offer a brief extemporaneous prayer, such as: "Dear God, please be with Mr. Jones. Help him when his dressings are changed today, and give him strength to face the uncertainties of tomorrow. Amen."

If the patient's religion is quite different from yours and you are uneasy about the differences, you can mention these feelings to your patient and offer to pray for him in your own fashion. Your intent and willingness to pray are more significant to most patients than your choice of words or the format of the prayer.

Supporting the Patient When His Faith or Beliefs Are Challenged

A patient's religious affiliation often influences certain aspects of his medical therapy, and this in turn can influence his treatment by the staff. Jehovah's Witnesses, for example, oppose the use of blood and will refuse blood transfusions during surgery or following an accident. Such a refusal will elicit a wide range of responses from the staff, ranging from ridicule or hostility through amazement and disbelief to complete support and understanding. These responses are in part determined by the patient's self-confidence and the strength of his convictions.

Two women, both Jehovah's Witnesses, happened to be admitted on the same day to the gynecological unit of a relatively small hospital. Each woman was scheduled for a hysterectomy, which usually involves the transfusion of at least 1 unit of whole blood. One woman told a nurse that she did not want a transfusion during surgery and refused to sign that portion of the operative permit. Because of the nurse's inadequate understanding and lack of sensitivity, the patient was quickly described (and labeled) as peculiar and a bit strange. The other patient was obviously familiar with the workings of a hospital and, upon admission, presented the head nurse with a paper, prepared by her lawyer, that described her position on use of blood. The patient's advance preparation, self-confidence, and legal support elicited a positive response from most of the staff.

Members of the Church of Christ, Scientist (Christian Scientists) believe that sickness and sin are faults of the mind. They believe that healing is a religious function, and the church has its own healers and sanitariums. Drugs and blood are not used; biopsies and extensive physical examinations are not done. A person may seek medical help for childbirth and fractures, but drugs are not used. Vaccinations are permitted when required by law. A devout Christian Scientist may live a long, healthy, and happy life and experience no significant conflict between his religious beliefs and current medical practice. Occasionally, however, an event occurs that could challenge his faith and his beliefs.

One such situation is that of a female Christian Scientist with advanced cancer of the breast. Because surgical intervention was not permitted, the cancer had destroyed the entire breast, exposing portions of the underlying muscle and bone. The patient probably entered the hospital either to learn a more effective way to care for the wounds or for help in clearing up the infection that is inevitable with such an extensive wound. Whatever the reason for her admission, such a hospitalization is difficult for both the patient and her family, but it is more tolerable when the staff is supportive, accepting, and nonjudgmental. It is *unprofessional and inexcusable* for any nurse or physician to criticize or blame the patient for her present condition. A "you brought it on yourself" attitude, whether expressed or merely implied, adds to the patient's psychological pain and suffering. She may already be tormented by doubts because her faith was not strong enough to avert the destruction of her body. Her family may be questioning the necessity of such suffering from a disease that can be cured through early detection and treatment.

Your task when caring for such a patient is to be supportive but nonjudgmental. You cannot tell her, "You did exactly the right thing. You were true to your re-ligion and God will take care of you"; nor can you imply or tell her that she was foolish to refuse medical treatment. You can best help to meet her spiritual needs by granting her *unconditional acceptance* by encouraging her and her family to discuss their spiritual concerns with each other and with their spiritual leader, and by helping her to sustain and possibly strengthen her faith in any way possible. Regardless of your own beliefs and feelings, *in a professional role* you must do everything in your power to enrich the quality of such a patient's spiritual life; *a nurse must never knowingly depreciate, weaken, or undermine the patient's faith.*

In some situations you will be confronted by conflicts between religion and medicine at a much earlier phase of the conflict. Even so, there are no easy answers to questions and dilemmas such as:

Who will provide medical care for a patient who refuses traditional therapy?

How can we reconcile the rights of parents and the rights of children when the parents, on religious grounds, will not permit a child to be treated in accordance with accepted medical practice?

How and by whom is a situation resolved when the patient's spiritual beliefs collide with various aspects of medical or nursing intervention?

You will be torn between a desire to see the patient benefit from current medical therapy and a desire to help the patient retain his faith and spiritual beliefs. Much soul-searching must take place before a nurse is able fully to attend to the needs and best interest of the patient.

Considering the Impact of Religion on Decision Making

Many significant decisions about health, illness, and death are influenced by the religious affiliation of the patient and his family. Decisions related to the following areas of concern are likely to be based on religious teaching and cultural norms:

- Prolongation of life by extraordinary means
- Care of the body after death
- Cremation
- Autopsy
- Donation of body parts (organ transplantation)
- Care of body tissue or an amputated limb
- Birth control
- Abortion
- Euthanasia
- Use of nontraditional or unproven therapies

Because any given medical activity is likely to be permitted by some religions and forbidden by others, it is important to know how a person's religious affiliation might affect the decisions he must make. Great sensitivity and skill may be needed to discern whether a certain course of action is freely chosen by the patient and family or whether it is prescribed by their religion. If a mutually acceptable decision cannot be reached because of religious requirements or spiritual beliefs, an alternative course of action or compromise will need to be arranged, with input from patient, family, physician, nurse, and spiritual advisor.

Including Members of the Clergy in Health Care Planning

In addition to traditional and expected activities such as the administration of sacraments, performance of rituals, and comfort of the dying and bereaved, members of the clergy can contribute in many other areas. A patient's clergyman may be able to:

- Help the patient and family accept a difficult diagnosis or poor prognosis
- Interpret explanations and instructions, especially when there are emotional, spiritual, language, or cultural barriers
- Act as a liaison between the patient and his family, the staff, the congregation, and the neighborhood
- Help locate resources, especially in rural areas, for problems related to such things as food, housing, and transportation

For a clergyman to help a patient and his family, he must be considered a member of the health care team, and he should on occasion be asked to participate in team conferences. The *clergyman cannot help unless he understands* the patient's diagnosis, present condition, planned therapy, and prognosis. Members of the staff should not give specific information about a patient to every member of the clergy who happens to ask, but with the permission of the patient and family, or at their request, the clergyman should be given the information he needs to function effectively. Young and inexperienced clergy may need to be reminded of the *confidential* nature of such information inasmuch as it will be of interest to other members of the parish or congregation who are likely to ask him about the patient.

Developing an Open-minded Attitude Toward Nonmedical Modes of Healing

The spiritual faith of many patients is a source of hope and strength as they undergo medical diagnosis and treatment. For them, medical and spiritual interventions are balanced and harmonious; they complement each other. Other patients who seem devoid of faith in higher power entrust their lives exclusively to the medical profession. A third group of patients turn, for one reason or another, from medical therapy to some form of spiritual healing.

A few of the many reasons for actively seeking a spiritual cure are:

The despair and frustration that occur when medicine is unable to effect a cure or give relief. Spiritual healing may be viewed, even by nonspiritual people, as a last resort when all else has failed.

Curiosity about a public invitation by a healer in the local newspaper.

The inspiration, teaching, or experience of a personal acquaintance.

A few faith healers may capitalize on the desperation of sick people to acquire money, prestige, or power; but many others are sensitive, gifted people endowed with an ability to use an unexplainable source of spiritual power for healing purposes.

Some patients have been healed by the ministrations of a single person. Others have been healed through the intercession of groups who have conducted lengthy prayer vigils. Some churches maintain an ongoing healing ministry as part of the work of the church. There are numerous organizations, such as Guideposts Magazine, in which the staff meet at a regular time each week to pray for those who have written or phoned to request such intercession and help. Many nurses are learning and using a technique, advanced by Dr. Dolores Kreiger, RN, called *therapeutic touch* that promotes healing and relieves pain and discomfort.

Some physicians reject the possibility of spiritual healing. They claim that instances of supposed healing are in reality instances of a mistaken diagnosis, a predictable remission of the disease, or a cure from an unexpected interaction between a combination of treatments. Other physicians and nurses will acknowledge that an unexplainable cure has taken place, and some believe that miracles can and do occur.

Some cures occur spontaneously and suddenly, often without any conscious awareness or searching by the patient. Other cures may be somewhat less dramatic. They are the culmination of months or years of work by dedicated people but are, in a way, no less miraculous. The person who discovers a new drug or develops a new surgical technique may have been inspired or given the courage and patience to persist by a spiritual power. The successful reattachment of a severed limb, the ability to see again through donated corneas, and the birth of a healthy baby conceived outside the mother's body—each of these is a miracle for the person involved.

Science can neither prove nor disprove the process of spiritual healing. You may be involved in related controversies over the years as it becomes increasingly apparent that medical science, in and of itself, is incapable of ensuring the health of humanity. Whenever a patient is attempting to meet his needs through some form of spiritual healing, there are several ways a nurse can help:

- By keeping an open mind. You cannot help your patient explore such issues if your mind is already made up and you are convinced that spiritual healing cannot or does not exist.
- By supporting the patient in his quest for healing. The patient has a right to rely on medical therapy, spiritual healing, or a combination of the two. You can serve as a liaison or intermediary among patient, family, clergyman, and members of the health care team.
- By helping the patient obtain the information needed to make informed decisions. Encourage him to obtain as much accurate data as possible. He should explore the possible consequences of any decision to decrease or discontinue medical treatment, using such questions as: If this surgery is not done, what is likely to happen? If chemotherapy is discontinued, what is the probable outcome?
- By supporting the patient and his family as each decision is made, regardless of whether you approve of the decision. Your input is appropriate during the decision-making process, but a nurse has no right to attempt to impose her opinions on the patient or his family. You may believe, for example, that a proposed trip to Lourdes in search of a cure is an irresponsible and unwarranted expense for a family on a limited budget. Once the decision to make the pilgrimage has been made, however, your task may be to help them plan how to minimize the risks for the patient and the stress of all concerned.

RITUALS, SACRAMENTS, AND PRACTICES

It is beyond the scope of this book to describe the details of each religion that are relevant to health and illness. A reference on major religions is included in the bibliography, and each nurse is professionally responsible for acquiring basic information about the religious groups found in her community.

Christian Sacraments

Baptism

Baptism is an initiatory rite of Christian churches. It is deemed necessary by the majority of Christian denominations, although there is considerable variance in the meaning ascribed to it and in the format of the rituals. For example, some churches sprinkle water on the head of an infant; others practice total immersion of an adult.

A valid baptism requires the use of water and the prescribed Trinitarian invocation, and can be performed by any person who is trying to do what the church requires. A newborn Catholic infant in danger of death must be baptized at once; if a priest is not available, a physician or nurse should baptize the infant. To do so, all that is necessary is to pour a small amount of water on the baby's head while saying, "I baptize you in the name of the Father, and of the Son, and of the Holy Spirit." A record of the baptism should be included in the baby's chart, and the family or priest should be informed that the baby was baptized. Catholics believe that an infant has a soul from the moment of conception, and therefore a fetus should be baptized unless it is obviously dead as evidenced by the presence of necrotic tissue.

The Eucharist

The Eucharist (also called Holy Communion or the Lord's Supper) is a central rite of Christian worship. It is a memorial activity that calls to mind the nature, life, and teachings of Jesus Christ and is based on his mandate at the Last Supper: "Do this in remembrance of me." The worshipper receives a bit of consecrated bread and wine or grape juice, or a thin wafer (the Host), which are called the elements of the Eucharist. These elements represent the body and blood of Jesus Christ. The Eucharist is celebrated in most Christian churches, but the frequency, nature, and distribution of the elements, the eligibility of worshippers, and the theological concepts vary greatly from denomination to denomination.

If a Protestant or Catholic patient is to receive Holy Communion, the nurse should ask what preparations, if any, are needed. Some religious groups require the worshipper to have fasted for several hours, although medication may be taken as needed. Some clergymen carry small communion sets that contain everything needed. Other prefer to use a communion set supplied by the hospital. It does not contain the elements but does include items such as a fresh white cloth for the bedside stand, a candle, a spoon, and a small glass.

The Eucharist provides an interesting example of the reciprocal relationship between spiritual matters and health care. Health care is sometimes modified to meet the patient's spiritual needs, but at other times, certain religious practices are modified because of health problems. During the early 1900s, for example, the area around Saranac Lake, New York, was a veritable mecca for patients with tuberculosis who had moved there to "take the cure." At that time, especially in rural Protestant churches, Holy Communion was celebrated with a large chalice, or common cup of wine. Tubercular worshipers sat at the rear of the church and, after drinking from the cup, carefully wiped the rim with a handkerchief before passing it to the next person. The public health problem of controlling the spread of the disease was minimized when the churches began to use individual cups instead of a common cup for the wine, and within a few decades, pasteurization and antibiotics had nearly eliminated the threat of tuberculosis. During the 1960s and 1970s, some Christian churches began to return to simpler forms of worship, including the breaking of a common loaf of bread and the use of a common chalice of wine for special worship services. Unfortunately, however, the symbolic simplicity of this sacrament has now been threatened, if not destroyed, by the discovery during the mid 1980s that AIDS might be spread by human saliva, and once again, the existence of a relationship between religion and health has been made manifest.

Anointing of the Sick

Prior to the changes instituted by the second Vatican Council in 1963, the Catholic sacrament of anointing of the sick was administered to a person only when death was imminent. The dying person was *in extremis,* and the sacrament was called *extreme unction* and was one of the last rites of the church for that person. The possibility of death is still the basis for this sacrament, but death need not be an immediate concern. The anointing of the sick is considered to be a source of strength or healing as well as a preparation for death. A person can be anointed whenever it seems possible that he might die from sickness or from old age, and he can be anointed more than once.

The anointing of the sick is sometimes preceded by confession and Holy Communion if the patient is dying. During the sacrament, the priest anoints several areas of the body with oil. An unconscious patient may be anointed if there is reason to believe that he would have desired the sacrament were he conscious. There is no comparable sacrament in general use in Protestant religions. Because the anointing of the sick (extreme unction or last rites) has been associated with imminent death for hundreds of years, many older Catholics still respond to this sacrament with fear or dread. The patient and family alike often think: "It must be pretty bad—they've called the priest to give me (or him) the Last Rites!" Before the administration of this sacrament, either the nurse or the priest may need to interpret its current use and meaning and thereby minimize unwarranted apprehension.

Jewish Obligations and Activities

Circumcision

Circumcision is practiced less often today than it was formerly. The circumcision of a *non-Jewish* infant is usually done a day or two after birth, before he leaves the hospital. The circumcision of a Jewish infant is done on the eighth day after his birth in a religious ceremony. If the baby is ill, the ceremony can be postponed. Occasionally, a formal, religious circumcision will be done on a hospitalized infant, and the nurse may need to make arrangements for the use of a private room and to facilitate arrangements between the rabbi, the family, the pediatrician, and nursing service.

Observance of the Sabbath

The Jewish Sabbath extends from sundown Friday to sundown Saturday. Orthodox Jews believe in strict observance of the Sabbath day and may refuse surgery and tests as well as other activities that require work by anyone on the Sabbath, such as eating freshly cooked food, being pushed in a wheelchair, or using the telephone. Certain holy days are strictly observed by many Jews and the manner in which a patient observes the Sabbath and the holy days should be assessed soon after admission.

Diet

The dietary practices of a Jewish patient depend on whether he is a Reform, Conservative, or Orthodox Jew. Most Jews do not eat pork or shellfish. The kosher diet of an Orthodox Jew uses meat that has been specially slaughtered, and follows prescribed guidelines for the preparation and use of meat and dairy products. A person can be excused from strict dietary restrictions when ill, and a conference between the patient, his rabbi, the dietitian, and the nurse may be beneficial in clarifying and resolving some of the complex issues involved. The dietary departments of many hospitals are well prepared to meet the needs of the Jewish patient who chooses to adhere to a kosher diet throughout his hospitalization.

PATIENT EDUCATION

Patient education related to spiritual needs is directed toward making sure that the patient knows that the quality of his nursing and medical care cannot be affected by his religious beliefs. The patient is not obligated to state his religious preference upon admission, and care may not be denied because of religious beliefs. Effective nursing care takes the patient's spiritual needs into account, but the ANA Code is specific in stating that nursing care is determined solely by human need, *irrespective* of national, ethnic, religious, cultural, political, or economic differences.

RELATED ACTIVITIES

1. If you have not already done so, visit a variety of churches and temples within the next few years so that you can more fully appreciate the vast differences in religious settings and backgrounds which can influence the spiritual needs of your patients. Try to visit a large cathedral, a small rural church, a non-Christian house of worship, and several different ethnic services. Note the similarities and differences in the use of symbols, rituals, music, and body language.

2. Regardless of the nature and intensity of your current belief system, begin to deveop a *noncritical, nonjudgmental* approach to the spiritual beliefs of your patients and their families. Learn to *listen* rather than talk, to *keep your opinions to yourself* even though you disagree, and to *think* carefully about what is being said. If this process is difficult because of your own strong convictions, practice for short periods of time until you can converse with a patient about his spiritual needs in a professional therapeutic manner.

SUGGESTED READINGS

Barry, Martha M: Dilemmas in Practice: ''The life of every creature''—a case of patients' rights. (Jehovah's Witnesses) *Am J Nurs* 1982 Sept; 82(9):1440–1442.

Damstugt, Don: Pastoral roles in presurgical visits. *Am J Nurs* 1975 Aug; 75(8):1336.

Dickinson, Sr. Corita: The search for spiritual meaning. *Am J Nurs* 1975 Oct; 75(1):1789–1794.

Fish, Sharon, and Judith Allen Shelly: Spiritual care: The nurse's role. Downer's Grove, IL, Inter-Varsity Press, 1978.

Heller, David: The children's God. *Psych Today* 1985 Dec; 19(12):22–27.

Highfield, Martha Farrar, and Carolyn Cason: Spiritual needs of patients: Are they recognized? *Cancer Nurs* 1983 March; 6(3):187.

Krieger, Dolores: *Foundations for Holistic Health Practices: The Renaisance Nurse.* Philadelphia, Lippincott, 1981.

Lawrence, Linda (PT Conversation with James Fowler): Stages of faith. *Psych Today* 1983 Nov; 17(11):56–62.

Pumphrey, John B: Recognizing your patient's spiritual needs. *Nursing 77* 1977 Dec; 7(12):64–70.

Ryan, Juanita: The neglected crisis (spiritual). *Am J Nurs* 1984 Oct; 84(10):1257–1258.

Stoll, Ruth I: Guidlines for spiritual assessment. *Am J Nurs* 1979 Sept; 79(9):1575–1577.

Part Six

Nursing Interventions for Physical Care and Comfort

26

Safety and Protection

Prerequisites and/or Suggested Preparation
There are no prerequisites for this chapter and no suggested preparation.

Safety is a shared responsibility. Each person, as soon as he is old enough to understand the concept of danger, must begin to assume some responsibility for his own safety. Small children must learn to protect themselves from sharp objects, poisoning, strangers, and fire, while teenagers must assume responsibility for coping with hazardous sports, drugs, and automobile or motorcycle accidents.

Neighborhood groups and various government agencies often set policies and oversee programs related to safety, but each citizen must assume his share of responsibility for safe streets, clean air and water, pure food, adequate fire protection, and safe working conditions. People with special training or in positions of power may have responsibility fo writing and enforcing laws and policies related to safety but in general, no one can "make" or "keep" another person safe.

People can protect themselves, however, only against those hazards of which they are aware. Public information and patient education form the basis for an adequate awareness of safety hazards. This information ranges from the warning on cigarette packages to children's programs on sexual abuse to guidelines for use in the event of a nuclear accident.

In some situations, a person or group of persons may be incapable of recognizing or responding to a threat of danger, and a more capable person must assume that responsibility, at least temporarily. Individuals who cannot protect themselves include persons who are very young, mentally retarded, comatose, senile, paralyzed, confused, or ill, as well as those who must live in a hazardous environment.

A nurse has a dual set of responsibilities. One set is shared with her neighbors and friends as a concerned citizen and the other set is unique because of her profession. A nurse can sometimes differentiate between her professional and personal responsibilities by determining whether she is involved in a given situation because she is a nurse, or because she is a citizen, a parent, a taxpayer, or a church member, for example. In most social situations, a nurse need be no more safety conscious than her fellow citizens; but in any life-threatening situation *of which she is aware* she is morally, and sometimes legally, obliged to do what she can to avert or minimize the danger.

An experienced nurse develops a "sixth sense" that enables her to be aware of hazards in the immediate environment even though she is participating in the situation as a spectator, guest, or in another capacity. A nurse seems to be always on guard, alert, and attentive, often without realizing it. Some of her observations may require no action at the moment but may, for example, prompt her to make a few strategic phone calls the following day. Other observations, such as seeing unattended children teasing a snarling dog in the park, would warrant immediate action.

A major goal of nursing is the prevention of illness and injury which includes protection from hazards and threats to safety. The scope and range of nursing interventions for safety are almost limitless. They range from the duties of a summer camp nurse to those of an industrial nurse in a steel mill, and from the interventions needed in a day nursery to those needed in a refugee center or intensive care unit.

In many aspects of nursing, patient safety is an overriding concern. It matters little how well-planned or efficient a procedure is if the safety of the patient is jeopardized. In many schools and institutions, an otherwise well-done procedure is rated unsatisfactory if the patient was unsafe at any time.

In nursing, the term safety includes both physical and psychological safety. A holistic approach to health requires a unified approach to body, mind, and spirit and all three must be safe if health is to be attained. The range of potential threats to an individual's safety is almost limitless, though only those hazards related to the *physical environment* are included in this chapter. Other hazards discussed in other chapters are: psychological trauma, physical abuse, surgical complications, infection, use of oxygen, back injury, drug misuse, eating disorders, immobility, electricity.

ENVIRONMENTAL SAFETY

The topic of environmental hazards is exceedingly complex because, in addition to universal hazards, such as toxic wastes, there are objects and activities that are safe for one person but not for another. This difference is determined in part by the person's *understanding and awareness* of potential danger, and in part by his *ability to cope* with the consequences. Many objects or activities must therefore be considered *neutral* until they are *viewed in a given context*. For example, a refrigerator on display in the window of an appliance shop is not a source of danger; an abandoned refrigerator poses little if any threat to an intelligent, rational adult. That same abandoned refrigerator, however, can cause death by suffocation to children playing inside it. It is appropriate, therefore, to focus on the *identification of potentially dangerous situations* rather than on specific objects or activities which might or might not be dangerous.

Individuals can learn to increase their awareness of hazards, and deliberate efforts should be made to encourage them to do so. They should be taught not only to recognize the threats of a given situation, but to generalize that knowledge to a wide variety of similar situations.

FALLS

Falls area leading cause of accidental injury and death, especially among the very young, the very old, and those who are weak and ill. The factors which contribute to falls are either personal or environmental. *Personal* factors are usually related to age, development, and physical condition. It is possible to compensate for deficits in these areas once they have been identified (see boxed material). *Environmental* factors which can contribute to falls include the floor, stairs, furniture, and equipment. Guidelines for reducing hazards from these sources are offered by a variety of insurance companies and health-related agencies.

One basic safety rule is this: *If a person is going to do it anyway, teach him to do it safely.* Therefore, if a child is a climber, teach him to manage heights safely. Give him some guidelines, such as "Make sure one foot is steady before you move the next one." Demonstrate to the little child how to do an activity safely. A creeping baby can come down stairs safely feet first on his hands and knees. A baby just learning to walk cannot walk down stairs, but he can learn to sit down on the top stair and come down one step at a time, using his buttocks and feet. Such a safety skill is important if there are no gates to keep him off the stairs, and is useful if a baby is too heavy for his caretaker to carry easily. This rule is valid for individuals of all ages, and for a large variety of activities, ranging from climbing trees or working on a roof to the use of matches or a sharp knife. If a feeble or elderly person persists in an activity which is potentially unsafe, help him discover a modification which will enable him to do it safely. Positive reinforcement and practice will be necessary to insure these kinds of safe behavior, regardless of the age of the individual or the type of activity.

Personal Factors Related to Falls

Baby
Falls in infancy are often caused by the caregiver's lack of awareness of a new motor skill. This may be evidenced by statements such as: "I didn't think he could roll over yet," or "I didn't know he could creep up those stairs."

Child
A child is often unaware of his own limitations. He may have no concept of danger and little fear of failing. Some children seem to be born climbers; they start climbing as young as 8 or 9 months of age and progress from chairs and tables to cupboard, refrigerators, porch rails, fences, and trees.

Aged Person
Some of the personal circumstances that contribute to an elderly person's falling arc (1) changes in balance, (2) poor eyesight, and (3) unsuitable clothing.

One reason for *poor balance* is that the elderly person's center of gravity gradually shifts forward. It is closer to the front of his base of support because his head and neck are held forward, his shoulders and back may be curved forward, and his entire torso may be tilted forward if there is any marked flexion of his hips. If he starts to lose his balance, he may be unable to regain it without assistance.

A person with poor balance can often maintain his mobility and independence with a tripod cane or a four-point cane. This type of cane is safer than a standard cane because it gives more support and because it stands in position ready for use it does not fall out of the person's reach. When a cane no longer gives adequate support, a walker will be needed.

Poor eyesight may keep a person from seeing small objects on the floor ahead of him. Night-lights should be used liberally throughout the home or hospital. A flashlight that is always at his bedside gives considerable comfort to many an elderly person. Living areas should be well-lighted both day and evening.

Unsuitable clothing such as loose dangling robes, floppy slippers, ill-fitting shoes or untied shoe laces increase the likelihood of falling. Clothing for the elderly person should be selected carefully, and altered as necessary for safety. If an individual can no longer reach down to tie his shoes, for example, he should be encouraged to switch to a loafer type of shoe rather than to loose slippers. Pants and robes should be shortened as needed. It may be necessary to shorten a long robe or gown as much as 2 or 3 inches across the front if a person leans forward very much.

Person Who Is Ill or Weak

A person may fall because of his physical condition or because of inadequate preparation for ambulation.

Physical Condition. A patient may fall for a variety of reasons such as weakness, hypotension, the effects of a new medication, dizziness, an electrolyte imbalance, fear, fatigue, or pain. A careful assessment will be needed to diagnose and treat the underlying condition, but it is of utmost importance that the nurse *take the patient at his word* if he feels at a given moment that he is about to fall. If a patient says, "I've got to sit down" or "I can't make it to the end of the hall," the nurse should help him back to bed or into the closest chair. If a patient has warned a nurse that he is incapable of doing what she has asked, *she could be held liable* if he fell and injured himself because she insisted that he complete a prescribed activity. The nurse's notes should describe the patient's condition and reactions in detail, and the nurse should report her inability to carry out the prescribed nursing or medical action.

Patients often feel weak or faint in the bathroom, therefore safety bars or grab rails should be installed over the tub, in the shower, and near the toilet (Fig. 26.1). In isolated or sound-resistant rooms, a push but-

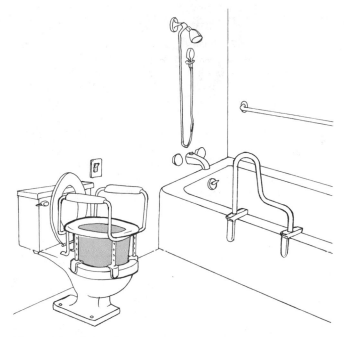

Figure 26.1 *Safety bars and grab rails. Note that the toilet seat is elevated for the safety of a person who cannot rise from a low seat.*

ton that will summon help should be accessible, clearly marked, and plainly visible at all times.

INADEQUATE PREPARATION FOR AMBULATION. After a period of immobility, a patient may fall because of the absence of an adequate progam of exercises to strengthen specific muscle groups which are needed for ambulation. Other falls are the result of inadequate teaching about the proper use of equipment such as crutches, a walker, or an artificial leg. Such preparation and teaching may be time consuming and difficult if the patient is fearful, confused, or disoriented; yet it is essential for the patient's safety. A patient on crutches who must go up and down stairs at home or work, for example, cannot be discharged safely until he has demonstrated his ability to use his crutches effectively in a variety of stair-climbing situations. The preparation for ambulation is described in detail in Chapter 27.

Environmental Factors that Affect Falls

The floor, the stairs, furniture, and equipment are environmental factors that affect falls. Most hazards in the average household or health care agency are easily removed or corrected if the persons involved are observant and concerned.

Floors

- Use nonslip wax whenever possible. If waxed floors are unavoidable, apply strips of nonslip material (such as that used on bathtubs) to the soles of shoes of an elderly or weak person.

- Avoid using scatter rugs. If they must be used, apply antislip rug tape or antislip powder to the back of each rug.
- Wipe up spilled liquids or food at once. In a hospital or other institution, wipe up the spilled substance yourself unless you can make provision for that area to be blocked off until the spill can be wiped up by housekeeping or maintenance personnel.
- Teach the patient and his family that newspapers and magazines are very slippery and to keep them off the floor.
- Teach children to keep toys out of the pathway of elderly persons.
- Position appliance cords and extension cords to prevent tripping.

Stairs

- Keep stairways well lighted.
- Install hand rails on at least one side, but preferably on both sides, of all stairways, open or enclosed.
- Use gates at top or bottom of stairs as needed to remind people who are weak or unsteady to seek assistance.
- Teach families to keep *all objects* off the stairs. A useful rule is: *Nothing but people on the stairs.* Place

a shelf or basket at both top and bottom to provide a routine place to put things to be carried up or down.

Furniture and Equipment

- Lock the wheels or casters of a wheelchair, bed, or stretcher when the patient is getting in or out.
- Replace the rubber tips on crutches, canes, and walkers when the tips become hard and smooth.
- Install an adequate number of grab rails next to the toilet, and the tub or shower.
- Place a nonslip mat in each tub or shower.
- Keep the hospital bed in *low position* when you are not giving care to the patient.
- Use side rails on the bed as indicated to insure patient safety.

Special Safety Measures

Side Rails

It is a mistake to assume that side rails will protect a patient from falling. Many adult patients view side rails as confining, punitive, or degrading. Some patients who feel this way will conform and passively accept the use of side rails, but others will resist their use in every way. Many patients have fallen as they climbed over the side rails or over the foot of the bed; it is questionable whether side rails should be used with a person who resists their use (Fig. 26.2). Side rails can *remind* an alert but weak patient not to get out of bed without

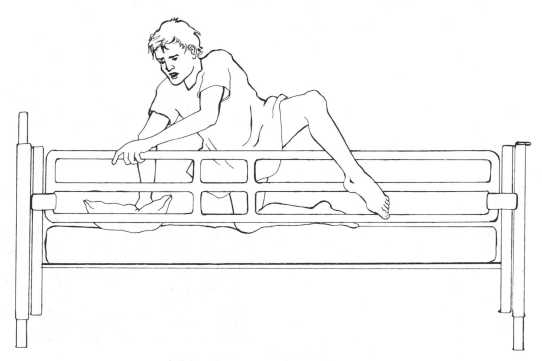

Figure 26.2 *An accident in progress.*

assistance and can keep a restless patient from rolling out of bed, but *side rails will not keep a patient in bed if he is determined to get out.*

Side rails contribute to patient safety when they:

- Remind the patient that the bed is narrow and often high
- Keep a semiconscious, restless, or confused patient from rolling off the edge of the bed
- Provide a support for a patient lying close to the edge during a treatment or while the bed is being made
- Serve as a grab rail for a weak patient to pull against to help turn himself and change his position

If hospital policy dictates the use of side rails for a given patient or if side rails have been ordered for that patient, they *must be used* for that patient even though the nurse's professional judgment deems their use unnecessary or unwise. A nurse who fails to follow established policy or fails to carry out a written order for side rails will be judged negligent. On the other hand, a nurse can be held responsible if a patient is injured because she *failed to inform* the appropriate people of the patient's negative reaction to the use of side rails.

A carefully detailed description of the patient's verbal and nonverbal reaction should be recorded in his chart and should be reported to the appropriate nursing and medical personnel. The reporting should be done immediately and if the nurse suspects that the patient might try to climb out, thereby injuring himself by falling or by dislodging vital monitors, drainage tubing, IV's, or other equipment.

Restraints

In this text, the word restraint refers to a device that limits a patient's *physical activity.* Social restraints and environmental restraints, such as quiet rooms or seclusion rooms, are used in psychiatric settings and are not discussed here.

A patient who must be restrained is often confused, disoriented, delirious, or otherwise unable to assume appropriate and necessary responsibility for his own safety and therapy. The purpose of a restraint is usually:

- To keep a patient from falling out of bed or from sliding out of his chair
- To protect a patient from his own actions, such as pulling out his IV or oxygen tubing, removing a dressing, or disconnecting a monitor
- To protect others from any aggressive or violent actions of the patient

The extent of the physical restriction caused by a restraint depends on the type of restraint used, which may be wrist, ankle, elbow, waist, jacket, or even a full-sheet restraint (Figs. 26.3 and 26.4).

LEGAL ASPECTS. Very few conscious patients are willing to be restrained. It is humiliating, demeaning, a loss of personal freedom, and at times an infringement of civil liberty. Any unwarranted use of restraints can be interpreted by the patient or his family as a form of imprisonment or involuntary confinement. The unwarranted use of restraints can be a basis for legal action. Any use of restraints, therefore, must be well justified on the basis of the *patient's safety and well-being* or the *safety of others.*

One of the most significant nursing responsibilities for the use of restraints is the *written description of the patient behavior* that necessitated the use of restraints and the alternatives that were tried. This documentation must show that restraints were indeed necessary to insure the patient's safety or the safety of others, so that there can be no basis for a claim that restraints were applied for the convenience of the nursing staff.

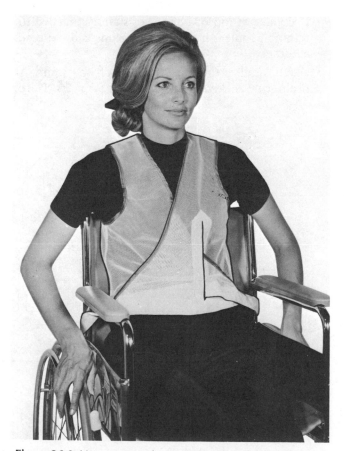

Figure 26.3 *Vest restraint for patient who may slide forward. (Courtesy of J. T. Posey Company, Arcadia, CA)*

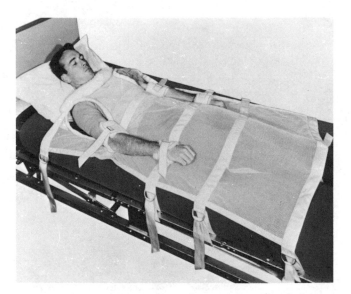

Figure 26.4 *A restraint net provides complete immobilization. It is sometimes needed in psychiatric settings, drug treatment centers, or emergency rooms. Note the padded straps and padding at the neck and shoulders. (Courtesy of J. T. Posey Company, Acardia, CA)*

The possible dangers and negative effects of restraints are so great that the need for their use must be *unquestionable*. In some institutions, the use of restraints is a nursing decision; in others, a physician's order is needed. It is important to understand agency policy and its relationship to state and local law as well as to the relevant nurse practice acts.

NURSING RESPONSIBILITIES. There are five major areas of nursing responsibility for the use of restraints: (1) assessment, (2) support of patient and family, (3) selection and application, (4) prevention of complications, and (5) charting.

Assessment

A careful assessment must be made of the need for and continued use of restraints. Because irrational or inappropriate behavior can be caused by a wide variety of things—fear, a new medication, pain, delirium from

---

Characteristics of an Acceptable Restraint

- Safe for the patient on whom it is applied.
- Strong enough to restrain the patient effectively.
- Constructed and applied so that it does not damage the skin and underlying tissue.
- Provides necessary control *without undue restriction*.
- Possible to release quickly in case of an emergency.

---

a high temperature—a patient should NOT be restrained solely on the basis of his overt behavior. The *cause* of the behavior should be identified or at least hypothesized, and alternative interventions tried before restraints are applied. For example, a frightened, delirious patient might not need restraints if some member of his family was always at his bedside. In some situations frequent reminders by an attentive paid sitter would avert dangerous behavior and be more acceptable to patient and family than the use of restraints. A change in medications will often alleviate the need for restraining a patient.

In addition to the initial assessments, an ongoing assessment is necessary to discover when the use of restraints can be *safely discontinued*. These assessments also provide the data for refuting any charges of unwarranted or unethical use of restraints.

Support of Patient and Family

The use of restraints is usually upsetting to both the patient and family, so a full explanation must be given when the restraints are first applied and repeated as often as necessary. A positive approach that describes the desired outcome is important, and each explanation should emphasize the fact that the patient is not restrained because of "bad" behavior. The use of restraints should not be viewed as a punitive action but as an action that will promote the patient's therapy and safety. This message must be conveyed by each nurse on every shift, both verbally and nonverbally, because the use of restraints can be devastating to a patient's self-esteem.

Because it is often impossible to evaluate the comprehension of an agitated, delirious, or confused patient, it is especially important that explanations be given frequently in the hope that the patient may hear and understand them. Such messages of empathy and caring are absolutely essential.

Selection and Application of Restraints

The restraint selected should provide essential safety with the least possible restriction (Figs. 26.5 and 26.6). Some patients need and welcome a gentle reminder to avoid a certain action, and the restraint can be applied with their full consent. Other patients will resist, and the restraint must be applied in such a way that injury will not result (Figs. 26.7 and 26.8).

The restraint must allow the patient to turn toward one side or the other. It is not safe to restrain a person in a spread-eagle position, flat on his back; he must be able to *turn his head and shoulders* to the side to prevent aspiration if he should vomit. If a patient is nauseated,

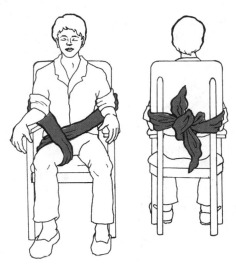

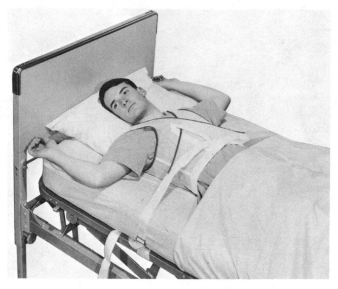

Figure 26.5 *Improvised restraint. A folded sheet around the patient's leg prevents him from sliding from the chair but does not restrict his chest expansion. (See also Fig. 26.6 below.)*

Figure 26.7 *The safety vest may be worn with the slot positioned in front for maximum security or in back for maximum movement. (Courtesy of J. T. Posey Company, Arcadia, CA)*

agitated, or completely restrained, check his condition every 15 minutes.

Wrist restraints may be used without ankle restraints just to remind the patient not to loosen a dressing or disturb an IV, for example, but *ankle restraints can never be used alone* for two reasons: (1) the patient can reach and release the ankle restraints if his hands are free; (2) he might forget about the ankle restraints, attempt to get out of bed, fall, and be caught up by the ankle restraints. For the same reasons, do not use restraints on only one side of the body.

If you are unsure about the safety of a restraint or a combination of restraints for a given patient, test them on another person, directing him to duplicate the patient's situation and see if he gets tangled up or if he can get out of the restraints.

When a patient is restrained to keep him from sliding out of his chair, make sure that the chair is comfortable and that it fits the patient (Chapter 29). Add

pillows and pads as needed because a restrained person is not able to change position and make himself comfortable.

Prevention of Complications

All the hazards of prolonged immobility are accentuated with a restrained patient, and all the precautions related to immobility must be observed (Chapter 29). Specific complications of extended or improper use of restraints include sensory deprivation, impaired circulation, joint stiffness, and injury to the skin.

Whenever a person in bed is restrained, it is important to provide as much sensory stimulation as possible to compensate for the decreased physical activity and decreased tactile stimulation. Whenever possible, raise the head of the bed at intervals during the day so that

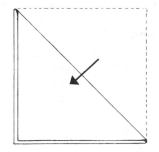
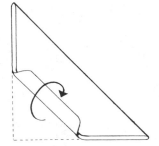
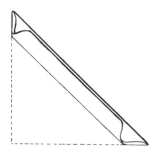

Figure 26.6 *A sheet is folded on the bias, as shown, to give some elasticity to an improvised restraint.*

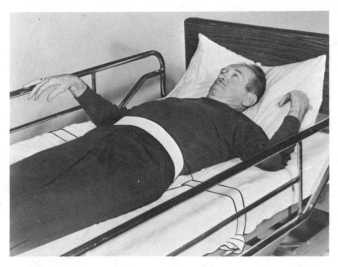

Figure 26.8 The safety belt is a gentle but effective reminder to the patient not to get out of bed. Patient may roll from side to side without restriction. (Courtesy of J. T. Posey Company, Arcadia, CA)

the restrained patient can look around and maintain or regain his orientation.

Check the patient's hands and feet every 1 to 2 hours for signs of impaired circulation such as cyanosis (blueness), pallor, or cold skin. Routinely check the tightness of each restraint. You should be able to insert a finger under a restraint that is tight enough to restrain but loose enough to insure adequate circulation to the hand or foot. Ask the patient about any discomfort, pain, or tingling sensations.

Use padding under wrist and ankle restraints to prevent irritation of the skin. Foam rubber over fabric is effective, but foam rubber should not be placed directly against the skin because it can cause sweating and maceration. Materials like absorbent cotton are not advisable because they tend to mat down and offer less protection than sheepskin or foam rubber.

General Guidelines for the Use of Restraints

- Reposition the patient's call bell as needed so that he can reach it while he is restrained.
- Fasten the straps of the restraint to the bed frame, NOT to the side rails. The tension on the straps would vary when the side rails were raised or lowered.
- Fasten the restraint in such a way that it can be released quickly. Example—tie it with a bow (where the patient cannot reach it) rather than a knot.
- Make the straps of wrist and ankle restraints slack enough to permit slight flexion of the knees and elbows, and to permit some movement of the extremities.

When using mitt restraints on a patient who is unlikely to flex, extend, and separate his fingers within the mitt, wrap his fingers with gauze to separate the adjacent skin surfaces and prevent sweating, irritation, and excoriation.

When wrist and ankle restraints are used, release each extremity and put it through its full range or motion at least every 3 or 4 hours. This must be done every 1 to 2 hours if the patient is elderly or arthritic, or has any other condition in which joints are likely to stiffen up quickly. While each restraint is off, check the condition of the skin. Apply lotion as needed and report any redness or irritation.

Permit and encourage the patient to do as much for himself as possible while each restraint is off. Some of his normal activities can and should be substituted for range-of-motion exercises. Even a confused patient, for example, is likely to be able to wash his face, with encouragement, when handed a washcloth. Such meaningful activity has *more psychological benefit* than range-of-motion exercises done by the nurse, and the *physiological* effect is at least equal. A patient might be able to brush his teeth, finish his bath, or even feed himself with help and supervision while his restraints are loosened.

It is important to *evaluate the patient's likely response* before releasing his restraints for exercise and skin care. If a patient seems agitated or unmanageable, the nurse should release only one arm or leg at a time, and should obtain assistance before removing a waist or jacket restraint to give back care. If, on the other hand, a patient seems relaxed and calmed by your presence, it may be feasible to release all restraints while you are at the bedside. It is important to remember, however, that *you are responsible* for the outcome whenever you remove restraints while there is still a valid order for their use.

Charting
Because of the inherent dangers of restraints and the ethical and legal implications of faulty or improper use, charting must be complete, explicit, and accurate. Each time the nurse cares for a restrained patient, she should chart the kind of restraints being used; the times at which they were removed and reapplied; the condition of the patient's skin, circulation, and range of motion; the patient's reaction to restraints; his behavior while they were off; and the intervals at which his condition was checked.

EQUIPMENT FAILURES

It is not so long ago that compresses, dressings, irrigating sets, and thermometers constituted the equipment needed for most nursing care. Now, many nurses are expected to use a wide variety of complex equipment, such as cardiac monitors, computers, and dialysis machines, in settings such as recovery rooms, intensive care units, and premature nurseries. If you choose to accept employment in such a setting, two basic assumptions should underlie your employment and subsequent practice:

Assumption 1. Before you use any piece of equipment, you will know how it works and how to operate it.

Assumption 2. When using any piece of equipment, you will know when it is *not working properly.*

Knowing How Equipment Works and How to Work It

Many of the machines in use in a hospital are vital to therapy and recovery; some are essential to life itself. Unless a technician is nearby at all times, you must understand the inner workings of each machine that you use—what the components are and how they work. The explanations required need not be complex. A few sentences will indicate whether the equipment contains a pump, gears, levers, valves, or whatever and whether it runs on centrifugal force, gravity, hydraulic pressure, or some other force.

Simple but complete printed operating instructions should be attached to every piece of equipment or be posted in a conspicuous place nearby. It is not enough to be told, "First you press this button, and then you turn that switch. If it doesn't seem to register, jiggle this knob until you can see the level of the fluid in this float." You can and should *refuse to assume responsibility* for the use of any machine about which there is inadequate information. Even when delegating the use of equipment to someone else, you must know how it works and what it is supposed to accomplish.

Knowing When Equipment Is Not Working Properly

Sometimes, reading gauges and checking equipment is as important a part of patient assessment as observing the patient himself. In fact, information on certain aspects of his condition can be obtained *only* from the gauges and monitors. Check each gauge and indicator for which you are responsible frequently enough to be able to detect any change in its operation. On one gauge, for example, if the needle is *not* moving or fluctuating, the gauge is broken. Another gauge or indicator may

be broken if the needle *is* moving. If the gauges are operating properly, any change in the readings indicates a change in the patient's condition.

Differences in such things as sound, rate of fluid flow, amount of drainage, and patient response can indicate a malfunctioning piece of equipment and should be checked at once. "I didn't notice" or "I didn't know what it was supposed to be doing" are inadequate excuses for jeopardizing a patient's therapy or his life.

You are responsible, in part, for seeing that the equipment you are using is properly maintained. Report such things as frayed cords, unusual sounds, weak tubing, variable pressures, or anything else that seems unsafe; then, *follow up on your report.* If an unsafe condition is not remedied, report it again and make sure that your action is noted, with the date, in the patient's chart so that you cannot be accused of ignorance of an unsafe condition.

Special problems are created whenever there is a power failure. All institutions have auxiliary power systems that light the corridors, stairways, operating rooms, and critical care areas. This permits staff to move about freely and life-saving activities to continue. Individual patient rooms may be without power for a time, however, and a top priority must be given to reassuring concerned and frightened patients. When you start work on a new unit, ask how the emergency power system operates and be sure you know how to operate any equipment that would have to be operated manually until full electrical power is restored.

A patient who is to be discharged from the hospital with a portable respirator, a home dialysis machine, or other essential equipment must know whom to call for repairs, whom to call in the event of a power failure, and what to do until the equipment is working again. In some areas the local power company will make special arrangements with people who are dependent on an uninterrupted supply of power.

POISONING

Poisoning is preventable. That is the message you must convey to the parents and grandparents of small children as you work with them in hospital, clinic, or home.

Assessment

Each family situation is different from others, and at least four pertinent assessments must be made before any effective teaching can be done. The areas to be assessed are (1) the attitude and understanding of the adults, (2) the habits and routines of the family, (3) the current storage of potential poisons, and (4) the characteristics of the child.

Attitude and Understanding of the Adults

Some parents have only a vague and limited understanding of the problem of accidental poisoning, and they may or may not be interested in learning about it. Some adults are knowledgeable, but for one reason or another are not motivated to make any changes in their own households.

Habits and Routines of the Family

The hazards of accidental poisoning are much greater in a family in which all manner of substances are left lying around than they are in a family that replaces every item after it has been used. A household in which small children are never left unattended is safer than a household in which children are unsupervised for long periods while the parents nap or watch television (see Table 26.1).

Current Storage of Potential Poisons

An assessment of current storage of potential poisons will indicate whether such things as cleaning supplies, insecticides, rat poison, and paint thinner are stored in secure, high cabinets or left on open shelves. In some homes the problem of safe storage is difficult to solve because there may be no safe storage areas in that house or apartment. It takes imagination and ingenuity to help a family child-proof a crowded household in which cabinets and closets are virtually nonexistent.

Characteristics of the Child

An assessment of each child will place him somewhere along a continuum between the child who is listless or noncurious, and the child who has "been into everything since he learned to creep."

Parents who have *purposely encouraged* curiosity, independence, and exploration by their toddler must be taught, or reminded, that these very attributes could lead to death by poisoning. Table 26.2 lists common plants that could tempt a toddler or young child to "investigate" by tasting. They must now lock up or move to a high place all substances that should not be touched or tasted, and must be vigilant when visiting,

TABLE 26.1 POISONING ACCORDING TO AGE AND PLACE

Age Group	Percent
Children under 5	72.4
Children 5 and over	12.6
Adults	15.0
Total	100.0
Place	
Kitchen	41.0
Bathroom	21.0
Bedroom	12.0
All other places	26.0
Total	100.0

Source: Central New York Poison Control Center, 1985.

TABLE 26.2 COMMON POISONOUS PLANTS

Type/Examples	Poisonous Parts
Houseplants	
Caladium	All
Diffenbachla (dumbcane)	All
English ivy	All
Philodendron	All
Poinsettia	Leaves, stem, sap
Garden Plants	
Castor bean	Bean, if chewed
Daffodil, jonquil	Bulb
Foxglove (digitalis)	Leaves, seeds, flowers
Hyacinth	Bulb
Larkspur (delphinium)	All, especially seeds
Lily of the valley	All
Narcissus	Bulb
Fruits/Vegetables	
Apple	Seeds
Apricot	Pit, leaves, stem
Mushroom	Some wild varieties
Potato	All but tuber
Rhubarb	Leaves
Ornamental Plants	
Azalea	All
Jessamine (jasmine)	All
Mountain laurel	All
Oleander	Leaves, stems, flower
Rhododendron	All
Field Plants	
Hemlock	All
Jimsonweed (thorn apple)	All
Trees/Shrubs/Vines	
Elderberry	Leaves, shoots, bark, root
Holly	Berries
Mistletoe	All, especially berries
Wisteria	All, especially pods and seeds

especially in homes inhabited by adults only. The grandparents' home, for example, may be dangerous if they are in the habit of leaving medicine and other hazardous items around.

Prevention

Families with small children should be taught to follow the guidelines listed below, plus any others that meet their special situations.

- Store only edible substances on lower shelves.
- Move nonedible items to high shelves or lock them up. Special child-proof temporary locks for cupboard doors are available in most hardware stores.
- Do not store *nonedible* liquids or solids in food containers such as milk cartons, peanut butter jars, or soft-drink bottles.
- Keep all medicine in a safe place (with child-proof caps whenever possible).
- As soon as a child is able to learn, start teaching him to differentiate between food and those things that must *never* be eaten or even tasted. Mr. Yuk and other warning stickers for children are available at many clinics and poison control centers and can be placed on containers of substances such as bleach, kerosene, and solvent (Fig. 26.9).

Table 26.3 shows the relationship between developmental level and the potential for poisoning.

Figure 26.9 *Mr. Yuk, the poison warning symbol of the National Poison Center Network, Children's Hospital of Pittsburgh.*

TABLE 26.3 POISONING RELATED TO DEVELOPMENTAL LEVEL

Age 0–5

Major cause of death in age group

< 1 year old: second highest incidence of poisoning; usually victim of mistake by parent or practitioner

2 year old: highest incidence of poisoning; often given by older sibling

Preschooler: can get to substances believed to be in safe places

> 4 year old: group experiences with poison common

Types of poison: pharmaceuticals, bleach, perfumes, lavatory cleaners, dishwashing products, plants

Age 6–12

Poisoning seldom accidental, sometimes suicide

Types of poison: medicines, gasoline, paint

Age 13–20

Poisoning commonly associated with suicide attempt or accidental overdose of experimental drug

Types of poison: drugs, alcohol, gasoline

Age over 20

Accidental inhalatin or ingestion as suicide attempt

Types of poison: gaseous products of bleach and ammonia combined drugs, ammonia, bleach, alcohol, lavatory cleaners

Treatment

The phone number of the nearest poison control center should be posted conspicuously near the telephone. Everyone in the family who is *old enough to use the phone* should know how to report a poisoning. Since uncertainty or confusion could result in a fatal delay of treatment, a poisoning drill in which members of the family practice ways to get help can be just as important as a fire drill.

If vomiting is recommended, it can be induced with a drug called *syrup of ipecac.* It is available without a prescription in all drugstores, and every family should have a small bottle of it on hand. The usual dose is 15 to 30 ml (1 to 2 T) depending on the age and size of the victim. It should be followed by at least 100 ml (½ cup), but preferably 2 or 3 cups, of water or other liquid. This is necessary to make sure that the victim vomits rather than merely retching if the stomach is empty except for the poison. Another 15 ml of ipecac can be given in 20 min if vomiting has not occurred.

If syrup of ipecac is not available, vomiting can be induced by pressing a blunt object against the back of

---

Guidelines for Reporting a Poisoning

- Make sure the phone number of the nearest poison control center is readily available.
- Give the following information:

    Name and age of victim

    Address

    Phone number

    Name or type of substance ingested (if known)

    Symptoms if any are apparent.
- LISTEN carefully for instructions.
- If you do not understand the instructions, *say so*. Caller should indicate his age if he is a child.

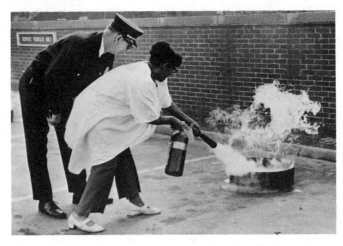

Figure 26.10 *A fireman supervises a nurse in the proper use of a small fire extinguisher.*

the victim's throat until he gags and vomits. Warm salt water will sometimes induce vomiting.

Vomiting should *not* be induced if a corrosive substance, such as an acid or a strong alkali has been swallowed. The esophagus will have been badly burned when the poison was swallowed and the act of vomiting will cause the damaged tissue to be burned again as the corrosive substance passes through the esophagus and mouth a second time. The corrosive substance must be neutralized at once as advised by the poison control center, and other emergency measures must be taken as soon as possible. As a rule, a lavage tube should not be passed to remove the contents of the stomach because of the danger of perforating the burned esophagus.

Vomiting should *not* be induced if the patient is unconscious or semiconscious or if his gag reflex is not present because there is danger that he might aspirate (inhale) the vomitus and poison into his lungs.

FIRE

Each situation involving a fire is distinctive, and a nurse's actions are influenced by the location, extent, and type of fire. Fire drills should be held at regular intervals, especially in an institution in which there are a large number of helpless or immobilized patients. You are responsible for knowing the exact location of exits, the location and operation of fire extinguishers, and the code used to inform the staff that there is a fire (Fig. 26.10). When you join an agency staff, check the procedure manual to determine the specific policies and course of action.

Families should know how to protect themselves from fire, and it is important for the community health nurse to encourage the use of smoke detectors and regular fire drills. Families should know how to cope with smoke—up to 80 percent of all deaths from household fires are caused by the inhalation of smoke and toxic fumes.

The bedrooms of invalids and young children should be identified with decals which can be obtained from the fire department. When searching in a smoke-filled house, firemen or other persons without a mask are likely to be crouching or crawling, so decals on bedroom doors should be relatively close to the floor.

Children should be taught to keep low, move toward the window for rescue, and *never hide* in a closet or under the bed. They should know that a fireman in full gear (face mask, protective suit, back pack with air tank) will look scary, especially at night, but they must *not* hide.

Although matches should be kept out of the reach of small children, an older child should be taught how

---

What to Do in Case of Fire

- If no one is in immediate danger, call the fire department.
- If a door is hot near the top (heat rises), don't open it.
- If there is smoke, creep along the floor for better breathing.
- If it is not safe to leave the room, stuff bedding (wet if possible), along the bottm of the door to keep smoke out.
- Cover your mouth and nose with wet cloths if possible.
- Move toward the window to await rescue.
- Report to prearranged meeting place outside the home.
- Never reenter a burning building.

What to Do If Clothing Catches Fire

- STOP! DROP! ROLL!
- Immerse burned area in *cold* water, or hold under running cold water. *Never* apply grease, butter, or ointment.
- Cover burns loosely with sterile or clean fabric, and transport victim to nearest medical care.

---

to handle matches safely. He can be given safe outlets for his normal curiosity about fire, such as lighting the family's holiday candles or starting the fire in the fireplace under close and qualified supervision.

Any child who seems *preoccupied with fire* or *unusually* fascinated by it should receive prompt, professional help. It is not safe to assume that he will "outgrow" an obsession with fire. In many cities specially trained members of the local fire department work directly with children or will make referrals to other qualified people (Fig. 26.11).

It is essential that no one, at home or in the hospital, be allowed to smoke while unattended if he is drowsy, confused, helpless, or sedated. In the hospital it may be necessary to enlist the help of the family or a paid sitter if members of the staff are unable to supervise adequately the smoking of an unsafe smoker. Even though smoking is injurious to health, withholding cigarettes from a chain smoker can increase his stress and tension and make his hospitalization unnecessarily difficult.

RADIATION

Danger from radiation ranges from the minimal danger from diagnostic x-rays through the potential hazards of nuclear medicine to the perils of a nuclear disaster. Anyone who works near a source of radiation should be concerned about appropriate safeguards, and nurses who care for patients receiving radiation therapy must learn to care for them safely. Nurses who live or work near a source of nuclear energy should have a basic knowledge of the effects of radiation on both people and the environment and should know, both as informed citizens and as nurses, what to do in the event of a disaster. Regardless of her personal views about the use of nuclear energy, a nurse's professional commitment demands that she be able to respond in an emergency to the physical and psychological needs of people in the community.

Radiation Therapy

Nuclear medicine involves the use of x-rays for both diagnostic tests and the treatment of cancer. Radiation affects all types of cells, but it has a special affinity for rapidly growing ones and is, therefore, used to destroy the proliferating cells of a tumor.

In the treatment of cancer, the *source* of radiation can be external or internal to the patient. The *external source* of radiation is an extremely high-powered x-ray machine that emits deeply penetrating gamma rays rather than alpha and beta rays, which have low penetrating

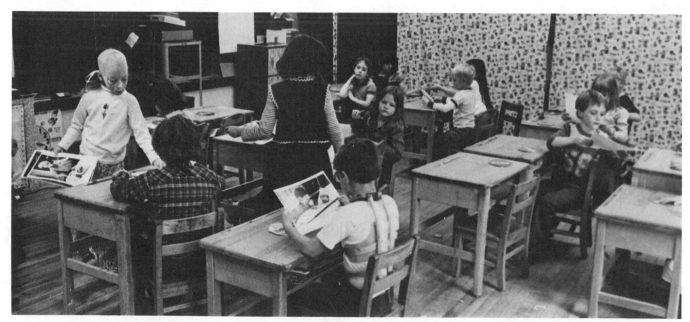

Figure 26.11 *Renee, still wearing her jobst, uses photographs of her experiences in the hospital burn unit to teach her classmates about fire safety.*

power. The gamma rays are directed toward the tumor and are focused as precisely as possible, but scattered rays will affect other areas of the patient's body as well as other people who are nearby. Danger to other people is decreased by shielding the machine in a basement room with thick concrete walls that absorb and block the rays. The patient should be informed that he will be left alone in the room during his treatment but that he will be constantly observed through a window or by a television monitor and that he will be able to talk with technicians and nurses outside the room.

The *internal sources* of radiation are radioisotopes that are administered in one of three ways: (1) given intravenously, (2) placed in a body cavity, or (3) implanted surgically into the tumor itself. Radioisotopes implanted in a body cavity or in the tumor are enclosed in tiny containers called beads, needles, seeds, or ribbons. These *contained radioisotopes* do not circulate through the patient's body and therefore are not present in body excretions and discharges. The only source of radiation is the radioactive implant itself. *Uncontained radioisotopes,* on the other hand, such as those given intravenously, circulate through the body and are present in blood, urine, feces, and vomitus, all of which must be handled as radioactive waste.

A patient who is receiving radiotherapy from an *external* source is not radioactive and poses no threat to other people. The patient whose body contains the *internal* source of his radiation therapy is radioactive, and safety precautions are necessary to protect those who care for him.

Safety Precautions

The factors that influence the nurse's safety and the safety of all others who come near the patient are time, distance, and shielding. The amount of exposure to radiation increases in proportion to the amount of *time* spent near the source of radiation, so it is imperative that the nurse plan ahead, work quickly, and keep her time with the patient to a minimum. Assignment to he care of the patient is often rotated among the staff so that no person receives excessive radiation.

Safety is enhanced by *distance* because the amount of radiation received drops sharply as distance from the source of radiation is increased. The amount of radiation at 4 feet from the source is only one-fourth of the radiation at 2 feet for example.

Shielding is critical for safety if the nurse must work close to a source of radiation for a period of time. Shielding is provided by wearing a lead apron and gloves and by using long forceps to handle contaminated dressings and other materials. Such materials are placed

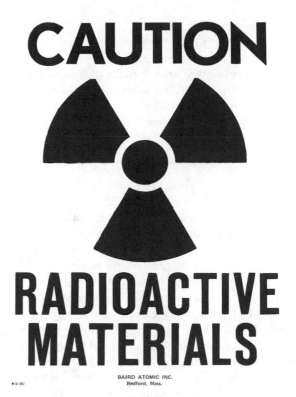

Figure 26.12 *Example of a warning sign posted by the radiotherapy department.*

in special containers for disposal as directed by the radiotherapy department.

Specific procedures and precautions are developed for each patient situation by the radiotherapy department and are based on the site of the implantation or source of internal radiation and on the characteristics and half-life of the radioisotopes being used (Fig. 26.12). One general policy is that a pregnant woman should not expose herself to radiation of any kind because the rapidly growing cells of the fetus are very susceptible to the effects of radiation.

Radiation therapy is physically and psychologically demanding of both patient and nurse, but meticulous attention to the guidelines and directions of the radiotherapy department can keep it safe for all concerned.

ASPHYXIATION

Asphyxiation is a condition in which a victim's intake of air is inadequate, and his body—especially his brain—suffers damage from lack of oxygen. The victim's inadequate air supply may be caused by an *inability to breathe air* that is readily available, or by a *lack of air.* An inability to breathe effectively enough to use the available air can be caused by such conditions as electric shock or chest injuries, while a lack of air is caused by a barrier between the air supply and a victim's lungs. Such barriers include a large piece of food (resulting in choking), water (resulting in drowning), or an airtight substance (causing suffocation). Asphyxiation because of a barrier which creates a lack of air is often preventable.

Choking

When an object is aspirated into the pharynx, larynx, or trachea, the victim's airway is partially or completely obstructed, causing acute resiratory distress. The object must be removed at once to allow oxygen to reach the lungs. Inadequate oxygenation of the blood will result in extensive or fatal brain damage within a very few minutes. The foreign object can be effectively expelled in many instances by a technique known as the Heimlich maneuver in which air is pushed from the victim's lungs with such force that the object is literally blown out of his airway by the outward rush of air. The victim then inhales spontaneously as soon as his airway is cleared (Fig. 26.13).

The object on which a victim chokes is most often a large piece of solid food, such as meat, but it could be a small toy, a large piece of hard candy, a balloon, or anything else a victim might put in his mouth which could block his airway. Since choking frequently occurs during a meal, whenever a person leaves the dinner table without an explanation, *someone should go after him* and stay with him until his safety is assured. When a person's airway is obstructed, no air can pass his vocal cords, so he is *unable to speak and ask for help.* Many people have died alone in a bathroom or restroom within a few yards of others who could have helped. In some restaurants, waiters and waitresses are trained in the use of the Heimlich maneuver, and posters explaining the procedure are posted in conspicuous places for the use of others.

Prevention of choking is based on careful teaching. The nurse and other adults should teach a child to keep *everything except food* out of his mouth, and both children and adults should be taught to cut solid food into small bites and chew it well. Children must learn not to run, jump, or bounce with food, candy, or large pieces of gum in their mouths. Every person should be taught that if he is choking, he should *stay with, or seek other people* and that he should point to his mouth and *signal distress* by putting his hand around his throat as if he were choking himself. A victim's inability to speak or even to cough will tell an observer that the person is *choking* and not having a heart attack.

Suffocation

A person's air supply can be shut off by anything that acts as a barrier between the air and his lungs. Common causes of suffocation include:

- An airtight compartment, such as an abandoned freezer
- A large plastic bag pulled over the head
- A cord, belt, or rope around the neck
- Snow, mud, sand, or water surrounding the head

Death from suffocation can occur very rapidly, or it can occur very slowly as in a mine disaster.

The prevention of suffocation involves teaching about four major sources of danger: airtight compartments, thin plastic, constriction of the neck, and being buried or covered. A few actions the nurse can take in each area are listed below.

Airtight Compartments

Teach people to remove doors of unused refrigerators and freezers, or render the doors inoperable.

Teach children *never* to crawl into an airtight box, stove, clothes dryer, or similar compartment.

Teach people that if they are trapped in a space with a limited air supply, they must try to stay calm and quiet because exertion and panic increase oxygen consumption.

Thin Plastic

Thin plastic near a person's face can be sucked against or into a victim's mouth every time he inhales. Children should not be allowed to play with thin plastic, such as dry cleaner bags, and thin plastic should not be used in place of a rubber sheet on a baby's crib.

Constriction of the Neck

Make sure that an infant cannot get his head between the spindles (bars) of his crib. The minimal safe distance between bars or slats is 2⅜ inches.

Teach people to keep cribs away from windows so children cannot play with venetian blind cords or drapery cords.

If an infant's garment has a drawstring at the neck, make sure it is knitted and flexible so it cannot tighten enough to strangle him.

In general, people need to be alert and think what could possibly happen in any given situation. In one situation a toddler who was put to bed with a sling on his arm and shoulder tried to climb out of his crib, became entangled in the sling, and strangled. Some

FIRST AID FOR
CHOKING

1 IMPORTANT: if victim can speak, breathe, cough, stand by but DO NOT INTERFERE

2 CALL AMBULANCE if victim cannot breathe, speak, cough.
Telephone_____

3 IF VICTIM IS CONSCIOUS:

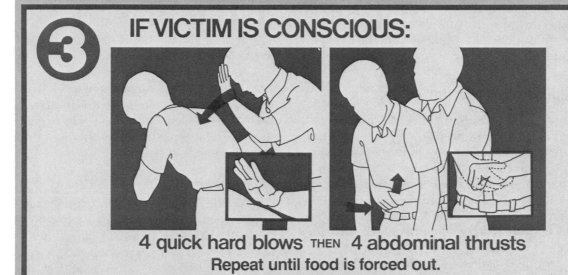

4 quick hard blows THEN 4 abdominal thrusts
Repeat until food is forced out.

IF VICTIM IS UNCONSCIOUS:

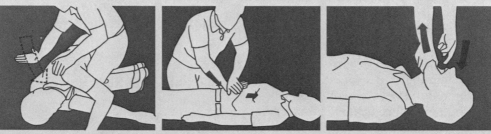

4 back blows THEN 4 abdominal thrusts THEN clear mouth
Repeat steps until food is forced out.
Do mouth-to-mouth or CPR as necessary.

Figure 26.13 First aid for choking. (Courtesy of the New York State Health Department.)
Note: Back blows are no longer recommended as part of the procedure in adults (1986).

types of baby harnesses and restraints for high chairs are also potentially dangerous.

Water, Snow, Mud, and Sand

Do not leave an infant or small child unattended in a tub or play pool even for a moment. Do not rely on flotation devices.

Teach children safe and acceptable behavior related to the beach, docks, farm ponds, brooks, and so forth.

Encourage use of slip-proof strips or a mat in the bathtub.

Encourage every person to learn to swim or to learn a flotation technique called *drown-proofing* (contact the Red Cross for details).

Teach children not to bury each other in snow or sand.

Teach children not to jump into high banks of snow or sand unless an adult is nearby.

Encourage construction workers to insist on proper safety precautions near excavations, and to avoid careless shortcuts.

Cardiopulmonary Resuscitation

The lungs of a person who has suffocated must be artificially ventilated by mouth-to-mouth resuscitation until he is able to breathe unassisted or until mechanical assistance is available. If his heart is not beating, cardiac compression is also needed. A combination of these two emergency measures is known as cardiopulmonary resuscitation (CPR). It must be initiated wihtin 3 to 5 minutes to prevent permanent brain damage from lack of oxygen.

CPR is a complex skill that is not learned from a book but through supervised practice on a lifelike model. Classes are conducted regularly and frequently by the American Red Cross and the American Heart Association. Many categories of health care workers are required to show evidence of certification in CPR as a condition of employment, and some hospitals now require all personnel, including physicians, to be *recertified each year*. You will probably need CPR certification before you are permitted to start some of your clinical rotations. A description of CPR is included in Appendix D, but you should seek training and certification as soon as possible.

In addition to insuring your own competency, it is important for you to encourage each patient and his family to acquire the skill as soon as possible. The classes are usually free of cost, and even children can become proficient enough to function in an emergency until help arrives.

PATIENT TEACHING

1. When a nurse is pressed for time, teaching about the patient's current condition usually takes priority over teaching about safety. To counteract this tendency, it is helpful to take a moment before interacting with a patient or family and to try to identify any potential hazards which might be relevant. For example:

What has this young mother of a toddler done to "child proof" her home to prevent poisoning?

What has this child been taught about electrical outlets and appliances?

Does this teenage baby sitter know CPR and how to manage in case of fire?

If you try to think of age-related hazards for each patient, you will begin to "think safety" and to incorporate relevant safety education into each patient's teaching plan.

RELATED ACTIVITIES

PICK A HAZARD AND TRY TO PREVENT IT. Use your own experiences and interests or the needs of your community, and identify a threat which could be eliminated. Then get involved in efforts to do so. Related activities might include:

making safety posters for the library or supermarket

speaking about falls at the senior citizen center

teaching a class for a troop of Scouts on the prevention and first aid for poisoning

writing a short article for the campus newsletter

Any list of contributions you could make would include activities with a wide variety of time commitments, which makes it possible for you to get involved to some degree despite a heavy academic schedule.

SUGGESTED READINGS

——— Test yourself: lightening. *Am J Nurs* 1980 July; 80(7):1300.

Berger, Mary Ellen, and Karl F Hubner: Hospital hazards: diagnostic radiation. *Am J Nurs* 1983 Aug; 83(8):1155–1159.

Brandeburg, Janice: Inhalation injury: carbon monoxide poisoning. *Am J Nurs* 1980 Jan; 80(1):98–100.

Conrad, Frances L: Tips for treating corrosive burns. *Nursing 85* 1985 Feb; 13(2):55–57.

DiFabio, Susan: Nurses' reactions to restraining patients. *Am J Nurs* 1981 May; 81(5):973–975.

Friedman, Freda, ed.: Restraints: when all else fails, there still are alternatives. *RN* 1983 Jan; 46(1):79–88.

Gassel, Thomas A, and J Richard Wuest: The right first aid for poisoning. *RN* 1981 March; 44(3):73–77.

Gaston, Susan F, and Lorna Lou Schumann: Inhalation injury: smoke inhalation. *Am J Nurs* 1980 Jan; 80(1):94–97.

Greenlaw, Jane: When leaving siderails down can bring you up on charges. *RN* 1982 Dec; 45(12):75–78.

Hassey, Karen: Demystifying care of patients with radioactive implants. *Am J Nurs* 1985 July; 85(7):788–792.

Isler, Charlotte: Hospital security: the burden is still on you. *RN* 1983 Aug; 46(8):54–58.

Jackson, Susan: Emergency! Dealing with burns. *RN* 1984 Oct; 47(10):35–39.

Jankowski, Carol B: Radiation emergency. *Am J Nurs* 1982 Jan; 82(1):90–96.

Jones, Marilee K: FIRE! *Am J Nurs* 1984 Nov; 84(11):1368–1371.

Lee, Patricia S, and Betty Jane Pash: Preventing patient falls. *Nursing 83* 1983 Feb; 13(2):118–120.

Lynn, Frances H: Incidents—Need they be accidents? *Am J Nurs* 1980 June; 80(6):1098–1102.

MacLean, Jill, et al.: Restraining the elderly agitated patient. *Can Nurse* 1982 June; 78(6):44–46.

Meth, Irving Marvin: Electrical safety in the hospital. *Am J Nurs* 1980 July; 80(7):1344–1348.

Murphy, Donna: Iodide—an rx for radiation accident. *Am J Nurs* 1982 Jan; 82(1):96–98.

Sumner, Sara M: Action stat: Electric shock. *Nursing 85* 1985 July; 15(7):43.

Sumner, Sara M, and Pamela Eaton Grau: Emergency! first aid for choking. *Nursing 82* 1982 July; 12(7):40–49.

Varricchio, Claudette G: The patient on radiation therapy. *Am J Nurs* 1981 Feb; 81(2):334–337.

Witte, Natalie Slocumb: Why the elderly fall. *Am J Nurs* 1979 Nov; 79(11):1950–1952.

Wyatt, Delia M: Are you prepared for a hospital fire? *Nursing 85* 1985 Feb; 15(2):51.

27

Prevention and Control of Infection

Section 1 Prevention of Infection

Section 2 Control of Infection

Prerequisites and/or Suggested Preparation
An understanding of the anatomy and physiology of the skin, basic knowledge of microbiology, and the concepts of epidemiology and the theory of multiple causation (Chapter 7) are prerequisite to understanding this chapter.

Section 1

Prevention of Infection

Humanity has always feared those diseases whose origin and mode of transmission were unknown. This is especially true when a disease such as AIDS seems to appear without warning, and when it occurs in epidemic form with a devastating outcome. In the past, such dread diseases have included bubonic plague, poliomyelitis, smallpox, and leprosy, and the afflicted people were likely to be cast out or rejected by society in an effort to reduce transmission of the disease.

Over the years, the incidence of communicable disease has been sharply reduced, and some diseases have been completely eradicated as a result of worldwide immunization programs. For example, the last case of smallpox *in the world* was located and treated in India by a team from the World Health Organization in the late 1970s.

INFECTION

Despite advances in the control of infectious diseases, problems of infection remain critical for several reasons. First, healthy people are now exposed to a wider range of diseases than ever before because of increased air travel. For example, whenever foreigners visit a remote area of the world, healthy natives can be exposed to diseases of civilization against which they have no immunity. A person in a highly communicable first stage of an undiagnosed disease can travel from city to city

within a few hours, exposing dozens of people in each place. These and other problems make it difficult to control the transmission of many infectious diseases.

In addition to the exposure of healthy people to a wider variety of organisms, the problem of infection control is compounded by the rising incidence of hospital-acquired (nosocomial) infections. The *Centers for Disease Control* (CDC)* estimates that 5 percent of all patients admitted to a hospital acquire an infection *while they are in the hospital*. These infections range from minor localized ones to life threatening or fatal systemic infections.

Nosocomial Infection

The term *nosocomial infection* refers to an infection that is acquired in a hospital. Such infections have always been present in hospitals, but in recent years several factors have made nosocomial infections a *major health problem* in the United States. First, the misuse or overuse of antibiotics has resulted in the development of virulent strains of microorganisms which are resistant to many antibiotics and are, therefore, virtually untreatable by drugs currently available.

Second, some hospitalized patients are afflicted with conditions that would have been fatal a few years ago. The treatment of these conditions is often complex and potentially dangerous, so the patient is at risk and susceptible to infection both because of the severity of his condition and the nature of the treatment. Examples of such patients include those who are undergoing kidney dialysis, organ transplants, and radiation therapy. The age of some of these patients places them in even greater jeopardy, for neither the very young nor the elderly have adequate natural defenses to fight a severe infection.

Third, a misplaced confidence in the power of antibiotics has developed over the years. The discovery of penicillin and subsequent "wonder drugs" resulted in a false sense of security because it seemed possible to

---

*The Centers for Disease Control (CDC) is a division of the Public Health Service of the US Department of Health and Human Services, Atlanta, Georgia. It is comprised of many centers and programs such as the Center for Infectious Diseases and the Hospital Infection Program which accounts for the fact that it seems to bear a plural name—the Centers for Disease Control.

treat almost any infection successfully. The ability to *prevent* infection suddenly seemed less important than the ability to *treat* infection. At the same time, the rigorous training in aseptic technique that had been required of all nurses was gradually relaxed. A mandatory 3- to 6-month experience in the operating room, for example, was dropped from many nursing programs, and the experiences which were substituted have not always instilled a comparable knowledge, skill, and valuing of sterile technique.

These factors—the increased virulence and resistance of organisms, the decreased resistance of some patients, the risk of infection that accompanies some treatments, and a laxity in aseptic technique—have combined to make nosocomial infections a major health hazard. Beyond the threat to life itself, a hospital-acquired infection may lengthen a hospitalization by days, weeks, or even months and can, as a result, be extremely costly in terms of the patient's time, energy, strength, loss of income, and disrupted family life. Nosocomial infections frequently result in legal action against the hospital, the physician, the nurse, or all three. Organizations such as the American Hospital Association (AHA) and the Centers for Disease Control (CDC) have established special commissions to study the problem. Some agencies have developed specially prepared infection control teams and in some places, the role of *nurse-epidemiologist* is emerging as a separate phase of nursing practice.

The Chain of Infection

Infections are spread when a sufficient number of *pathogenic* (disease producing) organisms are transmitted from an infected or contaminated source to a susceptible host. This host, in turn, becomes a reservoir of organisms which can then be transmitted to another susceptible person. This cycle of events is frequently likened to a chain with many links, the main ones being the source of infection, the transmission of the pathogens, and a susceptible host.

Before transmission to the host, pathogens are usually harbored in a reservoir that provides favorable amounts of food, moisture, darkness, and warmth. Growth and multiplication of organisms do not occur unless conditions are satisfactory, and many organisms, therefore, cannot survive in a clean, dry, sunny environment. The pathogens exit from the source of infection or reservoir via discharges from the respiratory, gastrointestinal, or genitourinary tract or via blood and infected tissue from a wound or break in the skin.

For infection to be spread, organisms must be transmitted from the source of infection to a susceptible host. The pathogens must survive the transmission *in suffi-*

cient numbers to overcome the resistance of the host's defenses. The pathogens are carried to the potential host by some vehicle such as air, contaminated food, water, insects, or contaminated objects or by direct contact between an infected person and the potential host.

Rats, flies, ticks, mosquitoes, and other vermin that carry pathogenic organisms are called *vectors*. Inanimate objects such as contaminated syringes, instruments, and soiled dressings that transmit pathogens are called *fomites*. Pathogens are also carried by air currents, especially in the droplets which are propelled forcefully by each sneeze or cough. In the hospital, the reservoir is likely to be a person (patient, visitor, or staff member). Individuals may be infected without showing any signs or symptoms of disease, and these people are called *carriers* or *colonized persons*.

Pathogens can enter the body through a break in the skin or mucous membranes or through a natural body orifice, such as the urethra, the vagina, and the mouth. These *portals of entry* can be created by injury, or by procedures such as surgery, intravenous therapy, and respiratory therapy. If the pathogens are sufficient in *number* and *virulence* to overcome the defenses of the host, infection occurs.

PREVENTION OF INFECTION

Infection can be prevented by interrupting the cycle in any of three ways:

1. Destroying or removing the source of infection
2. Decreasing susceptibility of the potential host by increasing his resistance to infection
3. Blocking transmission of the pathogens

Destruction or Removal of the Source of Infection

The *source of infection* can be removed by disinfection and sterilization of infected or contaminated objects, eradication of the disease (as with smallpox and polio, for example), proper disposal of waste and sewage, and destruction of pathogens within the patient's body through the use of antibiotics and other means.

Pathogenic organisms on inanimate objects can be killed or controlled in a variety of ways. *Sterilization* kills *all* organisms, pathogenic and nonpathogenic, and renders the object sterile. *Disinfection* kills most pathogenic organisms except spores. A disinfectant is a microbicidal chemical and is too irritating to be used on living tissue. An antiseptic is a microbistatic chemical that inhibits the growth of pathogens and can be used on humans.

Sterilization

The most efficient, economical, and widely used means of sterilization is *steam under pressure*. The temperature of free-flowing steam is the same as the temperature of boiling water, but in an autoclave the temperature of steam under pressure increases with the amount of pressure. A pressure of 15 to 17 lb increases the temperature of the steam from 100 degrees C to 121 to 123 degrees C (250–254 degrees F), which is high enough to destroy spores.

Articles to be autoclaved are wrapped in several layers of heavy fabric or strong, flexible paper. A temperature-sensitive tape is applied to each package before autoclaving. The tape changes color when sterilization is complete. Packages are autoclaved for 10 to 45 minutes depending on the size of the package, the method of wrapping, and other variables that affect the penetration of the steam. Packages are damp from the steam when removed from the autoclave and must be *dried under aseptic conditions* before they are handled and stored because a wet, porous paper cannot protect the contents from contamination.

Free-flowing steam is the same temperature as boiling water and will not kill spores. Many bedpan flushers conclude the cleansing process with a burst of steam. This does *not* sterilize the bedpan because the time is too short, usually not over 2 minutes.

Chemical compounds, such as alcohol and derivatives of chlorine, phenol, and iodine are used to disinfect large objects. In the home, chlorine is used to purify the water in swimming pools; and a chlorine bleach (such as Clorox) can be used to disinfect sickroom furniture and equipment. Other chemical solutions such as gluteraldehyde can sterilize articles that cannot be subjected to heat but which may be soaked.

Ethylene oxide, a gas, is used to sterilize objects that are sensitive to heat and/or moisture, such as plastic tubing, rubber, and some fabrics. In high concentrations this gas is toxic to humans, and the area in which it is used must be adequately ventilated.

Sunlight is cheap and available; but sterilization by ultraviolet rays requires at least 6 to 8 hours, and only those portions of the object or surface that are in direct contact with the sun's rays will be affected by the ultraviolet rays.

A combination of these methods of sterilization and disinfection is usually required in any given situation because of the many and varied objects and materials that are potential sources of infection.

Increasing Resistance to Infection

In addition to removing or destroying the source of pathogens, infection can be prevented by increasing the resistance of the potential host. This can be done by promoting or providing better nutrition, adequate rest and sleep, adequate exercise, a manageable level of stress, protection of the skin and mucous membranes, and adequate health care including immunizations and the appropriate use of antibiotics.

Blocking the Transmission of Infection

The prevention of infection by removing or destroying the source of infection, and by increasing the resistance of the potential host can be a complex, slow process and should be coupled with a more immediate solution to the problem: namely, *blocking transmission of the pathogens*. This is not a permanent solution because the possibility of infection will exist as long as there is a source of infection and a susceptible host. But, until a permanent solution is found, the patient can be kept safe by protecting him from pathogenic organisms.

Transmission of pathogens from the source of infection to a susceptible host is blocked by maintaining a state of asepsis. *Asepsis* means "to be without sepsis," in other words, without poison, without infection. Asepsis means the absence of *pathogens*. There are two categories of asepsis: medical asepsis and surgical asepsis. *Medical asepsis* is the absence of pathogenic organisms although nonpathogenic microorganisms are present. The process of maintaining a state of medical asepsis is called clean technique or medical aseptic technique (MAT).

Surgical asepsis is the absence of *all* microorganisms. The process of maintaining a state of surgical asepsis is called sterile technique or surgical aseptic technique (SAT).

Medical Asepsis

Medical aseptic technique is based on a sharp distinction between the concepts of *clean* and *dirty*. In the context of medical asepsis, an object or surface that is *free of pathogens* is clean. An object or surface which has been touched, or might have been touched, by pathogens is dirty (contaminated). Any object that has been used by a patient is considered contaminated because, for all practical purposes, there is no way of knowing whether or not pathogenic organisms are present. Bed linens, treatment trays, and thermometers are all considered contaminated after use. In the context of medical asepsis, the floor, doorknobs, water faucets, and sinks are dirty (contaminated).

In hospital utility rooms, various areas are designated as clean or dirty (contaminated). Fresh supplies are delivered, trays are opened, and treatments are prepared on clean surfaces, while used treatment trays are dismantled on dirty surfaces. Used equipment that is to be returned to the central supply department for cleaning and repackaging is rinsed free of all organic materials and then placed in a specially designated (dirty) cart or area.

Because waste products, including vomitus, blood, and other drainage, are emptied into the sink, the sink is obviously a dirty (contaminated) area. Other clean and dirty areas of the utility room which are not obvious must be identified so that they can be used properly. If one person contaminates a clean surface and fails to rectify the situation, the technique of all others using that surface will be faulty. Each succeeding person will mistakenly expect the formerly clean surface to be clean and will be using a contaminated surface as if it were clean.

Housekeeping

The housekeeping department is responsible for cleaning and disinfecting the utility rooms as well as all other areas of the hospital unit. The housekeeping department, with input from the nurse-epidemiologist and the maintenance department, establishes policies and routines for cleaning the walls, floors, windows, drapes, and all other components of the unit. It is often difficult to balance the necessary maintenance and cleaning of a unit with the needs of the patients and staff. For example, some floors that are easy to clean and polish are nonresilient and hard on the feet and legs of the staff. Some types of carpet decrease noise and are easy to walk on, but may be more difficult to clean. Carpets should not be used in such areas as a newborn nursery or an intensive care unit because the chances of soiling are great and proper maintenance would be very difficult.

The nurse is responsible for making sure that the patient's room and equipment are clean and sanitary even though parts of this responsibility may be delegated to others. In most hospitals, the housekeeping departments keeps the furniture clean, the window sills dusted, and the wastebaskets emptied. Should these things be left undone or be done inadequately, nursing must take action to resolve the issue because basic cleanliness is an integral part of medical asepsis.

The person who bathes the patient is responsible for cleaning the basin afterward, usually with a paper towel and soap or scouring powder. The person who empties the patient's bedpan, urinal, or bedside commode is responsible for rinsing it with cold water to remove all organic material. There is usually a water faucet on or near the patient's toilet for this purpose. If there is not, there is usually a large open hopper or a small closed bedpan flusher in the utility room. If a patient's bedpan is difficult to clean, the nurse may need to request a stiff toilet brush from the central supply department so that she and others can effectively clean the bedpan. If soiling of the hands is likely, disposable, nonsterile gloves should be worn to prevent gross contamination of the hands and to decrease the possibility of cross-contamination.

One of the most dangerous and offensive practices related to medical asepsis is that of grasping a bedpan under the rim when one is picking it up (Fig. 27.1). This practice is dangerous because the hazard is not obvious. The bedpan may look clean (on the outside), and you may fail to realize that by touching the inside, your hand will be every bit as contaminated as if it were visibly soiled with feces. Because the patient's bedpan is used by no one else, it is usually not disinfected or sterilized during his hospitalization, and the inside will thus be laden with pathogens, especially up under the rim. Keep your hands away from the inside of all bedpans, If you should accidentally touch the inside, *wash your hands more vigorously than usual, and take more time to wash them.*

Hospital policies vary with respect to responsibility for the cleanup of materials that are spilled in the patient's room and elsewhere on the unit. In some hospitals the housekeeping department assumes total responsibility for cleaning up spilled food, fluids, bath water, and so on, but the nursing department shares the responsibility for cleaning up blood, urine, and other body wastes. In some institutions the housekeeping de-

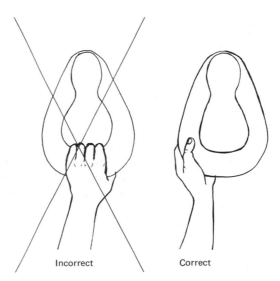

Incorrect   Correct

Figure 27.1 *The inside of a bed pan is grossly contaminated and should not be touched.*

partment will not remove spilled body fluids or wastes but will clean the area thoroughly as soon as it has been superficially wiped up. Needless to say, you must keep your uniform from becoming soiled while doing so and must wash your hands thoroughly afterward, as the floor may be heavily contaminated with pathogens. As with bedpans, if cleaning or handling contaminated surfaces or equipment is likely, disposable nonsterile gloves should be worn. You are responsible for observing and recording the color, consistency, and amount of the spilled drainage or excreta. It is important to chart the circumstances of the spill if the accident disrupted a treatment or test.

You are responsible for rinsing blood, drainage, and body wastes off any equipment you have used that is to be returned to central supply for cleaning and sterilization. Cold water is used for this because hot water coagulates protein and makes removal difficult. You are also responsible for the proper disposal of soiled dressings, drainage, sputum, and so forth.

The method of disposal must be both aseptic and esthetic. *Aseptic* disposal prevents the transfer of pathogens to any other object or surface except the interior of a proper trash can. *Esthetic* disposal does not offend any person's basic need for beauty, order, and cleanliness. Leaving a contaminated dressing in the patient's wastebasket is neither aseptically nor aesthetically acceptable.

Finally, you are responsible for the safety of your uniform. If it should become contaminated with material that might contain pathogenic organisms, change it if possible. If you cannot change your uniform, replace or cover it with a patient gown or scrub gown. This is vital even though your uniform may dry out and *look* clean. Although you may feel self-conscious and perhaps a bit foolish in a gown, *knowingly* wearing a contaminated uniform while caring for patients constitutes a serious act of negligence.

Handwashing

It was approximately 100 years ago in Vienna that Ignaz Semmelweis dramatically reduced the incidence of deaths from puerperal (childbirth) fever by insisting that physicians wash their hands before touching a new mother. Before this, it was common practice for a physician to come from the morgue or the bedside of an acutely ill patient and examine an obstetrical patient without washing his hands. Today, the CDC advises that *handwashing is the single most important aspect of the prevention of infection.*

Although some textbooks still insist that a nurse should always wash her hands between patients, it now seems that good judgment rather than a blanket rule should guide the nurse's actions. There are times when

hands *must be washed without fail,* but there are also times when it is not necessary, such as when passing oral medications, passing dinner trays, and taking oral temperatures with an electronic thermometer and disposable probe covers. Knowledge of the patients on the unit coupled with an understanding of medical asepsis will enable you to exercise good judgment with respect to handwashing in marginal situations.

All patients need to be protected from infection, but protection for some patients whose defenses are incomplete, impaired, or inadequate is an urgent, life-and-death matter. Such a patient must *never* be approached with unwashed hands. Examples of such patients include:

- A newborn infant with immature body defenses
- A patient with injury or damage to his skin (his first line of defense) as a result of burns, cuts, or a surgical incision
- A patient whose strength and resources have been depleted either by a long chronic illness or by an overwhelming acute illness
- A patient with a denuded body organ that is open to infection, such as the lining of the uterus after detachment of the placenta following delivery
- A patient whose body defenses have been altered by the effects of radiation, chemotherapy, or disease

You must wash your hands before you do a potentially risky procedure on *any* patient, such as changing the tubing of an indwelling catheter, changing a dressing, or instilling eye drops. The patient's defense system may be adequate, but the nature of the procedure poses a great risk of infection.

Hands must be washed *after* each treatment or procedure that involves *blood, discharges, or excreta.* Pathogens must be removed from your hands as quickly as possible to prevent their transfer to another patient and to protect yourself from infection.

Hands MUST Be Washed

- *After* any care involving blood, urine, vomitus, feces, sputum, drainage, exudate, and discharge
- *Before* every procedure for a patient whose body defenses are immature, impaired, or inadequate
- *Before* a risky procedure for *any* patient

Handwashing Procedure

1. Push your wristwatch and long sleeves up out of the way. If your hands are contaminated, use a dry paper towel to move your watch and sleeves.

2. Keep your hands and uniform away from the surface of the sink (Fig. 27.2). The inside of each and every sink is contaminated; you cannot know what has been emplied into or what has been washed there. If your hands touch the sink while you are washing them, rewash them. Do not let water splash from the dirty sink onto your skin; if it does, rewash your hands. The edge of the sink is contaminated; do not lean against it. If the sink in the utility room is too high for you or is too deep from front to back, find another sink which you can use without contaminating the front of your uniform.

3. Use plenty of soap and friction as you wash. Soap enhances cleansing by emulsifying fat and oil, and by lowering surface tension. Most soaps are effective if used with enough friction to loosen and remove the dirt and transient bacteria which are deposited on your skin as you care for patients. *Transient* bacteria may be pathogenic, but they stay on the *surface* of the skin and can be removed with lather and friction.

Resident bacteria, on the other hand, are embedded in the crevices of skin, nails, hair follicles, and sebaceous glands and are, therefore, inaccessible to lather and friction. Resident bacteria are normally present on the skin and are usually not pathogenic. Because scrubbing removes transient pathogenic bacteria but leaves resident nonpathogenic bacteria, the scrubbed skin is *clean but not sterile*. Skin cannot be sterilized and therefore must be covered with a sterile gown or gloves whenever sterility is required. Germicidal soaps are sometimes used in high-risk areas such as an operating room and a newborn nursery, but many of these soaps tend to make the skin dry and irritated with extensive use. Rough, dry skin is hard to cleanse properly and may crack, creating a health hazard for the nurse. The benefits of using a germicidal soap must be weighed against its undesirable side effects.

4. Wash your hands with abundant lather and brisk friction for 10 to 30 seconds, depending on the extent and type of contamination and the vigor with which

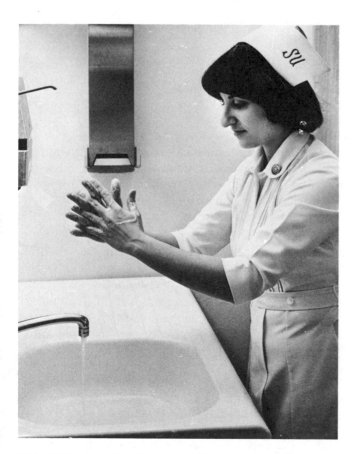

Figure 27.2 Keep hands and uniform away from the contaminated sink.

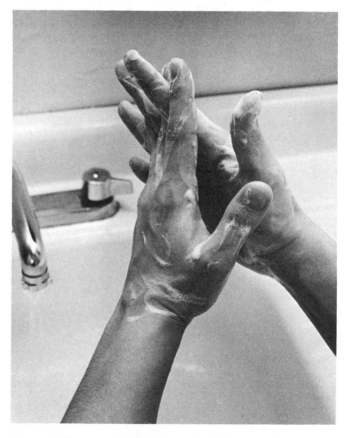

Figure 27.3 Interlaced fingers and brisk friction are necessary for effective handwashing.

the washing is done. Fingers should be interlaced so that lather and friction are applied to the sides of the fingers and the spaces between the fingers (Fig. 27.3). If your fingernails are short and were clean when you came on duty, they may not need any special attention. If they have become soiled, you may be able to clean them with the fingernails of the other hand and additional soap. If a supply of clean orangewood sticks is provided, they can be used if you are careful not to irritate or break the skin under or around the nail.

5. If you know that your hands were badly contaminated or if they are visibly soiled, rinse them and repeat the scrub. Because your hands were dirtier than your arms at the outset, they should be held lower than your elbows to keep the dirty water away from your arms. Once your hands are clean, they can be held at any height.

6. The faucets are grossly contaminated and cannot be touched with clean hands. Let the water continue to run while you dry your hands, and *then* turn off the faucets by using a *dry* paper towel (Fig. 27.4). A wet towel and wet hands will permit the transfer of pathogens by capillary action. If you accidentally touch the faucets, rewash your hands.

7. Drop the used towels into an *open* wastepaper basket or trash can (Fig. 27.5). If one is not available, you have two choices: you can take the used towels to an open container somewhere else, or you can use a dry paper towel to lift the lid of a covered container and then leave the dry towel on the lid of the container or carry it to an open container. If you accidentally touch the trash can or its lid, wash your hands again.

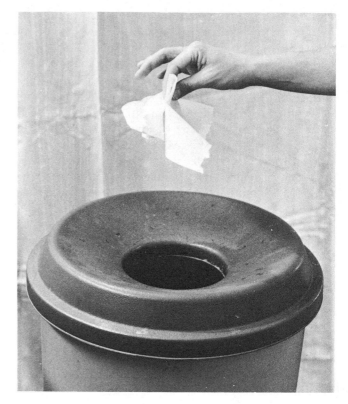

Figure 27.5 Keep hands clean while disposing of the paper towels.

If open wastepaper cans are not available, work through your head nurse to make sure that there is a large, open wastepaper container near every sink. Some institutions supply hot-air dryers instead of towels for drying hands, but paper towels are still needed when you turn off the faucets.

8. If the institution does not provide a dispenser with hand lotion, carry a sample-size bottle in your uniform pocket and use it regularly. Dry, chapped skin is likely to crack, leaving you vulnerable to infection.

A surgical scrub is similar to a medical scrub but is more intensive and thorough, and lasts 5 minutes. After a few minutes, the hands are cleaner than the arms and for the remaining scrub time, the hands are held above the elbows so that all water drains *away* from the hands. A sterile brush is often provided to increase the friction. The hands are held above the elbows as they are dried. Even a surgical scrub cannot sterilize the skin; the hands are *not sterile* and must be covered with sterile gloves before they touch anything that is to be kept sterile.

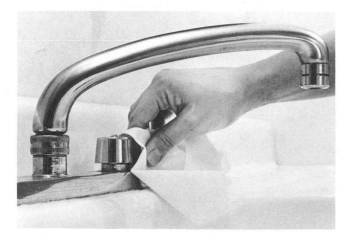

Figure 27.4 Turn off the faucet with a dry paper towel.

PROCEDURE 27.1

*Handwashing**

SUMMARY OF ESSENTIAL NURSING ACTIONS

1. Remove your wristwatch or push it up toward your elbow.
2. Keep hands and uniform away from contaminated surfaces of the sink.
3. Hold dirty hands *down* to keep dirty wash water from contaminating your arms and elbows.
4. Wash hands with *abundant lather and brisk friction* for 10–30 seconds, depending upon the type and extent of dirt or contamination.
   - Interlace fingers and wash all surfaces of fingers and hands.
   - Clean nails as needed.

5. After washing, hold clean hands *up* to let rinse water flow *away* from clean hands.
6. Dry hands with clean dry paper towel.
7. Drop towel into an open container.
   Rewash hands if you touch the trash container.
8. Use another clean DRY paper towel to turn off water faucet.
   THAT TOWEL IS NOW CONTAMINATED! Drop it into an open container.

*See inside front cover and pages 442–443.

Surgical Asepsis

Surgical aseptic technique (SAT) is the process of maintaining sterility throughout an operation, procedure, or treatment. Responsibility for the *initial sterility* of the equipment and supplies is assumed by the manufacturer or by the central supply department of the hospital. Responsibility for *maintaining sterility* is assumed by nurses and physicians.

Surgical asepsis is necessary when:

- The patient's skin has already been broken, either accidentally or intentionally during surgery
- The patient's skin will be incised or penetrated during a procedure such as surgery, a bone marrow biopsy, or an injection
- A sterile body cavity will be entered or penetrated during a procedure such as catheterization, lumbar puncture, or amniocentesis
- The patient has an immunological disorder that leaves him defenseless against an infection of any kind

Sterile technique is the process of assuring surgical asepsis by: (1) creating and maintaining a *sterile field* (work space) and (2) maintaining the sterility of all equipment and supplies. It is neither possible nor desirable for a nurse to memorize a set of rules for each and every situation involving surgical asepsis that might be encountered. Therefore, you must understand the principles that underlie surgical asepsis and that provide a basis for making decisions in a specific situation. The *principles* of surgical asepsis make it possible to de-

rive guidelines for the implementation of sterile technique.

If any principles of surgical asepsis are violated, a break in surgical aseptic technique has occurred and the sterile object or area has become contaminated. *An object is either sterile or it is contaminated;* it cannot be almost sterile or just a little bit contaminated. If there is any doubt or question, consider the object contaminated.

Putting On Sterile Gloves

1. Select gloves of proper size (size 6 and 6½ gloves are small; size 8 and 8½ gloves are large). If the gloves are too small and are stretched too tightly across your hands, they may rip or tear. If they are too big, the loose rubber or latex can be snapped or torn, thereby exposing your skin and possibly contaminating the sterile field. Gloves that are too large also decrease your manual dexerity.

2. If the gloves were commercially packaged, check the wrapper for directions, if any, on how to open the package.

3. Scrub your hands. Since there is always danger of tearing a glove, it is important to have the skin underneath as free of microorganisms as possible. Fingernails must be short, and all rings must be removed except for a perfectly smooth wedding band.

4. Remove the outer wrapper in accordance with the manufacturer's directions or in accordance with accepted procedure for opening a sterile package (see "Opening a Sterile Package," which follows).

5. If the gloves are prepowdered, proceed to step 7.

Principles of Surgical Asepsis and Guidelines for Their Application

PRINCIPLE 1. A STERILE AREA OR OBJECT REMAINS STERILE WHEN TOUCHED BY ANOTHER STERILE OBJECT

Guideline 1. Use sterile forceps or wear sterile gloves to manipulate articles on a sterile tray.

Guideline 2. Touch a sterile surface that is to remain sterile only with another sterile surface or object.

PRINCIPLE 2. A STERILE AREA OR OBJECT BECOMES CONTAMINATED WHEN TOUCHED BY ANY UNSTERILE OBJECT

Guideline 1. When the edge or rim of a sterile area is adjacent to or in contact with an unsterile surface, consider the edge or rim contaminated.

Guideline 2. If there is a tear or break in the covering of a sterile object, consider the contents contaminated. A break or tear in the cover allows the sterile object to be touched and contaminated by an unsterile object. In addition, the torn edges of the cover are considered contaminated because they are adjacent to the unsterile exterior of the package.

Guideline 3. Always keep the sterile area and sterile objects in view so that you can detect possible or actual contamination. Contamination can be caused by an unknowing person, a dropped object, flies, or a dangling bit of clothing or hair. Do not turn your back on a sterile tray or leave it unattended.

Guideline 4. Keep sterile objects above waist level to increase visibility and lessen the possibility of unintentional contamination.

PRINCIPLE 3. A STERILE OBJECT OR AREA BECOMES CONTAMINATED WHEN MICROORGANISMS ARE TRANSPORTED TO IT BY AIR CURRENTS OR GRAVITY

Guideline 1. Keep air currents at a minimum by avoiding any unnecessary movement of people, linen, curtains, and so forth.

Guideline 2. Do not reach across a sterile field. Particles of skin, hair, sweat, or clothing can fall onto the sterile field.

Guideline 3. Avoid laughing, coughing, sneezing, and excessive talking across a sterile surface. Droplets of moisture, saliva, or sputum will contaminate the field.

Guideline 4. Once a sterile tray has been opened, there is always a chance that it has been contaminated by air currents. Do not place unused articles from a sterile tray back with sterile supplies. Do not use them for another patient.

PRINCIPLE 4. A STERILE AREA OR OBJECT BECOMES CONTAMINATED WHEN CAPILLARY ACTION RESULTS IN CONTACT BETWEEN THE STERILE SURFACE AND A WET, CONTAMINATED SURFACE

Guideline 1. A sterile, porous material will serve as a barrier between an unsterile surface and a sterile object *only* if the material is *dry*.

Guideline 2. If a porous wrapper or barrier becomes wet, do not use the article inside the wrapper. When the wrapper or barrier is wet, moisture carries microorganisms by capillary action from any unsterile area through the wrapper to the sterile object, thereby contaminating it.

Guideline 3. Use a sterile, waterproof (nonporous) material as a barrier between a sterile object and an unsterile surface if there is a possibility of contamination from a wet surface by capillary action.

PRINCIPLE 5. A STERILE AREA OR OBJECT BECOMES CONTAMINATED WHEN GRAVITY CAUSES A CONTAMINATED LIQUID TO FLOW OVER A STERILE SURFACE

Guideline 1. When you do a surgical scrub, hold hands above level of elbows to keep water on arms from flowing back over clean hands.

Guideline 2. When you use transfer forceps that are kept in a disinfectant, keep the handles up and the wet ends down. This precaution prevents the solution from reaching the handles, becoming comtaminated by microorganisms on the handles, and flowing back to the sterile ends.

---

6. If a packet of powder is provided, open it and powder your hands to make the gloves slip on more easily. Do so over a waste container if possible, being careful not to contaminate your clean hands. Do not spill powder on the patient, equipment, supplies, or sterile field.

7. Open the inner wrapper and identify the right glove (Fig. 27.6a). Most right-handed people put the

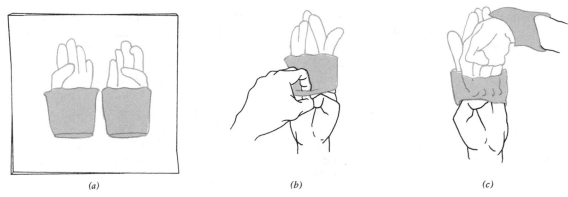

(a)   (b)   (c)

Figure 27.6 *Gloving technique (see text for description).*

right glove on first because then the gloved right hand can be used to put on the second glove, which is a bit more complicated than putting on the first one. Those who are left-handed may prefer to reverse steps 8 and 9.

8. Grasp the folded edge of the turned-down cuff of the right glove (Fig. 27.6*b*). Your left fingers and thumb should be touching only the *inside* of the glove, keeping the outside sterile. Slide your right hand into the glove, keeping your fingers straight. Do *not* attempt to adjust the cuff in any way.

9. Slide your gloved fingers under the cuff of the second glove (Fig. 27.6*c*). Lift the glove from the wrapper and slide your hand into it, keeping your gloved

thumb away from your bare wrist as you do so. Do not attempt to adjust the cuff unless your wrist is covered with the sleeve of a sterile gown; if you adjust the cuff, you increase the chance of contaminating your glove by touching your bare wrist, and it is not necessary for your wrists to be covered.

10. Adjust the fingers of the gloves until they fit smoothly.

11. If you are wearing a sterile, long-sleeved gown for use in the operating room or delivery room, you can turn the glove cuffs up over the cuffs of the gown, being careful not to touch the skin below the sleeve with your sterile gloves. If you are not wearing a sterile gown, do not attempt to adjust the glove cuffs.

PROCEDURE 27.2

*Putting on Sterile Gloves**

SUMMARY OF ESSENTIAL NURSING ACTIONS

1. Select gloves of proper size.
2. Inspect package for any evidence of prior opening or damage to package.
3. Scrub hands as indicated by the situation.
4. Open the package in accordance with the manufacturer's directions, or in accordance with accepted procedure for opening a sterile package.
5. Powder your hands unless the gloves were prepowdered by the manufacturer.
6. Maintain the sterility of the OUTSIDE of the gloves.
   - Pick up the right glove by grasping the folded edge of

the cuff (the inside of the glove). Touch NOTHING but the inside of the cuff as you slide your other hand into the glove.
   - Pick up the other glove by sliding your sterile gloved fingers *under* the cuff. Keep all parts of your gloved hand away from the inside of the other glove and your ungloved hand and wrist.
7. Adjust the fingers of the gloves until they fit smoothly. Do NOT try to adjust the cuffs which are next to your bare wrists.
8. Keep your eyes on the gloves at all times. If you are distracted, or think that you may have contaminated your gloves, remove them and start over again.

*See inside front cover and page 445.

Removing Gloves

1. Grasp the outside of the cuff of one glove and peel that glove off your hand (it will turn wrong side out as you do so). Drop the glove onto the used treatment tray or appropriate waste container.

2. Slip your ungloved fingers (which are clean) inside the cuff of the other glove (the inside is clean), and peel the glove off. Be careful not to touch the outside of the glove (which is contaminated) with your clean hand.

3. If the gloves are disposable, discard them with other contaminated materials. If the gloves are reusable, return them to central supply to be repackaged and sterilized.

Opening a Sterile Package

First of all, make sure that the *wrapper is intact and undamaged*. Then, if the item was commercially prepared and wrapped, proceed to read and follow any directions on the wrapper for opening the package (Fig. 27.7).

A package that was wrapped and sterilized by central supply is usually wrapped in flexible, tough paper or a double thickness of fabric. The paper wrapper is disposable; cloth wrappers are washed and reused. Cloth is much easier to unwrap because it folds easily and stays where it is placed, whereas paper tends to spring back and resist placement.

When a tray or other object is being wrapped, it is often placed diagonally on the wrapper, and each corner of the wrapper is then brought up and folded across the tray.

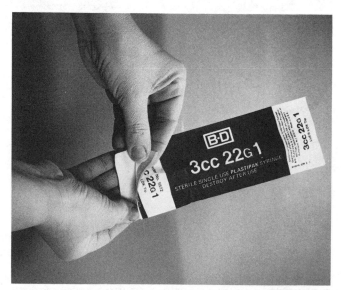

Figure 27.7 *Many sterile packages are opened by peeling the designated edges apart.*

Unwrapping a Tray or Other Object

1. Position the package in front of you so that the top corner of the wrapper is away from you, with the tip of the corner pointing toward you (Fig. 27.8a). This position enables you to open the furthest flap first, before the tray is uncovered, so there is no danger of contamination which might result from your reaching across a sterile field to lift up the farthest flap (Fig. 27.8b).

2. Take hold of flaps by pinching the outside of the wrapper.

3. Lift up the side flaps (Fig. 27.8c,d).

4. Open the flap nearest you (Fig. 27.8e). If space is limited, you may need to fold it back on itself, while the edges are still sterile, so that the corner does not fall against your uniform or some other surface. If sterile gloves are to be worn, leave the last corner in place over the tray to protect the contents from accidental contamination while you are putting on gloves. The last flap is still sterile and can be handled with your sterile, gloved hands.

Adding Items to a Sterile Tray

If fluids, such as an antiseptic, are to be added to the tray, remember that an object or area can be contaminated by capillary action through a wet wrapper between the sterile surface and a contaminated table or shelf even though the spilled fluid is sterile.

When you add fluids or objects from a covered container, hold the lid in your hand or place it sterile side (inside) *up* on a clean surface. The lid *never* goes sterile side down. It cannot be placed sterile side down on a sterile surface without contaminating that surface because the *outer edge* of the lid is not sterile. It cannot be placed sterile side down on an unsterile surface because the unsterile surface would contaminate it.

To add a dry item, such as an instrument, open the package and *drop* the item onto the tray *without shaking the package* and creating air currents. If the item is wrapped in cloth, open the package, expose the contents, and then gather the loose ends of the wrapper in your other hand to keep them from dangling and contaminating the tray as you reach over it to drop the item (Fig. 27.9).

When sterile supplies of any kind are to be added to a tray, remember that there is no set of rules to tell you how to do so. No two situations are alike, and no two procedures are done in exactly the same sequence. The single most important guideline is to *think, think, think, think!* Before each move or each decision that you must make, think about the principles of surgical asepsis. If the proposed action violates any one of the principles, stop and select another approach.

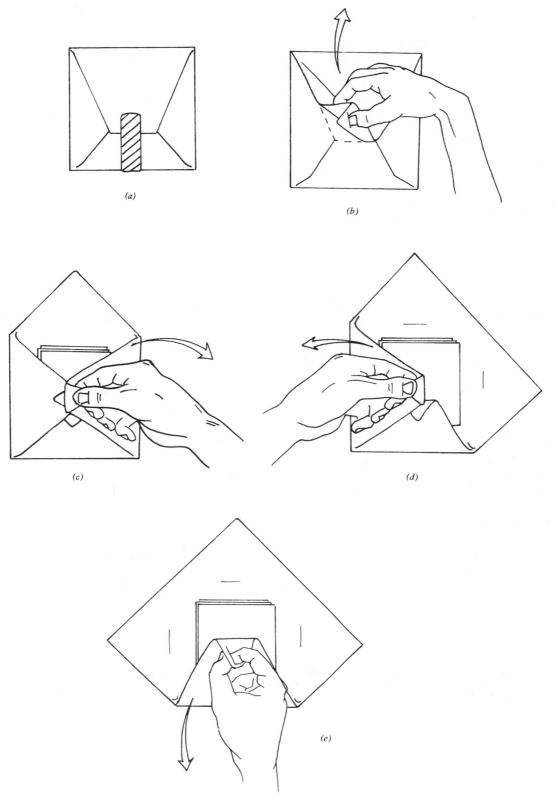

Figure 27.8 The steps in opening a sterile package (see text for description).

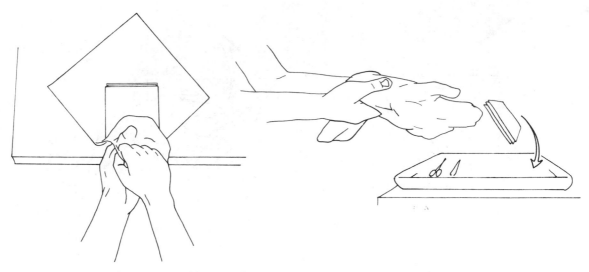

Figure 27.9 *Adding an object to a sterile tray (see text for description).*

PROCEDURE 27.3

Setting Up and Maintaining a Sterile Field*

SUMMARY OF ESSENTIAL NURSING ACTIONS

1. Select an appropriate workspace.
   - It should be clean, dry, uncluttered, free of drafts, within your line of vision while you work, and unlikely to become contaminated by the patient or another person brushing against it.
2. Make sure your assembled supplies are *complete*. (You cannot leave a sterile field to get a forgotten item.)
   - Include an extra item for any one that might easily become contaminated.
   - Make sure that a waste receptacle is within reach.
3. Check the wrapping of each sterile item, and discard the item if there is evidence that it has been torn, opened, or wet.
4. Teach the patient that he must not touch sterile items, or laugh, cough, or sneeze across the sterile field.

5. Decide whether the opened wrapper of a sterile tray or package will serve as the sterile field or whether you need a separate covering for the workspace.
6. Open wrapper or drape to create a sterile work surface.
7. Add sterile supplies or equipment *in accordance with the principles of surgical asepsis.*
8. Add sterile liquids *in accordance with the principles of surgical asepsis.*
9. Don sterile gloves when ready to handle sterile items (unless you plan to use forceps).
10. Maintain sterile techniques throughout the procedure.
    - Apply the principles of surgical asepsis to *each action you take* and *each decision you make.*

*See inside front cover and pages 445–449.

Section 2

The Control of Infection

INFECTION

The goals of infection control are the containment of pathogens, and the protection of your patient, yourself, and others. This is done by early detection of infection, and the use of appropriate aseptic and isolation techniques.

Early Detection

Every patient should be observed carefully upon admission and throughout his hospitalization for indications of any possible infection. The nurse has more contact with the patient than does the physician and is often the first person to detect the early symptoms of a developing infection.

A patient's skin should be assessed upon his admission and during baths and treatments for signs of *local infection* such as redness, swelling, heat, or pain around an incision, or a rash, pustule, or boil. Signs that might indicate a *generalized or systemic infection* include fever of unknown origin (FUO), undiagnosed diarrhea, purulent drainage, skin rash, foul odors, or signs of an

upper respiratory infection (URI) such as coughing or chest pain. Cloudy urine, body secretions which contain pus, and a foul odor to a normal body discharge, such as the menstrual flow, are other indicators of an infection. Such observations should be reported to the physician at once, and appropriate measures should be taken to protect other people. Because the nurse often notes the very early signs of infection, the infection is often confined and treated before it can be spread to anyone else.

The commonest nosocomial infections involve the urinary tract (43 percent), wounds (34 percent), the respiratory tract (16 percent), and the skin (4 percent). These figures indicate the areas of greatest susceptibility to infection and thus the areas that demand meticulous aseptic technique and careful observation.

Isolation

In the past, lack of knowledge about the origin and transmission of disease led to extensive and elaborate isolation procedures. Because people often did not know the cause or source of a disease, they tried to cover all possibilities by doing everything conceivable to contain an infection, from boiling the bed linens to fumigating the room with carbolic acid or sulfur.

Current isolation procedures are based on research findings and are designed to impose the least number of precautions that will be effective. An overdone and cumbersome procedure can be worse than none at all because it often leads to dangerous shortcuts. Guidelines for isolation procedures are provided by the CDC and by each hospital's infection control committee. In addition, many health care facilities now employ a *nurse-epidemiologist* whose main responsibility is the prevention and control of nosocomial infections.

Isolation Procedures

Isolation procedures are designed to *block the transmission of pathogenic organisms*. A variety of barrier (isolation) techniques, based on a knowledge of the agent, the mode of transmission, and the host, have been developed for this purpose.

The patient is either an agent or a susceptible host. If the patient has the infection, he is the *agent,* and isolation techniques are used to protect *other people*—

other patients, staff, and family. If a patient, such as a premature infant or a burned person, has limited defenses to combat infection, he is a *susceptible host,* and isolation techniques are used to protect *him* from infection.

The choice of an isolation technique is based on the *mode of transmission* of organisms from agent to host; isolation procedures vary depending on whether the pathogens are transmitted via blood, feces, contact with purulent drainage, or droplets of mucus.

The *underlying principles* of infection control do not vary, but isolation techniques must sometimes be modified to meet the reality of a given situation. For example, guidelines from the CDC advocate the use of a private room and bath for a patient with a disease such as diphtheria or meningitis. This is feasible and usually possible in a medical center, but it is an unrealistic recommendation for a patient in a remote native village. Just so, the *principles* of respiratory isolation do not change, but the *specific details* of respiratory precautions are different for a patient who conscientiously covers his mouth when he coughs than they are for a patient who is unable to cooperate in any way.

Types of Isolation

The 1985 guidelines from the CDC include seven types of isolation:

1. Strict Isolation
2. Contact Isolation
3. Respiratory Isolation
4. Tuberculosis (AFB) Isolation
5. Enteric Precautions
6. Drainage/Secretions Precautions
7. Blood/Body Fluid Precautions

The variations among these forms of isolation pertain to differences in the use of a gown, gloves, and mask as well as to differences in the handling of dishes, linen, equipment, body wastes, and dressings. The type of isolation instituted for a given patient is determined by the nature of the pathogens and their mode of transmission. Brief descriptions of the major modes of isolation are given here; detailed guidelines are available from each agency's procedure manual, from the hospital's infection control committee, and from the CDC.

Types of Isolation

STRICT ISOLATION

Strict Isolation is an isolation category designed to prevent transmission of highly contagious or virulent infections that may be spread by *both air and contact.*

Specifications for Strict Isolation

1. Private room is indicated; door should be kept closed. In general, patients infected with the same organism may share a room.
2. Masks are indicated for all persons entering the room.
3. Gowns are indicated for all persons entering the room.
4. Gloves are indicated for all persons entering the room.
5. Hands must be washed after touching the patient or potentially contaminated articles and before you take care of another patient.
6. Articles contaminated with infective material should be discarded or bagged and labeled before being sent for decontamination and reprocessing.

CONTACT ISOLATION

Contact Isolation is designed to prevent transmission of highly transmissible or epidemiologically important infections (or colonizations) that do not warrant strict isolation.

All diseases or conditions included in this category are spread primarily by close or direct contact. Thus, masks, gowns, and gloves are recommended for use by anyone in close or direct contact with any patient who has an infection (or colonization) that is included in this cate-

gory. In the case of *individual diseases* or conditions, one or more of these three barriers may not be indicated.

Specifications for Contact Isolation

1. Private room is indicated. In general, patients infected with the same organism may share a room. During outbreaks, infants and young children with the same respiratory clinical syndrome may share a room.
2. Masks are indicated for those who come close to the patient.
3. Gowns are indicated if soiling is likely.
4. Gloves are indicated for touching infective material.
5. Hands must be washed after touching the patient or potentially contaminated articles and before you take care of another patient.
6. Articles contaminated with infective material should be discarded or bagged and labeled before being sent for decontamination and reprocessing.

RESPIRATORY ISOLATION

Respiratory Isolation is designed to prevent transmission of infectious diseases primarily over short distances through the air (droplet infection). Direct and indirect transmission occurs with some infections in this isolation category but is infrequent.

Guidelines for Respiratory Isolation

1. Private room is indicated. In general, patients infected with the same organism may share a room.

2. Masks are indicated for those who come close to the patient.

3. Gowns are not indicated.

4. Gloves are not indicated.

5. Hands must be washed after touching the patient or potentially contaminated articles and before you take care of another patient.

6. Articles contaminated with infective material should be discarded or bagged and labeled before being sent for decontamination and reprocessing.

TUBERCULOSIS ISOLATION (AFB ISOLATION)

Tuberculosis Isolation (AFB Isolation) is an isolation category for patients with pulmonary TB who have a positive sputum smear or a chest x-ray film that strongly suggests current (active) TB. On the isolation card (for the patient's door), this category is called AFB (acid-fast bacilli) Isolation, to protect the patient's privacy.

Specifications for Tuberculosis Isolation (AFB Isolation)

1. Private room with special ventilation is indicated. Door should be kept closed. In general, patients infected with the same organism may share a room.

2. Masks are indicated only if the patient is coughing and does not reliably cover mouth.

3. Gowns are indicated only if needed to prevent gross contamination of clothing.

4. Gloves are not indicated.

5. Hands must be washed after touching the patient or potentially contaminated articles and before you take care of another patient.

6. Articles are rarely involved in transmission of TB. However, articles should be thoroughly cleaned and disinfected, or destroyed.

ENTERIC PRECAUTIONS

Enteric Precautions are designed to prevent infectious diseases that are transmitted by direct or indirect contact with feces.

1. Private room is indicated if patient hygiene is poor. A patient with poor hygiene does not wash hands after touching infective material, contaminates the environment with infective material, or shares contaminated articles with other patients. In general, patients infected with the same organisms may share a room.

2. Masks are not indicated.

3. Gowns are indicated if soiling is likely.

4. Gloves are indicated if touching infective material.

5. Hands must be washed after touching the patient or potentially contaminated articles and before you take care of another patient.

6. Articles contaminated with infective material should be discarded or bagged and labeled before being sent for decontamination and reprocessing.

DRAINAGE/SECRETION PRECAUTIONS

Drainage/Secretion Precautions are designed to prevent infections that are transmitted by direct or indirect contact with purulent material or drainage from an infected body site.

This newly created isolation category includes many infections formerly included in Wound and Skin Precautions, Discharge (lesion), and Skin Precautions, which have been discontinued. Infectious diseases included in this category are those that result in the production of infective purulent material, drainage, or secretions, unless the disease is included in another isolation category that requires more rigorous precautions.

Specifications for Drainage/Secretion Precautions

1. Private room is not indicated.

2. Masks are not indicated.

3. Gowns are indicated if soiling is likely.

4. Gloves are indicated for touching infective material.

5. Hands must be washed after touching the patient or potentially contaminated articles and before you take care of another patient.

6. Articles contaminated with infective material should be discarded or bagged and labeled before being sent for decontamination and reprocessing.

BLOOD/BODY FLUID PRECAUTIONS

Blood/Body Fluid Precautions are designed to prevent infections that are transmitted by direct or indirect contact with infective blood or body fluids. Infectious diseases included in this category are those that result in the production of infective blood or body fluids, unless the disease is included in another isolation category that requires more rigorous precautions, for example, Strict Isolation.

Specifications for Blood/Body Fluid Precautions

1. Private room is indicated if patient hygiene is poor. A patient with poor hygiene does not wash hands after touching infective material, contaminates the environment with infective material, or shares contaminated articles with other patients. In general, patients infected with the same organism may share a room.

2. Masks are not indicated.

3. Gowns are indicated if soiling of clothes with blood or body fluids is likely.

4. Gloves are indicated for touching blood or body fluids.

5. Hands must be washed after touching the patient or potentially contaminated articles and before you take care of another patient.

6. Articles contaminated with blood or body fluids should be discarded or bagged and labeled before being sent for decontamination and reprocessing.

7. Care should be taken to avoid needle-stick injuries. Used needles should not be recapped or bent; they should be placed in a prominently labeled, puncture-resistant container designated specifically for such disposal.

8. Blood spills should be cleaned up promptly with a solution of 5.25% sodium hypochlorite diluted 1:10 with water.

Isolation Categories of Selected Diseases and Conditions

Disease or Condition	Isolation Category
Abscess, minor or limited	Drainage/Secretion
AIDS	Blood/Body Fluid
Chickenpox	Strict
Cholera	Enteric
Decubitus ulcer, minor	Drainage/Secretion
Diphtheria	Strict
Gastroenteritis, salmonella	Enteric
Hepatitis, viral, type A	Enteric
Hepatitis B	Blood/Body Fluid
Impetigo	Contact
Major wound or burn infection	Contact
Malaria	Blood/Body Fluid
Meningitis	Respiratory
Mumps	Respiratory
Pneumonic plague	Strict
Rabies	Contact
Skin or wound infection, minor	Drainage/Secretion
Tuberculosis	Tuberculosis (AFB)
Whooping cough	Respiratory

Protective Isolation

Protective, or reverse, isolation is a term used to describe procedures which are designed to protect a patient who has a diminished or absent ability to combat infection. Such a condition can be caused by chemotherapy for cancer, immunosuppressive drugs for transplantation therapy, extensive burns, or a congenital defect of the immune system, for example.

Some hospitals protect such a patient by using a portable, clear plastic unit that encloses the patient and his bed. The nurse remains outside the unit and reaches through armholes with attached gloves to care for the patient. Because she does not enter the unit, gowns, gloves, and masks are not needed. The purified air that is circulated through the unit is under positive pressure to keep contaminated air from entering the unit. The patient can see what is going on around him, but opportunities for sensory stimulation are minimal, and direct human contact is very limited. Examples of such portable units are the Life Island and the Laminar Air Flow Room.

Some hospitals have created permanent protective isolation units in which the nurse, family, and staff wear sterile gowns, masks, caps, and gloves at all times. Such units permit more social interaction and sensory stimulation, including touching, than do the temporary units. In most hospitals, however, such units are impractical.

Recent studies show that since most immune compromised patients become infected by their own microorganisms, protective isolation in the absence of a sterile environment provides little additional protection, and it is believed that strict adherence to proper isolation precautions will provide as much benefit as current technology permits.

CARE OF THE PATIENT WHO MUST BE ISOLATED

It is not uncommon for a nurse who is learning to care for a patient in an isolation unit to focus her attention mainly on the isolation procedures. The procedures are complex and require careful attention, but it is essential that you concentrate on the *care of the patient*, not just on the care of the pathogens. Emphasis on the patient is possible when you have become competent and confident in using the techniques of isolation.

Needs of the Patient

A high priority should be given to the patient's psychological responses to the isolation precautions. The concepts of *isolation* and *being isolated* will elicit a variety of emotional responses from both the patient and his family, but adequate preparation and support can make the experience less difficult.

The patient should understand the isolation precautions to be used and the rationale for each. He needs to know what isolation can be like and that feelings of being neglected, left out, rejected, and lonely are not uncommon. If you have discussed with him the fact that such responses are likely to occur, he is more likely to be able to verbalize his own feelings with you because he will know that they are quite normal.

A patient in reverse (or protective) isolation may experience many of the feelings experienced by any other patient in isolation, but there is a difference. *Being protected* from the dangers of a possible infection is not the same as being a *source of danger to others*. The latter is likely to engender feelings of being dirty, unacceptable, or undesirable.

Another priority for nursing care is the *prevention of sensory deprivation*. Adequate sensory stimulation must be provided to counteract the sensory restrictions and resulting monotony of an isolated environment. This is especially important for infants and small children because optimal psychological growth and development cannot occur in the absence of appropriate stimulation. A child who lacks the physiological defenses to fight infection often spends months or even years in a protective isolation unit, and must be provided with an

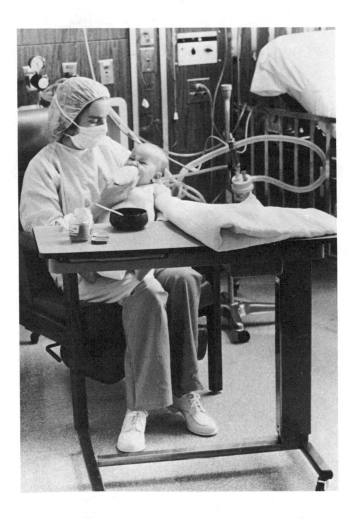

Figure 27.10 Holding and touching are especially important when isolation procedures are in effect and help to provide security and sensory stimulation even in this environment.

environment rich in opportunities for human interaction and intellectual stimulation. Such a child must be fondled, caressed, and played with even though the adult has to be garbed in sterile attire (Fig. 27.10).

Needs of the Nurse

Direct patient care often evokes psychological responses from the nurse that must be recognized and dealt with. Two of the most prevalent responses are related to *fear* and *resentment*.

Care of a patient in protective isolation can evoke fear of accidentally and unknowingly contaminating some part of the patient's environment, thereby endangering his life. The care of a patient with an infection or an infectious disease can also evoke a fear of personally contracting the disease. Even though your isolation technique is faultless, it is sometimes difficult

to dismiss the doubts and fears for your own safety that tend to creep into the situation.

The care of an isolated patient can also engender feelings of resentment ranging from mild irritation to anger. These responses can be provoked by stimuli such as:

The delay involved in having to don and remove a gown and gloves before each patient contact

The inconvenience of having to ask for, and sometimes wait for, assistance in carrying out some aspects of the isolation procedure

The feeling of being isolated from other patients and staff

The frustration of being confined in a unit for long periods with a patient who may be physically or psychologically difficult to care for

These feelings are usually intense if the nurse is assigned to an isolated patient for a number of days in succession. It is often necessary to negotiate a compromise between the *nurse's need* for relief and the *patient's need* for continuity of care by a familiar and trusted nurse.

ISOLATION TECHNIQUES

Special techniques and procedures which are used to control infection involve: the use of protective clothing, double bagging of contaminated materials, transportation of the patient, care of equipment, and ventilation.

Protective Clothing

Gown

An isolation gown is made of washable cotton or a disposable material. It opens down the back, extends below the wearer's knees, fastens at the neck and waist, and has snug-fitting wrist bands. It is worn with a cap and shoe covers in some settings.

PURPOSES. A *sterile* gown is worn in the operating room, in the delivery room, and in a protective isolation unit to keep *all* microorganisms from the patient. The outside of the gown is kept sterile; the inside is rendered unsterile by contact with the nurse's arms, hands, and uniform.

A (clean) gown is worn by a nurse to keep her uniform free of organisms when she cares for a patient with an infection or infectious disease. The outside of the gown is contaminated with infectious microorganisms; the inside is considered clean. Occasionally it is necessary for an isolated patient to leave his unit for special tests or treatments. In such situations, he wears a *clean* gown over his clothing to contain his pathogenic organisms and prevent the spread of his infection to others. The outside of the patient's gown is considered clean and the inside contaminated. This is the opposite of the condition of the nurse's gown as she works in the isolation unit.

The question that underlies the use of a gown is, "Who or what is being protected from what?"

- If the nurse's uniform is to be protected from the patient's pathogens, the nurse wears a clean gown.
- If the patient must be protected from all organisms, the nurse wears a sterile gown.
- If the people and the environment are to be protected from the patient's pathogens, the patient wears a clean gown over his clothing.

DONNING A GOWN. There is no special way to don a *clean* gown that is worn to protect your uniform; the gown is clean and your uniform is considered clean. Simply wash your hands thoroughly, and put the gown on. Then fasten the neck ties, overlap the back sections, and fasten the waist ties.

To don a *sterile* gown, you must cleanse your hands with a surgical scrub in preparation for putting on gloves after you are gowned. Because hands are never sterile, you cannot touch any part of the outside of a sterile gown except the neckband, a practice that is traditionally acceptable. The gown will be packaged with the neckband on top so that you can pick it up and let the gown unfold toward the floor. Carefully move your hands within the gown from the neckband to the inside of the shoulders and wiggle your hands and arms down the sleeves. You can manipulate the second sleeve by grasping it with the other hand while it is still covered by the first sleeve. Do not touch the outside of the gown with your bare hands. A person with gloved hands will help you by overlapping the back sections of your gown and fastening the ties.

REMOVING A GOWN. There are no microorganisms on a *sterile* gown. It poses no danger to the nurse, and there is no special way to remove it.

An *isolation gown* is never worn outside the patient's unit, so it must be removed before the nurse leaves the unit. A contaminated gown must be removed very carefully to prevent contamination of the nurse's arms and uniform:

1. Untie the waist ties so that you will not need to

touch them later with your clean hands. (Waist ties are considered contaminated.)

2. Remove your gloves, or wash your hands if gloves were not worn.

3. Unfasten the clean neckties with your clean hands. (The neckties have traditionally been considered clean even though the rest of the gown is contaminated.)

4. Slip your *clean hands under the clean neckband* and peel the gown down off your shoulders. *Do not touch the outside of the gown or let it touch your uniform.*

5. Roll the contaminated gown up, inside out, and discard it.

6. Wash your hands because they might have become contaminated as the gown was being removed.

REUSING A GOWN. The CDC recommends a *single-use technique* for gowns. A reuse technique should be used, therefore, only when resources are very limited and it is impossible for the nurse to obtain a clean gown each time she enters the isolated patient's unit. A reused gown, *properly handled,* is usually safer than no gown at all.

To remove a contaminated gown that must be reused, the following steps should be followed:

1. Remove your gloves or wash your hands before you unfasten the waist ties. Waist ties are considered contaminated, but they are clean in comparison to your grossly contaminated hands or gloves, and must be kept clean if the gown is to be reused.

2. Unfasten the contaminated waist ties.

3. Wash your hands again and unfasten the clean neckties.

4. Slip the clean fingers of one hand under the opposite wristband and pull the sleeve down over your hand.

5. Grasp the other sleeve with your covered hand and pull it off.

6. Take the gown off, making sure that the contaminated outside surface does not touch your clean hands or your uniform. The outside of the gown is contaminated; the inside is clean.

7. Bring the back edges together so that the gown is folded with the clean side in, and the contaminated side out.

8. Hang the gown up by the neck and shoulders in such a way that you can slip your clean hands inside it to don it the next time you need it.

To don a contaminated gown, the following steps apply:

1. Remember that only the inside of the gown and the neckband are considered clean. These are the only surfaces you can touch.
2. Pick the gown up by the neckband, carefully slip your hands inside the shoulders, and wiggle your hands and arms down the sleeves. You can manipulate a sleeve by grasping it with the hand that is still covered by the other sleeve.
3. Fasten the clean neckties with your still-clean hands.
4. Fasten the contaminated waist ties, realizing that your hands are now contaminated from doing so.

Masks

Masks filter both expired and inspired air and can be worn by either nurse or patient. Masks are worn by the nurse to prevent the droplet infection of an open wound, both during a dressing change and in the operating room, and when the nurse has a cold.

A mask is also worn by the nurse to protect herself from a patient who coughs and sneezes in her face and from infection by organisms that could become airborne during patient care. Both the nurse and the family wear masks for the protection of the patient in reverse isolation.

A mask can be worn by the patient to filter pathogenic organisms from his expired air while the nurse is caring for him, when visitors are present in his room, or while he is being transported to another department.

Masks are made of cotton, gauze, fiberglass, or paper. Some masks are effective; others are inadequate and give a false sense of security. A mask of thin or open gauze, for example, does not filter the air adequately, and a material that is too dense or rigid causes air currents and pathogens to flow under and over the mask.

A mask should be used only once and then be replaced by a fresh one; it should not be left dangling around the neck. A mask should be tied in a manner that causes it to conform to the contours of the face and that will keep it securely in place. Your mask should be untied with clean hands to protect your hair from contamination. Finally, a mask should be changed whenever it becomes wet because a wet mask permits the transmission of pathogens by capillary action and affords little or no protection. A mask might stay dry for as long as 1 to 2 hours in an air-conditioned operating room, or it might be wet after 10 minutes in a hot, humid patient unit. Guidelines for the use of masks should be based on careful research and should be specific to the material of the mask being used.

Gloves

Gloves are used as dictated by the prescribed type of isolation and are put on and removed in accordance with the directions in the first section of this chapter.

Double Bagging

Double bagging is a technique in which two bags are used to enclose contaminated equipment or supplies that are taken out of an isolation unit. A supply of inner bags is kept in the patient's unit; they are considered contaminated. Outer bags are stored outside the patient's unit and are therefore clean.

The fabric and material of the inner bag are determined by the type and expected treatment of the contents. For example:

For moist or wet dressings and equipment, use a waterproof inner bag.

For soiled linens, use a mesh bag or a water-soluble bag that dissolves when put in a washing machine.

For waste products that are to be incinerated, use a burnable inner bag.

For equipment that is to be autoclaved, use inner bags that can withstand the high temperatures of steam under pressure.

Items that are to be autoclaved or boiled should be rinsed thoroughly before they are bagged, to remove all protein that would coagulate at high temperatures and thereby coat and protect the pathogens.

The process of double bagging requires interaction between two people (Fig. 27.11). A helper stands outside the doorway of the patient's unit with her hands under the "cuff" of the clean outer bag, as you carefully lower the contaminated inner bag into the outer bag. You can touch the inside of the clean outer bag below the cuff as needed in order to insert the contaminated bag. The outside must be kept clean to prevent the spread of infection to the people who must handle the bag. After the clean cuff has been turned up and tied by the helper, the bag can be taken safely to the appropriate place for treatment of the contents.

Transportation of the Patient

Whenever it is necessary to transport an isolated patient from his unit to another department for a treatment or test, the following precautions must be taken to prevent the spread of infection.

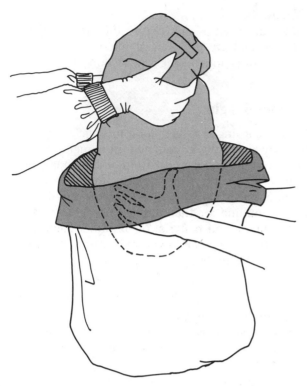

Figure 27.11 Double-bag protection against the spread of infection. The inner bag and the inside of the outer bag are contaminated (shaded areas). The outside of the outer bag is clean.

1. Prevent contamination of the stretcher or wheel-chair by covering it completely with a clean sheet.
2. Change or reinforce the patient's dressings as needed. Dress the patient in a clean gown; help him put on a mask if he is on respiratory precautions; and cover him with a clean sheet.
3. Notify the department to which the patient is being taken when the patient leaves his unit, and determine what precautions need to be taken on his arrival there.
4. When the patient returns, help him out of the wheelchair or off the stretcher in such a way that the vehicle does not become uncovered and contaminated.
5. If contamination does occur, cleanse the wheelchair or stretcher with a disinfectant before returning it to general use.

Care of Organic Wastes

If the patient is in a private room with a toilet, body wastes and uneaten food can be poured and scraped, without being splashed, into the toilet and flushed down the drain, because most municipal sewage disposal sys-

tems will render contaminated materials harmless. If there is no toilet in the room, waste materials can be dumped into a pail containing a disinfectant, and the pail can be emptied into a nearby toilet several times daily.

In primitive areas, contaminated materials can be buried at a distance from any water supply, or chloride of lime can be added to the materials which will render the pathogens harmless after several hours.

Care of Equipment

Whenever possible, all equipment needed for the care of the patient should be kept in his unit. When this cannot be done, you will need to devise ways to keep various pieces of equipment safe for general use. For example, you can protect a blood pressure cuff from contamination by slipping the sleeve of a clean gown over the patient's arm.

1. Spread the body of the gown over the bed linens and over the patient's chest.
2. Smooth the sleeve over the patient's arm, and then wrap the blood pressure cuff over the sleeve.
3. Remove the cuff without contaminating it and take it from the unit.
4. Disinfect the head of your stethoscope if it touched the patient's skin.

If there is no clock with a second hand in the room, place your watch on a clean paper towel so that it is visible; do not touch it while you take the patient's vital signs. Then either wash your hands before you pick the watch up, or pick it up with a paper towel or tissue and drop it into the clean hand of a helper.

Recent isolation guidelines no longer recommend the disinfection or special care of such things as money, books, mail, and games unless the item is visibly contaminated, because organisms do not live on a light, dry surface. Many textbooks and procedure manuals, however, still suggest that permission slips, consent forms, and other documents be placed between paper towels with only the place for the patient's signature exposed.

Ventilation

Some buildings are designed to provide negative air pressure in contaminated isolation units, and positive air pressure in reverse isolation units. Negative air pressure in an isolation unit means that clean air is drawn into the unit from the outside when the door is opened, and contaminated air does not flow out. This can be accomplished by an exhaust fan installed in the window or by a more elaborate central air-control unit.

Positive air pressure within a protective isolation unit means that purified, filtered air is brought into the room under enough pressure so that it flows out of the room when the door is opened, thereby preventing the flow of possibly contaminated outside air into the sterile environment.

Other Aspects of Infection Control

Teaching

Teaching related to the control of infection may involve a single person, a family, a neighborhood, or an entire community. During a flood or other disaster, for example, a community may need immediate information in order to cope with a contaminated water supply or disrupted sewage disposal. A crisis such as a "flu" epidemic calls for concentrated and coordinated action by a health care team to avert the mass infection of many citizens.

Case Finding

In addition to the early detection of infection and the use of appropriate barrier techniques, the nurse is often responsible for locating people with a given infection or people likely to become infected. The school nurse, for example, must often seek out children with pediculosis, scabies, or ringworm if the disease is known or suspected to be prevalent in her school. The community health nurse may be asked to make a follow-up visit to patients who have been discharged from a hospital unit that has had a large number of nosocomial infections.

If there is a high incidence of a certain disease in a given neighborhood or following a specific social event, the community health nurse may be asked to help locate potential victims. She may also be assigned the task of helping to locate the contacts of a patient with venereal disease.

Reporting

The laws and policies that regulate the reporting of infections are complex and frequently changed. Some infections must be reported only to the local health official or to the hospital's infection control committee; others must be reported to the state Department of Health or to the National Center for Disease Control. Some infections need be reported only if there is an epidemic, whereas a single case of another infection must be reported. For example, each one of the final cases of smallpox around the world had to be reported to the appropriate department of the World Health Organization.

Infections are reported in order to trace the spread of infectious diseases, to predict significant outbreaks or epidemics, to evaluate the effectiveness of existing infection controls, and to provide a basis for the development of new techniques, policies, and laws.

Research

Personnel at the CDC, members of infection control committees, and nurse-epidemiologists are some of the people engaged in research designed to improve the care of both people who have infections and those who are highly susceptible to infection. One such study, for example, showed that the respiratory droplets from a person with TB were not easily picked up by air currents after the particles had dropped. Therefore, the greatest danger of infection came from inhaling air within 3 ft of a TB patient's nose and mouth, while the *droplets were still airborne*. As a result of this information, current isolation techniques no longer consider everything in the patient's room contaminated, and the danger of inhaling infected droplets can be counteracted either by having the patient wear a mask to prevent the release of pathogens into the air or by having the nurse wear a mask to keep from inhaling infectious droplets.

PATIENT TEACHING

In a hospital situation, each patient must be taught how to help *protect himself from nosocomial infection*. He should be taught the rudiments of *medical asepsis*. He needs to know, for example, that hospital floors are contaminated, that he should wear slippers to protect his feet, and that objects from the floor should not be placed on his bed.

Each patient should be taught the elements of *surgical asepsis*. He needs to know how to cooperate during a sterile procedure, that he must not touch anything, and that he should not laugh, sneeze, or cough across a sterile field. Above all, the patient needs to know that he has a *right to speak out* if his health and safety are jeopardized by the faulty aseptic technique of any health care worker.

Much of this knowledge seems simple and commonplace, but it is unknown to many. You will need to sit down with the patient and his family and help them identify the factors which are relevant in their current situation and devise a feasible way to protect all those who are involved.

RELATED ACTIVITIES

Habits are hard to break, and unsafe techniques of medical asepsis are not likely to be permanently changed

Patient Teaching Related to Infection

To successfully protect themselves and others from infection, the patient and family need to know:

- How diseases are transmitted from one person to another
- How transmission of diseases can be blocked
- That the pathogens for each disease or set of symptoms have a specific portal of entry and exit
- How to prevent or eliminate sources of infection by such things as proper refrigeration, disposal of wastes, cleanliness, sanitation, and disinfection of sickroom equipment and supplies
- How to use basic sterile techniques in caring for wounds
- That hands must be washed *after* such activities as using the toilet, blowing one's nose, and changing diapers
- That hands must be washed *before* such activities as caring for a baby, giving an insulin injection, or dressing a wound
- That people with infections should be kept away from babies, small children, and old or debilitated people
- That resistance to infection can be increased by improved health, immunizations, and adequate medical supervision

by merely criticizing a nurse's performance. It is important, therefore, that you begin to develop a repertoire of motivational strategies which will enable you to work with your colleagues to prevent and control infection.

It is important (and often very easy) to identify faulty techniques and unsafe practices, but it is difficult to change those practices. An appropriate first step is to *get the facts.* Consult with the infection control nurse, or contact the Centers for Disease Control in Atlanta, Georgia, to determine whether the behavior you observed is truly unsafe or merely different from what you were taught.

If the technique or procedure is potentially unsafe, proceed with a combination of assertiveness, diplomacy, and tact. Avoid putting anyone on the defensive, and try to engage all involved persons in a process of mutual problem solving. Begin to read the journals of

nursing leadership and nursing management for hints on how other groups have solved similar problems in preparation for the time when you will be in a leadership position. In the meantime, perfect your own skills so that you can be an effective role model for others.

SUGGESTED READINGS

Anderson, David: AIDS: An update on what we know now. *RN* 1986; 49(3):49–56.

Bauer, Deborah: Preventing the spread of hepatitis B in dialysis units. *Am J Nurs* 1980 Feb; 80(2):260–261.

Brandt, Shirley L, and Patricia Benner: Infection control in hospitals: What are the challenges? *Am J Nurs* 1980 March; 80(3):432–434.

Hargiss, Clarice O, and Elaine Larson: Infection control—how to collect specimens and evaluate results. *Am J Nurs* 1981 Dec; 81(12):2166–2174.

Hargiss, Clarice O, and Elaine Larson: Guidelines for prevention of hospital acquired infections. *Am J Nurs* 1981 Dec; 81(12):2175–2183.

Jackson, Marguerite M, and Patricia Lynch: Isolation practices: A historical perspective. *Am J Infect Control.* 1985 Feb; 13(1):21–31.

Nadolny, Mary Diane: Infection control in hospitals—what does an infection control nurse do? *Am J Nurs* 1980 March; 80(3):430–431.

National Centers for Disease Control: *Guideline for Handwashing and Hospital Environmental Control, 1985.* Washington, DC, U.S. Government Printing Office.

National Centers for Disease Control: *Guideline for Isolation Precautions in Hospitals.* Washington, DC, U.S. Government Printing Office, 1983.

Nursing Photobook: *Controlling Infection.* Hicksville, NY, Skillbook Company, 1982.

O'Byrne, Carole: Clinical detection and management of postoperative wound sepsis. *Nurs Clin No Am* 1979 Dec; 14(4):727–742.

Palmer, Monica B: *Infection Control: A Policy and Procedure Manual.* Philadelphia, Saunders, 1984.

Solomon, Jacqueline, and Patricia Grant Higgins. Plague: alive, deadly, and all too easily misdiagnosed. *RN* 1983 Aug; 46(8):45–47.

Wood, Jacqueline: Exotic diseases—communicable, dangerous and, yes, possible! *Can Nurse* 1982 Feb; 78(2):18–22.

28

Sensory Status

Prerequisites and/or Suggested Preparation
Knowledge of the anatomy and physiology of the central and peripheral nervous systems is prerequisite preparation for this chapter. Suggested preparation includes an understanding of the basic concepts of health, stress, human needs, and individual development (Chapters 7, 8, 13, and 15).

An infant in an incubator, a child in an isolation unit, a young man in an intensive care unit, and an elderly woman in a monotonous nursing home all share a common danger—a potential alteration in their sensory status which will threaten both their psychological and their physical well-being. The sensory deprivation of a restricted environment can retard the normal development of the infant and child, the excessive stimuli of an intensive care unit can cause fatigue and delirium in the young man, and the elderly woman may succumb to deep depression and hopelessness.

These potential hazards can be averted by a holistic approach to nursing in which the nurse is as attentive to the mental and emotional needs of the patient as she is to the physiological needs. Since either sensory deprivation or sensory overload can cause serious psychological and physical problems, it is important for the nurse to do an early and thorough assessment of each patient's sensory status, and follow that assessment with vigorous nursing intervention.

ASSESSMENT OF SENSORY STATUS

Nursing care related to the patient's sensory needs must begin with an adequate assessment of his current status, followed by an evaluation of his immediate environment, and the potential risks to his well-being. Assessment of the patient's sensory status includes four major areas: (1) general appearance and behavior, (2) related health history, (3) psychosocial status, and (4) physiological function.

Collection of Data

The amount and kind of data collected about a patient's sensory status, and the sequence in which the data are sought, are influenced by the patient's condition, the nature of the environment, and the probable duration of the current situation. For example, data related to a comatose patient will of necessity be restricted to his *physiological* responses such as an assessment of his reflexes and his responses to painful stimuli. The *frequency* of assessing a comatose patient will depend upon whether the patient has just been brought into the emergency room, or has been in a coma for several months.

A thorough assessment of a patient's coordination, balance, cranial nerve function, and thought processes would not usually be warranted for a person in a dermatology clinic. On the other hand, a patient who has been described as confused needs an extensive assessment to determine whether the observed behaviors are caused by sensory deficits, disease, a drug reaction, unbearable stress, or environmental factors. Practical considerations of time and energy will also influence the extent of a given assessment.

Evaluation of Data

In order to be meaningful, the data collected must be compared with two standards: (1) the norm for a healthy person of the same age, and (2) the individual's usual or previous status. With respect to the first standard, it is important to know, for example, that a positive Babinski test (plantar reflex) is *normal* for infants up to the age of 1 year, but a positive Babinski is *pathological* in older children and adults.

In terms of the second standard, a description of a patient's current sensory status may be meaningless unless it can be compared with his previous sensory status. A state of confusion in a patient with a long history of mental illness has a different significance than a similar state of confusion in a person who was a clear and logical thinker until 1 week ago.

Information about *normal responses* to various tests of sensory status is available in textbooks and manuals, but information about a given patient's *prior status* can be obtained only from the patient, family and friends, or from earlier health records.

TYPES OF ASSESSMENTS

When assessing the sensory status of a given patient, the nurse first does a general, overall assessment followed by more specific psychosocial and physical assessments when indicated. This initial assessment includes an appraisal of the patient's appearance and behavior, and a relevant health history.

General Appearance and Behavior

This assessment may not be a separate activity—it can be done in conjunction with other nursing activities by an observant nurse who knows what to look for and who *consciously* makes detailed observations. The observations to be made are categorized below, and each category is followed by examples of adjectives which might be used to describe the patient:

> Posture: erect, slumped, lively, self-conscious, confident
>
> Grooming: clean, dirty, fashionable, disheveled, careless

Facial expression: alert, bewildered, dull, expressionless

Mood: fearful, angry, calm, cooperative, combative, sad

Movements: coordinated, awkward, balanced, clumsy, graceful

Observations of the patient's appearance and behavior will provide clues for more detailed assessments. For example, if the individual tends to drop things or knock things over, his cerebral and cerebellar function (coordination and balance) should be tested and his vision should also be tested since the problem could be caused by impaired depth perception or a limited field of vision.

Related Health History

An adequate health history will indicate areas of possible neurologic dysfunction which should be assessed in greater depth, and which will also indicate any need for possible safety precautions. If, for example, the patient gives a history of dizziness and fainting during the preceding few days, measures must be taken to protect him from injury and the staff from charges of neglect or malpractice if he should fall.

Not all nursing history forms or guidelines include an assessment of sensory status, but the professional nurse should be alert to indications that such an assessment is needed and be able to collect the necessary data. There is no correct or prescribed set of questions to be asked; the patient should be asked if he is experiencing, or has experienced, any of the following conditions:

Headaches

Weakness

Muscle spasms

Tremors

Syncope (fainting)

Vertigo (dizziness)

Tinnitus (ringing in ears)

Paresthesias (abnormal sensations)

Paralysis

Blurred vision

Recent injury

Anesthesia (loss of sensation)

Unconsciousness

Recent infection

For each affirmative response, it is important to determine the approximate date of onset, frequency of occurrence, duration, location, circumstances surrounding occurrences, and warning signs (if any).

In addition to asking about the topics listed above, it is especially important that the nurse ask the patient about any *changes* he has noticed, such as:

Changes in ability to perform everyday activities?

Changes in ability to concentrate, remember, express ideas?

Changes in mood, personality, relationships?

The last three areas of concern will help to direct the nature and scope of additional mental and emotional assessments which may be indicated.

PHYSIOLOGICAL ASSESSMENTS

Eight aspects of physiological function are commonly assessed by the nurse, although not all eight are assessed on every patient, nor on a single patient every time. These aspects are:

Level of consciousness

Pupils

Sensory function

Peripheral nerve function

Functioning of cerebrum and cerebellum

Motor strength

Reflexes

Cranial nerve function

The determination of which aspects of sensory function should be assessed is made by evaluating the data obtained from the health history, the patient's medical and nursing diagnoses, his progress to date, and his current condition.

Level of Consciousness

The first assessment to be made—the patient's level of consciousness—is often done quickly and informally. If the patient is alert and is talking coherently and sensibly, if his eyes are open, and he is making purposeful movements, he is fully conscious and no further assessment of consciousness is needed.

If there is reason to believe that the patient is *not* fully conscious, a detailed assessment should be made, using an objective tool such as the Glasgow Coma Scale.

Glasgow Coma Scale

For many years, a person's level of consciousness has been described by the use of adjectives such as alert or stuporous. The following six terms were commonly used:

Alert: fully responsive
Lethargic: drowsy but responds appropriately
Obtunded: responds slowly and dully
Stuporous: responds to commands
Semi-comatose: responds only to painful stimuli
Comatose: wholly unresponsive

These six terms were open to interpretation and as a result were imprecise and often confusing.

In 1974, the Glasgow Coma Scale was devised at the University of Glasgow to provide a standardized way of describing a person's level of consciousness. This scale assigns a score to each of three aspects of consciousness: visual, verbal, and motor responses. The resulting numerical score provides assessment data which are understandable and precise.

The advantages of the Glasgow Coma Scale are that it is *uniform* (the same rating is given by all observers), *quick* (numbers are used for charting and reporting), and *specific* enough to monitor fairly small changes in the patient's level of consciousness.

Using the Glasgow Coma Scale

To use the Glasgow Coma Scale, you determine whether or not a given response is testable, and then start with a mild or minimal stimulus. Since it is important to determine and record the patient's *best* score, it is necessary to start testing with the mildest stimulus possible. In a normal tone of voice, repeat your questions or commands as necessary. If the patient does not respond to this verbal stimulus, call the person by his first name, use a louder tone, and even shout before you proceed to apply a painful stimulus.

If the patient does not respond to loud, emphatic verbal commands, apply painful pressure. This can be done by pressing a blunt object such as a pen or pencil to the cuticle of the finger nail (the base of the nail where it meets the skin) or by pressing your finger in a circular motion over the patient's sternum. *Purposeful movements* in response to pain include withdrawing from the source of pain, or trying to push away the examiner's hand. It is important to apply the pain to a spot which the patient can reach; pinching the patient's calf or achilles tendon may not be a valid stimulus because the patient may be unable to reach those areas to try to brush the stimulus away.

When testing the patient's verbal responses, you need to individualize and vary your questions, especially if assessments are repeated frequently. The patient who is asked repeatedly "What is your name?" and "Do you know what day this is?" may become annoyed and refuse to answer and thereby receive a lower and inaccurate score. Orientation to time, place, and person can be determined by asking about visitors, what was eaten at the previous meal, and what is likely to happen later in the day.

If the patient curses in response to a painful stimulus, further testing is needed to determine whether it is an appropriate verbal response (with a score of 5) or whether the patient can utter only single, inappropriate words (score of 3).

When testing *motor responses*, it is wise to avoid the command "Squeeze my hand" because it is difficult to differentiate between a grasp reflex and obeying the

TABLE 28.1 GLASGOW COMA SCALE

Response	Behavior	Score
Eye-opening response	Opens eyes spontaneously, purposefully	4
	Opens eyes upon command to do so	3
	Opens eyes only in response to pain	2
	Does not open eyes at all	1
	Untestable (eyes bandaged or swollen shut)	U
Verbal response	Fully responsive and oriented	5
	Confused regarding time, place, or person	4
	Responds with inappropriate words, phrases	3
	Makes unintelligible sounds; moans, groans	2
	Makes no speech sounds at all	1
	Untestable (tracheotomy); other intubation)	U
Motor response	Moves limbs upon command	5
	Moves limbs purposefully in response to pain	4
	Flexes arms in response to pain*	3
	Extends arms in response to pain*	2
	Does not move at all	1
	Untestable (limb immobilized by cast, other)	U

The total score will range from 3–14 if all responses are testable. The *higher* the score, the *higher* the level of brain function.

*See Figure 28.1.

because different neurological conditions can yield the same overall score.

For example, the *total* scores of the following patients are identical, but the *different subscores* show that the nursing observations to be made, and the nursing care to be given, will vary, as will the medical diagnosis and treatment of each patient.

	PATIENT A	PATIENT B
Best eye-opening response	4	2
Best verbal response	1	2
Best motor response	2	3
Total score	7	7

Pupils

The assessment of a person's pupils is commonly called a *pupil check;* it assesses size and shape, reaction to light, and accommodation. Normal pupillary responses are frequently recorded as PERLA (*Pupils Equal Reactive to Light and Accommodation*) or PNERLA (*Pupils Normal in size and shape Equal Reactive to Light and Accommodation*).

Size and Shape

Pupils are examined first under normal lighting conditions. Pupils should be round and approximately equal in size. A normal adult pupil measures approximately 3.5mm. Pupils are smaller in infancy, dilate to maximum size in adolescence, and then become smaller in old age. Pupil size is an important diagnostic measure, and is also an indicator of changes in the patient's condition. A very constricted pupil is called a *pinpoint* pupil, and a very large pupil is called a *dilated* pupil; a marked difference in pupil size is a significant diagnostic finding. Accuracy in measurement and recording is essential, and many nurses who must do frequent pupil checks carry a small pocket-size card which enables them to compare a patient's pupil size with an accurate measurement (Fig. 28.2*a,b,c,*).

Reaction to Light

To test the pupil's reaction to light, move a penlight from the side of the patient's head toward the pupil to be tested. The pupil response is called a *direct light reflex,* and a normal pupil constricts briskly. The other pupil constricts slightly in what is called a *consensual light reflex.* Both pupils should be tested for the direct light reflex, and observed for a consensual reflex. Failure of one or both pupils to react to light indicates a serious pathological condition (Fig. 28.3).

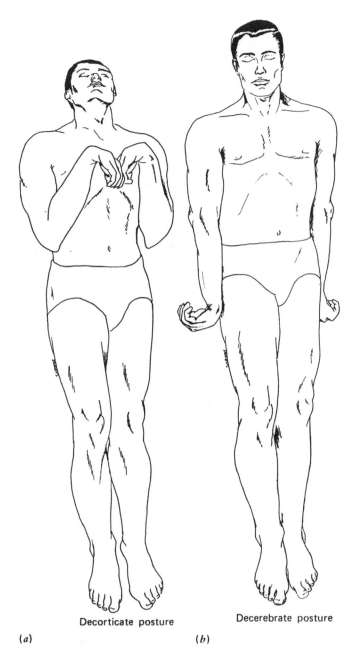

Decorticate posture   Decerebrate posture

(a)   *(b)*

Figure 28.1 *Decorticate and decerebrate posturing in response to painful stimuli. (a) Decorticate posture indicates damage above upper brain stem. Flexion of arms in response to pain equals score of 3 on Glasgow Coma Scale. (b) Decerebrate posture indicates damage to mid-brain and brain stem. Rigid extension of arms score a 2 on Glasgow Coma Scale.*

command. "Touch your chin" and "scratch your arm" are more useful commands.

An overall score of 14 indicates that the patient is fully conscious, while a patient with a score of 7 or below is usually considered to be in a coma. It is important to record the score for each subscale separately

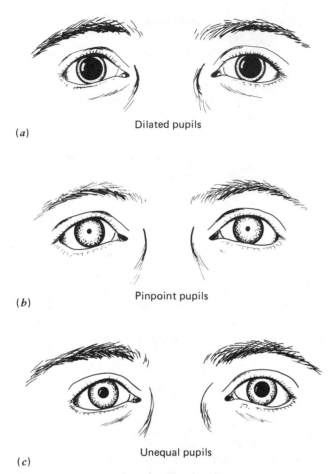

(a)

Dilated pupils

(b)

Pinpoint pupils

(c)

Unequal pupils

Figure 28.2 *Assessment of pupil size and shape.*
(a) Pupils are dilated, fixed, equal in size, regular in shape, and do not react to light. (b) Pupils are small (pinpoint), fixed, equal in size, regular in shape, and do not react to light. (c) Pupils are unequal in size, one or both may react to light and accommodation, depending upon underlying pathology.

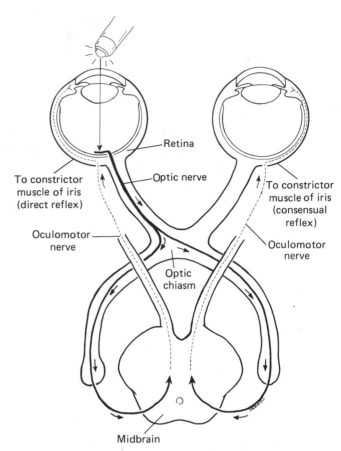

Figure 28.4 *Direct and consensual light reflex. Direct reflex: light shone directly on retina causes pupil of that eye to constrict. Consensual reflex: light shone into one eye normally causes pupil of other eye to constrict as a result of impulses sent across the optic chiasm.*

Accommodation

Accommodation is the adjustment of the eye for various distances, and is made possible by the eye's ability

Pupil size in millimeters

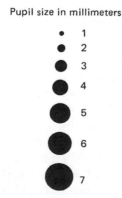

1
2
3
4
5
6
7

Figure 28.3 *Pupil size chart.*

to change the curvature of the lens in order to focus an image on the retina. Accommodation decreases with age. Accommodation is tested by holding your finger or a pencil in front of the patient, and asking him to follow it with his eyes as you move it toward him. The normal response is for his eyes to converge (cross) and the pupils to constrict as the object approaches his nose (Fig. 28.4).

Specific Sensory Functions

Vision

VISUAL ACUITY. Visual acuity (sharpness, clearness) is tested with standardized materials, the most familiar being the Snellen chart. The individual is positioned 20 feet from the chart, and asked to read down the chart until he can no longer read at least half the letters of a given line. A number at the edge of the chart indicates the distance at which a person with normal vision can read that line, and vision of the individual being tested is noted by recording both distances. For example, a person's vision is said to be 20/100 if at 20 feet he can read only the large letters which a person with normal vision can read at 100 feet.

A modified chart using only the letter E is used for children and illiterate persons. When this chart is used, the person is asked to indicate with his arms or fingers the direction in which the letter E is facing—up, down, right, or left.

VISUAL FIELDS. A person's field of vision refers to that portion of space which he can see without moving his eyes (Fig. 28.5*a,b*). The field of vision may be limited by a *central defect* which produces a blind spot in front of the person or by a *peripheral defect* which produces one or more blind spots at the edge of the field of vision. A central defect hampers reading or close work, while a peripheral defect creates a safety problem when a person is walking or driving.

To test peripheral vision, position yourself directly in front of the patient at eye level. Ask the patient to look straight ahead and cover one eye. Cover your eye opposite the one the patient is covering (e.g., his left eye, your right eye) so that your fields of vision are approximately the same. This will enable you to estimate the probable size of the patient's field of vision. Hold a finger at arm's length (outside the patient's field of vision) and slowly move your finger in until it enters the patient's field of vision. If your field of vision is normal, the patient should detect your finger at about the same point that you do. Check at least six points. Locate and record your findings in terms of the numbers on the face of a clock.

Hearing

WHISPER TEST. Ask the patient to cover one ear. Stand out of sight (so patient cannot read your lips), and whisper a few words. Normal response: the patient can repeat your message. Use different words to test the other ear.

If the whisper test indicates defective hearing, two additional tests are used.

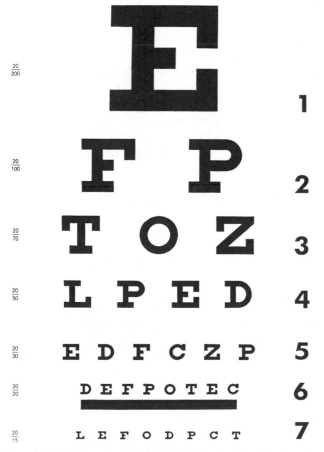

Figure 28.5(a) Standard Snellen Chart for testing visual activity.

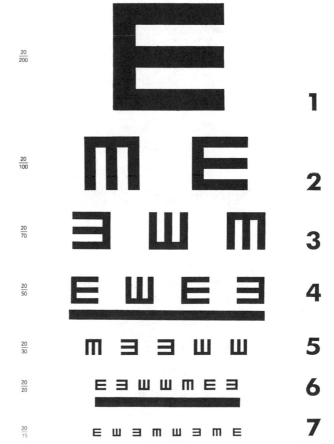

Figure 28.5(b) Modified Snellen Chart for children or illiterate persons.

RINNES TEST. This test compares the conduction of sound by air and bone. Place a vibrating tuning fork behind the ear over the mastoid process. When the patient can no longer hear the sound (bone conduction), move the tuning fork in front of the ear canal. Normal response: the patient can still hear it (air conduction).

WEBER TEST. This test assesses for lateralization of hearing. Place a vibrating tuning fork at the middle of the patient's forehead, and ask where he hears it, i.e., on one or both sides. Normal response: the sound is heard equally on both sides.

General Peripheral Nerve Function

A gross or preliminary assessment of peripheral nerve function is done by testing the patient's perception of pain, vibration, objects, and temperature.

Pain: Normal response is the ability to feel a pin-prick.

Vibration: Normal response is the ability to tell when the vibrations of a tuning fork stop.

Tactile discrimination: Normal response is the ability to recognize a familiar object such as a coin or key by *touch only*. This also tests the functioning of the cerebral cortex.

Temperature: (This is usually tested only if the person's perception of pain is abnormal.) Normal response is the ability to distinguish between hot and cold.

An inability to feel one or more of these stimuli indicates the need for more specific and detailed assessments.

Cerebellar Function

An initial, gross assessment of the cerebellum is done by testing the individual's coordination and balance.

Coordination

The factors which determine coordination are *accuracy, smoothness,* and *symmetry* of movement. Three commonly used tests of coordination are:

Close eyes and touch nose with alternating fore-fingers

Pat knees, alternating palms and backs of hands while gradually increasing speed

Walk heel to toe in straight line with eyes open

Balance

The *Romberg* test is used to test balance. Ask the patient to stand with his eyes closed and feet together. Stand close to the patient for safety in case he should lose his balance. The normal response is a *mild* swaying (negative Romberg sign).

Motor Strength

When you test for motor strength, it is not advisable to use the traditional hand grasp test because it may elicit a misleading strong grasp reflex. Two more reliable tests of motor strength are:

1. Ask the patient to close his eyes and extend his arms with palms up. If there is motor weakness, the palms will turn over and the arms will slowly drop.
2. Ask the patient to sit and hold his legs out for 10 seconds. If there is motor weakness, the affected leg will start to drop.

Reflexes

Plantar Response (Babinski)

With a moderately sharp object such as a key, stroke the side of the sole, from the heel up to the base of the little toe and then across the ball of the foot to the base of the big toe. The normal response after age 1: toes flex or do not move (negative Babinski). The pathological response: extension of big toe and fanning out of other toes (positive Babinski) (Fig 28.6).

Patellar Reflex (knee jerk)

Position patient with his knee bent and leg hanging freely. Place one hand on the patient's thigh and strike the tendon joint just below the kneecap with a reflex hammer. Normal response: knee extends and the quadriceps muscle contracts (Fig. 28.7).

Ankle Reflex (Achilles reflex)

Strike the achilles tendon with a reflex hammer. Normal response: plantar flexion (Fig. 28.8).

Biceps Reflex

Flex the patient's arm with the palm down and slightly lower than the elbow. Place your thumb in the antecubital space over the biceps tendon. Strike your thumb with the reflex hammer. Normal response: slight flexion of elbow and contraction of biceps muscle (Fig. 28.9).

Triceps Reflex

Flex the patient's arm with the palm slightly lower than elbow. Strike the triceps tendon just above the back of the elbow. Normal response: extension of elbow and contraction of triceps muscle (Fig. 28.10).

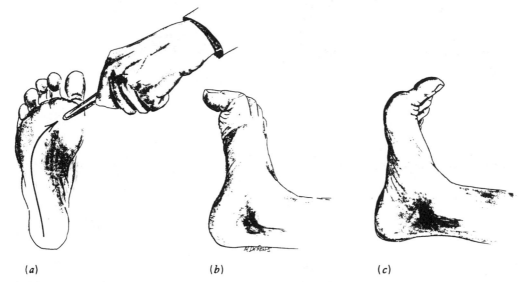

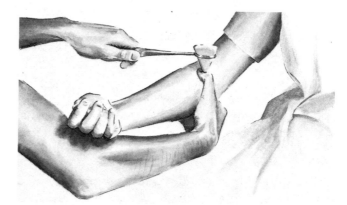

(a)   (b)   (c)

Figure 28.6 *Plantar response (Babinski). (a) Note direction of stroke. (b) Normal response (negative Babinski). (c) Abnormal response (positive Babinski).*

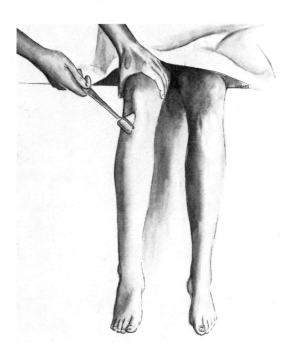

Figure 28.9 *Biceps Reflex. Normal response: contraction of biceps muscle and slight flexion of elbow.*

Figure 28.7 *Patellar Reflex (knee jerk). Normal response: quadriceps muscle contracts and knee extends.*

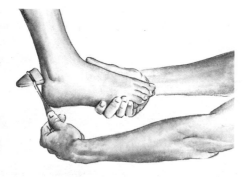

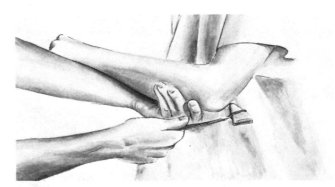

Figure 28.8 *Achilles Tendon Reflex. Normal response: plantar (downward flexion of ankle).*

Figure 28.10 *Triceps Reflex. Normal response: contraction of triceps muscle and slight extension of elbow.*

Notation System for Recording
Reflex Findings

> 0 = no response
> + = low response
> + + = normal response
> + + + = brisker than normal response
> + + + + = hyperactive, very brisk response

Cranial Nerves

I. Olfactory (smell)

Ask the patient to close his eyes and block one nostril. Place a familiar substance or object under the open nostril. Normal response: patient is able to detect odor. Use a different substance to test the other nostril.

II. Optic (vision)

Use tests for visual acuity and peripheral vision described above.

III. Occulomotor, IV. Trochlear, and VI. Abducens (eye movement)

Test the six cardinal fields of gaze by holding a pencil or finger directly in front of the patient. Direct him to hold his head still and follow the movements of the pencil with his eyes only. Move the pencil from the center outward in all six directions. Normal response: both eyes move together in all six directions.

V. Trigeminal (movement of jaw; facial and corneal sensation)

Movement of jaw: Ask the patient to move his jaw from side to side and up and down, and to clench his teeth. Normal response: the patient is able to do so.

Facial sensation: Have the patient close his eyes. Touch his forehead, cheek, and chin with a wisp of cotton. Normal response: he can discern when and where you are touching him.

Corneal sensation: This is not done routinely because it is very uncomfortable. When this test is indicated, you touch the cornea with a wisp of cotton. Normal response: blinking and tearing.

VII. Facial (facial expression; movement of eyelids)

Ask the patient to grimace (smile, frown, wrinkle his forehead, raise his eyebrows). Normal response: the ability to do so.

VIII. Acoustic (hearing)

Use tests of hearing described above.

IX. Glossopharyngeal, and X. Vagus (oropharyngeal sensations and motor function)

Gag reflex: touch the uvula (back of the throat) with a tongue depressor. Normal response: the patient will gag.

XI. Spinal Accessory (movement of head and shoulders)

Ask the patient to:

> Turn his head from side to side
> Lower his chin against resistance from your hand
> Shrug his shoulders while you push them down
> Push his forehead against your hand

Normal response: the patient is able to do so.

XII. Hypoglossal (movements of tongue)

Ask patient to stick out his tongue. Normal response: no tremor or sidewise deviation.

Ongoing Monitoring

After their initial assessment, patients with identified or potential sensory disturbances should be monitored at regular intervals. At least three *general* areas should be checked regularly, and if deficits are found, more specific testing should be done. The general areas to be monitored are: (1) LOC (level of consciousness), (2) ADL (activities of daily living), and (3) motor strength. In many instances, this monitoring can be done by carefully observing the way the patient responds to you, moves about, talks, and tends to his needs. If a deficit or change in status is noted or suspected, testing relevant to that deficit should be done promptly.

Vital Signs

Vital signs are not a routine part of the assessment of a patient's sensory status because a change in vital signs usually occur as a *consequence* of serious neurological dysfunction and not as a prelude to it.

SENSORY STIMULATION

The colorful mobile over an incubator and pictures on the wall in a nursing home are not placed there as decorations—they represent efforts to meet the patients' needs for sensory stimulation.

Sensory stimulation is a basic human need. It is essential for optimal psychological and physical development. Sensory stimulation promotes mental activity, fosters creativity, influences motivation, and prompts physical activity (Fig. 28.11).

Whether or not a person's need for stimulation is being met is determined by the quantity and quality of sensory input and by a person's ability to process the stimuli received. Sensory stimulation ranges along a continuum from *insufficient* stimulation (sensory deprivation) to *excessive* stimulation (sensory overload). Either extreme can produce disorganized thinking and uncomfortable feelings ranging from mild discomfort and confusion to panic and hallucinations.

It has been said that each person seeks *sensoristasis* (equilibrium of sensory function) just as he seeks homeostasis (equilibrium of physiological function). His need for sensory stimulation seems to be balanced by a need to protect himself from excessive stimulation. This balance is highly individualized; the amount of stimulation that is satisfying to one person can be excessive for a second person and boring for a third. A

person's tolerance for deviations from his preferred level of stimulation is influenced to some degree by his personality, inner resources, and preferred lifestyle.

Nursing Interventions

There are many nursing actions that will minimize the effects of undesirable levels of sensory stimulation. One of the most needed interventions is the initiation of more research studies to find ways to *prevent* both sensory deprivation and sensory overload, especially in short-term acute care settings. Such studies need not be expensive or complex, but should seek answers to such basic concerns as the following questions:

- How could input from nurses help the architects and decorators of health care facilities reduce both sensory deprivation and sensory overload?
- What questions could be asked of patients upon admission that would help to identify those who

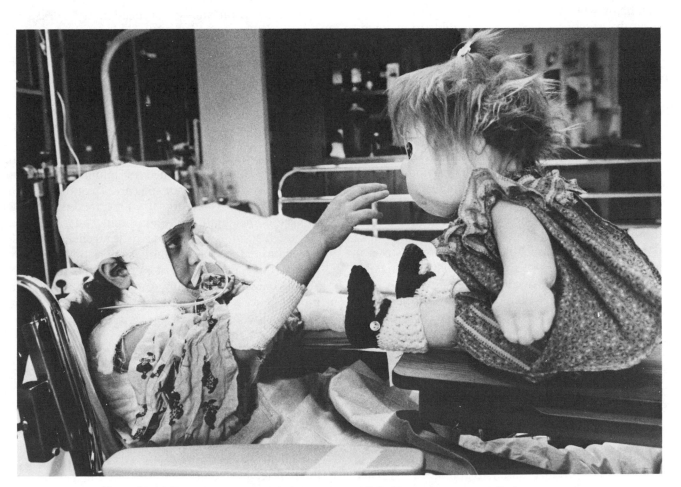

Figure 28.11 *Toys are an essential element in a child's life, and are especially important during a severe illness. Renee's tousled hair friend provides distraction from pain and discomfort, stimulates her mind and imagination, and is a source of comfort and reassurance.*

might be unusually susceptible to sensory deprivation or sensory overload?

- What kind of staff education programs would help nurses to modify coronary care procedures, for example, to reduce the incidence of such conditions as cardiac delirium?
- What patterns of patient-nurse communication are helpful and which are nonhelpful to a patient in either an overstimulating or a deprived environment?

Such nursing studies would provide a sound theoretical basis for making decisions about sensory deprivation and overload and would eventually result in improved nursing care.

SENSORY OVERLOAD

Stimuli that are excessive in number of intensity assault a person's senses and bombard him with sensations which he may be incapable of handling at the moment. The result, *sensory overload,* is comparable to blowing a fuse when electrical circuits are overloaded.

Causes

Sensory overload can occur at home, at work, at school, or in the hospital, and it is caused by the stimulation produced by an excessive number of people, objects, or activities in a limited space and time. The most frequently cited cause in nursing is the myriad of activities, equipment, and people in an intensive care unit. The noise of multiple monitors and machines; the scurry and flurry of dozens of nurses, technicians, physicians, and other workers; the bright lights; the strange odors; and the physical and psychological pain and distress all converge on the senses of an acutely ill and vulnerable patient, causing sensory overload. Even a relatively quiet nursing unit can overwhelm a patient who feels that there are too many health care workers, too many visitors, and too much equipment in too crowded a space. He is literally unable to take it all in, and he too suffers from sensory overload.

Symptoms

If the overload is moderate, the patient may simply look exhausted or give a verbal indication of his fatigue. If the overload is extreme or prolonged, the symptoms may produce either insomnia or excessive sleeping in an effort to withdraw from the barrage of stimuli. Other symptoms include disorientation, confusion, anxiety, and hallucinations.

Nursing Interventions

Everyone, sick or well, needs quiet moments at intervals throughout the day. This is hard to achieve in the hospital, and it can be equally difficult to achieve in some work and home situations. Some young mothers, for example, feel frantic and trapped by the incessant demands of their children; in fact some can find their only refuge in the bathroom.

The nursing interventions to alleviate sensory overload involve three types of activities. The nurse can (1) *block the input* of sensory stimulation, (2) help the patient *organize the stimuli,* or (3) teach him to *alter his response* to excessive stimuli.

Blocking Input

Any device or technique that can block the transmission of sensory stimuli is worthy of consideration when one is trying to reduce sensory overload. An eye mask or a folded washcloth across the patient's eyes, for example, will give relief from bright lights and the sight of incessant staff movement.

Earplugs, soft music via headphones, or "white sound" from a small fan will minimize confusing auditory stimuli; a deodorizer will reduce disturbing odors. A bad taste may seem like a minor problem to a healthy person, but a vile-tasting medication such as liquid potassium can seem like the last straw to a person who is nearly frantic from excessive stimuli. Every effort should be expended to make such medication palatable, thereby reducing sensory stimulation.

The stimuli of discomforts such as pain, nausea, and itching should be prevented or minimized by both medication and expert nursing care. Treatments can be scheduled to provide intervals of rest, and the number of visitors or length of visiting hours can be reduced. Although administrative and structural changes may be needed to reduce some stimuli, such as noise and confusing traffic patterns on a nursing unit, the nurse's attentiveness and ingenuity can do much to block the input of excessive stimuli.

Organizing Input

In addition to blocking as much excess stimulation as possible, you can help the patient to organize and make sense of the remaining stimuli. First of all, make sure that the patient knows whether it is day or night. In most settings, the normal changes in light and darkness throughout the day and night help to keep a person oriented. People who have been shipwrecked or imprisoned quickly try to devise a system for recording the passage of time and determining the date. Patients in an intensive care unit are often unable to do so; they are placed in windowless units with a constant level of lighting and are therefore unable to separate one day from another. If a patient is being fed intravenously he cannot even use the arrival of a breakfast or supper try to help him distinguish between morning and night (Fig. 28.12).

Whenever possible, institute a day-and-night cycle of lighting for the patient. If that cannot be done, make sure that you, the rest of the staff, and the family integrate data related to time and date into communications with the patient, even when he seems unresponsive. It may seem awkward to say, for example, "It's Tuesday morning, and it's crisp and cold outside—a typical September morning," but such an orientation can be as important as any other nursing action.

A patient will be less apprehensive and confused when he realizes that the ebb and flow of activity in the corridors is not random but is related to treatment schedules and changing shifts, when he knows that the beeping and clicking of machines have meaning for the staff, and knows that the strange sound heard each night is only the squeak of the rubber soles worn by an attendant on the night shift. Such sounds are easily distorted and misinterpreted by a patient who is fearful or disoriented.

A patient should be forewarned if environmental sounds might alarm him. He should be told, for example, that a patient in the next room is sometimes irrational so that an outburst of screaming from that room will not be so frightening. If there is another patient on the unit who repeatedly calls "Nurse, nurse," or "Help me, help me, please help me," the patient should know in advance that the other patient's cries are not being ignored by the staff and that he need not try to get out of bed to go and help the calling patient.

You can help the patient to make sense of the incoming stimuli by:

Listening carefully to the sounds the patient can hear and explaining any that are likely to be unfamiliar.

Watching for and explaining sights that could be upsetting to, or misinterpreted by, the patient,

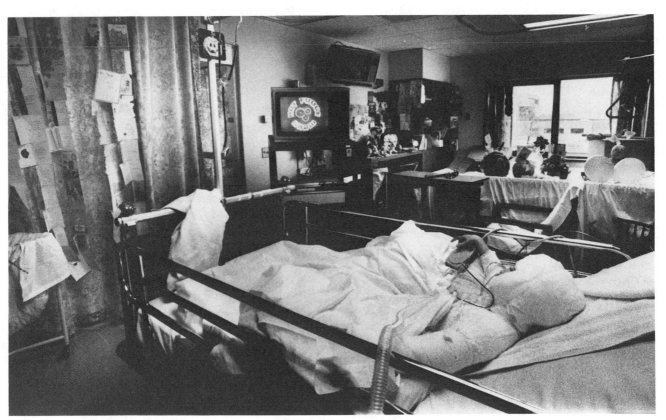

Figure 28.12 *Soon after surgery, while still swathed in bulky pressure dressings, Renee finds a measure of comfort in a favorite television program and an environment filled with the treasured possessions of a six year old. This picture illustrates the shift in nursing care from emphasis on a neat and tidy hospital unit to the structuring of an environment which provides sensory stimulation and satisfaction for the patient.*

especially those that are glimpsed only briefly or from a distance.

Explaining what you are doing and why in _simple, brief, and concrete_ terms. Explanations can be expanded at a later date, but long explanations at the moment often contribute to the sensory overload by adding even more information for the patient to process.

Altering Responses to Input

In addition to blocking some stimuli and helping the patient to make sense of the remainder, you can help the patient by teaching him to alter his responses to sensory input. There are a number of relaxation techniques that will help him to reduce his anxiety and tension despite continued sensory stimulation. The patient will still be aware of the stimuli but will be less upset by them. Some of these techniques were developed to help patients cope with pain or to promote relaxation during childbirth; others, such as transcendental medication (TM) are nonspecific. Some nurses prefer to adopt and use one specific technique; other nurses use selected elements of a number of techniques, depending on the nature and needs of the patient.

SENSORY DEPRIVATION

Sensory deprivation is a condition in which the available sensory stimulation is insufficient for a person's psychological well-being. The symptoms range from simple boredom and excessive sleeping to disorientation, confusion, anxiety, hallucinations, and illusions.

Under experimental conditions, subjects have been deprived of virtually all external stimuli for varying lengths of time. The subjects of such research are usually healthy young adults who know that they can drop out of the experiment at any time, and yet they each experience a variety of ill effects from sensory deprivation. In nonexperimental situations, the reduction of stimuli is usually less extreme, but the effect can be even greater because a patient is likely to be more susceptible to sensory deprivation than a healthy person might be.

Causes

The three main causes of sensory deprivation are: (1) inadequate sensory stimuli, (2) inability to receive stimuli, and (3) inability to process stimuli.

Inadequate Stimuli

Sensory deprivation can be the result of stimuli that are limited in quantity, quality, or both; the stimuli may be weak, infrequent, or monotonous. The adequacy of the stimuli may be unrelated to the condition of the patient's senses. He may have perfect vision and hearing, for example, bu sensory deprivation will occur if the stimuli are inadequate.

Inadequate sensory stimulation, often referred to as sensory restriction, can be caused by environmental conditions or by aspects of a patient's therapeutic regimen. _Environmental conditions_ that contribute to sensory restriction include:

Pale or colorless walls

Dim lights

Lack of either pictures or a window with a view

Absence of books, current magazines, newspapers, clocks, and calendar

A monotonous routine or schedule in which nothing interesting ever happens

Lack of social interaction

Aspects of therapy that contribute to sensory restriction include:

Immobilization in a cast, traction, circular bed, or Stryker frame

Isolation, either to protect others from the patient's pathogens or to protect the patient from possible infection

Bland diet, tube feedings, IV feedings

Restricted mobility because of IVs, monitors, oxygen, restraints, and so forth

Misplaced or undue emphasis on neatness, quiet, order, and rest

Inability to Receive Stimuli

A person who has an impairment of one or more sensory organs is said to have a _sensory deficit._ His contact with his environment, and the people in it, is incomplete, deficient, and interrupted. The environment may be rich with stimuli, but if one or more of his sensory organs is impaired to such an extent that it is not possible for him to receive sensory stimulation via some of the usual channels (sight, hearing, taste, touch, or smell), sensory deprivation will result. These sensory deficits can be caused by disease, injury, or a congenital defect and may be temporary or permanent.

Inability to Process Stimuli

Some people with normal sensory organs experience sensory deprivation in the midst of adequate stimuli because they are unable to assign a meaning to the stimuli around them. They are, in varying degrees, unable to use information effectively, to respond to stimuli appropriately, or to comprehend the meaning of certain objects and events. Some causes of an *inability to process* stimuli are:

Disease, such as stroke, brain lesion, high fever, or cerebral ischemia

Drugs, including central nervous system depressants such as narcotics and alcohol, stimulants, and hallucinogens

Decreased level of consciousness (coma or stupor)

Language barriers in the absence of a translator

Altered emotional states, such as anxiety or depression

Distortions of thought, including hallucinations (the occurrence of imagined events or the presence of imagined objects) and illusion (the misinterpretation of reality)

Variables That Influence the Effects of Sensory Deprivation

Regardless of cause, the impact and effect of sensory deprivation is influenced by the age and personality of the person, and the onset, extent, and duration of the deprivation. It has been well documented that adequate sensory stimulation is essential for the intellectual growth and psychological development of infants and children. Sensory stimulation also affects physical growth and development by motivating the infant to reach, gasp, explore, crawl, and climb to reach interesting and attractive objects.

Children, adolescents, and working adults are also affected by a nonstimulating environment, but the required activities of school, home, and work tend to keep them going. On the other hand, a retired or aged person whose world seems to be shrinking steadily is likely to become withdrawn, confused, or disoriented when sensory stimulation is reduced by a restricted environment, such as a dull and monotonous nursing home or a lonely apartment.

People who keep the radio or TV on constantly, who become bored easily, and who do not like to be alone are probably more likely to be upset by sensory deprivation than people who have the imagination and inner resources to tolerate or even enjoy a sensory-restricted environment.

Total sensory deprivation under experimental conditions produces a dramatic and obvious effect on the subject, but partial sensory deprivation over a long period of time can be even more damaging. A sudden onset of sensory deprivation such as accidental blindness is usually very upsetting to the person involved, but a gradual, almost unnoticed onset can be more devastating in the long run because the symptoms may develop slowly and be undiagnosed until the damage is severe and practically irreversible. Both the extent and duration of the deprivation are significant in predicting the possible effects of sensory deprivation.

Nursing Intervention

Nursing interventions related to sensory deprivation are based on at least three factors: circadian rhythm, change, and variety.

TABLE 28.2 IMPROVISED TOYS FOR HOME AND HOSPITAL

Suggested Use	Found at Home	Found in the Hospital
Water play	Measuring cups/spoons, sponges, margarine tubs/lids, squeeze bottles, funnel, coffee pot	Specimen cups/lids, disposable bulb syringe
Mobiles	Plastic cookie cutters, greeting cards	Baby picture from cereal or diaper box, magazine pictures, or cardboard
Nesting	Measuring cups/spoons, margarine tubs/lids, paper cups	Medicine cups, syringe containers, empty tape rolls
Stacking	Freezer containers	Drinking cups
Hiding	Empty margarine tubs/lids	Souffle cups, small boxes
Threading	Paper/ribbon rolls and tubes, shoe laces	Empty tape rolls and IV tubing
Textures	Pot scrubbers, sponges, cellophane tape	Cellophane tape, gauze
Shape identification	Plastic cookie cutters, sponges cut into shapes	
Banging	Pots, pans, wooden spoons	
Pull toy	Empty rolls, tubes	Cylinders
Tunnels, houses	Large appliance cartons	Large cardboard boxes

Adapted from: Verzemnieks, Inese L: Developmental stimulation for infants and toddlers. *AJN* 84:6 (June 1984) 749–752.

Circadian Rhythm

When days are monotonous, dreary, and indistinguishable one from the other, the patient may have no way to gauge the passage of time. In addition to the use of day-night lighting cycles, day-night clothing cycles should be instituted. In some nursing homes, for example, all patients who can be gotten out of bed wear street clothes during the day, and even bedfast patients wear different bed clothes during the daytime hours than they do at night.

Clocks and calendars should be accessible to all patients, and references to time and date should be made by family and staff throughout the day through comments such as "It's 5:30—the supper trays will be here soon" and "Today is Wednesday—the week is almost half over."

A small blackboard or memo board can help some patients keep track of events such as expected visits from out-of-town relatives, treatments, exercise schedules, and anything else that helps to make one segment of time different from another one.

Change

One of the most significant aspects of life is the element of change. Children grow taller, tomatoes ripen, patients get better, and the seasons change. The process of observing changes and making comparisons such as "the days are getting longer" or "the dog is getting lame" provide ongoing stimulation for people whose environment is restricted either in size or in scope.

The threat of sensory deprivation for a person who is sick or is housebound can often be counteracted by ensuring an ongoing series of changes within his environment. A window beside his bed or chair, one or more growing plants, or a pet will give him something to watch and keep track of. A hobby that grows and expands, such as a stamp collection, knitting, or writing to pen pals tends to keep a person interested and anxious to see what the next purchase, stitch, or letter will bring.

Variety

When people say "variety is the spice of life," it sounds as if variety were an "extra" or a bonus. On the contrary, variety is not a spice; it is a necessity for many people. People whose environments are limited and monotonous can be helped toward a richer and more satisfying life by increasing the variety of people, things, sensations, and ideas in their lives. This can be done in a number of ways as indicated by the following examples.

VARIETY OF PEOPLE

Refer the patient to a community day-care center, and then provide assistance as needed in having him get acquainted with others.

Arrange for volunteer groups such as Friendly Visitors, church members, or workers with Meals on Wheels to visit the patient's home on a regular basis.

Introduce the patient to others on the unit.

Take the patient to the hall or lounge several times daily and help him to get acquainted with other patients.

VARIETY OF IDEAS

Use radio and television *selectively*. When they are used indiscriminately for long periods, a person begins to listen passively, with no involvement or thought.

Check on the services of the local public library. Many libraries sponsor a mobile unit or home delivery service of some kind that enables homebound people to expand their ideas via books.

Converse with the patient about a variety of topics, such as news events, season of the year, or childhood memories. Unless he is upset by or unwilling to discuss a topic, pursue that topic as *long as possible*. The intent of your conversation is to stimulate the patient to think, and a format in which you touch lightly on first one topic and then another does not help a person to concentrate and does nothing to counteract confused or disorganized thinking. Pursuing any topic, from the picking of wild strawberries to favorite soap operas, will encourage the patient to remember, to explain, to listen, and to organize his thoughts. If he is helped to do this once or twice a day for 5 or 10 minutes, the variety and scope of his thoughts will have been expanded.

VARIETY OF SENSATIONS

Try to ensure variety in food, and in its seasoning, texture, and temperature. Food should be hot or cold and well seasoned, rather than bland and lukewarm.

Add color to the patient's unit with bright cushions, an afghan, or a wall hanging, for example.

Obtain a pass for the patient to be taken home for a visit or to go outdoors (in a wheelchair or on a stretcher if necessary).

Provide opportunities for the patient to touch as many surfaces during the day as possible. A healthy per-

TABLE 28.3 OPPORTUNITIES FOR INFANT STIMULATION IN THE HOSPITAL

Opportunity	Auditory	Visual	Tactile	Vestibular
Vital signs	Talk calmly	Play peek-a-boo	Touch and name body parts	Flex/extend arms and legs
Diapering	Sing a tune	Smile; make faces at baby	Sensations—wet, dry, soft	Rhythmic leg exercises
Bathing	Name body parts	Hide toy under washcloth	Water play	Encourage splashing
Feeding	Talk about food	Encourage baby to follow spoon with eyes	Sensations—warm/cool soft/firm food	Position in highchair or hold in arms
Treatments	Explain what is happening	Distract with empty package	Crush cellophane wrapper	
Nap time	Turn on music box	Darken room	Special toy in crib	Rock gently

Adapted from: Verzemnieks, Inese L: Developmental stimulation for infants and toddlers. *AJN* 84:6 (June 1984) 749–752.

son normally touches objects that are damp, dry, rough, smooth, dirty, clean, and so on, whereas a patient in bed may touch only his bed linen and the objects on his meal tray.

Touch the patient when you pause to talk with him and when he needs support and encouragement, not just when he is being bathed. The touch of a genuinely concerned person can be comforting, reassuring, and satisfying. (It is unfortunate that people seem unable to say of another person, "He wants to be loved," or "She wants to be caressed," although we can say easily that the dog wants his ears scratched or the cat wants to be petted.)

Because the manifestations of sensory deprivation and sensory overload are highly individualized, and because the symptoms are often similar, there can be no specific guidelines for nursing interventions. The most useful rule is probably "Try it and see what happens." If your patient responds in a favorable way, continue with your chosen interventions. If a given approach makes little or no difference or if it produces an adverse reaction, discontinue that approach and try a different one.

SENSORY DEFICITS

Alterations in Vision

There are four major causes of visual problems: (1) errors of refraction (focusing), (2) muscle imbalance, (3) disease, and (4) aging.

Problems Caused by Errors of Refraction

An error of refraction is a condition in which parallel rays of light are not brought into focus on the retina because of a defect or abnormality in the shape of the eyeball or in the refracting media of the eye. These conditions can be corrected with properly fitted lenses.

MYOPIA (nearsightedness). Myopia is a defect in which parallel rays of light converge and focus *in front* of the retina. Nearby objects are clearly visible, but more distant objects are blurred.

HYPEROPIA (farsightedness). Hyperopia is a defect in which light rays focus *behind* the retina, causing distant objects to be clear while nearby objects are blurred. *Presbyopia* is a form of farsightedness which accompanies advancing age due to loss of elasticity of the crystalline lens.

ASTIGMATISM. This defect is the result of an irregular curvature of the cornea which prevents rays of light from focusing sharply in a single point on the retina. As a result, there is no sharp focus and objects at any distance are blurred.

Problems Caused by Muscle Imbalance

STRABISMUS. Strabismus is a disorder in which one or both eyes deviates up or down, to the right or to the left. It is caused by one of the six oculomotor muscles being weaker or stronger than the others. It becomes apparent during early childhood, and can be treated effectively by drugs, exercises, or surgery. Strabismus should be corrected early because it can cause serious and permanent visual deterioration. Since the eyes are unable to focus on the same object, the brain receives two images. To avoid such visual confusion, the child learns to use only one eye. The vision in the other eye deteriorates from disuse, resulting in a serious condition called *amblyopia*. In some cases, the strabismus is not very noticeable, but the child may complain of headaches and have difficulty with schoolwork.

AMBLYOPIA ("lazy eye"). Amblyopia is characterized by reduction or dimness of vision in an eye in which there is no apparent pathological condition. The most frequent cause is disuse of the eye as a result of strabismus. Amblyopia accounts for approximately 25 percent of all eye problems in children and adolescents. If it is not treated, amblyopia results in permanent deterioration of the eye and loss of vision. It is imperative, therefore, that amblyopia be corrected before the age of 6 years. This is done by treating the strabismus and placing an eye patch over the good eye, thereby forcing the affected eye to function. Since amblyopia can be caused by strabismus which may be barely noticeable or missed entirely, it is important for all preschool children to have their vision tested by the age of 3 or 4 years.

Problems Caused by Disease

LOW VISION. Low vision is a term applied to faulty vision caused by a _pathological condition_ in the eye, in the visual pathways to the brain, or in receptor areas in the brain. This is in contrast to errors of refraction and problems of muscle imbalance in which the eye is essentially healthy. Low vision _cannot_ be corrected by conventional lenses, contact lenses, or reading glasses.

Low vision may be characterized by a central field defect, a peripheral vision defect, or both. Low vision may involve near or far vision or both. The condition may be congenital, or acquired as a result of disease such as a stroke, uncontrolled diabetes, hypertension, trauma, or a tumor.

Special devices, called low vision aids, are available but they are expensive. Such devices include hand-held or mounted magnifying lenses for near vision, telescopic lenses for far vision, and a video monitor for reading. Less expensive and more readily available aids include large-print books and magazines, recorded materials, ruled paper and felt tip pens for writing, adjustable lamps, reading stands, and special enlarged telephone dials.

Problems Caused by Aging

It is important not to blame all faulty vision after age 60 on the aging process, but there are a number of normal visual changes which must be taken into account as a person grows older. These changes include changes in focusing, light accommodation, depth perception, and the ability to distinguish colors.

Changes in the ability to focus on objects at various distances means that it takes an older person much longer to shift his gaze from a newspaper to a bird outside the window and back to the newspaper.

Changes in light accommodation make it difficult for an older person to accommodate to sudden changes in the intensity of light, such as going from shadow to sunlight, or from a brightly lighted room into a dim hallway. Any type of glare creates a problem, and this difficulty in accommodation to changes in light accounts in part for the problems of night driving.

Changes in depth perception mean that the person may be able to see an object clearly but be unable to tell how far away it is. Many behaviors which seem to indicate a lack of coordination are in reality problems of depth perception. The older person may bump into things because he cannot judge distances accurately. A messy eater may be unable to tell how far away the plate or cup is. Decreased depth perception can be dangerous for a person who must go up and down stairs, and it is advisable, therefore, to paint the bottom step a contrasting color.

Changes in the ability to distinguish similar colors can make it difficult for an older person to differentiate one object from another. For example, it can be hard to distinguish the wall, door, and doorway from each other if all are painted in shades of the same color, or to tell if one's slip is showing if the slip and dress are both pastel pink. This means that for many older people, brightly colored pillows, pictures, and clothing offer more sensory stimulation and enjoyment than do pastel objects.

Care of Eyes

EYE EXAMINATIONS. It has been estimated that half of all blindness is preventable. The American Academy of Ophthalmology recommends that a child's eyes be examined by the age of 6 months to make sure that there are no indications of eye disease, that the child can see with both eyes, and that the eyes are not crossed or turned (strabismus). This is especially important for babies at risk of impaired vision, namely those with a family history of early eye disorders and premature infants who were given oxygen (which can cause blindness if given in excessive doses). If a problem is suspected, the vision of a newborn infant can be tested by measuring the brain waves produced by the infant when he looks at patterns on a TV screen.

Every child should be tested for strabismus and amblyopia by the age of 3 or 4 years, as well as for distance vision. The latter can be done by a parent using a modified Snellen chart displaying only the letter E.

Young and middle-age adults usually attend to problems of vision because of the need to function effectively in school and on the job. Older adults, however, are likely to assume that diminished vision is an inevitable part of aging, and neglect to have their vision checked. In many instances, the decreased vision of an older person is due to an untreated cataract, undiagnosed glaucoma, or an uncorrected refraction error. The family, friends, or caretakers of an elderly person should be alert for signs of failing vision or eye problems, and make sure that the person is seen by an ophthalmologist. If the individual, young or old, is unable to pay for care and does not have health insurance, civic organizations such as the Rotary Club frequently sponsor screening programs, and nearly every city has free or low-cost eye clinics.

HEALTH CARE. When a visual problem is noted or suspected, an ophthalmologist should be consulted rather than merely having the person's eyes "checked" at an optical or eyeglass center. An ophthalmologist is a doctor of medicine who has had 3 to 5 years of additional training which enables him to diagnose and treat all diseases and conditions of the eyes. The ophthalmologist examines eyes in relation to the person's overall health and condition. An optometrist, on the other hand, is qualified to examine eyes *only* for errors of refraction, and to prescribe the appropriate lenses.

SAFETY. It is estimated that 90 percent of all eye injuries are preventable, and that approximately 45 percent of

TABLE 28.4 WHEN TO SEEK HEALTH CARE FOR THE EYES

Appearance

An eye that turns, or eyes that are crossed
Inflamed or watery eyes
Reddened, crusted, or swollen lids
Recurrent styes (infected sebaceous glands of eyelid)
Enlarged eyeball
Eye that appears cloudy
White spot on pupil

Behavior

Squinting, frowning
Tilting head, thrusting head forward
Shutting or covering one eye
Rubbing eyes excessively
Irritability associated with close work

Complaints

Itching, burning, scratchy feeling in eyes
Blurred or double vision
Dizziness
Inability to see blackboard or to read well
Headache or nausea after close work

them occur around the home, with the remainder occurring in connection with work or sports. Although eye injuries are easily prevented, over one million people suffer eye injuries each year. Safety precautions are clearly specified in most industries and some sports, but preventive measures around the home are more complex because of the wide variety of activities and ages of the persons involved. Each individual and family should be encouraged to assess its own situation and the specific risks involved, because what might be a real danger in one situation might be a negligible risk in another. For example, an emphasis on safety related to power tools is unwarranted in a home which does not have a workshop.

A few selected examples of commonly needed safety precautions are:

Teach children how to carry and manage pointed objects such as scissors, a pencil, or knife.

Make sure that a spray nozzle is directed away from your face before pressing it (e.g., hairspray, pesticide, cleaning agents).

Never let anyone stand in front of or beside a running lawn mower.

Wear protective goggles when spray painting or using a paint roller overhead.

Supervise children's play when they are using hard or sharp objects such as a metal toy rake, croquet mallet, or toy golf club, and when they are using objects which could be dangerous if thrown such as sand, blocks, or small metal cars.

FIRST AID. Since proper first aid for an eye injury can be the most vital step in saving someone's eyesight, professional and lay persons alike should know what to do in case of an accident.

The cardinal rule for treating a *speck or foreign particle* in the eye is *don't rub it!* Pull the upper lid out over the lower lid and blink a few times to let the lashes of the lower lid brush the particle off the inside of the upper lid. It may be difficult to know when the speck has been removed because discomfort and pain often persist after the object is gone. If the speck remains, or the pain persists for more than a few minutes, keep the eye closed and seek medical help (Fig. 28.13).

A *blow to the eye* is treated by applying an ice cold compress for at least 15 minutes. This will reduce pain and retard swelling. Blurred vision or a discolored eye could mean internal eye damage and an ophthalmologist should be seen at once (Fig. 28.14).

A *cut to the eye or lid* should be covered lightly with a bandage, and medical help should be sought at once. Never apply hard pressure to an injured eye or eyelid.

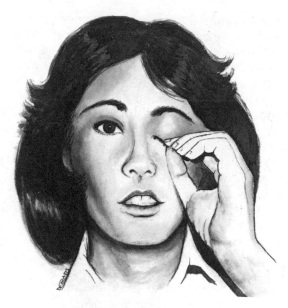

Figure 28.13 *First aid for speck in the eye: Don't rub it. Pull upper lid out and down over lower lid to promote mechanical removal of speck.*

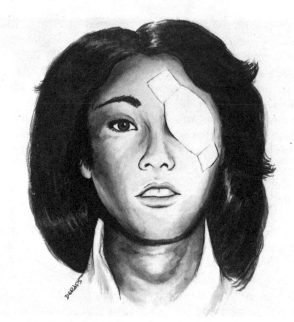

Figure 28.15 *First aid for cut to eye or lid: Cover lightly and seek medical help at once.*

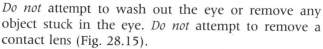

Do not attempt to wash out the eye or remove any object stuck in the eye. *Do not* attempt to remove a contact lens (Fig. 28.15).

A *chemical burn* is treated by flooding the eye with lukewarm water immediately. Use your fingers to hold the lids apart and keep the eye open as wide as possible. Pour water from a clean container or hold your head under a faucet. Flood the eye continuously and gently

for *at least 15 minutes*. The eye should be rolled about to flood all surfaces. Remove a contact lens to flood the surface underneath. Do not use an eye cup and do not bandage the eye. Seek medical help as soon as first aid measures are completed (Fig. 28.16).

USE OF EYEDROPS AND OINTMENTS. Since eyedrops and ointments are often prescribed for use in the home, lay

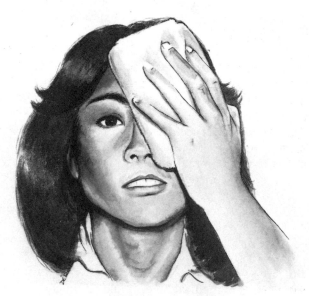

Figure 28.14 *First aid for blow to the eye: Apply ice pack for at least fifteen minutes.*

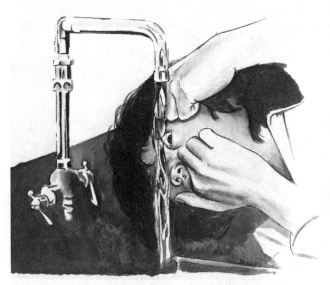

Figure 28.16 *First aid for chemical injury to eye: Flood with lukewarm water for at least fifteen minutes, then seek medical help.*

persons need to be taught how to administer them properly. The patient should be lying down or seated with his head tilted as far back as possible. Hold the eyedropper or tube of ointment in your dominant hand, and brace that hand against the patient's forehead so that if the patient moves his head, your hand will move with it and the dropper or tube will not injure the patient's eye.

With your other hand, pull the lower lid *down and out* to form a pocket for the medication. Place eyedrops in the center of this pocket. Place ointment in the pocket by squeezing a ribbon of ointment from the inner canthus of the eye (the angle nearest the nose) to the outer canthus of the eye. Have the patient close his eye, and with it still closed, look in all directions to distribute the medication over the entire surface of the eye.

An infant or toddler must be held or restrained for safety. If only one person is available, the child can be mummied by wrapping him securely in a small blanket or large towel. If the child fights the procedure by constantly moving his head, it is still possible for one person to give the medication safely by positioning the child between one's legs while sitting on the floor (Fig. 28.17).

INFECTION. When caring for a patient with an infected eye or eyelid, it is important to protect the other eye. The unaffected eye is bathed first, with a clean washcloth, washing from the inner canthus (the angle nearest the nose) toward the outer canthus. The affected eye is then washed in the same way, from the inner toward the outer canthus. Washing in this direction moves microorganisms away from the unaffected eye and away from the lacrimal ducts at the inner canthus. If the affected eye is unintentionally washed first, the washcloth should be discarded and a fresh one obtained before the other eye is washed.

UNCONSCIOUSNESS. If an unconscious patient keeps his eyes open, without blinking, the conjunctivae will become dry and susceptible to irritation and infection. The eyelids must be carefully washed, as often as necessary, to remove any crusts or exudate; and then the eyes should be closed and covered with eye patches. If necessary, the eyelids can also be taped shut to protect the conjunctivae. The patient's level of consciousness should be monitored carefully so the eye patches can be removed if there is a change; it would be frightening for him to regain consciousness and think he could not see.

CONTACT LENSES. There are three types of contact lenses in use: hard, soft, and gas-permeable. Hard lenses offer the advantages of good vision, ease of care, durability,

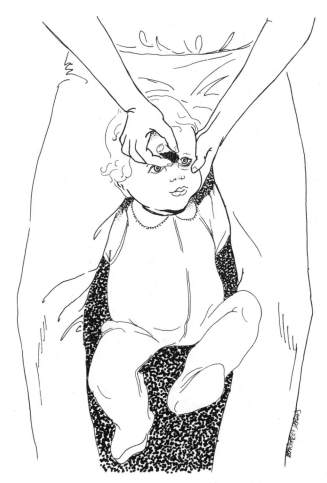

Figure 28.17 *One way to give eye drops safely without assistance.*

and low cost. Hard lenses are firm and non-pliable. They depend upon tears for lubrication and oxygenation of the cornea, and corneal abrasions can result if a person wearing hard lenses is unconscious and unblinking, especially if his eyes tend to remain open.

Soft contact lenses are more comfortable and easier to get used to, but there are three major disadvantages: (1) vision is less sharp; (2) bacteria can grow on the surface of the lenses, so the lenses must be disinfected regularly; (3) soft lenses are more easily damaged than hard lenses and must be replaced more frequently.

Gas-permeable lenses provide good vision, ease of care, and durability similar to that of hard lenses. These lenses are more flexible than hard lenses, allow a better flow of tears across the cornea, and, in addition, permit a higher level of oxygen transmission through the lens to the cornea.

The majority of patients are able to insert and remove their own contact lenses, but a patient who has become incapacitated by an accident or serious illness may be unable to do so. If a patient is unconscious or unable to answer questions when admitted to the hospital, his eyes should be checked for the presence of contact lenses. Some contact lens are difficult to detect, but can usually be spotted if a penlight is shone from the side across the patient's eyes. If present, the lenses should be removed, carefully identified as to right and left lens, and placed in a safe spot. (Because infection is the most serious complication of wearing contact lenses, wash your hands and trim your nails as needed before trying to insert or remove a patient's contact lenses.)

If contact lenses are not detected and are left in place for a number of days, irritation and damage to the cornea could result. Patients who are at risk for eye damage due to prolonged wear are persons with impaired judgment and an altered mental state as a result of psychiatric or psychological problems, substance abuse, or unconsciousness.

Hard lenses are removed by exerting enough pressure against the lower edge of the lens to tip the upper edge forward. The lens is then grasped by the upper edge and removed (Fig. 28.18). To insert a hard lens, moisten it with an appropriate wetting agent (not saliva), position it on the tip of your index finger, separate the eyelids, and place the lens directly over the cornea (Fig. 28.19).

To remove a *soft* contact lens, use your index finger to slide the lens from the cornea down over the sclera (the white portion of the eye); then pinch the lens slightly between your thumb and index finger to admit air under the lens. This will break the suction, and permit lens removal (Fig. 28.20).

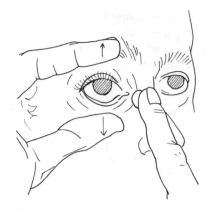

Figure 28.19 *Insertion of a hard lens.*

Before you insert a soft lens, always check to make sure that it is clear (not cloudy or smudged), and free of rips, lint, or specks. In addition, be very sure that it has not been turned inside out (Fig. 28.21). When the lens is pinched between the thumb and index finger, the edges should point inward. If the edges of the lens roll outward, it is inside out and must be reversed before being inserted. To insert the lens, place it on the tip of your index finger, separate the eyelids, and place the lens directly over the cornea (Fig. 28.22). Ask the patient if it is comfortable and if he can see clearly. If he cannot, rinse the lens and/or re-position it as needed. Also, be sure that you have not mixed up the right and left lenses.

ARTIFICIAL EYES. Upon admission, each patient should be asked if he has a prosthesis of any kind, such as an artificial leg or eye. If he has an artificial eye, he should

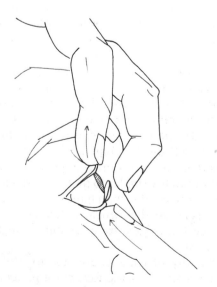

Figure 28.18 *Removal of a hard lens.*

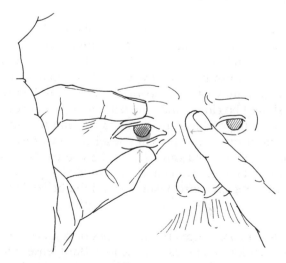

Figure 28.20 *Removal of a soft lens.*

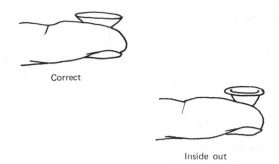

Figure 28.21 *A soft lens must be right side out before insertion.*

be asked to describe its care and what assistance (if any) he will need in order to care for it. With an emergency admission, the nurse should be alert to the possibility that the patient wears an artificial eye. The eye can be detected when the pupils are checked because the artificial eye will not react to light.

Some artificial eyes are permanently implanted and are not removed, although some type of periodic eye care is needed. Other types of artificial eyes are removed, washed, and replaced each day. If a patient is unable to explain what kind of prosthesis he has or describe its care, the nurse should consult with the family, notify his physician, or seek the advice of an ophthalmologist.

Helping the Visually Impaired Patient

A careful psychosocial assessment is the first step in helping a visually impaired person. It is necessary to

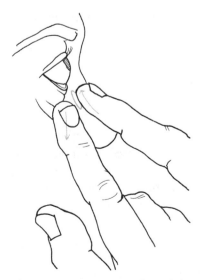

Figure 28.22 *Insertion of a soft lens.*

assess the person's feelings and attitudes about his difficulties before effective plans can be made to modify the environment or provide assistance with the activities of daily living. Depending upon the person's age and personality, the suddenness of onset, and the length of time he has had to become accustomed to his condition, the person may be matter-of-fact, angry, embarrassed, or frightened and timid because of his visual difficulties. An elderly person whose sight is failing rapidly may feel useless, depressed, and unwilling to try to do anything for himself. A person who was accidentally blinded may be so fearful and insecure that he is unwilling to leave the security of his bedside unit. Anger, frustration, and irritability may make it difficult to work with a young person whose career is being disrupted by impaired vision.

A thorough, sensitive, and ongoing evaluation of the patient's basic needs will indicate the areas in which help is most urgently needed. It is necessary to explore the cause and meaning of the patient's behavior before a valid diagnosis can be made, and appropriate plans made. A visually impaired person may resist leaving his room because of fear of falling, embarrassment, despair over the future, feelings of uselessness and little worth, or a desire for pity. In each instance, the nursing intervention would be entirely different in approach and content.

Therapeutic communication, therefore, is one of the first nursing actions to be taken with a visually impaired person. At the same time, three other aspects of care should be in progress: (1) provision of health care, (2) adjustment of the environment, and (3) maintenance of activities of daily living.

PROVISION OF HEALTH CARE. Health care for the visually impaired person includes regular eye examinations, the use of appropriate lenses or low vision aids, treatment of any underlying pathological conditions, psychological support, and counseling as needed.

ADJUSTMENT TO THE ENVIRONMENT. A satisfactory adjustment by a visually impaired person to his environment depends upon a proper orientation to it, and attention to both physical safety and psychological security. Depending upon the data provided by your psychosocial assessment of the patient and the severity of his visual impairment, proper *orientation* to a new environment includes any or all of the following nursing actions:

Encourage the patient to feel the size, shape and location of the bed, bedside stand, chair and other furniture.

Have him feel and practice using the bed controls, call bell, and any other equipment in his unit.

Walk with him to the closet, bathroom, nurse's station, lounge, elevators.

Make sure he knows where supplies such as soap, toilet paper, and towels are kept.

Measures to ensure the patient's *safety and security* include the following:

When helping the patient ambulate, let him take *your* arm rather than your taking his arm. *Lead* him, don't try to steer him.

Explain routines, time schedules, and procedures in advance of the event or activity.

Routinely check the patient's unit for potential hazards and remove any potential obstacles.

Keep all furniture and articles in the same place; do not move things without the patient's knowledge.

Increase the lighting as needed. Reposition lights to prevent glare, and provide an adequate night light.

Speak to the patient whenever you approach or leave him so that he knows whether someone is present or has left.

Explain, in advance, sounds which might be puzzling or frightening.

Communicate your findings and plans to other staff. Note on the Kardex any special arrangements made for or needed by the patient. Place needed information on the door of the patient's unit if feasible. Give other patients a sensitive and appropriate orientation to the patient's situation.

MAINTENANCE OF ACTIVITIES OF DAILY LIVING (ADL). The amount of assistance needed by the patient in eating, grooming, and managing his daily schedule will depend in part upon the duration of the visual impairment. If the condition has existed for a number of years, he is likely to have developed techniques for managing most of his daily activities, and will need only minimal assistance. On the other hand, if the impairment is recent, a great deal of teaching, encouragement, and problem solving will be required. If the onset was sudden, crisis intervention techniques followed by measures to reduce stress and develop new ways of coping will probably be needed before his problems can be tackled effectively.

If the visual impairment is severe, independence can be promoted by encouraging the use of a cane or guide dog. Such training is available through local organizations for the blind, and vocational rehabilitation is available to train visually impaired people for new jobs and careers.

Hearing Loss

Disease, injury, or congenital defects of the ear and associated nerves can cause a variety of pathological conditions including hearing loss, impaired balance, and distorted or abnormal sounds. Of these conditions, the one most likely to seriously affect a person's sensory status is a hearing deficit.

Hearing Deficits

A hearing loss may be either congenital or acquired. Some of the causes of an acquired hearing deficit are:

Injury from a sharp object, foreign body in the ear, or accident

Impacted wax (cerumen)

Disease such as measles, mumps, meningitis

Excessive noise, often industrial or work related

Drug toxicity, especially certain antibiotics

Chronic infection of the middle ear

Assessment of Hearing

The initial assessment of a person's hearing may be a routine hearing check done as part of a school health program or an examination done in response to complaints of the person or following an observation of the person's behavior.

Complaints by the individual (subjective data) include the following:

Decreased ability to distinguish one voice from another

Inability to locate the direction of sounds

Decreased ability to hear the sounds of birds and other high-pitched sounds

Humming, buzzing, ringing in the ears

Behaviors which may indicate a hearing loss are:

Inattention

Failure to respond to sound (may be the first indication of hearing loss in an infant)

Frequent requests for clarification

Inappropriate responses and interpretations

Tilting or turning head (same ear is always turned toward the speaker if there is greater loss in one ear than in the other)

HEARING TESTS. General or *gross tests* of hearing include the whisper test followed by the Rinnes and Weber tests if the whisper test suggests a hearing loss. These tests were described earlier as tests of sensory function.

Precise testing is done with a pure tone audiometer. This is an electronic instrument which produces pure tones of a known intensity in a headphone. The frequency and intensity of the tones can be varied by the examiner. The individual who fails a basic audiometric test is referred to an audiologist for more extensive testing.

Treatment of a hearing deficit may be medical, including removal of a foreign body or impacted wax, surgical, or mechanical (use of a hearing aid). Prompt treatment is important because in many instances permanent deafness can be prevented.

Additional assessments include a careful history of the patient and an analysis of the attitudes of both him and his family. It is important to determine whether the people involved are acknowledging, accepting, or denying the existence of a hearing problem.

Care of the Ears

SAFETY. Two of the most important aspects of safety are protection from both injury and excessive noise. *Injury* can be prevented by observing the following safety measures:

Teach children not to put anything in their ears! The old adage of "nothing smaller than your elbow in your ear" is still valid. The ears are self-cleaning and nothing is needed beyond cleaning the outer ear with a soapy washcloth. Parents should be taught to avoid the use of cotton-tipped swabs.

It is important not to blow one's nose too hard, and especially important not to close one nostril to increase pressure on the other one. Some authorities recommend keeping *both nostrils and the mouth* open when blowing the nose to reduce the pressure, because increased pressure can force contaminated material through the eustachian tube into the middle ear.

If the individual has a history of ear infections, it is advisable to protect the ears with ear plugs when diving and swimming.

Protection from a blow during some sports is afforded by protective headgear, such as that worn by a baseball player at bat.

Excessive and prolonged noise is one of the greatest hazards to hearing in industrialized civilizations. Federal and state safety regulations prescribe the use of protective ear plugs or helmets in some industries, but such equipment is not required in many settings with marginal or sporadic high level noise. Protective devices are considered a nuisance by many workers and consequently, by not using them, many workers suffer a gradual but permanent hearing loss over the years. Vigorous programs of regular testing and education are needed to combat this health problem.

Another cause of hearing loss is the excessive amplification of some music groups, both live and recorded. The day-in, day-out amplification via headphones can cause an insidious hearing loss which necessitates the need for an increasingly higher volume in order to hear all components of the recording. An occasional concert, even at a high decibel level, is probably less detrimental in the long run than long continued exposure to a slightly lower level of sound.

REMOVAL OF CERUMEN. Impacted cerumen (wax) must *not* be removed with an object such as a toothpick or bobby pin because of the danger of puncturing or otherwise injuring the ear drum. A cotton tipped applicator should *not* be used because it tends to force the wax deeper into the ear canal.

Hard and impacted wax must be first *softened* and then gently flushed out with lukewarm water. Wax can be softened by the instillation of a few drops of hydrogen peroxide, glycerine, mineral oil, or a commercial preparation. It may be necessary to repeat the treatment several times a day for a few days until the wax is soft enough to be rinsed out. A small, soft rubber ear syringe (bulb syringe) is used to direct a *gentle* flow of tepid water against the side of the ear canal.

The water should be at approximately body temperature because either warm or cool water in the ear can make the person feel dizzy. The water should be directed against the side of the ear canal because, if it is directed into the center of the canal, it tends to force the cerumen back into the ear canal.

A recent innovation in the removal of cerumen is the use of a dental instrument (such as Water Pik) to produce a steady, gentle flow of water. Both the temperature and the amount of pressure are easily regulated and maintained.

Some people produce larger than normal amounts of cerumen, which must be removed several times a year, while others never need to have it done. Regardless of the frequency, careful attention must be paid to the removal of ear wax because in many instances, hearing losses have been corrected by the removal of impacted cerumen.

Effects of Hearing Loss

The impact of a hearing loss depends in large part upon the patient's age at the onset and the severity of the loss. If the hearing loss was present at birth or occurred within the first few years of life, the development of speech will be markedly impaired, with serious impact upon the individual's social interaction, communication, and education. Unless adequate training is given, all aspects of the child's life can be restricted and limited. In the absence of adequate testing and diagnosis, the child may be considered retarded and treated accordingly.

When the hearing loss develops later in life, especially when it develops slowly, psychological problems may be of paramount importance. The individual is likely to feel depressed, isolated, and insecure. He may be frustrated and angry when he cannot understand what is being said and may become paranoid because he thinks people are talking about him. Some people are embarrassed and would rather guess than ask for something to be repeated. The deaf person may appear to be aloof, uncooperative, inattentive, or slow witted because of his failure to respond to statements which he in fact does not hear.

Any moderate to severe hearing loss poses a threat to the individual's safety because he is unable to hear an approaching car, fire alarm, warning shout, or important directions. Parenting is difficult for those who cannot hear a baby's cry, and job and career opportunities are limited.

Helping the Hearing Impaired Person

Three major types of nursing intervention are:

> To promote good ear care and adequate audiometric testing
>
> To promote the use of compensatory techniques
>
> To facilitate communication

Promoting Good Health Care

The person with an actual or suspected hearing loss should be referred to an audiologist for precise and specific testing and diagnosis, and to an ear, nose, and throat specialist (an otolaryngologist) whenever he has a medical problem. He must be taught appropriate safety measures in order to protect his residual hearing.

Promoting Compensatory Techniques

One of the greatest barriers to compensating for a hearing loss is the resistance of the individual. This resistance may be due to embarrassment, apprehension, or denial of the problem. Denial may be caused by fear of social stigma, ignorance, inadequate testing and diagnosis, and possibility of losing one's job, financial concerns, or family attitudes. One of the most significant and difficult nursing interventions, therefore, is to help the patient and his family accept the reality of the situation and develop a positive approach to the problem.

> ### Ways to Compensate for a Hearing Loss
>
> - Develop the ability to lip read
> - Learn sign language
> - Install a *visual* fire alarm system
> - Install specially adapted telephone equipment
> - Acquire a dog trained to assist the hearing-impaired person
> - Watch closed captioned television programs
> - Obtain a properly fitted hearing aid

HEARING AIDS. A hearing aid requires a significant psychological and financial investment and represents a major decision on the part of the individual, and of his parents if he is a child. Many people unfortunately suffer grave disappointment and financial loss because they have purchased an improperly fitted or poor-quality hearing aid, or because they have unrealistic expectations.

Guidelines for the purchase and use of a hearing aid include the following:

- Obtain a prescription from a competent audiologist based upon careful testing and diagnosis. A hearing aid should *never* be purchased on the advice of a door-to-door salesman, an advertisement, or an over-the-counter salesperson.

- Purchase the hearing aid from a reputable firm which will provide both service or repairs of the aid, and instruction in its use.

- Describe one's needs and the intended use of the hearing aid to both the audiologist and the salesperson. (The type of hearing aid needed and its adjustments may vary depending upon whether its primary use will be to use the telephone, listen to TV or radio, listen to conversation or music, participate in groups, or listen in large meetings.)

- Make sure that the individual can manage the adjustments and controls. The parts of a hearing aid are tiny, and a person with limited vision or poor manual dexterity may find one type of aid much easier to manage than another. The ability to operate one's own hearing aid is important for a child who has a strong developmental need to become independent.

- *Don't judge the hearing aid prematurely!* It often takes a considerable length of time to become accustomed to the device itself, and to the new world of sounds which have not been heard in a long time, or may have never been heard before. It is important to remember that even the person's own voice will sound different. Use the hearing aid for *short* periods of time at first, and seek help from the supplier promptly before frustration overshadows the hope of success.

- Orient others to the need for changed ways of communicating. It will take a while for people who have been accustomed to speaking loud to alter their manner of speaking.

Facilitating Communication

The many things which can be done to facilitate communication with a deaf person can be grouped into four categories. These are: position and visibility of the speaker's face, rate and tone of voice, conversational clues, and the use of supplemental materials.

POSITION AND VISIBILITY OF THE SPEAKER'S FACE. Since vision is often used by a deaf person as a supplement to his auditory perception, it is absolutely essential that he be able to see the speaker clearly. Specific guidelines include the following:

Move in front of the patient to get his attention. Touching him will startle him.

Make sure that your face is adequately lighted. (Do not stand with your back to the main source of light because your face will be in shadow and the patient will see only your silhouette.)

Make sure that your mouth is visible. Don't smoke or chew gum while talking, and keep your hands away from your mouth. This is especially important for a lip reader, but nearly every hearing-impaired person gets some information from the movements of the speaker's mouth.

Do not try to converse with a deaf person while standing behind him, to the side, or in another room.

Be sure that the person is wearing his glasses or contact lenses and that they are clean.

RATE AND TONE OF SPEAKER'S VOICE. Guidelines related to the speaker's voice can be summarized in two words: *low* and *slow*. Since high-pitched sounds are harder to hear, it is helpful to use a lower tone of voice, especially with older people. This phenomenon accounts for the puzzled comments of families that an individual seems to be able to hear whispers ("things he isn't supposed to hear") but fails to respond to much ordinary conversation.

The rate of speech should be slower than normal. It is important to reduce any background noise, such as the radio or TV, or to move away from a noisy crowd to a quieter spot.

CONVERSATIONAL CLUES. It is helpful for the hearing-impaired person to know what the conversation is or will be about. An introductory statement such as "I've been thinking about" or "I'd like to teach you about . . . this morning" will enable the individual to orient himself to the topic and will reduce the chances of his missing the first few sentences. In a rapidly moving conversation, such as at the dinner table, it is considerate for people to announce abrupt shifts in conversation in some way.

When an individual misses a point or asks for clarification, his embarrassment will be reduced if the speaker paraphrases the material rather than repeating it verbatim.

USE OF SUPPLEMENTAL MATERIALS. It can be very helpful to supplement your spoken messages with written materials, pictures, and non-verbal messages such as facial expressions and gestures. It is especially important to write down any unfamiliar words or phrases, such as anatomical and medical terms.

Patient teaching of the hearing-impaired person is an extremely challenging nursing activity and will require much ingenuity, patience, and sensitivity.

SENSORY DISTURBANCES

Seizures

The terms *epilepsy* and *epileptic seizures* refer to disorders of cerebral function characterized by sudden brief attacks of altered consciousness, motor activity, or sensory phenomena. An epileptic seizure can be frightening to watch, and throughout history, there have been varying degrees of stigma associated with a person afflicted with seizures.

Epilepsy may be either idiopathic or acquired. *Idiopathic* epilepsy (also called primary or genetic epilepsy) has an unknown etiology, and accounts for the majority of cases. *Acquired* epilepsy (also called symptomatic or secondary epilepsy) can be caused by head trauma, infection, toxic substances, metabolic disorders, cerebral hemorrhage, cerebral edema, or tumors. It can also be caused by brain damage at birth and may not become apparent until later in life.

The international classification of epileptic seizures includes two broad categories: partial and general. A *partial* (focal motor) seizure is the result of a *localized* electrical disturbance in the brain, and the symptoms depend upon the area of the brain involved.

General seizures affect the entire brain and produce the types of seizures most commonly associated with epilepsy.

Absence (petit mal) seizures are characterized by the sudden onset of a staring spell and lack of responsiveness. There is a momentary pause in an activity, then it is resumed. The seizure lasts only about 10 seconds or less, and is easy to miss or misinterpret. Absence or petit mal seizures commonly appear between the ages of 5 and 12 years and continue into the teens.

Tonic-clonic (grand mal) seizures are the type most commonly associated with the term epilepsy. The patient may or may not experience an *aura* which is some type of warning sensation before the seizure is noticeable. The first observable sign is often a blank stare followed by a low cry and loss of consciousness. The *tonic* phase is evidenced by increased muscle tone which produces a rigid flexed posture followed by a rigid extended position. The *clonic* phase produces rhythmic bilateral jerks which are rapid at first and then become further apart. The extremities jerk violently and the patient's jaws are clenched. There is increased salivation which is often forced through the clenched jaws, causing the patient to froth at the mouth. There are respiratory spasms, and 10 to 15 second periods of apnea. The patient may bite his tongue, and be incontinent of urine or feces. As the paroxysms subside, the muscles become flaccid (limp). The patient may fall into a deep sleep, or may awaken in a confused or drowsy state.

Intervention During a Seizure

An epileptic seizure is *self-limiting;* the two most important responses are to *stay calm* and *stay with the patient!* It is essential that you stay with the patient in order to: (1) protect the patient from injury, and (2) observe the patient carefully.

PROTECTION OF THE PATIENT. The patient must be protected from aspiration, asphyxiation, and injury. Injury most commonly results from violent motor activity and includes bruises, lacerations, muscle strain, and broken bones.

OBSERVATION OF THE PATIENT. If this is a first seizure, or the type of epilepsy has not been diagnosed, your observations will be important. Note the initial signs of the seizure, the onset, progression and duration of the motor activity, any injuries which may have been sustained, and the manner of recovery.

As the seizure ends, decide whether to cover the patient and let him sleep, or help him wake up and pull himself together. Reorient and reassure the patient. If this is the first seizure he has ever had, he will be extremely frightened. If this is the first seizure after a long absence of seizures, he will be greatly upset at the prospect of his condition being out of control. Help him

---

Insuring Safety During a Seizure

1. Lower the patient to the floor. Don't try to move him unless he is in danger from a nearby hot radiator, stairs, sharp edges, etc. Move nearby chairs or other hard objects.

2. Protect the patient's head with padding, a pillow, or your lap.

3. Loosen clothing around neck, and if possible, position patient on side or turn head to side if possible. In the hospital, insert a soft oral airway or padded tongue depressor in the patient's mouth if there is time before the tonic phase begins. Once the patient clenches his jaw, *do not* try to open his mouth or try to force anything into it. You are likely to break his teeth. ·

4. *Do not try to forcibly restrain* the patient. Trying to restrain the patient increases the danger of injury from the violent muscle spasms. If protection from a nearby hazard is needed, use a very gentle loose restraint.

5. Reassure the patient. The sense of hearing is the last sense to go, so talk calmly to him even though he will not be able to answer you.

6. Allay the anxiety of onlookers. Assure them that the seizure will end soon and that no emergency action is needed.

---

wipe his face, and protect him from embarrassment as much as possible if he has been incontinent.

Talk with the patient, family, or others to obtain as much of a history as possible. Get medical help if it seems warranted, and refer the patient to a doctor if the condition is new or uncontrolled.

Diagnosis of the cause and type of epilepsy depends upon accurate descriptions of the seizures by family, onlookers, or professional persons. Diagnostic testing includes a complete neurological examination, skull x-ray studies, computerized axial tomography (CAT scan), electroencephalogram (EEG), lumbar puncture, and blood studies. *Treatment* is based on the treatment of the underlying cause, education of the patient and family, and the use of anti-epileptic drugs which will enable the person to lead a normal life.

Febrile Convulsions

Children between the ages of 6 months and 5 years are subject to convulsions associated with a high fever (104 degrees F, [40 degrees C] or higher). The convulsions resemble tonic-clonic (grand mal) seizures and are a fairly common childhood disorder. If there is no evidence of neurological dysfunction, the child is observed carefully and subsequent fevers are treated promptly with antipyretic drugs and cooling measures. If the seizures recur, especially in the absence of a fever, the child should be evaluated for epilepsy.

Organic Brain Syndrome

Organic brain syndrome (OBS) is the term applied to a cluster of symptoms caused by changes in the physical structure or physiological functioning of the brain. These changes alter the patient's mental status and result in observable emotional and intellectual behaviors.

The symptoms associated with organic brain syndrome are so diverse that they are frequently dismissed or attributed to aging, a psychiatric condition, a personality quirk, or just a phase. In reality, these symptoms frequently have an identifiable cause which is usually treatable and often curable. In such cases, painstaking detective work will prevent the patient from needless suffering and misery.

A few of the many changes in mental status which can result from organic brain syndrome include: loss of energy, depression, irritability, insomnia, confusion, anxiety, decreased intellectual functioning, changes in mood and personality, apathy, and delirium. Organic brain syndrome is a complex phenomenon which is beyond the scope of this textbook, but it is *essential* that even beginning practitioners recognize its existence and avoid the pitfall of misinterpreting obvious changes or underestimating the significance of subtle changes in patient behavior. Some of the important causes of organic brain syndrome are categorized in Table 28.5.

PATIENT TEACHING

Of all the innumerable possibilities for patient teaching related to sensory status, three points merit special attention because each one will significantly affect the quality of life of the persons involved.

TABLE 28.5 ORGANIC BRAIN SYNDROME

Possible Causes	Examples
Metabolic disorder	Diabetes; hypoglycemia
Convulsive disorder	Epileptic seizure
Neoplastic disease	Brain tumor
Degenerative brain disease	Alzheimer's disease
Cerebrovascular disease	Stroke; arteriosclerosis
Pressure on brain	Head injury; hemorrhage
Infectious disease	Meningitis; encephalitis
Nutritional disease	Pernicious anemia; pellagra
Drug toxicity	Alcohol; heavy metals; side effects of prescribed drugs

1. The hearing and vision of an infant should be assessed regularly by parents until they know whether or not the child hears with both ears and sees with both eyes. Subsequent assessments should be made by a professional person if a problem is discovered or suspected, and treatment should be started at once. A child will *not outgrow* a problem of hearing or vision.

2. Changes in the mental status of an older person should *not* be attributed to the aging process because, in many instances, such changes are caused by medications or treatable physical conditions which may be as yet unsuspected or undiagnosed.

3. Adequate sensory stimulation is important at all ages but is crucial for infants, children, and older people. Sensory stimulation is essential for the intellectual and psychological development of babies and toddlers; parents should be taught that toys, play, being read to, and other forms of attention from adults is a *necessity*, not an optional activity. Sensory stimulation is essential for older persons in order to maintain mental alertness, motivation, meaning, and purpose to life.

RELATED ACTIVITIES

It is not possible for a healthy person in a lively environment to fully appreciate the impact of sensory deprivation but it is possible to catch a glimpse of such an existence by engaging in the following experiments.

1. Pretend that you have just been blinded and that the doctors do not know yet whether this condition will be temporary or permanent.

Choose a typical day and blindfold yourself for at least 12 hours and preferably 24 hours. During this time, do each of the following: (1) dress and groom yourself, (2) eat with other people, (3) go outdoors, (4) attend class, (5) enter a public building, and (6) ride in a car or bus if possible. (Protect yourself from any potential danger by asking a friend to accompany you as needed.)

It is important that the blindfold not be removed for any reason. If an emergency makes this necessary, start over again at another time. If the experience of being blind is brief, it will seem like an interesting game, and the reality of blindness will never be sensed.

Throughout this experiment, pay close attention to your emotional reactions, and the way in which these responses influence your choice of activities, your reactions to other people, and your usual ways of handling stress and problems.

Make careful note of the things people did that were helpful, and the things you *wish* someone had done to help you, because these actions will be similar to the nursing interventions which will increase your skill as a professional nurse.

2. Borrow or buy an effective set of ear plugs and wear them for an entire day. Focus your attention at frequent intervals on your *emotional* reactions to the various situations in which you find yourself.

SUGGESTED READINGS

Bozian, Marguerite W, and Helen M Clark: Counteracting sensory changes in the aging. *Am J Nurs* 1980 March; 80(3):473–476.

Campbell, Emily B, Margaret A Williams, and Susan M Mlynarczyk: After the fall—CONFUSION. *Am J Nurs* 1986 Feb; 86(2):151–154.

Clark, Barbara: What to do when your patient lets slip his grip on reality. *Nursing 84* 1984 July; 14(7):50–56.

Cohen, Stephen, and Sr. Erica Bunke: Sensory changes in the elderly (programmed instruction). *Am J Nurs* 1981 Oct; 81(10):1851–1880.

Cohen, Stephen, and Elizabeth Harris: Mental status assessment (programmed instruction). *Am J Nurs* 1981 Aug; 81(8):1493–1518.

Curtis, Patricia: Our pets, ourselves. *Psych Today* 1982 Aug; 16(8):66–67.

Dodd, Marylin J: Assessing mental status. *Am J Nurs* 1978 Sept; 78(9):1501–1503.

Francis, Gloria: The therapeutic use of pets. *Nurs Outlook* 1981 June; 29(6):369–370.

Freeman, Catherine C, and Elizabeth A Hefferin: Are you out of touch with your patients? *RN* 1984 April; 47(4):51–53.

Hanawalt, Ann, and Kathy Troutman: If your patient has a hearing aid. *Am J Nurs* 1984 July; 84(7):900–901.

Heller, Barbara R, and Edward B Gaynor: Hearing loss and aural rehabilitation of the elderly. *Top Clin Nurs* 1981 April; 3(1):21–29.

Hellman, Hal: Guiding light. *Psych Today* 1982 April; 16(4):22–28.

Jones, Cathy: Glasgow coma scale. *Am J Nurs* 1979 Sept; 79(9):1551–1553.

Joyce, Christopher: Space travel is no joyride. *Psych Today* 1984 May; 18(5):30–37.

Krieger, Dolores: Therapeutic touch: The imprimatur of nursing. *Am J Nurs* 1975 May; 75(5):784–787.

Krieger, Dolores, et al: Therapeutic touch: Searching for evidence of physiological change. *Am J Nurs* 1979 April; 79(4):660–666.

Lindenmuth, Jane E, Christine S Breu, and Jean A Malooley: Sensory overload. *Am J Nurs* 1980 Aug; 80(8):1456–1458.

Ludewick, Ruth: Assessing confusion: a tool to improve nursing care. *J. Gerontal Nurs* 1981 Aug; 7(8):474–477.

Meer, Jeff: The light touch (effects of lighting). *Psych Today* 1985 Sept; 19(9):60–67.

Norman, Susan: The pupil check. *Am J Nurs* 1982 April; 82(4):588–591.

Norman, Susan, and Thomas R Browne: Seizure disorders. *Am J Nurs* 1981 May; 81(5):984–994.

Pines, Maya: INFANT-STIM: It's changing the lives of handicapped kids. *Psych Today* 1982 June; 16(6):48–53.

Sandoff, Ronni: A skeptic's guide to therapeutic touch. *RN* 1980 Jan; 43(1):24–31.

Stern, Elizabeth J: Helping the person with low vision. *Am J Nurs* 1980 Oct; 80(10):1788–1790.

Vernberg, Katherine, Janine Jagger, and John A Jane: The glasgow coma scale: how do you rate? *Nurse Educator* 1983 Autumn; 8(3):33–37.

Verzemnieks, Inese L: Developmental stimulation for infants and toddlers. *Am J Nurs* 1984 June; 84(6):749–752.

Walleck, Constance Anne: A neurological assessment procedure that won't make you nervous. *Nursing 82* Dec; 12(12):50–57.

Welch, Judith, Judith Taylor, and Beth Quinn: Emergency! Dealing with eye injuries. *RN* 1984 March; 47(3):53–54.

Wisser, Susan Hiscoe: When the walls listened. *Am J Nurs* 1978 June; 78(6):1016–1017.

Wolanin, Mary Opal: Physiologic aspects of confusion. *J. Gerontal Nurs* 1981 April; 7(4):236–242.

29

Physical Activity

Prerequisites and/or Suggested Preparation
The basic concepts of anatomy and physiology plus an introductory understanding of pathophysiology (Chapter 12) are prerequisite to this chapter. The principles of stability and balance (Chapter 11) are basic to Section Three of this chapter.

Section One

Exercise and Ambulation

The benefits of physical activity are well documented, and increasing numbers of people are trying to include some form of exercise in their daily routines. This trend is accompanied by increased opportunities for people of all ages and lifestyles to find a satisfying form of physical activity. Such opportunities include physical fitness clubs, aerobic dance classes, family-centered hiking and biking trails, preschool gymnastic programs, senior citizen exercise classes, and the Special Olympics for retarded persons.

Physical activity is especially important during illness. Not only do the physiological and psychological benefits of exercise contribute to the healing process, but exercise can actually prevent many of the complications associated with illness.

Whenever there is a possibility that physical activity might adversely affect the patient's condition, the amount and type of activity will be prescribed by the physician in consultation with the physical therapist. In the absence of any such restrictive conditions, however, the patient's physical activity is usually a nursing responsibility.

OVERVIEW OF CHAPTER

Nursing responsibilities and interventions related to physical activity are so extensive that this chapter is divided into three sections: (1) exercise and ambulation, (2) protection from the hazards of immobility, and (3) methods of moving and lifting patients safely. The sections are designed to be read in sequence, and Sections Two and Three each presume an understanding of the preceding section.

BENEFITS OF EXERCISE

The *physical* benefits of exercise and ambulation include increased cardiac output and improved circulation, fuller chest expansion and deeper respiration, improved tone of abdominal muscles, less likelihood of constipation, more complete emptying of each kidney pelvis, improved appetite, increased muscle tone and strength, and the maintenance of joint mobility.

The *psychological* benefits of exercise and ambulation include an increased sense of well-being and a different perspective of one's situation. A walk in the hall or a trip to the physical therapy department provides a change of environment, interaction with different people, and increased sensory stimulation in general. In some settings, group exercise programs provide an opportunity for increased social contacts.

Not only does the presence of physical activity yield physiological and psychological *benefits*; the absence of physical activity produces physiological and psychological *harm*.

REASONS FOR INADEQUATE ACTIVITY

An initial assessment of a patient's musculoskeletal status begins with a careful observation and analysis of his ability to perform the activities of daily living. While you are admitting or caring for a patient, you can observe his ability to walk, sit, stand, balance, lean over, reach, and grasp. You need not ask him to demonstrate these activities specifically; his ability can be assessed initially by watching him do such things as reach over and tie his shoes, comb his hair, handle the newspaper, walk to the bathroom, or reach to pull down the window shade. If he is unable to do any of the activities that can usually be done by a person of his age and general condition, a more detailed analysis of his ability will be needed to determine whether the limitations are due to lack of spirit, strength, structure, or range of motion.

Lack of Spirit or Motivation

Depression, despair, apathy, or hopelessness will diminish a person's spirit and his desire to move about. He may be *physically capable* of performing all the activities of daily living but *lack the motivation* to do so. If a patient's lack of spirit is not due to his general physical condition or to the effects of medication, a psychiatric consultation or referral may be needed as a resource for other members of the health care team.

Lack of Strength

If a patient attempts to perform the activities of daily living but is unable to do so, he may be lacking in strength. He might be weak from a systemic illness such as influenza, or his muscles may be weak from disuse. He may have poor muscle tone (atony) or his muscles may have wasted away and decreased in size (atrophy). If *lack of strength* is the cause of the patient's limited activity, efforts must be made to analyze the precise nature of the problem which could be, for example, a neurological disorder, a potassium deficiency, or the aftereffects of pneumonia, each of which requires a different and specific therapy.

Structural Defects

The activity of a patient can be limited by *structural or skeletal problems*. The absence of a body part, whether congenital or acquired, is an obvious problem, whereas the problems of movement following a spinal fusion are less observable.

Some skeletal problems are identified by comparing the patient's present condition with his previous condition as shown in earlier x-ray films and records. Other skeletal problems can be identified by comparing the patient's body, or some part of it, with the normal size and shape of that body part.

Lack of symmetry in the two sides of a patient's body could indicate a nonsignificant finding such as a slight difference in shoulder elevation, but it could also indicate a serious problem. If the gluteal folds of an infant are not symmetrical, for example, the infant may have a congenitally dislocated hip; and if the pants or skirt of a preteen child do not hang evenly, a careful back examination might disclose the presence of scoliosis (Fig. 29.1).

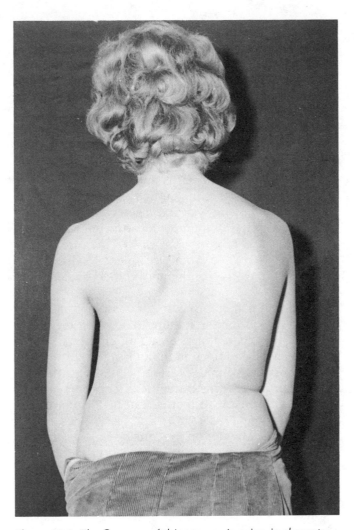

Figure 29.1 *The* S *curve of this woman's spine is characteristic of scoliosis.*

Limited Range of Motion

Some patients will be strong and anxious to move and exercise but will be held back by a limited range of motion. This limitation may be due to a disease process such as arthritis, or it may be the result of a previously developed contracture. Proper medical management of the disease process, including the use of analgesics if needed, plus physical therapy can halt a worsening of the limitation and will maintain or possibly increase the patient's current range of motion.

Restrictions Related to Therapy

In addition to personal deficits of motivation, strength, structure or range of motion, a patient's activity may be limited by restrictions imposed by the physician or another external force. A new brace, phlebitis, an inability to manage crutches, or orders for complete bed rest after a heart attack can limit a patient's ability to exercise and ambulate.

ROLE OF PHYSICAL THERAPIST

The physical therapist is responsible for diagnostic and therapeutic measures related to a patient's musculoskeletal system. The physical therapist evaluates the patient's musculoskeletal status and prescribes the therapy appropriate for a diagnosed condition, such as hemiplegia following a stroke. The evaluation is done either in the physical therapy department or at the patient's bedside if he cannot be moved because he is in traction, for example. Some treatments and exercises are done by the physical therapist; others are taught to the patient, family, or staff.

The physical therapist also acts as a consultant or resource person for the nursing staff when they need help with a patient, and a consultant or referral service is usually available to community health nurses.

The nurse is responsible for helping each patient maintain or increase his current level of muscle strength and joint movement so that he can perform his activities of daily living (ADL). The nurse is also responsible for follow-up activities on the nursing unit. A brief session in the physical therapy department each day is usually inadequate; each patient needs an opportunity to practice what he has learned at intervals throughout the day. If the physical therapist does not send periodic reports to the nursing unit with suggestions for practice between sessions, you will need to take the initiative and seek the information you need for planning the nursing aspects of the patient's program of exercise and ambulation.

TYPES OF EXERCISES

There are five major types of exercise: passive, assistive, isometric, isotonic, and resistive. The choice of exercise depends on the condition and ability of the patient and on the desired outcome.

Passive Exercises

Passive exercises are done *by the nurse or physical therapist* for a weak or helpless patient, to maintain his joint motion and flexibility. The patient is a passive recipient of these exercises. Because he does not contract his muscles or expend any energy, the exercises will *not* maintain or increase his muscle strength.

Active Exercises

Active exercises are done by the patient in order to maintain or increase muscle strength. Four common categories of active exercise are: assistive, isometric, isotonic, and resistive.

Assistive Exercises

Assistive exercises are active exercises in which the patient initiates each movement and continues it *to the limit of his ability*. The nurse or therapist then helps him to complete it. The patient's active participation helps to maintain muscle strength, and the completion of each movement by the nurse ensures the maintenance of joint motion.

In some situations, the assistance is not provided by a person but by devices such as slings or pulleys. These devices support enough of the weight of the body part being exercised for the patient to be able to complete the exercises (Fig. 29.2).

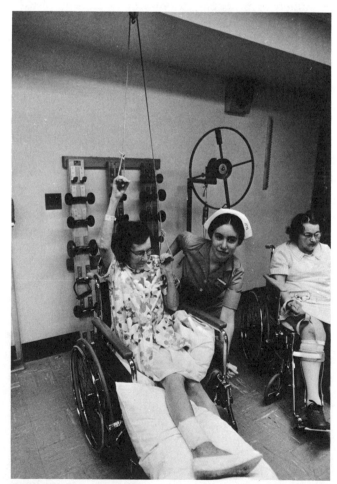

Figure 29.2 *An assistive exercise in which the patient pulls with one arm to passively exercise the other.*

Isometric Exercises

Isometric (or static) exercises are done by the patient and will maintain muscle strength and aid venous return. These exercises are active exercises in which there is increased muscle tension but no change in the length of the muscle. Because the muscle does not shorten, there is no joint movement, and isometric exercises therefore will not maintain joint function.

Isometric exercises are called *muscle-setting exercises*. Muscle groups which are commonly "set" (tensed) during illness in preparation for ambulation are the gluteal, abdominal, quadriceps, and gastrocnemius.

Isotonic Exercises

Isotonic exercises are probably the most familiar and widely used type of exercise. They are active exercises in which one or more muscles contract and a body part is moved. When done regularly, these exercises maintain joint function and increase muscle strength.

Resistive Exercises

Resistive exercises cause the involved muscles to act *against an opposing force*. The muscle actively tries to overcome the resistance, and muscle strength increases quite rapidly. Resistance can be provided by a person who holds or restrains the arm or leg, or it can be provided by weights attached to the body part being exercised.

MAINTENANCE OF JOINT FUNCTION

The statement "I'm stiff from sitting so long," often heard after a long class or meeting, is an indication of the tendency for unused joints to stiffen up. When a person is ill, he is likely to lie quietly without moving for extended periods and may as a result become stiff very quickly. A person with arthritis, for example, can lose considerable joint mobility if he becomes ill and does not move about for a few days.

The flexor muscles are stronger than extensor muscles, and the joints of an inactive person are gradually pulled into a flexed position unless preventive measures are taken. If the flexion is not counteracted by exercise and protective positioning, contractures develop and the joints become frozen in a flexed position. In extreme situations this process culminates in a permanent fetal position.

It is essential to maintain joint flexibility because contracted or immobile joints make protective positioning difficult or impossible. As a result, it is hard to relieve pressure over bony prominences and to protect the patient from pressure sores. Adequate skin care is difficult because, when joints are inflexible, it is not possible to separate the skin folds adequately, especially in the perineal area. If a person is in a curled or fetal position, chest expansion is restricted, and changes in abdominal pressure make elimination difficult.

Normal activities of daily living are difficult or impossible when joints are stiff and immobile. Contracted fingers restrict the function of the hand. Footdrop prevents a normal gait. A "frozen shoulder" makes it impossible to reach overhead.

Failure to maintain a full range of motion throughout an illness can lead to tragic complications for any patient who is comatose, has a history of orthopedic problems or arthritis, is confused, apathetic or depressed, or is on bedrest. Maintenance of joint function must be given *top* priority for such patients because the prevention of contractures is a nursing responsibility.

Assessment

As soon after admission as possible, a careful assessment should be made of the range of motion of any patient whose joints are deemed to be in danger of becoming stiff and contracted. This initial assessment provides the baseline data necessary for planning nursing care and evaluating its effectiveness.

Two skills are related to an assessment of a patient's range of motion: the ability to handle each joint in a way that is safe and comfortable for the patient, and the ability to communicate one's findings.

Handling of Joints

Some patients can demonstrate the range of motion of each joint for you, especially if you show or describe the movement you want to observe. In general, however, the patients about whom you are concerned may not be able to do this and you will need to manipulate each joint to determine its present range of motion.

Safety and comfort for the patient depend on your knowledge of the normal range of motion for each joint so that you do not attempt to move a joint beyond its normal range. Safety and comfort also depend on your ability to hold and manipulate each joint. The two basic ways to support a joint are cupping and cradling (Fig. 29.3). *Cupping* means to cup your hands and use them to hold the joints being assessed or exercised. *Cradling* means that your hand supports the underside of a joint while the distal portion of the patient's arm or leg rests on your forearm.

Both cupping and cradling meet the criteria for safe and comfortable manipulation of an extremity:

- The extremity is supported at the joints
- The "belly" of the muscle is not grasped
- All movements are controlled, slow, and smooth

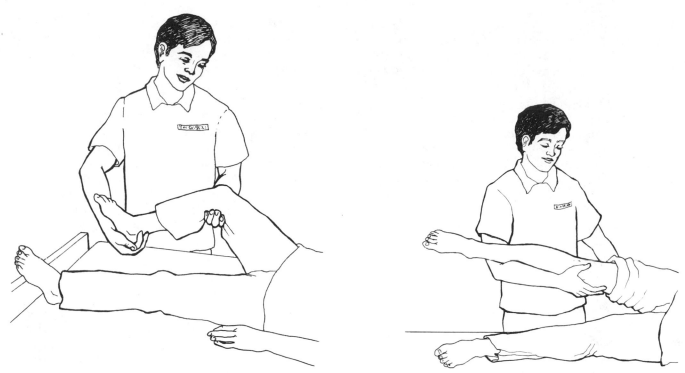

Figure 29.3 *Safe and effective methods of support during range of motion activities.* Left: *Cupping.* Right: *Cradling.*

Assessment of Joint Motion

The extent of a patient's range of motion is determined by moving each joint, or asking the patient to move each joint, through every movement possible for that joint. If the patient's joint can be moved easily and completely through each possible movement, he has a *full* range of motion in that joint. If one or more movements cannot be completed, he has a *limited* range of motion for that joint.

When the patient is moving his own joints, he will stop when he has reached the limit of movement for a joint. When *you* are manipulating the patient's joints, you will need to determine when his limit has been reached. There are three cues to the limit of a patient's range of motion:

The patient will give a *nonverbal* message of discomfort. Watch his face and hands as you work.

He will give a *verbal* message of discomfort; he will tell you that it hurts.

You will *feel* a resistance, a stiffness, or a restriction as you approach the limit of a movement.

The point at which you receive a verbal or nonverbal message of discomfort or feel resistance marks the limit of the range of motion for that joint. This point is often indicated by the number of degrees from a neutral position (considered to be 0 degrees).

Communication of Findings

The precise use of correct terminology adds to the authority and credibility of your data and enables other members of the health care team to know the patient's range of motion clearly. There is a great difference between the significance your colleagues attribute to one notation that a patient "can't move his arm very far from his body" and another notation of "left-arm abduction 30 degrees." Both phrases mean approximately the same thing, but the latter is precise and professional.

When you assess your patient's range of motion, ask him about any observed limitations because it is important to differentiate, for example, between a new and developing limitation of elbow movement and a limitation that has been present since a childhood accident 30 years ago.

Range of Motion Exercises

ROM exercises are done several times daily to maintain joint flexibility. *Passive ROM exercises* are done by the nurse for a patient who is unable to do any part of them for himself (Fig. 29.4). Since the patient expends no energy, passive ROM exercises can maintain joint function but cannot maintain or increase muscle strength.

Passive ROM exercises can be done as a separate

Terms that Describe Range of Motion

- Distal: farthest from the trunk or from the center of the body
- Proximal: closest to the trunk, or center of the body
- Abduction: away from the midline of the body
- Adduction: toward the midline of the body
- Flexion: bending a joint
- Extension: straightening a joint
- Hyperextension: movement beyond full extension
- Rotation: turning in a circular motion around a fixed point
- Circumduction: moving the distal end of a bone in a circle while the proximal end remains stationary (the movement of the bone forms a cone)
- Pronation: turning the palm toward the back of the body, or toward the feet when arms are extended out in front of the body; the position of hands when the person is lying prone (face down) with arms at sides, or when standing in a relaxed position
- Supination: turning the palm toward the front of the body, or away from feet when arms are extended out in front of the body
- Inversion: turning the sole toward the midline of the body
- Eversion: turning the sole away from the midline of the body
- Internal rotation: rotating toward the midline of the body
- External rotation: rotating away from the midline of the body

Active ROM exercises maintain joint function and also contribute to the maintenance of muscle strength in proportion to the amount of participation by the patient. The exercises are *assistive* if the patient is helped to complete part of each movement; they are *isotonic* if the patient does each one without help.

Active ROM exercises should be incorporated into the patient's ADL as quickly as possible both to give meaning and purpose to the exercises and to teach the patient how to continue exercising at home without having to set aside lengthy exercise periods. Regardless of whether the exercises are active or passive, the exercises done should be checked against an overall list of exercises in order to prevent any omissions. ROM exercises should be done smoothly, comfortably, rhythmically, and regularly. The movements for exercising each joint are shown in Fig. 29.5.

MAINTAINING OR INCREASING MUSCLE STRENGTH

Moving About in Bed

Patients should be encouraged to move and to keep moving about in bed. It is usually easier to *maintain muscle strength* than it is to try to regain it once it has been lost. A patient should *turn himself* and *move himself* whenever possible, when the bed is being made or treatments given unless such activity has been specifically prohibited.

There are several pieces of equipment that will help a patient to move himself, but the single most important factor in self-help is time. Often, a weak or partially disabled patient does not move himself or turn himself simply because the nursing staff is rushed or impatient and does not give him time enough to do so. It takes considerable time and patience to teach a pa-

nursing intervention or can be incorporated into other nursing activities. Shoulder flexion can be done when the patient's arm is washed, for example, and hyperextension of the hip can be done each time the patient is placed in a protective side-lying position.

PROCEDURE 29.1

*Providing Passive Range of Motion Exercises**

SUMMARY OF ESSENTIAL NURSING ACTIONS

1. Know the purpose of the range of motion exercises (are they a nursing measure to maintain joint motion, part of prescribed therapy to prevent or treat contractures, etc.).

2. Incorporate exercises into other activities such as the bath whenever possible.

3. Support each joint in a manner which is both safe and comfortable for the patient.

- Support the underside of each joint of the extremity being exercised.
- Never grasp the "belly" of a muscle.

4. Use slow, smooth, rhythmical movements.

5. Continually assess the patient's response to the exercises.
   - *Watch* for non-verbal messages of discomfort.
   - *Listen* for verbal indications of discomfort or pain.
   - *Feel* for resistance, restriction, or limitation of movement.

*See inside front cover and pages 495–496.

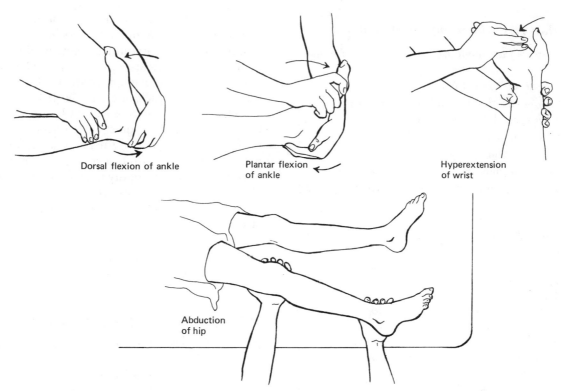

Dorsal flexion of ankle

Plantar flexion of ankle

Hyperextension of wrist

Abduction of hip

Figure 29.4 *Examples of passive range of motion exercises being done by the nurse.*

tient to move himself, but the benefits outweigh the cost. For one thing, it simply does not make sense to move and turn a patient hurriedly and then return at a later time to teach him exercises to regain the strength lost by not moving himself.

Many patients do not need side rails for safety but use them as grab rails when turning from side to side and to hold themselves on their sides for treatments or bed making. If a patient is confused or has a diminished level of awareness, you may need to remind him each time he needs to turn to reach for the side rail, and wait for him to do so.

A trapeze attached to an overhead frame (known as a Balkan frame) will enable the patient to change position, to get on and off the bedpan, and to lift himself a few inches off the bed for back care if he cannot turn on his side. The use of a trapeze strengthens the *biceps* muscles, which are used to flex the elbows and lift a weight; the use of a trapeze will *not* strengthen the triceps muscles, which are needed to extend the elbows for using a walker or crutches.

A patient who finds it hard to rise to a sitting position in bed may be able to do so with the help of a long piece of rope or braided fabric tied to the foot of the bed for him to pull against. This can be especially helpful at home, when the head of the bed cannot be

raised to bring the patient to a sitting position and when there is no trapeze or side rail.

Exercises to Prepare for Ambulation

Quadriceps Setting

For a person to walk and to get up out of a chair, the large muscles of the thigh (the quadriceps) must be strong enough for him to extend his knees and stabilize them. A patient with weak quadriceps often complains of wobbly knees or shaky legs. He cannot get out of a chair without assistance, step up on a curb or stair, or walk with confidence. He cannot use good body mechanics to pick things up because he cannot rise to a standing position from a stooped position. A person with weak quadriceps cannot manage crutches or a walker if he has the use of only one leg or foot. Exercises to strengthen the quadriceps muscles, therefore, are some of the most important of all exercises done to prepare for ambulation.

Quadriceps setting is an isometric exercise in which the muscle is set (tensed) with almost no movement of the knee or leg. Some patients can learn to do the exercise when directed to tense their thigh muscles or pull their kneecaps toward their head, but many patients are unable to follow those directions.

ELBOW

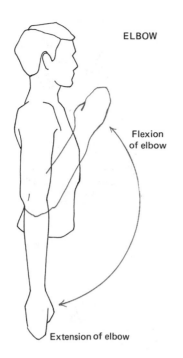

Flexion
of elbow

Extension of elbow

KNEE

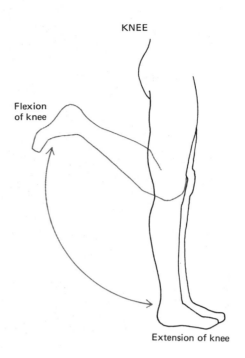

Flexion
of knee

Extension of knee

HIP

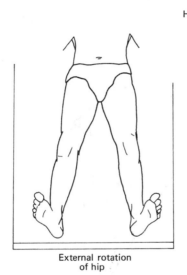

External rotation
of hip

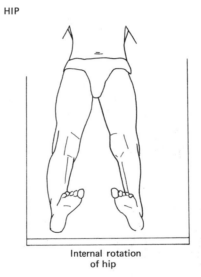

Internal rotation
of hip

NECK

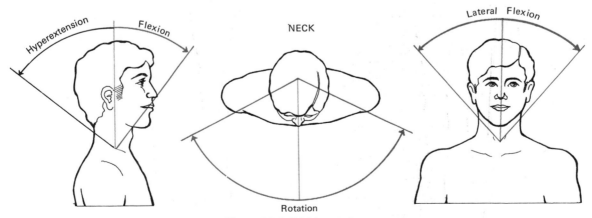

Hyperextension

Flexion

Rotation

Lateral Flexion

Figure 29.5 ROM exercises.

ANKLE

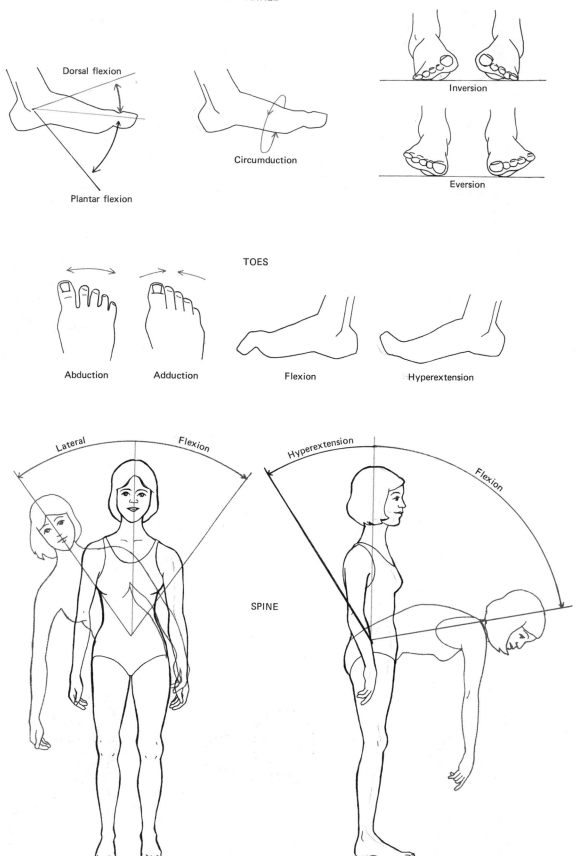

Dorsal flexion

Plantar flexion

Circumduction

Inversion

Eversion

TOES

Abduction

Adduction

Flexion

Hyperextension

Lateral

Flexion

Hyperextension

Flexion

SPINE

Figure 29.5 (cont.)

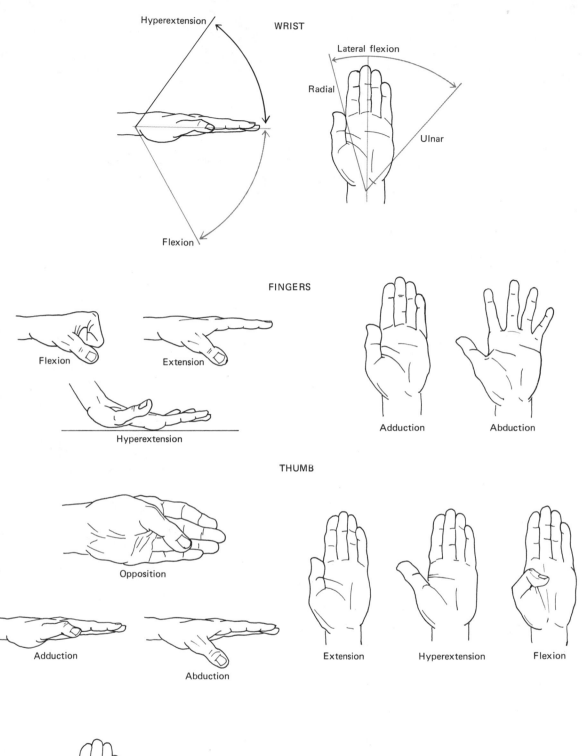

WRIST

Hyperextension

Lateral flexion

Radial

Ulnar

Flexion

FINGERS

Flexion

Extension

Hyperextension

Adduction

Abduction

THUMB

Opposition

Adduction

Abduction

Extension

Hyperextension

Flexion

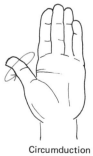

Circumduction

Figure 29.5 *(cont.)*

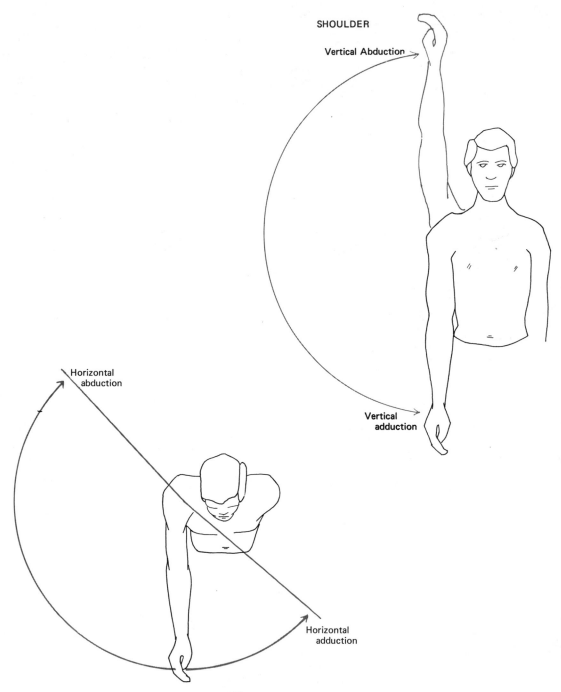

Figure 29.5 (cont.)

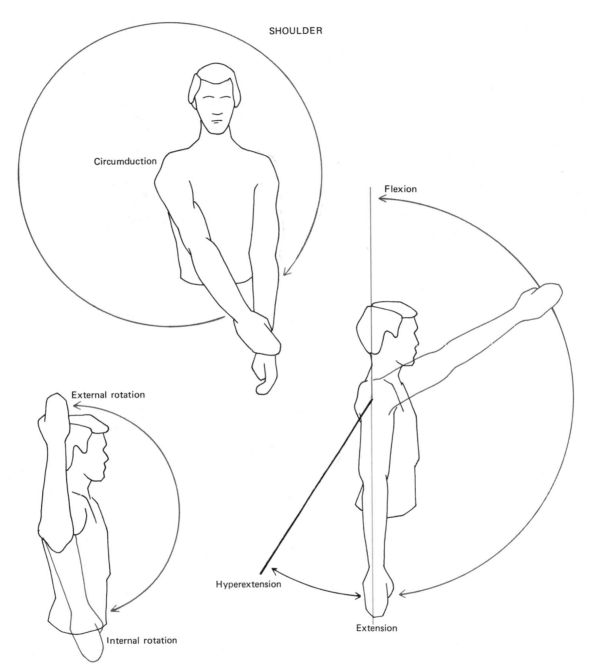

SHOULDER

Circumduction

Flexion

External rotation

Internal rotation

Hyperextension

Extension

Figure 29.5 *(cont.)*

HIP

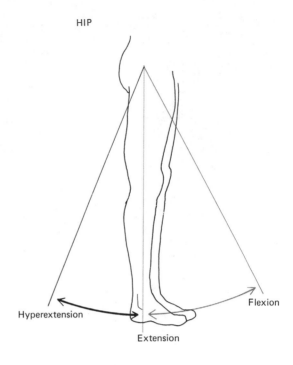

Hyperextension

Extension

Flexion

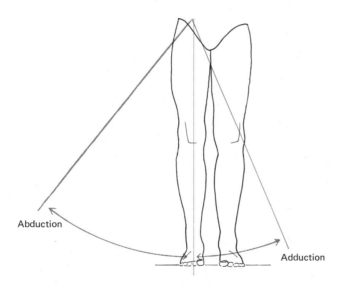

Abduction

Adduction

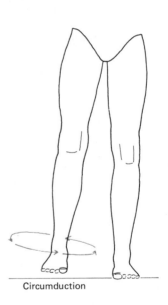

Circumduction

Figure 29.5 *(cont.)*

To teach a patient to set his quadriceps, place your hand under his knee and ask him to *press the back of his knee against your hand.* If the patient's quadriceps are extremely weak, the movement produced by the exercise may be *almost imperceptible,* and it may be several days before he can recognize the feeling of a tensed quadriceps muscle.

When teaching quadriceps setting to a patient, it is important that you keep your other hand away from the top of his knee or thigh. When directed to press his knee against your hand, the patient may become confused by the pressure of two hands. He might logically wonder "Which hand?" and just as logically press against your upper hand.

Help the patient establish a schedule for doing his quadriceps setting exercises, such as upon awakening, while waiting for lunch, while watching the evening news, and before falling asleep. Help him to set a mutually acceptable standard of performance based on his strength and motivation. An example of an acceptable standard is: "Tense your muscle and hold it for a count of 5. Do this five times for each leg each exercise period."

The quadriceps can also be exercised while the patient is sitting in a chair by slowly extending the knee and holding the foot and lower leg up for an agreed-upon count. A physical therapist often makes the exercise more difficult by adding weights (resistance) to the patient's foot or ankle. This active isotonic exercise then becomes a resistive exercise and thus increases muscle strength more rapidly.

Exercises to strengthen the quadriceps muscles are important for patients who have been sedentary for years, who have been or are going to be on bed rest for a long time, or who will need increased strength in one leg. The exercises are an important way for an athlete, for example, to maintain a high level of muscle strength while bedfast.

Lift-ups

To use crutches or a walker effectively, a patient must have enough strength in his *triceps* to extend and stabilize his elbows while he lifts or shifts his body weight. (Pulling on an overhead trapeze or the side rails is done with the *biceps* muscles; it does *not* strengthen the triceps muscles.) Some young, athletic people are able to do push-ups from a prone position to strengthen their triceps, but most older people, especially those who are ill, cannot do so and must do lift-ups instead.

Help the patient to a sitting position on the edge of the bed or in a chair, then teach him to try to lift his buttocks off the bed or chair by pressing down with his hands. A person with short arms cannot do this exercise until large books or blocks of wood are placed beside each hip for him to push on. Help the patient set up a schedule for doing lift-ups based on his condition and the urgency of his need for increased muscle strength.

Preparation of Hands

Some patients do not have enough strength in their hands to grip crutches or a walker effectively, but they can increase the strength and often the mobility of their hands by squeezing rubber balls regularly for gradually increasing periods of time.

The size of the ball depends on the size of the patient's hands. A solid sponge-rubber ball about the size of a tennis ball is satisfactory for most adults. The resistance of the ball increases the effect of the exercise and the patient's hands will ache after exercising unless he starts *slowly* and increases the time gradually. Gripping the ball five to 10 times with the entire hand is followed by digging each fingertip, one at a time, into the ball for five to 10 times each. The patient should gradually increase the exercise until he is gripping the ball and exercising each finger 25 to 50 times once or twice a day.

Dangling

Any problems related to orthostatic hypotension, such as dizziness or faintness, must be prevented or overcome before a patient can ambulate with confidence and pleasure. A susceptible patient should be raised to a sitting position several times each day with his feet lower than his body. (See Section 2 for more detailed information about orthostatic hypotension.)

DEVICES AND EQUIPMENT FOR AMBULATION

Patients who have limited use of one or both legs or who are weak and unsteady on their feet must rely on the support of a walker, cane, or crutches.

Walker

A walker offers the greatest support of all the commonly used aids to ambulation. It is made of aluminum tubing and is therefore lightweight and easy to handle. It does not tip or fall out of reach as a cane or crutch might do. Walkers are available in sizes to fit anyone from a toddler to a very tall adult, and many are adjustable. A walker should be high enough so that the patient does not have to bend over or lean forward to use it.

The patient should be taught to lift the walker, set it ahead a few inches, and then step up to it. This series of movements, "Lift, set ahead, walk up," "Lift, set ahead, walk up," should be verbalized, repeated, and practiced until the patient does it automatically.

A patient should *not* be taught to slide the walker along the floor because although this practice may be feasible on a smooth, polished floor, it is *not safe* on other surfaces. A patient who has gotten into the habit of sliding his walker is likely to continue to do so on a rough surface, and the walker will tip over if the front legs catch on a rug or threshold, or in a crack in the sidewalk.

The patient should be taught to *pick up his feet* when he walks; he should not shuffle, and he should wear shoes instead of slippers. The legs of the walker should have rubber tips to prevent slipping. Walkers with casters are available, but they are hard to control and should be used only in special situations. Some walkers have a swing-down seat that enables a patient to sit down and rest as needed. People who use a walker at work or for shopping often devise a way to carry a variety of needed items by attaching a bag, or a bicycle basket to the front of the walker.

Crutches

The three commonly used types of crutches are the axillary (or underarm) crutch, the elbow-extension or platform crutch, and the Loftstrand (or Canadian) crutch. The wooden axillary crutch is the cheapest and is preferred for short-term use. The elbow-extension crutch is used by patients whose wrists are weak or painful. Loftstrand crutches are often used by people with a permanent disability. A clamp grips the user's forearm, gives added support, and keeps the crutch from falling. The absence of an axillary bar on a Loftstrand crutch eliminates any danger of nerve damage from pressure on the radial nerve in the axilla.

Measurement

To be safe and efficient, axillary crutches must be exactly the right length, and are measured in either of two ways.

1. With the patient lying on his back, measure from his axilla to the bottom of his heel and add 2 inches to that distance.

   The extra 2 inches makes the crutch long enough to reach to the front and sides of the patient's feet for a good base of support.
2. With the patient standing with his shoes on, measure from the anterior fold of the axilla to a point 6 in to the side of his foot. The patient should be measured in the shoes he will wear while using the crutches. The crutch length should include the rubber tip and the rubber underarm pad, if used.

When a correctly measured crutch is in position for use, two fingers can be inserted between the axillary bar and the patient's axilla. If the crutch is too long, the pressure of the underarm bar on the radial nerve in the axilla will cause an injury called *crutch palsy* or crutch paralysis. Patients are often taught to use crutches that are unpadded to discourage the tendency to lean on the axillary bar. Sponge-rubber padding is often added later for a patient who stands with his crutches held under his arms.

In addition to the *overall length* of an axillary crutch, the *height of the handgrip* is important. Both of these dimensions are adjustable on a well-made crutch, and this is an important feature of crutches for a growing child. The handpiece should be adjusted so that the patient's elbow is *slightly flexed.* If the hand grip is too low, the radial nerve can be damaged even if the overall crutch length is correct, because the extra length between the handpiece and the axillary bar can force the bar up into the axilla as the patient stretches down to reach the handpiece. If the handgrip is too high, the patient's elbow is sharply flexed, and the strength and stability of his arms are decreased.

Gaits

Except in settings such as an emergency room or college infirmary, a physical therapist usually assumes responsibility for prescribing the gait to be used by a patient. If, however, a physical therapist is not available, you may have to assess the situation and teach the patient the gait that seems most appropriate.

FOUR-POINT GAIT. A four-point gait is used by people who are able to bear some weight on both feet, such as a person with cerebral palsy or arthritis. This gait approximates a normal, reciprocal walking pattern: right crutch then left foot, left crutch then right foot. It is a very safe and stable gait because the patient moves only one foot or one crutch at a time, leaving three of the four points always in contact with the floor or ground.

TWO-POINT GAIT. A two-point gait is a more rapid version of a four-point gait and requires the patient to move a foot and the opposite crutch simultaneously (right foot and left crutch, then left foot and right crutch). Like the four-point gait, it is used by people who can move both feet and bear weight on both feet. Both gaits help to maintain muscle strength because the muscles of the lower leg and thigh are used.

THREE-POINT GAIT. A three-point gait is used by a person who has the full use of only one leg. It is the gait used by a person with a broken leg or sprained ankle, for example. With this gait, the affected leg and both crutches are moved forward, and then the good leg is advanced. The crutches act as a *substitute* for the non-weight-bearing leg. This is in contrast to the two- and four-point gaits, in which the crutches are a *supplement* to the patient's legs.

SWING-TO AND SWING-THROUGH GAITS. The swing-to and swing-through gaits are very rapid gaits that can be used by a person whose legs are paralyzed but able to bear weight. After both crutches have been moved ahead, the person lifts his body and swings both legs up to or through the crutches. A person who used this gait develops strong upper-arm and shoulder muscles, but the leg muscles become or remain weak and atrophied because the legs are not used except for weight bearing.

Patient Teaching

Children and young adults usually learn to handle crutches easily and quickly, but patients who are less strong and agile may need extensive teaching and practice. A person who is fearful and apprehensive about using crutches must learn to *balance* with them before he tries to walk with them.

To help such a patient, help him stand with his back against the wall or some high, flat object. Show him how the crutches should be held, and then hand them to him. Have him first position the crutch tips about 4 in in front of each foot, and then move them about 4 in to the side to obtain a broad base of support.

Next, have the patient *sway* from side to side and *lean* forward a little to get the feeling of the handgrips. He can then progress to picking up first one crutch and then the other. When he feels confident of his ability to balance himself, demonstrate the gait he will be using and let him take a step or two.

Before his discharge, the patient should be able to manage his crutches while getting into and out of his bed and a chair and be able to go up and down stairs and steps, both with and without a railing. These skills are usually taught by a physical therapist, but in a small hospital or an emergency room, the nurse may need to teach the patient. If you are working in such a setting, consult the hospital's procedure manual or an orthopedic textbook for details of the skills a patient must learn, and practice them yourself before trying to teach them.

Canes

A cane provides support for a person who has the use of both legs but is weak and unsteady. A traditional straight cane with a curved handle or a walking stick will suffice for many people, but a tripod cane or a four-point cane offers more support for a person who loses his balance easily and frequently. These canes will stand alone beside a bed or chair and are useful for elderly people who find it difficult to lean over to pick up a fallen cane.

PREPARATION FOR PHYSICAL ACTIVITY

There are a number of determinants of the success of a patient's exercise program. Some of these are comfort, timing, and clothing.

Comfort

A patient cannot be expected to participate eagerly or even willingly in any kind of physical activity if he is in pain or other discomfort, or if he expects the scheduled physical activity to cause him pain or discomfort. A careful assessment of his situation will help to identify real or potential stressors such as pain, nausea, fatigue, worry, or despair. If a patient is reluctant to exercise or ambulate, some of the following interventions are likely to be helpful:

- Explore the patient's feelings about exercising.
- Explain as often as necessary the benefits to be gained from exercising.
- If pain is a problem, give his prescribed analgesic about 20 minutes *before* the scheduled exercise or ambulation.
- Whenever possible, promise to honor the patient's request to stop when he feels that he cannot tolerate any more activity, and then *keep that promise.*

In some situations, the exercise or activity is essential for the prevention or treatment of a potentially disabling condition and must not be cut short. If so, explain to the patient why the exercise must be completed in the face of pain and discomfort.

Try to understand what exercise or ambulation means to the patient. It may represent his return to an uncertain future, his inability to deny any longer the reality of his situation, or pressure to do something that seems far too difficult. A patient's feelings, such as frustration at being weak, anger over an amputated leg, or denial that his paralysis is permanent may make him reluctant to try to exercise or ambulate (Fig. 29.6).

Timing

The success of an exercise program will be influenced by the patient's circadian rhythm and his personal habits. It may be unrealistic to expect a sick person who is an "owl" or a "night person" to function well during an 8:30 am session in physical therapy each day, and a conference with the physical therapist could result in an afternoon or late-morning appointment.

Personal habits and preferences are also influential and should be taken into account whenever possible and appropriate. If an elderly patient has watched a certain television program for many years or has always taken a quick nap after lunch, it might be advisable to let him continue to do so if feasible rather than insist that he exercise during that particular time.

Clothing

In addition to being comfortable, clean, and attractive, the clothing of a patient who is about to exercise or

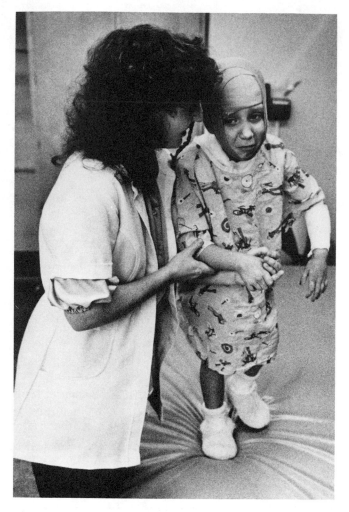

Figure 29.6 *Therapist Gabby Libbard tries to encourage Renee as she explains that exercise is essential even though the donor sites are extremely painful.*

ambulate should be safe and nonrestrictive. If the patient is going to walk, he should wear shoes, not slippers, because shoes provide support and promote a better walking posture than do slippers.

Clothing should be trim and tailored; loose, floppy robes, gowns, or pajamas are not safe for a person who is just learning to use crutches or a cane because he is likely to get tangled up in them. Clothing that is baggy conceals the outline of the patient's body and makes it difficult for the nurse or therapist to evaluate his posture and gait.

EVALUATION OF AMBULATION

There are three standards against which the patient's ambulation should be measured: normal standing gait and posture, the patient's previous posture and gait, and any expected deviations related to his current condition.

The patient should be walking with his head erect and his back straight. His feet should be lifted with each step; and his walker, cane, or crutches should be used correctly. The patient's previous manner of ambulation must also be taken into account, however. It is unrealistic to expect an elderly person to stand erect if he has not done so for many years. You may need to consult a member of the family to determine whether the patient's current posture is the same or worse than it was before.

You will also need to take into account the stage of the patient's illness or convalescence. If you remember that almost every surgical patient initially *leans forward* to reduce tension on his sutures and incision, you will not be as insistent on an erect posture for a patient one day after chest or abdominal surgery as you will be for the same patient a week later.

Reminders to walk correctly can sound like nagging to a patient who feels that he is already doing his best. This can be alleviated by trying to ignore faulty movements and by giving *positive reinforcement* for each improvement. Remarks such as "That's good; keep your head up," "That's right; lower your eyes, not your head, to see the floor," and "You are lifting each foot a bit higher today" will, by repetition, teach the patient the way he should walk.

PROCEDURE 29.2

*Helping a Patient to Ambulate**

SUMMARY OF ESSENTIAL NURSING ACTIONS

1. Assess patient's strength and motivation.
2. Decide on the amount and type of assistance which may be needed for the patient's safety and psychological security. Obtain a walker, walking belt, services of a helper, etc., as needed.
3. Set a realistic and mutually acceptable goal for ambulation.
4. Select a time for ambulation when patient is not already tired from other activities.
5. Ascertain need for pain medication if ambulation may be painful.
6. Mentally review process of managing a falling patient (p. 419).

*See inside front cover and page 507.

7. Prepare patient for ambulation.
   • Put on shoes or very *sturdy* slippers.
   • Help patient look and feel as attractive as possible.
   • Take necessary equipment into account. (patient's catheter, need for a rolling IV pole, etc.)
8. Give appropriate encouragement and praise.
9. During ambulation, seek frequent feedback from patient.
   • Check pulse, note respiration as indicated.
   • Believe patient if he says he cannot walk any farther and take appropriate action.
10. Make plans for strengthening exercises as indicated by patient's response to ambulation.

Section Two

Immobility

HAZARDS OF IMMOBILITY

The use of prolonged bed rest as a therapeutic measure has changed considerably since World War II. Before that time, surgical patients were kept in bed for several weeks after abdominal surgery, and new mothers were not allowed out of bed until 7 to 10 days after delivery. Because prolonged bed rest was thought to be necessary, it naturally followed that the resulting complications were considered unfortunate but inevitable. Weakness and fainting were expected when a patient was first allowed out of bed, and a long period of convalescence was anticipated. Postoperative pneumonia and blood clots were dreaded but common complications. The incidence of phlebitis of the leg was so common in bedfast mothers after childbirth that it was called *milk leg* because symptoms usually appeared about the time the mother's milk came in.

During World War II, army physicians were forced by limited space, personnel, and other resources to get seriously wounded men up and out of bed more quickly than anyone had thought possible. Unexpectedly and surprisingly, the incidence of postoperative complications decreased; and within a decade or two, the concept of *early ambulation* had spread to civilian hospitals. As a result of this and other advances, it is now possible for a patient to enter an in-and-out surgery unit in the morning for the repair of a hernia, for example, and go home that afternoon.

Studies have shown that *early ambulation is helpful* and that *prolonged bed rest is harmful* to the majority of patients, not just to surgical and obstetrical patients. Adequate rest is a basic physiological need that must be satisfied, but the need for rest must be balanced against the body's equally urgent need for exercise and activity. A body cannot function properly if either need is unsatisfied while the other is met to excess. Elimination, circulation, respiration, thinking, feeling, and all other body processes are disturbed and distorted either by excessive bed rest or by unreasonable exercise.

Extra rest is needed in certain situations to decrease the oxygen and energy requirements of the body and to permit the repair and healing of body tissue. A fractured bone, for example, must be immobilized in a cast or traction to ensure undisturbed healing, and a damaged heart must have its load lessened for a period of time. A person with a very high fever is unable to meet the energy requirements of both the fever and physical activity and is usually confined to bed until the fever subsides, although he may be allowed out of bed to use the bathroom.

In general, however, the potential dangers of prolonged immobility are so great that no patient is permitted to lie motionless all day unless activity would endanger his life or therapy at the moment. Patients who are weak, in pain, or seemingly too sick to be moved are lifted out of bed and positioned in a comfortable chair for short periods several times a day. It sometimes seems cruel or heartless to an observer, but the benefits to the patient far outweigh his momentary discomfort.

Some patients are immobilized not for the treatment of a current illness but as the end result of a paralyzing accident or a disease such as muscular dystrophy. The hazards of immobility are similar for all patients, however, regardless of the cause; and the purpose of this section is to help the nurse protect an immobilized patient from the preventable complications of prolonged inactivity.

Because the human body is a system composed of many interdependent subsystems, it is not possible to discuss the effects of immobility in terms of one system alone. Impairment of one system affects one or more other systems, and nursing actions taken to prevent or treat any single effect of immobility will alter other body responses as well. Bed exercises, for example, might be initiated primarily to maintain joint motion, but the increased muscle activity affects the metabolism of calcium and subsequently the skeletal system. At the same time, the cardiovascular and respiratory systems are influenced by the exercises, as evidenced by an increased pulse rate and an increased rate and depth of respiration. The intensity and effect of these changes depend on the age and condition of the patient and the type and duration of the immobility.

PRESSURE ULCERS

Prolonged pressure over any area of the body in which a bone is near the surface will cause a pressure sore because pressure over a bony prominence shuts off the circulation to that area, thereby causing death of the tissue (necrosis). Common sites are the areas over the sacrum, heels, ankles, hips, and scapulae as well as over prominent vertebrae (Fig. 29.7). Pressure sores are also called bed sores and *decubitus* ulcers (from the Latin word for lying down).

When a patient sits or lies in one position for an extended time, his body weight compresses the skin and underlying tissue between any bony prominences and the surface of the bed or chair (Fig. 29.8). As circulation to the area decreases, the cells receive inadequate oxygen and nutrients; waste products are not carried away, and the cells soon die.

Pressure sores can be caused by *any* object that compresses the underlying tissue—a mattress, chair seat, a buckle or other part of a brace, a splint, or tight restraint. Small children are likely to poke things down under their casts, and constant vigilance and ingenuity are needed to prevent them from doing so. A teaspoon or a tiny toy wedged under a cast creates an area of great pressure, and a pressure sore can develop unnoticed. The amount of damage depends on the amount and duration of the pressure. *Duration* is the most significant contributor; low pressure for a long time is more detrimental than intense pressure for a brief time.

Types

A pressure sore is categorized as either superficial or deep. A *superficial* (cutaneous) pressure sore begins with a reddened area of skin, which gives the warning signals of ischemia (inadequate blood supply), namely *pain, tingling, and numbness.* An active person responds to these warning signals by changing his position enough to relieve the pressure, thereby averting damage to the tissue. A person who is acutely ill, in pain, paralyzed, sedated, comatose, or confused is unable to respond to the warning signals and does not move, leaving the pressure unrelieved. In such situations the responsibility for detecting pressure points and relieving the

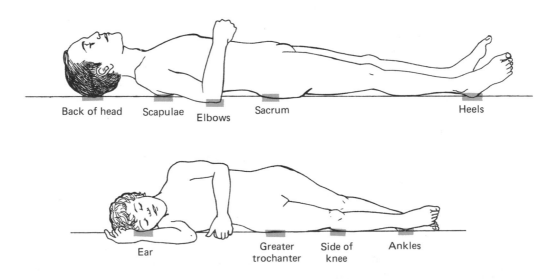

Figure 29.7 Common sites for pressure sores.

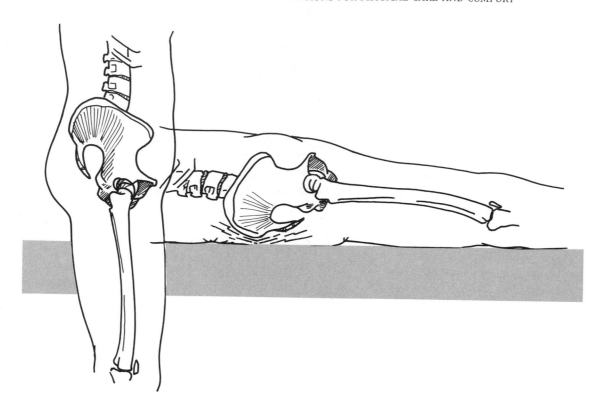

Figure 29.8 *Compression of tissue between the mattress and a bony prominence shuts off circulation to the area and if not corrected, causes injury to the tissue.*

pressure must be assumed by the nurse until the patient is capable of doing so.

The reddened skin over a pressure point is injured, but initially it is still alive and it may be able to heal itself *if the pressure is relieved and circulation is restored.* If, however, the area of reddened skin is damaged by further pressure, friction, or any other trauma, the skin breaks down and the area is open to infection. Once the skin is broken, a shallow, saucerlike crater develops and enlarges quite rapidly. An untreated superficial pressure sore will become steadily deeper and deeper until the underlying bone is exposed. The speed with which the pressure sore enlarges is determined by the physical condition and resistance of the patient, whether or not the pressure has been relieved, and whether or not the area is infected or clean.

The early symptoms of a *deep* pressure sore are often not visible on the patient's skin; there may be no area of reddened, irritated skin. A deep pressure sore is begun by a shearing force that causes underlying layers of tissue to move in opposite directions. A *shearing force* can be created when the head of a patient's bed is raised and he slowly slides down toward the foot of the bed. His body weight is pulling him down, but his

skin may be sweaty and stuck to the damp sheet. His skin is held in contact with the sheet by friction, but his subcutaneous tissue moves with his body. In the process, small capillaries are stretched until they tear and decrease circulation to the area (Fig. 29.9). The damage caused by separated layers of tissue and torn capillaries may be indicated by a hard lump, purplish discoloration, and tenderness. Accumulated waste products from this inflammation and injury must be discharged from the body somehow, and so the area of necrosis extends toward the surface of the body and breaks through the skin.

Necrotic Slough

Many pressure sores contain a patch of dead tissue that is attached to living tissue. This black necrotic tissue is called *slough* and must be removed to promote healing. The slough can be removed by surgical debridement, by the application of proteolytic enzymes that destroy necrotic tissue, or by the use of specially prepared dressings that adhere to the slough and pull it off when the dressing is removed.

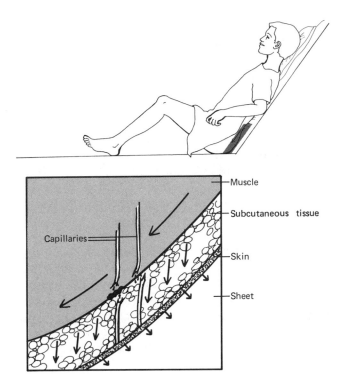

Figure 29.9 Top: a shearing force can be created over the patients' sacrum when he slides down in bed. Bottom: cross section of tissue over sacrum showing lines of force and tension. Note the torn capillaries which disrupt circulation to the area.

Labels in figure: Muscle, Subcutaneous tissue, Capillaries, Skin, Sheet

Contributing Factors

Pressure is the precipitating cause of a pressure sore, but there are a number of other contributors such as nutritional status, weight, circulation, and condition of skin. Poor nutritional status places a patient at risk. A vitamin C deficiency results in capillary fragility; a negative nitrogen balance prevents the early repair of small injuries to the skin and underlying tissues. Thinness predisposes a patient to pressure areas over body prominences because there is little or no fatty tissue to absorb the pressure, while obesity greatly increases the amount of weight and pressure exerted on the bony part.

One person who is especially at risk is one who is paralyzed from a spinal cord injury but who is independent enough to take care of himself at home. Because he is unable to feel any warning signals and because there is no nurse to check for pressure areas, he must be taught to use a mirror to examine the underside and lower portion of his body at frequent, regular intervals. Poor circulation results in lack of oxygen to the cells, and the lack of adequate oxygen decreases the cells' ability to respond to injury. A patient whose general condition is deteriorating rapidly is at risk, as are elderly patients.

Any condition that destroys or weakens the integrity of the skin increases the possibility of a pressure sore. Some of these conditions are:

Friction, which can remove the protective epithelial layer of the skin

Dehydration, which results in the loss of elasticity and resilience of the skin as well as dry, easily irritated skin

Maceration, which results in soft, fragile, water-logged skin—a condition caused by prolonged contact with urine, perspiration, or other moisture

Prevention and Treatment

There is no single, specific effective treatment for a pressure sore. Over the years, treatments have ranged from the application of gentian violet, insulin, goldleaf, and granulated sugar to the use of maggots, sawdust beds, sheepskin pads, skin grafting, and hyperbaric oxygen. Each of these treatments has been somewhat successful, but in many instances the reasons for success are unknown. Careful research might indicate that success is proportional to the vigor with which the pressure sore is treated. For example, the frequency of any treatment influences the frequency with which the patient must be turned so that the treatment can be done. The pressure is relieved each time, and it could be that this frequent and regular relief of pressure is more significant than the nature of the substance that is applied. In fact, a Dr. Vilan of Paris is credited with the observation that "you can put anything you like on a pressure sore except the patient."

Because there is no specific and quickly effective treatment, a patient who develops one or more pressure sores is subjected to weeks or even months of pain, restricted activity, and expense. It therefore behooves the patient, family, nurses, and all other health care workers to do everything possible to *prevent* the development of a pressure sore. Prevention of pressure sores is a nursing responsibility, and the incidence of pressure sores in a given institution is a measure by which the quality of nursing care can be evaluated.

The conditions that predispose a patient to pressure sores, such as thinness, are often the same ones that make it difficult to heal them, and the nursing measures used to prevent pressure sores are very similar to the measures used to treat them. The purposes of both prevention and treatment are:

Relief of pressure over bony prominences

Increased circulation to the area

Assurance of an adequate diet

Protection of the skin and granulation tissue

The nursing measures taken for prevention and treatment are so similar they need not be discussed separately. If many of the nursing measures used to treat pressure sores had been used with equal vigor upon admission for each patient at risk, the pressure sores might never have developed.

Relief of Pressure Over Bony Prominences

The patient's position must be changed every 1 to 2 hours depending on the patient's physical condition. If the patient is unable or unwilling to move himself, that responsibility must be assumed by the nursing staff. A written, specific schedule must be followed without fail on all three shifts because for some patients, the negligence of a single nurse on a single shift can undo the accomplishments of all staff on the preceding shifts.

Since pressure sores are caused by concentrated pressure over a small area, prevention and treatment are aimed at distributing weight and pressure evenly over the patient's entire body surface. This is done by the use of special mattresses and pads. Detailed information on protective positions and the use of special equipment is presented at the end of this section.

Increased Circulation to the Area

Any measure that stimulates circulation to the tissue around a pressure sore will increase the supply of nutrients for the cells and will remove accumulated waste products.

Any reddened area of skin should be treated as a potential pressure sore, and a reddened area over a patient's sacrum, for example, should be granted a top priority for nursing care. It is important to observe whether or not the redness disappears with massage. Redness caused by brief or light pressure will fade when the pressure is removed and normal circulation to the area is restored. Extensive pressure results in tissue damage and produces a redness that does *not* fade with massage and relief of pressure. Massage can be vigorous if the skin seems intact and strong, but it must be gentler if the skin seems fragile and delicate. Lotion should be used for dry skin while alcohol is useful in drying and toughening soft, oily, or macerated skin. It is essential to report and chart the presence, size, and appearance of any reddened area including whether the skin is intact and whether the redness disappears with massage.

Exercise, including passive bed exercises, will stimulate circulation of the blood to some degree in all parts of the body.

Its effect is limited in tissue over areas that do not move, such as over the sacrum, but exercise can increase circulation to pressure areas over ankles, heels, and elbows. Exercise tends to contribute to a sense of well-being, which in turn contributes oftentimes to a willingness to move about a bit more.

A local application of heat will stimulate circulation to an area around an actual or potential pressure sore. A physician's order is needed in some institutions.

Adequate Diet

A high-protein diet is necessary for tissue building and repair. Sufficient vitamin C is needed to ensure adequate capillary strength. The fluid intake should be increased as needed until optimal skin turgor (elasticity and resiliency) are attained in order to increase resistance to skin irritation and injury.

Protection of Skin and Granulation Tissue

Protection of tender skin or a newly healed area of skin can be one of the most significant nursing measures because excellent progress in preventing or treating a pressure sore can be undone by a single rough or careless movement. The skin or granulation tissue can be protected by the avoidance of friction, protection from irritating substances, and prevention of infection.

AVOIDANCE OF FRICTION. Gentleness, coupled with a knowledge of body mechanics and the properties of friction, will enable the nurse to move and turn a patient without trauma to his skin or to a pressure sore. A turning sheet must be used for each patient who has a pressure sore or is at risk. Linens should not be pulled or yanked or twitched out from under him. He should not be allowed to lie on crumbs or wrinkles, and the rim of the bedpan should be covered with a folded towel or disposable pad so that his skin will not stick to it.

The list of potential irritants is long indeed. Let it suffice to say that friction or being stuck to an object such as a bedpan can remove portions of fragile skin, remove a newly formed scab, or damage newly healed tissue and so should be avoided in every way possible.

PROTECTION FROM IRRITATION. Tender but unbroken skin can be given some protection from friction and moisture by the application of a substance such as tincture of benzoin. This is a brown liquid that forms a tough coating on the skin. When using tincture of benzoin, it is extremely important that you allow it to dry thoroughly. Before it dries, it is sticky; if it comes in contact with the patient's gown or sheets, it will cause the fabric to stick to the patient's skin and will injure the skin when the fabric is peeled off. Air dry the area for 15 to 20 min or use a heat lamp to speed the drying, then dust the tincture of benzoin lightly with talcum powder before you allow the area to be pressed against sheets or clothing.

Another protective substance is zinc oxide ointment. This is a very thick, white paste that can be used to cover a pressure sore and give it some protection from urine and feces. Zinc oxide is the base for many of the commercial preparations used to prevent diaper rash. Since it is available without a prescription and is relatively inexpensive, it is suitable for home use.

PREVENTION OF INFECTION. A *clean* pressure sore is slow to heal and hard to treat; an *infected* pressure sore presents almost insurmountable nursing and medical problems. Three major ways to prevent infection are:

1. *Conscientious handwashing* before you give care to the patient, thus protecting him from pathogens from other patients.
2. Meticulous hygiene for the patient, especially if he is incontinent of urine or feces. His skin must be kept clean and dry at all times.
3. Sterile technique as indicated when you treat the pressure sore.

METABOLIC CHANGES

During periods of immobility, tissue is being broken down faster than it is built up; the processes of *catabolism* exceed those of *anabolism*. Stores of protein are depleted, and a condition of negative nitrogen balance develops. A negative nitrogen balance indicates that protein is being lost from the body more rapidly than it is taken in, and body stores of protein must be replenished for tissue building and healing.

It is often difficult to ensure an adequate intake of protein because the patient may be suffering from anorexia (loss of appetite) or nausea, and feel unable to eat. High-protein foods often satisfy a person's appetite before he has eaten enough to fulfill his nutritional requirements, and, therefore, a high-caloric diet may be ordered instead. Such a diet may be more palatable, and the use of carbohydrates will spare the body's protein. Ways to prevent or compensate for negative nitrogen balance are described in Chapter 33.

Disuse Osteoporosis

During a period of immobility, calcium is lost from bone, which then becomes porous, fragile, and brittle. This process of decalcification of bone results in *osteoporosis* (porous bone). It occurs during immobility because a major regulatory mechanism is not functioning. Normally, musculoskeletal stresses balance the ratio of bone formation and bone absorption. The stress of weight bearing and the pull of muscle against bone stimulate *bone-building* (osteoblastic) activity. During periods of immobility, the absence of stress and pull on the bone results in increased *bone-absorbing* (osteoclastic) activity; calcium is excreted, and the bony matrix becomes thin and porous. The process of decalcification is usually reversible if the patient becomes mobile, but it may become pathological if enough bone and minerals are lost. *Disuse osteoporosis* is a serious problem for people who are permanently immobilized or who are becoming increasingly immobile from arthritis, for example.

Disuse osteoporosis cannot be prevented or treated by simply increasing the patient's intake of calcium because the excess calcium is excreted and can result in painful calcium deposits in joints or contribute to the formation of renal calculi (kidney stones). Disuse osteoporosis is prevented and treated by *maintaining musculoskeletal stress* during the period of immobility, and by *early ambulation*. Each patient should be taught to press his feet against the footboard of his bed as if he were walking and to push with his legs and pull with his arms to move himself about in bed.

If the immobility is expected to be lengthy or permanent, a device such as the tilt board is used. The patient is strapped to the board, which is then raised to a vertical position so that his feet, legs, and vertebrae are bearing weight even though he is unable to walk or stand alone.

MUSCULOSKELETAL COMPLICATIONS

Any condition, physical or psychological, that keeps a patient from exercising enough to maintain joint flexibility and muscle strength can cause *contractures* and *muscle atrophy*. This process starts within a day or two in susceptible patients.

Contracture

A *contracture* is an abnormal shortening of a flexor muscle resulting in a stiff, flexed joint. Changes occur in the muscle and soft tissue around the joint. The loose connective tissue becomes dense and solid through a process called fibrosis, and flexion of the affected joint may become permanent.

Because flexor muscles (those that flex) are stronger than extensor muscles (those that extend), failure to exercise and fully extend a joint at regular intervals allows the flexor muscles to draw the joint gradually into a flexed position. An immobile patient whose joints have not been exercised gradually assumes a rigid, fetal position with permanently flexed hips, knees, shoulders, and elbows. The condition of a patient confined to a wheelchair will eventually be complicated by permanently contracted hips and knees if those joints are not exercised *regularly* and *fully*. His joints become "frozen" into a sitting position.

Failure to exercise an immobile patient's ankles and to support his feet in an anatomically correct position will cause a condition called *footdrop,* whereby one or both of the patient's feet are drawn into a position of plantar flexion which frequently becomes permanent. In this position, the patient cannot touch his heel to the floor because of the shortened Achilles tendon, and extensive physical therapy and braces may be needed before the patient can walk again. *Footdrop can be prevented* by exercise and proper positioning, and its occurrence in any patient suggests nursing negligence or malpractice.

Muscle Weakness and Atrophy

Muscle atrophy is a condition characterized by decreased muscle size, tone, and strength. Lay people describe atrophic muscles as being shrunken and wasted away. Decreased muscle strength starts as a weakness that is noticeable after only 1 or 2 days of bed rest. Weakness leads to decreased endurance and decreased ability to tolerate exercise, which often causes the patient to become even less active. Decreased activity leads, in turn, to more weakness and, unless the cycle is broken, muscle atrophy results. The old adage *Use it or lose it* is as true for muscle strength as it is for any other body function.

It is often difficult to convince a weak patient that exercise, not rest, is needed to gain strength, and many families who are caring for a patient at home will succumb to his plea that he is too weak to exercise. *Passive exercise* (done by the nurse for the patient) will maintain *joint motion,* but *active exercise* (done by the patient) is necessary to maintain or increase *muscle strength.* Active bed exercises are absolutely essential in preparing a patient for ambulation at a later date, especially if he will need strength in specific muscles to manage equipment such as crutches or a walker.

RESPIRATORY PROBLEMS

One of the greatest hazards of immobility is *hypostatic* pneumonia, which is caused by the *stasis* (pooling) of pulmonary secretions. Because these secretions provide a good medium for bacterial growth, stasis increases the risk of pulmonary infection. Pooled pulmonary secretions also inhibit the diffusion of oxygen and carbon dioxide in the alveoli. An active person breathes deeply

from time to time during the day and also normally coughs up any secretions that might accumulate.

During a period of immobility, however, chest expansion is limited by weakness or pain, pressure of the bed against the chest, and the weight of the upper arm when the patient is lying on his side. Breathing while a patient is lying down takes approximately twice the effort that breathing when he is standing up does. The patient's lack of activity deprives him of any stimulus to breathe deeply. The result of all these factors is shallow breathing and inadequate lung expansion.

Hypostatic pneumonia is prevented by measures that cause the patient to expand his lungs fully and that prevent the pooling of any secretions. An alert patient can be taught to expand his lungs by breathing deeply at frequent, regular intervals. A confused person or a child will need to be reminded and supervised. A weak or comatose patient will probably need the assistance of some mechanical respiratory device.

The pooling of secretions is prevented by frequent turning and changing of the patient's position. Some patients can assume responsibility for turning themselves every 1 or 2 hours, but others must be turned by the nurse. This is usually combined with the turning and repositioning that must be done every 1 or 2 hours to prevent bed sores.

In addition to turning a patient from side to side, you should position him in an upright position several times a day unless it is contraindicated. Care must be taken to keep the patient from sliding down in bed and creating a shearing force that might cause a deep pressure sore. While he is in a sitting position, the patient should cough hard enough to cough up any secretions that might have accumulated in his lungs (Chapter 32).

CHANGES IN ELIMINATION

Urinary Elimination

A major cause of urinary problems during a period of immobility is the pooling of urine in the pelvis of the kidney. Gravity drains the kidney pelvis when a person is standing, but it does not do so when the person is lying down. Because the kidney pelvis is not completely drained, urine accumulates and favors the formation of kidney stones from the extra calcium taken from the bones as a result of disuse osteoporosis. Normal amounts of calcium are kept in solution by the citric acid in the urine, but excessive amounts may be precipitated out of solution, especially if the urine has become slightly alkaline as a result of bed rest.

Renal calculi (kidney stones) are less likely to occur if the patient is turned frequently to promote drainage of the kidney pelvis and to prevent the stasis of urine. The patient should be ambulated as soon as possible or, if he will be immobile for a long time, he should be brought to an erect position with some device such as a tile board or special bed. Fluids should be forced to dilute the concentration of calcium, and in some cases the pH of the urine should be lowered by means of diet to ensure the acidity that will help to keep the calcium in solution.

Intestinal Elimination

Constipation is a common complication of immobility because, in addition to the basic causes of constipation such as changes in diet and routine, the effects of medications, and lack of privacy, the muscles used in defecating are weakened by prolonged bed rest. The general loss of muscle tone that accompanies immobility affects the abdominal muscles, the diaphragm, the muscles of the pelvic floor, and the sphincter muscles. Weakness and loss of tone in these muscles contribute to the development of constipation.

The *excessive* straining likely to accompany constipation can be extremely dangerous to a patient who has very high blood pressure or who has had a stroke, a heart attack, or recent eye surgery, and it must be prevented.

CARDIOVASCULAR EFFECTS

Four frequently encountered effects of immobility on the cardiovascular system are: increased workload of the heart, orthostatic hypotension, increased incidence of thrombus formation, and increased use of the Valsalva maneuver.

Increased Workload of the Heart

With a patient in a recumbent position, blood from the legs increases the normal venous return to the heart, which causes an increase in cardiac output, stroke volume, pulse rate, and overall work load. In general, these increases are *physiological* (not pathological) effects of immobility and are not considered complications, although the effect of a recumbent position on the workload of the heart may need to be evaluated for patients with various kinds of heart trouble.

Orthostatic Hypotension

When a person who has been recumbent for an extended time first assumes an erect position, he may faint as a result of a drop in BP (orthostatic, or postural,

hypotension). This is caused by a decreased ability of the autonomic nervous system to maintain an even distribution of blood throughout the body when it is in an erect position. Blood tends to pool in the lower parts of the body, and the resulting decrease in blood circulating through the head and upper body causes the person to faint. The exact mechanism of this phenomenon is not known.

The problem of orthostatic hypotension can be minimized by elevating the head of an immobilized patient several times a day unless this is contraindicated, by raising him to a standing position as soon as possible, and by ambulating him at the earliest opportunity. When a patient who has been on bed rest for more than a few days is to get out of bed for the first time, he should be brought to a fully erect position *slowly* and by stages. For example, the nurse might first help him to sit up in bed supported by the raised head of the bed, then to sit on the edge of the bed with his feet and legs lower than his body, and finally, to stand beside the bed.

Elastic (Ace) bandages or elastic stockings will help to prevent the pooling of blood in the legs and will aid the return of venous blood to the heart. If the problem of orthostatic hypotension is severe, a pressure bandage across the abdomen will help prevent pooling of blood in the lower part of the body. If the patient will be on bed rest for an extended period of time, a tilt board or circular electric bed is often used in conjunction with elastic stockings and abdominal pressure to retain the body's ability to maintain its blood pressure when erect and to decrease the probability of orthostatic hypotension when the patient is finally ready for ambulation.

Increased Incidence of Thrombus Formation

Prolonged bed rest can contribute to the process of thrombosis (the formation of a blood clot in a blood vessel) by producing one or more of the conditions that predispose to clot formation. Immobility slows the circulation of venous blood, and the resulting stasis creates a situation that favors the development of a clot whenever the intima (the lining) of a vein is injured in any way. Prolonged or intense pressure that compresses the vein is likely to damage it, and a slow or stagnant venous blood flow past the injury fosters clot formation. Clots are more likely to form when damage to the intima and stasis of the blood are accompanied by changes in the coagulability of the blood as a response to surgery, trauma, drugs, or disease.

Pulmonary Embolism

It is important to protect patients from thrombosis because of the risk of a pulmonary embolism. If a *thrombus* should be dislodged from its original site, it becomes an *embolus* and it travels through the veins of the leg and trunk. These veins become increasingly larger and terminate in the inferior vena cava. The clot then passes through the heart and enters the pulmonary artery. When the clot reaches an artery small enough to block its further passage, it obstructs that artery and prevents all blood flow beyond that point. A large clot can obstruct a large artery, shutting off circulation to a large portion of the lung. A major interruption of the blood flow through the lung drastically changes the circulation of blood to and from the heart and can be fatal. If only a small pulmonary artery is blocked, the heart is not significantly affected. The involved lung tissue dies, but it is replaced with scar tissue.

Pain and tenderness in the calf can be early symptoms of *thrombophlebitis* (inflammation of a vein with clot formation), and the calf should *not be massaged* until the condition has been evaluated because of the danger of dislodging a clot and causing a pulmonary embolism.

Causes of Pressure and Injury

Some of the most common causes of injury to deep veins are:

Prolonged pressure of the mattress on the calf of the leg

Prolonged pressure on the popliteal vein when the knee-gatch of the bed is raised or the knees are flexed on pillows

Pressure of the tibia of one leg on the calf of the other leg

Compression of the femoral vein by weight of pelvis and upper leg

Pressure on the popliteal space from the edge of the seat of an ill-fitting, too-high chair or wheelchair

Prevention of Thrombus Formation

Measures that prevent the pooling and stasis of venous blood and damage to the vein will help to decrease the likelihood of clot formation. Such measures include the following nursing actions:

- Use a protective side-lying position to keep pressure of the upper leg off the lower leg
- Provide frequent changes of position to avoid prolonged pressure on a deep vein
- Avoid pressure on the popliteal space from the knee-gatch of the bed, pillows, chair seat, or sitting with legs crossed
- Promote return of venous blood from legs by use of elastic stockings or bandages

- Stimulate return of venous blood by contracting leg muscles through active exercises while in bed or chair
- Elevate the patient's legs when he is sitting in a chair

Increased Use of the Valsalva Maneuver

The *Valsalva maneuver* occurs whenever a patient makes his thorax rigid and holds his breath while straining to defecate or while using his arms and upper trunk to move himself about in bed. During this maneuver, his intrathoracic pressure is increased, which decreases the blood flow to his heart. When the patient lets his breath out, the intrathoracic pressure decreases and there is a sudden surge of blood to the heart. This can be dangerous for a person whose heart cannot compensate for the suddenly increased workload.

This maneuver occurs at intervals throughout the day with active people, but its use increases in a patient who is bedfast, especially if he is constipated. Its occurrence can be reduced by:

- Preventing constipation
- Teaching the patient to avoid straining
- Permitting the patient to use a bedside commode rather than a bedpan as soon as possible
- Encouraging a cardiac patient to accept or ask for help in moving himself about in bed

PSYCHOSOCIAL EFFECTS

The *physiological* effects of immobility are relatively consistent and predictable from patient to patient, but the *psychosocial* effects are highly individual and depend on the patient's response to his immobility. Some of the circumstances that influence his responses are the onset, cause, and duration of the immobility; his developmental level; and his perception of the impact on his life.

The patient may react to the psychosocial stressors of immobility with anger, depression, anxiety, denial, grief, or any of the responses that characterize his own reaction to stress.

PROTECTIVE POSITIONING

A patient in bed who cannot or will not change position must be protected from pressure sores and contractures. When a patient lies in bed in an unprotected position for extended periods of time, the muscles of the body relax and gravity tends to pull the body into an "easier" position. In a back-lying position, for example, the legs roll outward into a position of external rotation, and the feet drop from an upright position to one of plantar flexion. If these movements are not corrected, the hip and ankle joints develop crippling contractures.

Each of the three basic positions—back-lying, side-lying, and prone—protects certain specific areas of the body but at the same time poses a hazard to other areas if used exclusively. A side-lying position, for example, relieves pressure on the patient's back and heels but creates pressure on his hips, shoulders, and ankles, and since a person tends to curl up when lying on his side, this position also contributes to flexion contractures of his hips, knees, and elbows.

Patients who cannot or do not move about in bed require continuous *protective positioning* in order to avoid the musculoskeletal complications of bed rest, and they must be repositioned every 1 or 2 hours for maximum protection. A written schedule of position changes is often included in the nursing care plan for a patient and is written in the Kardex or the written nursing care plan for all to follow.

Protective Back-lying Position

The protective back-lying position (Fig. 29.10) closely approximates the anatomically correct standing position, and the characteristics of both are:

Head, trunk, and legs. Good alignment with no lateral flexion and no deviation from the midline of the body

Back and neck. Extended, with no flexion of spinal column

Legs. Parallel (no abduction or adduction)

Knees. Relaxed and extended, but no hyperextension

Feet. Parallel, at right angles to legs, with toes pointing straight ahead or straight up

Complications that result from continued use of an unsupported, unprotected back-lying position are: flexion of the spine and neck (which produces a sunken chest and forward-held head), flexion of the hips, external rotation of the hips, external rotation of the hips, and plantar flexion of the ankles.

Preventing Flexion of the Hips, Spine, and Neck

Flexion of the hips, spine, and neck is caused by the improper use of pillows or by a too soft, sagging mattress and springs. It can be prevented by the cautious use of pillows and the use of a bedboard. In the home,

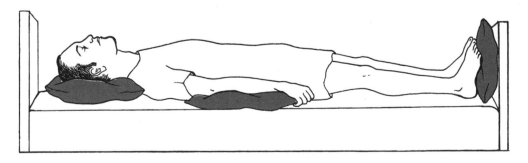

Figure 29.10 *Protective back-lying position.*

a piece of plywood can be cut to size and slipped between the mattress and a soft or sagging spring. Some families who are concerned about the prevention of back problems and the promotion of good posture have plywood under every mattress in the home. Folding bedboards are available for use in travel.

In the hospital, a one-piece bedboard would interfere with the action of the bed's adjustable springs and would not permit the head of the bed to be raised. Therefore, a sectional bedboard is used. Slats of wood about 3 inches wide that extend from one side of the bed spring to the other are encased in heavy fabric that keeps them together yet permits them to be rolled or unrolled for insertion or storage. An orthopedic ward will have bedboards on nearly every bed, but they must be requisitioned on other units.

One or two pillows may be used to support the patient's head and neck in a *neutral* position (neither flexed nor hyperextended). The patient's chest should be *fully expanded,* and the pillows under the head and neck should extend down under the shoulders as needed to achieve this position.

Preventing External Rotation of the Hip

An unsupported hip tends to roll *outward* (external rotation) and if left in that position for an extended period of time, a permanent contracture of the hip develops. If a patient lies quietly without changing position for hours on end, he will need the protection of a *trochanter roll.* A trochanter roll changes the position of the leg and hip by lifting the greater trochanter which causes the leg to roll from a position of external rotation back to a neutral position.

A trochanter roll is made by folding a sheet or blanket so that its width extends from the patient's *waist* to his *knee.* One end of the folded sheet is placed *all the way* under the patient's lower back and thighs. If the sheet is inserted only part way under the patient's back, the ends of the folds are uncomfortable and create uneven pressure against his back, which contributes to the development of pressure sores.

The loose end of the folded sheet is rolled under, *toward the mattress* (Fig. 29.11). If it is rolled up and away from the mattress, so that the finished roll lies on top of the sheet, the trochanter roll will soon unroll and become useless. Once the folded sheet is in place, the end of the roll is rolled under until the patient's *foot* assumes an *upright position.* You will not see any change in the position of the hip itself. If the roll is too small to be effective, unroll the end of the sheet and insert more material.

The rotation of the leg back to a neutral position seems to occur almost at the end of the process of making the trochanter roll; it is not seen as a gradual movement throughout the process. A trochanter roll is properly placed when the patient's *patella* (kneecap) and *toes* point *toward the ceiling* (Fig. 29.11). The roll is rather bulky and looks uncomfortable, but it is not. Have a friend or classmate make one for you so you can see how it feels, and practice making them for people of various heights and weights. Each time you practice, direct your "patient" not to move his leg and to let the pressure of the trochanter roll bring the leg to a neutral position.

On occasion, you may see a person attempt to control external rotation by placing a sandbag or other heavy weight against a patient's ankle. It will momentarily hold the foot in what appears to be a neutral position, but very quickly the foot and leg will slide away from the sandbag into an adducted position in which the leg can once more become externally rotated. External rotation of the leg is the outward sign of external rotation of the *hip* and must therefore be *corrected at the hip,* not the ankle.

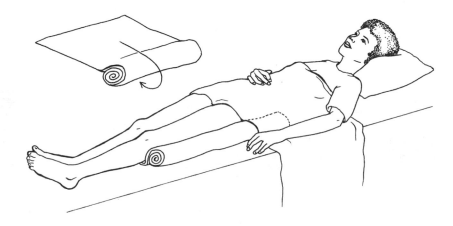

Figure 29.11 *Trochanter roll in place to prevent external rotation of the hip.*

PROCEDURE 29.3

*Making a Trochanter Roll**

SUMMARY OF ESSENTIAL NURSING ACTIONS

1. Fold a sheet or bath blanket so that the folded width will extend from patient's waist to knee.
2. Position one end completely under the patient's body and remove all wrinkles.
3. Roll the other end *toward* the mattress and away from patient's hip.
4. Continue rolling the fabric along the patient's leg and hip until the patella (kneecap) and toes point directly toward the ceiling.
   - Include additional fabric in the roll if necessary.
5. If both hips need to be supported in a neutral position, *center* the folded sheet under the patient's body and include enough extra fabric in the roll on each side to bring each hip into a protected position.

*See inside front cover and page 520.

Preventing Footdrop

Footdrop is a deformity in which the ankle is contracted into a position of plantar flexion; the patient may be unable to touch his heel to the floor when he tries to walk. The prevention of footdrop is a nursing responsibility and should be started upon admission for patients who are neither active in bed nor ambulatory. Prevention is cheap and effective, but the treatment of footdrop is expensive and often ineffective.

The position of plantar flexion is confusing because the opposite position is also a position of flexion—dorsal flexion. (Some texts refer to this position as *extension* of the ankle because the ankle looks as if it were extended.) When the foot moves toward the dorsal (top) surface of the foot, the ankle assumes a position of *dorsal flexion*. When the foot moves toward the plantar (bottom) surface of the foot, the ankle assumes a position of *plantar flexion*. It may help you remember the difference between the two to connect plantar flexion (toward the sole) with plantar warts, which occur on the sole, or with planting one's feet firmly on the ground.

Footdrop is prevented in two ways: (1) by removing pressure from the dorsal surface of the foot and (2) by supporting the plantar surface of the foot. Pressure is removed from the dorsum of the foot by keeping the weight of the bedclothes off the feet. In the hospital, this is done by placing a footboard under the bedding to support its weight. The footboard must extend at least an inch beyond the patient's toes in order to be effective. In the home, if a regular footboard is not available, any object that is *higher than the length of the patient's feet* can be used, such as a serving tray, cookie sheet, or piece of plywood.

Removing the weight of the bedding affords only partial protection against footdrop; the pull of gravity on the feet must be counteracted. This is done by *supporting the plantar surface* of the feet. In the hospital, it is usually possible to position the footboard against the patient's feet; one piece of equipment keeps the bedding off the dorsal surface *and* supports the plantar surface at the same time (Fig. 29.12).

If the footboard is not adjustable and can be placed only at the end of the mattress, a footbox is used to fill the space between the patient's feet and the footboard. The footbox is covered with a sheet or bath blanket to provide a comfortable, warm surface for the patient's feet. If for some reason the patient's knees are flexed, the angle of the footboard or footbox must be adjusted to correspond to the angle of the patient's feet.

In the home, a carton, box, suitcase, chair cushion, footstool on its side, or other object can be used to support the patient's feet. If the object used to support the feet extends above the toes, a separate footboard is not needed to support the weight of the bedding.

In the hospital, when a footboard or a footbox is requisitioned, it is delivered to the nursing unit and is sometimes set on the floor. If so, it must be cleaned with soap and water or a disinfecting solution before it is placed in the patient's bed. This is especially important if the patient has an incision or an open lesion. If the footbox or footboard is removed while the bed is being made, it must be placed on clean newspapers or some other clean surface so that it will not need to be cleaned again before it is replaced in the patient's bed. Equipment such as footboards should be cleaned carefully between patients.

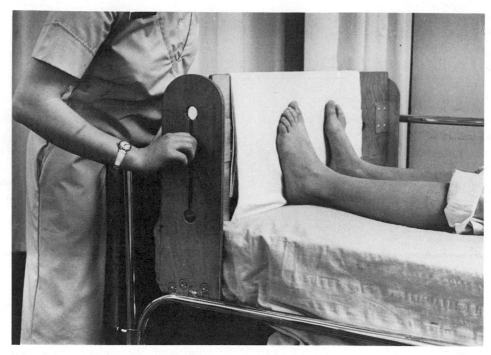

Figure 29.12 *An adjustable footboard can be slid toward the head of the bed to fit a short person and adjusted to the correct anatomical foot position.*

PROCEDURE 29.4

Using a Protective Back-lying Position*

SUMMARY OF ESSENTIAL NURSING ACTIONS

1. Position patient on his back with body in good alignment (no lateral flexion or twisting of spine).
2. Protect neck and spine from undue flexion.
   - Place bedboard under mattress if needed because of patient's weight, diagnosis, and/or soft or sagging springs and mattress.
   - Position pillow under head *and* shoulders to keep neck in good alignment.
3. Protect ankles from footdrop.
   - Support sole of foot with covered box or footboard.

*See inside front cover and page 519.

- Keep weight of bedding off patient's toes and dorsal surface (top) of foot.
4. Protect hips from external rotation if necessary because of patient's condition.
   - Use trochanter roll to keep hips in neutral position with knees and toes pointed toward the ceiling (see Procedure 29.3).
5. Protect skin from irritation.
   - Make sure lower bedding is tight and wrinkle free.
6. Ask patient if position is comfortable; make any adjustments which are feasible and safe.

Protective Side-lying Position

A side-lying position is familiar and comfortable for many patients, and it is used to relieve pressure on the patient's sacrum, heels, scapula, and the back of his head. Unless the patient is positioned properly, however, a side-lying position substitutes another set of problems for the ones it relieves. The weight of the upper arm can restrict the chest expansion of a weak patient, the width of the lower shoulder can produce lateral flexion of the neck, and the pressure of the upper leg on the calf and thigh of the lower leg can interfere with circulation in that leg.

A protective or supported side-lying position (Fig.

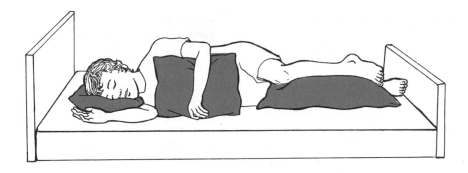

Figure 29.13 *Protective side-lying position.*

29.13) prevents the occurrence of these problems and can be evaluated by the following criteria:

- Upper shoulder and hip are over lower shoulder and hip; body is in good alignment; torso is not twisted
- Upper arm is supported by pillows as needed to prevent pressure on chest
- Upper leg is parallel to mattress (no adduction of hip) and supported on pillows with no pressure on lower leg
- Head and neck have enough support to prevent lateral flexion of neck
- Lower arm is in a comfortable position

Positioning a Patient on His Side

To position a patient on his side, first move him on his back to the edge of the bed away from the direction he will be facing when positioned. If he is left in the center of the bed and then turned to his side, he will be too near the edge of the bed for safety, and there will be no room for the pillows needed to support his upper arm and leg.

Next, *cross* the patient's legs in the *direction of the turn.* When he is turned, the weight of the upper leg falling toward the mattress will help pull the patient over onto his side. If it is feasible, teach the patient to grasp the side rail and pull to help turn himself. After the patient has been turned onto his side, stand behind him and either slide your arms under his hips or use a pull sheet to pull his hips toward you. A movement of only an inch or two helps to stabilize the patient and adjust the skin and subcutaneous tissue under the patient's hip. Use good body mechanics to protect your back as you do this.

The patient's head should be supported with a pillow equal to the width of his shoulder to prevent lateral flexion of the neck. One or two pillows should be used as needed to support the weight of the patient's upper arm. Care must be taken to keep the pillows away from

the patient's face if the room is hot, or the patient feels claustrophobic and closed in by too many pillows.

The position of the patient's lower arm depends on the condition of the elbow. If he has full range of motion in that elbow, his forearm can rest on the mattress under the pillow that is beneath his head. If the range of motion is limited, the forearm will need to rest on top of one of the pillows; the patient will be unable to lay it on the mattress.

Before the upper leg is positioned on pillows, it is advisable to take this opportunity to *hyperextend the hip* several times (Fig. 29.14). Hyperextension is part of a

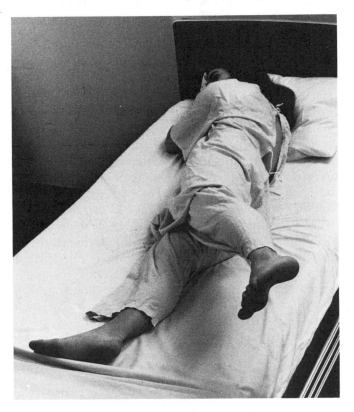

Figure 29.14 *This patient is able to hyperextend her hip without the assistance of the nurse.*

normal walking gait, and can be done in bed only with the patient in a prone or side-lying position. (The lower hip cannot be hyperextended until the patient is turned to the other side.)

One or two pillows are used to support the patient's upper leg from groin to ankle. Three or more pillows may be needed if he is very tall. Enough pillows should be used to prevent adduction of the upper leg; the entire length of the leg should be parallel to the mattress.

In the home, the patient's upper leg can be supported on a long thick piece of foam rubber rather than on numerous pillows. The foam rubber should be about 36 inches long (depending on the length of the patient's flexed leg), 18 inches wide, and 4 to 6 inches thick (depending on the width of the patient's hips). The width can be trimmed until a regular pillow case can be pulled over each end; it is not necessary to make a special case. Many people with back problems routinely support the upper leg to prevent adduction whenever they assume a side-lying position.

When the patient has been positioned, grasp his shoulder and hip and gently move his body back and forth to check the stability of his position. He may need a pillow at his back unless the room is so hot that he cannot tolerate the warmth of another pillow. Tuck one edge of the pillow under the patient's back, and firmly roll the other edge *under toward the mattress*. It will *not* stay in place and will *not* support the patient if it is rolled up, away from the mattress.

If a patient has a pressure sore, a heat lamp is often used to stimulate circulation and promote healing while he is in a protective side-lying position.

Positioning a Patient With a Fractured Hip

When moving or turning a patient following the repair of a fractured hip, it is imperative to *prevent adduction* of the affected hip and leg. Whenever a person's leg is moved toward or past the midline of the body, there is outward pressure on the head of the femur. If you cross one of your legs over the other, you can feel an outward pressure in the hip of that leg. It is possible to dislocate a fractured hip by adducting it; therefore, the patient must be moved in such a way that there is not even a momentary adduction of the hip. (For more information, see Procedure 29.5, Logrolling.)

When the patient is turned *onto his affected hip*, there is no problem of adduction. Gravity and the weight of the affected leg pull it away from the midline toward the mattress, and there is no adduction. The mattress

splints and limits the movement of the hip. When you turn a patient to his unaffected side, however, care must be taken not to let the affected leg (the upper leg) drop toward the midline. First of all, teach the patient that his affected hip and leg must be supported at all times during each and every turn so that he can share the responsibility for safeguarding his hip.

If a helper is available, have her hold the affected leg in a neutral or slightly abducted position while you turn the patient and place the necessary number of pillows under the affected leg. You may need more pillows than you would expect because the weight of the leg compresses the pillows and can let the leg drop into a position of adduction.

If a helper is not available, you will have to position the pillows while the patient is still lying on his back before he is turned. Place as many pillows between his legs as needed to support the affected leg and hip. Then, while the patient is rolling onto his side, move the affected leg *and* the pillows at the *same time* (Fig. 29.15). Later on, as the patient gains strength, it will be possible just to support the affected leg while the patient turns himself and then to position the pillows at the completion of the turn.

Because the patient with a fractured hip is often elderly and susceptible to pressure sores and other dangers of immobility, it is important to turn him regularly but with constant vigilance to prevent adduction and possible dislocation of the affected hip.

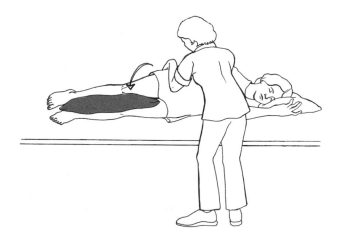

Figure 29.15 *Moving a patient with the leg supported to protect a fractured hip (see text for explanation).*

PROCEDURE 29.5

Logrolling*

SUMMARY OF ESSENTIAL NURSING ACTIONS

1. Know the reason why this procedure must be used to turn the patient.
2. Secure the assistance of two or three nurses, depending upon the size, weight, and condition of the patient.
3. Slide patient to the edge of the bed *while keeping the body in perfect alignment* (no lateral flexion of spine and neck).

*See inside front cover and page 524.

4. Prepare patient for turn.
   - Have small pillow ready to slip under head to prevent lateral flexion of neck when patient is on side.
   - Position pillow between legs to prevent adduction of hip when patient is turned.
5. Roll patient to side using pull sheet if indicated.
6. Check alignment of patient and make any necessary adjustments.

PROCEDURE 29.6

Using a Protective Side-Lying Position*

SUMMARY OF ESSENTIAL NURSING ACTIONS

1. Move patient on his back to side of bed opposite the direction he will be facing when positioned on side.
2. If patient is able to help turn, put up a side rail on side of bed patient will be facing.
3. Cross patient's legs in direction of turn.
4. Turn patient onto side.
   - Encourage patient to grasp side rail or edge of mattress to help pull self onto side.
   - Use pull sheet as needed to turn helpless patient.
5. Stand behind patient, reach under patient's hips and pull them toward you until patient's torso is stable and comfortable.
6. Use enough pillows to meet following criteria:

*See inside front cover and page 523.

   - Head and neck are aligned with spine and supported to prevent lateral flexion of neck.
   - Upper arm is supported to prevent pressure on chest.
   - Lower arm is in comfortable position.
   - Upper leg is parallel to mattress and supported to prevent abduction of hip and pressure on lower leg.
   - Body is in good alignment; torso is not twisted.
7. Tuck pillow firmly behind patient's back for support as needed.
8. Make sure there are no wrinkles under patient in clothing or sheets.
9. Make any adjustments needed to fulfill *purpose* of side-lying position (to facilitate conversation with visitors, relieve pressure, promote drainage, watch television, etc.).

Protective Prone Position

A protective prone position relieves pressure on the patient's back and sides, but many patients find, or expect to find, the position difficult or uncomfortable. A patient may be reluctant to assume a prone position because he or she:

Will have, or expects to have, difficulty breathing

Has not been in a prone position for years

Finds it painful to turn the neck

Has been left in a prone position too long on previous occasions

Finds it painful to lie on the abdomen if it hyperextends the back

Is so stooped that it is uncomfortable or painful to be forcefully straightened by a prone position

Some of the objections to a prone position are invalid with respect to a *protective* or *supported* prone position. If the patient is *properly positioned,* he will be relatively comfortable even the first time and will become more comfortable with each succeeding positioning. The nurse can help the patient accept the prone position by positioning him with skill, keeping the first few periods very short, and turning him promptly at the agreed-upon time.

Positioning a Patient in a Prone Position

Before moving a patient into a prone position, the nurse should explain the procedure even though the patient may seem unresponsive. It is wise to anticipate as many areas of reluctance as possible, to describe the way you plan to prevent or minimize any potential discomfort, and to discuss the patient's concerns with him.

1. Move the patient as close to the edge of the bed as possible. Use a pull sheet and get extra help if the patient is apprehensive, heavy, or helpless. He must be at the *edge* of the bed before the turn so that he will be in the *center* of the bed at its conclusion.

2. Cross his ankles in the direction of the turn, placing the leg nearer the side of the bed over the leg closer to the center of the bed.

3. With the patient still on his back, position the arm nearer the center of the bed with the *palm against his thigh*. As he is turned onto his abdomen, he will roll over that arm, but any discomfort will be brief and minimal. Do *not* attempt to get the patient's arm out of the way by placing it over his head. Such a position could injure the patient's shoulder as he rolls over it or when you try to position it after the turn. There is no comfortable or *safe* way to bring that arm to his side after he is on his abdomen, especially if his range of motion is limited in any way.

4. Ask the patient to face away from the direction of the move and maintain that position during the turn so that his face will not be buried in the mattress.

5. If the patient has large or tender breasts or has any lower back problems, position a pillow between the patient's midriff and hips. The pillow *cannot* be put in place later; it *cannot* be inserted after the patient has been turned (Fig. 29.16).

6. If the patient is alert, ask him to reach for the edge of the bed or side rail and help to pull himself over. If he is not alert, position the arm and hand nearer the edge of the bed by his side out of the way.

7. Roll the patient onto his abdomen and immediately check the position of his face and neck.

8. Pull his lower arm out from under his body as needed and make him comfortable (Fig. 29.17).

9. Adjust the pillow under the abdomen as needed.

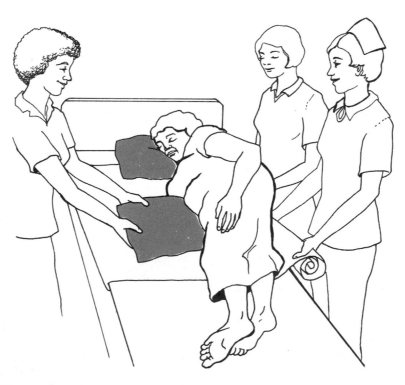

Figure 29.16 *Placement of a pillow to protect a patient with large breasts or a lower back problem before turning to a prone position.*

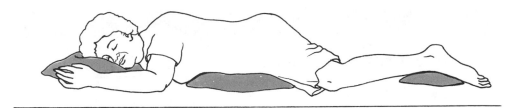

Figure 29.17 *Protective prone position.*

Add other small pillows or pads under the head or shoulders as needed for good alignment and comfort.

10. Position the patient's feet to prevent footdrop, which can result from pressure against the dorsal surface of the foot. If he is tall, let his feet hang over the end of the mattress. Place a folded towel over the edge of the mattress to cushion the corded edge and to lift the feet enough so that his toes do not touch the frame of the bed. If his feet do not reach the foot of the bed, elevate his lower legs on pillows. The number of pillows needed depends on the length of the patient's lower leg and size of his feet. His knees should rest on the mattress, and his feet should be almost at right angles to his legs.

11. Cover the patient and place the bell cord within reach.

12. Return *promptly* at the designated time. If the patient is apprehensive or uncomfortable, he may tolerate this position poorly, especially if he is left for an unnecessarily long time. The protective prone position is an extremely important position because, in addition to relieving pressure on the patient's back and sides, it is the only position that ensures *full extension* of the patient's hips.

Semiprone Position

The semiprone position is used for patients who cannot tolerate a prone position. It relieves pressure on the patient's back and sides, but his hips are not fully ex-

tended (Fig. 29.18). The patient's head, shoulders, and hips are well aligned; there is no twisting of his spine. His upper arm, thigh, and trunk are supported by pillows, and a small pillow is placed under his head as needed. The patient may find it a bit uncomfortable to have an arm behind his back, but he may become used to it, especially if the position is used regularly at fairly frequent intervals.

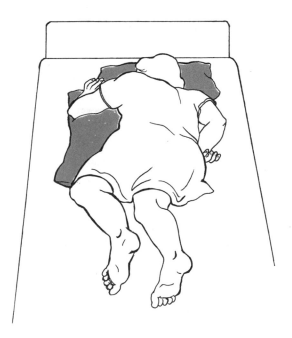

Figure 29.18 *Protective semiprone position.*

PROCEDURE 29.7

*Using a Protective Prone Position**

SUMMARY OF ESSENTIAL NURSING ACTIONS

1. Try to anticipate and relieve any patient anxiety about lying in a prone position.
2. Secure adequate help from staff or family unless patient is able to help self.
3. Move patient as close to edge of mattress as feasible.
4. Position patient for the turning:
   - Position arm nearest center of bed with palm against thigh.
   - If indicated by patient's condition or body build, position pillow in center of bed between patient's midriff and hips.
   - Cross patient's ankles in direction of turn.
   - Help patient turn face AWAY from direction of turn.

*See inside front cover and page 526.

- If patient is able to help, raise side rail so he can pull against it with upper arm.
5. Roll patient toward center of bed and *immediately* make sure that his head and neck are comfortable.
6. Make any adjustments needed for patient comfort.
   - Place small pillows or pads under head and shoulders.
   - Reposition arms for comfort.
   - Adjust pillow under abdomen if one was used.
7. Protect ankles against footdrop.
8. Question patient about comfort and make further adjustments as indicated.
9. Return promptly at designated time to move patient from prone position.

PROTECTIVE EQUIPMENT

Special beds, pads, and mattresses are often used to prevent or treat some of the complications of immobility. Pads and mattresses that distribute the patient's weight help to prevent pressure ulcers, and mechanical beds and frames that change the patient's position help to prevent or alleviate problems of the cardiovascular and musculoskeletal system.

Pads and Mattresses

Air Mattresses

One of the devices used most frequently to prevent or treat pressure ulcers is the *alternating pressure pad*. This pad is placed between the mattress and the bottom sheet and consists of lengthwise compartments that alternately inflate and deflate about every 5 minutes, thereby relieving pressure on different parts of the patient's body every few minutes. The flow of air through the compartments is created and controlled by a small electric pump.

Sheepskin

In addition to evenly distributing the patient's body weight, a sheepskin keeps the skin dry. It permits the circulation of air across the skin and prevents or reduces maceration. The resilient texture of sheepskin decreases any shearing force and minimizes skin abrasion from friction.

The sheepskin is placed on top of the bottom sheet, in direct contact with patient's skin, and either natural or synthetic sheepskin can be used. Natural sheepskin

must be washed *with care* to prevent damage to the wool fibers, and it is usually not practical for use under an incontinent patient. Synthetic sheepskin is easy to launder and can be used for patients with drainage and discharge.

Water Mattresses

A water-filled mattress will distribute the patient's body weight evenly over a large area, but it also introduces several new problems. Many experts think that the patient's pelvis rides low and that this position fosters contractures of the hip and ineffective drainage from an indwelling catheter. The movement of the water makes some treatments difficult, while the semiweightlessness bothers some patients. The legs are usually close together (adducted), and it may be necessary to place a pillow between the patient's knees to protect the inner surfaces from pressure sores. More research and study on the use of water beds is needed to validate or refute various opinions about them.

Foam-rubber Pads

Large, mattress-size foam-rubber pads can be placed between the patient's mattress and the bottom sheet. Pressure on bony prominences is relieved, but the absence of a smooth, firm surface under the sheet makes it more difficult to move and turn the patient.

Small pieces of foam rubber are used to pad and protect elbows, heels, and other areas, sometimes in conjunction with an elbow or heel protector (Fig. 29.19). When foam rubber is used under a patient's heel, the heel is lifted off the mattress, and care must be taken to prevent hyperextension of the knees; it may be nec-

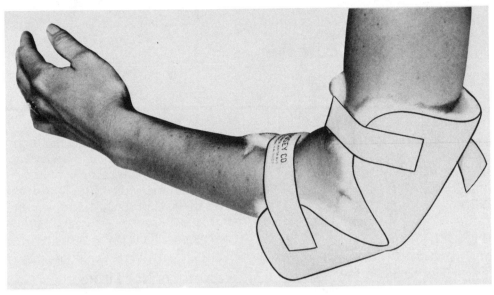

Figure 29.19 *Sheepskin elbow protector. (Courtesy of J.T. Posey Company)*

essary to place a small pad under the patient's knees for protection.

Rings and Doughnuts

Inflatable or sponge-rubber rings should *not* be used to relieve pressure over a bony prominence, such as a heel or sacrum, because, while pressure is relieved at the center hole or opening, pressure *around* that area is increased. The pressure of the ring itself can decrease circulation to the original pressure area and deprive those cells of oxygen and nutrients.

Special Beds and Frames

One mechanical device for turning a patient consists of identical, canvas-covered frames, about the size of a stretcher, that are attached to a supporting structure (Fig. 29.20). The patient is positioned on one frame and is covered by the second one. The frames are fastened together, and with the patient sandwiched between them, the frames are rotated 180 degrees so that the patient is turned over. The upper frame is removed, and the patient is made comfortable until it is time to be turned again.

The frames are narrow and seem restrictive to the patient, but they are invaluable in caring for patients whose body alignment must be maintained at all times and for patients who are completely immobilized. The patient can be turned from a prone to a supine position with no friction against the skin, no disturbance of skeletal alignment, and minimal physical exertion by the nurse. Sections of the canvas covering are removable so that the patient can use the bedpan and a small section at the end can be removed so that the patient, when lying on his abdomen, can read, or feed himself if he has the use of his arms. These frames, regardless of the name of the manufacturer, are often called *Stryker* frames, just as most people call facial tissues *Kleenex*. Each frame is different, and directions for its use should be attached to it.

A circular electric bed permits the patient to be placed in either a prone or a supine position, and in addition, enables the patient to be raised to an erect position. An erect or nearly erect position helps to prevent orthostatic hypotension, counteracts disuse osteoporosis by permitting weight bearing on the long bones, facilitates deep breathing and full expansion of the lungs, and promotes drainage of the kidney pelvis.

In the absence of a circular bed, a tilt board can be used to obtain the benefits of bringing the patient to an erect position.

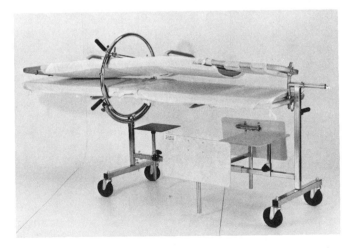

Figure 29.20 *A Wedge Turning Frame. (Courtesy of Stryker Frame Company, Kalamazoo, MI)*

Section Three

Transfer Techniques

BODY MECHANICS

Moving and lifting a helpless patient from bed to stretcher or chair is one of the most hazardous tasks in nursing; the incidence of back strain and injury is high for three reasons. First, nursing is one of the few professions in which workers are expected to move objects weighing from 100 to 200 lb a number of times a day. Second, some nurses either lack adequate knowledge of body mechanics or fail to apply their knowledge to nursing. Third, nurses often take dangerous shortcuts, assuming, "It won't happen to me," or "I'm too young (or healthy) to have back trouble."

Muscles and Balance

A human figure, standing with feet together, is theoretically as unstable as any other tall object of equal dimensions. In reality, the stability of a human is increased by continual muscular activity. When the body starts to lean or sway in any direction, the muscles on the opposite side of the body contract to hold the body upright and keep it from falling.

When a person is working in a position that causes his *line of gravity to fall outside his base of support,* these muscle contractions become intense. Fatigue and strain will result unless the center of gravity is brought back over the base of support or unless the base of support is enlarged enough to extend it out under the center of gravity and stabilize the body.

Preparation for Lifting

When the movements of lifting are analyzed, five distinct movements are evident, and they should precede the actual lifting: (1) stabilizing the pelvis, (2) lengthening the midriff, (3) enlarging the base of support, (4) lowering the center of gravity, and (5) bringing the weight to be lifted over the base of support or as close to it as possible before you try to lift it.

Stabilizing the Pelvis

When the pelvis is properly balanced, the line of weight bearing passes through the body of each lumbar vertebra. If the muscles that support the pelvis are weakened by prolonged poor posture, fatigue, or ill health, the pelvis tips forward. In this position, the lumbar curve is increased, the weight of the upper trunk is not supported evenly by the bodies of the lumbar vertebrae, the abdomen protrudes, and the positions of the chest and head are distorted (Fig. 29.21).

To correct this situation, a person must consciously tip his pelvis back by contracting his abdominal and gluteal muscles. There are several ways to describe this tilting movement: (1) the foremost part of the upper pelvis (the anterior superior iliac spine) is tilted back toward the spinal column; or (2) the movement is like the one a person makes instinctively when he tries to avoid a spanking. In addition to consciously assuming this position before lifting, a person may need to do some conditioning exercises to develop enough muscle tone to tilt and stabilize the pelvis. In combination, these movements are sometimes called "putting on the internal girdle."

Lengthening the Midriff

The midriff—the area between the sternum and the umbilicus—should be fully extended. If the midriff is allowed to sag, the rib cage is lowered and the abdo-

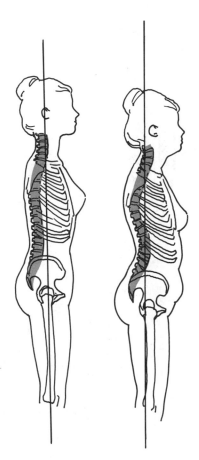

Figure 29.21 *Comparison of the effects of pelvic positions.* Left: *pelvis in proper position.* Right: *pelvis tilted forward.*

men protrudes more than usual. The normal curves of the spine are exaggerated.

When a person assumes a long midriff, three things happen: (1) the abdomen is flattened (which helps maintain good pelvic position); (2) the curves of the spine assume a good physiological alignment; and (3) with the rib cage raised, the chest is moved up and out and the lungs can be fully expanded without difficulty.

Enlarging the Base of Support

The object to be lifted is usually in front or nearly in front of the lifter, so the direction of movement will be mainly back and forth rather than from side to side. Therefore, in relation to a standing position, the base of support should be *considerably enlarged* from *front to back* and slightly enlarged from side to side.

Lowering the Center of Gravity

The center of gravity can be lowered by flexing of the knees and hips. The forward foot should be placed flat on the floor while the rear foot is positioned on its toes.

Body weight should be evenly divided between the feet, so that, in leaning forward to pick up the object to be lifted, the trunk will remain over the enlarged base of support.

Bringing the Weight to be Lifted Over the Base of Support or as Close to It As Possible

The closer the weight, the shorter the time the lifter will be unstable before getting the weight over his base of support. Because the center of gravity shifts toward any *additional* weight, the lifter's line of gravity may fall outside his base of support momentarily as he lifts, but this time of relative instability can be greatly shortened by moving the object to be lifted as close as possible to his base of support before he starts to lift.

Lifting

Lifting involves two powerful groups of muscles, the gluteal muscles and the quadriceps. The gluteal muscles contract to extend (straighten) the hips, and the quadriceps extend the knees. As these muscles contract, they permit the legs to straighten and the body to stand upright. The fibers of the long, thin muscle of the back, the sacrospinalis, can stabilize the back and keep it erect, but they should *not* be called upon to lift.

Figs. 29.22 and 29.23 show the comparative size of the sacrospinalis, and the quadriceps and gluteal muscles.

Disregarding for the moment such important aspects of lifting as base of support, center of gravity, and line of gravity, you can see that a stooping position with back straight is preferable to a bending position on the basis of *muscle size* alone.

When you lift an object up to a high shelf or lower it from a high shelf, the additional weight and extended height make the body more difficult than ever to balance. Many people tend to stand on tiptoe with feet together in this situation, and as a result, the center of gravity is high and the base of support extremely small. To minimize these conditions, the lifter should stand as close to the shelf as possible so that the weight of the object is transferred quickly from the shelf to the arms and over the base of support. It is best to use a

---

Safe Lifting Posture

- Pelvis stabilized and midriff lengthened
- Head erect
- Base of support enlarged
- Trunk inclined forward from hips
- Entire body as close to object to be lifted as possible

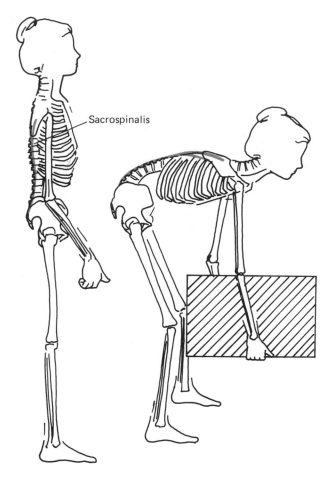

Figure 29.22 _Improper lifting using the sacrospinalis muscle._

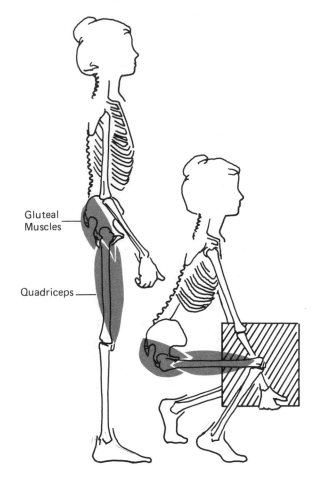

Figure 29.23 _Safe lifting using quadriceps and gluteal muscles._

step stool or box to avoid having to stand on tiptoe with a small base of support.

MOVING AND LIFTING PATIENTS

Patients are moved from their beds for a variety of reasons, and preparation for any such move must be based on a careful assessment of the _total situation_ because the basic problem of moving a heavy weight (the patient) is often compounded by the presence of such things as tubes or a cast, and by psychological conditions such as fear and apprehension.

Assessment of the Patient's Condition

First of all, assess how the patient's physical condition may affect the process of moving him. A patient in a body cast may be able to use both arms and one or both legs to help himself, but a patient who has just had a heart attack may be unable to help in any way.

Special problems in moving are posed by a patient with numerous tubes and attachments. Specific isolation precautions must be taken when you are moving a patient who is currently isolated because of an infection, and a patient with severe pain may need to have his move timed to follow his pain medication.

Very careful assessments and plans must be made before moving an extremely heavy person (250 to 350 lb or more) to ensure safety for both patient and nurse. To avoid embarrassing the patient and to maintain his confidence in the staff, most deliberations and discussions of the best way to move him should take place _outside_ the patient's room.

Preparation for Moving and Lifting

There are certain necessary preparations common to all moves and transfers regardless of the move to be made, the method to be used, or the ability of the patient to participate.

Preparation of the Patient

When you are ready to move the patient, explain what you are going to do and why. Explain how you plan to move him, why you have chosen that method, and how he can help. If you are short, thin, or otherwise small of stature, you can retain the patient's confidence in you by explaining that your chosen method of lifting will be both safe and comfortable regardless of your physical size.

Preparation of Furniture and Equipment

After explaining the move, make any necessary physical preparations as follows:

1. Raise the bed from the low position to a comfortable working height.
2. Because the patient's skin is easily injured by friction, tighten the lower linen as needed to give a smooth, wrinkle-free surface, thereby reducing friction as the patient is moved.
3. If the patient's skin is damp and sticky, dry and dust it with cornstarch or talcum powder to decrease friction during the move.
4. Lock the wheels of the bed and the stretcher or wheelchair. If the wheels on either the bed or stretcher cannot be locked, have a helper hold the bed and stretcher together while the patient is moved from one to the other.

Preparation of the Nurse

Before each move, consciously review the body mechanics of lifting and take time to properly do the following *before* starting to lift:

1. Establish a wide base of support
2. Stabilize your pelvis
3. Lengthen your midriff
4. Lower your center of gravity
5. Bring the object to be moved (the patient) as close to your base of support as possible

No matter how rushed you may be, this preparation cannot be safely overlooked or omitted.

USING A HYDRAULIC LIFTER

A hydraulic lifter (Fig. 29.24) is used for two reasons: (1) to lift a patient safely and comfortably and (2) to protect from injury the people who must lift the patient. Of the two reasons for using a hydraulic lifter, the second is usually more important because, although there are other ways to lift a patient safely, they

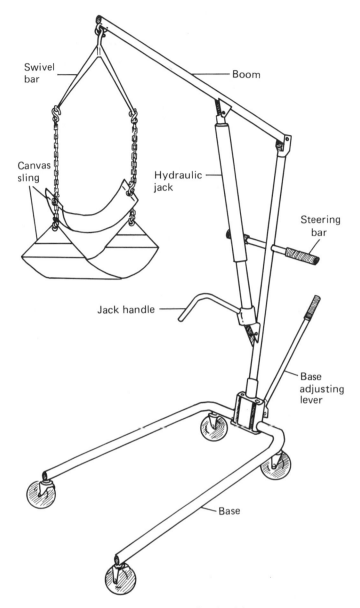

Figure 29.24 *Hydraulic lifter.*

are often *dangerous for those who must do the lifting.* There is no other way to lift a heavy, helpless patient from bed to chair, for example, that is safe for *you and your helper.* A hydraulic lifter does not necessarily save time, nor does it always reduce the number of people needed to lift the patient. It does, however, protect the lifters from the threat of backstrain, back injury, and hernias.

To use a hydraulic lifter effectively, you must:

1. Understand how it works (Chapter 11)
2. Practice using it
3. Explain its use to the patient
4. Make sure you have someone to help you

Practicing with the Lifter

Once you understand how the hydraulic lifter works, practice until you are *confident* of your ability to use it in a variety of situations. Practice lifting a large or heavy classmate or a fellow employee until you know exactly what the lifter can and cannot do. Many patients are frightened by this method of lifting because a hydraulic lifter does not look especially strong and sturdy and because the thought of being swung through the air by it is a bit unnerving. Practice *being lifted* until you can anticipate possible concerns and apprehensions which a patient may have.

Preparation of Patient and Helper

Before you bring the lifter into the room, explain to your patient why you are going to use it. He should know that a lifter is used for *your* safety as well as for his comfort and safety because otherwise he might refuse to have it used on the grounds that he finds it comfortable to be lifted by several nurses. Explain the procedure, and describe what it will feel like to be lifted in this way.

You will need at least one helper because it takes one person to operate the lifter and one person to guide and steady the patient as he is swung through the air. If the helper is not familiar with the use of a hydraulic lifter, explain its operation before you enter the patient's room.

Placement of the Slings

The patient should be rolled to his side, held there by the helper while you place the fabric sling under him, and then rolled back onto the sling. A one-piece sling is safest and gives the patient a feeling of security (Fig. 29.25), and it is available with a wired head support.

If separate back and seat slings are used, they must be carefully positioned. The top edge of the back sling should be near the level of the patient's axilla. The placement of the seat sling depends on the width of the sling and length of the patient's thigh. Ideally, the sling should reach from just above the popliteal space to the center of his buttocks. If the sling is narrow, it should be placed just below the gluteal fold so that, when he is in a sitting position, he is in the same position on the sling as a child is on a swing seat. If the sling is too close to the knees or too far under his buttocks, he will either slide off frontward or fall back between the slings.

Next, attach the chains or straps to the sling or slings and lift the patient several inches off the bed to test the placement of the sling (Fig. 29.26). Make any adjustments needed to ensure the patient's safety. If the lifter

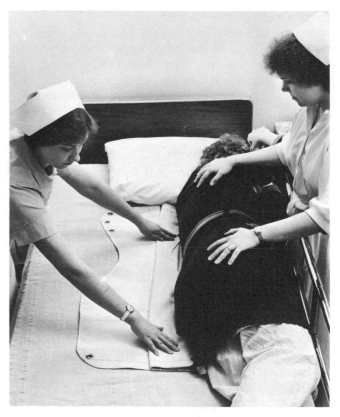

Figure 29.25 *Placing a one-piece sling for a hydraulic lifter under the patient.*

has chains and if it is to be used frequently for that patient, indicate the adjustment you found most satisfactory by marking the appropriate link of the chain with string or adhesive tape or by noting it on the Kardex.

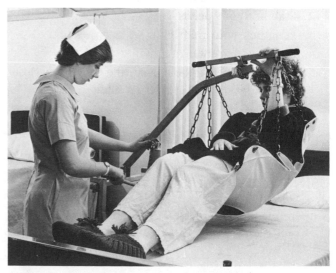

Figure 29.26 *The nurse checks the placement of the sling before moving the patient away from the bed.*

Moving the Patient

The patient may keep his arms inside the sling or may hold onto either the chains or the swivel bar. When you are certain that he is both comfortable and safe, proceed to lift him until the seat sling clears the bed. The helper should slowly turn the patient to *face* the lifter as you move it away from the bed. Adjust the base of the lifter to fit around the chair. As you move the lifter toward the chair, the helper should steady the patient, keep the swivel bar from spinning, and position the patient well back over the chair seat when you reach the chair with the lifter (Fig. 29.27).

Tell the patient when you are ready to lower him. If he is not properly positioned on the chair seat, raise him a few inches, and reposition him. Then lower the boom enough to detach the straps or chains and move the lifter away. The sling is *left in place*, ready to be reattached when the patient is to be lifted back to bed.

If the patient is lifted onto a stretcher or other flat surface instead of into a chair, the slings can be removed to protect his back from wrinkles. It is not possible to remove and replace slings under a patient in a sitting position, but the sling can be pulled tight and smooth under the patient before you leave him.

Special slings are available with a hole in the seat portion of the sling to permit the use of a toilet or commode. A hydraulic lifter can be used to lower a patient into the bath tub, and some models are designed to lift a patient into and out of a car. Some mechanical patient lifters are not hydraulic but instead have a ratchet mechanism similar to that of a car jack. Their use and operation is very similar, however, to that of a hydraulic lifter.

USING A PULL SHEET

When a patient needs to be moved toward the head of the bed or onto a stretcher, the process can be damaging to his skin and joints. When a patient is lying in bed, his body weight presses his skin against the lower sheet so tightly that considerable friction is created whenever he is pulled across the sheet. This friction can irritate and excoriate fragile or tender skin. It can damage the sensitive skin of a reddened pressure area and can destroy a new tissue that may have started to fill in a pressure ulcer (bedsore). Each break in a patient's skin is dangerous whether it be a crack, a scraped area, or the destruction of new tissue, because it provides a portal of entry for pathogenic organisms.

Protecting the Skin From Friction

Friction between a patient's skin and his bed linen can be avoided by use of a pull sheet when moving him up in bed, or from bed to stretcher. A *pull sheet* is a draw sheet or folded bed sheet that is placed under the patient for use in moving or turning him. When the patient is moved on a pull sheet, all friction occurs

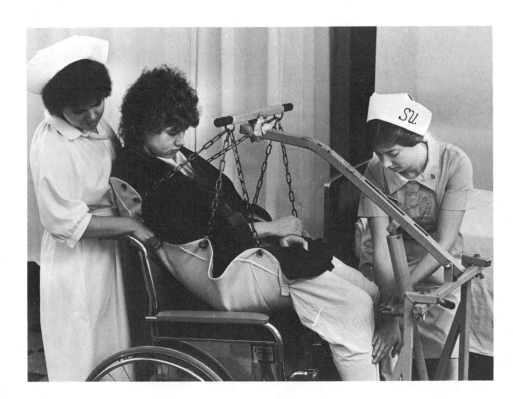

Figure 29.27 *One nurse guides the patient into the wheelchair while the other nurse lets the sling down and protects her legs and feet.*

PROCEDURE 29.8

Using a Hydraulic Lifter*

SUMMARY OF ESSENTIAL NURSING ACTION

1. Make sure you know how to use the lifter BEFORE you take it into the patient's room.
2. Get someone to assist you; do NOT try to use the lifter alone.
3. Position slings under the patient.
4. Attach lifter chains to slings.
5. Lift patient several inches off bed to test placement of slings and functioning of lifter.
   - Make any necessary adjustments for comfort and/or safety *while the patient is still positioned over the bed.*

6. Direct your helper in guiding the movement of the patient while you operate the lifter.
7. *Slowly* lower the patient into chair or onto stretcher.
8. Check the position of the patient; lift him a bit and readjust his position as needed until he is both safe and comfortable. Make sure that the slings beneath him are not wrinkled.
9. Detach chains and move lifter out of the way.
10. Make sure signal cord, drinking water, and other desired items are within reach.

*See inside front cover and pages 533–535.

---

between the pull sheet and the sheet beneath it. There is no friction between the pull sheet and the patient's skin. The patient's skin is pressed firmly against the pull sheet but does not move across it.

A pull sheet must be *strong* enough to support the patient's weight, *wide* enough to give support from his shoulders to his knees, and *long* enough to leave sufficient material on each side of his body for the nurses to grasp as they move him. A large bed sheet folded in half or an *extra* draw sheet can be used. (A draw sheet is a cotton half-sheet used over a rubber draw sheet which is placed across the center of the bed to protect the mattress.) It is not advisable to untuck the regular draw sheet and use it as a pull sheet, because each time the patient is moved and the draw sheet is moved, the rubber sheet is partially uncovered and is in contact with the patient's skin.

The patient who needs a pull sheet is usually not very active in bed, and the cotton pull sheet can often be left in place. It is not tucked in; the ends are neatly rolled up next to the patient ready for use.

If the patient is *extremely* heavy, his body weight will increase the friction between the pull sheet and the sheet beneath it, making it very hard to move the pull sheet. In such a situation, the nurse can requisition a piece of heavy plastic sheeting (at least 2 feet by 3 feet) to place under the pull sheet each time the patient is moved. This provides a slippery surface across which the pull sheet will move easily. The plastic sheet usually cannot be left in place because it tends to wrinkle under the patient if he moves about. In warm weather, it can cause the patient to perspire, and it would make positioning difficult to maintain whenever the head of the bed is elevated.

Protecting the Muscles and Joints

In addition to protecting the patient's skin from abrasion, the use of a pull sheet protects his muscles and joints from pressure and strain. When a pull sheet is not used, the patient is subjected to uneven pulls and pressures as parts of his body are grasped tightly while he is pulled or tugged toward the head of the bed or onto a stretcher. Nurses and attendants sometimes hurriedly slip an arm under each axilla of a helpless patient, for example, and pull against his shoulders to move him up toward the head of the bed. Considerable pressure must be used to move the patient's weight (100 to 200 lb) across a soft surface and will be most uncomfortable for the patient. When a pull sheet is used, the pressure needed to move the patient is evenly distributed across his body by the sheet, and he is not subjected to localized pressure against a muscle or joint.

Conditions That Require the Use of a Pull Sheet

- Fragile, tender skin
- Reddened pressure areas that are potential pressure ulcers
- Open pressure ulcers
- Healing pressure ulcers
- Bruised, burned, or excoriated skin
- Painful joints (arthritis, cancer of the bone)
- Generalized pain or discomfort
- Extensive dressings that could be loosened by friction

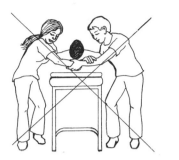
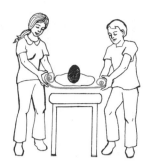

Figure 29.28 *The use of a pull sheet permits good body mechanics and protects the nurses from back strain.*

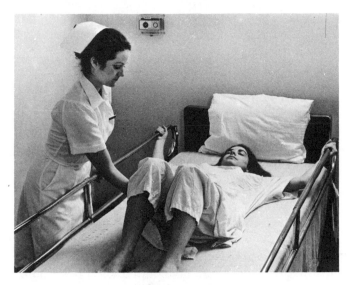

Figure 29.30 *The nurse positions the patient's legs before a move toward the head of the bed (see text for description). Note the position of the pillow.*

The use of the pull sheet ensures the safety and comfort of the patient, but it is of equal importance to the safety of the nurse. The pull sheet makes it possible for you to keep your center of gravity over your base of support and to use protective body mechanics as you move the patient up in bed or from bed to stretcher (Fig. 29.28, above). When a pull sheet is not used, you must lean over the bed to get a good grasp on the patient or to get your arms under him (Fig. 29.28, above). The few minutes it takes to put a pull sheet in place can prevent an accumulation of minor back strains that can result in a disabling back injury.

MOVING A PATIENT TOWARD THE HEAD OF THE BED

When a patient is correctly positioned in bed, his hips are directly over the *hinge* that permits the head of the bed to be raised and lowered (the *break* in the bed). Whenever the head of the patient's bed is raised, the patient begins to slide toward the foot of the bed; and soon the break in the bed is under his chest, not under his hips. As a result, the normal curvature of his spine is distorted and his chest is sunken. In addition to causing muscular and skeletal problems, this position makes respiration difficult and can be detrimental to a patient with respiratory problems.

It is necessary, therefore, from time to time to move the patient toward the head of the bed and to reposition him in an anatomically correct position. Because it takes less energy to move a person or a heavy object along a flat surface than it does to move him up an incline (Fig. 29.29), the first step in the process is to *lower the head of the bed* unless it is contraindicated, as it may be for certain patients with respiratory or neurological disorders.

Helping a Patient Who Can Lie Flat

If a patient can lie flat, the first step in moving him is always to lower the head of the bed. Subsequent steps depend on the patient's ability and willingness to help himself. If a patient can use *both his arms and his legs,* he will need minimal assistance once the head of the bed has been lowered. He can grasp the headboard of the bed, an overbed trapeze or side rails, and pull while he pushes with his legs. If he has *limited use of his arms or legs,* ask him how much and what kind of help he needs. It is very important to encourage a patient to do

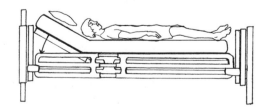
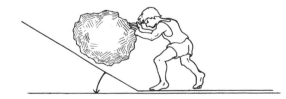

Figure 29.29 *The figure on the right dramatizes the amount of effort it takes to move a patient up in bed when the head of the bed is elevated. The rock and the patient are of equal weight, and the angles of the hill and bed are equal.*

as much as he can for himself because the exertion of moving will help to counteract the dangerous effects of immobility (Fig. 29.30).

Helping a Patient Who Cannot Lie Flat

If a patient who has to be moved toward the head of the bed is unable to breathe while lying flat, he will have to be moved to a sitting position. If he is able to sit on the edge of the bed with his feet on a chair, you can lower the head of the bed and help the patient wiggle along the edge of the bed toward the head, lifting first one buttock and then the other until his hips are over the break in the bed. A patient may be able to use an overhead trapeze bar to keep himself in a semisitting position while the head of his bed is lowered and several nurses move him toward the head of the bed.

If the head of the bed cannot be lowered and the patient cannot help himself, a hydraulic lifter should be used. There is no way in which nurses can safely lift an adult in a sitting position up toward the head of the bed without mechanical assistance when the head of the bed must be kept raised.

Moving a Helpless Patient

Any patient who is extremely weak, comatose, paralyzed, in severe pain, on strict bed rest because of a cardiac problem, or immobilized with a cast or traction cannot move himself up in bed and must, therefore, be moved by the nurse whenever he has slid toward the foot of the bed.

Moving With a Pull Sheet
The pull sheet method of moving a helpless patient toward the head of the bed is preferred because it is safe for both the patient and nurse.

Moving Without a Pull Sheet
A *helpless* patient should *not* be moved without a pull sheet unless he has healthy, intact skin and is not in pain. He should *not* be moved without a pull sheet unless the number and strength of the nurses are adequate to protect each nurse from back injury. If the patient is heavy, four persons will be needed—two for his head and shoulders and two for his hips. The steps of the procedure are similar to those of the pull sheet method.

1. Explain to the patient what you are going to do and why, even if he seems unresponsive.
2. Lower the head of the bed, adjust the pillows, and flex the patient's knees.

> ### *Moving a Patient Toward the Head of the Bed With a Pull Sheet*
>
> 1. Explain to the patient what you plan to do and why. Do so even if the patient seems unresponsive.
> 2. Lower the head of the bed and put a pull sheet in place unless one is already in position.
> 3. Adjust the pillows as needed. Remove them if the patient can lie completely flat. If the patient is very small or light in weight and there is any possibility of his being moved so fast or so far that he might bump his head, place a pillow in front of the headboard (Fig. 29.30).
> 4. Ask the patient if he can support his head during the move. If so, ask him to bring his chin down toward his chest at the start of the move. If not, position the pull sheet so that his head will be supported by it or ask an extra assistant to support the patient's head.
> 5. Flex the patient's legs (or ask him to do so), bringing his heels as close to his buttocks as is comfortable (Fig. 29.30). If the patient cannot keep his legs in this position, brace them with a pillow or ask a helper to support them. The legs of an adult constitute a large percentage of his body weight, so when you move his feet and legs toward the head of the bed *before* his body is moved, the weight of his legs can be subtracted from the total weight to be moved. The legs need not be manipulated during the move because the force of gravity will pull them down as the patient's body is moved.
> 6. Check the position of the patient's hips with respect to the break in the bed to determine how far he needs to be moved.
> 7. Position at least one person on each side of the bed (two if the patient is extremely heavy). Stand close to the bed to keep your center of gravity and base of support as near to the weight to be moved as possible.
> 8. With the head of the bed down and the patient's knees flexed, stabilize your pelvis and, on the count of three, slide the patient toward the head of the bed.
> 9. Check the position of the patient's hips and repeat the move if necessary.
> 10. Tighten the lower bedding and replace the patient's pillows. If the pull sheet is to be left in place, remove all wrinkles and roll the ends up next to the patient.

3. Position your feet. Because you need to face the patient and lean over the bed in order to get your arms under the patient, your feet will of necessity be almost at right angles to the bed. They will need to be separated front to back to bring your base of support as close to the weight to be lifted as possible. Your feet also need to be separated from side to side to permit you to shift weight in the direction of the move.

PROCEDURE 29.9

Moving a Patient Toward the Head of the Bed with a Pull Sheet*

SUMMARY OF ESSENTIAL NURSING ACTIONS

1. Protect your back by getting enough people to help you before starting to move the patient.
2. Prepare for the move.
   • Lower the head of the bed unless contraindicated.
   • Make sure the pull sheet is in position; it should support patient's head if patient is unable to do so.
   • Remove or reposition pillows as needed.
   • Flex patient's knees.
   • Position your feet parallel to the side of the bed.

   • Stabilize your pelvis.
   • Decide who will give the verbal signal to move patient.
3. At the signal, slide pull sheet and patient toward head of bed.
4. If the patient's hips are not positioned over break in bed, repeat the move.
5. Straighten pull sheet and bottom sheet, replace pillows as the patient desires or as needed to support the patient in a protective position.

*See inside front cover and page 538.

---

4. Place your arms under the patient's hips and shoulders; stabilize your pelvis; and, on the count of three, slide the patient toward the head of the bed, *lifting as you slide* him to reduce friction as much as possible.

5. Check the position of the patient. It is often necessary to repeat the moves because, if the patient is heavy, each attempt may move the patient only a few inches.

MOVING A PATIENT FROM BED TO STRETCHER

Many patients can move themselves from bed to stretcher with minimal assistance if given enough time, and many prefer to do so because they can then control any movement that causes discomfort or pain. It usually takes longer for a patient to move himself, and there is a temptation for busy staff members to rush in and bodily move the patient. This is usually not in the best interest of the patient, and any decision to lift or pull a patient from bed to stretcher should be made on the basis of the patient's inability to move himself rather than the impatience of the staff.

Four commonly used means of transfer from bed to stretcher are: patient roller, three-man lift, hydraulic lifter, and pull sheet. The hydraulic lifter (previously explained) should be used whenever another method might jeopardize the safety of either nurse or patient.

Patient Roller

A patient roller, or roller bar, consists of a series of long metal rollers supported by a flat, metal frame and cov-

ered with fabric. When a roller bar is placed under a patient, his weight can then be transferred from bed to stretcher by rollers so he can be moved without lifting him. No fewer people are needed for this method than for the other methods of transfer, but the nurse's risk of back injury is markedly reduced.

To use a roller bar for transferring a patient from bed to stretcher, the procedure is to:

1. Position a pull sheet under the patient unless one is already in place.
2. Using the pull sheet, move the patient toward the edge of the bed nearest the stretcher.
3. Turn the patient to his side with the pull sheet and position the roller bar behind his back under the pull sheet. Roll the end of the pull sheet up toward the patient as needed to keep it from getting under the roller bar.
4. Position the stretcher beside the bed and lock the wheels. Bridge any difference in levels with one or more pillows placed end to end.
5. Adjust the position of the roller bar so that it spans the space between the patient and the stretcher.
6. Use the pull sheet to lower the patient back down onto the roller bar.
7. Move the patient across the roller bar onto the stretcher. Work quickly because the rollers are uncomfortable to lie on. One person uses the pull sheet to pull the patient across the rollers while another person on the far side of the bed keeps the pull sheet taut. A third person must support the patient's head and shoulders when a short version of the roller bar is used.

8. Move the stretcher away from the bed and, with someone standing on each side of the stretcher to keep the patient from falling, turn him onto his side and remove the roller bar.

9. Straighten the lower linen and make the patient comfortable with pillow and blankets.

10. Put up the side rails of the stretcher or fasten the safety straps.

Three-man Lift

One of the safest ways to transfer a patient from bed to stretcher is by the three-man lift, or three-man carry. This method is safe for the nurse because the weight each nurse is lifting is over her base of support. During this carry, the patient is raised and lowered primarily by flexion and extension of the knees and elbows, so there is minimal risk of back strain if the nurses keep their backs straight. The method is also safe and com-

fortable for the patient because he is not subjected to friction against his skin, and his body alignment is not distorted.

The stretcher is usually placed at right angles to the foot of the bed, with the head end of the stretcher next to the bed. This placement is the most efficient, but the stretcher can be placed anywhere, even out in the hall, as long as there is room enough for the lifters to walk while carrying the patient. If for any reason the wheels on the stretcher cannot be locked, the stretcher must be braced against a wall or held in place by a helper. *Never* attempt a three-man lift with an *unsecured* stretcher.

The position of each lifter is determined by the size and strength of the person. The shoulders of an adult male patient are broad and heavy, so they are carried by the person with the longest arms (usually the tallest person). The weight of a female patient is often centered in her hips, which should be carried by a strong person. The shortest person usually carries the feet and legs because they can be held lower than the head and

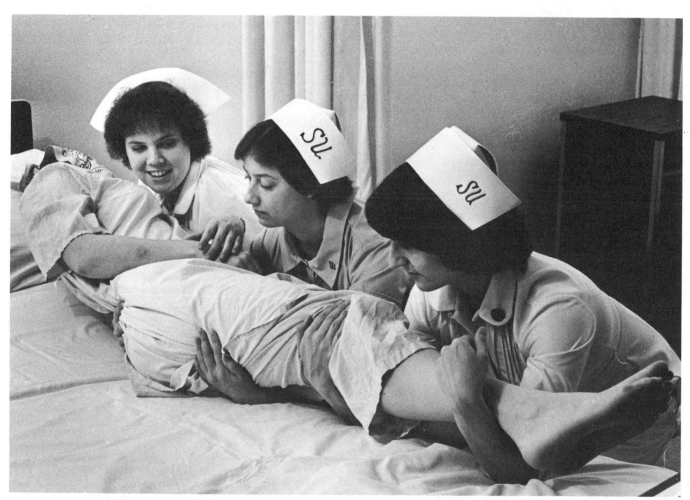

Figure 29.31 *The first step of a three-man lift. In this team, the nurse on the left gives the signals throughout the lift.*

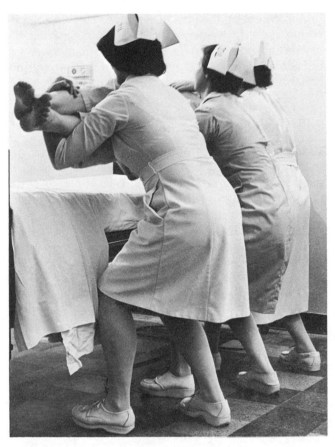

Figure 29.32 *Note the protected backs of the nurses and their wide bases of support in this second step of a three-person lift.*

Sequence of Steps for Three-man Carry

1. With your knees bent and back straight, reach under the patient and pull him to the edge of the bed (Fig. 29.31).
2. Keeping your knees bent and your back straight, with *elbows on the bed,* roll the patient onto your chest (Fig. 29.32).
3. Straighten your knees and stand erect. Evaluate the position of your hands and arms. Make any desired adjustments *before* you step away from the bed.
4. Pivot and walk to stretcher.
5. Keeping the patient *against your chest* and keeping your back straight, bend your knees and lower your body until your elbows rest on the stretcher (Fig. 29.33).
6. Extend your arms slowly and let the patient roll away from your chest onto his back.
7. Remove your arms, make the patient comfortable, and either put up the side rails of the stretcher or fasten the safety straps securely.

body. Each end person should place his inner arm close to the center person's arm in order to help carry the weight of the body.

The patient's arms are positioned at his sides or folded across his chest. He should be asked if he can help to support his head and neck. If not, the person carrying the patient's shoulders must assume responsibility for doing so.

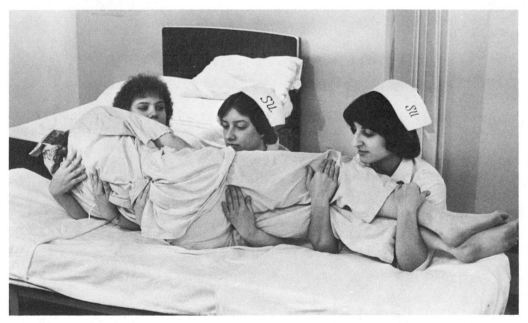

Figure 29.33 *Elbows on the stretcher support the weight of the patient as she is lowered onto the stretcher in the fifth step of a three-person lift.*

A stretcher is narrow, so the patient will probably be centered on it and will not need to be moved. When you transfer the patient back to bed, however, he will be lowered onto the mattress at the side of the bed and must then be moved toward the center.

Because the effectiveness of the three-man carry depends in part on teamwork, one person should give a signal for each step of the procedure so that movements are synchronized for a smooth maneuver. If all three lifters are familiar with the carry and if each person understands which movement is to be executed with each count, the leader merely counts to six. If the carry is not familiar to one or more of the lifters or if they do not remember which movement corresponds to each count, the leader should give simple directions instead of counting to six, for example:

- Pull to edge
- Roll to chest
- Stand up
- Pivot and turn
- Elbows to mattress
- Lower arms

Agreement on the type of signals to be given and by whom should be reached before all of you enter the patient's room. A discussion of these matters at the bedside may make you appear uncertain and will not enhance the patient's confidence in your competence.

Pull Sheet

To transfer a patient from bed to stretcher with a pull sheet, three or four people are needed depending on the weight of the patient. A pull sheet is placed under the patient, unless one is already in use, and the patient is moved to the edge of the bed. The stretcher is positioned against the bed, and the wheels are locked.

To move the patient from bed to stretcher, two persons reach across the stretcher and grasp one end of the pull sheet. If the patient is unable to support his head, one of these persons will need to do so. A third person kneels on the bed beside the patient and grasps the other end of the pull sheet (Fig. 29.34). On a count of three, the kneeling person *lifts* the patient enough to reduce the friction while the other two persons pull the patient onto the stretcher.

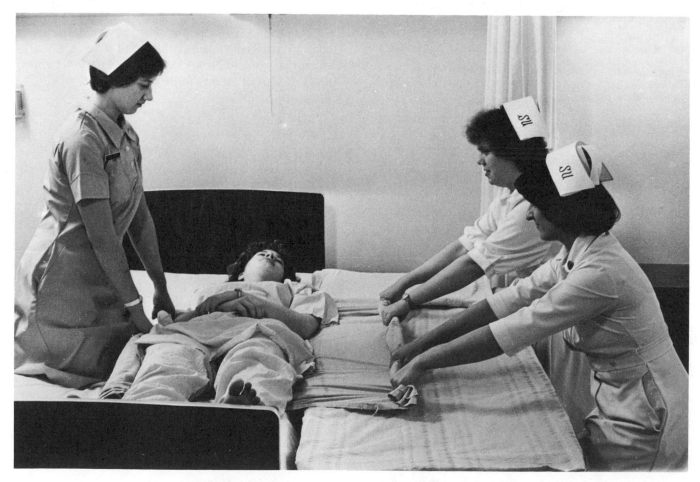

Figure 29.34 *A pull-sheet transfer can be safe when done correctly.*

This method of moving a patient to and from a stretcher is probably the one most frequently used, partly because no equipment is needed and partly because it seems simple. Most workers have seen this method used and feel confident of their ability to use it, whereas many people need to practice using a hydraulic lifter or a three-man carry before they feel confident enough to use them.

The pull sheet method is the *most hazardous* of the commonly used transfer techniques in terms of the nurse's safety.

In this procedure, two of the three people involved are required to pull while leaning across a stretcher, thereby risking muscle strain and lower back injury. The third person is subject to similar injuries because she is expected to lift while kneeling on an unstable, soft surface.

As the patient is pulled toward the stretcher, the person kneeling on the bed is liable to be pulled off balance. The likelihood of this is reduced by anticipating the problem, moving one knee forward, shifting body weight to that knee, and releasing your grip on the pull sheet before you are pulled off balance. These movements are difficult because they must be done almost simultaneously.

You maintain medical asepsis during this procedure by kneeling on a clean sheet or towel to protect your uniform from contaminated or soiled bed linens and to protect clean bed linen from any pathogens that might be on your uniform.

Ways to Protect Nurse When Transferring Patient With Pull Sheet

IF YOU MUST REACH AND PULL

Stabilize your pelvis

Widen your base of support (position one foot under the stretcher)

Keep your back as straight as possible

Lower your body by flexing your knees and hips

Pull with your arms, not your back

Bring the end of the pull sheet close to you before you pull so as to minimize reaching beyond your base of support as you pull

IF YOU MUST KNEEL AND PULL

Keep your back straight and stabilize your pelvis

To lift the patient, *extend your hips* which automatically elevates your body, if your arms are not moved and your back is kept straight, lifting your body with your hips will automatically lift the patient too

Insist that a second person kneel beside you and lift with you if the patient is heavy

HELPING A PATIENT OUT OF BED AND INTO A CHAIR

The majority of patients are encouraged to get out of bed several times a day. The hazards of bed rest and immobility are so great that patients cannot be permitted to remain in bed for extended periods of time. Pain, discomfort, weakness, and apprehension often make getting out of bed a stressful experience for the patient, and you must provide both psychological and physical support.

Before getting a patient out of bed, you will need to obtain the patient's robe and shoes or slippers and a blanket for his knees if the room is cold or drafty or if they are needed for privacy and modesty. If you know or suspect that the patient will be very weak and unsteady on his feet, you may want to place a strong belt around his waist to provide a convenient place to grasp and support him. Commercial belts with handles, called *ambulation belts* or *walking belts,* are available (Fig. 29.35), but any wide leather belt works very well.

Some patients are unable to stand but would benefit from being out of bed at regular intervals, so a hydraulic lifter is used to lift them from bed to chair and back again. Nearly every hospital has at least one lifter and even though it may be annoying to have to track it down each time you want to use it, the lifter makes it possible for a helpless patient to be gotten out of bed with no risk to himself or his nurse.

Placement of Chair

Before you help a patient into a chair, review his physical capabilities, and position the chair accordingly. If the patient has the use of both arms and both legs, placement of the chair is optional, although it is usually convenient to place it beside the bed near the foot. If the patient is unable to use one arm, one leg, or both, the chair must be positioned parallel to the bed and placed so that, when the patient is sitting on the edge of the bed, the chair is *beside his stronger side.* With the chair in this position, the patient reaches for the chair with his strong arm and steps away from the bed with his strong leg while his weaker side is supported by the bed (Fig. 29.36a,b). In such situations, placement of the chair is very specific. Depending on the arm or leg involved and side of bed to be used, there is only one possible position on each side of the bed that will satisfy the criteria of a chair *next to the stronger side;* on one side of the bed, the chair will be beside the head of the bed while on the other side it will be next to the foot. Whenever possible, the patient should get out of bed on the side of his stronger arm and leg so he can "lead" with his stronger side and his weaker side can "fol-

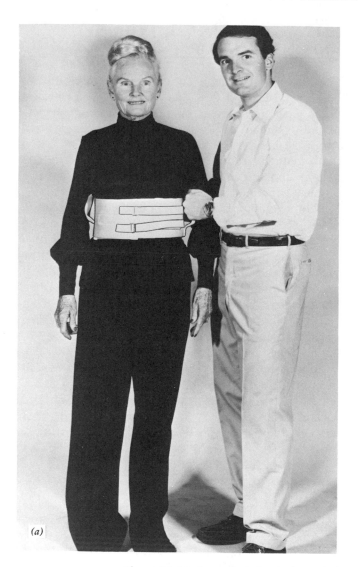
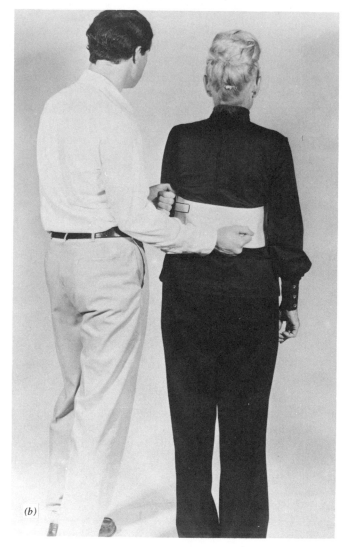

(a) *(b)*

Figure 29.35 *An ambulation belt can help ensure patient safety while walking. (Courtesy of J.T. Posey Company)*

low." In this way, his weaker or affected side does not get in the way of his stronger or unaffected side, and the weight of his weaker side does not have to be pushed across the bed by his stronger side (Fig. 29.36c,d).

Helping the Patient to a Sitting Position

Once the chair, clothing, or any necessary accessories are ready, the nurse can help the patient move toward the side of the bed, then bring him to a sitting position by *raising the head of the bed,* and helping him swing his legs over the side. In this position, you can put his robe and shoes or slippers on him, as well as a walking belt if one is to be used.

If the patient is able to bear weight on one foot only, that foot should be dressed with a sturdy shoe or slipper

and the other one dressed differently to remind the patient not to step on it. Some patients have no difficulty remembering which foot to use, but some elderly or confused patients need a simple reminder, especially if there is no pain or discomfort to remind them.

In the home, the head of the bed probably cannot be elevated to help the patient rise to a sitting position. Do not attempt to compensate by pulling or trying to lift the patient to an upright position. Instead, teach the patient to roll onto his side by pulling on the edge of the mattress with his far hand and foot. Then, while lying on his side, he should get both feet over the side of the mattress and raise up on his lower elbow while pushing on the mattress with his upper hand.

Given *enough time*, and with someone nearby to prevent falling, most patients can bring themselves to a

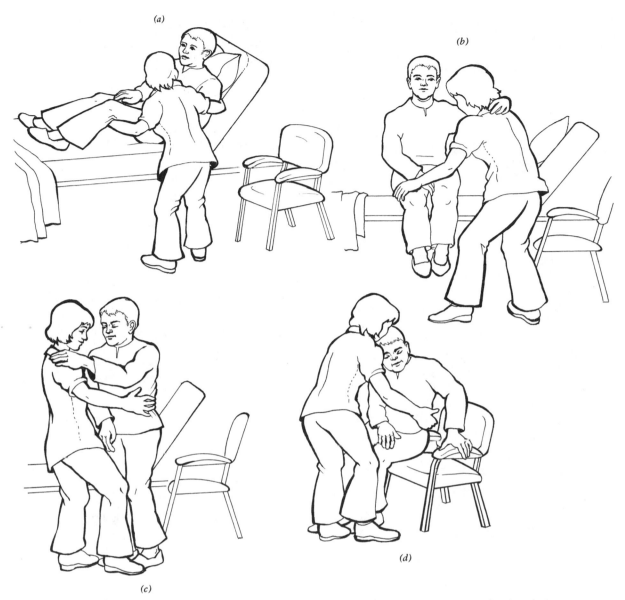

Figure 29.36 *Getting a patient out of bed when one side of the patient is weak. The chair has been positioned so that he can reach for it with his stronger arm.*

sitting position and should be encouraged to do so. You can help if need be by helping the patient to position his arms and legs. Although this method often looks awkward and difficult, it is less strenuous for most patients than trying to rise to a sitting position from a supine (back-lying) position. The procedure is *time consuming* when the patient is weak or just learning to do it, but the exercise that results is invaluable in helping the patient to regain or maintain his strength.

While the patient is still sitting on the side of the bed, ask him how he feels. Some patients experience a drop in blood pressure when coming to an erect position (orthostatic hypotension), especially the first time they get out of bed. If the patient mentions lighthead-

edness, dizziness, sweating, or faintness, help him to lie down again until the symptoms are relieved, and check his blood pressure, pulse, and respiration as indicated by his subsequent symptoms.

Helping the Patient to Stand

If you have any doubts about the patient's ability to stand and then sit down in the chair, make sure that a helper is present *before* you ask the patient to stand (Fig. 29.37). Teach the patient to reach for and hold onto the back or arms of the chair, the edge of the bed, the bedside stand, or any other stable object rather than holding exclusively onto the nurse. You can help by using your knee to brace the patient's knees to keep them from buckling as he stands beside the bed. If the patient needs additional support, you can grasp his belt or place your arms under his axilla with your palms over his shoulder blades.

If the bed is high and cannot be lowered, lock the wheels of the bed and then help the patient to slide slowly over the side of the bed until his feet touch the floor, keeping him informed of his progress with indications such as "only 6 more inches" or "only an inch or two more." *Do not use a footstool* unless you are positive that it will not tip over, and that the patient can step down from it (which a weak person may be unable to do).

Never use a footstool for a person who has the use of only one leg. If a person who is unable to bear weight on one of his legs because of surgery, a cast, or paralysis, for instance, tries to use a footstool, he will find himself standing on one foot on a footstool with no way to get to the floor except to jump.

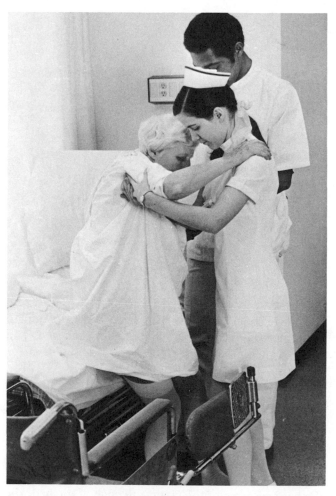

Figure 29.37 *To insure a weak patient's safety, the chair is positioned and extra help is available before the patient gets out of bed.*

Helping the Patient Into the Chair

The nurse can help the patient to get into the chair by teaching him to:

1. Back up until the backs of his legs touch the front edge of the chair seat
2. Slide one foot back under the chair to enlarge the base of support and increase stability
3. Lean forward slightly as he sits down to keep from tipping backward or sitting down before his hips are well back in the chair

Checking the Fit of the Chair

In most hospitals you will need to use whatever chair is available, whether or not it fits the patient. You should, therefore, check to see what modifications, if any, are needed to ensure the patient's comfort and safety. A properly fitting chair should enable the patient to sit in such a way that the following criteria are met:

- Feet are flat on the floor
- Ankles, knees, and hips are flexed at right angles
- Back and thighs are fully supported by chair
- There is adequate space behind the knees
- The weight-bearing line of head and neck and trunk passes through the pelvis

If the chair is *too low*, the patient's knees and hips are sharply flexed, and the lower part of the back is unsupported. The weight-bearing line of head and trunk does not pass through the pelvis (Fig. 29.38).

If the chair is *too high*, the patient's feet are not flat on the floor and there is likely to be pressure on his popliteal nerves and blood vessels (Fig. 29.39).

If the chair is *too deep*, the lower back is not supported, and the weight-bearing line of the head and trunk does not pass through the pelvis (Fig. 29.40).

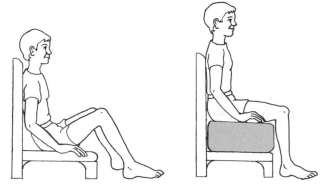

Figure 29.38 *Modification necessary for a chair that is too low.*

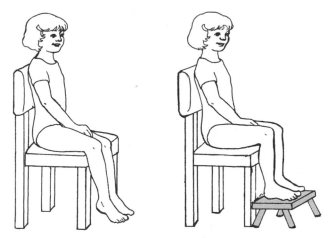

Figure 29.39 *Modification necessary for a chair that is too high.*

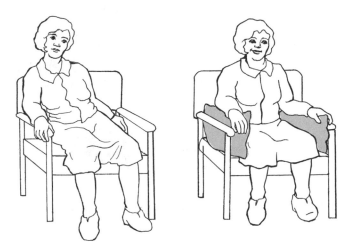

Figure 29.41 *Modification necessary for a chair that is too wide.*

If the chair is *too wide*, or if the arms are too low, the patient must lean to one side or the other for support (Fig. 29.41).

Modifying the Chair to Fit the Patient

Most problems of chair fitting can be corrected by the judicious use of pillows or folded blankets and a foot rest. It is important to evaluate the relationship between patient and chair because the comfort of a patient affects his willingness to get out of bed again and because poor sitting posture can be physiologically detrimental. The patient who is most severely affected by a badly fitting chair is the patient who is *least able to do anything about it*, such as a feeble, confused, or paralyzed patient. He may be unable to shift his position to get comfortable, and he may be unable to get himself back to bed. He is unable to help himself, and it is an unconscionable act of negligence to put a helpless patient in a badly fitting chair and leave him there for hours in the name of therapy.

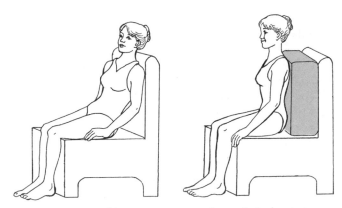

Figure 29.40 *Modification necessary for a chair that is too deep.*

Teach your patient to *stimulate the circulation in his legs* while sitting by intermittently pressing his feet against the floor, as if he were rocking. If the patient's ankles tend to swell after he has been sitting for a while, this can often be prevented by elevating his feet and legs to promote the return of venous blood. The leg rest should be slightly lower than the seat of the chair and should support the feet and entire length of the lower leg. If only the feet are supported, the knees drop into a position of *hyperextension*, which is both uncomfortable and dangerous, especially for a patient with arthritis or any other joint problem (Fig. 29.42).

For safety's sake, the patient's call bell must be placed within his reach. If there is a possibility that he might try to get up and fall, an appropriate restraint may be necessary. Drinking water, tissues, and something to read should be accessible.

Helping the Patient Back to Bed

When the patient is ready to go back to bed, the nurse can help him plan how he will manage. Only as a last resort should your body provide the support needed by a weak or heavy patient. Instead, teach him to make the following preparations before he tries to stand:

1. Place one foot back under the chair to enlarge his base of support
2. Move his hips closer to the front edge of the chair
3. Straighten his knees and hips as he pushes with the foot that is under the chair
4. Lean forward *slightly* to maintain balance

Teach the patient how to use the arms of the chair, the edge of the bed, or any other steady object to help

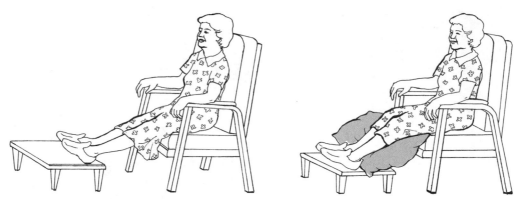

Figure 29.42 *One way to prevent hyperextension of the patient's knees when the feet are elevated.*

himself rise from the chair. Give him *plenty of time.* Getting up may seem to take him forever, and it is hard to watch a patient struggle to get up. It may take three or four attempts, but if you teach him how to manage his body movements, getting up by himself will help him maintain or regain his strength and self-confidence. Patients who are terminally ill cannot be expected to regain lost strength and agility, but they can *maintain* some degree of strength and independence.

Do not attempt to get an extremely weak patient back to bed alone unless the bed can be in a low position. If the bed is high, a footstool may be needed and the patient may be unable to get up on the footstool and then pivot to sit on the edge of the bed without considerable assistance. You will need to ask someone to help you keep the patient from falling. It is often helpful to raise the head of the bed so the patient can lean against it.

When the patient is seated on the edge of the bed, remove his robe and slippers, have him lean against the raised head of the bed, and then help him lift his legs onto the bed (Fig. 29.43). Finally, adjust the head of the bed to the desired height, move the call bell back to the bed, and leave the patient feeling comfortable.

USING A WHEELCHAIR

A wheelchair has two main purposes: to transport a person from one place to another, and to enable a person who cannot walk to live a good and full life. When a wheelchair is used in a hospital for transportation only, little if any attention is paid to the size or features of the wheelchair. Use is high, partly because of hospital policy that often requires every patient regardless

---

PROCEDURE 29.10

Helping a Patient From Bed to Chair

SUMMARY OF ESENTIAL NURSING ACTIONS

1. Check with patient and/or staff to determine whether or not you will need assistance in helping patient out of bed. If so, make sure helper is present *before* you start.
2. Position chair so that it is on patient's strongest side when he is sitting on edge of bed.
3. Assist patient to a sitting position on edge of bed. Whenever possible, do so by raising head of bed.
4. Put on patient's shoes or slippers and robe.
5. While patient is still sitting on edge of bed, check for any

indications of orthostatic hypotension (dizziness, faintness, change in pulse rate).

6. Lower bed, Do NOT use a footstool. If patient's feet do not touch floor, ease patient over edge of bed *slowly* with assistance or helper until feet reach the floor.
7. Assist patient to pivot, and back up until back of knees touch seat of chair.
8. When patient is seated, check fit of chair and modify it for comfort and safety.
9. Make sure patient can reach signal cord, water, and other items he may need.

*See inside front cover and page 543.

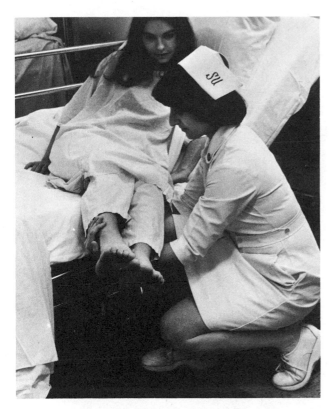

Figure 29.43 Note the good body mechanics of the nurse helping a patient back to bed.

of physical condition to be admitted, discharged, and taken for diagnostic tests or treatments via wheelchair and partly because many patients are too ill to walk. Because the demand for wheelchairs is high and the supply is sometimes low, the hospital worker may consider himself fortunate to find one for the patient to use, and he is not often concerned about its size or specifications.

This approach is acceptable when the patient will not be sitting in the wheelchair for more than a few minutes, but it will not suffice when the patient must spend many hours in the chair each day. The child who uses a wheelchair in school and the employee who works from his wheelchair, for example, are dependent on a proper fit and the presence of essential features in order to participate in activities of daily living.

Selection

The person who uses a wheelchair all day usually has a neurological, muscular, or skeletal disorder and has problems with strength, movement, and balance. The wheelchair must fit well enough to *support* the patient and to *compensate for deficiencies* in strength and move-

ment. Four measurements related to the support and balance of the patient are: the width and depth of the seat, the height of the arms, and the distance from the seat to the footrest. Standard sizes fit the majority of people, from a 30 lb 3-year-old to a tall man weighing 225 lb, but additional sizes can be ordered.

In addition to the fit of the chair, careful attention must be paid to the specific needs of the patient. His daily activities and his physical environment must be carefully assessed before his chair is selected or designed. Examples of questions that must be answered are: How high and wide is the table or desk he will be using? How large is the space around his toilet? Would it help to have a removable arm on the wheelchair? If so, which one? Does he have the strength to move his own chair? Is an electric chair necessary or desirable?

Many other such factors are included in the assessment. For example, weight and compactness are important if the wheelchair must be put into and taken out of a car a number of times a day. If the patient is able to use only one arm to propel the wheelchair, it will go in circles unless it has a one-wheel drive. The optimal size and placement of wheels are determined by the size and angle of the steps, curbs, and ramps that will be routinely encountered.

You may be involved in the patient's decision to rent or buy a wheelchair. Rented chairs are usually equipped with basic features and are useful for patients who will be afflicted with minimal or moderate dysfunction for a limited time. Any patient with a severe disability should have his own chair, even though it is a major expense. A wheelchair that meets the patient's needs will cost from $500 for a simple, well-fitted chair to over $2,000 for an electric chair with minimal features. You may need to teach the family about sources of financial help, such as the Easter Seals and March of Dimes funds, especially for children who outgrow their wheelchairs every few years.

The patient should be encouraged to participate in community life as fully as desired and possible. Families and friends can be taught how to check the physical aspects of the auditorium, store, or restaurant the patient wants to visit either by phone or in person (preferably in person). The family member or friend should check access to the building itself, and to emergency exits, rest rooms, telephone, and the areas that are of particular interest to the patient. If a person is denied access to a public building because of physical barriers to the use of a wheelchair, he should bring the situation to the attention of his local community action group. Institutions and agencies that accept federal funding for any part of their programs must make those programs accessible to everyone.

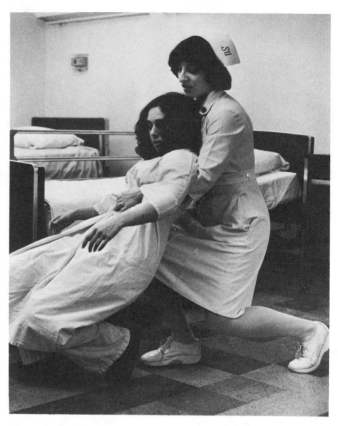

Figure 29.45 *Lowering a falling patient to the floor in a way which protects both patient and nurse.*

PROTECTING A FALLING PATIENT

At some time or another during your career, a patient will start to fall and you will be tempted to try to catch him before he reaches the floor. You *cannot* do so *safely* and should not even try. It is usually not possible to

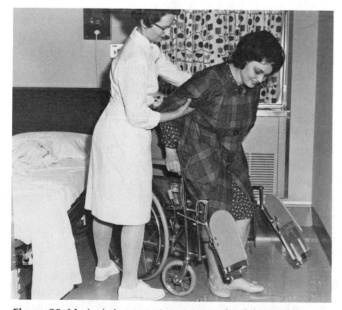

Figure 29.44 *Assisting a patient into a wheelchair. The wheels are locked, and the foot and leg supports have been moved out of the way.*

keep an adult from falling, and the risk of back injury from trying to do so is very great. Instead, your efforts should be directed toward protecting the falling patient from injury.

If a patient suddenly feels faint and starts to fall, put your arms around his waist, separate your feet to give a broad base of support, extend your leg, and let him slide slowly down your leg to the floor (Fig. 29.45). As he slides, bend your knees to lower your body. When the patient is safely on the floor, assess his condition and decide whether to help him to his feet, call for assistance in getting him up, or wait for a physician to come and examine him.

If it seems advisable to have the patient examined by a physician at once, make him as comfortable as possible with a pillow and with a blanket if the room is cold or drafty. If the patient seems able to get to his feet, teach him to roll over, get on his hands and knees, and then rise to a standing position. It will help to place a chair next to him so he can use it for support as he starts to rise.

If the patient is unable to get to his feet, a hydraulic lifter should be used to pick him up and carry him to his bed. If the patient weighs less than 100 lb, a three-man carry might be used with great caution, but it is difficult to use good body mechanics while lifting a bulky, heavy object from the floor. Patients and families should be taught that, whenever an adult falls at home, he should be made comfortable on the floor until help arrives if his condition seems serious. If the person seems able and anxious to get up, the family should teach him to get onto his *hands and knees* and then use a *chair* for support to help him rise from his hands and knees. It is usually difficult if not impossible for a weak or elderly person to rise to a standing position directly from a back-lying position.

PATIENT TEACHING

Two of the most important topics for patient teaching are exercise and body mechanics. Teaching about the need for regular exercise is important because, for many people, it is no longer a routine part of everyday life—it must be a planned activity. Children must be taught that gym classes 2-3 times a week cannot provide enough exercise for normal growth and health, and that regular vigorous exercise should be substituted for some of the recreational time spent with television and computers. A strong commitment to exercise must be developed throughout childhood and adolescence in preparation for good health habits as an adult. Exercise is often more difficult and less satisfying for elderly people, especially those who are homebound, but they must be taught that many potential health problems can be averted or postponed by a daily exercise program.

Back problems account for much absenteeism and misery, and preventive teaching should begin during childhood before faulty posture and poor body mechanics have become habitual. Small children normally squat down to pick things up, and such behavior should be reinforced and retained. Adolescents and young adults need to learn that they are *not* too young for back strain and injury, and that a conscious effort must be made to protect one's back at all times. Many people afflicted with 'a bad back' need considerable support in coping with the problem because it is difficult to ask for help in carrying groceries, lifting a heavy child, or managing heavy objects at work when one looks perfectly healthy.

RELATED ACTIVITIES

Your professional career can be threatened or limited by failure to use good body mechanics as you care for patients. It is somewhat difficult to evaluate your own body mechanics because you tend to lift properly whenever you are thinking about it, so it is advisable to seek the help of a colleague. Ask that person to observe you unannounced and unobtrusively for a period of time and then cite instances in which your body mechanics were good as well as instances in which they were potentially dangerous. Make a conscious effort to make your body mechanics consistently good, and then ask for a second series of observations in order to evaluate your progress.

SUGGESTED READINGS

Exercise and Movement

Agee, Barbara L, and Christine Herman: Cervical logrolling on a standard hospital bed. *Am J Nurs* 1984 March; 84(3):314–318.

Ciuca, Rudy, Jennie Bradish, and Suzanne M Trombly: Passive range-of-motion exercises: a handbook. *Nursing 78* 1978 July; 8(7):59–65.

Cohen, Stephen and Gigi Viellion: Patient assessment: examining joints of the upper and lower extremities (programmed instruction). *Am J Nurs* 1981 April; 81(4):763–786.

Cohen, Stephen, and Gigi Viellion: Teaching a patient how to use crutches (programmed instruction). *Am J Nurs* 1979 June; 79(6):1111–1126.

Dehm, Michael M: Rehabilitation of the cardiac patient: the effects of exercise. *Am J Nurs* 1980 March; 80(3):435–440.

Devney, Ann M: Bridging the gap between inhospital and outpatient care. *Am J Nurs* 1980 March; 80(3):446.

Gandy, Ethel D, and Gretchen Veigh: Help the amputee stand on his own again. *Nursing 84* 1984 July; 14(7):46–49.

Hoepfel-Harris, Jean A: Improving compliance with an exercise program. *Am J Nurs* 1980 March; 80(3):449.

Leinweber, Eileen: Belts to make moves smoother. *Am J Nurs* 1978 Dec; 78(12):2080–2081.

Milazzo, Vicki: An exercise class for patients in traction. *Am J Nurs* 1981 Oct; 81(10):1842–1844.

Owen, Bernice Doyle: How to avoid that aching back. *Am J Nurs* 1980 May; 80(5):894–897.

Reeder, Jean M: Help your disabled patient be more independent. *Nursing 84* 1984 Nov; 14(11):43.

Robertson, Carolyn: Clear the exercise hurdles for your diabetic patient. *Nursing 84* 1984 Oct; 14(10):58–63.

Simpson, Carol F, and Glenda R Dickinson: Exercise: Adult arthritis. *Am J Nurs* 1983 Feb; 83(2):273–274.

Thomassen, Pauline F: Helping your scoliosis patient walk tall. *RN* 1984 Feb; 47(2):34–37.

Winslow, Elizabeth Hahn, and Therese M Weber: Rehabilitation of the cardiac patient: progressive exercise to combat the hazards of bed rest. *Am J Nurs* 1980 March; 80(3):440–443.

Immobility

Ahmed, Mary Cooke: Op-site for decubitus care. *Am J Nurs* 1982 Jan; 82(1):61–64.

Byrne, Nancy, and Marjorie Feld: Overcoming the red menace: preventing and treating decubitus ulcers. *Nursing 84* 1984 April; 14(4):55–57.

Getz, Patsy A, and Bonnie M Blossom: Preventing contractures: the little "extras" that help so much. *RN* 1982 Dec; 45(12):45–48.

Kerr, Janet C, Shirley M Stinson, and Mary Lou Shannon: Pressure sores: distinguishing fact from fiction. *Can Nurse* 1981 July/Aug; 77(7):23–28.

Lucke, Kathleen, and Connie Jarlsberg: How is the air-fluidized bed best used? *Am J Nurs* 1985 Dec; 85(12):1338–1340.

Malkiewicz, Judy: A pragmatic approach to musculoskeletal assessment. *RN* 1982 Nov; 45(11):57–62.

Morley, Margaret: 16 steps to better decubitus ulcer care. *Can Nurse* 1981 July/Aug; 77(7):29–31.

Phipps, Marion, et al.: Staging care for pressure sores. *Am J Nurs* 1984 Aug; 84(8):999–1003.

Sanchez, Divina G, Betty Bussey, and Marie Petorak: How air-fluidized beds revolutionize skin care. *RN* 1983 June; 46(6):46–48.

Shannon, Mary L: 5 famous fallacies about pressure sores. *Nursing 84* 1984 Oct; 14(10):34–41.

Stoneberg, Carla, Nancy Pitcock, and Catherine Myton: Pressure sores in the homebound: one solution. *Am J Nurs* 1986 April; 86(4):426–428.

30

Hygiene and Grooming

Prerequisites and/or Suggested Preparation
The basic concepts of nursing process, medical asepsis, sensory stimulation, physical activity, and immobility are prerequisite to this chapter. (Chapters 17, 27, 28, and 29, respectively).

THE PATIENT'S BATH

The patient's bath is one of the significant activities of the day because of its psychological implications and physiological effects. Bathing is an important activity for the patient who can bathe himself; his ability to do so may represent progress toward improved health, or it may be one of the last things he is still able to do for himself.

The patient who cannot bathe himself may react to his dependency with anger, anxiety, resentment, worry, passive resignation, or calm acceptance. Regardless of the nature of the patient's emotional reaction and the way in which he expresses (or fails to express) that reaction, being bathed by a nurse is stressful.

A patient's reaction to being bathed by another person will be influenced by his age, his past experiences, and the nature of his illness or condition as well as by the age, attitude, and skill of the nurse. Some people find it comforting to be bathed by a sensitive, caring nurse. For others, being bathed is the last straw, the ultimate indignity.

A patient may be acutely embarrassed if the nurse is young and of the opposite sex. In the home, many adults find it extremely difficult to be bathed by a son or daughter. If the patient's condition has progressively worsened, the need to be bathed may seem to indicate that there is no hope for recovery.

TYPES OF BATHS

The type of bath and the extent of patient participation depend on the goals of the bath and on the condition and needs of the patient.

Shower or Tub Bath

A patient who is steady on his feet, not subject to periods of dizziness or fainting, and without any cast or dressing that must be kept dry is often permitted to take a tub bath or shower. This is usually a nursing decision; but in some institutions a doctor's order may be needed.

The tub room or shower should be equipped with handrails and grab bars, a nonskid rubber mat or safety strips on the floor of the tub or shower stall, a chair for the patient to use while dressing, and an emergency bell for summoning help if needed. There should also be an "occupied" sign to hang on the door because the door should *never* be locked for privacy.

In addition to the patient's toilet articles and fresh clothing, some type of bath mat is needed. In the hospital, the floor has been contaminated by the shoes of many nurses and attendants, and the organisms must be kept away from the patient. Anything that will not soak through may be used: a regulation bath mat, a heavy towel, thick newspapers, or a plastic-backed incontinent pad. Any of these will promote medical asepsis and help protect the patient from a nosocomial infection.

Modifications of Tub Bath

If the patient is not strong enough or agile enough to step over the side of the tub and lower himself into the water, he may be able to manage with the aid of two chairs or a hydraulic lifter.

USING TWO CHAIRS. When two chairs are used, one chair is placed in the tub (Fig. 30.1). The patients sits on the chair outside the tub, pivots his body on the chair seat, and swings his legs over the side of the tub. He then stands up in the tub, pivots, and sits down on the chair in the tub. The patient is then able to soak his feet; and even though he is not actually sitting in the water, he is able to use plenty of water for washing himself (in contrast to the small amount of water available for a bed bath) and to retain a large measure of independence despite his weakness or lack of agility. At home, a person who is weak or unsteady should bathe only when there is another adult at home and within earshot of the bathroom, ready to help in case the patient needs assistance.

USING A HYDRAULIC LIFTER. In many hospitals and long-term care facilities, hydraulic lifts are used to lower a weak or helpless patient safely into a tub of water. Canvas slings are positioned under the patient *before* he is taken to the bathroom. In the bathroom, the slings are attached to hooks on the boom (arm) of the hydraulic lifter, and the nurse or attendant carefully swings the patient over the tub and gently lowers him into the water. This method of bathing a weak or helpless patient permits a more thorough cleansing of the skin, provides the sensory stimulation of warm water, and gives the esthetic satisfaction of a "real bath." The nurse is legally and morally responsible for the safety of the patient and must be both skillful and knowledgeable with respect to the use and proper functioning of the hydraulic lifter (see Chapter 29).

The nurse is responsible for maintaining the patient's modesty and privacy, and the patient should be wearing a hospital gown or be covered with a large towel as much of the time as possible.

Bed Bath

Bed Bath Taken by the Patient

Many patients who are confined to bed are able to bathe themselves although some will need considerable

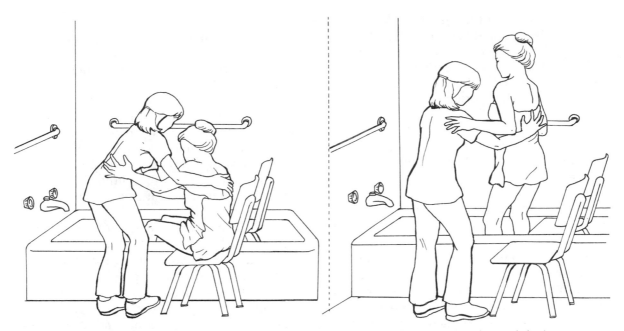

Figure 30.1 *The two-chair method makes it possible for a weak person to take a tub bath or shower.*

assistance. For example, an elderly woman who is very weak and shaky must exercise in order to gain strength; she needs a bed bath but should be encouraged to bathe herself, with *as much assistance as needed.*

EQUIPMENT. The nurse assembles the equipment, explains to the patient what he is to do, and explains what she will do to assist. Minimal equipment includes a towel, a washcloth, soap, a basin of water, and a clean gown or pajamas. The patient's comb, brush, deodorant, talcum powder, lotion, equipment for oral hygiene, and any other grooming aids should be placed within easy reach of the patient.

A soft, absorbent, cotton-flannel bath blanket is used to cover the patient during the bath. It provides warmth and privacy and permits the top bedding to be removed or fanfolded to the foot of the bed so it will not get wet. If available, a second towel is placed under the body part being washed to protect the bottom bedding from getting wet.

PROCEDURE. Because a small amount of water cools rapidly, fill the basin with *hot* tap water and carefully place it where it will not tip over. Suggest to the patient that he wash his face, arms, chest, abdomen, and if possible, his legs. Explain that you will return to refill the basin with fresh, hot water and will wash and rub his back at that time, after which he can finish his bath. Some patients will understand the phrase "finish your bath"; others will need more explicit directions such as "wash between your legs," "wash your private parts," or "wash your genitals." It is important that the patient

know there will be an opportunity for this part of the bath; if he does not know, he is likely to wash his genitals and rectal area after his legs, leaving you with a soiled cloth for his back. The genital and rectal areas are washed last for esthetic and sanitary reasons. Many agencies provide only one washcloth; therefore, the cleanest body parts are washed first and the genital and rectal areas are washed last.

While washing the patient's back, sacrum, and buttocks, carefully inspect the skin for any reddened areas that might indicate the beginning of a pressure sore. After you have rubbed the patient's back, tell him you will leave the unit for a few minutes to give him some privacy while he finishes his bath.

At the conclusion of the bath, wash and dry the basin, put away the patient's toilet articles and grooming aids, and make the bed as described later in this chapter.

PATIENT'S NEED FOR PRIVACY. Unnecessary exposure of the patient's body is a threat to his psychological safety and security. With the exception of small children and confused or irrational people, most people are modest and prefer to keep their bodies covered in the presence of strangers. No nurse has the right to violate that modesty. No one has the right to embarrass another person even though that person may submit without a word, thereby giving the appearance of acceptance. Patients often do not protest an invasion of privacy because they erroneously assume that all nurses are indifferent to exposure, nudity, and lack of modesty. Some patients do not protest violations of their privacy because they fear that they will be teased, ridiculed, or thought naive and old fashioned. They *need* the services of the nurse, and therefore they try to be "good patients" and do what seems to be expected of them. A common remark is "I was always a modest person until I came to the hospital."

During the bath, the patient's body should be covered with a towel or bath blanket, or if need be, the sheet. The unit curtains should be pulled, the room door closed, or both.

PATIENT RELUCTANCE TO BATHE. A patient may be reluctant to bathe himself because of fear, lack of energy, or depression.

A thorough assessment might indicate that the patient is afraid to move enough to bathe himself because he fears that "a clot might break loose," "my incision might split open," or "the IV might infiltrate again." Careful teaching could help the patient reconcile his fears with reality and with the benefits to be gained from moving about while bathing.

Human energy is finite, and the amount of energy available to a sick person may be very limited indeed. A careful nursing assessment might reveal that the patient who feels unable to bathe himself simply *does not have enough energy*, for example, to feed himself, go for chemotherapy, visit with family members, ambulate twice a day, and bathe himself. If the goals of the bath are examined in the context of the overall plan for meeting patient needs, a bath given by the nurse may be an extremely appropriate way to conserve the patient's energy.

The fact that you believe a patient needs to be bathed does not mean that you must do the actual bathing; it may be more appropriate to delegate the activity to an aide, an orderly, or a family member. But even if you are unable personally to bathe each of your patients who needs to be bathed, your assessment and professional judgment will enable you to *direct the activities* and *focus the attention* of the person who will do the actual bathing. For example, you can say to that person, "Try to talk with Mr. Jones while you bathe him and find out how he feels about going home to his daughter's. He sometimes gets talkative during a backrub when he is not facing you," or "Miss Evans seems mad at the world in general lately. She is refusing her medication and treatments, but won't say why. Listen carefully—you may be able to pick up some clues that will let us know how to help her."

Bed Bath Given by the Nurse

A bed bath is given by the nurse when the patient is comatose, confused, feeble, paralyzed, very young, or immobilized. A patient who is on *strict bed rest* after a heart attack must also be bathed by the nurse.

REACTIONS OF THE NURSE. Giving a complete bed bath is often stressful for the nurse as well as for the patient. If you were reared in a family in which there was minimal physical contact or in a family in which there was considerable emphasis on modesty and privacy, you are likely to be uncomfortable while handling a patient's body. Much of this discomfort will dissipate in time as you focus on the purposes and goals of the procedure and as you attempt to put your patient at ease.

You will eventually be able to bathe the majority of patients with confidence and comfort, but a few will continue to make you feel uneasy because they either remind you of significant people you have known or because they are about your own age. It is sometimes difficult to bathe a person who represents power or authority, such as a teacher, priest, or physician. If physical contact with patients continues to make you uncomfortable, it is important that you seek help from an instructor, counselor, or therapist because touching is an integral part of nursing, and is essential to your professional expertise.

You will undoubtedly experience some embarrassment as you bathe your first helpless patient. A helpless patient cannot bathe his own genitals, and you must do so for him. Your discomfort may be minimal if the patient is comatose or a child; but if the patient is alert and yet unable to bathe himself because of weakness, paralysis, or immobility, your discomfort may range from moderate to severe. Later in this chapter, ways to minimize this embarrassment are discussed.

SAFETY OF THE NURSE. If the height of the patient's bed is adjustable, raise it to a height that enables you to work without bending over and then move the patient to the side of the bed closer to you. This will permit you to work in an effective, safe position, you will not need to lean or bend over, and your center of gravity will remain over your base of support.

If the patient is large or heavy, do not try to reach across the closer leg to wash the far leg; instead, move to the other side of the bed. It will take an extra moment or two to do this, but a large leg can weigh 40 lb or more and is far too heavy to be lifted from the opposite side of the bed.

In the patient's home, an ordinary bed can be elevated on blocks of wood to a comfortable working height *if the patient is bedfast*. If, however, the patient is sometimes able to get out of bed, it is not safe to elevate the bed. In such a situation, you can protect your back by kneeling beside the bed as you bathe the patient. Teach

PROCEDURE 30.1

*Giving a Bed Bath**

SUMMARY OF ESSENTIAL NURSING ACTIONS

1. If possible, bathe patient at the time he normally bathes.
2. Provide for patient comfort and safety throughout bath.
   - Adjust temperature of room as needed.
   - Keep patient covered to prevent chilling.
   - Fill basin with *very* warm water as it cools quickly.
   - Keep bed linens dry.
3. Make sure bath is esthetically and psychologically acceptable.
   - Protect the privacy of the patient.
   - Wash cleanest areas of the body first.
   - Use separate wash cloth for genitals or wash them last.
   - Encourage patient to participate in bathing.
4. Make sure bath is effective.
   - Know the reason the patient is being bathed.

- Use long firm strokes.
- Use appropriate amount of soap; rinse thoroughly.
- Wash genitals thoroughly; make sure you can see what you are doing.
- Soak feet, especially if you plan to trim patient's toenails.
- Work rapidly enough to complete bath without tiring the patient.
5. Incorporate range of motion exercises into movement of all extremities.
6. Make careful assessments throughout the bath.
   - Assess mental status, respiration, range of motion, pain, hydration, emotional status, and knowledge of illness or condition.
7. Utilize the bath as an opportunity for patient teaching and/ or therapeutic communication.

*See inside front cover and pages 557–574.

---

the family to keep a pad or cushion handy to protect the knees of those giving care to the patient. You will also need to kneel when bathing a patient in a bathtub. In the hospital, kneel on a towel or newspaper to keep your uniform clean and uncontaminated.

Whether you are standing or kneeling, the bath is a fairly long procedure, so protect your back by lengthening your midriff, stabilizing your pelvis, and keeping your center of gravity over your base of support.

PARTIAL BATH. In the event of serious understaffing, partial baths are given. A partial bath includes washing the patient's face and hands; giving thorough back, rectal, and genital care; plus attention to deep folds of skin as needed. A partial bath does *not* mean superficial attention to all parts of the body; it means *thorough care to selected parts* of the body.

GOALS OF THE BATH

An effective bath can meet many basic needs if it is used as a *significant nursing intervention* rather than merely a routine procedure. An effective, well-planned, and skillfully given bath will accomplish several of the following purposes or goals:

- Protect against infection by helping to maintain the integrity of the skin

- Promote activity that stimulates respiration and circulation
- Help to maintain joint function
- Promote rest, relaxation, and comfort, both physical and psychological
- Provide a period of sensory stimulation
- Maintain or increase the patient's level of self-esteem

The goals set for a bath will differ from patient to patient and from day to day, and the goals you set for a given patient will determine the activities that are most appropriate for that patient for that particular bath.

Selection of Goals for Bath

As soon as you have acquired enough information about the patient to assess his current needs, you will be in a position to decide what can be accomplished through the bath and its associated activities. For example, if your patient is a frail woman with a fractured hip who seldom turns over in bed because of arthritis, a primary nursing goal will be the *prevention of pressure ulcers* and the *maintenance of joint mobility,* and the activities of the bath will be directed toward this end.

If, however, the patient is an obese person who is perspiring profusely and is currently incontinent of feces, the goals for the bath will be, among other things, to *cleanse the skin* in the rectal area and perineal areas, to

TABLE 30.1

Goal for Bath	Outcome Criteria
Maintain integrity of skin	Skin is clean, supple, and intact.
Stimulate respiration and circulation	Patient increases chest expansion during bath. If circulation was poor, color improves and extremities are warmer than before bath.
Maintain joint function	Joint function is not decreasing; range of motion is maintained or is gradually increasing.
Promote relaxation	Physiological signs of anxiety and stress are decreased; patient may fall asleep after back rub.
Provide sensory stimulation	Patient may show increased response to stimuli, more spontaneous movements, increased communication, and less apathy or withdrawal.
Increase self-esteem	Patient looks and acts more self-confident; may say something like "Now I feel human again," or "Now I'm ready to face the world."

Activities Which Contribute to the Attainment of Goal 1

- Using an appropriate cleansing agent
- Cleansing deep folds of skin
- Giving adequate genital care
- Checking for pressure areas
- Giving special skin care as needed
- Giving an effective back rub
- Providing adequate mouth care

---

reduce body odor, and to *prevent excoriation of the skin* in deep folds such as the groin. The goals for another patient who is anxious, tense, and generally uncomfortable may be to *promote rest and relaxation* through providing a warm bath, a soothing back rub, therapeutic communication, and relevant patient teaching.

The baths of these three patients will have many activities in common, but the *primary* focus, goals, and evaluation of effectiveness will be different for each.

Outcome Criteria for Bath Goals

Given the goals for a specific patient, you will need to establish the outcome criteria for these goals just as you would for any other procedure. For each goal, there must be one or more indicators of success. Some goals, such as maintenance of joint mobility, are difficult to evaluate on a day-to-day basis, and progress or success can be noted only over longer periods of time.

GOAL 1: TO MAINTAIN THE INTEGRITY OF THE SKIN AND MUCOUS MEMBRANES

Cleansing Agents

If the skin is *oily, sweaty, or dirty,* use soap to cleanse the skin, rinse it thoroughly, and dry it by rubbing briskly.

Dead epithelial cells will be rubbed off; if the patient is black or heavily tanned, these cells may resemble dirt on the washcloth or towel.

If the skin is *dry, irritated, or fragile,* use little or no soap, rinse thoroughly, and gently pat dry with the towel. A neutral, superfatted soap can be used if soap is necessary. An occasional bath with baby lotion or another similar preparation will refresh the patient while protecting the skin from further irritation and drying.

Cleansing Deep Folds of Skin

The deep folds of skin in the groin, under the breasts, or under a pendulous abdomen provide the warmth, darkness, and moisture essential for the growth of bacteria. These areas are therefore susceptible to irritation, excoriation, and infection and are a source of foul body odors. Meticulous cleansing will prevent or deter the onset of these uncomfortable and embarrassing conditions.

It is important to lift the breast, abdomen, or other tissue with one hand until you can see the entire fold. Look for any signs of inflammation or infection.

The treatment of any abnormal condition will depend on the *nature and severity of the condition.* If the area is moist with perspiration and is slightly red, a light dusting of cornstarch or talcum powder will help to keep the area dry. If the skin folds are deep, it may be necessary to tuck a piece of facial tissue, or soft fabric into the folds to separate the skin surfaces, absorb moisture, and permit healing of any irritation or excoriation. If the skin surfaces are irritated, a light application of vaseline will reduce friction and soothe the irritated skin, but if the skin fold looks infected, it should be reported to the physician because an antibiotic ointment may be needed.

Some people are susceptible to inflammation and infection of the navel, which is accompanied by a disagreeable odor. These individuals find that it is important to cleanse the navel with an alcohol swab every few days.

Genital Care

The skin and mucous membranes of the rectal area, perineum, and external genitalia are susceptible to irritation from vaginal and urethral discharges, perspiration, urine, and fecal matter. If these areas are kept scrupulously clean and dry, the tissues will remain healthy. In fact, an *absence of odor* from the genitalia, and the *presence of healthy, normal perineal skin* are two indicators of *expert* nursing care.

When bathing the genitalia, there are no substitutes for warm water and soap, a soft washcloth, and adequate visualization of the area. This part of the bath is fraught with potential embarrassment, and there is a rather natural tendency for the nurse to want to wash without looking or to hand the washcloth to the patient, no matter how incapacitated he may be. Such measures are never effective and are in fact dangerous because the rest of the staff will *assume* that rectal and genital care have been given. They will continue to assume so until: (a) some conscientious nurse inspects the area, (b) the patient eventually reports the resulting irritation and discomfort, or (c) the odor becomes very noticeable.

To give genital care, place a towel under the patient's buttocks and arrange the bath blanket or another towel so that the genitalia can be exposed while the rest of the patient's body remains covered. Then, with a warm, wet, soapy washcloth, thoroughly wash all surfaces and folds of skin. There is no way to do this without actually handling and looking at the genitalia. The labia must be separated to wash the inner surfaces, and the penis and scrotum must be lifted to wash beneath them.

In some situations, it might be helpful to begin the process of genital care by saying to the patient, "I'm going to finish your bath (or "wash between your legs" or "wash your penis and scrotum") now. We may both feel a bit uncomfortable about it. Is there anything I can do to make it easier for you?"

Because the penis contains erectile tissue, the physical stimulation of washing it may cause an erection. The normally flaccid penis becomes engorged, hard, and erect. This phenomenon can occur as spontaneously as the erection of a mother's nipple when her baby is put to breast. It can occur at any age and is likely to take place without sexual desire or erotic overtones. For a time following some spinal cord injuries, any stimulation of the skin of the lower abdomen or thighs of a male patient may cause a reflex ejaculation of seminal fluid and an abnormal, persistent erection of the penis (called priapism). A careful explanation of these physiological responses, coupled with sensitivity and acceptance by the nurse, will help the patient cope with these unexpected and embarrassing reflexes.

If an erection should occur during the bath, it cannot be ignored. The nurse can see it and the patient can feel it. It is helpful if the nurse has thought through ahead of time the possible responses that might be made. You might, for example, excuse yourself, saying that you will be back in a few minutes to finish the bath. You might remain at the bedside, visiting with the patient as you wait for the erection to subside.

Protecting a Body Cast

The edges of a plaster body cast will deteriorate if they become wet and soiled. The nurse should always examine the lower edges of a body cast carefully as she bathes a patient's genitalia and should notify the physician if the cast has become soft or moist because it may be necessary to change it.

One way to protect the cast from moisture and soiling, and the underlying skin from maceration, is by proper placement of the patient on the bedpan, using as many pillows as necessary to prop the cast into an optimal position. The edges of the cast are sometimes covered with a thin plastic material, or waterproofed with shellac, varnish, or liquid plastic, and these protected surfaces should be washed with soap and warm water during the bath. The nurse should wash and thoroughly dry the skin under the edge of the cast if there is space enough to do so.

Protecting the Urinary Meatus

It is important to protect the urinary meatus from possible infection; therefore, that area is washed *before* the rectal area, while the washcloth is still as clean as possible. In an uncircumcised male, the prepuce, or foreskin, covers the end of the penis. Smegma, a cheesy substance secreted by the sebaceous glands, tends to collect under the loose folds of the foreskin, and you will need to retract the foreskin gently until the end of the penis is exposed (Fig. 30.2). The foreskin is replaced after the penis has been thoroughly washed, rinsed, and dried. This is done to prevent constriction and possible impaired circulation. The scrotum is rather sensitive, but it must be washed thoroughly. If the patient is perspiring, a dusting of cornstarch or talcum powder will help absorb moisture and protect the scrotum from irritation.

The female urinary meatus can be protected from infection by always cleansing that area of the genitalia first. Bath time is an opportune time to teach a female patient, adult or child, to wipe from front to back after using the toilet or bedpan, using each piece of toilet tissue only once. A woman who is obese or who has only a limited range of motion, cannot do this. She cannot reach from behind to wipe from front to back,

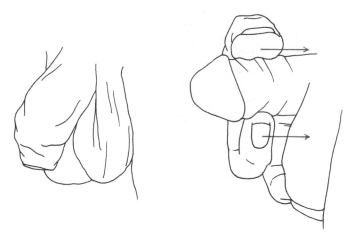

Figure 30.2 *Left: Uncircumsized penis. Right: Retraction of the foreskin for cleaning the meatus.*

so she must be taught to wipe or wash the front of her genitalia first, and then wipe or wash her rectal area.

If a patient has an indwelling urinary catheter, it is extremely important to cleanse the section of the catheter which is adjacent to the urinary meatus. The nurse should very gently pull the catheter out about ½ inch. That portion of the catheter is likely to be ringed with mucus, bits of tissue, and bacteria, which would increase the probability of a urinary tract infection. The meatus and the part of the catheter that is next to it should be washed with clean, soapy water and rinsed thoroughly. It can then be sponged or swabbed with an antiseptic solution if so ordered.

Feminine Hygiene

The term feminine hygiene was probably coined by manufacturers before the advent of explicit advertising, and it refers to menstrual hygiene, douching, and the control of odors originating from the genitalia.

Menstruation can be a stressor for a woman who is hospitalized, and will be even more stressful if her customary supplies are not readily available. An immobilized or incapacitated patient will be embarrassed at not being able to care for herself, but the nurse can reduce this stress by *anticipating* the need for a tampon or napkin change so that the patient is not put in the position of repeatedly having to request it.

Careful attention must be paid to the needs of a patient who cannot recognize or verbalize her needs, such as an unconscious, confused, or severely retarded woman. The amount of menstrual flow, the type of protection used, the frequency of the change, and the activity of the patient will determine how often the perineal area needs to be washed. Premoistened tissues, such as those used for diaper changes, can be more efficient than washcloths for frequent perineal care.

Special sensitivity and empathy will be needed for a young girl who menstruates for the first time while hospitalized. She may be as young as 9 or 10 years of age, and she may or may not have been prepared by her mother or another person. In addition to appropriate physical care, considerable psychological support and teaching may be needed. A careful assessment of her knowledge and emotional response to menstruation will indicate the type of teaching needed.

A small amount of white or colorless mucus discharge from the vagina is normal and is easily wiped away with toilet tissue. A daily or twice-daily washing with soap and water usually keep the area clean and free from odor. If the vaginal discharge is copious, purulent, or irritating to the skin, or has a foul odor, a physician should be consulted. Young girls who have been sexually active or are ignorant about sex may fear that any vaginal discharge is indicative of venereal disease. They need to be taught that there are many possible causes of vaginal discharge, that prompt diagnosis and treatment are important, and that if the discharge is caused by venereal disease, confidentiality will be assured.

Sprays developed to control perineal odors have proven hazardous to women whose skin is sensitive to one or more of the ingredients. Reactions have ranged from mild skin irritation to severe excoriation, loss of pubic hair, and extensive scarring. The liberal use of soap and water remains the safest and most effective way to prevent odors and feel clean.

Pressure Areas

The bath provides an opportunity for the nurse to examine all areas of the patient's body for red or broken areas of skin. Even if the patient bathes himself, it is the nurse's responsibility to check the integrity of his skin if his condition gives her reason to believe that he might be susceptible to skin breakdown. Reddened areas should be massaged lightly but firmly enough to stimulate circulation to the area. An increased blood supply will bring more nutrients and oxygen to the area, which will promote healing and help prevent further damage to the tissues. Red or broken areas should be reported immediately, and preventive measures, such as regular changes of position, should be instituted at once. The patient needs to be told of the problem so that he can *participate knowledgeably* in the prevention of skin breakdown.

Special Skin Care

Prickly Heat Rash

During hot weather, infants and adults alike may be afflicted with heat rash. The affected skin can be soothed by sponging it with a solution of baking soda and water or giving a tub bath of one-half box of soda in a tub of lukewarm water. After bathing, the skin should be air dried or gently patted dry; rubbing will stimulate more itching and discomfort. Despite the heat of the day, an infant with prickly heat rash is often more comfortable wearing a cotton knit shirt than he is without one, for the shirt absorbs perspiration.

Diaper Rash

The by-products of decomposing urine and feces are extremely irritating to the skin and will cause damage ranging from a mild diaper rash to extensive excoriation with permanent scarring. The infant and the incontinent adult must be kept clean and dry, with prompt and vigorous treatment of any breaks in the skin. Diaper rash can be prevented by a *thorough* washing and rinsing of diapers and pajamas, by thorough and frequent cleansing of the buttocks, perineum, and groin; and by protecting the skin with a light application of petroleum jelly. There are a number of commercial preparations available for the prevention and treatment of diaper rash, all of which are rather expensive, especially for families with limited budgets. Zinc oxide ointment (the basic ingredient of most commercial diaper rash preparations) is heavy and thick and will coat and protect skin that has already been afflicted. If the patient's urine is dark and concentrated, it is important to increase his intake of water, because dilute urine is less irritating to delicate and irritated skin.

Giving a Back Rub

A back rub may be a luxury for a patient who is ambulatory or convalescent and able to move about freely in bed, but it is an *absolute necessity* for a patient who is either unable or unwilling to change position frequently. An effective back rub for this patient is psychologically relaxing and is also physiologically stimulating to the skin and underlying muscles. The warmth and increased circulation of blood to the area *relieves muscle tension, removes waste products,* and *brings increased amounts of nutrients to the cells.*

A back rub can vary in complexity from the commonsense approach of a concerned family member to the intricate manipulation of a professional masseur. To give a back rub, first raise the bed to the high position or kneel beside a low bed, then move the patient to the edge of the bed closer to you. Position him on his side with his back toward you, making certain that his head, neck, and extremities are comfortable. Next, place a towel lengthwise on the bed next to the patient and tuck the edge under him to keep the bottom sheet dry.

Warm a small amount of lotion in your hands because cold lotion startles a patient and causes him to tense the muscles in his back—the very ones you are trying to relax. Begin to rub by combining long strokes and circular movements. All movements should be symmetric, slow, even, and rhythmic. It is good to ask the patient which movements are most relaxing or most effective in relieving discomfort or pain. The tips of your fingers may be satisfying across his shoulders, for example, while the heel of your hand may be most effective at the base of his spine.

In general, long, slow, firm strokes with even, steady pressure are used along the spine, while circular, kneading movements are effective over the sacrum, buttocks, and shoulders (Fig. 30.3). A back rub should not be short, abrupt, or routine; a token rub accomplishes little or nothing. The back rub is one of the most symbolic yet therapeutic of all nursing interventions; it is a nonverbal expression of concern and caring.

Special attention should be paid to any reddened areas, whether reddened by pressure over a bony prominence such as the scapula or sacrum or whether reddened from wrinkled sheets or crumbs. Some of the redness may fade as the area is rubbed and circulation to the surrounding tissue is improved. The exact location, dimension, and description of any red or broken area of skin which persists after the back rub should be reported and charted.

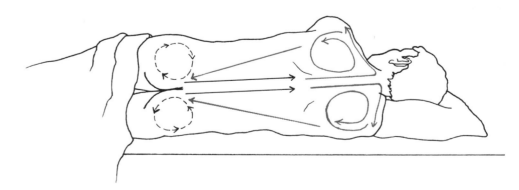

Figure 30.3 Schematic drawing of the direction of hand movements for a back rub.

At the conclusion of the back rub, wipe off any excess lotion and, if the patient desires it and it is available, dust on a little talcum powder. Tighten the lower bedding and leave the patient to rest.

Special Back Care

If a patient is especially vulnerable to pressure sores, you may find the phrase "special back care" written on the Kardex. Interpretations of such an order may range from simply giving more than one back rub per day to a rigorous and detailed program of back care. Such care might include, for example, frequent massage, regular changes of position at frequent intervals, and the use of a heat lamp to increase circulation to the area.

If hospitals and nursing homes were staffed for optimal patient care, there would be no need to order "special back care" because back care would be accorded a top priority. It would be as inconceivable to omit back care as it would be to forget a patient's meal. But since staffing is seldom optimal, it is especially important to identify those patients who are *vulnerable to pressure sores* and to give them effective back care during each bath and at bedtime.

Caring For the Patient's Mouth and Teeth

Although the condition of a person's mouth affects his self-esteem, nutrition, speech, and general well-being, nursing has seldom been actively involved in dental health. The relationship between nursing and dentistry has been and still is less direct than the relationship between nursing and medicine.

Opportunities for collegial relationships between nursing and dentistry are limited, but there are a number of ways nurses can contribute to the dental health of their patients. Three areas of responsibility are (1) assessment, (2) mouth care, (3) and patient teaching.

Assessment

Some patients, for one reason or another, are likely to contract diseases of the teeth and gums, and such patients are said to be *at risk*. It is unrealistic to expect a nurse to assess the mouth of every patient for whom she is responsible, and when time is limited, it is better to do a *thorough* mouth assessment on patients at risk than to do a superficial assessment on every assigned patient.

PEOPLE LIKELY TO BE AT RISK. Factors which place a patient in jeopardy are related to age, diagnosis, treatment, and physical and psychological condition. Careful assessments should be made on:

- Patients who are dehydrated
- Patients who are unable to eat or drink
- Patients who have leukemia or who are receiving chemotherapy
- Patients who are receiving oxygen or drugs such as atropine which are very drying to mucous membranes
- Patients who are unable to care for their own mouths and are dependent on the care of others, including patients who are confused, comatose, very young, retarded, depressed, or incapacitated

---

PROCEDURE 30.2

Giving a Back Rub*

SUMMARY OF ESSENTIAL NURSING ACTIONS

1. Protect your back by raising bed to high position.
   - If this is not possible, kneel beside the bed.
2. Position the patient near side of bed closer to you.
   - If feasible, position patient on his abdomen.
   - If patient is not comfortable in that position, or it is contraindicated, position patient on his side.
3. Expose patient's entire back, including the sacrum.
4. Warm lotion before using it.
5. Rub back with strokes that are slow, symmetric and rhythmic.

6. Ask patient for feedback about places that need rubbing, strokes that feel especially good, and special preferences.
7. Make sure that your interaction with the patient is consistent with the purpose of the back rub. Ex: Talk with patient if purpose is to provide sensory stimulation or distraction from pain. Be relatively quiet if purpose is to soothe, calm, and relieve tension.
8. Continue back rub long enough for it to be effective.
9. Dry patient's skin, powder it if desired, and reposition patient as needed for comfort and safety.

*See inside front cover and page 561.

A patient may not fit any of the above categories, but an assessment of his mouth is warranted if he has halitosis (bad breath); if his teeth are obviously broken, dirty, and neglected; or if he has pain in his teeth or gums when he eats. You may not be able to assess his mouth immediately because he may be extremely sensitive about the condition of his mouth and might take offense at such an action. Diplomacy and tact will be needed as you seek to learn whether the condition of his mouth is the result of a deep fear of dentists, lack of money, or some other reason.

ASSESSMENT OF THE MOUTH. The only equipment needed for assessment is a small flashlight and a tongue depressor, which is used to depress the tongue or hold it aside to permit examination of other areas of the mouth.

The areas of the mouth to be assessed and the characteristics of normal and abnormal conditions are shown in Table 30.2.

Mouth Care

The giving of mouth care is one of the most significant of all nursing interventions, yet it is frequently assigned a very low priority, for understandable reasons. Mouth care can be unpleasant, difficult, distasteful, and downright repulsive. A community health nurse may find, during a routine visit, for example, that a healthy but forgetful 85-year-old patient who lives alone has developed halitosis and discover that she has apparently forgotten to remove and clean her dentures for several weeks. The process of cleaning the patient's dentures and her mouth may be repulsive, but it must be done. A nurse cannot in good conscience leave a patient with a dirty mouth any more than she can leave an incontinent patient in a wet or soiled condition.

Mouth care is an important activity that can be satisfying to both patient and nurse when it is done thoroughly and with the tact and sensitivity that will minimize the patient's embarrassment.

HELPING A PATIENT WITH MOUTH CARE. An assessment of the patient's ability to participate will determine the type of equipment and assistance the nurse will need to provide. A patient who is ambulatory is likely to be completely self-sufficient regarding the care of his teeth or dentures, but other patients will need varying degrees of assistance. A patient who cannot go to a wash basin or sink will need to substitute a cup of water and an emesis basin. If a patient cannot or does not expectorate, you will need equipment for suctioning. If mouth care is painful for a patient as a result of chemotherapy, for example, it may be necessary to give an analgesic or apply a topical anesthetic before starting to give mouth care. All such equipment or assistance should be assembled and in readiness before mouth care begins.

GUIDELINES FOR GIVING MOUTH CARE. Even when a unit is short of staff and assignments are heavy, each patient should have mouth care every morning and night. If the nurses are unable to provide this very basic care, it should be delegated to others except for those patients with special conditions of the mouth, such as recent oral surgery.

Although each patient situation is different, the following guidelines outline an approach to mouth care applicable to a majority of circumstances.

- Explain what you plan to do and how you plan to proceed (even though the patient gives no evidence of hearing you). Tell the patient how he can help as you go along; be specific ("Keep your head turned to the side" or "Please hold the basin").
- If your patient is comatose, has a poor or absent cough and gag reflex, or cannot expectorate, make

TABLE 30.2 ASSESSMENT OF MOUTH

Area	Normal Appearance	Abnormal Appearance
Lips	Pink, smooth, moist	Cracked, dry, blistered (cold sores, fever blisters)
Tongue	Firm, medium red, moist, freely movable	Coated (fuzzy, white), shiny, beefy red, dry, cracked, with ulcers or sores
Mucous membranes of mouth	Pink, moist	Red, shiny, ulcerated, blistered
Gums (gingivae)	Firm, pink, moist, close to teeth	Swollen, spongy, beefy red, bleeding, pus present, receding, discolored
Teeth	Shiny, clean, intact or repaired	Dull, dirty, with cavities, with teeth missing or broken, with some teeth loose, or unable to wear dentures
Saliva	Thin, watery	Thick, viscous, scant, mucoid, profuse (patient may be drooling)

sure that suction equipment is within reach and in good working order. The rubber catheter or suction tip should be clean, and ready for use. A container of water is needed to rinse saliva and dentifrice from the catheter. A rubber-tipped bulb syringe can be used both to flush the mouth with small amounts of fluid and to suction fluids from the mouth, and is especially useful in a patient's home when a suction machine is not available.

- Position your patient in the safest and most comfortable position possible as determined by his condition and therapy. The relative safety of commonly used positions is:

  Safest. Side-lying or back-lying with *head raised.* Most comfortable; presents least danger of aspiration.

  Safe. Side-lying with head of bed flat. Comfortable but not as safe. Place pillow at patient's back as needed to *maintain side-lying position.*

  DANGEROUS. Back-lying with head of bed flat. Patient may aspirate fluid or foamy dentifrice. Have suction equipment available. Used only when patient *cannot be turned* to his side or cannot have his head raised.

- After patient has been positioned, place inner curve of the emesis basin against patient's lower jaw.

- Ask patient to open his mouth. If he does not respond, open his mouth by exerting gentle pressure on his chin and mandible (his lower jaw). If he cannot or will not keep his mouth open, ask an assistant to hold it open with a padded tongue depressor. (You cannot do so because you will need both hands to give mouth care.)

  To pad a tongue depressor, wrap gauze around one end, leaving the other end uncovered as a handle. For extra strength, use two tongue depressors. Cover the gauze completely with adhesive tape to keep any loose threads out of the patient's mouth and to keep it from getting wet and soggy. Some people cannot tolerate the sensation of cloth in their mouths and react to it as other people do to the screech of chalk on a blackboard. Adhesive tape, especially plastic tape, makes a padded tongue depressor tolerable.

  Do not put your finger in a patient's mouth unless his jaws are held apart by a padded tongue depressor. You could be bitten, and a human bite is considered more dangerous than an animal bite.

- Use a toothbrush to clean your patient's mouth unless it is contraindicated because of oral surgery, trauma, or open lesions. Other devices, such as prepackaged commercial swabs, will not remove dental plaque. You can estimate their probable effectiveness by imagining what it would feel like to clean your own mouth with a cotton swab. If the use of a toothbrush is prohibited for medical reasons, a toothette can be used. This is a small cube of foam rubber at the end of a stick.

  The effervescent action of hydrogen peroxide will help to loosen particles of food and debris. It is sometimes mixed with an equal amount of mouthwash to add a refreshing taste.

- Mouth care should be given frequently enough to ensure a clean, moist, comfortable mouth. For some patients, mouth care in the morning and evening is sufficient; for others, mouth care must be given every 1 to 2 hours.

- Mouth care is most effective when it is an integral part of the overall nursing regimen. It is not an isolated activity, and it cannot be fully effective unless the patient has adequate nutrition and an optimal fluid intake.

PROCEDURE 30.3

*Giving Mouth Care**

SUMMARY OF ESSENTIAL NURSING ACTIONS

1. Talk to patient throughout the procedure even if he is comatose or unresponsive.
2. Position the patient for *safety* and *comfort*.
3. If patient is unconscious, has a poor gag reflex, or cannot expectorate, have suction equipment ready.
4. Select cleansing materials on the basis of patient preference, availability, and agency policy.
5. Use a toothbrush rather than swabs unless it is contraindicated by the condition of the patient's mouth.

6. Adjust the amount of pressure used for cleaning to the health of the patient's mouth (be *very gentle* if mouth is sore from chemotherapy, for example).
7. NEVER PUT YOUR FINGERS IN THE PATIENT'S MOUTH.
   • Use padded tongue depressors if necessary to keep patient's mouth open.
8. Use assessments made during mouth care to plan frequency and type of care needed in the future.

*See inside front cover and pages 562–563.

CARE OF DENTURES. A patient who has dentures or removable bridgework will need a covered denture cup in which to store his dentures at night and whenever he is not wearing them, such as during surgery. In a hospital, small waxed containers with snap-on lids are provided and should be *labeled* with the patient's name and room number.

In the hospital or nursing home, dentures are probably the patient's most expensive and valuable possession, and they should thus be *properly safeguarded* at all times. Dentures are *very expensive and difficult to replace* because a mold or cast of the patient's mouth must be made. It can take several weeks to make new dentures, and it is embarrassing for a patient to be without teeth during this time.

CLEANING DENTURES. Dentures can be brushed with a regular brush and toothpaste, or they can be soaked overnight in an effervescent cleansing solution. An inexpensive cleaning solution can be prepared at home by adding 1 teaspoon household bleach (such as Clorox) and 2 teaspoons softening agent (such as Calgon) to ½ glass (4 oz) cool water. Chlorine bleach tends to be corrosive and may *seriously damage dentures* so Calgon (*never* Calgonite) must be added as an anticorrosive agent.

When cleaning a patient's dentures, the nurse should place a washcloth or towel in the basin to cushion the impact if they should drop.

Patient Teaching

A detailed assessment of the patient's knowledge and attitudes toward dental health will be needed before the nurse can make *specific* plans for teaching, but some possible areas for teaching include:

• The value of *preventive* dentistry. It is *not* true that "your teeth have to go, sooner or later" or that "you lose a tooth with every baby."
• The characteristics of a good dental program. Good dental care includes regular brushing and the use of dental floss, with visits to the dentist every 6 to 12 months for cleaning, scaling (removal of tartar), and inspection for cavities or other problems. Low-cost or free dental clinics are available in many places. The first visit to the dentist should be made by the age of 3 years at the latest because cavities can develop as early as 18 months of age. Some dentists refer very young children, or children with special problems, to a *pedodontist* (a specialist in children's dentistry).

TOOTHBRUSHING. Brushing across the teeth merely forces food and bacteria into the spaces between the teeth and brushing toward the gums can force food and bacteria under the gums. Teeth should therefore be brushed *away* from the gums, toward the biting or chewing surfaces of the teeth.

The selection of a dentifrice is a personal matter, although the use of fluoridated paste is often recommended by dentists. A mixture of table salt and baking soda makes an effective yet inexpensive dentifrice. Some families add a little oil of peppermint for flavoring. (This mixture should not be used by people on a salt-restricted diet.)

Patients and families should check the effectiveness

of their brushing from time to time by using disclosure tablets, which can be obtained from their dentists or through the local dental society. These tablets stain dental plaque red when they are chewed; hence, any red that remains after a typical brushing indicates areas where brushing did not remove all dental plaque.

USING DENTAL FLOSS. Dental floss is used to remove dental plaque and bits of food from the spaces between the teeth and from adjoining tooth surfaces. Floss is slippery and hard to hold when it is moist with saliva so the ends are wrapped around a finger on either hand to give a secure grip on the floss. This requires a piece of floss 12 to 15 inches long even though only a few inches are actually used to floss the teeth. The hands are positioned so that 1 to 2 inches of floss is held taut between them (Fig. 30.4). The floss is pulled against first one side and then the other of each tooth in turn and moved up and down each surface to remove plaque and debris. Care must be taken when working the floss down past a tight spot between two teeth because, when the floss is forced beyond the restricted space, too much force can cause it to suddenly hit and injure the gum. Some dentists recommend unwaxed rather than waxed floss because it is softer and may cause less damage to the gums. The patient should be cautioned against harsh back-and-forth movements that could lacerate the gum. Bleeding may occur during the first few flossings.

Depending on the condition of the mouth, the particles of food or debris and clumps of bacteria may or may not be large enough to be visible on the used dental floss. The fact that food and debris are not al-

ways visible on the floss does not mean that they are not being removed by flossing.

Floss can be worked under some parts of fixed or permanent bridgework, but an extremely tightly fitting bridge may require another method of cleaning, such as water under pressure from a Water Pik, for example. People with fixed braces or wires to hold a fractured jaw in place for healing will not be able to floss, and they too will need an alternative method of cleaning between the teeth. Halitosis is one indication that more intensive cleaning is needed around fixed bridgework, braces, and wires.

Flossing should be done daily; if teeth are tight and food tends to become trapped between them, flossing should then be done more often. With practice, teeth can be thoroughly flossed in about 1 minute, which is a very minimal investment of time for so important a health practice.

Flossing should *not* be decreased or stopped if a patient notices that his gums are inflamed and swollen or are beginning to recede, or if any teeth seem loose. On the contrary, flossing should be done more thoroughly than ever, and the patient should see a dentist at once, preferably a *periodontist* (a specialist in gum diseases).

Inclusion of the Dentist in Health Care Planning

The patient's dentist should be included in planning care for any patient whose mouth has been affected by his illness or whose mouth is the source of his problems. If the patient does not have a dentist, a referral can be made to a nearby dental clinic or dentist.

The nurse is often in a position to promote the inclusion of dental care in the overall health care of *people with special problems.* Such people include those with problems of limited income, geographical isolation, and lack of transportation; those confined to bed or a wheelchair or in an institution; and those who are especially mobile, such as street people, runaway children, and migrant workers. Each of these underserved groups needs access to the services of a dentist, and nurses may be able to help promote a closer relationship between dentistry and the overall health care delivery system.

Dentist's Contribution to Health Care

Among the many functions of a dentist, five are especially important: (1) the prevention and treatment of caries (cavities), (2) diagnosis and treatment of periodontal disease, (3) early diagnosis and treatment of malocclusions, (4) early detection of tumors and disease, and (5) replacement of missing teeth.

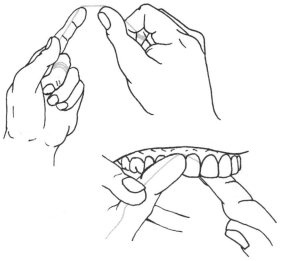

Figure 30.4 *Dental floss must be taut to remove debris from between the teeth. The position of the hands will vary with the location of the tooth.*

CARIES. Caries is thought to be caused by the interaction of a number of factors rather than by a single agent. The enzymes present in saliva, plus bacteria from dental plaque on the teeth, plus refined sugar and carbohydrates, act together to increase the acidity of the mouth. Increased acidity erodes or dissolves susceptible enamel and dentin, thereby permitting bacterial invasion and decay.

Prevention of cavities is aimed at interrupting this process by removing one or more of the conditions which contribute to cavities as follows:

- Remove the dental plaque. This is a dense film of bacteria on the teeth that interacts with sugar to produce cavities. It can be removed by brushing and the use of dental floss. If plaque is not removed, it will calcify and form tartar (calculus).
- Reduce intake of refined sugar or reduce its effect by brushing immediately after eating.
- Increase resistance of enamel to decay by fluoridation of water, application of fluorine to the teeth, or the use of a fluoridated toothpaste.

Treatment of cavities involves removal of decayed material and filling the space with amalgam (silver), porcelain, plastic, or gold.

PERIODONTAL DISEASE. Diseases of the gums and tissues surrounding the teeth are especially common after middle age. They range from a minor inflammation of the gums resulting from poor oral hygiene to a painful deterioration of the gums followed by the loosening and eventual loss of teeth. Periodontal disease can be caused by poor oral hygiene and inadequate dental care, by systemic conditions such as leukemia, and by chemotherapy.

Treatment is difficult, lengthy, and painful. It involves, among other things, vigorous excavation and cleaning of the teeth below the gum line by the dentist and meticulous daily oral hygiene at home. Treatment often extends over a period of weeks or months.

MALOCCLUSION. The problems created by crowded or crooked teeth or by a malformed jaw are both functional and cosmetic. The uneven pressures of a faulty bite exert a tremendous force upon the teeth or portions of teeth that touch each other and render those teeth more susceptible to subsequent problems. Malocclusions often affect speech, and distortions of the jaw and teeth can be damaging to a person's self-esteem.

Evaluation and treatment should be started early. Some children require only simple braces but others need fixed braces or even oral surgery. No person, child or adult, with a serious malocclusion should forego treatment for financial reasons alone. Treatment is often classified as a type of rehabilitation, and clinics and financing are frequently available from state or federal funds.

TUMORS AND DISEASE. *Early detection* of cancer of the mouth increases the success of treatment. It is not uncommon for a dentist to refer to a specialist a patient who had failed to do anything about "that little sore on the side of my tongue" which had been present for a number of months. Any ulcer or sore in the mouth that does not heal should be brought to the dentist's attention.

MISSING TEETH. Proper nutrition is difficult to achieve when a person is partially or completely edentulous (without teeth). A patient should be encouraged to obtain new well-fitting dentures if his are broken, lost, or ill-fitting. Financial aid is often available through social service agencies, Medicare, or other health insurance.

Bridges and partial plates (dentures) are important, not only because they permit a person to chew properly but because the replacement teeth keep the natural teeth from shifting out of place, into the space left by the missing teeth. If a child loses a tooth prematurely, either naturally or as the result of an accident, a spacer tooth should be used to maintain that space until the permanent tooth grows in or until a permanent replacement has been prepared and put in place.

If a tooth is accidentally loosened and knocked out, it should be located, rinsed off, and either reinserted into the tooth socket or kept moist in some other way. The individual should then be taken to the dentist at once because, in some cases, it is possible to implant the tooth successfully.

GOAL 2: TO STIMULATE RESPIRATION AND CIRCULATION

One of the significant tasks related to this goal is that of teaching the patient the advantages of increasing his respiration and circulation, thereby helping him to value it as an important goal, one toward which he is willing to strive with your help. Many of the complications of bed rest can be prevented or minimized by activities that stimulate respiration and increase circulation. If these activities can be combined with the bath, the patient need not be disturbed to do a variety of special exercises and will therefore be assured longer periods of rest throughout the day.

Encourage the patient to do as much of his bath as he is psychologically and physically able to do. One patient might be able to slowly bathe himself if you hand him the hot, soapy washcloth and then rinse it for him. Another patient may be able to wash his face and then, when rested, do a thorough job of washing his genitals when handed the prepared washcloth. The amount of participation will vary from day to day. The nurse's task is to communicate the benefits of increasing amounts of activity without ever suggesting or implying a reluctance to bathe the patient.

Encourage the patient to turn over by himself as you prepare to rub his back or make his bed, unless this is contraindicated.

If the patient has bathed and turned himself, he may not need to do any specific exercises to improve his respiratory function. If not, encourage him to cough, turn, and deep-breathe at intervals throughout the bath (see Chapter 32 for details).

If your assessment indicates that the patient is not moving because of pain and discomfort, the bath may be an excellent time to teach the patient effective ways to cope with pain.

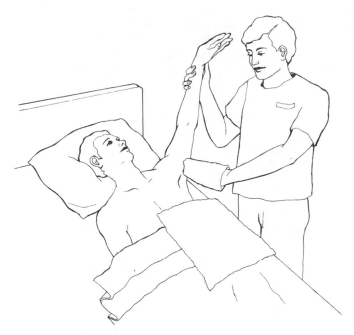

Figure 30.5 *Range-of-motion exercises can be incorporated into the bath.*

GOAL 3: TO MAINTAIN JOINT FUNCTION

In health, each joint is exercised at intervals throughout the day as a person engages in the activities of daily living. For example, flexion of the shoulder occurs whenever a person reaches to pull down a window shade, to get something from a high shelf, or to put on a pullover sweater. Unfortunately, there are few such movements demanded of the patient in bed. Unless these movements are programmed into the bath, joint motion begins to diminish rather quickly and may soon become limited, especially if there is a history of arthritis or other muscle or joint pathology.

As each body part is washed, either by you or by the patient, make sure that each joint is put through its full range of motion (see Chapter 29). When the axilla is washed, for example, a common tendency by both patient and nurse is to hold the arm only a few inches from the body and to manipulate the washcloth into the resulting small space. A more therapeutic way to wash the axilla is to flex the shoulder so that the arm is raised overhead (Fig. 30.5).

The person who bathes himself usually finds it easier to do so with the head of the bed raised. If, however, *you* are going to bathe the patient, the head of the bed should be lowered during the bath unless it is contraindicated. This is especially important if the patient lies curled up or has been in the Fowler's position for the greater part of the day. When the bed is flat, the patient's body can be fully extended during the bath to

counteract the flexion of major joints during the rest of the day.

After rubbing the patient's back, or while making the bed, help the patient to *hyperextend each hip* eight or 10 times. This movement is an important part of a normal walking gait and can be done *only* when the bed is flat and the patient is lying on his side or abdomen.

GOAL 4: TO PROMOTE RELAXATION

If the promotion of relaxation is a major goal for the bath, it must be the focus throughout the entire bath. The patient needs to know your intent is to help him relax, and all your nonverbal cues must support this intention. There can be no subtle messages of being rushed. If you are pressed for time with a heavy assignment, you may need to substitute a partial bath for the full one you had planned to give; but that partial one must be unhurried. Whenever possible, organize your work so that the majority, if not all, of the patient's treatments are done before the bath. Then, after a soothing, therapeutic back rub, the bed can be made and the patient left free to doze or sleep.

Since psychological concerns are as likely to interfere with rest and relaxation as are physical discomforts, your communication during the bath may be directed toward the relief of anger, fear, hostility, worry, or anxiety. It may be directed toward teaching the patient new ways to relax, to cope with tension, or to manage the psychological aspects of his pain. On the other hand, if your assessment indicates that the patient is simply *physically exhausted,* you can help him most effectively by *not talking,* and by letting nonverbal ministrations convey your concern and caring.

GOAL 5: TO PROVIDE SENSORY STIMULATION

For some patients, Goal 4 (relaxation) may be incompatible with Goal 5 (stimulation) and you may find it necessary to choose between these goals on a given morning.

Many patients who are depressed, apathetic, or confused need to be stimulated, roused to greater awareness of their surroundings, and helped to respond more fully to the people around them. For these patients, the bath should be a time of increased sensory stimulation.

First of all, make certain that you foster optimal sight and hearing. Make sure that the patient's eyeglasses or contact lenses are clean and in place as needed during the bath. It is difficult for a patient to respond to you if he cannot see you clearly. Increase the visibility in the room by opening blinds, raising shades, or turning on the lights as needed. If the patient has a hearing aid, make sure it is working and positioned properly in his ear. There can be little effective increase in the level of awareness if one or more of the usual channels of communication are inoperative.

Orient the patient as often as necessary to time, place, and person. In the monotony of most hospitals and extended care facilities, it is difficult for patients to keep track of people, time, and events. Each day seems like the one before it, and members of the staff may seem to merge into a monotonous parade of people.

The patient may seem slow or hesitant about participating in his own care. Clear, concise directions will give the person who is depressed, preoccupied, or anxious a chance to *focus his attention and attempt each activity* before you move in and help him complete the task. For example, instead of a general direction such as "Now you can wash your face," it may be more helpful to say to some patients, "Here is your washcloth; wash your eyes first. Now your ears," and so on. This approach requires considerable patience because it is time consuming; but even though you could do each task for the patient in half the time, you must let him do as much as possible if the goal of the bath is sensory stimulation.

The bath itself should be brisk (yet gentle) and stimulating. The warmth of the water, the friction of the towel, the movement of each extremity—each of these provides stimulation for the patient. In addition, the taste of mouthwash, the odor of cologne, the feel of hand lotion, plus the sight of the nurse's face and the sound of her voice all provide valuable sensations.

Stimulate conversation during the bath by selecting a few topics likely to be of interest to the patient and *pursuing them in some depth.* The patient cannot participate in a conversation if the nurse flits from one topic to another before he can organize his thoughts enough to respond. Above all, even when the patient seems semiconscious or comatose, interact with him throughout the bath *as if he were fully alert and capable of comprehending every word spoken.* The sense of hearing is the last sense to fail, and many a patient has, upon regaining consciousness, been able to repeat many things spoken in his presence during a time when he was supposedly not aware of anything.

GOAL 6: TO MAINTAIN OR INCREASE SELF-ESTEEM

You know from experience that the way you look (or the way you think you look) affects the way you feel. When a healthy person is confident and pleased with his appearance, his energy, enthusiasm, and abilities seem to be enhanced. Many tasks seem less formidable, and things seem to go better. The same phenomenon occurs during periods of sickness or ill-health; a patient who has not been feeling well will often seem transformed by a shampoo and a haircut, cosmetics, or shave, and an attractive gown or pajamas. Self-confidence regarding his physical appearance contributes to his overall self-esteem and enables him to interact more easily and effectively with staff and family (Fig. 30.6). Conversely, a patient who is embarrassed by his appearance cannot interact with members of the health care team or his family on an equal footing any more than a nurse could feel confident and assertive in a rumpled, shapeless uniform with dirty, disheveled hair and an offensive body odor.

This goal—to maintain or increase the patient's self-esteem—may be the hardest of all to reach because the significance of grooming is affected by culture, values, and habit. You will need considerable diplomacy, tact, and sensitivity to communicate to the patient that you are caring, not criticizing.

Hair

Assessment of Hair and Scalp
As you care for the patient's hair, examine the condition of both hair and scalp. In health, the hair is usually clean, shiny, untangled, and evenly colored, and the

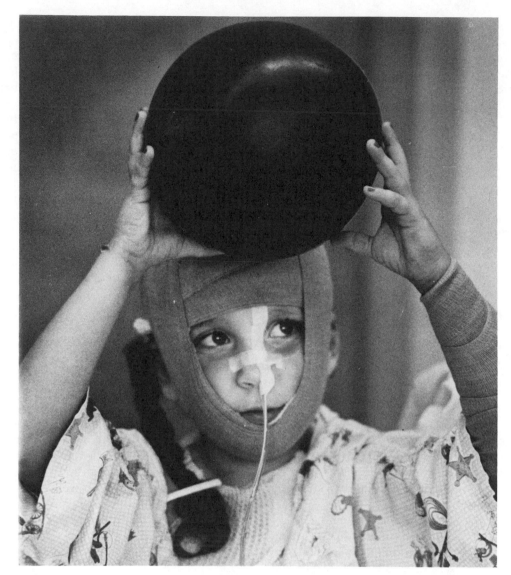

Figure 30.6 *Both Renee's mother and the nursing staff realize that a young girl needs to feel pretty. Note Renee's gaily printed gown, the neat braid and colored barrette, and her bright nail polish.*

scalp is clear. Deviations from normal would include hair that is dirty, dull, matted, unusually thin, coarse, or infested with lice, and a scalp that is scaly, irritated, infected, or bald in places. If your observations detect an unusual or unhealthy condition, you will need additional data. The patient's physical status, diagnosis, or therapy may be responsible for the condition of his hair. Before questioning the patient, look for obvious clues and answers. For example, dirty, uncombed hair and a scaly scalp may be the result of the patient's depression and apathy coupled with lack of attention from an overworked staff. Hair loss may be one of the anticipated side effects of drugs used to treat cancer. If you are unable to account for the condition of the hair or scalp, matter-of-factly describe your observations to the patient and ask if the condition is normal for him or if it represents a change.

Care of the Hair

The self-esteem of any person, regardless of age, is affected by the condition of his hair, and a sick person is especially vulnerable to low self-esteem if his hair is dirty and unkempt.

Many patients are able to manage the care of their hair if given minimal assistance and encouragement by the nurse. The patient can be helped to shampoo his hair at reasonable intervals, either in the shower or at the sink in his room, and many agencies have portable hair dryers that can be requisitioned for a patient's use. Some hospitals and long-term care facilities provide the services of a barber and a beautician. For some patients, a pass to leave the hospital long enough to visit the hairdresser may be an important part of therapy and recovery.

When a patient's activity is restricted, or when a patient is weak, confused, or very young, care of his hair becomes a nursing responsibility. The patient's hair should be combed or brushed as often as necessary to keep it looking attractive and should be arranged attractively in a style that is familiar and satisfying to patient and family. For example, an elderly woman who normally wears her long hair in a bun should wear it that way in the hospital. There are times when the long hair of an acutely ill patient must be braided to expedite nursing care, but this should be a *temporary* measure (unless a coronet of braids is the customary hairstyle). The hair of an elderly patient should *not* be arbitrarily braided for convenience, tied with ribbons, and then described as "cute." This lack of sensitivity can be as damaging to the self-esteem of an older woman as would putting the hair of an incapacitated young businesswoman who was expecting a visit from a business associate into pony tails, and expecting her to feel good about her "cute" appearance.

TANGLED HAIR. Regular and thorough brushing will usually keep a patient's hair free from tangles. You may, however, encounter a patient whose hair has not been adequately cared for and find yourself confronted with a mass of snarled hair. In such a situation there are three things that will make caring for this hair tolerable for both nurse and patient:

1. Do not attempt to remove all the tangles in one session. Work on the hair at short intervals because the process will be tiring for both of you and uncomfortable for the patient.
2. Protect the patient's scalp from pain and discomfort. Use your fingers to separate a small lock of hair. Grasp it firmly with one hand and begin to brush or comb the *loose* end of the lock. Do *not* start to brush or comb at the scalp end of the lock. Hold the lock of hair *between the comb and the scalp* so that any pulling from the comb will be absorbed by your fingers before it reaches the scalp. If the hair is extremely tangled and there is a great deal of pulling, it helps to wrap the lock around your finger to lessen the pulling on the scalp (Fig. 30.7).
3. Moisten the locks with a cotton ball and alcohol or water to free badly tangled strands of hair. In some situations, a very small amount of oil is effective. The latter is feasible only if it is possible to shampoo the hair at once or if the pillow and

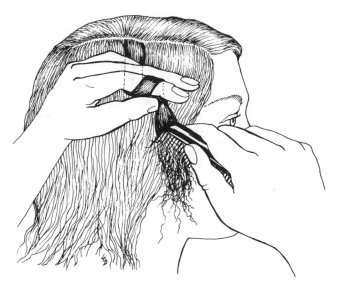

Figure 30.7 *Technique for reducing the discomfort of combing snarled hair.*

bedding can be protected from oil until it can be washed off.

Occasionally, you will see a patient whose hair is so matted that you are tempted to cut it. This is rarely necessary if the nursing staff or the family will conscientiously work on the hair at *frequent short intervals.* Except to permit emergency treatment of the head or scalp, a patient's hair should *not* be cut without permission, preferably *in writing,* from the patient or family.

SHAMPOOS. Once the hair is free of tangles, it should be shampooed, and a regular program of hair care should be initiated. Care of the hair is a nursing responsibility, but in some acute care settings, a physician's order is needed in order to shampoo the hair of patients with certain conditions.

Most patients can be taken by stretcher or wheelchair to a convenient *clean* sink (not the "dirty" or contaminated sink in the utility room). You will need a plastic shampoo tray or waterproof sheeting, a hose spray, shampoo, a washcloth to protect the patient's eyes or ears, and a liberal supply of towels. The patient's brush and comb should be washed before the shampoo in preparation for combing and arranging the clean hair.

You will need to give a bed shampoo if a patient is in traction, for example, and cannot be taken to a sink (Fig. 30.8). In addition to the equipment listed above, you will need large pitchers of water and a pail to catch the water from the plastic tray or a trough made from waterproof sheeting. Short hair can be towel dried, but

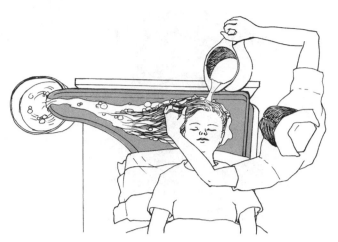

Figure 30.8 *In-bed hair shampoo.*

a hair dryer or blower is helpful if the patient has long or heavy hair.

CARE OF VERY CURLY OR KINKY HAIR. If the patient's hair is kinky or very curly, ask the patient or family what type of hair care is most effective and satisfying. As a rule, you should *not* wet such hair without asking the patient. Moisture will *increase* the kinkiness and make it more difficult to manage. Water also restores the curliness or kinkiness of hair that has been temporarily straightened by a hot comb or iron. A very coarse comb, or pick, will be needed to care for an Afro style. Some black patients prefer a tightly braided hairstyle that obviates the need for the hair to be combed each day. A black person may have very dry hair and his scalp will need frequent application of oil, petroleum jelly, or a special commercial preparation, especially after a shampoo.

Common Problems

DANDRUFF. A certain number of dead cells are normally shed by the scalp each day and are removed by brushing, combing, and the ordinary movements of the head and hair.

Excessive *pityriasis* (dandruff) indicates an abnormally dry scalp or, in some situations, an infectious process. Vigorous, regular brushing plus massaging the scalp with baby oil or petroleum jelly before a shampoo will usually relieve the condition. When you are treating the scalp, the hair should be parted into small sections so that the oil (or medication) is applied directly to the scalp, not to the hair. For severe cases of dandruff, a medicated shampoo may be warranted.

LOSS OF HAIR. *Alopecia* (loss of hair) can be gradual or sudden, complete or partial. It is caused by disease,

drugs, age, trauma, or radiation. Hair is also lost by shaving of the head before brain surgery. One of the unfortunate aspects of both brain surgery and chemotherapy is the total or partial loss of hair, and even though the patient was probably told about this when he consented to the treatment or surgery, the actuality of losing his hair can be devastating. The magnitude and significance of the loss will depend to a large degree on the age, sex, and personality of the patient. For example, many small children are not self-conscious about their loss of hair, but adolescents are usually very sensitive about their baldness; girls should be fitted for a wig as soon as possible or helped to keep their heads covered with attractive scarves or kerchiefs. The nurse will need to assess carefully the patient's reaction to the loss of hair and respond accordingly. The patient is likely to manifest behaviors characteristic of grief and loss in general as well as those related to a marked change in body image (see Chapter 24).

In addition to psychological support, several specific interventions are needed. First of all, the patient needs to know that the hair *will* grow back, although the color may be different if the hair loss was due to chemotherapy. Itching may be a problem as the hair begins to grow, especially if the hair was shaved off. The scalp and new hair shafts must be kept clean, soft, and supple. The patient's head and new hair must be washed often enough to remove any dirt, perspiration, and dead epithelial cells. In hot weather, this will need to be done more frequently for patients wearing wigs than for those wearing cooler scarves or kerchiefs. As the stubble or blunt ends of shaved hair begin to grow, you may need to soften the shafts of hair with baby oil or petroleum jelly from time to time. (A similar prickly discomfort usually occurs after pubic hair has been shaved before perineal or genital surgery, and similar softening measures are needed.)

The incidence of hair loss among patients with leukemia is high because they are usually treated with chemotherapy. Because the patient's defense mechanisms have been altered, both by the disease and by the treatment, he must be protected from infection. One potential source of infection for these patients is a scalp that has been scratched by dirty fingernails. Therefore, in addition to ensuring adequate cleanliness of the patient's hair and scalp, you will need to teach him to keep his fingernails short and clean and to avoid scratching his scalp hard enough to break the skin. If the patient is a child, confused, or irresponsible, the nurse or family must assume responsibility for adequate care of his nails. Some patients avoid the problem of potential infection by scratching an itchy scalp with a soft brush rather than their fingernails.

Care of the patient's wig depends on whether it is

made of natural hair or synthetic fibers, and the manufacturer's directions for care should be followed.

INFESTATIONS OF LICE. Although pediculosis (lice) is most commonly associated with poor hygiene and unsanitary living conditions, any person can become infested, either through direct contact with another person or from a comb, hair, clothing, or other article containing lice.

Head lice (pediculosis capitis) are found in the hair. *Crab lice or pubic lice* (pediculosis pubis) are found in hair-covered areas of the body such as the pubes, axillae, beard, or eyebrows. *Body lice* (pediculosis corporis) do not adhere to the body but infest the clothing.

Head lice are small, gray, and difficult to see. Their presence is detected by small, light colored, oval particles on the hair that differ from dandruff in that they are *not* loosened by brushing or combing the hair. These particles are the *nits* (eggs) that are deposited on the shafts of the hair. Other indications of head lice are complaints of itching or scratching by the patient and the presence of scratches on the scalp, especially around the ears and hairline. The treatment of head lice consists of shampooing the hair with a medication such as Kwell and then using a fine-toothed comb to remove any remaining nits. If a person, usually a child, is infested repeatedly, other classmates or members of the family are probably infested and in need of treatment.

Low-income families may find the cost of a commercial medication such as Kwell prohibitive and may try to substitute a home remedy such as turpentine. The community health nurse must help the family obtain a safer remedy, because turpentine is very irritating, will burn a sensitive scalp and the eyes, and is flammable.

Pubic lice are difficult to treat because pubic hair is usually heavy and dense. Pubic lice are treated by shaving the hair off the affected area or by applying a medication that is left in place for 12 to 24 hours and then removed by bathing. The patient with pubic lice is advised to inform his sexual partner, if any, of his condition so that treatment can be sought as needed.

A complete bath and clean clothing and linen usually suffice as the treatment for *body lice,* inasmuch as the lice adhere to clothing and are removed with it. Infested clothing should be bagged until laundered.

SUPERFLUOUS HAIR. *Hirsutism* (superfluous hair) is a problem for some women, but the mere presence of facial or body hair cannot automatically be assumed to be a problem. A woman's feelings about body or facial hair are affected by her age, race, sexuality, and the current attitudes of society as reflected in magazines and television. Because of wide differences among women, you will need to assess the situation carefully to note any cues that would indicate that body or facial hair is a problem for a given patient. Since the patient may be embarrassed, you may need to take the initiative and make an overt verbal response to any cues you receive from the patient.

Superfluous hair can be removed by shaving or by using a depilatory, in either cream or lotion form. Hair can also be permanently removed by electrolysis. The facial hair that sometimes appears after menopause may be unnoticeable if it is bleached. Regardless of the method of removal preferred by the patient, it is important that provision be made for this aspect of personal hygiene.

Men should be allowed and encouraged to shave themselves in accordance with their usual routines unless shaving is contraindicated for medical reasons, such as the need for complete bed rest after a heart attack. If a patient is unable to shave himself, it is the nurse's responsibility to arrange for someone else to do so.

When caring for a patient who is receiving anticoagulant therapy, it is important to maintain the integrity of the skin. The blood-clotting mechanisms of the patient on anticoagulant therapy have been altered by drugs such as heparin and warfarin, and even a small cut can be serious. Assess the patient's understanding of anticoagulant therapy and the effects of the drug he is taking. If the patient is not fully aware of the potential danger of hemorrhage, obtain the information you need and use the bath time to teach him how to protect himself during his day-to-day activities. An electric razor is safest for this patient, although an experienced and skilled person could use a safety razor. Under *no* circumstances should a patient on anticoagulant therapy use a straight razor.

Body Odors

An offensive body odor can nauseate and sicken even a healthy person and can be demoralizing to a patient. Common sources of bad odors in the patient's unit include decomposing urine or feces in unemptied or poorly washed receptacles, vomitus, intestinal gases, purulent drainage from wounds, improperly discarded dressings, and bloody or purulent discharge, especially from cancer of the cervix or uterus.

Odor control starts with prevention, and careful housekeeping will eliminate the source of many odors. Bedpans, urinals, commodes, and emesis basins should be promptly emptied and cleaned. Soiled and bloody dressings should be removed from the patient's unit as soon as they are taken off the patient. Meticulous genital care must be given to the patient who has cancer of the uterus.

When odors persist despite every effort to eliminate

the source, deodorizers and deodorants must be employed. If your patient's condition results in offensive odors, the control of these odors can be one of your most difficult nursing tasks. Everyone who enters the unit is immediately aware of the odor, so there is nothing to be gained by ignoring the problem or pretending it does not exist in an attempt to protect the patient from embarrassment. The problem should be overtly acknowledged; possible solutions should be voiced by all concerned, and vigorous efforts must be made to find the most effective solution. Some success has been achieved by giving the patient an oral medication containing chlorophyll. Effective room deodorizers use either an electrostatic device or a porous material such as charcoal to absorb odors. Sprays that attempt to mask the odor often make the situation worse. Simple measures such as opening the windows and airing the room, even in winter, are helpful.

Nails

A patient needs assistance in caring for his nails if his vision is poor, his hands tremble, his hands are stiff or painful, he cannot reach his feet, or he is weak and incapacitated. Fingernails and toenails are easier to cut safely if they have been soaked in warm, soapy water for at least 15 to 20 minutes. Nail clippers or curved nail scissors are more efficient than bandage scissors. The nails of an infant who is scratching his face and eyes should be cut with special baby scissors that have round safety tips instead of sharp points. Toenails should be cut straight across, rather than in a curve, to help prevent ingrowing. If the nails are thick and horny, they may need to be cut with surgical instruments or by a podiatrist.

The fingernails of some patients should be kept short either for safety or for esthetic reasons. The patient's nails should be short if he is irrational and restless and there is danger of his scratching himself or others, if there is a possibility that bacteria lodged under his fingernails might come in contact with an incision, sterile dressing, or open wound, or if he is incontinent of feces and prone to get fecal matter under his fingernails. One general guide for the length of a patient's fingernails is that they should not be visible beyond the fingertips when the hand is held palm up (pronated).

In addition to his toenails, a patient may have corns or calluses that need attention. A referral to the agency's podiatrist within a few days after admission should be part of that patient's *preparation for future ambulation.*

Diabetic Foot Care

The skin of the diabetic's feet and legs is easily injured and is very slow to heal because of poor circulation and disturbed metabolism. Proper hygiene is one of many aspects of the special care that is needed by diabetics. The patient must be taught to wash his feet and legs carefully and gently, but if his hands are unsteady or his vision is impaired, he should *not* attempt to cut his own toenails. Corns and calluses should be treated by a podiatrist.

In many agencies nurses are not permitted to cut the toenails of a diabetic patient because of the risk of injuring the tissue and the subsequent danger of infection. In such instances it is the nurse's responsibility to refer the patient to a *podiatrist.* You can facilitate the work of the podiatrist by making sure that corns, calluses, and toenails are softened by soaking before his visit.

If you are planning to cut a diabetic patient's toenails, first soak his feet for *at least 15 to 20 minutes.* Make sure that both the patient's foot and your hands are supported and steady, that the lighting is adequate, and that you have assembled the appropriate instruments, such as toenail clippers or toenail cutters. Bandage scissors will *not* do; the straight blades are neither effective nor safe.

Clothing

It is not enough for a patient's clothing to be clean and functional; it must be *psychologically comfortable.* Whenever possible, the patient should wear clothing that closely resembles his usual attire. In some pediatric units, for example, children who can be out of bed are dressed in jeans and T-shirts rather than pajamas. If the condition of a female patient is such that she must wear a short, open-back gown, she can still look and feel attractive because many department stores now carry a line of lovely gowns that open down the back.

A new robe, gown, or pajamas will boost the morale of some patients, but others find security and comfort in old, familiar clothing. The nurse's task is to assess the situation carefully enough to differentiate between the patient who is inwardly embarrassed by an old garment and the patient who feels comfortable and very secure in an equally disreputable one.

CARE OF THE PATIENT'S ENVIRONMENT

The Patient's Unit

A minimal patient unit contains a bed, a bedside stand, a wastebasket, a chair, and an overbed table, all of which are enclosed by a curtain, plus a locker or drawer space for clothing, and a bathroom down the hall. Newer hospitals and more expensive accommodations usually have an easy chair, a television, and a sink in the room, plus a bathroom in many semiprivate rooms. A private room will have a private bath, a telephone, and sometimes a desk and shelves.

On admission, the patient is issued a package of supplies, which includes a washbasin, a soap dish and soap, an emesis basin, a toothbrush and small tube of toothpaste, a comb, a pitcher for drinking water, and a plastic tumbler. In many hospitals the patient is charged for these items and takes them home when he is discharged. These supplies are kept in the bedside stand, along with a bedpan plus a urinal for a male patient.

As soon as a patient is admitted, he consciously or unconsciously begins to stake out his own territory. The patient in a private room needs to do nothing but unpack and settle in, but the process is more complex for patients in semiprivate or ward accommodations. These patients seek answers to questions such as: "How much of this space is mine?" "Which locker or drawer is mine?" and "Which chair should my visitors use?" To the staff, the patient's unit is just one of many similar units, but not so to the patient; the space allotted for his use is temporarily his world. His space will be the only place he has in which to eat, sleep, bathe, entertain visitors, receive treatments, transact business, worship, and anything else he chooses or is required to do.

The patient's reaction to his immediate environment (his unit) will be influenced by his age, culture, past experience, and personal habits. To a patient who is accustomed to overcrowded living conditions with little privacy, even a crowded four-bed ward may seem spacious and lonely. On the other hand, a teenager who spends a great deal of time alone in his room may be very upset by the lack of privacy in the hospital.

It is important to assess the patient's response to his room or unit because, although there may be little or nothing that you can do to change it physically, your understanding of his reaction will help to explain some of his subsequent behavior.

The appearance of a patient's room or unit reveals much about the patient. The nonverbal messages from a unit in which there are no flowers, no personal possessions, and no cards are very different from the nonverbal messages of a room in which there are plants, flowers, notepaper, books, plus the patient's own radio and travel alarm clock.

Of course, the patient's room or unit also reveals a great deal about the staff, and the condition of the room and its equipment indicates the standards and priorities of the nurse who is currently caring for the patient. Such things as uneaten food, an unemptied emesis basin, or a soiled dressing in an open wastebasket suggest that the nurse either does not understand the importance and interrelatedness of medical asepsis, orderliness, and

the patient's well-being, or does not care enough to provide the patient with an environment that is sanitary and esthetically acceptable.

Cleaning the Patient's Unit

The housekeeping department is responsible for the daily cleaning of the room and some of its furniture, and for a thorough cleaning of the unit between patients. The bathroom is cleaned, the wastebasket is emptied, and the floor is dusted each day. The floor and window sills are washed periodically. The housekeeping employee is *not* responsible for the care of the patient's personal possessions, so the bedside stand is seldom cleaned because it is usually covered with the patient's belongings. In some hospitals an occupied bed is not dusted by a housekeeping person, although the other furniture is cleaned as needed.

Nursing Responsibility for the Unit

Nurses are responsible for two categories of items in the patient's unit: the equipment and supplies used by the nurses (see boxed material), and the personal possessions of the patient.

The patient's response to his immediate environment may be based on his need to be in control and make decisions, his anger at being in the hospital, his need for the security of consistency and routine, a compulsive need for orderliness and neatness, or any one of a dozen other reasons.

The value systems of nurse and patient may differ with respect to cleanliness and neatness, and this can be a source of conflict, expressed or unexpressed. A messy or casual nurse may be annoyed by a meticulous patient who seemingly nags and harps at her about the

---

Criteria for Maintenance of the Patient's Unit

- Used dressing trays, discarded gloves, and so forth are removed at the conclusion of each treatment.
- Spills are wiped up as quickly as they occur.
- The bedpan, the urinal, and the commode are emptied promptly, rinsed thoroughly, and covered until needed.
- Equipment no longer needed is removed.
- Extra supplies are piled neatly if they cannot be stored out of sight.
- IV poles and other surfaces are not cluttered with unused pieces of adhesive tape or old tags and labels.
- Uneaten food is removed and not allowed to accumulate.
- The wastebasket is emptied *immediately* if soiled dressings, sanitary napkins, or other refuse has been dropped into it.

condition of the room. A nurse who values cleanliness and neatness may be quite intolerant of an untidy patient. Both patients might be justified in saying, "I'm paying for this room and I want it cleaned up (or left just the way it is)!"

If a patient is ambulatory, the nurse usually assumes very little responsibility for his possessions, but if the patient is weak, confused, or confined to bed, the nurse must assume responsibility for the condition of his immediate environment. Dead flowers should be removed, old newspapers taken out, and the top of the bedside stand straightened and damp-dusted with a wet paper towel.

You can offer to help the patient straighten his bedside stand, but a nurse should never rearrange, remove, put away, or discard *anything* without the consent of the patient if he is alert enough to understand her. He may want to keep that empty candy box as a remembrance of the friend who sent it, and he may be saving all his little plastic medicine cups for his granddaughter's playhouse.

Making the Patient's Bed
Of all the items in a sick person's environment, his bed is among the most important. In addition to its importance to the patient's territoriality, space, and psychological security, the bed can, if it is properly made, contribute to his physical comfort and safety. Four essential criteria for effective bed making are:

- The patient is protected from cross-infection
- The patient's skin is protected from irritation
- The patient's feet are protected from footdrop
- The finished appearance is esthetically pleasing

In addition, bed making is effective when the nurse is protected from muscle strain and unnecessary fatigue.

PROTECTING THE PATIENT FROM CROSS-INFECTION. Three basic rules for preventing the spread of infection are:

1. *Keep all linen off the floor.* A piece of clean linen that touches the floor is contaminated and should be discarded. Soiled linen should be placed on a chair or in a laundry bag or hamper, not on the floor.
2. *Keep soiled linen away from your uniform.* Linen that has been soiled with drainage, blood, pus, feces, or urine may contain live pathogens that can be transferred to your uniform and carried to another patient.
3. *Do not shake the bedding.* Air currents can carry

pathogenic organisms from one patient unit to another.

PROTECTING THE PATIENT FROM SKIN IRRITATION. The patient's skin is a major defense against various physiological and environmental hazards and must, therefore, be kept intact. Major threats to the integrity of the skin from the bed are:

- *Maceration and softening of the skin* from prolonged contact with damp sheets
- *Interrupted or disturbed blood flow through the skin* over areas of concentrated pressure from wrinkles
- *Irritation of the skin* from bleaches and other products used in the laundry

The patient's skin can be protected from these hazards by keeping the sheets *dry* and *free from wrinkles.* Place an absorbent mattress pad or flannel blanket under the bottom sheet to absorb perspiration and keep the patient's skin dry. Tighten the bottom sheet frequently enough to keep it free from wrinkles.

Skin irritation from laundry products such as detergents and bleach is often noticed first on the patient's elbows if he presses them into the sheets when he turns over and moves about.

Irritation of sensitive skin can be prevented by using specially prepared linen. This linen may be referred to as untreated, allergy free, or any one of a variety of other terms. It is usually not ironed, and the finished bed will not look crisp and attractive. The linen is safer and more comfortable, however, and serious skin damage can usually be averted by the *prompt and consistent* use of untreated linen.

PROTECTING THE PATIENT FROM FOOTDROP. Footdrop is a hazard when tightly tucked bedding pulls a patient's feet into a position of plantar flexion. Some patients need the extra protection and support of a footboard, but *all* patients need adequate toe room. This is provided by making a toe pleat in the upper bedding and by letting the spread and top sheet hang loose over the side of the bed.

PROTECTING THE NURSE FROM MUSCLE STRAIN AND FATIGUE. You can protect your back by raising the bed to a comfortable working height. If the height is not adjustable, kneel or squat so that you can *keep your back straight* while making the bed. Avoid reaching and making unnecessary trips around the bed by first making the half of the bed closer to you, and then walking to the other side to make that half. Use protective body mechanics throughout the procedure, keeping your back straight and your pelvis tilted back as you work.

Making an Unoccupied Bed

The amount of linen needed depends on whether the bed is being remade for the same patient or whether it has been stripped and washed and is being made up for a new admission.

Guidelines for making an unoccupied bed include:

- Position the bottom sheet so that the bottom hem just barely reaches the end of the mattress. This allows *as much sheet as possible to be tucked under the head end* of the mattress and will keep the sheet in place when the head of the bed is raised.
- Miter the corners at the head of the bed, and tuck the sheet under the side of the mattress (Fig. 30.9).
- Position the top sheet so that the top hem just barely reaches the head end of the mattress. This allows as much sheet as possible to be tucked under the foot of the mattress. Do not tuck this sheet in yet.
- Position the spread so that the top hem is a few

inches below the head end of the sheet. Turn the end of the sheet back over the end of the spread. Tuck the foot ends of both the sheet and the spread under the end of the mattress.

- Miter the corners at the foot of the bed, *handling the spread and sheet together,* as if they were one piece of fabric.
- Make a toe pleat to provide adequate space for the patient's feet (Fig. 30.10). To make a pleat, grasp all layers of upper bedding (sheet, blanket if any, and spread) 12 to 15 inches from the foot of the bed. Stand at the foot of the bed and with one hand at each side of the bed, lift the bedding to make a long tent about 4 to 6 inches high across the bed. Fold the top of the tent toward the foot of the bed, making a 2-inch to 3-inch pleat. Remove any wrinkles, leaving the foot of the bed neat and tidy.
- Put on the pillowcase, keeping the pillow away from your face. This is especially important if the

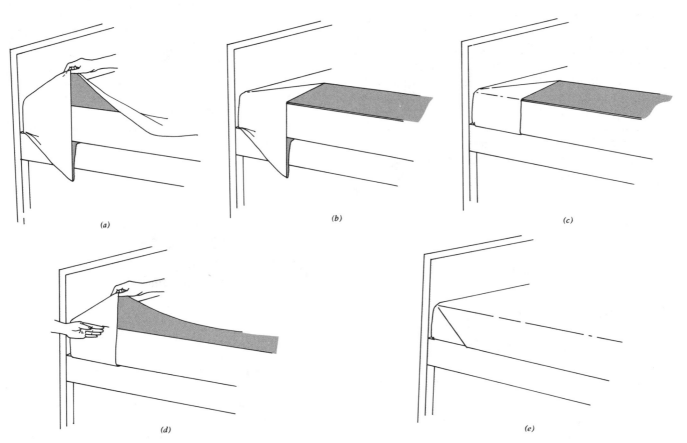

Figure 30.9 *Making a mitered corner. (a) Lift the edge of the sheet until it is perpendicular to the edge of the mattress. (b) Fold the sheet back along the edge of the mattress. (c) Tuck the lower triangle of the sheet under the mattress. (d) Hold the sheet firmly against the upper edge of the mattress while bringing the edge of the sheet down over the side of the mattress. (e) Tuck the edge of the sheet under the mattress.*

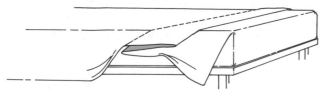

Figure 30.10 Toe pleat (see text for explanation).

patient has an *infection or undiagnosed illness.* Grasp the pillowcase at the center of the end seam (Fig. 30.11a) and pull it back over your hand like a huge mitten (b). (This turns the pillowcase inside out.) Grasp the end of the pillow with your covered hand (c) and pull the case down over the pillow (d). Work the corners of the pillow into the corners of the pillowcase, and align the side seams of the pillowcase with the side seams of the pillow.

- Fanfold the upper bedding to the foot of the bed so that it is out of the way when the patient is ready to get back into bed.

THE POSTOPERATIVE BED. When a patient goes to surgery, his bed is made in such a way that he can be easily transferred from stretcher to bed and then covered quickly. The top sheet and spread are fanfolded either to the far side of the bed or to the foot of the bed so that almost the entire surface of the mattress is exposed and ready to receive the patient.

The need for additional preparation depends on the type of surgery, the type of anesthesia, and whether the patient is coming directly from the operating room or from the recovery room. Some patients vomit postoperatively as they recover from anesthesia, and the head of the bed should be protected by waterproof material plus an absorbent covering. Little or no prepa-

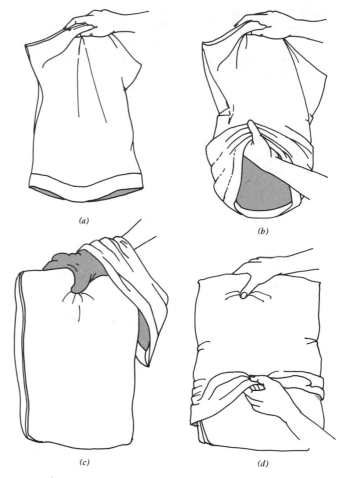

Figure 30.11 Putting on a pillowcase (see text for explanation).

ration of the bed is needed if the patient has spent a period of time in the recovery room, though absorbent pads are often placed where drainage might occur.

PROCEDURE 30.4

*Making an Unoccupied Bed**

SUMMARY OF ESSENTIAL NURSING ACTIONS

1. Maintain medical aseptic technique at all times.
   - Wash hands as indicated by the situation.
   - Keep all linen off floor.
   - Do not shake linen and create air currents.
   - Keep used linen away from your uniform.
   - Keep pillow away from your face when putting on pillowcase.

- Dispose of used linen according to school or agency procedure.
2. Use protective body mechanics; raise adjustable bed to high position.
3. Conserve energy; make minimal trips around the bed.
4. Conserve linen; reuse linen when appropriate.

*See inside front cover and page 577.

Making an Unoccupied Bed*

5. Make sure finished bed meets the following criteria:
   - Sheets are straight on bed (sides of sheets are parallel to sides of mattress).
   - Sheets are centered on bed (same amount of sheet hangs down on each side).
   - Corners are made precisely.

- Bottom sheet and drawsheet are TIGHT and WRINKLE FREE.
- Edges of pillowcase are parallel to edges of pillow.
- Pillowcase is wrinkle free.
- End of spread and folded edge of top sheet are about 4 to 6 inches from head of bed.
- Toe pleat is adequate in size and neatly made.

*See inside front cover and page 577.

Making an Occupied Bed

To make an occupied bed, the patient is positioned on one side of the bed while the nurse makes the other. He is then moved to the freshly made portion while she makes the remaining side of the bed.

An occupied bed must be made in such a way that the comfort and safety of the patient is maintained throughout the procedure. Comfort can be assured by (1) keeping the patient covered for warmth and privacy, and (2) repositioning the pillow under his head as he is turned from side to side. Safety is assured by raising the side rail on the far side of the bed to keep the patient from falling out of bed and to give him something to pull against as he is turned.

Guidelines for making an occupied bed include:

- Raise the bed to a comfortable working height.
- Remove the top bedding after covering the patient for warmth and privacy.
- Position the patient comfortably and safely on one side of the bed, facing the edge of the bed. Loosen the lower sheet and roll it up close to the patient's back, along the center line of the bed.
- Place the center fold of the fresh bottom sheet along the center line of the bed, under the roll of soiled linen. Tuck the first half of the fresh sheet in as if making an unoccupied bed.
- Help the patient turn back over the center roll of linen onto the fresh sheet. Pull out the soiled bottom sheet and tuck in the fresh one.
- Put the top sheet and spread on the bed and tuck them in. Replace the used pillowcase with a fresh one.

When you make an occupied bed, it is important to remember that slow, ineffective motions can be tiring or irritating to the patient. It is essential, therefore, to practice making an occupied bed until you can make one quickly and skillfully without tiring the patient, and so that the finished product is medically aseptic, free from wrinkles and esthetically pleasing.

PROCEDURE 30.5

*Making an Occupied Bed**

SUMMARY OF ESSENTIAL NURSING ACTIONS

1. Keep patient comfortable and covered throughout the procedure.
2. Use side rails as needed for patient safety and/or to help patient turn self from side to side.
3. Maintain any position which has been ordered for the patient.
4. Avoid disruption of any tubes, traction, or other equipment.

*See inside front cover and page 579.

5. Maintain medical asepsis throughout procedure. See examples listed for making an unoccupied bed (Procedure 30.4).
6. Conserve energy.
7. Conserve linen.
8. Work rapidly enough to avoid tiring the patient.
9. Make certain the finished bed meets the eight criteria for an acceptably made unoccupied bed (Procedure 30.4).

PATIENT TEACHING

It is important for the patient and his family to know that a bath does more than get a person clean. For some people, this message can be conveyed through apparently casual conversation which incorporates mention of exercise, skin care, self-esteem and social interaction. Other people will profit from a more structured discussion of the bath. For example, the family who is caring for a patient at home may need to be carefully taught that a bath provides sensory stimulation, increases circulation and respiration, counteracts some of the effects of immobility or limited mobility, conveys concern and caring, and improves self-esteem. Patient and family alike should be encouraged to plan on frequent baths in order to obtain these benefits even though the patient "isn't dirty."

RELATED ACTIVITIES

1. In order to understand some of the concerns of a patient who must be bathed by another person, imagine that both your hands are bandaged following moderate burns. How do you think you would react to being bathed (including genital care) by: (1) a nurse your own age, (2) a nurse of the opposite sex, and (3) a member of your family?

2. In each hypothetical situation, how do you think each of you would respond? What would help make the situation more tolerable for you?

SUGGESTED READINGS

Barsevick, Andrea, and Jane Llewellyn: A comparison of the anxiety-reducing potential of two techniques of bathing. *Nurs Res* 1982 Jan/Feb; 31(1):22–27.

Bersani, Gayle, and William Carl: Oral care for cancer patients. *Am J Nurs* 1983 April; 83(4):533–536.

Drury, Dolores A, and Betty J Reynolds: Foot care for the high-risk patient. *RN* 1982 Nov; 45(11):46–49.

Feustel, Delycia A: Pressure sore prevention—aye, there's the rub. *Nursing 82* 1982 April; 12(4):78–83.

Forbes, Karen, and Shirlee A Stokes: Saving the diabetic foot. *Am J Nurs* 1984 July; 84(7):884–888.

Giorella, Evelyn Clark: Give the older person space. *Am J Nurs* 1980 May; 80(5):898–900.

Graham, Sue, and Margaret Morley: What 'foot care' really means. *Am J Nurs* 1984 July; 84(7):889–891.

Grier, Marion E: Hair care for the black patient. *Am J Nurs* 1976 Nov; 76(11):1781.

Hayter, Jean: Territoriality as a universal need. *J Adn Nurs* 1981 March; 6(2):79–85.

Maagdenberg, Anna Marie: The "violent" patient (territoriality and personal space). *Am J Nurs* 1983 March; 83(3):402–403.

MacMillan, Kathleen: New goals for oral hygiene. *Can Nurse* 1981 March; 77(3):40–43.

Mangieri, Dorothy: Saving your elderly patient's skin. *Nursing 82* 1982 Oct; 12(10):44–45.

Maxwell, Mary B: Scalp tourniquets for chemotherapy—induced alopecia. *Am J Nurs* 1980 May; 80(5):900–902.

Ramos, Linda Yoder: Oral hygiene for the elderly. *Am J Nurs* 1981 Aug; 81(8):1468–1469.

Rubin, B Anne: Black skin: Here's how to adjust your assessment and care. *RN* 1979 March; 42(3):31–35.

Schweiger, Joyce L, John W Lang, and James W Schweiger: Oral assessment: how to do it. *Am J Nurs* 1980 April; 80(4):654–657.

Sykes, Julie, et al: Black skin problems. *Am J Nurs* 1979 June; 79(6):1092–1095.

Welch, Deborah, and Keith, Lewis: Alopecia and chemotherapy. *Am J Nurs* 1980 May; 80(5):903–905.

Welch, Lynne Brodie: Pediculosis at summer camp. *Am J Nurs* 1979 June; 79(6):1073.

Wells, Ruthann, and Kathy Trostle: Creative hairwashing techniques for immobilized patients. *Nursing 84* 1984 Jan; 14(1):47–51.

Zuenick, Martha: Care of an artificial eye. *Am J Nurs* 1975 May; 75(5):835–837.

31

Fluid and Electrolyte Balance

MaryAnn Middlemiss

Section 1 *Regulation of Body Fluids*

Section 2 *Maintenance and Restoration of Fluid Balance*

Prerequisites and/or Suggested Preparation
A basic knowledge of anatomy and physiology, the principles of physics related to fluid flow and osmosis (Chapter 11), and the pathophysiology of edema, thrombosis, and phlebitis (Chapter 12) are prerequisite to understanding this chapter.

Section One

Regulation of Body Fluids

The status of a patient's fluid and electrolyte balance is one of the primary indicators of his physical condition. In health, a person's fluid output is proportional to his fluid intake, and the chemical components of his blood and other body fluids are within normal limits.

If the balance of either body fluids or electrolytes is disrupted, a variety of signs and symptoms quickly become evident, and the nurse's assessment of this imbalance guides and directs her nursing interventions. For example, when the nurse observes that a patient has poor skin turgor, dark concentrated urine, and a degree of mental confusion, she will deduce that his fluid intake is inadequate and that certain electrolytes are unbalanced; unless it is contraindicated, she will intervene to increase his fluid intake at once.

BODY FLUID

The term *body fluid,* in the context of fluid and electrolyte balance, refers to intracellular, interstitial, and intravascular fluids. These types of fluids are compartmentalized by cell membranes and the walls of blood vessels; but the water, electrolytes, nutrients, and wastes of these fluids are readily exchanged across the membranes from one compartment to another.

Fluid balance is achieved and maintained when the volume and composition of the fluid in each compartment are within normal limits.

Body fluid has the following essential functions:

- It transports materials to and from cells (both wastes and nutrients).
- It acts as the solvent for the solutes that are essential for cell function.
- It provides a medium for cell metabolism.
- It maintains blood volume.
- It influences body temperature.

Body fluid is divided into two main categories: *intra*cellular fluid (ICF) and *extra*cellular fluid (ECF). *Intracellular* fluid is contained within the cells of the body and is composed of water, protein, and large amounts of potassium (K+) and phosphates plus small quantities of other substances (Table 31.1). Although ICF is compartmentalized within trillions of body cells, it is described and analyzed as if it were contained within one single cell or one single fluid compartment.

Extracellular fluid includes all body fluid outside the cell. It includes both intravascular and interstitial fluid. It flows through the blood vessels as plasma (the intravascular fluid) and surrounds each cell (the interstitial fluid). ECF is composed of water and large amounts of sodium (NA+), chlorine (CL−), and bicarbonate (HCO₃) plus other substances (Table 31.1).

ICF constitutes about 70 percent of a person's total body fluid; the remaining 30 percent is ECF. About four-fifths of the ECF is located between the cells (interstitial fluid), while approximately one-fifth is located within the blood vessels (intravascular fluid).

TABLE 31.1 BODY FLUIDS CONTENT

	Extracellular Fluid	Intracellular Fluid
Na^+	142 mEq/L	10 mEq/L
K^+	5 mEq/L	141 mEq/L
Ca^{++}	5 mEq/L	< 1 mEq/L
Mg^{++}	3 mEq/L	58 mEq/L
Cl^-	103 mEq/L	4 mEq/L
HCO_3^-	28 mEq/L	10 mEq/L
Phosphates	4 mEq/L	75 mEq/L
SO_4^{--}	1 mEq/L	2 mEq/L
Glucose	90 mg%	0–20 mg%
Amino acids	30 mg%	200 mg% (?)
Cholesterol, phospholipids, and neutral fat	0.5 g%	2–95 g%
PO_2	35 mm Hg	20 mm Hg (?)
PCO_2	46 mm Hg	50 mm Hg (?)
pH	7.4	7.0

Source: Guyton AC: *A Textbook of Medical Physiology.* ed 6. Philadelphia, WB Saunders, 1981, p. 41.

Intracellular fluid = 70 percent of total body fluid

Extracellular fluid = 30 percent of total body fluid

   Interstitial fluid (24 percent of total body fluid)

   Intravascular fluid (6 percent of total body fluid)

Plasma is used for the laboratory analysis of body fluids for two reasons: (1) it is accessible and (2) intravascular fluid (plasma) and interstitial fluids are almost identical except for colloid particles in the plasma (plasma proteins). Intracellular fluid (ICF) is not accessible enough for *direct* laboratory analysis, but it can be studied indirectly by virtue of the fact that each change in ECF produces a corresponding change in ICF, and vice versa.

SOLUTIONS

Because all body fluids are composed of water plus dissolved or suspended substances, they are solutions and, as such, conform to the laws of physics that govern the properties and characteristics of solutions. A *solution* is a mixture of two or more substances, one of which is a liquid. The proportions of the substances can be varied up to the limits of solubility. The liquid is the *solvent,* and the substance that is added is the *solute.* If the solute interacts with the solvent and udnergoes a chemical change, that substance is said to be *soluble* in that liquid. If the solute is unchanged by contact with the solvent, it is insoluble in that liquid. A solution that contains a relatively small amount of solute is a weak or *dilute* solution. One that contains a relatively large amount of solute is a strong, or *concentrated,* solution. When no more solute can be dissolved by the solvent, the solution is *saturated.*

Measurement of Concentration

The concentration of a solution can be expressed in terms of the proportionate weights or volumes of solute and solvent. For example, 1 gram of sugar in 100 grams of water yields a 1 percent solution, and 1 cup of sugar in 4 cups of water gives a 1:4 solution. Such expressions of concentration are adequate for use in such activities as cooking or canning fruit and even for the preparation of some oral or external medications, but they are not precise enough for analyzing body fluids. The chemical composition of cellular and extracellular body fluids, such as plasma, must be maintained within a *very narrow range* of values; any marked deviation would jeopardize a person's life.

When fluids are taken by mouth, the human body is able to process both concentrated and dilute solutions, but when fluids are given intravcnously, they must be either compatible with, or equivalent to, the composition of normal body fluids. Determinations of equivalency and compatibility must be made at a *molecular* level to achieve the necessary precision and accuracy. These calculations of concentration are based on the chemical, osmotic, or hydrogen-ion activity of the solute.

Chemical Activity as a Measure of Concentration

An *electrolyte* is a chemical substance such as salt (NaCl) that breaks up into electrically charged ions when placed in a solvent such as water. This process is termed ionization or dissociation. Ions that carry a negative charge, such as CL^-, are called anions; and ions that carry a positive charge, such as Na^+, are called cations. Non-electrolytes are substances such as glucose and plasma proteins that do not ionize and that are electrically neutral. The major functions of electrolytes are:

   Promotion of neuromuscular irritability

   Maintenance of body-fluid osmolality

   Regulation of hydrogen-ion balance

   Movement of body fluid between fluid compartments

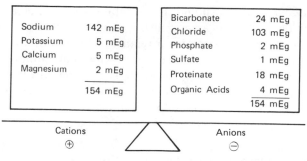

Sodium	142 mEq	Bicarbonate	24 mEq	
Potassium	5 mEq	Chloride	103 mEq	
Calcium	5 mEq	Phosphate	2 mEq	
Magnesium	2 mEq	Sulfate	1 mEq	
		Proteinate	18 mEq	
	154 mEq	Organic Acids	4 mEq	
			154 mEq	

Cations ⊕   Anions ⊖

Figure 31.1 *The cations and anions of extracellular fluid balance each other when their chemical activity is expressed in milliequivalents.*

The total number of cations and the total number of anions in plasma must be equal (154 each) (Fig. 31.1), and any attempts to prevent or treat an imbalance of the patient's electrolytes must be based on laboratory analysis of his current fluid and electrolyte status.

The unit of measurement of chemical activity is the milliequivalent (mEq). It represents the number of cations available to combine with anions. The combining power of a molecule is not based on its molecular weight because chemicals with the same molecular weight can have different combining powers, while other chemicals with different molecular weights can have the same combining power. For example, 23 mg sodium, 39 mg potassium, 20 mg calcium, and 4,140 mg proteinate each carry one electrical charge and are therefore equal in terms of chemical activity. This is why *equivalent weights* are used as a basis for comparing one compound with another.

The quantities of electrolytes in the body are so small that 1 mEq (1/1000 of an equivalent weight) is used as the unit of measurement. One mEq equals one electrical charge, and one mEq of any electrolyte equals one mEq of any other electrolyte even though the weights needed to produce that charge are different. The concetration of a solution can be expressed in terms of the number of milliequivalents per liter (mEq/L).

The analogy that can be used to clarify this concept is related to horsepower. A person who needs a 75-horsepower motor to run his motorboat cannot find the best motor by weighing each motor. Several motors of the same weight can have different horsepower, while motors of differing weights can have the same horsepower. To select an appropriate motor for a boat that requires 75 horsepower, the person must compare only 75-horsepower motors regardless of their size, shape, or weight. In similar fashion, combining power expressed in milliequivalents is a more useful comparison of potential chemical activity than molecular size or weight.

Osmotic Pressure as a Measure of Concentration

Another basis for comparing the concentration of solutions is osmolality. The *osmolality* of a solution is equal to the total number of dissolved particles of solute per unit of solvent. These particles are called *osmols* and can be either electrolytes or non-electrolytes. The osmol is the basic unit of measurement of osmotic pressure. The number of particles of solute in the body is so small that the milliosmol is used for measurement instead of the osmol, and osmolality of body fluids is expressed as milliosmols per liter (mOsm/L).

Osmotic pressure is created when there is a difference in the osmolality of the solutions on each side of a semipermeable membrane. *Osmosis* is the movement of water across a membrane in an effort to equalize the concentrations of two different solutions (Fig. 31.2). Water moves from the least concentrated solution toward the more concentrated solution in an effort to dilute it. Water leaves the solution that has the fewest dissolved particles of solute in order to dilute the solution with the greatest number of dissolved particles. Osmolality is the relationship between the number of particles of solute and the volume of solvent (mOsm/L). The addition of more solvent to a strong solution as a result of osmosis dilutes that solution and reduces its osmolality.

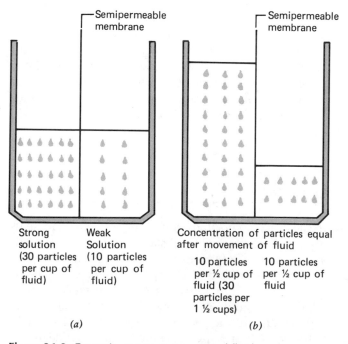

Strong solution (30 particles per cup of fluid)   Weak Solution (10 particles per cup of fluid)

Concentration of particles equal after movement of fluid

10 particles per ½ cup of fluid (30 particles per 1 ½ cups)   10 particles per ½ cup of fluid

(a)   *(b)*

Figure 31.2 *Osmosis causes movement of fluid across a semipermeable membrane from a weaker to a stronger solution. Movement of fluids stops when the solutions are of equal strength (b).*

Osmotic pressure decreases as the difference between osmolalities of two solutions decreases, and the movement of water across the membrane ceases when the concentrations have been equalized. Osmotic pressure is sometimes described as the cumulative attraction of particles for water, with the particles in the higher of two concentrations exerting the greater attraction for water and drawing the water to that side of the membrane.

Osmotic pressure can be measured by the number of millimeters of mercury that must be applied to the more concentrated solution to hold back the movement of water from the weaker solution. It is the amount of pressure that would be needed to block the equalization of solutions with different osmolalities.

Changing the Concentration of a Solution

The concentration of a solution can be changed by *movement of the fluid* (the solvent) or by *movement of the particles* (the solute). *Fluid* is moved in or out of a cell or blood vessel by the processes of osmosis and filtration; *particles* are moved by diffusion, filtration, or an active transport mechanism.

Movement of Fluid

The movement of fluid between blood vessels, interstitial spaces, and intracellular spaces is necessary for the transfer of nutrients, wastes, and body-regulating chemicals and hormones. This movement is made possible by osmosis and filtration. Differences in the osmolality of plasma, interstitial fluid, and intracellular fluid regulate the speed and direction of the movement.

MOVEMENT OF BODY FLUID BY OSMOSIS. Plasma, interstitial fluid, and intracellular fluid each have an osmolality of approximately 300 mOsm/L. With reference to body fluids, a solution that contains more than 300 particles is said to have high osmolality, or hyperosmolality. A solution that has fewer that 300 mOsm/L is described as having low osmolality, or hypo-osmolality. The commonly used terms for these concentrations are *hypertonic* and *hypotonic*.

An *isotonic* solution has the *same* osmolality as extracellular fluid and therefore, it can be given intravenously without altering the osmolality of the plasma. Some bottles of IV fluids are labeled by the manufacturer in terms of osmolality (mOsm/L), but other fluids are labeled in terms of percentage of solute in the solution. A. 0.9 percent solution of salt is isotonic, for example, and is referred to as *normal saline* solution. When a cell is in contact with an isotonic solution, the osmolalities of the solutions on each side of the membrane are equivalent, and there is no movement of water

across the membrane. When a cell is in contact with a *hyper*tonic solution, the ICF is less concentrated than the hypertonic solution. Water is drawn from the less concentrated fluid in the cell in an attempt to equalize the osmolality of the two fluids. As water is lost from the cell, the cell shrinks. If the difference in fluids is great enough, this process (*crenation*) will continue until the cell is destroyed.

A cell surrounded by a *hypo*tonic solution has a higher osmolality than the hypotonic fluid and must absorb fluid to achieve an equilibrium with the surrounding fluid. If the difference in concentration is great enough, the cell will continue to absorb water and swell until it bursts.

It is important to note that, although all body fluids have approximately the same osmolality (300 mOsm/L), there is a slight but significant difference. The osmolality of interstitial and intracellular fluid is 302.2mOsm/L, while the osmolality of plasma is 303.7mOsm/L, a difference of 1.5 mOsm/L. This is due to the presence of colloidal particles in the plasma.

This slight difference (about 0.05 percent) between the osmolality of plasma and that of interstitial fluid is important. The increased osmotic pressure of the plasma pulls fluid into the blood vessels and counteracts the tendency of the blood pressure to force fluid out of the blood vessels, thereby enabling the body to maintain its required blood volume.

MOVEMENT OF BODY FLUID BY FILTRATION. In addition to movement by osmosis, fluids move from one compartment to another by *filtration*. In response to the laws of physics, fluids flow from an area of greater pressure to one of lower pressure. Hydrostatic pressure is the pressure exerted by a column of water, and it is a force that causes a fluid to flow through a membrane (filtration). In a closed system this pressure can be increased by the addition of a positive pump that forces fluid through the membrane. In the body, the heart serves this purpose and creates enough blood pressure to force intravascular fluid (plasma) out of the arterioles and into the interstitial spaces. Blood pressure is also a controlling force in the filtration processes of the kidneys.

The permeability of the membrane, or filter, determines whether only the solvent, or the solvent plus part of the solute, can pass through it. In industry, for example, it is possible to select a filter that will filter out one, two, or all of the various solutes. In the body, the permeability required of any given membrane is determined by the function or purpose of that membrane.

The hydrostatic pressure (blood pressure) inside an arteriole is greater than the pressure outside the arteriole, so water and some solutes are moved through the walls of the blood vessel into the interstitial spaces around the cells. The pressure on the movement of fluids is modified by the osmotic pressure created by plasma proteins. This force is called the colloid osmotic pressure, or *oncotic* pressure. Whereas hydrostatic pressure pushes fluid out of the blood vessels, oncotic (osmotic) pressure pulls fluid into the blood vessels. Hydrostatic pressure minus colloid osmotic (oncotic) pressure equals the filtration pressure. The oncotic pressure of plasma is approximately 22 mm Hg. This means that it takes a force equal to 22 mm Hg to counteract the pull of plasma proteins.

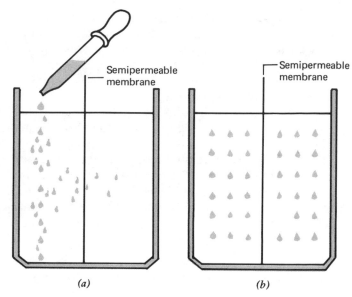

Figure 31.3 *Diffusion of particles across a semipermeable membrane. Diffusion stops when dispersion of particles is equal (b).*

FILTRATION PRESSURE OF CAPILLARIES

	Hydrostatic Pressure of Blood		Osmotic Pressure of Plasma Proteins		Filtration Pressure
Arteriole	32 mm Hg	−	22 mm Hg	=	+10 mm Hg (fluid leaves arteriole)
Venule	12 mm Hg	−	22 mm Hg	=	−10 mm Hg (fluid enters venule)

Movement of Particles

The movement of both water and solute is important in the regulation and balance of fluid and electrolytes. Whereas water is moved by osmosis and filtration, *particles of solute* are moved by diffusion, filtration, and active transport.

DIFFUSION. Diffusion is the dispersion of dissolved substances throughout a gas or liquid until the particles are evenly distributed. This process can be demonstrated by adding a few drops of food coloring to a glass of water. The particles of coloring diffuse throughout the water until it is evenly colored. Particles of solute will diffuse across a cell membrane if the membrane is permeable enough (Fig. 31.3). The difference in concentration on each side of a membrane is called the *diffusion gradient;* the larger the gradient, the more rapid the movement of particles.

Oxygen (O_2) and carbon dioxide (CO_2) are examples of molecules that can diffuse through the pores of a cell membrane. There is more O_2 in arterial blood than there is in interstitial and intracellular fluid, so O_2 diffuses out of the arterioles into the interstitial fluid and into the cells. The concentration of CO_2, however, is greater in the cells than it is in the blood, so CO_2 diffuses out of the cells and into the venules.

Diffusion can occur in conjunction with osmosis. The particles diffuse across a membrane from the most concentrated solution to the least concentrated solution while the water moves by osmosis in the opposite direction. Both processes stop when the concentrations have been equalized.

FILTRATION. Dissolved particles can be forced through a membrane by hydrostatic pressure if the membrane is permeable enough to permit their passage.

ACTIVE TRANSPORT. Particles move easily and passively from a concentrated solution to a more dilute solution by diffusion or filtration. Under certain circumstances, however, particles must be moved in the opposite direction, from a dilute solution to a more concentrated one. Transport of the sodium ion is one example of such a situation. Extracellular fluid normally has a high concentration of sodium ions (140 mEq/L) in contrast to a very low intracellular fluid concentration of only 10 mEq/L. Sodium ions therefore diffuse across the cell membrane into the cell. If unchecked, this process would result in a potentially hazardous change in concentrations, producing a low serum sodium concentration and an elevated celluar sodium level.

To prevent such abnormal levels, the sodium ions that diffuse across the membrane into the cell must be returned to their rightful extracellular compartment. This movement from a low concentration of sodium toward a higher concentration is difficult and requires energy. The process is called *active transport*. The mechanism is not yet clearly understood, but it is believed that a chemical carrier exists for each substance that must be transported. The substance is attached to its carrier, carried through the cell membrane, and detached from the carrier on the other side. The process of transporting sodium ions from ICF back to interstitial fluid is often referred to as a *sodium pump,* and it involves a carrier substance called *adenosine triphosphate* (ATP).

The processes of the sodium pump also transport potassium ions in similar fashion but in the opposite direction, back from the low concentrations of ECF to the normally high concentration within the cell. A number of other electrolytes and nonelectrolytes require active transport, and the amount of energy and type of carrier needed for each depend on the characteristics of the particle to be transported and of the cell membrane, and on the osmolalities of the solutions involved.

FACILITATED DIFFUSION. *Facilitated diffusion* is a process that involves the use of a carrier substance to move a particle such as glucose through a membrane; the process is very similar to active transport except that it is passive. It cannot move particles against a chemical or molecular gradient. Active transport can move particles "up hill" from a low to a higher osmolality, for example, but facilitated diffusion can only move particles "down hill" from a high to a lower osmolality.

Movement of Body Fluid by the Lymphatic System

The lymphatic system provides an additional route for the return of fluid and protein from the interstitial spaces to the blood. Lymphatic channels carry excess interstitial fluid from almost all areas of the body through the thoracic duct, which empties into the venous circulation at the junction of the internal jugular and subclavian veins.

Proteins and some other large particles cannot pass directly from interstitial fluid back into the blood vessels and must be carried through the lymphatic system for reentry into the vascular system. If this process were halted, the accumulated proteins would rapidly increase the osmotic presure of the interstitial fluid, and the fluid balance would be so seriously disrupted that death could ensue in about 24 hours.

The lymphatic system has numerous functions, but none is more important than the transfer of protein molecules from interstitial fluid back to the blood. Hence, any blockage of either the lymph channels or the lymph nodes by disease or injury causes severe swelling (edema) of body parts distal to the blockage.

REGULATION OF FLUID VOLUME

The volume of body fluid depends on age, percentage of body fat, and the balance between intake and output

of fluid. Body fluid constitutes approximately 75 percent of an infant's total body weight. This percentage decreases to approximately 60 percent of an adult's weight and declines even further during old age. Fat cells contain almost no water, and obesity can decrease the percetage of body water to as low as 45 percent of body weight. Day-to-day variations in fluid volume depend on fluid intake, fluid losses, and distribution of fluid throughout the body.

Fluid Intake

Approximately two-thirds of a person's daily intake of water is obtained from the water and other liquids he drinks, and nearly one-third is derived from the water content of the food he eats. A small amount is released as a by-product of the oxidation of food.

The oral intake of water is controlled primarily by the thirst center in the hypothalamus, which is probably stimulated by dehydration of its neurons. The thirst center can be activated by a number of conditions. One such condition is a decrease in ECF volume as a result of hemorrhage or of acute cardiac failure and decreased cardiac output. Another condition that causes thirst is intracellular dehydration. This occurs when hyperosmolality of ECF draws fluid from the cells. An IV injection of hypertonic saline or glucose, for example, will cause intense thirst within a few seconds.

Dryness of the mouth, whether from a drug such as atropine or from breathing through the mouth, will cause a person to drink even though the sensation is not the same as the sensation of thirst. Stimulation of the thirst center is inhibited by drinking and also by fullness of the gastrointestinal tract, probably as a result of pressure on peripheral sensory receptors.

Fluid Loss

Water is lost from the body in urine, sweat, and feces plus insensible loss through the skin and lungs.

Through Skin and Lungs

The water lost through the skin and lungs is termed *insensible* because the person is insensitive to the loss; he is not aware of its occurrence. Diffusion of water through the skin is *slowed* by the cornified layers of the skin; but when these outer layers of skin are destroyed, as by burns or abrasion, for example, water loss can increase from the normal 350 cc/day to 3,000 to 5,000 cc/day. The amount of water lost in the form of sweat varies with body temperature, environmental temperature, and exercise; and that amount can also markedly affect the fluid balance of the body.

Through the Gastrointestinal Tract

Over 7 L of water is transferred across the membranes of the gastrointestinal (GI) tract and reabsorbed every 24 hours. This fluid includes saliva, bile, pancreatic juice, and intestinal secretions. Of this large amount, normally only 100 to 200 ml is lost in feces, but significantly larger amounts are lost when a patient is vomiting or has diarrhea.

Through the Kidneys

The processes of glomerular filtration and tubular reabsorption in the kidneys make possible the regulation of both water and electrolytes. These processes are primarily controlled by two hormones: the *antidiuretic hormone* (ADH) and *aldosterone,* although the amount of fluid lost as urine is also affected by drugs, injury, and diseases such as diabetes and uremia.

ANTIDIURETIC HORMONE. The osmoreceptor-antidiuretic hormone system maintains the osmotic pressure of extracellular fluid through its effect on the production of urine. Any *increase* in the osmolality of ECF stimulates the hypothalamus to produce ADH. Such an increase in extracellular osmolality can be caused by water loss, blood loss, medications, and physiological responses to pain, injury, or other stress. ADH causes the kidney to reabsorb water in order to dilute the high concentrations of solutes in the ECF, thereby reducing its osmolality. (The antidiuretic effect is directly opposite the effect of a diuretic, which increases the output of urine.) As a result of this antidiuretic activity, the osmoreceptors of the hypothalamus sense the decreased osmolality of the ECF and respond by slowing the production of ADH. The antidiuretic effect ceases, and a diuretic action can begin. If this changeover did not occur, water would continue to be reabsorbed; the concentration of the ECF would become increasingly dilute, and its osmolality would fall below normal. The release of ADH, therefore, produces an anidiuretic effect on the kidney. The production of urine is markedly slowed, and water is retained while solutes continue to be excreted. The decreased amount of water makes the urine darker and more concentrated.

The *inhibition* of ADH, on the other hand, permits diuresis, and the amount of water lost can rise to five to 15 times normal. This loss of water causes ECF to become concentrated, and as a result, osmolality of the ECF increases. The osmoreceptors of the hypothalamus are then stimulated to produce ADH, and the cycle continues.

Hypo-osmolality of ECF, which inhibits the production of ADH, can be caused by excessive water intake and a resultant increase in blood volume as well as by cold, diuretics, alcohol, and diabetes. The ways in which these factors reduce the osmolality of the ECF are complex; but in each case, the kidney rids the body of excess water and brings the osmolality of the ECF back to normal. The production of ADH is inhibited, less water is reabsorbed by the kidney, and there is an increased amount of dilute urine.

ALDOSTERONE. Aldosterone is a hormone secreted by the adrenal cortex; it regulates the reabsorption of sodium by the tubules of the kidney. This hormone is extremely important inasmuch as sodium constitutes 90 percent of all the extracellular cations, and any significant loss of sodium ions would seriously alter the osmotic pressure of the extracellular fluid. Such an alteration would affect the transfer of solute and water between extracellular and intracellular fluid.

Among the many circumstances that stimulate the secretion of aldosterone by the adrenal cortex are sodium depletion or excessive potassium in the ECF, and any kind of great physical stress such as extreme exercise or extensive burns. Any condition characterized by the loss of sodium and a resulting decrease in sodium ion concentration stimulates the production of aldosterone. This stimulates the reabsorption and conservation of sodium ions by the kidney. In addition to the regulation of sodium concentrations, an aldosterone feedback mechanism regulates the concentration of potassium by a method that is exactly opposite to the one used to regulate sodium.

FLUID IMBALANCE

Body fluids are balanced when the net difference between fluid intake and fluid losses produces a state of hydration that is adequate for all body processes. When either an excess or a deficit of water occurs, a state of imbalance exists, and regulatory processes immediately try to regain a homeostatic condition.

Excess water volume inhibits thirst, and causes a decreased production of ADH and aldosterone. As a result, the intake of fluid slows, there is increased production of dilute urine, and less sodium is reabsorbed until normal fluid balance is regained.

Decreased water volume excites thirst and stimulates the production of ADH and aldosterone. As a result, fluid intake increases; more sodium is reabsorbed, more water is retained, urine is more concentrated, and less urine is produced until normal fluid balance is regained.

Dehydration

Dehydration is a condition in which there is a deficit of extracellular fluid, followed by an osmotic shift of intracellular fluid into the extracellular compartments in an effort to equalize the osmolalities of the two fluids. As a result, there is both an intracellular and an extracellular fluid volume deficit, and the overall effect is called dehydration.

Dehydration can be caused by an inadequate fluid intake, by excessive fluid losses, or by an electrolyte imbalance. Dehydration can occur very rapidly in infants and young children because body fluids constitute a larger percentage of their body weight, thereby giving greater impact to any shift in the volume, distribution, or osmolality of body fluid. Elderly people are also susceptible to dehydration because they have proportionately less body fluid and therefore have little reserve for use in a crisis.

The signs and symptoms of dehydration are listed in Table 31.2. The nursing care of a dehydrated patient is based on correction of the underlying causes and relief of the symptoms. Nursing interventions specific to fluid and electrolyte imbalance are included in Section 2 of this chapter.

Overhydration

Overhydration (fluid excess) is a condition in which the volume of ECF exceeds the needs of the body. It is seen less frequently than dehydration because it usually does not occur unless kidney function is impaired. Normally, when the blood volume becomes too great, the cardiac output and arterial pressures increase. This increases filtration through the kidneys, causing an increased loss of fluid (urine) from the body, thereby returning the blood volume to normal.

Overhydration is often referred to as *circulatory overload*. The overload, or excess of body fluid, can be caused by kidney failure (decreased output), excessive or too-rapid administration of IV fluids (increased input), or excessive retention of sodium. When a circulatory overload occurs, it usually constitutes a medical emergency because it can cause a potentially fatal *pulmonary edema*. The patient develops cyanosis, dyspnea, moist rales, and frothy sputum. Unless it is treated effectively, fluid oozes out of the distended pulmonary blood vessels into the lungs. The alveoli fill with fluid, and the patient literally drowns in his own body fluid.

ELECTROLYTE IMBALANCE

The clinical manifestations of electrolyte imbalances are complex because they rarely occur in isolation. Electrolytes and fluids are so interrelated that the imbalance

TABLE 31.2 ASSESSMENT OF HYDRATION

Areas to be Assessed	Dehydration	Optimal Hydration	Overhydration
Skin Turgor	Pinched up skin returns to normal very slowly	Pinched up skin returns to normal very quickly	
Texture	Dry, rough	Supple, smooth, not dry	Flushed, moist
Lips, mucous membranes	Dry, cracked	Pink, moist, smooth	
Mucus secretions (ex., saliva)	Viscous, thick, ropey		Thin, watery
Weight	Rapid weight loss	Weight steady	Rapid weight gain
Vital signs	↑ Respiratory rate ↑ Temperature ↓ BP		Tachycardia ↑ BP
Circulation	Soft, compressible veins; veins re-fil slowly	Veins refill quickly	Distended neck veins
Urine	Scant, dark, concentrated		Dilute, pale amber color, amount
Specific gravity	Increased	Normal (1.003–1.030)	Decreased
Mentation	Confused, disoriented		Headache, confusion, convulsions, coma
Respiration			Cough, dyspnea, shortness of breath, cyanosis, rales
Other	Thirsty		

↑ = Increased
↓ = Decreased

of one electrolyte is usually accompanied by the imbalance of body fluids and other electrolytes.

It is not feasible in an introductory text to present a comprehensive picture of electrolyte imbalances. In this chapter, imbalances of sodium and potassium are described very briefly; for a fuller description, and for material related to other electrolytes, it will be necessary to consult a medical-surgical nursing text.

Sodium Imbalances

Sodium is the principal cation of *extra*cellular fluid. The normal plasma level of Na$^+$ is 142 mEq/L (in contrast to an intracellular Na$^+$ level of 10 mEq/L). *Sodium deficiency* (*hypo*natremia) is indicated by a plasma sodium level below 137 mEq/L and is usually caused by the loss of Na$^+$ from the body, sometimes coupled with inadequate intake of Na$^+$. Sodium losses can be the result of excessive perspiration, gastrointestinal losses from vomiting, diarrhea, or gastric suction, or the loss of body fluid from massive burns. The signs and symptoms of hyponatremia may be the result of excessive loss of sodium or an excessive gain of water. Clinical signs of hyponatremia are dependent upon the cause. These signs include a postural drop in blood pressure and decreased fullness of neck and hand veins. Decreased blood volume brings less blood to the kidneys, and the production of urine is decreased, a condition called *oliguria*. Medical treatment includes IV therapy to restore a normal sodium concentration.

Sodium excess (*hyper*natremia) is indicated by a plasma sodium level above 142 mEq/L and may be caused by decreased water intake; ingestion of unusually large amounts of salt; administration of excessive amounts of saline solutions; by diseases such as heart trouble and kidney disease that disrupt fluid regulation; or by the administration of cortisone, which causes the retention of sodium and water. Other symptoms include dry, sticky mucus membrane, rough dry tongue, restlessness, and lethargy which may progress to coma. In *hyper*natremia, sodium accumulates in the ECF, especially interstitial tissue, and water follows. The symptoms of hypernatremia include distention of neck veins, excessive and rapid weight gain, pitting edema, and dyspnea because of pulmonary edema. Treatment includes restricted sodium intake and a careful regulation of water intake until a normal concentration of sodium is achieved.

Potassium Imbalances

Potassium is the major intracellular cation. The normal intracellular level is 142 mEq/L, whereas the normal extracellular level (the plasma level) is only 4 mEq/L.

A major function of potassium is the regulation of the resting membrane potential of nerve and muscle cells, and an imbalance of K$^+$ ions produces disordered muscle and nerve function.

Potassium *deficit* (*hypo*kalemia) is indicated by a plasma K$^+$ level below 4 mEq/L and is most often caused by loss of K$^+$ through the kidneys or GI tract. It can also be caused by the prolonged use of IV fluids that do not contain an amount of K$^+$ equivalent to that which the patient would normally receive through his food. Loss of K$^+$ through the kidneys is caused by diuretic therapy, endocrine disorder, kidney disease, or by physiological responses to the stress of surgery, crushing injuries, or burns. Losses from the GI tract are the result of vomiting, diarrhea, or gastrointestinal suctioning without replacement of the K$^+$ lost.

Signs and symptoms of hypokalemia are related to its effect on neuromuscular and cardiac function. These symptoms include generalized muscle weakness, cardiac arrhythmias, decreased activity of the intestinal tract, shallow respirations, and apathy. Because some of these symptoms are initially mild and are sometimes discounted as minor complaints, it is important to check the serum K$^+$ level of all patients who are at risk.

Treatment is based on the administration of oral or intravenous potassium and on the provision of a diet that contains adequate amounts of potassium.

Potassium *excess* (*hyper*kalemia) is indicated by plasma K$^+$ in excess of 5.6 mEq/L. The kidneys are normally able to excrete any excess potassium, so hyperkalemia is not common. It can occur in patients with acute kidney failure or with chronic kidney failure severe enough to require hemodialysis.

If, however, an intravenous infusion containing potassium is administered too rapidly, a potentially dangerous hyperkalemia may result. If the potassium excess is great enough, hyperkalemia will precipitate a cardiac arrest.

HYDROGEN-ION IMBALANCES

The hydrogen-ion balance of the body refers to that balance which is compatible with life. Because an acid has a high H$^+$ concentration and a base (an alkali) has a low H$^+$ concentration, the hydrogen-ion balance is often referred to as the acid-base balance. The acid/base ratio in the body is 1:20, that is, 1 part carbonic *acid* (H$_2$CO$_3$) to 20 parts *base* bicarbonate (HCO$_3$). The quantities of carbonic acid and bicarbonate can vary greatly as long as an exact 1:20 ratio of acid to base is maintained. When a 1:20 acid-base balance is maintained, the pH of arterial blood is 7.4. A pH of 7.0 is neutral, so arterial blood is slightly alkaline.

If the acid/base ratio is altered, the pH of the blood

is altered and a state of acidosis or alkalosis results. A pH of arterial blood *below* 7.4 (below normal) indicates acidosis; a pH above 7.4 indicates alkalosis. The pH normally deviates up to 0.05 in either direction, giving a normal range of from 7.35 to 7.45. Any greater deviation is pathological, and if the pH of arterial blood falls below 7.0 or rises above 7.8, death ensues very quickly.

Samples of arterial blood are used to assess acid-base balance. The pH of interstitial fluid and venous blood is about 7.35. It is slightly more acidic than arterial blood because the excess CO_2, which will be excreted by the lungs, combines with body water to form carbonic acid. Other body fluids have widely differing pH values: urine, 6.0; intracellular fluid, 6.9 to 7.2; bile, 5.0 to 6.0; and gastric secretions, 1.0 to 2.0.

pH is the symbol for a *negative* logarithm of hydrogen-ion (H^+) concentration, and it is important to remember that there is an *inverse* relationship between H^+ concentration and pH. That is, the higher the H^+ concentration, the more acidic the solution and the lower the pH. Conversely, the lower the H^+ concentration, the more alkaline the solution and the higher the pH. Because an acid has a high H^+ concentration, it releases hydrogen ions and is called a hydrogen *donor*. An alkaline solution (a base) has a low H^+ concentration, and it attracts or accepts hydrogen ions. It is a hydrogen *receiver*.

Regulatory Mechanisms

The body strives to maintain its acid-base balance by means of chemical buffers and by the action of the lungs, the cells, and the kidneys, which serve as physiological buffers.

Chemical Buffers

An acid-base buffer is a chemical that can combine with any acid or base that is added to body fluids. The source of the acid or base may be a drug, an excess of acidic or alkaline food or drink, or the by-product of a metabolic process. Acid-base buffers keep the pH of body fluids within normal limits and functions only when excessive acid or base is present. One such buffer present in all body fluids is the bicarbonate buffer. It occurs as a bicarbonate of sodium, poassium, calcium, or magnesium.

The bicarbonate buffer includes both carbonic acid (H_2CO_3) and a bicarbonate ion (HCO_3^-), and therefore it can either absorb or release hydrogen ions. If a strong acid is added to a solution containing a bicarbonate buffer, the acid releases a hydrogen ion to the bicarbonate ion (HCO_3^-) of the buffer because acids are hydrogen donors.

$$H^+ + HCO_3^- = H_2CO_3$$

Bicarbonate   Carbonic acid

The strong acid that was added to the solution is thereby converted to carbonic acid, which is very weak, keeping the solution from being strongly acidic. Carbonic acid is unstable and almost immediately dissociates into CO_2 and H_2O.

When a strong base is added to a solution containing a bicarbonate buffer, the base absorbs hydrogen from the carbonic acid portion of the buffer because bases are hydrogen receivers. The result is water and a neutral bicarbonate salt.

Two other buffer systems of the body involve phosphate and plasma protein and function in a manner similar to the bicarbonate buffer system. Such chemical buffers are, in a sense, the body's first line of defense against an acid-base imbalance because their reactions are almost instantaneous. These reactions are relatively short-lived, however, and other regulatory mechanisms must then take over.

Lungs

The relationship of the lungs to acid-base balance is complex and cyclical. Any change in the acid-base balance of the body alters the depth and rate of respiration, while, at the same time, an intense change in respiration can modify the acid-base balance. The lungs give off CO_2 and thereby regulate the *carbonic acid* portion of the bicarbonate buffer system; the *bicarbonate ions* are regulated by the kidney.

EFFECT OF HYDROGEN-ION IMBALANCE ON RESPIRATION. When there is a high H^+ concentration (excessive acid) in the body, the bicarbonate buffer system reacts with it to produce carbonic acid (H_2CO_3), which dissociates into CO_2 and H_2O. This action is rapid and the lungs can alter the plasma pH within a matter of minutes. The excess CO_2 stimulates the respiratory center to increase the rate and depth of respiration in order to blow off the excess CO_2.

Conversely, a low H^+ concentration (excessive base) in the body reduces the rate and depth of respiration in an attempt to conserve CO_2. The lungs react to changes in the body's acid-base balance within several minutes, but they regulate only the carbonic acid level of the blood. The regulation of bicarbonate ions must be assumed by the kidney.

EFFECT OF RESPIRATION ON HYDROGEN-ION BALANCE. Increased ventilation (hyperventilation) causes CO_2 to be blown off more rapidly than it is formed. The carbonic acid level of the blood drops, the H^+ concentration decreases, the blood becomes less acidic, and the pH rises.

Decreased ventilation (hypoventilation) means that less CO_2 is blown off. CO_2 accumulates in body fluids, the H^+ concentration increases, the blood becomes more acidic, and the pH falls.

Cells

Hydrogen ions are transported back and forth across cell membranes as needed by the processes of diffusion and filtration. It takes several hours for significant shifts to occur in response to a hydrogen-ion imbalance.

Kidneys

The lungs are unable to compensate for pH disturbances when there is severe pulmonary dysfunction, and under these conditions, compensation must be accomplished by the kidneys.

Kidneys regulate the bicarbonate ions of the body's bicarbonate buffer system. When the H^+ concentration of extracellular fluid is elevated, the kidneys excrete H^+ and retain bicarbonate ions. When the H^+ concentration of ECF is too low, H^+ is added to it in exchange for sodium, and bicarbonate ions are excreted. Renal compensation for imbalances is slow, and may take hours or days.

Types of Imbalance

There are two types of hydrogen-ion imbalance: acidosis and alkalosis. *Acidosis* is characterized by an increased H^+ concentration and a lowered pH. *Alkalosis* involves a decreased H^+ concentration and a raised pH. Each type of imbalance can be either respiratory or metabolic in origin. *Respiratory* acidosis or alkalosis is caused by an alteration in carbonic acid levels in the blood; *metabolic* acidosis or alkalosis is caused by altered bicarbonate levels.

Respiratory Hydrogen-ion Imbalance

Respiratory *acidosis* is caused by *hypo*ventilation and results in increased CO_2 levels which increase the level of carbonic acid. A slight degree of respiratory acidosis can be caused by a person holding his breath, but the accumulated CO_2 will stimulate his respiratory system and cause him to breathe involuntarily. Significant respiratory acidosis is caused by obstructed respiratory passages, chronic lung disease, damage to the respiratory center, pneumonia, and any interference with an exchange of gases between the blood and the alveoli. Medical treatment involves control or correction of the underlying pathology and improvement of ventilation.

Respiratory *alkalosis* is caused by *hyper*ventilation.

CO_2 is blown off more rapidly than it is produced, resulting in a decreased plasma H_2CO_3 content. Respiratory alkalosis can result from hyperventilation caused by hysteria, anxiety, strenuous exercise, high altitudes, and any drug or condition that overstimulates the respiratory system. Treatment includes sedation as needed and the administration of CO_2. A person can obtain CO_2 by rebreathing his own expired air from a paper bag held over his nose and mouth.

Metabolic Hydrogen-ion Imbalance

Metabolic acidosis and alkalosis are imbalances other than those caused by an excess or deficiency of CO_2 in body plasma. Although metabolism, as well as respiration, involves CO_2, carbonic acid from dissolved CO_2 is called a respiratory acid; whereas other acids, whether from metabolism or ingestion, are called metabolic acids.

Metabolic acidosis results from either an accumulation of metabolic acids or a loss of alkali (deficit of bicarbonate ions) in the extracellular fluid. An accumulation of metabolic acids can be caused by kidney failure with the resulting inability to excrete excess acids and by overproduction of metabolic acids in conditions such as uncontrolled diabetes and starvation. A deficit of bicarbonate ions (loss of alkali) can be caused by severe diarrhea or by vomiting the contents of the GI tract *below* the stomach. The contents of the stomach are acidic, but the rest of the GI tract is alkaline; and the loss of the contents of the lower GI tract results in a significant loss of bicarbonate ions.

Metabolic acidosis results in central nervous system depression. Early symptoms include headache, confusion, and drowsiness, followed by stupor and coma if the blood pH falls below 7.0. There is often a sweet, fruity (acetone) odor to the breath. Respirations are rapid and deep (known as Kussmaul respirations).

Metabolic acidosis results in arterial blood gases which have a lowered pH and a decreased level of bicarbonate. The body's method of compensation includes the excretion of H^+ and the conservation of HCO_3^- by the kidney as well as the release and blowing off of CO_2 by the lungs.

Medical treatment includes treatment of the underlying cause and, when necessary, administration of a bicarbonate solution, correction of any fluid imbalance, and a low-protein, high-carbohydrate, high-calorie diet.

Metabolic *alkalosis* occurs less frequently than metabolic acidosis and is caused by excessive intake of alkaline drugs or food resulting in an excess of bicarbonate ions in the plasma. Metabolic alkalosis can also be caused by the excessive use of diuretics, excessive gastric suctioning, and vomiting of gastric contents *only* with no vomiting of alkaline intestinal contents.

Metabolic alkalosis results in overexcitability of the central and peripheral nervous systems. The peripheral nerves are involved first, and the symptoms include restlessness, dizziness, tingling of the fingers and toes, and twitching of the extremities, followed in severe cases by tetany or convulsions. Tetany is characterized by muscle spasms, which can be fatal if the muscles of respiration are involved. Tetany develops because alkaline body fluids slow the ionization of calcium; then, when the concentration of calcium ions drops, the nervous system becomes increasingly active and irritable. Respirations are slow and shallow, as the lungs try to conserve CO_2.

In metabolic alkalosis, arterial blood gases indicate an elevated pH (7.45 or more) and an increased level of bicarbonate. The body's attempts to compensate include excretion of HCO_3^- and retention of H^+ by the kidneys, and retention of CO_2 by the lungs.

Medical treatment of metabolic alkalosis includes the correction of the underlying cause, replacement of fluids lost by vomiting and diarrhea, use of IV solutions and medications such as ammonium chloride, and the correction of potassium and calcium deficits. Calcium ion concentration is further regulated by the parathyroid gland.

IMPLICATIONS FOR NURSING

The conditions of acidosis and alkalosis are exceedingly complex because the signs and symptoms of one condition frequently duplicate the body's compensatory responses to another condition. It is often difficult, therefore, to know whether the physical condition of a patient represents the early signs of one type of acid-base imbalance or the compensatory mechanism and the end result of an opposing imbalance. The complexity of these conditions warrants continual study and necessitates an integrative approach to the nursing care of patients with an imbalance of body fluids of electrolytes.

Section Two

Maintenance and Restoration of Fluid Balance

Identification of Patients at Risk

Assessments

Regulation of Oral Fluid Intake

Intravenous Therapy
  Administration
  Equipment
  Sites
  Solutions
  Rate of Administration
  Complications
  Assessments Related to IV Therapy
  Basic Procedures
  Patient Responsibility

Fluids by Central Venous Route

Administration of Blood
  Transfusion Reactions
  Nursing Responsibilities for Administration of Blood
  Starting a Blood Transfusion
  *Nursing Responsibility in the Event of a Transfusion
    Reaction*

Measurement of Fluid Intake and Output

The physician prescribes the *treatment* for diagnosed fluid and electrolyte imbalances, but there are five aspects of care which are *nursing* responsibilities. The nurse is responsible for the identification of patients at risk, assessments related to fluid balance, regulation of oral fluid intake, administration of IV therapy, and measurement of fluid intake and output.

IDENTIFICATION OF PATIENTS AT RISK

There are at least five categories of people who are in danger of developing fluid or electrolyte imbalances. These categories are composed of persons who:

Have limited access to fluids

Are losing fluids and electrolytes

Have an altered intake of food

Have an altered intake of electrolytes

Have predisposing conditions

Limited Access to Fluids

It always comes as a shock to discover that a badly dehydrated patient would willingly have increased his fluid intake had he had the opportunity to do so. Many patients have a low fluid intake because they either do not realize that a greater intake is needed or do not have access to the necessary fluids.

Patients who may be *unaware of a need for more fluids* include people who are depressed, apathetic, semiconscious, confused, or developmentally disabled. Patients whose fluid intake may be inadequate simply because *fluids were not accessible* are people who are weak, paralyzed, restrained, confined to bed, very young, or very old. These people are often unable to exercise one of life's most basic rights: to be able to drink when one is thirsty.

It is not uncommon for the medical and nursing staff to be puzzled by a patient's symptoms—such as mental confusion, for example—only to discover belatedly that he is dehydrated. In one such situation a nurse assigned to an elderly patient was told that he did not seem responsible, that he should be restrained in his chair, and that he seemed to like to look out the window. The nurse discovered that, by turning his chair toward the window, the staff had inadvertently positioned him with his back toward his bedside stand and his drinking water. His mental confusion had seemed to increase with each passing day, and he was, as a result, more carefully restrained "for his own protection," making him less able to get a drink. The less he drank, the more dehydrated he became, and the more intense was his lethargy, apathy, and mental confusion. As soon as the cycle was broken, his fluid intake increased, his mental confusion decreased, and there was no longer any need to restrain him.

Other people who may suffer from an inadequate fluid intake are those who are *NPO (nothing by mouth) for a series of diagnostic tests.* While each nurse in turn may prepare the patient properly for the tests that are to be done on her shift, no one may notice that, as a result of a *series* of correct and proper preparations, the patient has had little opportunity to drink. This can be a serious problem for an elderly patient who has limited fluid reserves, and it is also likely to happen to the "good" patient who thinks, "If I'm supposed to be able to drink they'll bring me a drink."

Loss of Fluids and Electrolytes

Any person who is losing fluid other than normal amounts of urine and sweat is in danger of developing fluid and electrolyte imbalance. Such losses occur as the result of hemorrhage, large draining wounds and burns, a colostomy or ileostomy, heavy and prolonged perspiration, gastric or intestinal suction, repeated enemas, vomiting, and diarrhea. Prolonged or severe vomiting and diarrhea are especially serious in infants, small children, and elderly people and can lead to potentially fatal dehydration and electrolyte imbalances *within a few days.*

Altered Intake of Food

A well-balanced diet plus an adequate fluid intake tends to ensure protection against fluid and electrolyte imbalance in the absence of any pathological condition. An unbalanced diet—one that contains disproportionate amounts of carbohydrate, protein, fat, or fluid—is a potential source of danger. Such diets include concentrated tube feedings, high-protein feeding to promote healing, imbalanced weight reduction diets and other fad diets. Serious fluid and electrolyte problems will result from malnutrition, near-starvation, and prolonged fasting.

Altered Intake or Regulation of Electrolytes

A person's food and fluid intake may be balanced and adequate, but manipulation of his electrolytes, either intentionally or unintentionally, can place him at risk. This manipulation or alteration of electrolytes can result from a low-sodium diet, diuretic therapy, taking incompatible medications, failure to take prescribed medications as ordered, self-medication, or faulty administration of electrolytes via IV fluids.

Predisposing Conditions

Some people are vulnerable because of conditions that predispose them to fluid or electrolyte imbalance. Such conditions include chronic kidney disease, congestive heart failure, diabetes, prolonged immobility, and ascites.

ASSESSMENTS

It is important to know the signs and symptoms of each specific type of fluid and electrolyte imbalance, but it is even more important to know which areas should be assessed *before* an imbalance has developed. These areas should be assessed for two reasons. First, it is important to learn what is "normal" for a given patient. For example, it is advisable to know the amount of his *usual* fluid intake before prescribing an amount

TABLE 31.3 ASSESSMENTS RELATED TO FLUID BALANCE

Area of Concern	Aspects to Be Assessed
Intake and output	Total amount of fluid taken in and lost, and the relationship between the two
Urine	Concentration (check specific gravity if urine is very pale and dilute or very dark and concentrated)
Weight	Gain or loss (a change of more than 0.5 kg (1.1 lb) in 24 hours usually indicates a gain or loss of *fluid;* changes related to caloric intake are usually slower)
Tissue	Condition of mucous membranes of mouth, turgor of skin, filling of peripheral and neck veins, and presence of edema (puffy eyelids, swollen fingers or ankles, swelling over sacrum)
Respiration	Rate and depth, presence of dyspnea, or moist rales
Mentation	Increase or decrease in level of consciousness, presence of confusion, or headache
Muscle tone	Weakness, twitching, flaccidity (flabbiness), spasms

of fluid that would supposedly constitute an increased intake. Second, these areas should be assessed regularly so that any change can be noted and evaluated as soon as possible (Table 31.3).

REGULATION OF ORAL FLUID INTAKE

The majority of people maintain an adequate fluid balance by drinking whenever they are thirsty. Under certain conditions, however, criteria other than thirst are used to determine how much a person can or should drink, and his fluid intake must be increased or restricted accordingly.

Increased Intake

A person's fluid intake must be increased whenever he is losing larger-than-normal amounts of fluid, when he is in danger of developing urinary tract stones, or when he has an infection or fever. The amount of fluid prescribed depends on the age, size, and condition of the patient. The phrase "force fluids" usually means an intake of about 2,500 to 3,000 ml (2-½ to 3 qt) per day for an adult.

The most important aspects of increasing fluid intake are the person's preference, choice of fluids, and pacing. Within the limits of any dietary restrictions, such as a low-sodium or a diabetic diet, the fluids should be as varied or monotonous as the patient desires. Some people have a few favorite fluids and will drink these until the prescribed amount is reached. For example, a coffee drinker who must increase his fluid intake by 1,000 ml per day may prefer to drink an extra six or seven cups of coffee (even if it must be decaffeinated) rather than a variety of juices or other fluids. Other people find it very difficult to drink when they are not thirsty and can manage to do so only when provided a wide variety of tempting liquids, including gelatin, sherbet, ice cream, and ice pops, if permitted.

When fluid intake must be greatly increased, it is imperative that nurse and patient work together to prepare a schedule which, if followed, will ensure that the prescribed fluid intake is achieved within each 24-hour period. The total amount of fluid prescribed, less the amount of fluid normally taken with meals, equals the amount of fluid to be scheduled throughout the day. This amount, divided by the patient's number of waking hours, indicates the *amount to be taken each hour.*

Many patients prefer to drink more fluids during the day than are scheduled and little or none during the evening so they will not have to get up during the night to urinate. Other patients, who are normally wakeful during the night do not share this concern.

Every patient, *adult or child,* should know his fluid goal for the day and should know at any time during the day whether or not his fluid intake is on schedule. Given a chart, even a small child can cross out a picture of a cup of milk, a glass of juice, or an ice pop as it is finished.

If a patient is not achieving his scheduled intake, he must be helped and encouraged to drink throughout the day because it is extremely difficult for a patient who is not thirsty to make up a large fluid deficit at the end of the day. Children can often be tempted to drink from novel containers or utensils. The opportunity to drink through a straw, drink directly from a soft drink bottle, use a doll teapot and little cups, spoon water from a dish, or play at being a baby and drink from a baby bottle will often capture the imagination of a child and help him to drink more fluid (even though such tactics may seem unnecessary to some adults).

Restricted Intake

It is sometimes necessary to restrict, either completely or partially, a patient's oral fluid intake. A patient may be ordered NPO for a short period before surgery, before certain diagnostic tests, or while he is nauseated and vomiting. Oral fluids may be limited or severely restricted for extended periods when a patient is unable to produce and excrete adequate amounts of urine because of kidney disease. When fluids are severely limited for any length of time, the patient's thirst may begin to symbolize deprivation, neglect, or abuse; and his physical and psychological discomfort can cause him to beg for or even "steal" a drink. Patients have been known to drink bath water, water from flowers or other patients, and even their own urine in frantic efforts to relieve their thirst. The problem of restricted intake and other problems related to kidney failure are averted for some patients by kidney dialysis; but when such therapy is not possible, nursing measures to minimize the discomfort of thirst are essential. Such measures include the careful timing and rationing of permitted fluids, good mouth care, and the use of illusion and diversion. They are described below.

Timing and Rationing

Because eating distends the stomach and tends to decrease thirst for 1 to 2 hours, it is advisable to curtail the amount of fluid served with meals if the patient concurs, thereby increasing the amount available at other times. It is especially important to help the patient spread his allotted intake over the entire day. This is done by removing all stimuli that tempt him to drink a large amount at once, such as a full pitcher of water at his bedside. Sweet, salty, and dry foods stimulate thirst and should be omitted from the diet.

Mouth Care

Good oral hygiene is needed to prevent an accumulation of thick mucus and dried secretions in the mouth. Decreased or absent salivary secretion can also cause *parotitis* (inflammation of the parotid glands) or *stomatitis* (inflammation of the mucous membranes of the mouth). Some authorities recommend the use of hard candy and chewing gum to stimulate the secretion of saliva, but others think the overall long-term effect of such measures is increased thirst and dryness of the mucous membranes.

The agents used for mouth care must be carefully evaluated because some solutions, such as lemon juice and glycerine, are initially refreshing but tend to increase thirst and dryness after a short period of time.

Illusion

Measures that give the illusion of larger amounts of fluid are useful. Receiving a *small glass completely filled* often makes a person feel more satisfied and less deprived than receiving a large glass only half full. A small glass of chopped ice looks like a lot of fluid, but the *liquid* volume of ice is only about half that of an equal volume of water. It is necessary to melt and measure the water obtained from a specific number of ounces of chopped ice before serving a similar portion to a patient because the size of the ice chips will affect the amount of water produced when the ice melts.

Very cold liquids tend to inhibit the desire to drink. A person is usually unable to drink as much as he could if the liquid were warmer, but he may feel temporarily satisfied. This phenomenon makes possible the practice at some fairs, for example, of offering fairgoers "All the milk you can drink—FREE." The milk is served at a temperature only a few degrees above freezing; although it tastes delicious, a person is unable to drink more than a small amount of it.

A patient may find it helpful to hold water in his mouth for a few moments and then spit it out. The satisfaction and the relief of discomfort may last no longer than 15 to 20 minutes, so this measure may need to be repeated at frequent intervals. Needless to say, this option can be offered only to those patients who will not swallow the water.

Diversion

Diversion is useful in helping a patient who is preoccupied with his thirst and his desire to drink. An engrossing hobby, game, or conversation with others can help him forget his discomfort and distress for at least a little while.

When a patient's kidney function requires a severe curtailment of fluid and he is unable to control his urge to drink, he will require the help and assistance of external controls. In extreme situations he must be denied access to all sources of water and other fluids, and the nursing staff and his family must monitor his activities.

INTRAVENOUS THERAPY

Fluids are given intravenously when a patient is physically incapable of taking adequate liquids by mouth, or when his situation prohibits fluid by mouth. Fluids are also given intravenously when a patient needs rapid correction of either a fluid or an electrolyte imbalance. Intravenous therapy is administered to:

Restore or maintain fluid volume
Restore or maintain electrolyte balance
Meet the nutritional needs of the patient
Supply one or more of the components of blood
Facilitate the administration of drugs

Administration

The physician prescribes the solution that is to be infused and in some situations may actually start the IV.

In other situations, a specially trained nurse may do so. Some large institutions maintain an IV therapy department with a team of technicians who are responsible for all IV infusions throughout the hospital. Nurses usually add the subsequent bottles of solution as ordered, but the IV team is called whenever a problem develops. State law and institutional policy determine the circumstances under which a nurse is permitted to start an IV and to add medications or a unit of blood.

Nursing Responsibilities

Regardless of who orders and starts the IV, the nurse is largely responsible for the safety of the procedure and for the comfort of the patient.

SAFETY. The safety of an IV infusion depends on sterility of the procedure, accuracy of administration, early detection of untoward effects, and preservation of the patient's usable veins.

COMFORT. It is very important to remember that, for most patients, an IV is never routine. An IV may confirm a patient's fear that his condition is very serious; it may be viewed as an additional hazard and a source of infection or other complications. If the IV is being given to make up a fluid or nutritional deficiency, it may be perceived by the patient as punishment for not eating or drinking enough. For many patients, concern over the functioning of the IV equipment is a constant stressor and source of anxiety. Some patients dare not move while an IV is running for fear of disturbing the needle or doing something else wrong. Because of concerns such as these, the nurse must be sensitive to the patient's *psychological comfort* or discomfort with respect to IV therapy.

The patient's *physical comfort* will depend on the extent to which his mobility is restricted and the condition of the IV site. Depending on the location of the venipuncture, the patient will need varying amounts of assistance to move, turn, and exercise without dislodging the needle. Whenever possible, he should be encouraged to ambulate, using a portable IV pole on casters. If it is necessary to restrain the patient to keep him from pulling out the needle and injuring the vein, he should be released from the restraint at regular intervals for periods of supervised movement, exercise, and skin care.

An IV infusion that is running properly should not be uncomfortable. Therefore, complaints of pain or discomfort should be investigated to rule out a serious problem such as infiltration of fluid or irritation of the vein and incipient thrombophlebitis. Some drugs, such as potassium, are extremely irritating to the wall of the vein and are painful if the IV is allowed to run too fast.

It may be necessary, therefore, to slow the rate in order for the patient to be able to tolerate the infusion. Because of the variables and the complexity of IV therapy, any discomfort can indicate a serious problem, and each and every complaint should be thoroughly investigated at once.

Equipment

The equipment needed to start and administer an IV infusion includes:

A container of IV fluid

Tubing and a needle

Some means of regulating the rate of flow

A place to hang the container of fluid

A tourniquet, antiseptic, and adhesive tape (Fig. 31.4).

Fluid Containers

Intravenous fluids are vacuum packed in sterile glass bottles or plastic bags that usually contain 250, 500, or 1,000 ml. Glass containers have two openings; one opening permits fluid to flow out, while the other lets air flow in to equalize the pressure as fluid is removed. Both openings must be uncovered when an IV is started.

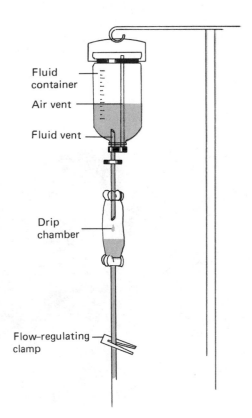

Fluid
container

Air vent

Fluid vent

Drip
chamber

Flow–regulating
clamp

Figure 31.4 *Basic intravenous setup consisting of fluid container, tubing with drip chamber, and clamp.*

Since plastic bags are collapsible, there is no need to equalize the pressure in order to prevent a vacuum; the bag simply collapses as the fluid drains out, and a second opening for air is not needed.

Needles

IV needles are made of either steel or flexible plastic. The choice of needle depends on the age and size of the patient, the site to be used, and the condition of the vein. A steel needle is used when the vein is difficult to enter, and a needle with side pieces, called a *butterfly* needle (Fig. 31.5, top), is used when it is difficult to stabilize the needle and hold it in place. A flexible plastic catheter permits more movement of the extremity and is often used when the IV site is near a joint.

A steel needle is often used in conjunction with a plastic catheter, and the set is referred to as an *intracath* (Fig. 31.5, bottom) or an *angiocath* (middle). The catheter is threaded through or attached to a rigid needle; after the venipuncture, the needle is withdrawn, leaving the flexible catheter in place.

Tubing

IV tubing is transparent so that fluid levels and the presence of air bubbles or blood can be seen. One end of the tubing has an attachment for the needle and is kept covered until attached to the needle. The other end has a sharp, rigid, hollow spike that is pushed into the appropriate opening in the container of fluid.

A number of inline devices are often included or can be attached to the tubing to increase the precision of administration or the versatility of the setup. Such devices include a filter when blood is given and attachments that permit the addition of medications or the

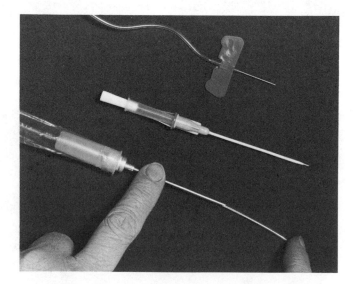

Figure 31.5 *Intravenous needles.* Top: *butterfly needle.* Middle: *angiocath.* Bottom: *intracath.*

addition of a second bottle containing another type of IV fluid.

Regulators

The rate of flow of an IV can be regulated manually or by an infusion pump. Manual control involves the use of one or more clamps and a drip chamber in the tubing (Figure 31.4). The drip chamber enables the nurse to count the number of drops per minute and to increase or decrease the rate by adjusting the clamp on the tubing.

An infusion pump is an electronic device that automatically controls the infusion drop rate. The infusion pump can be adjusted to regulate the flow of fluid through various kinds of IV equipment, and it is essential that it be adjusted in accordance with the brand of equipment being used. For example, if the pump is set for use with fluids and tubing from one manufacturer, it must be reset before it can accurately regulate fluid through equipment from another manufacturer. It has an automatic shutoff and an alarm that sounds when the fluid container empties or when the selected infusion rate is not being maintained. Battery-operated rate meters are also available. Infusion pumps are used in pediatrics, intensive care units, and for any patient who is especially vulnerable to circulatory overload.

Sites

The selection of a site for venipuncture depends in part on the condition of the patient's veins and on his need for IV therapy in the future. The selection of a site is not usually a problem for a person with healthy veins who will need IVs for only a few hours or a few days. The choice of a vein can be critical, however, for a patient who must undergo long-term IV therapy or who has veins that are fragile and sclerosed from frequent or continued IV's.

When there are several possible sites, the following criteria for selection are used:

- The vein should be easily accessible (near the surface of the body).
- The site should *not* be over a joint. Such a site requires immobilization of the joint to prevent displacement of the needle and causes patient discomfort.
- The *nondominant* hand or arm should be used to give the patient as much freedom and independence as possible.
- The smaller, *distal* veins should be used before the larger, proximal ones. For example, the back of the hand should be used before the forearm, and

both should be used before the antecubital space in the elbow. If the proximal vein site is damaged or rendered useless, the more distal part of that vein cannot be used.

Preferred sites are the dorsum of the hand and the forearm for children and adults, and the veins of the scalp for an infant. These sites permit maximum movement for the patient and save the larger veins for future use.

When the superficial veins are no longer usable or are not accessible because of a cast or dressings, it may be necessary to use a deeper and less accessible vein. A surgical incision is made in the vein, and a fine, radiopaque catheter is threaded into the vein and held in place with a suture or two. This method of entering a vein is called a *cut-down* and is used for long-term therapy. The sub-clavian vein is a common site with the catheter threaded into the superior vena cava.

The choice of a site is affected by the condition of the patient's extremities. The use of a paralyzed arm or leg is debatable because, although its use for an IV would not be restrictive or uncomfortable for the patient, it would be potentially dangerous inasmuch as he could not feel and report the early indications of a complication.

A patient who has had a radical mastectomy should not have an IV in the adjacent arm because lymphatic drainage from that arm is likely to have been surgically disrupted if the lymph nodes in the axilla were involved. Such disturbance of lymphatic circulation is liable to cause swelling that could interfere with venous circulation throughout the arm.

During prolonged IV therapy, the physician or the IV team may quite literally begin to run out of places to start an IV, and every effort must therefore be made to "save" each usable vein. The objective of such efforts is to keep the needle or catheter patent (open) because, when an IV ceases to function, it is usually necessary to restart it in a different vein. To preserve the integrity of each vein for as long as possible, the nursing staff should do the following:

- Check the position of the needle and the flow of solution frequently to make sure that the needle is still positioned properly in the vein.
- Immobilize the extremity if necessary to keep the needle in the proper position.
- Move and turn the patient carefully so that the IV tubing does not become kinked or caught under his body, shutting off the flow of fluid.
- Do not let the IV tubing sag below the level of the needle. If this happens, blood will flow from the

vein back into the tubing unless the container of fluid is raised or the rate of flow is increased to compensate for the level of the tubing and to prevent the backflow of blood.

- Do not let the container of fluid run dry. If there is going to be a brief delay in adding the next container, *slow the rate of flow* to keep the small amount of remaining fluid from running in too fast.
- Have a container of an approved fluid ready for use if the prescribed fluid is infused before the next one has been ordered. An order for this action is often abbreviated KVO (keep vein open). The interim fluid (often normal saline solution) is run at the slowest rate that will keep the vein open, usually about 10 ml/h.

Solutions

IV fluids are categorized as isotonic, hypertonic, or hypotonic. An *isotonic* solution has the same osmolality as plasma and interstitial fluid. It can be added to intravascular fluid without affecting its osmolality and without causing fluid to shift into or out of the cells. Isotonic fluids are used to replace or maintain blood volume. Commonly used isotonic fluids are 0.9 percent NaCl, which is called *normal saline* (NS), and 5 percent dextrose in water (D_5W), called *5 percent D and W.*

A *hypertonic* solution has an osmolality greater than that of extracellular fluid. An IV infusion of a hypertonic solution increases the osmolality of ECF and causes intracellular fluid to shift out of the cells in an attempt to dilute the more concentrated ECF. It causes the cells to shrink. Examples of hypertonic fluids are D_5NS (5 percent dextrose in normal saline), $D_{10}W$ (10 percent dextrose in water), and $D_{10}NS$ (10 percent dextrose in normal saline). (Note that D_5NS is hypertonic, while D_5W is isotonic. A solution of normal saline is already isotonic, so the addition of 5 percent dextrose increases its osmolality and makes it hypertonic.)

A *hypotonic* solution has an osmolality lower than that of ECF. An IV infusion of a hypotonic solution decreases the osmolality of the ECF, which then moves toward the cells to dilute the more concentrated ICF. The cells absorb fluid and swell, thereby replacing any fluid lost through dehydration. Examples of hypotonic solutions include one-half strength normal saline (0.45 percent saline) and less than 5 percent dextrose in water.

Lactated Ringer's is an isotonic solution of H_2O, Na^+, K^+, Cl^-, Ca^+, and lactate. It is used as an alkalinizing solution.

Dextran is a polymer of glucose solution in which the molecules are too large to pass through the capillaries readily. Dextran holds water in the vascular system and maintains the blood volume. It is used as a plasma extender or plasma substitute; it is not used as a food.

Rate of Administration

The prescribed rate for an IV infusion depends on:

Age and size of the patient
Urgency of the need for the fluid or drug
Nature of the fluid
Cardiac and renal status of the patient
Size of the vein being used
Reaction of the patient to the infusion

The rate of an infusion is designated in two ways: the number of *milliliters per hour* and the number of *drops per minute.* The physician's written order will specify either the number of milliliters per hour, or the total number of hours allotted for the complete infusion of the prescribed fluid. If the order specifies total hours for infusion, the nurse must calculate the number of milliliters that must be infused each hour to accomplish this. If, for example, a patient is to receive 3,000 ml of fluid in a 24-hour period, the fluid must run at a rate of 125 ml/hour.

$$\frac{\text{Total amount of solution}}{\text{Total number of hours}} = \frac{3,000 \text{ ml}}{24 \text{ hours}} = 125 \text{ ml/hour}$$

To make certain that all staff can tell whether or not the IV fluids are being infused according to schedule, a *time tape* or *flow strip* is attached to the IV bottle. This strip of paper or tape indicates the hour at which the IV was started, the amount that should have been administered at the end of each succeeding hour, and the hour at which the IV should be finished (Fig. 31.6).

The IV infusion must be *on schedule at all times* because there is no way in which it can be speeded up safely. Administration that is too rapid exposes the patient to the risk of circulatory overload, which is a serious threat to cardiac function. Circulatory overload can be fatal to an infant or a small child, an aged person, or a patient in a state of cardiac or renal failure.

To achieve the calculated hourly rate of administration, it is necessary to know the rate per minute so that the flow can be adjusted from time to time as needed to keep on schedule. The rate per minute represents the number of milliliters per minute but is measured and recorded in drops per minute because drops are easily counted and regulated. The calculations of this rate is based on the *drop factor,* which is equal to the number of drops in each milliliter of solution.

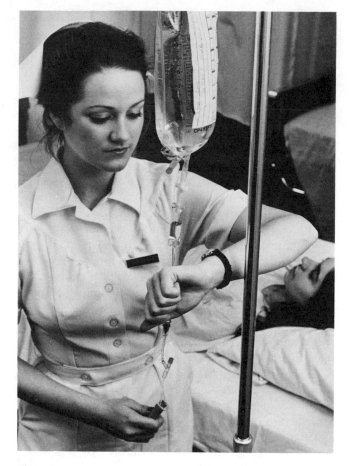

Figure 31.6 *Nurse regulates the drops-per-minute rate of fluid flow. Note the flow strip on the container of fluid.*

The drop factor is determined by the size of the opening at the bottom of the drip chamber of the IV set; the larger the opening, the larger the drop of fluid and the fewer the number of drops in a milliliter of fluid. Each manufacturer prints the drop factor for his equipment either on the IV set itself or on the carton in which it is packaged. The more common drop factors are 15 drops/ml, 20 drops/ml, and 60 drops/ml.

The drop-per-minute rate can be determined by dividing the milliliters-per-hour rate by 60 to obtain the milliliters-per-minute rate, and then multiplying that number by the drop factor to get the drop-per-minute rate.

Two formulas are needed to determine the drop/minute rate:

Step 1 $\dfrac{\text{ml/hour}}{60} = \text{ml/minute}$

Step 2 $\text{ml/minute} \times \text{drop factor} = \text{drops/minute}$

Sample Problem

What is the drop/minute rate for an IV scheduled to run at 125 ml/hour with a drop factor of 20 drops/ml?

Solution:

Step 1 $\dfrac{ml/hour}{60} = ml/minute$

$\dfrac{125}{60} = 2.1 \ ml/minute$

Step 2 $ml/minute \times drop factor = drops/minute$
$2.1 \times 20 = 42 \ drops/minute$

This patient's IV should therefore be adjusted so that it flows at a rate of 42 drops/minute in order to achieve the prescribed rate of 125 ml/hour.

Rate adjustments are made by loosening or tightening the clamp on the tubing, and it is likely that the nurse will need to make several small adjustments to obtain the correct rate of flow. The rate of flow is timed with a second hand after each new adjustment.

The calculation and maintenance of the correct rate of flow is one of the most critical aspects of IV therapy. Because any of a number of variables will alter the rate of flow, it is necessary for the nurse to stop by the bedside and count the number of drops per minute at regular intervals. Many of the variables are discussed in Chapter 11. These laws of physics should be studied or reviewed so that you can adjust the equipment of an IV infusion in a manner that will achieve the prescribed rate of flow safely.

The variables that influence the rate of flow include size of needle, diameter of tubing, viscosity of fluid, height of fluid container, and the venous BP of the patient. Kinks and compression of the tubing can obliterate the patency of the tubing and stop the flow of fluid. Raising or lowering the patient's bed can alter the rate of flow.

Complications

Infiltration

Infiltration of IV fluid into the interstitial spaces of the tissue around a vein occurs whenever the tip of the needle or the intravenous catheter punctures the wall of the vein, allowing fluid to accumulate *outside* the vein. Infiltration should be suspected whenever an IV slows or stops running. Other indications of infiltration are discomfort or pain, and localized swelling at the site. The skin in the area usually feels cool to the touch and looked blanched (pale or white).

It is common practice to test for infiltration by lowering the container of IV fluid below the level of the needle and watching for a backflow of blood. If there is a backflow of blood, the needle is supposedly in the vein; if no blood appears in the tubing, the point of the needle is considered to be outside the vein. This test is not reliable because a backflow of blood can occur when the level of the needle is not entirely outside the vessel wall; some fluid can be escaping into surrounding tissues while some is flowing into the vein. Furthermore, this test is not reliable because the absence of a backflow of blood does not always indicate infiltration; it may mean that the bevel of the needle is pressed against the vessel wall, thereby blocking any backflow.

Two reliable signs of infiltration are swelling at the site and an IV that still drips when a tourniquet is applied to the extremity (Mitchell, 1977). If the needle is properly positioned in the vein, the application of a tourniquet will increase the venous pressure enough to check the flow of the IV fluid. If, however, the point of the needle is outside the vein, the IV fluid can continue to run despite increased pressure within the vein.

In addition to being uncomfortable and often painful, an infiltrated IV can be dangerous because some drugs, such as antimetabolites (anticancer drugs) and potassium, cause necrosis (death of tissue) and sloughing of the involved tissue. Thus, when an IV stops running and infiltration is suspected, it is important to check the patency and pressure of the IV setup. Causes—other than infiltration—of slowed or stopped flow of fluid through the tubing and needle are:

Kinked tubing

Compressed tubing (the patient may be lying on it)

Improperly adjusted clamp (it may be closed too tightly)

Inadequate hydrostatic pressure (it may be necessary to raise the container of fluid)

Faulty position of the extremity (the needle may be pressed against the wall of the vein)

All of these possibilities should be checked and the equipment adjusted to confirm the suspicion that the IV has infiltrated before calling the physician or a member of the IV team to come and restart the IV in a different site.

Phlebitis

Inflammation of the vein (phlebitis) at the site of an IV can be caused by *mechanical* irritation of the vein by the tip of the needle or catheter, or by *chemical* irritation from drugs or electrolytes. Phlebitis is characterized by the classical signs of inflammation: heat, pain, swelling, and redness. The symptoms of phlebitis, therefore, are warmth, tenderness, and a slight swelling at the site of the IV and redness along the vein, which feels cordlike.

Treatment includes changing the site of the IV and applying hot packs for comfort. In addition to providing comfort, hot packs increase circulation to the area, thereby speeding the transport of nutrients to the area for healing and the removal of waste products from the site. Notify the doctor and arrange for the IV to be restarted in a different site.

Embolism

Two types of emboli are associated with IV infusions: thromboembolism and air embolism.

THROMBOEMBOLISM. A thrombus (blood clot) can be caused by the roughening of the endothelial surface of the vein by an IV needle coupled with a slower-than-usual flow of blood past the roughened area and past the tip of the needle. If the blood clot breaks loose, it is carried by the blood through the venous circulation until it becomes lodged in a blood vessel. If the clot is large enough to obstruct circulation in a vital organ such as a lung, the thromboembolism is very serious indeed. One or more clots can form at the tip of the needle whenever an IV is unintentionally slowed or stopped, and they will obstruct any further flow of IV fluid. Some physicians, nurses, and technicians try to keep the vein usable by forcing fluid from a syringe through the needle in a effort to dislodge the clot. This action is dangerous if the clot is large, and it is therefore prohibited in some institutions. If the clot is small enough to be dislodged by a small amount of pressure, such as the pressure from 2 ml (½ tsp) of sterile normal saline in a hypodermic syringe, the clot is so tiny that it poses little danger as a pulmonary embolism. If more pressure is needed, the clot is large, and attempts to dislodge it could be dangerous.

AIR EMBOLISM. The possibility of a fatal air embolism from air bubbles in a patient's IV tubing has been consistently emphasized, but the hazard is usually exaggerated. The danger of such a complication is minimal because, although it is not possible to study the phenomenon experimentally, it has been calculated that the amount of air needed for a fatal embolism is greater than the total volume of the IV tubing, which is usually not over 5 ml (Mitchell, 1977).

Air bubbles in a patient's IV tubing do, however, pose a serious psychological hazard. The presence of one or more bubbles can raise a patient's level of fear and apprehension to an almost intolerable level. It is important, therefore, to run enough fluid through the tubing to remove all the air *before* attaching the tubing to the needle. This action will prevent stress for the patient and family and will also protect the patient who has an undiagnosed cardiac defect that might make

him more vulnerable to the possible effects of an air embolism.

Circulatory Overload

The overly rapid infusion of IV fluids can produce a *circulatory overload* (hypervolemia) in infants, children, elderly people, and in patients with circulatory and renal problems. The early symptoms of excess fluid are headache, dyspnea, shortness of breath, and a dry cough that later becomes productive of a frothy sputum as fluid begins to accumulate in the lungs. Venous distention occurs which is especially noticeable in the neck veins. The pulse becomes rapid, and the respiratory rate and BP are increased.

A number of things can cause an overly rapid infusion of IV fluid. A curious child or confused adult can open the drip regulator. A simple friction clamp can become caught in the bedding or on the bed frame and be dislodged. A nurse or technician sometimes increases the rate of flow in an effort to "catch up" when the administration of an IV is behind schedule and then fails to slow it down again to the prescribed rate.

Circulatory overload is such a dangerous complication that every effort must be expended to prevent its occurrence. The rate of flow can be preset in some types of IV equipment, but in the absence of such a safeguard, there are a number of ways to protect the patient. Some of these protective actions are:

- Position the flow regulator so that it cannot be reached by irresponsible or confused persons or become caught in the bedding
- Always use a flow strip to monitor the rate of infusion
- Check the actual rate of infusion against the scheduled rate at frequent intervals
- Do not infuse the fluid at a rate faster than ordered. Do not try to "catch up" when administration has been too slow unless an increased rate has been ordered *in writing* and unless you are in almost constant attendance
- Check the condition of especially susceptible patients at frequent intervals
- If the patient's circulatory status is precarious, use *small containers of fluid* rather than the usual 1 L size to minimize the possibility of an accidental overly rapid infusion

Assessments Related to IV Therapy

The assessments described below should be made whenever a nurse first assumes responsibility for the care of a patient with an IV and then at intervals throughout her shift or assigned time with him. It is not safe to omit any of these assessments on the assumption that they were probably made earlier by the person who started the IV or added the last bottle of fluid. If there was an error, of either mission or commission, the nurse then on duty would share responsibility for the error if she failed to notice the mistake or problem and thereby perpetuated it. Three areas to be assessed are the patient, the fluid, and the equipment.

The Patient
Although the importance of assessing the patient seems obvious, a nurse could enter a patient's unit, check the level of his IV fluid and possibly the rate of flow, and leave the unit without even glancing at the patient. If he happened to be lying on his side, with his back to the IV, he could be experiencing a severe reaction, of which the nurse would be unaware.

It is important to make at least a cursory assessment of the patient each time you check his equipment. Even a quick assessment will provide basic data related to rate and depth of respiration, presence of dyspnea or cough, level of consciousness, and any symptoms that might indicate an adverse reaction to the fluid, medications, or rate of flow.

The IV site should be inspected at regular intervals for temperature, color, and the presence or absence of swelling. The use of the single question "How does your arm feel?" gives the patient an opportunity to report and describe any discomfort, such as pain, that might be an early sign of some complication.

The Fluid
Check all labels on the container of fluid to make sure the patient is receiving the right fluid. The fluid itself should be crystal clear; there should be no cloudiness, sediment, or discoloration in it. The level of the fluid should be appropriate for the current hour, as determined by the flow strip on the container.

The Equipment
The following assessments should be made at frequent, regular intervals:

RATE OF FLOW. Count the number of drops per minute; or, if an infusion pump is being used, determine the rate of flow from the machine gauge. If the rate of flow is too slow or too fast, check the height of the container of fluid and adjust it as necessary before you proceed to make other adjustments.

TUBING. Tubing should not be kinked, compressed, or dangling below the level of the mattress. There should be no tension on it; the patient should be able to move and turn without pulling on it.

DRIP CHAMBER. The drip chamber should be partially filled with fluid.

DRIP REGULATOR. The regulator should be out of reach of any person, child or adult, who does not understand the importance of the prescribed rate of flow.

Basic Procedures

Preparing IV Fluids
The initial steps in preparing IV fluids include: (1) checking the physician's written order; (2) obtaining a container of the prescribed fluid; (3) examining the bottle of fluid for possible cracks and the fluid itself for cloudiness, sediment, or discoloration that might indicate contamination; and (4) labeling the container. The label should include the patient's name and the number of that container (such as No. 1 of 4 that have been ordered) as well as the name and dose of any medications that have been added.

The nurse should then calculate the *hourly rate of flow* and prepare and attach a flow strip to the container so that all staff can tell whether or not the rate of administration is on schedule. Finally, she must calculate the *drops-per-minute rate* so that she can regulate the rate of flow as soon as the IV has been started. *All calculations should be done with paper and pencil*, and another person should check them as needed to ensure accuracy.

Preparing an IV Setup
Select the appropriate IV setup and check the package for rips, tears, punctures, dampness, or other damage that would permit contamination of the contents. If a package has been opened or damaged in any way, the contents should not be used. Next, open both the package and the container of fluid, and attach the tubing to the container, using sterile technique. When the container of fluid is opened, a characteristic sound should be heard when the vacuum in the container is broken. The sound differs, depending on whether a glass bottle or plastic bag is opened, but it is still evident that a vacuum has been broken. If this sound is not heard, the fluid should not be used.

Push the sterile spike at the end of the tubing into the correct opening. Make sure the clamp on the tubing is closed to keep the fluid from running out. Then hang the container of fluid so that you can use both hands to remove the air from the tubing. Remove the protector from the end of the tubing, keeping both the protector and the end of the tubing sterile. Open the clamp and let fluid run through the tubing into a basin to remove all bubbles of air. Close the clamp and replace the protective cover over the end of the tubing.

Starting an Intravenous Infusion

Each hospital has an accepted procedure for starting an IV, and the person designated for this task will indicate what assistance, if any, is needed. The following guidelines are related to the kinds of assistance that may be expected of you.

Identify the patient, using his hospital identification band, before the IV is started. (He should already have been told the purpose, expected benefits, and duration of the prescribed IV.) The person starting the IV (physician, member of an IV therapy team, or specially prepared nurse) will select a site and apply a tourniquet. The tourniquet occludes the venous return of blood and makes the vein more prominent and accessible. The skin is cleansed with an antiseptic such as Betadine, the needle is inserted, and the tourniquet released.

The intravenous tubing is attached to the needle, and the clamp is opened enough to let the fluid flow slowly. The needle is taped in place, and the tubing is looped and taped to the skin so that any pull or stress will be on the tubing and not on the needle (Fig. 31.7). The person who starts the IV may regulate the rate of flow or may ask the nurse to do so in accordance with the rate indicated by the physician's order.

Changing Containers

Well *before* it is time to add more IV fluid, you should have the next container of fluid available and labeled with the patient's name, room number, the number of

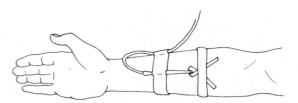

Figure 31.7 *An example of taping that prevents dislodging of the IV needle and tubing. Avoid encircling the arm with tape. Snug wrapping can restrict circulation.*

that container of fluid (such as the second or third of a series) plus the name and amount of any drugs, vitamins, or electrolytes that have been added to the fluid.

To add the new container, slow the rate of flow as much as possible without stopping it, then remove the spike from the empty container and quickly insert it into the full container, keeping the spike sterile. Work quickly so that the drip container does not empty and so that the normal rate of flow can be resumed without delay.

Discontinuing an Infusion

The nurse is usually responsible for removing the IV needle or catheter when all the prescribed fluids have been administered. This action involves the following steps:

• Check both the physician's written order and the patient's identification band before discontinuing an IV. It is costly in terms of time and patient discomfort to have to restart an IV that was removed prematurely or in error.

PROCEDURE 31.1

Setting Up for an IV*

SUMMARY OF ESSENTIAL NURSING ACTIONS

1. Check label of container against doctor's order.
2. Label bottle with patient's name, room number, drip rate, medication, and in accordance with agency policy.
3. Take the labeled bottle, IV set, tourniquet, armboard, cleansing agent, and adhesive to the patient's room.
4. IDENTIFY THE PATIENT.
5. Open the IV set using sterile technique.
6. Uncover the opening(s) in the IV fluid bag or bottle.
7. Insert the spike end of the tubing into the appropriate opening.

8. Move the clamp along the tubing until it is positioned just below the drip chamber, and close the clamp.
9. Hang the fluid bottle or bag on an IV pole.
10. Squeeze and release the drip chamber until it is half full of fluid.
11. *Maintaining sterile technique,* uncover the free end of the tubing, loosen the clamp, and let enough fluid run through tubing into a container to remove the air from the tubing.
12. Tighten the clamp and replace the protective cap on the end of the tubing.
13. Assist the person starting the IV as needed.

*See inside front cover and pages 605–606.

- Take an alcohol sponge or sterile gauze square and an adhesive bandage such as Band-Aid to the patient's bedside.
- Shut off the IV so that any remaining fluid will not run onto the bed linens when the needle or catheter is withdrawn.
- Loosen the adhesive tape without dislodging the needle, which would be uncomfortable for the patient and might injure the vein.
- Apply pressure over the needle with the sterile gauze square or alcohol sponge with one hand, and withdraw the needle with the other.
- Maintain pressure over the site until any bleeding stops and apply the Band-Aid.
- If a catheter was used, examine the tip to make certain that it is intact. This is important because the fine, flexible tip could have been damaged or weakened during insertion. If the tip seems to be irregular instead of smooth, save the catheter and report your observation to the physician or IV team.
- If the patient's extremity was immobilized during the IV and is stiff from disuse, help him to flex the joints and move the extremity, and encourage him to continue exercising it.
- Chart the time and reason the IV was discontinued, the amount of fluid absorbed, and any pertinent data about the condition of the patient.

Changing the Patient's Gown

The process of changing a patient's gown while an IV is running is complicated, but it is often necessary to do so, especially when the patient is perspiring profusely, vomiting, or incontinent. Gowns that snap along the shoulder seam are convenient for both patient and nurse, but any gown can be changed safely. (See boxed material.)

Guidelines for Changing a Gown With an IV Running

1. Remove the sleeve from the patient's *noninvolved* arm. Keep him covered with the top sheet.
2. Remove the IV bottle or container from the pole.
3. Slide the second sleeve off the patient's arm and over the tubing and bottle, keeping the container of fluid at its original height to maintain the prescribed rate of fluid flow.
4. Rehang the fluid container and discard the gown.
5. Unfold the fresh gown and identify the sleeve that must be slipped over the IV setup.
6. While you are facing the front of the gown, slide your arm up into the sleeve from the lower edge of the sleeve toward the neck of the gown.
7. With the sleeve on your arm, grasp the fluid container with that hand and remove the container from the pole. Use your other hand to pull the sleeve off your arm, over the container and tubing, toward the patient's arm.
8. Rehang the container of fluid.
9. Slip that sleeve over the patient's arm and shoulder. Insert the second arm into the second sleeve and tie or fasten the gown.
10. Check and, if necessary, adjust the rate of flow of IV fluid before doing anything else.

When a gown is changed, three precautions are important: (1) do not dislodge the needle, (2) do not kink or disconnect the tubing, (3) keep the container of fluid at approximately its usual height.

Changing the Patient's Position

Whenever the patient turns or is helped to turn in bed, there is a possibility that the needle will be dislodged

---

PROCEDURE 31.2

Discontinuing an IV*

SUMMARY OF ESSENTIAL NURSING ACTIONS

1. Clamp the tubing to stop the flow of IV fluid and/or shut off the IV pump.
2. Remove the arm board if one was used.
3. Open package containing an alcohol sponge or sterile gauze square.
4. Loosen and remove the adhesive tape *without dislodging the needle.*

5. Apply light pressure over the needle with the alcohol sponge or gauze square, and withdraw the needle.
6. Apply firm pressure until any bleeding stops. Apply a Band-aid.
7. Chart the amount of IV fluid absorbed and/or the amount of IV fluid remaining in accordance with agency policy. Indicate the reason the IV was discontinued.

*See inside front cover and pages 606–607.

or the tubing will be disconnected by rough and careless movements. Therefore, *before* the patient is turned, make sure the tubing is free and that it will not be pulled, kinked, compressed, or subjected to strain of any kind during the move. Advise the patient of any precautions to be taken.

If there was any accidental pull on the tubing during the move, check the security of the tubing connections and tighten them as needed. Check the drip rate after the patient has been repositioned and adjust it if necessary.

Patient Responsibility

The patient should be taught that a properly administered IV is not uncomfortable and that he should report either of the following conditions to the nurse at once:

- Pain, discomfort, or swelling at the venipuncture site
- General discomfort or new symptoms that might indicate a systemic reaction to the IV fluid or drugs being administered.

In addition, both the patient and his family should be taught to report the following conditions promptly:

Blood in the tubing
Leaking or disconnected tubing
A nearly empty bottle
An unusually rapid drip rate
An extremely slow or absent drip

FLUIDS BY CENTRAL VENOUS ROUTE

Fluids may be administered by a central venous route. A large vein like the juglar, innominate, or sub-clavian is selected. A catheter is placed through the skin and into one of these veins, and then threaded carefully into the superior vena cava. The insertion of the catheter is done under strict aseptic conditions. The procedure is the same as for the insertion of a central venous pressure line. Fluids and special highly concentrated formulas may be administered by this route. Different catheters are being manufactured for administration of different types of fluids. These catheters may have multiple lumens available for various uses; such as drawing blood and administering fluids. Each lumen must be clearly labeled so that the correct use of the lumen is carefully designated. One complication which accompanies this particular method of infusing fluids is in-

fection. Careful inspection and cleansing of the catheter is described in the hospital procedure manual and should be carefully adhered to by the nurse. Sterile technique is used in changing the dressing.

ADMINISTRATION OF BLOOD

The administration of blood is often the only course of action for treating both serious disorders of the blood and hemorrhage from trauma or disease. The process is exceedingly complex but relatively safe provided adequate safeguards are employed.

Problems related to blood transfusions are caused by improper collection, analysis, and storage of the blood, by careless administration of the blood, or by the patient's physiological response to the blood itself. Complications include hemolytic, allergic, and bacterial reactions; circulatory overload; buildup of citrate or potassium; and occasionally an infectious disease such as hepatitis, malaria, or AIDS.

Transfusion Reactions

A *hemolytic reaction* is the most serious and life-threatening of all transfusion reactions and occurs when a patient receives incompatible (mismatched) blood. Symptoms are caused by the *destruction of red blood cells* (hemolysis), and they include chills, fever, shock, and kidney failure. Death may ensue unless emergency medical care is started at once. Hemolysis is evidenced by hemoglobinemia (free hemoglobin in the plasma) and hemoglobinuria (free hemoglobin in the urine).

An *allergic reaction* is distressing and uncomfortable for the patient but rarely fatal. The exact cause is not known, but the blood donor may have taken drugs or eaten food to which the recipient is allergic. Symptoms include hives, mild edema, nasal congestion, and bronchial wheezing. The transfusion is usually slowed if the reaction is mild, or stopped if it is severe. Medications to relieve the symptoms are administered.

A *bacterial or a pyrogenic reaction* is not common, and severe reactions or fatalities because of contaminated blood are rare as a result of improved aseptic procedures for collecting and storing blood.

Nursing Responsibilities for Administration of Blood

In most settings, nurses assume a major responsibility for the safety of each patient who receives a blood transfusion.

Some aspects of blood administration such as the

collection, laboratory analysis, and storage of blood are beyond the control of the nurse, but the nursing staff is responsible, at least in part, for any error in the actual administration of blood to the patient. The nurse also is responsible for the prompt and detailed assessment of any untoward physiological reactions of the patient.

The details of an approved and safe procedure will vary from setting to setting, but the following responsibilities of the nurse are relatively consistent from one agency to another.

Identification of the Patient

The physician writes the order for typing and cross-matching the patient's blood with a potential donor's blood from the blood bank. If a sample of the patient's blood and the blood that has been selected as a likely match prove to be compatible in every way, the record of this typing and cross-matching initiates a long process of detailed record keeping. When properly done, it is possible to trace each unit of blood from donor to recipient and to verify compliance with each precaution and safeguard along the way.

The laboratory is responsible for guaranteeing that each unit of blood to be administered to a given patient is compatible with the sample of that patient's blood that was received by the laboratory. The nursing staff is largely responsible for ensuring that the blood is administered to the patient for whom it was intended.

Each agency should have a rigorous procedure that will ensure the verification of all data related to the administration of blood. Such data include the reports of all laboratory tests; the final report of the cross-matching including the name of the donor, the patient's name, blood type, hospital number, and hospital location; and data from the label of the unit of blood to be administered. Every form and every label for each step of the process should bear the same identifying number. In some settings the patient's hospital ID number is used throughout the process. If for some reason the patient's identification band has been removed, the laboratory technicians will not supervise the use of that blood. In most settings two or more registered nurses, or a nurse and a physician, must verify the accuracy of all identifying data independently of each other and must sign appropriate documents to certify that this was done. All such documents become part of the patient's record.

If there is any discrepancy whatsoever in the numbers or other identifying data, the blood should be returned to the blood bank at once. If the situation cannot be easily and completely resolved, the whole process must be repeated, starting with blood typing and cross-matching.

Starting a Blood Transfusion

State law and agency policy determine the procedure for starting a transfusion. In many institutions the physician must perform the venipuncture and start the administration of the first unit of blood or blood products, but in most settings a registered nurse is permitted to add a unit of blood to an IV infusion of fluids or to add another unit to an ongoing transfusion of blood.

Blood is more viscous than other IV fluids and a large needle (18 or 19 gauge) must be used in order to permit the passage of red blood cells without damage to their structure, and to permit an adequate rate of flow. The person who hangs a unit of blood is responsible for checking it for bubbles, clots, or any abnormal appearance of the blood. If there has been any destruction of the red blood cells (hemolysis), the plasma will look reddish rather than clear yellow. The container of blood should be *gently* inverted to remix the plasma and the red blood cells that settle to the bottom upon standing. The container should *not* be shaken because such agitation will damage the red blood cells. The person who hangs a unit of blood is responsible for making sure that a filter is in place between the blood and the tubing to remove any possible fibrin clots or collections of white blood cells.

Guidelines for Administration

TEMPERATURE. Blood should be used cold, preferably within 30 minutes after being taken out of the refrigerator. If administration is delayed for any reason, the blood should be returned to the blood bank for proper storage to prevent destruction of the blood cells. The blood need not be warmed before use except for administration to newborns or to patients who might be susceptible to cardiac arrhythmia from massive transfusions of very cold blood. In most situations the blood is sufficiently warmed as it passes through the tubing en route to the patient's body.

RATE. Because transfusion reactions occur most frequently during the first 10 to 15 minutes, the initial rate of infusion should be *very slow*. A rate no greater than 25 ml/15 minute will minimize the number of red blood cells received by the patient while he is being observed for possible adverse reactions. Reactions can occur after as little as 10 ml of blood has been administered. If no reaction occurs during the first 10 to 15 minutes, the rate can be increased to the rate ordered by the physician for the remainder of the infusion. In general, a unit of whole blood (450 ml) can be administered in 1-½ to 2 hours. A slower rate may be needed if the patient has circulatory or renal problems, and a faster rate may be needed if the patient has suffered a severe blood loss. In an emergency, a unit of blood can be infused in less than 10 minutes by using a pressure pump system to deliver the blood rapidly. In any instance, a unit of blood must be transfused in less than 4 hours to minimize the dangers of red blood cell hemolysis and bacterial growth at room temperature.

ADDITIVES. *No medications should be added to blood. No solution except normal saline should be used in conjunction with a transfusion.* This means that the fluid which precedes the unit of blood and which is in the tubing when the blood starts to flow must be normal saline, and only normal saline can be added to the IV setup after the blood has been administered. Any solution containing calcium, for example, can cause clotting, whereas a solution containing dextrose will cause hemolysis of the red blood cells. Such reactions seldom occur when these solutions are given by a separate IV infusion because then the solutes are *rapidly dispersed* throughout the bloodstream rather than slowly interacting with a static unit of blood.

Observation of the Patient

Because some of the early symptoms of a transfusion reaction may resemble symptoms of the patient's existing illness or condition, they can be differentiated only by a careful analysis of any *changes* that become apparent after the transfusion has been started. It behooves the nurse, therefore, to assess the condition of the patient just prior to any administration of blood. Baseline data related to temperature, respiration, pulse, blood presure, and color of skin and nails will provide a basis for later comparison. Changes in vital signs can be detected only when measurements have been taken before the transfusion was started and again during the first 15 minutes of the procedure. Two sets of vital signs are needed to determine the presence and degree of any change.

An assessment of the patient's status in general, plus the presence or absence of pain or other discomfort, will help you to determine whether his difficulty in breathing during a transfusion might be related to the transfusion or whether it had started several hours earlier.

Rather than trying to memorize the symptoms associated with each specific transfusion reaction or complication, you should assess your patient frequently enough throughout the transfusion to be able to detect *every change* in his condition, especially during the first 15 minutes.

The process of assessment must be repeated with

> ### Signs and Symptoms Related to Transfusion Reactions
>
> - Chest pain or a heavy feeling in the chest
> - Difficulty breathing (dyspnea) wheezing, shortness of breath, dry cough
> - Abrupt change in one or more vital signs such as a drop in BP, chills, fever
> - Allergic responses such as hives, itching (pruritus), and rash (urticaria)
> - A burning sensation along the transfused vein
> - Sudden sharp pain in the back or flank

---

each unit of blood because the error-free, safe administration of one unit does not guarantee the safe administration of subsequent units.

Assessment of the patient during the early part of a transfusion is especially important when the patient is unable for any reason to tell the nurse if he suddenly feels bad or to describe his symptoms. An infant or a comatose or confused patient is at great risk during a transfusion unless the nurse is especially observant and attentive.

Support of Patient and Family

To the patient and his family, a blood transfusion can be either a welcome and accepted therapy or a frightening and dreaded experience. Many patients have heard, through the media or from people they know, about people who have had serious or fatal reactions to the accidental administration of mismatched blood, and they fear that it might happen to them. Fears do not necessarily subside when a blood transfusion is over because of the publicity surrounding the rare instances of the transmission of AIDS through a transfusion.

The patient and family both need to know, before the actual transfusion, that blood has been ordered and why. There should be ample opportunity for questions, and a chance to discuss feelings and reactions. Some people are forbidden by their religious beliefs to receive blood while others are merely uneasy or apprehensive about doing so.

A blood transfusion is never a routine procedure, but the assessments you make relative to the possibility of a reaction must appear to be routine to avoid alarming the patient and family. They must not suspect the depth of your concern about safety during a transfusion. Your approach to the patient, therefore, must be based on vigilance, calmness, and empathy.

Nursing Responsibility in the Event of a Transfusion Reaction

Before a transfusion is started, you should always determine your legal and professional responsibility in that particular setting and plan your course of action in advance of any possible reaction. A slow or ineffective response could be fatal for the patient.

Your course of action will be determined by the state nurse practice act and by agency policy as well as by the reality of the situation. If, for example, there is a physician on the nursing unit, you would slow the rate of the transfusion and summon the physician at once. If, however, no physician is immediately available, you should stop the flow of blood and add a container of normal saline to keep the IV line and needle open and ready for use.

The physician may decide, after a careful physical assessment, to continue the blood transfusion. If so, the patient must be observed closely throughout the procedure.

If the transfusion is not continued, the following steps are usually taken:

1. The container of blood is returned to the blood bank with the blood administration set still attached.
2. A blood sample from the other arm and a urine specimen are also sent.
3. A written description of the incident is entered in the patient's chart which includes the time and

---

FLUID INTAKE INCLUDES

- All liquids taken by mouth, including foods that become liquid when melted, such as ice cream, sherbet, gelatin, and cracked ice
- All IV fluids including blood and blood derivatives
- Tube feedings
- Parenteral feedings
- Fluid instilled into a body cavity
- Irrigating fluid that has been *retained* rather than being expelled from the body

FLUID OUTPUT INCLUDES
- Urine
- Vomitus
- Liquid stool
- Perspiration
- Drainage from drainage tubes or a suction machine
- Insensible losses from skin and lungs

---

amount of blood transfused, the patient's reaction, the physician's name, and a precise description of each event that took place.

MEASUREMENT OF FLUID INTAKE AND OUTPUT

Accurate measurement of a patient's fluid intake and output provides the data necessary for making decisions about his *fluid balance*. The degree of balance or imbalance between intake and output helps to assess kidney function and to determine whether fluid intake should be increased or decreased, and it provides a basis for the prescription of drugs to regulate fluid balance.

Both patient and nurse must know the reasons for measuring intake and output. Some of these reasons are:

- To evaluate the relationship between intake and output
- To monitor progress toward the prescribed intake
- To determine how soon and how much the patient urinates after surgery
- To determine whether or not the patient can drink enough to warrant discontinuing the administration of IVs

Knowledge of the reasons for measuring intake and output does not affect the data obtained, but it does affect the subsequent nursing actions. For example, a daily oral intake of 1,200 ml may mean that the patient must more than double his intake if he is to reach a prescribed intake of 2,500 ml per day, and vigorous nursing action may be needed to help him reach that goal. In another situation, an identical intake of 1,200 ml in 24 hours could indicate the need for restricted fluids if the patient's urinary output has fallen to 350 ml for the same period of time.

Intake and output measurements are nearly always ordered together, but in many situations one of them may be more important than the other. Measurements of intake and output are usually totaled and charted at the end of each 8-hour shift, but in cases of severe kidney failure, for example, the measurements must be taken every 1 to 2 hours.

The measurement of some fluids can be done by using the markings on the container. Cartons of milk are labeled with the number of ounces per carton; containers of IV fluids are calibrated in milliliters; and many urinary collection bags are marked with lines that indicate the number of milliliters at a given level. Fluids in uncalibrated containers must be measured.

Intake

Nearly every institution has charts or reference tables that indicate the number of milliliters in each of the most commonly used containers, such as the cup, bowl, and glass on the dinner trays and the patient's bedside water pitcher. In the home, the capacity of each container should be measured and written down for future reference.

It is important to ask the patient how much he has had to drink. It is not safe to assume, for example, that if the water pitcher is half empty, the patient drank one-half of the pitcher of water. It may have been only three-quarters full to start with, or the patient may have used most of it to water his plants.

Output

Because the nurse empties (or supervises the emptying) of all containers of body fluids such as suction bottles, urinary drainage bags, and the bedpan or urinal of a patient confined to bed, these measurements are usually accurate.

Some patients who are on intake and output measurements are given bathroom privileges (BPR) with the expectation that they will collect and measure their own urinary output accurately. These patients must be taught to use a urinal or bedpan in the bathroom instead of the toilet, empty the urine into a graduated measuring device, and record the amount on the I&O measurement (intake and output) record sheet, which is posted in or near the patient's unit. All patients on I&O measurement must also be taught to keep urine and feces separate in order to permit the accurate measurement of urine. A special container, frequently called "a hat," may be used to measure urinary output. It is made to fit under the toilet seat and is comfortable and convenient.

PATIENT TEACHING

For a patient and his family to participate effectively in the prevention or treatment of a fluid or electrolyte imbalance, they must understand:

- How to measure and record oral fluid intake and urinary output.
- The need to observe and report the signs of potential or possible imbalance such as prolonged vom-

iting or diarrhea, edema, scanty or profuse urine, and a *rapid* change in weight.
- The importance of following a prescribed diet and the dangers of fad diets.
- The necessity of compliance in taking prescribed medications and the dangers of self-medication.

SUGGESTED READINGS

Regulation of Body Fluids

Baker, Wendy L: Hypophosphatemia. *Am J Nurs* 1985 Sept; 85(9):999–1003.

Elbaum, Nancy: Hypercalcemia. *Nursing 84* 1984 Aug; 14(8):58–59.

Folk-Lighty, Marie: Solving the puzzles of patients' fluid imbalances. *Nursing 84* 1984 Feb; 14(2):34–41.

Glass, Linda B, and Cheryl A Jenkins: The ups and downs of serum pH. *Nursing 83* 1983 Sept; 13(9):34–41.

Guyton, Arthur C: *Textbook of Medical Physiology.* ed.6. Philadelphia, Saunders, 1981.

Maxwell, Mary B: Pedal edema in the cancer patient. *Am J Nurs* 1982 Aug; 82(8):1225–1228.

Metheny, Norma Milligan, and WD Snively: *Nurse's Handbook of Fluid Balance.* ed. 3. Philadelphia, Lippincott, 1979.

Quinlan, Margo: Edema: what really causes it—how to control it. *RN* 1984 April; 47(4):55–57.

Quinlan, Margo: Solving the mysteries of calcium imbalance: An action guide. *RN* 1982 Nov; 45(11):50–100.

Maintenance of Body Fluids

Anderson, Marjorie A, Saundra N Aker, and Robert O Hickman. The double-lumen hickman catheter. *Am J Nurs* 1982 Feb; 82(2):272–273.

Arthur, Gwen M: When your littlest patients need IVs. *RN* 1984 July; 47(7):30–35.

Bjeletich, Joan, and Robert O Hickman: The hickman indwelling catheter. *Am J Nurs* 1980 Jan; 80(1):62–65.

Blood Therapy (continuing education feature): *Am J Nurs* 1979 May; 79(5):925–948.

——— Rutman, Roanne, et al: Screening donors and the phlebotomy procedures.

——— Kazak, Aldona: Processing blood for transfusion.

——— Collins, Laura C: Preventing and treating transfusion reactions.

——— Buickus, Barbara A: Administering blood components.

———Thomas, Susan F: Transfusing granulocytes.

——— Parker, Anita Lynne: Massive transfusions.

Cohen, Stephen, Jeanne Elizabeth Blust, and Norma Bukna Manos: Fundamentals of IV maintenance (programmed instruction). *Am J Nurs* 1979 July; 79(7):1274–1287.

Feldstein, Arlene: Detect phlebitis and infiltration before they harm your patient. *Nursing 86* 1986 Jan; 16(1):44–47.

Haughey, Brenda: CVP lines: monitoring and maintaining. *Am J Nurs* 1978 April; 78(4):635–638.

Johnston-Early, Anita, Martin H Cohen, and Kathleen S White: Venipuncture and problem veins. *Am J Nurs* 1981 Sept; 81(9):1636–1640.

Keithley, Joyce K, and Kay E Fraulini: What's behind that IV line? *Nursing 82* 1982 March; 12(3):33–42.

Lawson, Millie, Joseph C Botlino, and Kenneth B McCredie: Long-term IV therapy: a new approach. *Am J Nurs* 1979 June; 79(6):1100–1103.

Leser, Deborah Rimmer: Synthetic blood: a future alternative. *Am J Nurs* 1982 March; 82(3):452–455.

Madden, Kathleen, and Lance Adams: Autotransfusion: now it's saving lives in the ED. *RN* 1983 Dec; 46(12):50–53.

Masoorli, Susan Thomas, and Sharon Piercy: A life saving guide to blood products. *RN* 1984 Sept; 47(9):32–37.

Masoorli, Susan Thomas, and Sharon Piercy: A step-by-step guide to trouble-free transfusions. *RN* 1984 May; 47(5):34–42.

Masoorli, Susan Thomas: Tips for trouble-free subclavian lines. *RN* 1984 Feb; 47(2):38–39.

Mascaro, Jane: Managing IV therapy in the home. *Nursing 86* 1986 May; 16(5):50–51.

Nelson, Ramona, and Helen Miller: Keeping air out of IV lines. *Nursing 86* 1986 March; 16(3):57–59.

Ostrow, Lynne Stanton: Air embolism and cental venous lines. *Am J Nurs* 1981 Nov; 81(11):2036–2038.

Querin, Janice Johnson, and Linda Dixon Stahl: 12 simple, sensible steps for successful blood transfusions. *Nursing 83* 1983 Nov; 13(11):34–43.

Runquist, Barbara, Joyce Aspinall, and Lucy Hibbard: A new approach for problem IV dressings. *RN* 1984 June; 47(6):49–51.

Steel, Jennifer: Too fast or too slow—The erratic IV. *Am J Nurs* 1983 June; 83(6):898–901.

Wilkes, Gail, Paula Vannicola, and Paulette Starck: Long-term venous access. *Am J Nurs* 1985 July; 85(7):793–795.

32

Respiration and Circulation

Prerequisites and/or Suggested Preparation
A basic knowledge of the anatomy and physiology of the respiratory and circulatory systems, pathophysiology (Chapter 12), and techniques of percussion and auscultation of the chest (Chapter 18, Section 5) are prerequisite to this chapter.

The ultimate purpose of respiration is the oxygenation of body cells and the elimination of excess carbon dioxide from the body. This goal cannot be accomplished by the respiratory system alone since the gases must be transported to and from the most remote cells of the body by the circulatory system. The functions of the respiratory and circulatory systems are so interrelated that, in some contexts, it is inappropriate to try to consider them separately. This chapter, therefore, includes both respiration and those aspects of circulation that affect the transportation of gases to and from the body cells.

OXYGENATION

Although no cell of the body can survive without oxygen, the cells of the brain are especially sensitive, and cerebral anoxia (lack of oxygen) results in brain damage within approximately 5 minutes. Biologic death usually occurs within 10 minutes.

The oxygenation of body cells depends on the combined actions of both the respiratory and the circulatory systems. The action of the respiratory system alone is not sufficient, for two reasons. First, an adequate supply and intake of oxygen cannot oxygenate the cells unless it reaches them, anymore than plentiful food in a grocery store can nourish a family a few miles away unless the food is transported to them. Second, the organs of the respiratory system cannot function unless the circulatory system supplies them with blood. If, for example, the blood supply to the lungs were cut off, the cells of the lungs would soon die from lack of oxygen, making respiration impossible.

The interdependence of the circulatory and respiratory systems is demonstrated dramatically during either cardiac or respiratory arrest. During cardiac arrest, blood is no longer pumped to the brain. As a result, the respiratory center in the brain fails, and the person stops breathing. During respiratory arrest, breathing ceases, and the blood cannot be oxygenated. Because the cells of the heart muscle cannot survive for long without oxygen, when respiration fails, the heart soon fails.

The interdependence of these two systems is the basis for instituting *coordinated cardiopulmonary* resuscitation in an emergency rather than providing artificial ventilation and cardiac compression as separate entities. A skilled rescuer, even when working alone, can quickly institute cardiopulmonary resuscitation, thereby restoring both circulatory and respiratory function.

RESPIRATORY PROCESSES

Respiration is the transportation both of oxygen from the atmosphere to every cell of the body, and of carbon dioxide from each cell out to the atmosphere. The phases of this process are delineated in various ways by different authors. This text uses four phases to describe the processes of respiration: (1) pulmonary ventilation, (2) diffusion, (3) circulation, and (4) regulation.

Pulmonary ventilation is the movement of air in and out of the lungs, between the atmosphere and the alveoli. *Diffusion* is the movement of oxygen and carbon dioxide between the alveoli and the blood, and between the blood and the cells. *Circulation* is the transport of oxygen and carbon dioxide by blood and other body fluids to and from the cells. *Regulation of respiration* refers to the neural and chemical control of all phases of respiration.

Pulmonary Ventilation

Anatomical Structures

The anatomical structures involved in ventilation are the diaphragm, the external muscles of inspiration and expiration, and the organs depicted in Fig. 32.1.

NOSE. The nose has three important functions: (1) The nose filters the air before it reaches the lungs. Foreign particles are trapped by fine hairs (cilia) and are expelled by sneezing or blowing the nose. (2) The nose moistens air before it reaches the lungs. Water is picked up by the air as it passes over the moist mucous membranes. This prevents dry air from reaching the lungs, where it would dry the alveolar membranes and interfere with both diffusion and respiratory defense mech-

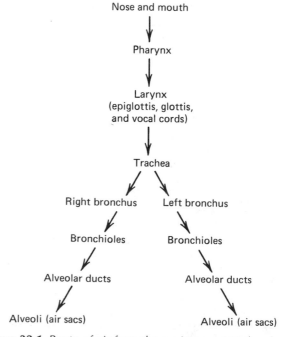

Figure 32.1 Route of air from the environment to the alveoli.

anisms. (3) The nose warms incoming air. As air flows through the nasal passages, it is warmed to body temperature. This prevents cold air from reaching the lungs, where it would cause vasoconstriction of capillaries and interfere with gas exchange. In addition, the increased warmth enables the air to carry more moisture.

LARYNX. The larynx contains the vocal cords and epiglottis, which protect the lungs in two ways. First, these structures close during the act of swallowing and prevent food, liquids, and nasal secretions from entering the lungs. This is a reflex action that can be depressed by unconsciousness, neurological disease, or local anesthesia. Second, the vocal cords and epiglottis close before a cough. This action allows enough pressure to build up in the lungs to produce the high expiratory flow of air that is needed to expel secretions and foreign matter. The rate of a forceful cough has been estimated to be from 75 to 100 miles/hour.

TRACHEA, BRONCHI, AND BRONCHIOLES. The trachea contains 13 C-shaped cartilage rings that prevent collapse of the airway. The trachea bifurcates (branches) into the right and left bronchi. The right bronchus is more in line with the trachea, while the left bronchus branches off at almost a 90 degree angle. As a result, it is easier to pass a suction catheter into the right bronchus than into the left, and foreign matter is more likely to pass through the straighter right bronchus into the right lung than it is to find its way into the left lung.

The bronchi, which have firm cartilage walls, branch into bronchioles that have smooth *muscle* walls. This means that the bronchioles can collapse during a spasm, such as an asthmatic attack, for example, because there is no cartilage to help keep them open.

Bronchioles are lined with cilia and mucus. Any foreign matter that enters is trapped in mucus and propelled by cilia back through the increasingly larger airways to the trachea, where is is finally expelled by coughing.

ALVEOLI. Each bronchiole eventually branches into alveoli. The alveolar epithelium secretes a substance called *surfactant,* which decreases the surface tension of fluids lining the alveoli, thereby permitting full expansion of the lungs. The alveoli of some infants do not secrete enough surfactant, and the resulting high surface tension pulls on the walls of the alveoli, causing them to collapse. This condition is called *hyaline membrane disease,* or infant respiratory distress syndrome.

The function of the estimated 250 million or so alveoli is the exchange of oxygen and carbon dioxide between the air and the capillaries. Each of these gases flows from an area of high concentration to an area of low concentration. Therefore, because inspired air has a higher concentration of oxygen than does the blood, oxygen flows (diffuses) from the alveoli into the blood. Venous blood has a higher concentration of carbon dioxide than air, so carbon dioxide diffuses from blood into the alveoli. These gases diffuse through both the capillary wall and the adjacent alveolar wall.

Ventilation Processes

INSPIRATION. Inspiration is an active process caused by the contraction of the diaphragm and muscles of the chest. Because the diaphragm is dome shaped, any amount of contraction pulls it down, thereby increasing the space in the thoracic cavity above it. This increased chest space lowers the pressure within the chest, which in turn lowers the pressure in the lungs and alveoli. When the pressure in the alveoli drops below the atmospheric pressure of the environment, air flows into the respiratory tract and fills the lungs.

Minimal inspiration will occur when the *intra-alveolar pressure is approximately 3mm Hg less than the atmospheric pressure.* Because atmospheric pressure changes with altitude, intra-alveolar pressure is not constant and is simply written − 3 mm Hg. At sea level, atmospheric pressure is 760 mm Hg, and an intra-alveolar pressure of −3 mm Hg would equal 757 mm Hg. Forced inspiration, in contrast to minimal inspiration, can create an intra-alveolar pressure as low as − 80 mm Hg.

EXPIRATION. Expiration is usually a passive process. It normally occurs when the diaphragm relaxes and rises and when the chest muscles relax, causing the size of the thoracic cavity to decrease. As chest size decreases, pressure within the chest increases. When the intra-alveolar pressure rises to approximately 3 mm Hg above the atmospheric pressure, air flows out of the respiratory tract. When expiration is forced by actively contracting the abdominal muscles, the intra-alveolar pressure may rise to + 100 mm Hg or more.

Ventilatory Function Tests

The effectiveness of expiration and inspiration is measured by tests made with a spirometer and a recording device. A spirometer is an instrument that contains a floating drum that moves up and down in response to changes in pressure as the patient breathes through his mouth into a mouthpiece. Each fluctuation of the drum is recorded in ink on a moving strip of paper (Fig. 32.2).

Each test measures a specific aspect of ventilation, and it is often necessary to use the results of a variety of tests to obtain a complete picture of overall ventilatory function. Lung volumes are affected by height, weight, age, and sex. ''Normal'' values are based on the lung volumes of young adult men.

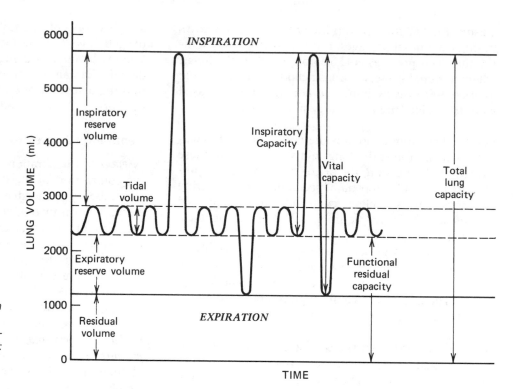

Figure 32.2 *Respiratory excursion during normal breathing and during maximal inspiration and maximal expiration. (From Guyton AC: Textbook of Medical Physiology. Ed 6. WB Saunders Co., 1981)*

Tidal volume (TV) is the amount of air inspired or expired with each breath during normal, quiet breathing. The average TV is about 500 ml (Figure 32.2). Of this amount, about one-third is *dead-space* air (the air in the upper air passages that never reaches the alveoli and therefore has minimal effect on respiration). TV is affected by position and is increased by activity and fever.

Minute respiratory volume equals the total amount of new air that is moved into the lungs in 1 minute, which is the TV times the respiratory rate. Based on a rate of 12 breaths per minute and a normal tidal volume of 500 ml, the minute respiratory volume for a young adult man is 6,000 ml (or 6 L). This volume also is increased by activity and fever.

Inspiratory reserve volume (IRV) equals the amount of air that can be inspired after (at the end of) a normal inspiration (about 3,000 ml). The *expiratory* reserve volume (ERV) equals the amount of air that can be expired after a normal expiration (about 1,100 ml) (Fig. 32.2).

Residual volume (RV) is the volume of air remaining in the lung after maximum expiration (about 1,200 ml). This air prevents the lung from collapsing after expiration (Fig. 32.2).

Vital capacity (VC) is the maximum amount of air that can be expired after a maximum inspiration (about 4000–6000 ml) (Fig. 32.2).

$$VC = IRV + TV + ERV$$

Total lung capacity (TLC) equals the amount of air in the lungs after maximum inspiration (about 5,800 ml) (Figure 32.2).

$$TLC = RV + VC$$

or

$$TLC = RV + IRV + TV + ERV$$

Both VC and TLC are decreased in restrictive lung diseases.

Timed vital capacity is the percentage of the vital capacity that can be expired in 1, 2, and 3 seconds. This volume is decreased in obstructive respiratory diseases.

Diffusion

Diffusion is the movement of particles across a semipermeable membrane from an area of high concentration to an area of low concentation. In respiration, there are two aspects of diffusion: (1) the exchange of gases between the alveoli and the pulmonary capillaries across the alveolar and capillary walls, and (2) the exchange of gases between the systemic capillaries and the body cells across the capillary and cell walls.

A dissolved gas creates a pressure against a membrane as it tries to diffuse across the membrane. The amount of pressure created by any gas depends on the concentration of that particular gas in the solution, even though other gases may be dissolved in the same solution. The pressure (P) of a dissolved gas is written Po_2, Pco_2, and so on.

The pressure of a dissolved gas depends on the proportion of that gas to the total volume of gases. It is calculated by multiplying its percentage of the total volume of gases by the pressure of the atmosphere at sea level (which is 760 mm Hg). For example, if the mixture is 40 percent oxygen, the pressure exerted by the oxygen equals 40 percent $\times$ 760 mm Hg, or 304 mm Hg. Inasmuch as the total pressure is 760 mm Hg, the oxygen is responsible for only part of that pressure (304 mm Hg), and the force the oxygen exerts against the semipermeable membrane is thus called a *partial pressure*. The notation Po_2 therefore indicates the partial pressure of oxygen in a given mixture.

The rate of diffusion across a membrane depends on the partial pressures of gas on each side of the membrane (the greater the difference, the more rapid the exchange of gas) and on the permeability, thickness, and total surface area of the membrane.

Blood gas analysis is a test which provides the most accurate means of assessing respiratory function. Respiratory insufficiency is usually expressed in terms of the levels of CO_2 and O_2 in the blood. Normal arterial oxygen pressure (PaO_2) is 80 to 100 mm Hg, while normal arterial carbon dioxide pressure ($PaCO_2$) is 35–40 mm Hg.

Circulation

The circulation phase of respiration includes the transportation of freshly oxygenated blood to all cells of the body and the transportation of deoxygenated blood back to the lungs. This is a two-step process involving both the pulmonary and the systemic circulation. The *pulmonary circulation* carries blood to and from the lungs for the intake of O_2 and the discharge of CO_2, while the *systemic circulation* carries the blood to and from each cell of the body (Fig. 32.3). If either portion of the circulatory system is deficient, the entire system will be less effective in meeting the needs of the body. If the *pulmonary system is defective*, the blood carried to the cells *cannot* be properly oxygenated. Even if the systemic circulation is excellent, the body cells cannot receive sufficient oxygen if the circulation to and from the alveoli was faulty. On the other hand, the pulmonary circulation can be efficient, but if the systemic circulation fails, the well-oxygenated blood may never reach the cells of the body.

Pulmonary Circulation

The pulmonary arteries and veins constitute the pulmonary circulation, and their function is to circulate blood to and from the alveoli for the exchange of O_2

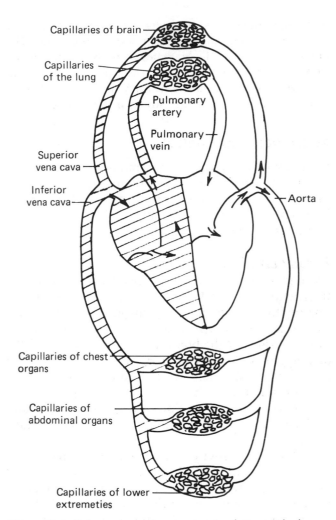

Figure 32.3 *Pulmonary and systemic circulation. (Black = pulmonary circulation, white = systemic arterial circulations, shaded = systemic venous circulation)*

and CO_2. The pulmonary arteries and veins are *not* part of the systemic circulation; they do not nourish and sustain the cells of the body as do the arteries and veins of the systemic circulation.

The pulmonary artery brings deoxygenated blood to the lungs. CO_2 diffuses from the capillaries into the alveoli, and O_2 diffuses from the alveoli into the capillaries. The oxygenated blood is then carried by the pulmonary vein to the heart. It is important to remember that, whereas the arteries of the systemic circulation carry oxygenated blood, the reverse is true of the pulmonary circulation. The pulmonary arteries carry deoxygenated blood from the heart to the lungs, and the pulmonary veins carry freshly oxygenated blood to the heart.

Systemic Circulation to the Lungs

The cells of the lungs are nourished by the systemic circulation, just as are all other cells of the body. The bronchial arteries and veins, which are part of the systemic circulation, supply the tissues of the lungs. The bronchial artery and its branches carry oxygenated blood from the aorta to all parts of the lung and bronchial tree, while the bronchial veins carry deoxygenated blood from the lung tissue to the superior vena cava.

Regulation and Control

Each of the three phases of respiration (ventilation, diffusion, and circulation) has its own specific regulatory mechanisms. The control of ventilation and circulation is described here; the regulation of diffusion is discussed in Chapter 31.

Regulation of Ventilation

The regulation of ventilation depends on the control of the rhythm, rate, and depth of respiratory movement. The rhythm of expiration and inspiration is controlled by the nervous system. The respiratory center, located in the medulla of the brainstem, sends impulses to the diaphragm by the phrenic nerve and to the muscles of the chest and abdomen by other motor nerves. Failure of the respiratory center—as a result of injury, drugs, or disease—stops the rhythmic cycle of respiration, and prolonged artificial respiration is then needed to maintain life.

Although the rhythm of respiration normally continues almost unchanged year after year, the *rate* and *depth* of respiration fluctuate widely—almost minute by minute—in response to the changing needs of the body. These changes are dictated by the demands of exercise, body temperature, speech, emotional reactions, drugs, disease, and other factors. Because the goal of respiration is to maintain the proper concentrations of O_2, CO_2, and hydrogen ions in body fluids, it is reasonable that the rate and depth of respiration are regulated by the levels of these substances in the body.

It would seem that the cellular need for oxygen would be the basic regulator of ventilatory rate. This does occur in some situations when the alveolar air cannot provide enough oxygen for transport by the hemoglobin. This would occur at high altitudes, for example, or in a disease such as pneumonia. In such cases, the lack of oxygen stimulates chemoreceptors located near the junction of the carotid artery and the aorta. These chemoreceptors stimulate the respiratory center whenever the Po_2 falls below 60 mm Hg. This regulatory mechanism is not the major control of needed ventilation, however, because the hemoglobin is usually saturated with oxygen, and changes in the level of oxygen in the blood do not therefore significantly affect the rate of respiration. Under most conditions, the Po_2 levels of the body are regulated by the hemoglobin-O_2 buffer

system and by blood flow to the tissues rather than by ventilation.

The *most powerful regulator* of the rate and depth of pulmonary ventilation is the *level of CO_2* in the blood. Whenever the activities of the body create an increased demand for O_2, those same activities produce an increased level of CO_2, and the respiratory center is stimulated to increase the rate and depth of respiration to blow off the excess CO_2. (The relationship between respiration and the regulation of both CO_2 and hydrogen-ion concentration was described in Chapter 31.)

Regulation of Circulation

Influences on the circulation of blood to and from the cells of the body are BP and heart action. BP is determined in part by the volume of circulating blood and by the condition of the blood vessels. A significant decrease in blood volume from hemorrhage, for example, will lower BP and decrease the flow of blood to the cells. Vasoconstriction increases BP and, within normal limits, promotes adequate circulation, but a narrowing of the lumen of the arteries by arteriosclerosis can markedly decrease the flow of blood to the area.

The efficiency of any circulatory system depends on the efficiency of its pump; and in humans, adequate circulation depends on effective heart action. One indicator of heart action is cardiac output, which is determined by multiplying the stroke volume by the number of beats per minute. The heart of a healthy adult normally ejects about 70 ml from each ventricle with each contraction, and a heart rate of 65 beats/minute therefore yields a cardiac output into the systemic circulation of approximately 4,500 ml/minute. An equal amount of blood is simultaneously ejected into the pulmonary circulation. Cardiac output increases and circulation is improved by anything that increases the heart rate, such as exercise, or anything that increases the stroke volume, such as cardiac drugs.

RESPIRATORY PROBLEMS

Pathological conditions related to respiration are described in this chapter only as a background for discussing assessment of the respiratory and circulatory systems and as a basis for understanding some of the nursing interventions related to respiration. A full explanation of these conditions can be found in medical-surgical nursing texts.

Ventilatory Dysfunction

Abnormal lung conditions can be classified into two main categories, restrictive and obstructive. The problems associated with restrictive lung conditions are primarily those of inspiration, whereas problems associated with obstructive lung conditions are largely those of expiration.

Restrictive Lung Conditions

A *restrictive* lung condition is present when expansion of the lungs is impaired and inspiration is limited or hampered. This can be caused by decreased elasticity of the lungs, restricted movement of the chest, or both. The signs and symptoms of restrictive lung diseases include:

- An increase in the effort needed to breathe
- Rapid, shallow breathing
- An inability to maintain normal arterial blood gas pressures when the disease is severe
- A decreased vital capacity and total lung capacity

A restrictive lung disease may be asymptomatic (without symptoms) when the patient is at rest, but shortness of breath will occur with fever, exercise, stress, or any other form of exertion or extra demand.

The major causes of restrictive lung disease are neurological, muscular, and skeletal. *Neurological* causes include central nervous system tumors or trauma, which interfere with respiratory control, or peripheral nervous system dysfunction, such as myasthenia gravis, which interferes with the innervation of respiratory muscles.

A major *muscular* cause of restrictive lung disease is muscular dystrophy, which is characterized by a progressive weakness of respiratory muscles. *Skeletal* causes usually involve an alteration in the ability to expand the thoracic cage. This can be the result of a vertebral abnormality such as curvature of the spine, or a trauma such as fractured ribs. Thoracic surgery constitutes a type of trauma, and postoperative pain causes the patient to splint his chest and fail to breathe deeply.

Conditions that prevent the full downward movement of the diaphragm during inspiration are ascites, obesity, and the later stages of pregnancy. The downward movement of the diaphragm is less impaired when the patient is in an upright rather than a supine position, and a semi-Fowler position may be needed to permit sleep and rest.

Another category of restrictive lung diseases includes *diffuse pulmonary disease,* which produces fibrosis (scarring) of lung tissue. The normally elastic tissue of the lungs may also be replaced by scar tissue after radiation therapy to the lungs, and as a result of a group of "dust diseases" such as silicosis and asbestosis.

Obstructive Lung Conditions

Obstructive lung conditions are the result of chronic obstruction of airflow through the lungs because of spasm of the airways, structural changes in the airways, or an accumulation of mucus or other matter. The signs and symptoms of obstructive lung conditions include:

- *Increased resistance to airflow, especially during expiration.*
- *Difficulty in coughing productively.* The patient is often unable to generate a high enough flow of air to move secretions because the airways either collapse or are obstructed.
- *Increased susceptibility to respiratory infections* because secretions cannot be coughed up and the dark, moist, warm, and stagnant environment of the pooled secretions is a good medium for bacterial growth.
- *Decreased vital capacity and decreased expiratory reserve* volume because the airflow becomes obstructed before the patient can expire completely.
- *Increased total lung capacity and residual volume* because air is trapped behind (distal to) the obstructed airways.

The major category of obstructive respiratory disease is called *chronic obstructive pulmonary disease* (COPD). It is also called chronic obstructive airway disease (COAD) and chronic obstructive lung disease (COLD). This disease includes such conditions as emphysema, asthma, and chronic bronchitis. Another obstructive disease is cystic fibrosis. This is a disease of childhood, as the patient rarely reaches adulthood because of pulmonary complications caused by accumulations of thick, viscous mucus in his lungs.

Combination Disorders

The distinctions between restrictive and obstructive diseases are not always clear, and they often overlap. For example, a tumor can interfere with full expansion of the lungs during inspiration as well as interfering with outflow of air during expiration. Thoracic surgery may initially cause restrictive pulmonary function owing to pain, but an obstructive problem may develop because of an accumulation of secretions in the lungs.

Circulatory Dysfunction

Circulatory problems that are closely related to respiration can be either cardiac, vascular, or a combination of the two. One of the commonest cardiac problems is congestive heart failure. The inability of the left side of the heart to contract effectively causes pulmonary congestion, which interferes with the diffusion of gases across the alveolar membranes. The resulting pulmonary congestion contributes to right-sided heart failure, which results in disturbed venous circulation.

Vascular conditions that interfere with circulation include atherosclerosis, phlebitis, peripheral vascular disease, and the occlusion of a blood vessel by an embolus.

ASSESSMENTS

There are many assessments related to respiration, and it is important to be able to select for use those that are *relevant to a given patient*. In many nursing situations it is neither feasible nor necessary to do a complete respiratory assessment on each patient. Some data, such as a respiratory history, for example, may already have been obtained by the physician or respiratory therapist, and some of the other assessments are unnecessary if the patient has no respiratory problems. The nurse selects from the commonly needed assessments *those which are likely to be significant* in either planning or evaluating nursing care. These selections are based on the purpose of the assessment and the condition of the patient.

Purpose

Assessments related to respiration are made for the following reasons:

- To obtain the data needed to plan nursing care. If, for example, the nurse's assessment indicates that a patient's chest is clear and that he has been able to cough up any existing secretions, there is no need to intervene. If, on the other hand, the patient seems unable or unwilling to cough and has moist rales in his chest, it is important to teach him at once how to deep-breathe and to cough with minimal discomfort. He may also need postural drainage, which would be ordered by his physician.
- To determine areas in which patient teaching is needed.
- To evaluate the effectiveness of nursing care given.
- To evaluate changes in the patient's symptoms and condition. Both in the hospital and in community health, for example, assessments are made as a basis for deciding whether or not to call the physician.
- To identify potential health problems.

Assessment, therefore, gives a basis for action, whether it be planning care for assigned patients in a medical center or deciding what to do about the complaints of a patient in an isolated, rural home.

People Who Need Regular Respiratory Assessment

- Patients with preexisting pulmonary disease such as emphysema or asthma.
- Smokers and ex-smokers
- Postoperative patients who have had chest or abdominal surgery (they often do not deep breathe or cough well because of postoperative pain)
- Patients with tracheostomies or laryngectomies because the normal defense mechanisms of the upper respiratory tract have been bypassed by the surgery
- Patients with depression of the CNS and possibly the respiratory center as a result of intracranial disease, injury, or narcotic overdose
- Patients with muscle weakness from spinal cord injuries, neuromuscular disease, or general debilitation who may not have the strength to deep-breathe and cough properly
- People who have decreased resistance to infection as a result of radiation or chemotherapy for treatment of cancer, or great stress
- People with deformities of the chest wall that prevent effective use of the respiratory muscles
- People with restricted downward movement of the diaphragm owing to ascites, abdominal distention, or obesity (not usually a problem during pregnancy because those women are usually relatively young and in general good health)
- Patients with existing circulatory problems, such as peripheral vascular disease or congestive heart failure

Identification of Patients To Be Assessed

In addition to patients whose current diagnosis or symptoms indicate a need for respiratory assessment, patients who are vulnerable and at risk for respiratory problems should be assessed regularly.

The more predisposing conditions which are present in any one person, the greater the risk for that person and the more urgent the need for regular respiratory assessments. For example, the risk of pulmonary problems is much greater for an elderly, debilitated smoker who has just had chest surgery, than it is for a middle-aged nonsmoker who has been in good health but must now undergo the same type of chest surgery.

There are, in general, three types of nursing assessments to be made: (1) observations, (2) respiratory history, and (3) physical examination of the patient.

Observations To Be Made

Posture and Position

Patients with certain respiratory disorders often assume *typical* or *characteristic* postures. A patient with chronic obstructive pulmonary disease (COPD), for example, characteristically leans forward while sitting and places his hands on his knees or his elbows on the arms of the chair or a table. This position props up his clavicles and gives more space in his thoracic cavity.

It is not sensible to try to memorize a number of such postures, because some of them, though typical, are seldom encountered. It is, therefore, important to describe, in some detail, *any posture that a patient assumes frequently.*

Facial Expression

A patient may look drawn and tired, for example, because of the physical exertion of walking and moving when short of breath, or he may look anxious or frightened because of air hunger or dyspnea.

Neurological Status

Changes in alertness as well as personality can be caused by an abnormal pH, Po_2, or Pco_2 of blood. These changes can progress from anxiety and restlessness to increased irritability, confusion, or drowsiness, and finally to stupor or unconsciousness.

Speech

A patient may be able to speak only a few words or sentences before he begins to gasp for breath or to wheeze or cough.

Color

Oxygenated hemoglobin is red, whereas deoxygenated hemoglobin in blue. *Cyanosis* is a bluish tinge to the skin and mucous membranes and is caused by an increased amount of reduced (deoxygenated) hemoglobin. It is a *late sign* of respiratory distress and does not usually appear until the arterial Po_2 is 45 mm Hg or less (the normal level is 80 to 100 mm Hg). Cyanosis is most visible in areas that are highly vascular and thin skinned such as the lips and nailbeds. The nurse should also check under the patient's tongue or inside his cheeks, because cyanosis can usually be detected in these areas regardless of skin color.

Extremities

The patient's hands and feet should be warm and pink if his circulation is adequate. Cold, white skin usually indicates inadequate arterial blood flow to the area, while cool, blue or purplish skin indicates a poor venous return. Edema of fingers or ankles suggests a circulatory or electrolyte disturbance. *Clubbing* of the fingers is the enlargement of the tip of the finger plus a decrease in the angle at the base of the nail and is caused by a chronic decrease in the oxygen saturation of blood supplying the fingers. The femoral, popliteal,

or dorsalis pedis pulses, or all three, should be palpated whenever poor circulation of the feet and legs is suspected.

Respiratory History

It is often advisable to question the patient about his respiratory status to obtain data that are not readily observable and to gain insight into the patient's reaction to his illness. Six areas to be assessed include: dyspnea, cough, sputum, pain, occupation, and use of tobacco. This information is obtained by talking with the patient, *provided the information has not already been obtained by another person.*

Dyspnea

The patient's perception of his own shortness of breath or his difficulty in breathing is usually communicated most clearly when it is stated in terms of activities of daily living (ADL). General, vague phrases such as ''awfully short of breath'' and ''real hard to breath'' are less useful than precise descriptions such as ''I have to stop and rest part way up the stairs,'' ''I have to sleep sitting up now,'' or ''I can walk about a block and then I have to stand still and catch my breath.'' The nurse's questions should help the patient describe how much he can do before symtoms appear, how long the symptoms last, and what, if anything, relieves them.

Cough

The presence of a cough indicates irritation of the air passages. The aspects to be assessed include the frequency and duration of the cough, what triggers the cough (such as exercise, eating, lying down), the effect of body position, time of day, or irritants such as cigarette smoke or cold air, the characteristics of the cough, and how it is relieved.

Sputum

The amount and characteristics of the patient's sputum must be determined in order to make a diagnosis and to evaluate the patient's response to therapy. The points to assess are:

- *Consistency* (thick or thin? watery or viscous?)

Phrases Used to Describe a Cough

- Productive (sputum is raised)
- Hacking (frequent, not usually severe or productive)
- Paroxysmal (sudden, prolonged episodes of forceful coughing)
- Explosive or brassy (usually harsh and unproductive; sometimes shrill and strident)

- *Amount* (may range from 1 to 2 teaspoons to a pint or so daily. If the patient has not been using a sputum container, it will be necessary to estimate the amount.)
- *Color* (may range from clear to white, yellow, or green, depending on the organisms present and the length of time it has remained in the lungs)
- *Blood* (may be blood tinged or contain large amounts of blood from a hemorrhage. Bright red blood is from an arterial source, dark red blood from a venous site. A patient is usually frightened by bloody sputum and tends to seek medical help quickly.)

A sputum specimen will be needed to identify any causative organism. To get a good specimen, the nurse should collect the first sputum that is raised in the morning. This is done by having the patient take three deep breaths, hold the last breath, and cough deeply and forcefully, using the abdominal muscles.

Pain

There are no pain receptors in the lung tissue itself, but pain can emanate from the chest wall, pleura, or upper respiratory tract. The amount of pain experienced is difficult to measure, so an assessment of it should describe the relationship between the pain and activity, indicating what causes it and what, if anything, relieves it.

Occupation

Certain occupations are likely to lead to restrictive lung diseases if the worker inhales the dust over a prolonged period of time. Some of these disease conditions and their causative agents are:

Farmer's lung	Fungus from wet hay
Anthracosis	Coal dust
Asbestosis	Mining, textile, and roofing products containing asbestos
Silicosis	Silica from mining, metal grinding, and pottery

Use of Tobacco

Patients who smoke or have smoked in the past are more susceptible to lung diseases such as COPD or lung cancer and to pulmonary complications postoperatively or during a period of immobility.

Physical Examination of the Chest

The chest is examined in an orderly fashion, starting with inspection, followed by palpation, percussion, and auscultation. One side is compared with the other throughout the examination; any differences in size, symmetry, and sound are noted. Provision must be made to ensure privacy because the patient must be undressed; it is not possible to adequately examine the chest while the patient is clothed.

Landmarks

Some of the landmarks used as reference points when examining the chest are shown in Fig. 32.4. The sternal angle is especially important because it is the landmark for locating and numbering the ribs. The sternal angle (angle of Louis) is the angle formed where the slanting, bony ridge of the manubrium joins the body of the sternum. The second rib is attached to the sternum at this angle. To locate all othe ribs, count up or down from the second rib.

The dome of the diaphragm and the base of the lungs are about the level of the fifth rib (Fig. 32.5). The bifurcation (branching) of the trachea is found slightly below the sternal angle in front of and below the ridge of the scapula in back.

Inspection

The size and shape of the chest, as well as the rate and rhythm of the patient's breathing, are assessed by inspection.

SIZE AND SHAPE OF CHEST. The normal adult chest is oval shaped, with a lateral diameter that is greater than the anterior-posterior diameter. The chests of normal infants, adults with emphysema, and normal aged people are rounder (more barrel-shaped). A *funnel* chest can be identified by a depression of the lower portion of the sternum. A *pigeon breast* is caused by an elevation or forward displacement of the sternum, which is made more prominent by grooves in each side of the anterior chest wall.

The patient's back and posterior chest should be inspected for symmetry of the chest walls and alignment of the vertebrae. The right and left shoulders, scapulae, and hips should be level. One high shoulder or hip, one scapula more prominent than the other, or any distortion or displacement of the vertebral column may indicate a curvature of the spine. *Scoliosis* is a lateral curvature that is especially common in adolescent girls. *Kyphosis* (hunch back) and *lordosis* (sway back) are anterior-posterior curvatures. Some patients have more than one curvature, which severely limits respiratory capacity.

RATE AND RHYTHM OF BREATHING. The patient's respiratory rate should be within normal limits and regular. *Inspiration is normally about two-thirds as long as expiration.* The normal respiratory rate for adults is 16 to 20

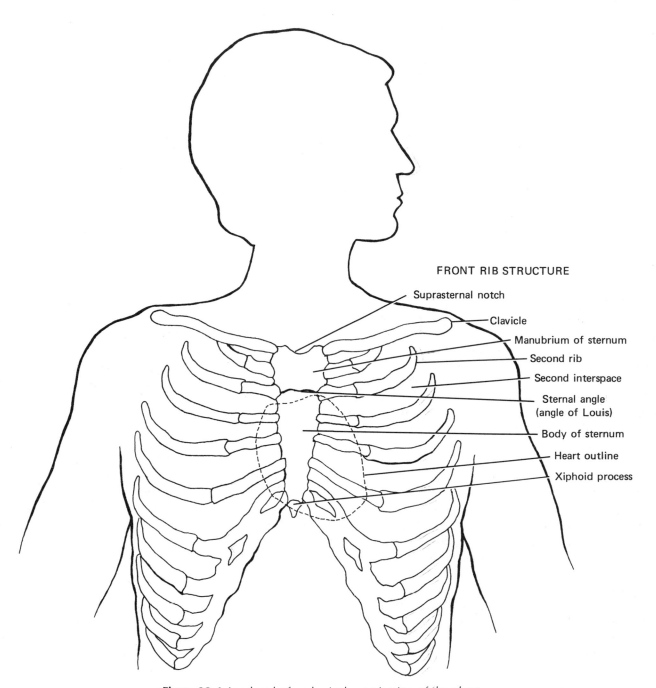

FRONT RIB STRUCTURE

Suprasternal notch
Clavicle
Manubrium of sternum
Second rib
Second interspace
Sternal angle
(angle of Louis)
Body of sternum
Heart outline
Xiphoid process

Figure 32.4 *Landmarks for physical examination of the chest.*

breaths/minute, although an athlete may have a rate as low as 12 to 14/minute. A normal infant breathes up to 44 times/minute.

The ratio of respiratory rate to pulse rate is about 1:4, which means that a respiratory rate of 16 is often accompanied by a pulse rate of 64. A change in body temperature causes a corresponding change in both respiratory and pulse rates. An increase in body temperature of 1 degree C causes the respiratory rate to increase by 4 breaths/minute and the pulse rate to in-

crease by 16 beats/minute. The respiratory rate of an adult with a temperature of 39 degrees C (2 degrees above normal) would increase about 8 breaths/minute as his increased metabolism makes it necessary to blow off more CO_2.

The chest should be observed for any retraction of the interspaces during inspiration or bulging during expiration. Both are abnormal and are seen with conditions such as emphysema, asthma, or an obstructed airway.

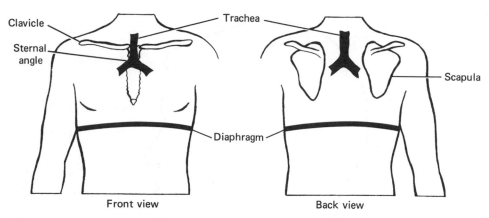

Figure 32.5 *Location of the diaphram and the bifurcation of the trachea, front and back views.*

Palpation

Palpation is used to assess areas where pain or tenderness has been reported, to assess any observed abnormality such as a lump or mass, and to assess chest expansion.

To assess respiratory excursion (chest expansion), place your hands around the base of the patient's rib cage with your thumbs touching his spine. Ask the patient to take a deep breath, and as his chest expands, your thumbs will move apart. When chest expansion is symmetrical and both lungs are expanding equally, your thumbs will move an equal distance from the midline.

Palpation is also used to assess *fremitus,* the vibrations from speech that are transmitted from the airways and lungs through the chest wall. These vibrations are called both vocal fremitus, because they occur when the patient speaks, and tactile fremitus, because they can be felt with the palm of the hand. They are felt on the posterior chest wall when the patient says "ninety-nine." If fremitus is faint, ask the patient to lower the pitch of his voice (deepen it) or speak louder. With practice, you will learn to recognize normal fremitus and can then detect increased or decreased fremitus, both of which are abnormal.

Percussion

Percussion is used to determine whether areas of the chest are fluid filled, air filled, or solid. The percussion sounds of normal air-filled lung tissue change from resonant to dull when fluid is present. *The thorax should be resonant* except for areas of cardiac dullness, liver dullness, and gastric tympany.

Percussion is also used to determine the level of the diaphragm. Inasmuch as the space above the diaphragm (the air-filled lungs) sounds resonant and the area below the diaphragm sounds dull, the point at which the percussed chest sounds change from reso-

nant to dull marks the level of the diaphragm.

To assess *diaphragmatic excursion,* have the patient take a deep breath and mark his skin at the level of the diaphragm at maximum inspiration. Then ask the patient to exhale forcefully and mark the level of the diaphragm at maximum expiration. Measure the distance between the two marks. A normal excursion is 5 to 6 cm.

Auscultation of the Lungs

Auscultation is done to assess the flow of air through the passages of the respiratory tract and to assess the condition of the lungs and pleura. Two types of sounds will be heard: *breath* sounds and *adventitious* (abnormal) sounds. Both must be distinguished from any extraneous sounds created by the movements of the patient or the friction of bedding against the stethoscope tubing.

BREATH SOUNDS. There are three types of breath sounds: vesicular, bronchovesicular, and bronchial. You can learn these by repeatedly listening to your own chest. *Vesicular* breath sounds are soft and low pitched. They are normally heard over most of the lung, and the length of inspiration is greater than the length of expiration.

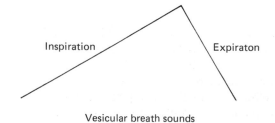

Vesicular breath sounds

Bronchovesicular breath sounds are medium in pitch and intensity (loudness). They are heard over the bronchi (over the sternum and between the scapulae). Inspiration and expiration are of equal length.

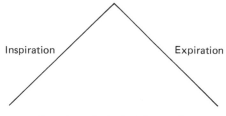

Bronchovesicular breath sounds

Bronchial (tubular) breath sounds are loud and high pitched. They are heard over the trachea, but not normally heard over the lungs. Expiration is longer than inspiration.

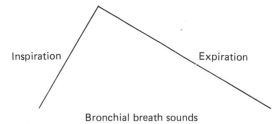

Bronchial breath sounds

Breath sounds decrease when the air flow is decreased because of shallow breathing related to pain, occlusion of a bronchus, or muscular weakness. Breath sounds are diminished when the sounds are muffled by fluid or by excess tissue (from obesity) between the lungs and the stethoscope.

ADVENTITIOUS SOUNDS. *Rales* are separate, noncontinuous sounds produced by the movement of moisture in the airways, especially during inspiration. Fine rales are heard in small air passages and sound like the fizz of a carbonated beverage or the sound produced by rolling a lock of hair between your fingers in front of your ear (Bates, 1979). Medium rales are heard over larger passageways. Coarse rales are bubbling, gurgling sounds produced by secretions in the trachea; they are often referred to as a "death rattle." Rales usually sound different after the patient has coughed.

Rhonchi are continuous sounds produced by air that is forced through passageways that are narrowed by thick secretions, edema, inflammation, or other obstructive conditions. They are often most prominent during expiration. *Wheezes* are high-pitched, hissing sounds heard over small passages. Sonorous rhonchi are low-pitched sounds heard over large airways. Rhonchi may sound different after the patient has coughed.

Friction rubs are crackling, grating sounds produced by inflammation of the pleura. The inflamed surfaces are rough and produce a grating sound when they rub together. This sound can be simulated by placing the palm of one's hand over one's ear and rubbing the back of that hand with the other palm. Friction rubs are usually accompanied by pain, especially during deep breathing.

Auscultation of the Heart

The valves of the heart open and close at different times in the cardiac cycle. When the valves are open, there is normally no audible sound. The closure of each valve, however, produces a specific, identifiable sound.

Each cardiac cycle includes two major sounds, which are often referred to as "lub-dub." The "lub" is the first heart sound and is called S_1. It is associated with the closure of the mitral and tricuspid valves, which close at approximately the same time at the beginning of ventricular systole and the start of the cardiac cycle. S_1 is longer, softer, and lower pitched than the second heart sound. It is best heard at the apex or lower tip of the heart, which is called the point of maxium impulse (PMI).

The "dub" is the second sound and is called S_2. It indicates the closure of the pulmonary and aortic (semilunar) valves, which occurs at the beginning of diastole, when the ventricles of the heart begin to fill again. S_2 is shorter and higher pitched than S_1 and is heard best over the top of the heart.

The interval between S_1 and S_2 represents ventricular systole, and the interval between S_2 and S_1 represents ventricular diastole. These intervals are normally silent and should be carefully assessed for the presence of unusual sounds. Occasionally people will have irregular blood flow and blood currents through stiffened or incompetent valves, causing murmurs. Loud murmurs in systole and all murmurs in diastole are considered pathological.

Third and fourth heart sounds are sometimes heard, but not as frequently or easily as S_1 and S_2. Heart sounds are sometimes split. This means it may be possible to detect two components of one of the heart sounds. Splitting is not uncommon in S_2.

Heart sounds are auscultated not over the anatomical location of the valves but in the auscultatory area (area of auscultation) for each sound (Fig. 32.6). S_1 and S_2 can be heard in all four areas, but S_1 is heard best in the mitral area, whereas S_2 is best heard in the aortic and pulmonic areas.

Locations of Auscultation for Heart Sounds

Area of Auscultation	Location
Aortic area	Right second intercostal space, close to sternum
Pulmonic area	Left second intercostal space, close to sternum
Tricuspid area	Left fifth intercostal space, close to sternum
Mitral area	Left fifth intercostal space, midclavicular line

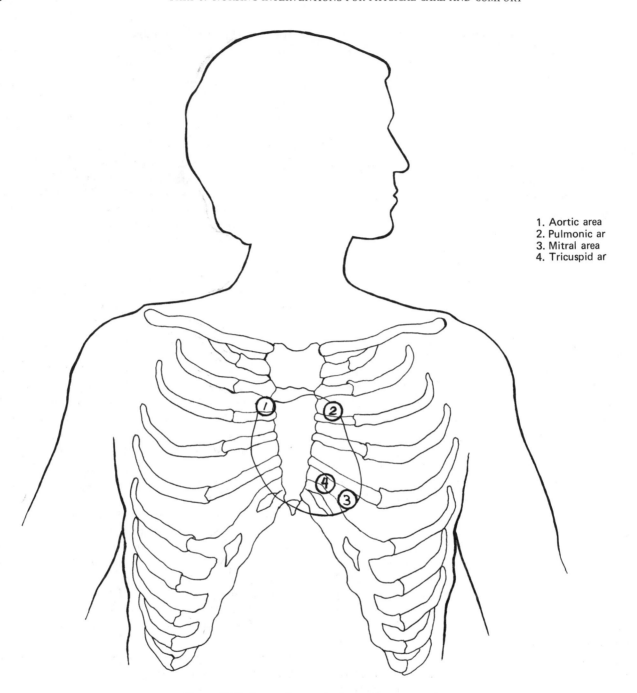

1. Aortic area
2. Pulmonic ar
3. Mitral area
4. Tricuspid ar

Figure 32.6 Areas of auscultation of heart sounds.

The key to successful auscultation lies in listening *to one thing at a time*. It is frequently helpful to close your eyes. Identify S_1 and S_2, listen to them separately, and then compare them. When these sounds are familiar, focus first on systole (which follows S_1), then on diastole (which follows S_2), and listen for extra sounds and murmurs during these normally quiet intervals.

NURSING INTERVENTIONS

As the technology and procedures for meeting the needs of patients with respiratory problems have become more extensive and complex, many hospitals have established respiratory therapy departments. These units are staffed by specially trained therapists and technicians

Normal Adult Chest Findings

- Inspection

    Lateral diameter greater than anterior-posterior diameter

    No deformities of ribs or spine

    No retraction or bulging of interspaces

- Palpation

    No areas of tenderness

    No lumps or masses palpated

    Respiratory excursion symmetrical

    Normal fremitus

- Percussion

    Entire thorax resonant except for areas of dullness over heart and liver

    Diaphragmatic excursion normal

- Auscultation of the lungs

    Breath sounds normal

    Vesicular sounds over most of thorax

    Bronchovesicular sounds over large bronchi

    No adventitious sounds (no rales, rhonchi, or pleural friction rubs)

- Auscultation of the heart

    Heart sounds normal

    S_1 and S_2 audible in all areas; S_2 louder than S_1

    Systole and diastole silent, without murmurs

who administer prescribed treatments, monitor and maintain equipment, and evaluate patient progress.

Such specialization can improve patient care *if* there is optimal communication and cooperation between the departments of nursing and respiratory therapy. Whenever nurses cease to assume responsibility for the respiratory needs of their patients and the entire responsibility is shifted to respiratory therapists, patient care is fragmented, and serious deficiencies are likely to develop. The problems that arise are related to patient and family teaching, assessment of patient progress, scheduling of treatments, continuity of care throughout all three shifts, medications, and plans for discharge. It is important, therefore, to coordinate the efforts and expertise of respiratory therapists and nurses.

Nursing interventions related to respiration include measures that promote adequate ventilation, circulation, and diffusion. These interventions are determined by medical orders, nursing orders, and an ongoing assessment of the patient.

NURSING MEASURES TO PROMOTE VENTILATION

The nursing measures commonly used to promote pulmonary ventilation include: (1) deep breathing and coughing, (2) positioning and ambulation, (3) postural drainage, (4) vibration and percussion, (5) humidification, and (6) maintenance of an artificial airway.

Coughing and Deep Breathing

When thoroughly and conscientiously done, coughing and deep breathing can prevent serious and life-threatening complications such as postoperative pneumonia, and can also alleviate existing conditions. Coughing and deep-breathing exercises are prescribed to fully aerate the lungs and to help move any secretions from the alveoli and tiny passageways toward the large air passages, from which they can be expelled. Coughing and deep breathing should be used prophylactically for all high-risk patients, especially those who are immobilized or who have been anesthetized, and should be instituted at once for any patient when auscultation of his chest reveals adventitious sounds such as rales.

Coughing and deep breathing are among the most significant of all nursing measures because secretions that are allowed to accumulate in the lungs can result in life-threatening conditions.

Deep Breathing

Secretions flow by gravity from the upper to the lower portions of the lungs where the secretions tend to pool (accumulate), especially if respirations are shallow. Shallow respirations tend to aerate only the upper part of the lungs, and therefore, deep respirations with full expiration and inspiration are needed to ventilate the lower portion of the lungs and to help move secretions so that they can be removed by coughing.

Results of Inadequate Ventilation

Accumulated secretions in the lungs:
- Provide an excellent medium for bacterial growth
- Make respiration less efficient and increase the work of breathing
- Can occlude the airways and cause atelectasis (airless, collapsed alveoli)
- Interfere with air movement throughout the lungs and with gas exchange in the alveoli
- Make it difficult for a patient to maintain a normal level of blood gases

The *depth* of breathing can be increased in two ways. First, it can be increased to some extent by use of the intercostal muscles to expand the upper chest, thereby increasing the air flow to the upper lobes. Second, the depth of breathing can be increased significantly by contraction of the diaphragm. This increases the depth (or length) of the thorax, expands the capacity of the chest, and greatly increases the flow of air to the base of the lungs.

Diaphragmatic breathing is taught most easily with the patient in the supine position, but the patient should then be taught to do it in both a sitting and a standing position so that he can breathe deeply each hour regardless of his position. Whenever possible, deep breathing should be taught well in advance of surgery so that learning can take place without the added stress of postoperative pain. The patient should be able to deep breathe effectively without assistance and have begun to develop strength in his abdominal muscles *before surgery*. He should be committed to breathing deeply postoperatively, and it should be so familiar to him that he can do it as directed while still groggy from the anesthesia.

PURSED LIP BREATHING. Sometimes a patient should be taught to inhale through his nose and exhale through his mouth with his lips pursed. During inhalation, the nose warms, filters, and moisturizes the inspired air. Exhaling through pursed lips, as if blowing gently at a candle, is beneficial for several reasons. It prolongs expiration and tends to convert the rapid, ineffectual, shallow breathing of some patients into slower, deeper breathing that promotes a more complete emptying of the lungs. Some chronic lung disorders cause the airways to lose their resilience and cause some of them to collapse during expiration. When airways collapse, air is trapped, and the patient feels short of breath because he cannot exhale effectively. Pursed-lip breathing creates enough back pressure to keep the air passages open and to promote a slower, more relaxed pattern of breathing.

Alternative Ways to Promote Deep Breathing

Attentive nursing care coupled with effective patient teaching will ensure adequate ventilation for most patients. In some situations, however, it may be necessary or desirable to use mechanical devices to assist or motivate the patient.

BLOW BOTTLES. Blow bottles are a device that promotes forced expiration as the patient attempts to blow hard enough to displace colored water from one bottle to another through a connecting tube. The procedure is repeated every 1 to 4 hours, and the patient is encouraged to try to displace more water with each breath every time he tries. He can blow water back and forth between bottles, and receive immediate feedback concerning his efforts as he watches the colored fluid rise and fall.

In the absence of blow bottles, similar results are obtained by having the patient blow through a straw into a half-filled soft-drink bottle or tall glass. The number and size of the bubbles that are formed indicate the force of the patient's expiration. Even small children with respiratory problems can be taught to blow bubbles, and they often delight in doing so.

INCENTIVE SPIROMETER. There are many types of spirometers on the market, but they are all *designed to promote inspiration* and to *provide a visual or auditory incentive* for inspiring. The patient is instructed to inspire as deeply as possible through the mouthpiece. If the inspiration is adequate, a light will go on, small balls will be forced into the air, or some other type of feedback

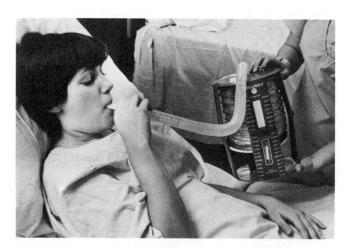

Figure 32.7 *One type of incentive spirometer used to promote adequate respiration.*

Guidelines for Teaching Diaphragmatic (Deep) Breathing

1. With patient in a supine position, place your hand on his abdomen.
2. Ask him to push his abdomen up against your hand during *inspiration*. To do this, he must pull down (contract) his diaphragm, which pushes the abdominal contents up against your hand.
3. During *expiration*, he should let his abdomen relax.
4. This exercise should be done slowly and deeply and should be repeated at least 10 times/hour.

will be provided. The incentive spirometer is used every 1 to 4 hours. Some spirometers are disposable and can be taken home by the patient (Fig. 32.7).

INTERMITTENT POSITIVE PRESSURE BREATHING. An electrically powered positive pressure machine can be used to force air or oxygen into the patient's lungs during inspiration. When a preset pressure or volume is reached, the air flow stops and the patient expires passively. Such machines can be used to assist ventilation or to completely control ventilation for a patient who is comatose from a head injury, narcotic overdose, or other condition. The overall management of intermittent positive pressure breathing (IPPB) therapy is complex, and in many institutions the treatments are given by a member of the respiratory therapy team.

Coughing

The purpose of coughing is to expel secretions from the lungs to permit free passage of air and adequate exchange of gases. An effective cough is always preceded by a deep breath. After a deep inspiration, the epiglottis and the vocal cords are closed, and air is trapped in the lungs. The abdominal and intercostal muscles contract, the diaphragm rises, and the intrapulmonary pressure may reach 100 mm Hg. When the pressure has reached its peak, the epiglottis and the vocal cords open, and air is expelled at a high velocity, carrying secretions and other foreign matter with it. It is essential, therefore, that the patient's cough be *preceded* by an inspiration deep enough to build up a column of air behind the secretions that are to be expelled.

It is easiest for the patient to cough in an upright position because that position promotes a lowering of the diaphragm, which permits increased pressure to be generated. Teaching must be done preoperatively so that there is ample opportunity for practice *before* the patient with a painful incision has to cough.

Each patient should be taught to cough following the sequence listed below:

1. Slowly take three deep, diaphragmatic (abdominal) breaths.
2. Hold the last breath for a few seconds.

3. Cough three times before inspiring again, a procedure know as triocough—three coughs on one breath.
4. Cover the mouth with several thicknesses of tissues during each cough.

The coughs must be forceful enough to move secretions from small airways up into increasingly larger airways, from which the secretions can be expelled. As a result of this movement of secretions, rales are likely to sound different after the patient has coughed.

If pain, from abdominal or thoracic surgery, for example, interferes with a patient's ability to cough effectively, it may be necessary to medicate him before he tries to cough and to teach him how to splint and support the painful site. You can splint the area by standing behind the patient and placing your palms on each side of the incision, or the patient can press a folded blanket or pillow against his abdomen for support during the cough. Some patients are frightened both by the pain and by their fear that coughing will tear open the incision, and much gentleness and patience is needed as the patient tries to cough effectively (Fig. 32.8).

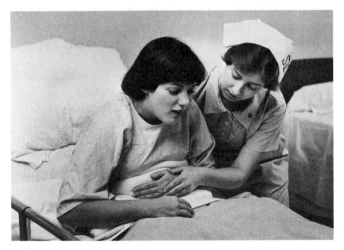

Figure 32.8 Physical and psychological support are necessary when coughing is painful.

PROCEDURE 32.1

Helping a Patient to Cough, Turn, and Deep Breathe*

SUMMARY OF ESSENTIAL NURSING ACTIONS

1. If patient has not been previously instructed, teach him the benefits and necessity of coughing, turning, and deep breathing at regular intervals.
2. Help patient to sit upright unless it is contraindicated.
3. Instruct patient to take three deep abdominal breaths and hold the last one for a few seconds.
4. Direct the patient to cough as deeply as possible two or three times.
5. If the patient has an incision, show him how to splint it with his hands or a pillow to reduce the pain and/or relieve his anxiety about injuring the incision.
6. Repeat the procedure once or twice with encouragement and appropriate praise.
7. Assist the patient back to a comfortable position with a reminder to turn from side to side at frequent intervals.
   • If the patient is unable or unwilling to turn by himself, return at designated intervals to help him do so.

*See inside front cover and page 631.

Alternative Ways to Stimulate Coughing

If a patient cannot cough after taking deep breaths, there are several cough-stimulating techniques that can be tried. The nurse or the patient can apply pressure with a thumb over the trachea just above the manubrial arch at the top of the sternum. This creates an artificial obstruction that triggers coughing. Pressure should not be enough to cause retching or vomiting. Another technique requires the patient to exhale completely. As he nears the end of the expiration, encourage him to keep exhaling. This builds up the Pco_2 and may trigger a cough reflex.

Suctioning is used as a last resort to induce coughing when a patient is unable to cough productively and has secretions in his lungs. Suctioning is uncomfortable for the patient and carries with it the risk of possible infection. A physician's order is needed. A suction catheter can sometimes be used without suction to induce coughing because the presence of the catheter in the trachea may be enough to stimulate the cough reflex. Sometimes the coughing that results will move the secretions toward the trachea but not enough to expel them, and then the secretions must be suctioned out.

Positioning and Ambulation

Frequent repositioning or ambulation of the patient is often needed to prevent the respiratory complications caused by the accumulation and stasis of secretions and inadequate aeration of the lungs. When the patient is lying down, expansion is limited in the portion of his chest that is pressing against the mattress, and failure to move and turn him frequently causes any secretions that are present to collect in the dependent (lower) portion of his lungs.

Considerable ingenuity is needed to make a dyspneic or orthopneic patient comfortable. A high Fowler position is often needed, and a patient with orthopnea may find it necessary to sleep in a chair. Upright positions make breathing easier because gravity keeps the abdominal contents from pushing up against the diaphragm and impeding inspiration. An upright position also relieves or prevents any compression of the thorax by the mattress.

All patients, whether high risk or not, should turn or be turned from side to side every 2 hours unless this is contraindicated. They should be out of bed in a chair for 20 minutes, two to three times daily, and ambulated two to three times daily unless this is contraindicated.

Postural Drainage

Postural drainage is a treatment in which the patient assumes a series of positions that will promote drainage of secretions from his lungs, especially the middle and lower lobes. When a person is in an *upright* position, the upper lobes drain by gravity, but there is no way to drain the lower lobes. Special positions are therefore necessary to allow secretions to drain from the lower lobes up into the large bronchi and trachea, where the secretions can be coughed up (Fig. 32.9).

Postural drainage is ordered for patients who have excessive or thick secretions and for those who are unable to cough effectively. Postural drainage is contraindicated for patients whose vital signs are adversely affected by changes in position and for most patients with cardiac conditions.

Postural drainage is done as often as necessary to keep the lungs clear, usually from one to four times daily. It is usually done before breakfast because secre-

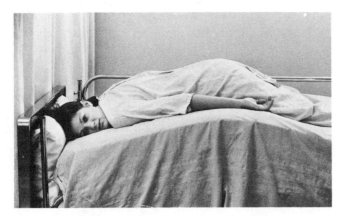

Figure 32.9 One position that will promote gravity drainage of secretions from the lungs.

tions pool in dependent parts of the lungs during sleep. Clearing the lungs of these accumulated secretions makes breathing easier and therefore makes it easier for the patient to eat breakfast. Postural drainage is not done directly after meals because it might cause vomiting. It is usually done at bedtime so that breathing will be easier when the patient lies down to sleep.

The duration of each position is determined by the patient's condition and his response to the treatment. When a patient can be made comfortable in the prescribed positions, when the secretions are being drained passively by gravity, and when only one or two lobes need to be drained, a given position may be maintained for as long as 20 minutes. But when a patient is acutely ill or tolerates the treatment poorly, when postural drainage must be combined with percussion and vibration of the chest (see below), or when many areas must be drained and many postural changes are necessary, each position can be maintained for only a few minutes.

The specific areas of the lungs that need to be drained are identified during physical examination by percussion and auscultation of the chest, and by x-ray films. When the treatment is done prophylactically, as part of the daily care of a child with cystic fibrosis, for example, every section of every lobe is drained during each treatment. The positions used to drain each lobe or section of a lobe are prescribed by the physician or the physical therapist, and effectiveness is assessed by repeated percussion and auscultation, and by x-ray examination.

As with all other procedures, postural drainage must be thoroughly explained to the patient. He should be medicated for pain as needed before the treatment is started and then helped to assume each prescribed position. The patient is encouraged to use diaphragmatic breathing to expand the lower lobes of his lungs fully

and to promote drainage. Because the purpose of the treatment is the removal of secretions, the patient is encouraged to cough, and must be provided with adequate tissues and a waste container, such as a paper bag. If the patient is left alone during postural drainage, *his bell cord must be within reach.* Mouth care is essential at the end of the treatment to remove all traces of coughed-up secretions.

Assessment is an integral part of postural drainage, both to identify the areas that need to be drained and to evaluate the effectiveness of the treatment. In addition to auscultating the patient's chest, the nurse should take the patient's vital signs and check his color before the treatment is started. As the secretions move through the respiratory tract and as the patient tries to cough them up, his respiration can be affected. It is important, therefore, to watch the patient's face for any change in color and to note any shortness of breath or change in rate of pulse or respiration. The treatment should be stopped if there is any marked change in the patient's condition. The patient's lungs should be auscultated both before and after postural drainage, and any differences in rales or rhonchi, for example, should be described and recorded.

Vibration and Percussion

Vibration and percussion are manipulations of the patient's chest that are often used in conjunction with postural drainage to increase the flow of secretions. The action can be likened to the process of shaking and hitting a bottle containing a thick substance to move it toward the neck of the bottle. Vibration and percussion treatments are ordered by the physician and are usually given by the respiratory therapist or the nurse, although family members are often taught the procedure as an adjunct to postural drainage.

Percussion is done with the hand in a cupped position. With your elbow and shoulder relaxed, alternately extend and hyperextend your wrist for a period of 1 or 2 minutes, striking the patient with your cupped hand each time. Each blow is intended to dislodge a mucus plus or thick secretions. The treatment can be uncomfortable, so it is done through the patient's clothing or a towel (Fig. 32.10).

Percussion is done over the spots designated by the physician or the respiratory therapist; it is not done over sensitive areas such as the spine, kidneys, spleen, sternum, or breasts. It is important to watch the patient closely because dislodged mucus plugs or thick secretions could occlude an airway and increase his respiratory difficulties. Percussion is usually followed by vibration.

Vibration is used to speed the movement of secre-

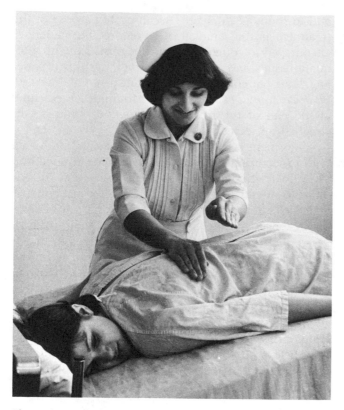

Figure 32.10 *Percussion is used to increase the effectiveness of postural drainage.*

tions that have been loosened by percussion. The nurse does this in the prescribed spots by placing the heel of one hand on the back of the other hand. With your hands on the patient's thorax at the prescribed points, ask the patient to take a deep breath and expire slowly through pursed lips. As he expires, lean forward with your arms straight and vibrate (jiggle or shake) the area under your hands for the duration of the expiration. This is repeated for four or five expirations. Vibration is done *only during expiration,* and is not done to the sensitive areas mentioned above. Observe the patient for any adverse effects and assist the patient to deep breathe and cough up the loosened secretions.

Humidification

Humidification is, in the context of respiration, the process of increasing the water content of air or oxygen to decrease the viscosity of thick secretions, thereby making their removal easier.

A gas is saturated when it is holding the maximum amount of water vapor it can hold at a given temperature. The capacity of a gas to hold water vapor increases with temperature. As air enters the nose, it is warmed and therefore able to hold more water vapor.

Because the warmed air can hold an increased amount of moisture, it absorbs moisture from the mucous membranes, so that, by the time it enters the alveoli, it is warmed to 37 degrees C and fully saturated. If the inspired air is dry, considerable moisture will be absorbed from the mucous membranes of the nose and mouth, leaving these surfaces dry, uncomfortable, and more susceptible to infection or irritation.

Cilia are the hairlike projections of the cells that line the respiratory tract from the nose to the bronchioles. They are 3 or 4 μ long (1 μ = 1/25,000 inch), and their major function is to carry mucus toward the pharynx, from which it is either expectorated or swallowed. The cilia normally beat at a rate of approximately 300 strokes/minute, but this rate is slowed by smoking, narcotics, sedatives, anesthesia, and emotional stress. When ciliary activity is decreased, mucus transport is slowed and the mucus is exposed to the air for a longer period of time. Dry, cool air absorbs water from the mucus, making it more viscous, and thereby slowing its transport even more. As a result, the mucus becomes very thick, and difficult to move. Therefore, it is likely to be retained or trapped in air passages, where it can obstruct them.

Additional moisture, from sources outside the patient's body, must be provided for patients who are dehydrated or whose mucous membranes are already dry and also for patients with thick or copious secretions. Humidification is also needed by a patient with a tracheostomy or other artificial airway because the warming and moisturizing mechanisms of the nose are bypassed when air enters the trachea directly.

Adequate humidity of inspired air can be maintained in two ways, either by keeping the patient's mucous membranes moist or by adding moisture to the air or oxygen before it is inspired. The mucous membranes of the patient's nose and throat are kept moist by forcing of fluids, either orally or intravenously, so that he is fully hydrated. The mucous membranes can also be kept moist by addition of water to the air before it is inspired, because moist air takes less moisture from the lining of the respiratory tract. Water can be added to the air by means of a humidifier or a nebulizer.

A *humidifier* is a device that forces a gas (either room air or oxygen) through sterile water so that it picks up water vapor and becomes more humid. Many different types are available, and they can be operated either at room temperature or at a higher temperature, which will increase the humidity. Some humidifiers for use in the home do not force air through water but instead expose a large, wet surface to the air. The water evaporates from the wet surface, enters the air, and thereby increases the moisture content of the air.

In the home, it is sometimes necessary to increase

the humidity of the air very rapidly to relieve the respiratory distress of a child with the croup, for example. You can do this in the bathroom by running hot water in the shower or by boiling pans of water in the kitchen with the kitchen doors closed.

A *nebulizer* is a device that produces a mist, or foglike suspension, of liquid particles in air or oxygen. The smaller the particles, the deeper they are able to penetrate the respiratory tract before they settle out of the inspired air.

Maintenance of an Artificial Airway

An *artificial airway* is used to maintain a patent (open) airway when the patient's upper air passageway has been occluded by injury, tumor, swelling, or another obstructive condition. An artificial airway also permits the use of a respirator or another source of mechanically controlled ventilation, and facilitates the suctioning of thick secretions that the patient is unable to cough up.

An *endotracheal tube* is used for short periods of time (from a few hours to a few days) and is inserted through the patient's nose or mouth. When an airway is needed for a longer period of time, a *tracheostomy tube* is inserted directly into the trachea through a surgical incision at the level of the second or third cartilaginous ring. The decision to use an artificial airway is made by the physician; and except in an emergency, the tube is inserted and removed by the physician.

Endotracheal Tube

An endotracheal tube is inserted through the patient's mouth or nose, and must be taped securely to the patient's face to keep it in place. If the tube is inserted through the patient's mouth (an orotracheal tube), special precautions may be needed to protect the tube and the patient's teeth if he tries to bite it.

The patient can have nothing by mouth while an endotracheal tube is in place; therefore, mouth care is vitally important. Because the tube passes between the vocal cords, the patient is unable to speak, so alternative methods of communication must be established at once if the patient is conscious. The patient may write messages, point to letters or pictures, or nod Yes or No to questions asked by others. Both the patient and his family will need frequent explanations and reassurance.

The patient's chest must be assessed at regular intervals. If the tube is properly positioned, both sides of the chest should be ventilating. If the tube has slipped down into one of the mainstem bronchi, it will obstruct the other bronchus and there will be decreased breath sounds on that side. A suspicion of improper placement should be confirmed by x-ray film. Auscultation of the chest is done frequently to assess the need for suctioning and to detect any changes that might indicate the development of complications.

Removal of an endotracheal tube (a process called *extubation*), either accidentally or intentionally, can be hazardous because of the possibility of aspiration, tracheal or laryngeal trauma, edema, or spasm following removal. The patient must therefore be observed closely for signs of respiratory distress following extubation.

Tracheostomy Tube

If intubation is needed for longer than a day or two, a tracheostomy tube is safer and more comfortable for the patient despite the fact that an incision is necessary for insertion. A tracheostomy tube rather than an endotracheal tube is used when the patient has suffered burns, surgery, or other trauma to his face and when his neck cannot be hyperextended for insertion of an endotracheal tube because of cervical injuries.

Because the tracheostomy tube is inserted below the vocal cords, expired air cannot reach or pass through the vocal cords, and speech is impossible. A patient who has a permanent tracheostomy is eventually taught how to block his tube intermittently to permit some form of speech, but the person with a new tracheostomy is faced with a major crisis. If intubation was done to alleviate a respiratory emergency, *someone should stay with the patient* until he is responsive enough to understand what has happened to him and until he is familiar with the communication system that will be used. The psychological ramifications of a tracheostomy, either temporary or permanent, can be almost overwhelming and must be granted a high priority among nursing interventions.

HAZARDS RELATED TO INTUBATION. In addition to being assured of some means of effective communication, the patient must be protected against infection. Inspired air now bypasses the upper respiratory tract where it would have been warmed, filtered, and moisturized. Under most atmospheric conditions, humidification is needed to protect the mucous membranes because a dry mucous membrane is more susceptible to trauma and infection than a moist one. The transfer of pathogenic organisms by air currents must be avoided because the air enters the lungs directly, with no filtering by the cilia to trap microorganisms and other foreign matter. The tracheostomy incision is treated like any other surgical wound, and *sterile technique is essential* whenever the stoma (the surgical opening) is cleansed and dressed. The skin around the tube is cleansed with sterile water and hydrogen peroxide to loosen both moist and dried secretions. An antibiotic ointment is sometimes used,

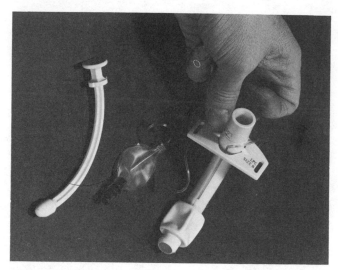

Figure 32.11 *Tracheostomy tube and obturator. Obturator (left) is placed inside tracheostomy tube (right) before insertion in the patient's trachea and is then removed. The blunt end of the obturator guides the tube through the incision. Center: a device used to inflate and deflate the cuff at the lower end of the tracheostomy tube.*

and the area is covered with a specially prepared, divided sterile dressing, often referred to as pants.

Both endotracheal and tracheostomy tubes are available with a cuff (Fig. 32.11, right) that can be inflated to fill the space between the tube and the trachea and prevent any leakage of air around the tube. When a high pressure cuffed tube is being used, it must be deflated at regular intervals to prevent damage to the trachea. Continuous pressure against the walls of the trachea interferes with circulation to the tissues, thereby causing pressure sores. Newer types of low-pressure cuffs do not need to be deflated.

Obstruction or accidental displacement of either an endotracheal or a tracheostomy tube is an *emergency,* for asphyxiation can occur very rapidly. Equipment for coping with such an emergency must therefore be kept in the patient's unit at all times.

Suctioning

The suctioning of an intubated patient to remove accumulated secretions is a complex task that should be attempted only after careful preparation and under competent supervision. Briefly, a few of the most important guidelines are:

- *An intubated patient is very susceptible to respiratory infections.* Therefore, a sterile catheter should be used each time he is suctioned. In situations in which this is not possible, the catheter should be rinsed after use with sterile water, soaked in an antiseptic solution until the next use, and exchanged for a sterile catheter every 8 hours. A sterile glove is worn on the hand used to manipulate the catheter.

- *Suctioning removes air as well as secretions from the lungs.* Therefore, before each suctioning, the patient must be adequately oxygenated by deep breathing or by the administration of oxygen. He should not be suctioned for longer than about 5 seconds with reoxygenation. If a clock with a second hand is not readily accessible, hold your breath each time you suction, then stop suctioning *before* you are completely out of breath, because the patient's ability to go without air is shorter than yours.

- *No suction should be used during the insertion of the catheter.* Suctioning in the absence of secretions tends to pull the catheter against the wall of the tracheostomy tube or against the lining of the trachea or bronchus and may damage those surfaces.

Premature suction is avoided or prevented either by the use of a special switch or device on the suction machine or by a Y connector on the tubing. The openings at the bottom and one arm of the Y connector are attached to the suction catheter and the suction tubing. The other arm is open and permits a flow of air which breaks the suction. When suction is needed, this second arm of the Y is covered with your thumb, the intake of air is blocked, and suction is created.

- *Consult the hospital procedure manual or other detailed procedure manual, and secure qualified supervision before suctioning an intubated person for the first time.*

PROCEDURE 32.2

*Suctioning a Patient**

SUMMARY OF ESSENTIAL NURSING ACTIONS

1. Recognize the indicators of a need for suctioning (rapid or distressed breathing, rasping or gurgling respirations, moist rales, and so on).
2. Determine whether or not a specific amount of suction has been prescribed.
3. Determine whether equipment and supplies at bedside are complete. If not, obtain them.
4. Raise head of bed to semi-Fowler position unless this is contraindicated.
5. Maintain sterile technique throughout procedure.
6. Estimate distance catheter should be inserted, and lubricate tip with sterile water or saline.
7. Insert catheter gently WITHOUT SUCTION.

- For nasopharyngeal suction, insert catheter through whichever nostril is likely to be more patent. If resistance is encountered, try the other one. DO NOT USE FORCE.
- For oral suctioning, insert catheter along one side of mouth to minimize gagging.

8. Apply suction and withdraw catheter slowly while rotating it back and forth. Total suctioning time should not exceed 10–15 seconds.
9. Rinse catheter with sterile saline or water.
10. Encourage patient to breathe deeply and cough.
11. Check respiratory status; use stethoscope as indicated.
12. Repeat suctioning, deep breathing, and coughing until airway is clear.

*See inside front cover and page 636.

NURSING MEASURES TO PROMOTE CIRCULATION

Poor circulation can be caused by a number of pathological conditions related to heart, blood volume, or blood vessels. Examples of such conditions include, respectively, heart failure, hemorrhage, and thrombophlebitis. Any measures designed to improve circulation by treating such disease conditions fall within the realm of medical practice and must be ordered by the physician. Other measures, however, can improve circulation by treating not the disease but the *body's response to a disease process*. Such treatments fall within the scope of independent nursing action, although the physician is often consulted. Circulation can be improved either by increasing the flow of blood to and through an area of the body, or by promoting the return of venous blood to the heart.

Measures To Increase the Flow of Blood

The flow of blood to and through an area of the body can be increased by exercise and heat, and also by decreased use of vasoconstrictors such as coffee and tobacco.

Exercise

The amount and type of exercise employed will be determined by the *condition* and *needs* of the patient. For example, exercise is obviously an inappropriate and unsafe way to improve the circulation of a patient who has just suffered a heart attack or whose blood volume is low because of hemorrhage. Exercise is also unsafe if a patient has thrombophlebitis from which a thrombus might break loose and produce a dangerous embolism.

Examples of Ways to Increase Circulation

- A patient confined to bed can:
  - Turn over in bed frequently
  - Do active ROM exercises
  - Do quadriceps setting exercises
  - Push against the footboard with a walking motion
  - Bathe and groom self
- A person who sits for long periods can:
  - Push against the floor as if rocking in a rocking chair
  - Raise and lower feet and legs at regular intervals (a form of quadriceps setting)
  - Move ankles in a circle
  - If able to walk at all, stand and take at least a few steps every hour
- A person who is able to walk should:
  - Walk several times daily (around his room, up and down the hall, or outdoors when possible) until he begins to tire
  - Incorporate a full program of ROM exercises into his activities of daily living (ADL)

Exercise is an appropriate way to increase circulation that is inadequate because of narrowed or constricted blood vessels or as a result of a patient's failure to move about. If a patient is unable to move, passive range-of-motion exercises and frequent turning by the nurse are essential. If a patient is able to move, the amount and type of appropriate exercise depends upon his condition.

Heat

Unless contraindicated, heat is often used to increase circulation to and through an area. A person with poor circulation, especially peripheral vascular disease, should minimize vasoconstriction of his feet by wearing warm footwear, including bed socks at night if needed.

Measures to Promote Venous Return

Some circulatory problems are due to poor venous return from the feet and legs, which causes dependent edema, venous stasis, or both. An important method of promoting venous return from the legs is by the use of elastic antiembolism stockings. These stockings support the veins and help prevent the pooling of venous blood in dilated blood vessels. They are often referred to as TEDS, the trade name for *t*hrombo*e*mbolitic *d*isease *s*tockings.

Everyone, especially those persons with circulatory problems, should avoid any pressure or constriction such as that created by tight elastic on knee-length hose or pressure on the popliteal space from the seat of an ill-fitting chair. A person who must stand for long periods should shift his weight from one foot to the other to contract the muscles of calf and thigh and stimulate venous return. A person who sits for long stretches of time should be taught to elevate his feet as needed to prevent dependent edema in his feet and ankles.

Buerger-Allen Exercises

Many people with poor circulation in their legs are advised to do Buerger-Allen exercises, which were developed as a treatment for a peripheral vascular disease called Buerger's disease. In these exercises, circulation is enhanced by alternately raising and lowering the legs, which tends to fill and empty the veins. The patient lies on the bed with his legs and feet elevated until the skin blanches. This usually takes 2 to 3 minutes. The back of a chair tipped upside down makes a good leg rest. The patient then lowers his legs over the side of the bed for several minutes and exercises his ankles for several minutes until his feet are pink. Finally, he lies flat with his legs flat on the mattress for 3 to 4 minutes. The time for each position depends on the time needed for each color change. This color change must be watched

for and timed until the time needed for the change has been established. The three steps are usually repeated five to ten times every 6 to 8 hours.

NURSING MEASURES TO PROMOTE DIFFUSION

Oxygen Therapy

Oxygen is administered to treat conditions in which a patient is unable to achieve or maintain a normal arterial Po_2. A low blood level of oxygen (hypoxemia) can be caused by a variety of conditions, both acute and chronic, including airway obstruction, acute heart failure, acute respiratory failure, pulmonary edema, shock, and pneumonia.

The concentration of oxygen in room air is approximately 21 percent. The concentration of oxygen that is administered to a patient ranges from 21 percent to 100 percent, depending on the needs of the patient and the type of equipment used. *Oxygen is a medication* prescribed by the physician, and the dose must be as carefully regulated as that of any other therapeutic substance. Too little oxygen is ineffective, but too much can be dangerous. Many adults are blind today because, as premature infants, *before the hazards were known*, they were given high concentrations of oxygen, and suffered retrolental fibroplasia as a result.

The amount of oxygen that is actually inspired by the patient varies with the rate of flow (liters/minute), the type of equipment used, and the patient's rate and depth of ventilation. Various devices, such as a flow meter and an oxygen analyzer, are used to measure the concentration of oxygen being delivered to a patient. The effectiveness of oxygen therapy is monitored by analysis of the patient's arterial blood gases. The normal Po_2 is 90 to 100 mm Hg.

Equipment

There are many different methods of administering oxygen, the most common of which are described here. These methods include the use of a nasal cannula, nasal catheter, face mask, tracheostomy collar, croupette, or oxygen hood.

A *nasal cannula* is probably used most frequently. It consists of a length of flexible plastic tubing that slips around the patient's head, with two soft prongs about ⅝ inch long that fit into his nostrils. The advantages of the nasal cannula are that it is inexpensive, disposable, easy to use, comfortable, and does not interfere with eating, drinking, or talking.

A *nasal catheter* is a soft rubber or plastic catheter that is inserted through a nostril until the tip lies just above the uvula. It can be seen when the patient lifts his uvula by saying "aah." The catheter is taped to the patient's face, is rather uncomfortable, and must be changed from nostril to nostril every 8 to 12 hours to prevent irritation of the mucous membrane. It does not interfere with talking or eating.

It is difficult to regulate with precision the amount of oxygen actually received by the patient through a nasal cannula or nasal catheter because it is affected by whether the patient breathes through his mouth or his nose. A *simple face mask* covers the patient's nose and mouth. The amount of oxygen received depends on the fit of the mask as well as the rate of flow, and the patient's rate and depth of ventilation. The main disadvantages are that the mask must be removed for eating and talking, and it seems very confining to some patients.

A *Venturi face mask* permits a specified percentage of oxygen to be administered accurately (Fig. 32.12). The Venturi principle is: any constriction in the diameter of a tube creates a change in the velocity and pressure of a gas as it passes through the constriction. In a Venturi oxygen mask, when 100 percent oxygen passes from a narrow tube into a larger section of tubing, the resulting change in pressure draws room air into the mask through holes on each side. The rate of flow of room air is controlled by the size of the holes, and adapters are available that will yield a precise concentration of oxygen to the patient, usually between 24 percent and 40 percent. The disadvantages of the Venturi mask are the same as the disadvantages of any face mask.

A *tracheostomy collar* delivers humidified oxygen directly to a patient's tracheostomy tube. A *croupette* is a tentlike apparatus that fits over an infant in a crib to provide both oxygen and humidity. An *oxygen hood* fits

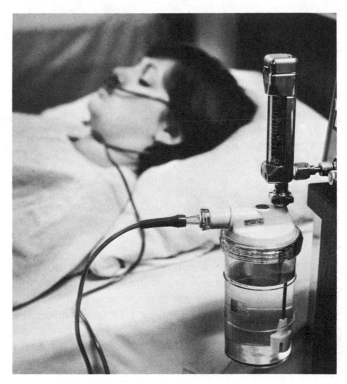

Figure 32.13 *Supplemental oxygen should always be humidified to prevent drying and crusting of mucous membranes within the respiratory tract.*

over the head of a child or an adult to provide a high concentration of oxygen and humidity (Fig. 32.13).

When a patient is unable to ventilate enough to benefit from the administration of oxygen, a mechanical ventilator (respirator) must be used in conjunction with oxygen to assist ventilation and maintain the Po_2 level above a minimum of 60 mm Hg.

Nursing Responsibilities

ADMINISTRATION. In many settings, the oxygen equipment is set up and started by the respiratory therapy department, but the nursing staff is then responsible for the subsequent administration. This includes checking the dose of oxygen (the rate of flow, the concentration of O_2, or both) at regular intervals, checking the functioning of humidifying equipment, and monitoring the rate and depth of the patient's respiration. Careful planning is often needed to ensure that the patient receives optimal benefit from the oxygen. This means that a patient who is receiving oxygen intermittently (prn) or whose face mask must be removed for meals must be given oxygen at the time of greatest exertion. If, for example, a patient with a face mask is to be gotten out of bed and into a chair for a meal, the mask should not be removed *before* he gets out of bed, even

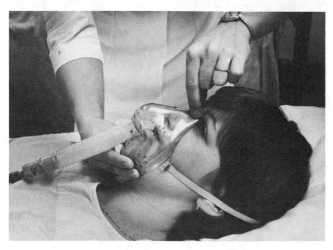

Figure 32.12 *Venturi mask, which allows the administration of a very accurate dosage of oxygen.*

though it must be removed shortly afterward so he can eat. He needs oxygen during the activity of moving from bed to chair; it is more beneficial to *prevent hypoxemia* than it is to try to relieve the after effects of oxygen deprivation. A patient who has been directed to use oxygen prn at home needs to be taught, for example, to use oxygen while making a bed rather than using oxygen afterward to relieve the distress that follows exertion with inadequate oxygen intake. There is nothing to be gained by trying to do without oxygen when there is a physiological need for it.

If a patient who is using a face mask needs continuous oxygen, a nasal cannula can be substituted for the mask at meal time.

SAFETY. The safety of the patient and others must be ensured when oxygen is being used. Oxygen will not explode, but *oxygen supports combustion* and substances that are safe in room air become highly flammable in concentrated oxygen. For example, oil is not used on oxygen equipment because a spark can ignite oil in the presence of 100 percent oxygen.

THERE CAN BE NO SMOKING IN THE AREA. "No Smoking" signs must be posted and rigidly enforced. All matches and, if necessary, all smoking materials must be removed from the patient's unit.

Static electricity must be prevented because sparks ignite easily in oxygen. Oils or other flammable substances such as ether should not be used in the area. All electrical plugs, outlets, and equipment must be grounded, and poorly insulated or frayed cords cannot be used.

PSYCHOLOGICAL CONSIDERATIONS. Whenever possible, patient teaching should precede the use of oxygen, for both patients and families are often distressed by a fear that the oxygen will explode or by a belief that oxygen is used only when a patient is critically ill or getting worse. It is important, therefore, that the patient and family be given ample time and opportunity to express their feelings and concerns.

In noncritical situations, people often worry that the patient will become dependent on the use of oxygen, and the nurse will have to explain that the patient's need for oxygen is determined by analysis of his arterial blood gases and that the use of oxygen will be adjusted accordingly.

If oxygen therapy is to be discontinued or the patient is being weaned from oxygen after a very long period of use, a calm, relaxed environment is necessary because excitement, stress, and tension will increase his need for oxygen. Oxygen should not be suddenly discontinued before a period of exertion such as physical therapy or on a day when the patient is having an important diagnostic test or many visitors. Someone should remain with him for a time when the oxygen is first discontinued. If this is not possible, his call bell should be placed within easy reach, or he should be wheeled into the hall near the nurse's station so that his respiratory status can be readily assessed and so that he will not feel anxious or frightened without his oxygen.

PROCEDURE 32.3

Administering Oxygen*

SUMMARY OF ESSENTIAL NURSING ACTIONS

1. *Insure safety from fire when oxygen is in use.*
2. Check equipment for comfort and effectiveness.
   - Adjust elastic band of cannula for proper fit.
   - Change nasal catheter regularly to avoid irritation of nares.
   - Make sure that face mask fits snugly.

3. Check the rate of flow of oxygen; keep it at the prescribed concentration or number of liters/minute.
4. Keep adequate amount of water in humidifying equipment.
5. Anticipate and attend to psychological needs of patient and family.
6. Assess patient's respiratory status at regular intervals.

*See inside front cover and pages 639–640.

Complications

The overuse or misuse of oxygen can produce a variety of serious complications, including respiratory depression, oxygen toxicity, atelectasis, and retrolental fibroplasia.

RESPIRATORY DEPRESSION. In healthy people, an *increased* Pco_2 stimulates respiration in order to blow off the excess CO_2. The *reverse* is true for patients with chronic respiratory disease, however. These patients retain CO_2, and their *usual* Pco_2 level is thus higher than normal (hypercarbia).

For such patients, the stimulus to breathe no longer comes primarily from their Pco_2 and they breathe in response to a decreased Po_2 (hypoxemia). Any abrupt administration of oxygen elevates the Po_2, thereby reducing the patient's stimulus to breathe. This results in hypoventilation or even apnea (cessation of breathing). Patients who have, or are suspected of having, chronic hypercarbia should be given *low doses of oxygen* and observed carefully, and their blood gases should be monitored closely.

PULMONARY OXYGEN TOXICITY. Prolonged exposure to a high concentration of oxygen can damage lung tissue by causing alveolar edema or hemorrhage, hyperplasia (overgrowth) of alveolar linings, early fibrosis, or pulmonary congestion. Such damage interferes with the exchange of gases in the alveoli and as a result, ever-increasing amounts of oxygen must be administered to maintain an adequate Po_2. Inasmuch as the safe dose of oxygen has not yet been established—in terms of either concentration or duration of exposure—it is important to avoid possible toxicity by keeping the use of oxygen to the lowest possible dose that will maintain an adequate Po_2.

ATELECTASIS. Room air contains approximately 80 percent nitrogen, and as nitrogen is not absorbed from the alveoli by the blood, the nitrogen pressure in the alveoli helps to keep the alveoli fully expanded. When a patient is receiving high doses of oxygen, the oxygen replaces nitrogen, and the percentage of nitrogen may drop from 80 percent to 50 percent or less. Because most of the oxygen is absorbed and there is less non-absorbable nitrogen to keep the alveoli expanded, the alveoli may collapse, especially if other pulmonary problems, such as pooled secretions, are present. Because oxygen cannot be absorbed through collapsed, airless alveoli, hypoxemia develops.

In addition to observing patients for signs of hypoxemia and atelectasis, nursing care of patients receiving oxygen should include prophylactic measures such as deep breathing and coughing plus frequent change of position to prevent any pooling of secretions.

RETROLENTAL FIBROPLASIA. Premature infants are especially susceptible to fibrosis in the chamber of the eye behind the lens (the retrolental chamber), and the damage can result in blindness. The eyes of adults can be damaged also.

SUGGESTED READINGS

Bates, Barbara: *A Guide to Physical Examination,* Ed 2, Philadelphia: Lippincott, 1979.

Beller, Linda Cissel, and Kathryn L Neunaber: The 'simple' valsalva. *Am J Nurs* 1986 April; 86(4):398–399.

Brown, Iva: Trach care? take care—infections on the prowl. *Nursing 82* 1982 May; 12(5):44–49.

Bolton, Margie E: Hyperbaric Oxygen Therapy. *Am J Nurs* 1981 June; 81(6):1199–1201.

Buschiazzo, Linda: What's new in CPR? *Nursing 86* 1986 Jan; 16(1):34–37.

Callahan, Mary: COPD makes a bad first impression, but you'll find wonderful people underneath. *Nursing 82* 1982 May; 12(5):68–72.

Carroll, Patricia Fuchs: Caring for ventilator patients. *Nursing 86* 1986 Feb; 16(2):34–39.

Cohen, Stephen, and Sara Wells: Nursing care of patients in shock: fluids, oxygen, and the intra-aortic balloon pump (programmed instruction). *Am J Nurs* 1982 Sept; 82(9):1401–1422.

Cohen, Stephen, and Sara Wells: Nursing care of patients in shock: evaluating the patient (programmed instruction). *Am J Nurs* 1982 Nov; 82(11):1723–1746.

Cohen, Stephen, and Madonna Stack: How to work with chest tubes. (programmed instruction) *Am J Nurs* 1980 April; 80(4):685–712.

Cross, Malinda: Dissolving the threat of pulmonary embolism. *RN* 1984 Aug; 47(8):34–41.

D'Agostino, Janet S: Set your mind at ease on oxygen toxicity. *Nursing 83* 1983 July; 13(7):55–56.

Darovic, Gloria O: Ten perils of mechanical ventilation . . . and how to hold them in check. *RN* 1983 May; 46(5):37–42.

Dennison, Robin: Cardiopulmonary assessment: How to do it better in 15 easy steps. *Nursing 86* 1986 April; 16(4):34–39.

Doyle, Jeanne E: All leg ulcers are not alike: managing and preventing arterial and venous ulcers. *Nursing 83* 1983 Jan; 13(1):58–63.

Erickson, Barbara Ann: Detecting abnormal heart sounds. *Nursing 86* Jan; 16(1):58–63.

Fahey, Victoria A: An in-depth look at deep vein thrombosis. *Nursing 84* 1984 March; 14(3):34–41.

Fuchs, Patricia L: Streamlining your suctioning techniques (3 parts). *Am J Nurs* 1984 May, June, and July. Part 1: Nasotracheal suctioning. May; 14(5):55–61. Part 2: Endotracheal suctioning. June; 14(6):46–51. Part 3: Tracheostomy suctioning. July; 14(7):39–43.

Fuchs, Patricia: Before and after surgery—stay right on respiratory care. *Nursing 83* 1983 May; 13(5):47–50.

Fuchs, Patricia L: Getting the best out of oxygen delivery systems. *Nursing 80* 1980 Dec; 10(12):34.

Harper, Rosalind W: *A Guide to Respiratory Care: Physiology and Clinical Applications*. Philadelphia, Lippincott, 1981.

Humbrecht, Barbara, and Eileen Van Parys: From assessment to intervention: how to use heart and breath sounds as part of your nursing care plan. *Nursing 82* 1982 April; 12(4):34–42.

Ivancin, Lois A: Healing those frustrating stasis ulcers. *RN* 1983 Aug; 46(8):38–40.

Marcenek, Margaret Boyle: Hypertension: what it does to the body. *Am J Nurs* 1980 May; 80(5):928–933.

Maxwell, Mary B: Dyspnea during lung cancer. *Am J Nurs* 1985 June; 85(6):672–677.

McConnell, Edwina A: Fitting antiembolism stockings. *Nursing 78* 1978 Sept; 8(9):67–71.

Miller, Patricia Gonce: Assessing C.V.P. *Nursing 85* 1985 Sept; 15(9):44–46.

Mims, Barbara C: You *can* manage chest tubes confidently. *RN* 1985 Jan; 48(1):39–44.

Mizuki, June A: It takes top-notch teamwork once a ventilator-dependent patient decides . . . There's no place like home. *Am J Nurs* 1984 May; 84(5):646–648.

Nielson, Lois: Assessing patients' respiratory problems. *Am J Nurs* 1980 Dec; 80(12):2192–2202.

Pfister, Shirley: Respiratory arrest—are you prepared? *Nursing 82* 1982 Sept; 12(9):34–41.

Rifas, Ellene: How to listen in on breath sounds. *RN* 1984 March; 47(3):30–33.

Summer, Sara M, and Vicki Lewandowski: Guidelines for using artificial breathing devices. *Nursing 83* 1983 Oct; 13(10):54–57.

Taylor, Dolores Lake: Assessing breath sounds. *Nursing 85* 1985 March; 15(3):60–62.

Weaver, Terri E: New life for lungs . . . through incentive spirometers. *Nursing 81* 1981 Feb; 11(2):54–59.

Wimsatt, Ruth: Unlocking the mysteries behind the chest wall. *Nursing 85* 1985 Nov; 15(11):58–63.

33

Nutrition

Rosalinda T. Laqua

Prerequisites and/or Suggested Preparation
An introductory course in nutrition, and knowledge of the basic processes of pathophysiology (Chapter 12) are prerequisite to understanding this chapter.

Food has different meanings for different people, and it is often associated with special occasions such as weddings, funerals, and certain religious ceremonies. Food is used to show love, the denial of food is often used as punishment, and the anxious person uses food to momentarily relieve his anxieties. It is important, therefore, for the nurse to understand and appreciate the ways in which these psychological and sociological factors influence a person's food habits before she can effectively meet his nutritional needs.

Each person's level of nutrition is the result of eating habits which are determined in part by one's cultural heritage, ethnic group, religion, and social environment. Food idiosyncrasies and food preference patterns are established during early childhood, and they usually become increasingly rigid as a person ages. Eating habits are also affected by agriculture, weather conditions, transportation, and the person's economic status.

NUTRITION

Simply stated, nutrition is the study of food in relation to health. Nutrition deals with the physiological needs of the body for specific nutrients, the ways and means of supplying these nutrients through adequate diets, and the effects of failure to meet nutrient needs. A *nutrient* is any chemical substance needed by the body for one or more of the following functions: providing heat or energy, building or repairing tissues, regulating body processes, and making essential substances such as enzymes and hormones. Nutrients are broadly classed as carbohydrates, proteins, fats, vitamins, and minerals. An adequate diet consists of a balance of these nutrients and water, which serves as a solvent and means of transport for both nutrients and the waste products that result from the use of food.

CATEGORIES OF NUTRIENTS

Carbohydrates

Carbohydrates are the most readily available source of energy and the primary source of calories in most diets. Starches, sugars, and cellulose are familiar forms of carbohydrates from plant foods. Carbohydrates in the body occur chiefly as glucose (physiologic sugar) and glycogen (animal starch). Starches and sugar supply the body with a relatively inexpensive and important source of energy, and each gram of carbohydrate yields approximately 4 kilocalories (k cal). Starches and sugars also exert a *sparing action* on behalf of protein in the body. Protein is not used as a source of energy when sufficient carbohydrate is available to supply the body's needs. The energy needs of the body take precedence over other needs. Glucose is the sole source of energy for the brain and is indispensable for the functional integrity of nervous tissue. Therefore, a steady supply of glucose from the blood is essential for the proper functioning of these tissues.

Although *cellulose* is not digested and is not a source of energy for humans, it provides bulk in the intestinal tract and stimulates the peristaltic movement of the gastrointestinal tract. Cellulose and other indigestible forms of carbohydrate are more commonly referred to as roughage or dietary fiber. There has been considerable interest in cellulose (fiber) in recent years; lack of dietary fiber may be related to the etiology of common diseases of the colon, such as diverticulosis, constipation, and cancer. By affecting stool bulk, softness, and transit time, dietary fiber is thought to play a role both in reducing the exposure of the intestinal mucosa to possible carcinogenic substances in the feces and in lessening colonic pressure that may lead to diverticulosis. Dietary fiber has also been found to lower blood glucose and cholesterol levels.

Carbohydrates provide about 45 to 55 percent of the day's calories in typical American diets. Foods such as pastas, breads, cereals, legumes, potatoes, and corn are good sources of starch; they also contain varying amounts of protein, minerals, and vitamins. Refined sugar, syrups, and many candies and sweets are pure carbohydrate and contain little of the other nutrients. They are referred to as "empty calories" because they contribute nothing but calories. On the other hand, unrefined cereals and many fruits and vegetables contain dietary fiber and other nutrients. The fiber intake of the average American adult is estimated at about 20 grams (g) per day. This amount is much less than the fiber consumption in the early 1900s because of the decrease in the consumption of potatoes, fruits, cereals, dry peas, and beans. A dietary fiber intake of 25 to 40 gm per day is desirable for optimal gastrointestinal function.

Although cellulose is now a recognized food additive, powdered cellulose does not have the same functional characteristics as the cellulose that occurs naturally in foods, and many people could improve their diets by eating more complex carbohydrate foods. Table 33.1 lists the fiber content of common foods.

Proteins

The biological role of protein is unique: protein truly merits its name, which originated from a Greek word, *proteios*, meaning "to take first place." An important function of protein is its role in tissue synthesis, which is essential for the growth and maintenance of body

TABLE 33.1 DIETARY FIBER CONTENT OF SOME FOODS*

Food	Serving Size	Dietary Fiber (g)	Food	Serving Size	Dietary Fiber (g)
Fruits			*Vegetables*		
Apple	1 med	3.2	Asparagus	4 spears	0.9
Apricots	3	2.4	Beans, baked	1 c	18.6
Banana	1 med	5.9	Green beans	1 c	3.5
Cherries	10	1.3	Broccoli tops	1 c	5.6
Cranberries	½ c	2.3	Brussel sprouts	1 c	6.5
Dates, dried	10	7.0	Cabbage, shredded	1 c	1.9
Figs, dried	2	18.5	Carrots	1 c	3.2
Grapes, green	20	1.1	Cauliflower	1 c	2.5
Mangoes	1	4.5	Celery	1 stalk	0.7
Cantaloupe	¼ melon	2.5	Cucumber	6 slices	0.2
Honeydew	¼ melon	2.7	Lettuce	1 c	0.8
Orange	1 med	4.5	Mushrooms	1 c	1.8
Peach	1 med	2.1	Onion	1 small	1.4
Pear	1 med	3.1	Peas	1 c	11.3
Pineapple, canned	1 c	2.2	Pepper, sweet	1 c	0.9
Pineapple, fresh	1 c	1.9	Potato, boiled	1 med	1.4
Plums	2	2.5	Spinach	1 c	3.5
Prunes, dried	4	5.2	Tomato	1 med	3.0
Raisins	½ c	5.4			
Strawberries	1 c	3.3	*Breads and Cereals*		
			White bread	1 slice	0.8
Nuts			Whole-wheat bread	1 slice	2.4
Almonds	10	3.6	All-Bran	½ c	9.9
Brazil nuts	10	5.4	Cornflakes	1 c	2.8
Peanuts	½ c	5.7	Grape Nuts	1 c	5.3
Peanut butter	2 T	2.1	Rice Krispies	1 c	1.4
			Shredded wheat	1 biscuit	3.0
			Special K	1 c	1.7

*All foods fresh unless stated otherwise.
Source: Slavin, JL : Dietary Fiber. *Dietetic Currents,* 10 (c):31, 1983.

tissues. Adequate protein must be included in the child's diet for growth to occur, because where total protein intake is inadequate, growth is impeded or even stopped.

In adults, an insufficient intake of protein produces a wasting of tissue as body protein is broken down over a period of time. The body does not store protein in the same way or to the same extent that it stores fat and carbohydrate. Although all organs and tissues store protein to a limited extent, the stored protein is more appropriately termed *labile tissue protein.* This means that the protein reserve is in a dynamic state and is constantly being broken down *(catabolism)* or resynthesized *(anabolism).*

Protein is a structural component of all living cells and is found in muscles, nerves, bones, teeth, skin, hair, nails, blood, and glands. Almost all body fluids contain protein. All enzymes, antibodies, and some hormones like insulin, thyroxine, and adrenalin are composed of protein. Enzymes catalyze the chemical reactions in the body, whereas hormones are essential for regulating various body processes. Antibodies are a part of the body's defense mechanism to fight infection and to provide maximum resistance to infectious agents. This protection applies to microbial as well as toxic chemical substances.

Protein is a regulator of blood pH, osmotic pressure, and water balance. The *amphoteric* nature of protein helps maintain the body at a pH that is slightly alkaline. That is, if body fluids contain excess acid, the proteins function as a base; whereas if body fluids contain excess alkali, the proteins can function as an acid. Plasma proteins, particularly albumin, are important in maintaining the normal osmotic pressure of body fluids. Edema results when plasma protein level is low as a result of a protein deficiency.

When used as a source of energy, protein provides about 4 k cal/gm. Fat and carbohydrate should be the main source of energy, not protein, because protein is needed for many other important functions in the body.

Proteins are found in both animal and plant foods. Animal protein sources include beef, veal, pork, poultry, fish, eggs, milk, and cheese. Plant proteins are found in legumes, wheat, and corn. Approximately 12 to 15 percent of the day's calories should be derived from protein, and at least one-third of the protein intake should come from animal sources. Animal proteins are of high quality and are said to be *complete* proteins. A complete protein contains all the essential amino acids in amounts sufficient to maintain life and promote growth. Vegetable proteins are called *incomplete* because they do not contain all the essential amino acids and cannot by themselves support life or growth. Vegetable proteins can, however, be combined with small amounts of complete proteins or with each other to create a complete assortment of amino acids in the amounts needed for tissue synthesis. Protein requirements in vegetarian diets can be met by combining complementary plant proteins to achieve the necessary balance of essential amino acids. The four basic types of vegetarian diets are:

1. *Lacto-ovo-vegetarian.* Milk, cheese, and eggs are taken, in addition to cereals, legumes, vegetables, and fruits. There is no problem securing adequate protein with this diet.

2. *Lactovegetarian.* Only milk and cheese are used to supplement an all-vegetable diet. Milk products add complete protein and enhance the amino acid values in vegetable proteins.

3. *Pure vegetarian (vegan).* Foods of plant origin are eaten, without restrictions as to kind. Careful planning is required to achieve combinations that provide the necessary amounts of the essential amino acids. A deficiency in vitamin B_{12} may occur because that vitamin is present only in animal foods.

4. *Fruitarian.* Plant foods eaten are restricted to fruits, nuts, honey, and grain. The likelihood of protein inadequacy is much greater in this diet than with other vegetarian diets.

The recommended daily protein allowance for a normal adult is 0.8 gm/kg body weight. Protein requirements vary with age, body size, physiological condition (growth, pregnancy, and lactation), type of protein in the diet, adequacy of caloric intake, and state of health. Protein needs are greater during stress and other conditions of increased nitrogen breakdown (protein catabolism), such as burns, surgery, fever, and acute infections. Merely staying in bed for several days will put a person into *negative nitrogen balance* (a state in which more nitrogen is being excreted than is being consumed). Depletion of body protein can lead to poor wound healing, anemia, increased susceptibility to infections, and decreased ability to fight complications. It is important, therefore, to make sure that the diets of ill and convalescent people contain liberal amounts of protein.

Fats

Fat is the body's most concentrated source of energy. It provides 9 k cal/gm in contrast to the 4 k cal/gm of carbohydrates and proteins. The term *fat* is often used interchangeably with the term *lipid,* which includes a heterogeneous group of compounds related to the fatty acids. The fatty acid called *linoleic acid* is essential for growth and for the prevention of certain types of dermatitis in infants.

Fats serve as carriers of the fat-soluble vitamins, A, D, E, and K. These vitamins are not soluble in water but are miscible with the fats and oils in foods. In the stomach, fats depress gastric secretion and slow emptying time, thus providing a feeling of fullness and satisfaction after a meal.

Body fat is stored in special adipose (fatty) tissue. This storage of fat is a reserve source of energy for times when food intake is insufficient to meet the body's needs. Adipose tissue also helps to hold the body organs and nerves in position and protect them against traumatic injury and shock. The subcutaneous layer of fat insulates the body and thereby serves to preserve body heat and maintain body temperature. The gustatory (taste) value of fats also deserves to be mentioned.

The recommended intake of fat is 30 to 35 percent of the total calories, although typical Americans obtain about 45 percent of their calories from fat. Rich sources of fat include meats, butter, margarine, cream, cheese, and salad dressings. Other sources of fat are far less obvious. These so-called hidden fats occur as marbling or small deposits of fat in the muscle of high-quality meat. Milk, nuts, olives, and avocados are other sources of hidden fat. Although fats are widely available in animal foods, some plants are also valuable sources of oils. Most cooking oils are made from plant sources such as olives, corn, soybeans, safflower, and cottonseed.

There is considerable interest in the topic of consumption of fat and cholesterol (a type of lipid compound found only in foods of animal origin) because dietary fat and cholesterol have been associated with the causation of atherosclerosis and coronary heart disease. The cholesterol content of a typical American diet is about 600 to 700 mg per day. A cholesterol intake of 300 mg or less is recommended by the American Heart Association. Found only in animal sources, cholesterol is present in large amounts in egg yolks, liver, and organ meats. It is present in smaller amounts in the fat of meat, whole milk, cheese, and ice cream. Fruits, vegetables, and cereals contain no cholesterol. Table 33.2 shows the cholesterol content of some foods.

TABLE 33.2 CHOLESTEROL CONTENT OF SELECTED FOODS

Food Item	Size of Serving	Mg Cholesterol per serving
Brain	3½ oz	2082
Sweetbreads	3½ oz	466
Kidneys	3½ oz	375
Liver	3½ oz	300
Egg	1 large	273
Lobster	3½ oz	200
Oysters	5–8 medium	200
Shrimp	3½ oz	150
Crab	½ cup	100
Beef, med. fat	3½ oz	125
Beef, lean	3½ oz	95
Chicken, dark meat	3½ oz	95
Chicken, white meat	3½ oz	70
Veal cutlet	3½ oz	90
Lamp chop	3½ oz	70
Pork, ham	3½ oz	58
Halibut	3½ oz	75
Haddock	3½ oz	60
Salmon	3½ oz	35
Tuna, in oil	3½ oz	25
Tuna, in water	3½ oz	55
Butter	1 tbsp	36
Milk, whole	1 cup	35
Milk, 2% fat	1 cup	18
Milk, skim	1 cup	4
Cheese, cheddar or cream	1 oz	30
Cottage cheese, cream	½ cup	17
Cottage cheese, low fat	½ cup	9

From: Pennington, JA, and Church, HN: Bowe's and Church's *Food Values of Portions Commonly Used.* ed. 14. Philadelphia, J.B. Lippincott Co., 1985.

Vitamins

Vitamins are a group of organic substances that are present in food in minute quantities. They are needed by the body to promote growth and maintain life, and they vary widely in chemical structure and functions. Many act as coenzymes for specific reactions in the metabolism of nutrients and the release of energy from carbohydrates, proteins, and fats. Often called "accessory food factors," vitamins do not provide calories for energy.

Vitamins are classified into two groups on the basis of solubility: (1) the fat-soluble vitamins—A, D, E, and K and (2) the water-soluble vitamins—B complex and C. The members of the B-complex vitamin group are vitamin B_1 (thiamin), B_2 (riboflavin), vitamin B_6 (pyridoxine), vitamin B_{12} (cobalamin), niacin, folic acid, biotin, and pantothenic acid. The fat-soluble vitamins are absorbed along with dietary fats, and therefore, any substance or condition that interferes with the absorption of fats also interferes with the absorption and use of these vitamins. The fat-soluble vitamins can be stored in the body to some extent; and unlike the water-soluble vitamins, they are not normally excreted in the urine.

As a general rule, vitamins are widely distributed in many foods consumed by humans. No food contains all the vitamins, but a varied diet containing all the food groups will provide all the vitamins required for optimal health. The use of vitamin supplements is not necessary for a well-nourished person who eats a balanced diet. Vitamin supplements are recommended only as a therapeutic measure in the treatment of some illnesses or to correct an existing deficiency condition caused by a faulty diet. Vitamin supplements not only are expensive but may present a serious hazard to health. The issue of megavitamin supplementation is discussed later in this chapter.

Specific deficiency diseases occur when the intake of vitamins is inadequate. A deficiency in vitamin A results in night blindness and xerophthalmia, for example, and a deficiency in vitamin D impairs the absorption of calcium and causes rickets in children and osteomalacia in adults. Thiamin deficiency results in beriberi, and scurvy results when vitamin C is deficient.

Fat-soluble Vitamins

VITAMIN A. Vitamin A has several important functions in the body. Widely recognized as the vitamin that prevents night blindness, vitamin A is a component in the visual cycle that enables one to see in dim light. In children, vitamin A promotes optimal bone and skeletal growth.

Vitamin A is necessary for the normal maintenance

of the epithelial cells that line the body surfaces, including the intestines and skin, and that form the body's main barrier to infections. Without vitamin A, the epithelial cells become dry and flat and eventually harden to form scales that slough off. This process is called keratinization. In the eye, the tear ducts dry, robbing the eye of its cleansing and lubricating action and allowing infection to set in. The cornea becomes dry and hard, and this condition, called xerophthalmia, can lead to blindness in extreme vitamin A deficiency.

In the respiratory tract, ciliated epithelium in the nasal passages dries up, the cilia are lost, and a barrier to infection is thus removed. The mouth and salivary glands become dry and cracked, allowing invading organisms to multiply. The skin becomes rough and scaly with small papular eruptions around the hair follicles. This condition, called *follicular hyperkeratosis*, is commonly described as goose bumps or goosepimples.

There are few food sources of vitamin A. The vitamin is found only in animal foods, chiefly liver, egg yolk, and butter. Yellow and green vegetables and fruits such as squash, carrots, spinach, and apricots contain carotene, a provitamin that can be converted to vitamin A in the body. Other sources are products such as milk and margarine that are commercially fortified with vitamin A.

Excess vitamin A, or hypervitaminosis A, can cause toxic reactions such as violent headaches; nausea, peeling and thickening of the skin; coarse, sparse hair; and swelling and pain of long bones. The level at which vitamin A becomes toxic varies from one person to another. Massive doses of the vitamin should not be taken without a physician's prescription and supervision.

VITAMIN D. Vitamin D promotes the development of normal bone and teeth. Its primary function is to facilitate calcium and phosphorus absorption from the intestine and their deposition in bone tissue. A deficiency in vitamin D results in rickets in children and osteomalacia in adults. Rickets is characterized by soft and fragile bones, delayed dentition and closure of the fontanelles, bowlegs and knock-knees, beadlike protrusions on the ribs (rachitic rosary), swollen and enlarged joints, and a potbelly from weak abdominal muscles. Osteomalacia is common among women who have had a series of pregnancies combined with a low vitamin D intake and little exposure to the sun. The condition is characterized by a rheumatic type of pain in the pelvis, lower back, and legs and by softening and tenderness of bones. Involuntary twitches, muscle spasms, and a susceptibility to bone fracture occur with a severe lack of vitamin D.

Excessive intake of vitamin D from food is unlikely.

There are few natural food sources other than fish-liver oils and milk fortified with vitamin D. Vitamin D is not present in plants. Self-prescribed high-potency pharmaceutical preparations and excessive intake of concentrated fish-liver oils are the two common causes of vitamin D toxicity. Excessive intake of vitamin D produces toxicity, resulting in demineralization of the bones and deposition of calcium in soft tissues. Other toxic effects are nausea, diarrhea, vomiting, and weight loss. Continued overdose of the vitamin can result in renal damage, uremia, and death in severe cases.

The body is able to make vitamin D when the skin is exposed to sunlight. The energy provided by the ultraviolet rays of the sun converts 7-dehydrocholesterol, a lipid compound present under the skin, to the active vitamin. Clouds, fog, ordinary glass, clothing, and any other element that filters the sunlight will impede the irradiation of 7-dehydrocholesterol and the manufacture of vitamin D.

VITAMIN E. The public is often confused about the role of vitamin E because, although it was initially designated the antisterility vitamin, the reproductive function of this vitamin is seen only in rats. In humans, vitamin E functions as an antioxidant. It protects the fat in red blood cells from oxidation, thus preventing hemolysis (breakdown) of erythrocytes. Vitamin E also prevents the oxidation of vitamins A and C and the unsaturated fatty acids, enabling these essential nutrients to perform their specific functions in the body.

Vitamin E deficiency in adults is rare, although hemolysis of erythrocytes has been reported in infants. Good food sources are vegetable oils, unmilled cereals, and green leafy vegetables. Except for egg yolk, liver, and milk, animal foods are poor sources of the vitamin. Because of its antioxidant property, vitamin E is used in the food industry as an additive to prolong the shelf life of prepared foods. Even though vitamin E has not shown toxic effects, prolonged intake of large doses may be more toxic than is presently known. A large dose of vitamin E interferes with the functioning of vitamin K and can prolong the clotting of blood. High intakes of vitamin E also reduce the serum thyroid hormone and elevate the serum triglyceride in women.

VITAMIN K. Often called the antihemorrhage vitamin, this vitamin is involved in the process of blood coagulation, mainly in the formation of prothrombin. A deficiency in vitamin K results in delayed blood clotting in adults and hemorrhagic disease in newborn infants. Synthesis of vitamin K by intestinal bacteria is the body's main source of the vitamin, although it is also found in dark green leafy vegetables, egg yolk, and liver. A dietary deficiency of this vitamin has not been seen, inasmuch as it is synthesized in the intestines. A conditioned vitamin K deficiency may result, however, from diseases in which fat absorption is impaired, such as sprue and celiac disease, and also from sulfonamide or antibiotic therapy, which destroys intestinal bacteria and prevents synthesis of the vitamin in the intestines. Menadione, the synthetic form of vitamin K, has been known to be toxic, causing vomiting and hemolytic anemia.

WATER-SOLUBLE VITAMINS

THIAMIN. Vitamin B_1, or thiamin, is a component of a coenzyme that is required in the formation of energy from carbohydrate and fat. Thiamin also helps maintain normal appetite, regulates muscle tone of the GI tract, and maintains normal functioning of the nervous system. Early signs of thiamin deficiency are loss of appetite, constipation, irritability, depression, and general weakness. Severe thiamin deficiency is clinically recognized as *beriberi.* In children, beriberi has a rapid onset and can cause death within a short period of time; in adults, it takes a more deliberate course. Beriberi is manifested in two forms: dry beriberi, a form characterized by progressive paralysis and mental confusion; and wet beriberi, a form characterized by pitting edema and swelling of the tissues owing to fluid retention. The heart muscle also becomes edematous, and heart failure may result if the thiamin deficiency remains uncorrected. The chief sources of thiamin are yeast, pork, liver, and other glandular organs, whole grains, and enriched cereals and breads.

Intolerance to large doses of thiamin has been reported and is presumably due to simple chemical toxicity, principally through the formation of excessive amounts of histamine.

RIBOFLAVIN. Also called vitamin B_2, riboflavin is an essential component of the flavoprotein coenzymes that are essential for normal cellular oxidation. The vitamin also promotes growth and development, maintains normal skin tone and vision, and converts the amino acid tryptophan to niacin, another of the B vitamins. A deficiency of riboflavin results in *ariboflavinosis,* a condition characterized by fissures at the corners of the mouth (angular stomatitis), cracks on both upper and lower lips (cheilosis), and inflammation of the tongue (glossitis) with a characteristic magenta color. Symptoms of ariboflavinosis are not confined to the mouth and tongue. The eyes become sensitive to the light, a condition called *photophobia,* and vascularization of the cornea from riboflavin deficiency may lead to complete opacity of the cornea.

Milk is the best source of riboflavin. Other food sources are eggs, meats, green vegetables, and whole grain cereals. Because riboflavin is destroyed by ultraviolet light, the riboflavin content of milk is reduced when milk is marketed in clear glass bottles. Milk should be stored in tinted glass bottles or in plasticized cartons if it is likely to be exposed to direct sunlight to avoid destruction of riboflavin. There is no known toxicity for riboflavin.

VITAMIN B_6. Vitamin B_6 is a term given to three compounds known as pyridoxine, pyridoxal, and pyridoxamine. The vitamin functions as a coenzyme in the metabolism of amino acids and essential fatty acids; it is also necessary for the production of urea and the conversion of the amino acid tryptophan to niacin, a B vitamin. Pyridoxine is used therapeutically to control the nausea and vomiting of pregnancy and to alleviate the peripheral neuritis that may be caused by the use of isoniazid, an antituberculosis drug. Pyridoxine is found mainly in plant foods; pyridoxal and pyridoxamine are found in foods of animal origin. A dietary deficiency of vitamin B_6 is not common, although a conditioned deficiency may be induced by certain drugs and antagonists of the vitamin. Deficiency symptoms include nausea and vomiting, loss of appetite, weight loss, general weakness, and seborrheic dermatitis around the nose and mouth. Injection of large doses (100 mg) of pyridoxine can produce a hypnotic effect such as sleepiness.

VITAMIN B_{12}. Vitamin B_{12}, or cobalamin, has several functions and is particularly important for the normal development and maturation of the red blood cells, the normal functioning of nervous tissue, bone marrow, and the GI tract, and the metabolism of carbohydrate, protein, and fat. Vitamin B_{12} is widely distributed in minute amounts in foods of animal source, but plant foods are practically devoid of the vitamin. A dietary deficiency of vitamin B_{12} is therefore seen only in strict vegetarians. A conditioned deficiency, known as pernicious anemia, may result from a gastrectomy or from a lack of *intrinsic factor,* a chemical substance in normal gastric juice that facilitates the absorption of vitamin B_{12} in foods. The symptoms of pernicious anemia include a general feeling of weakness and fatigue, a smooth and sore tongue, cracked lips, abdominal discomfort, and coldness of the extremities. Pernicious anemia stemming from lack of intrinsic factor requires the injection of vitamin B_{12} on a regular basis.

Vitamin B_{12} has been found to be effective in the treatment of several types of macrocytic anemia other than pernicious anemia, including the anemia associated with sprue and chronic liver disease, and in the treatment of peripheral neuritis associated with diabetes, chronic alcoholism, and cirrhosis of the liver (Albanese, 1980). Whether a deficiency of vitamin B_{12} is present in these conditions remains unknown.

NIACIN. Nicotinic acid, or niacin, is a constituent of two coenzymes that are involved in the release of energy during the metabolism of carbohydrate, protein, and fat. Niacin is also essential to normal growth and health of the skin, the normal functioning of the GI tract and the nervous system, and the synthesis of fatty acids. Food sources of niacin include meats, poultry, fish, green vegetables, and whole grain and enriched cereals.

Prolonged niacin deficiency results in *pellagra,* a condition characterized by the "three D's": dermatitis, diarrhea, and dementia. The dermatitis that develops is bilateral and symmetrical. Skin rashes appear on both sides of the body when areas such as the hands, feet, cheeks, and neck are exposed to sunlight. The skin looks dry, scaly, and hyperpigmented. In addition to diarrhea, other digestive disturbances include nausea and vomiting, an inflamed tongue that is bright red or scarlet, and a sore mouth with angular cracks and fissures. Dementia is manifested by insomnia, irritability, confusion, hallucinations, and delusions of persecution. These disturbances may become so severe that the patient is hospitalized due to mental illness.

Nicotinic acid, when used in large amounts to lower blood cholesterol and to induce cerebrovascular ataxia, can cause transient side effects such as burning and tingling sensations, flushing of the skin, throbbing of the head, and vasodilation.

FOLIC ACID. Also referred to as folacin, folic acid functions in the transfer of single carbon units from one compound to another and serves as a coenzyme in various intracellular reactions. Together with vitamin B_{12} and vitamin C, folic acid is necessary for the regeneration of red blood cells. It is used to treat tropical sprue and macrocytic anemia. The vitamin can be toxic in large doses.

Folic acid is widely distributed in plant and animal foods. Liver, whole grains, and dark green leafy vegetables are good sources. A dietary deficiency is not common in healthy people who eat a normal diet. Folic acid deficiency may, however, be induced by some drugs such as phenytoin (Dilantin, an anticonvulsant), oral contraceptives, barbiturates, and some chemotherapeutic agents. A folic acid deficiency may develop secondary to disease, as in sprue and leukemia. Folic acid deficiency is characterized by macrocytic anemia, oral lesions, inflammation of the tongue, diarrhea, and other gastrointestinal disturbances.

BIOTIN. There are five forms of biotin that occur in food and have activity in the body. Biotin is involved in carbon dioxide fixation, which is an important mechanism in cellular synthetic reactions. It is essential for the release of energy from carbohydrates, for the synthesis and oxidation of fatty acids, and for the deamination of amino acids for the release of energy from proteins. Dietary biotin deficiency is rare; the vitamin is widely distributed in foods. Biotin deficiency can, however, be induced by a large intake of raw egg whites. A substance in raw egg whites, called avidin, can combine firmly with biotin and make it unavailable to the body, producing a syndrome known as *egg white injury.* This condition is characterized by scaly dermatitis, muscle pains, and general malaise. The avidin in raw egg white is inactivated by heat. It is not advisable to eat raw eggs in large quantities.

PANTOTHENIC ACID. Derived from a Greek work that means "from everywhere," pantothenic acid is universally present in all foods. Particularly rich sources are organ meats and whole grain cereals. This vitamin is a component of coenzyme A, which functions in several energy-related metabolic reactions in the body. It is also necessary for hemoglobin formation and the synthesis of fatty acids, cholesterol, and some steroid hormones. Pantothenic acid deficiency in humans is unlikely to occur unless induced by an antagonist. Deficiency signs include abdominal discomfort, decreased gastric secretion, burning sensation in the feet, cramping of leg muscles, and poor motor coordination. Induced pantothenic acid deficiency also results in the loss of the body's ability to produce antibodies.

VITAMIN C. The functions of vitamin C, or ascorbic acid, in the human body have not been completely defined, although several functions have been identified. It promotes the formation of collagen; maintains the elasticity and strength of normal capillary walls; facilitates the absorption and use of iron; stimulates the conversion of folic acid to its metabolically active form, folacin; and helps to protect the body against infections. Good food sources are citrus fruits, strawberries, cabbage, tomatoes, green peppers, and potatoes.

A number of factors, including smoking, the use of oral contraceptives, and wound healing increase the need for vitamin C. A deficiency in vitamin C results in *scurvy,* a condition characterized by swollen and bleeding gums, petechial or cutaneous hemorrhages, pain and tenderness of thighs and joints, poor wound healing, and anemia.

Excessive and prolonged intake of vitamin C can lead to iron overload and, when it is excreted in the urine, can cause the formation of urate and oxalate stones. It can also produce a false positive test for sugar and a false negative test for occult blood in the stool. Symptoms similar to scurvy develop when a high dose of vitamin C is suddenly discontinued after the body has adjusted to the high intake. It is therefore important to gradually reduce the high intake over a period of 10 to 14 days.

The role of vitamin C in preventing or overcoming infections has been the subject of controversy during the past decade, and evidence to support the hypothesis that massive doses of vitamin C will prevent and cure the common cold is still lacking. The vitamin should be viewed as giving some protection, rather than as providing complete insurance, against infections.

Minerals

Minerals are the substances remaining in food after water and the carbon-containing compounds (carbohydrate, protein, fat, and vitamins) have been removed. These inorganic elements are needed daily by the body in small amounts to perform vital functions. Minerals make up about 4 percent of body weight. In general, the role of a mineral in the body is classified as either structural or regulatory. The function of a mineral is structural when the mineral is an integral part of cells, tissue, or a substance such as vitamins, hormones, and enzymes. Examples are iodine in the hormone thyroxine, sulfur in hair, iron in hemoglobin, cobalt in vitamin B_{12}, and chloride in the hydrochloric acid of gastric juice. Calcium, phosphorus, fluoride, and magnesium are structural constituents of bones and teeth. Regulatory functions of minerals include maintenance of water and acid-base balance, transmission of nerve impulses, regulation of muscle contraction and relaxation, growth of body tissues, and catalysis of numerous biological reactions.

Minerals are classified as either macrominerals or microminerals (trace elements). The classification is based on the relative amount or weight of the various minerals in the body. The macrominerals are calcium, phosphorus, potassium, sodium, sulfur, chloride, and magnesium. The microminerals, or trace elements, are iron, fluoride, iodine, chromium, cobalt, copper, zinc, manganese, and selenium. As a total group, minerals are available in fruits and vegetables, meats, milk, eggs, cereals, water, and nearly all other foods except such refined foods as granulated sugar and oils.

Calcium

Calcium is a major mineral constituent of the body and makes up 1.5 to 2.0 percent of body weight. Of this amount, 99 percent is present in bones and teeth; the remaining 1 percent is found in soft tissues and body fluids and serves a number of functions not related to bone structure. Calcium is important in blood coagulation, transmission of nerve impulses, contraction of muscle fibers, and activation of enzymes. Calcium deficiency results in rickets in children and osteomalacia in adults. Good food sources include milk, cheese, and other milk products (except butter), and some green leafy vegetables.

Chloride

Although widely distributed in the body, chloride is highly concentrated in the cerebrospinal fluid and the gastrointestinal secretions, especially in gastric juice. It is commonly combined with sodium in the extracellular fluid and with potassium in the intracellular fluid. Chloride is important in the maintenance of acid-base balance and in the regulation of osmotic pressure. Food sources are table salt, meats, milk, and eggs. Chloride deficiency occurs only after prolonged vomiting, profuse sweating, diarrhea, or excessive loss of extracellular fluid.

Chromium

Chromium is an essential trace mineral occurring in minute amounts in the blood and various tissues. It is present at birth, and the amount in the body declines with age, depending on the dietary habits and the amount of chromium in the water supply. It plays a role in carbohydrate metabolism by increasing the effectiveness of insulin, hence facilitating the transport of glucose into the cells. It is also implicated in the development of kwashiorkor and marasmus (see "Hospital Malnutrition"), and sclerotic aortic plaque.

Meats, cereals, fruits, and vegetables are good sources of chromium. Marginal or overt chromium deficiency may contribute to diabetes mellitus, atherosclerotic heart disease, and a severe protein deficiency state.

Cobalt

As an integral part of vitamin B_{12}, cobalt is needed for blood formation and the prevention of pernicious anemia. It is present in animal tissues as cobalamin and is also present in large quantities in plants, especially green leafy vegetables.

There is some evidence that large intakes of cobalt, such as in cobalt therapy, can be toxic and can cause proliferation of otherwise normal cells in bone marrow, muscle, and the thyroid gland. There is no known toxicity with cobalt intake from food sources.

Copper

The body contains about 100 mg of copper concentrated in the liver, spleen, kidneys, and heart. It is needed for the metabolism of iron and the maturation of red blood cells. Copper may also play a role in cancer, the healing of wounds and repair of connective tissue, and the metabolism of cholesterol.

Copper is widely distributed in foods and rich sources are liver, kidneys, shellfish, nuts, and legumes. Although dietary copper deficiency is unlikely to occur, excess loss of copper through kidney dialysis and the long-term use of parenteral nutrition deficient in copper can cause growth retardation, disturbances in bone development, and anemia similar to that of iron deficiency.

Fluoride

Current interest in this trace mineral is centered on its role in the prevention of dental caries and osteoporosis. Fluoride is present as a normal constituent in all diets, being widely but unevenly distributed in foods. Fluoridation of drinking water at 1 to 1.5 parts per million is recommended. Excessive intake of fluoride results in a condition called *dental fluorosis*, or mottling of the teeth.

Iodine

About 80 percent of the total iodine in the body is in the thyroid gland; the rest is present in blood, hair, skin, and other tissues. Iodine is an important constituent of the thyroid hormones, thyroxine and thyronine, which are necessary in the regulation of normal basal metabolic rate (BMR). A deficiency in this mineral results in simple goiter. Food and water provide iodine in the diet in various amounts depending on the iodine content of the soil. Seafoods are the richest sources; the most practical source is iodized table salt.

Iron

More than half of the iron in the body is found in the hemoglobin of red blood cells; the rest is present in muscle myoglobin and in various oxidative enzymes such as the cytochromes and oxidases. It is stored in the tissues as ferritin and hemosiderin. Iron is necessary for the prevention of nutritional anemia and plays an important role in respiration and tissue oxidation. The hemoglobin of red blood cells and the myoglobin of the tissue cells are vital for oxygen transport to the cells and storage within the cells. Important dietary sources are liver, lean meat, molasses, nuts, dried fruits, and whole grain and enriched cereals.

Magnesium

Magnesium is concentrated in bones and teeth. It promotes the retention of calcium in tooth enamel, thus increasing resistance to dental caries and loss of teeth. Magnesium activates enzymes involved in the release of energy from carbohydrate, protein, and fat; and it plays a role in muscle contractility, nerve irritability,

and acid-base balance. Magnesium deficiency is rare because it is widely distributed in foods. Milk, whole grains, nuts, and green vegetables are especially rich sources. Conditioned magnesium deficiency has been observed in chronic alcoholism, kwashiorkor, burns, and in surgical patients maintained on parenterally administered fluids for long periods of time.

Manganese

Manganese is needed for normal bone development; it is a component of arginase, an enzyme required for the body's manufacture of urea. It also enhances the production of the thyroid hormone thyroxine and the utilization of the vitamin thiamin. Main food sources are whole grains, legumes, leafy greens, meats, and seafoods. The human requirement for manganese has not yet been established; only a few cases of manganese deficiency has been reported in humans. The symptoms of deficiency are weight loss, dermatitis, and change in hair color.

There is no toxicity from dietary manganese even at very high intakes. If inhaled after prolonged exposure to dust, as in the case of miners, manganese can accumulate in the liver and the central nervous system and produce symptoms resembling Parkinson disease.

Phosphorus

Next to calcium, phosphorus occurs in the second-greatest quantity in the human body. About 90 percent of the body's phosphorus is deposited as inorganic phosphate (in combintion with calcium) in the bones and teeth; the remainder is found in the soft tissues, especially striated muscles, where it performs an important function. Phosphorus is a constituent of the buffer system and helps regulate the pH of the blood. It interacts with calcium to give rigidity to bones and teeth, helps regulate osmotic pressure, is a component of nucleic acids, transports fatty acids as phospholipids, and is a constituent of coenzymes involved in fat and carbohydrate metabolism.

All foods rich in protein and calcium are also good sources of phosphorus. These include milk, cheese, meats, legumes, whole grain cereals, and leafy green vegetables.

Dietary phosphorus deficiency is not likely to occur if protein and calcium intakes are adequate. However, ingestion of large amounts of antacids, such as aluminum hydroxide, can lead to phosphorus deficiency, resulting in low blood phosphate level (hypophosphatemia), muscle weakness, malaise, and bone pains.

Potassium

Potassium plays a key role in maintaining the proper osmotic pressure of the cell. It is the chief cation in the intracellular fluid; only a small amount is present in the extracellular fluid under normal conditions. Potassium also helps regulate acid-base balance, transmits nerve impulses, and acts as a catalyst in many biological reactions, especially those involving the release of energy and the formation of glycogen and protein. It is widely distributed in many foods. The amount present in the normal diet is more than sufficient for minimal potassium needs. Although deficiency from diet is unlikely to occur, potassium deficiency may result from prolonged diarrhea, abnormal kidney function, diabetic acidosis, and renal disease. Symptoms of deficiency are weakness, nervous irritability, mental disorientation, and cardiac irregularities.

Sodium

Sodium is the chief cation in the extracellular fluid and exerts a force opposite to that of potassium in the intracellular fluid. It plays a crucial role in maintaining equilibrium between extra- and intracellular fluids. Sodium also regulates the osmotic pressure and acid-base balance; transmits nerve impulses; facilitates the absorption of various nutrients, including glucose; and aids in relaxing contracted muscle in the presence of potassium. Dietary lack is unlikely to occur because sodium is easily supplied by table salt and many foods. Sodium depletion in the body may occur, however, as a result of conditioning factors such as excessive sweating or vomiting, burn, diarrhea, and other disorders marked by loss of body fluids. Sodium deficiency is characterized by muscular cramps, weakness, and possible vascular collapse and coma in severe deficiency.

Sulfur

Sulfur, a trace mineral, is a structural component of cells and is highly concentrated in hair, nails, cartilage, and skin. It is also a structural part of the B vitamins thiamin, pantothenic acid, and biotin and of the amino acids cystine, cysteine, and methionine. Sulfur occurs in most food proteins, and the need for this mineral is met when the protein supply is adequate.

Zinc

Zinc is found in minute amounts in hair, skin, nails, bones, liver, kidneys, muscles, pancreas, spleen, and testes. It is essential for growth and is involved in many enzymes as a cofactor for their metabolic action. Zinc is also needed for the action of insulin, the hormone that regulates carbohydrate metabolism. Plant and animal foods that are good sources of protein are the best sources of zinc. Zinc deficiency results in dwarfism, delayed wound healing, delayed sexual maturity, and loss of the senses of taste and smell. Zinc deficiency may be due to inadequate dietary intake or increased loss from the body, as in burns and kidney dialysis.

Water

Water is vital to life, second only in importance to oxygen. Approximately two-thirds of the total body weight is water. Humans can survive only a few days without water but can live for several weeks or longer without food. A 20 percent loss of body water causes death.

Water performs various functions in the body. All chemical reactions take place in the presence of water. Water acts as a solvent and a medium of transport for the nutrients and waste products that result from the ingestion, digestion, and assimilation of food. Water is the major constituent of essential body fluids, including blood, saliva, digestive juices, and perspiration. In the blood, water is the medium for transporting compounds throughout the body. As a constituent of saliva and digestive juices, water serves as a lubricant to promote the movement of food and the elimination of waste products. Water also serves as a lubricant for joints, and it helps regulate the body temperature. Overheating of the body is prevented by the evaporation of water from the lungs and the skin.

Water is supplied by fluids in the diet and by many foods that have a high water content, particularly fruits and vegetables. Another source of water comes from the oxidation of foods in the body. This is known as metabolic water, or water of combustion, and amounts to about 300 to 400 ml daily.

Under normal conditions, a daily intake of 1 ml water/k cal is generally considered sufficient. This means about 2 to 2½ L (quarts) of water daily for most adults eating a normal diet. The need for water is increased in hot climates and whenever body water is lost by excessive perspiration, vomiting, burns, fever, and other pathological conditions that increase the need for water over and above the normal requirement. Chapter 31 discusses water balance and control in greater detail.

NUTRITION AND THE LIFE CYCLE

Infancy

The study of nutrition encompasses the entire life cycle. The first 12 months of life are characterized by the most rapid rate of growth and development, causing an infant's nutritional needs to merit special attention. The total caloric needs of an infant gradually increase from about 350 to 500 k cal/day at birth to about 1,000 kc at 1 year of age. Milk provides all the calories during the first few weeks of life. Cereals, fruits, eggs, vegetables, and meat provide the remaining calories when they are added to the infant's diet. Normal infants who are breastfed or are given the standard 20 k cal/1 oz formula will generally adjust their intake to meet their energy needs.

The *protein* requirement during infancy is higher per kilogram of body weight than that of the older child or adult. During the first 6 months of life, the infant needs about 2 gm/kg body weight. The amount of protein relative to the body weight gradually decreases until adulthood, when the protein need is about 1 gm/kg body weight.

Childhood

The nutritional requirements of the preschool child are an extension of his needs in infancy. The primary concern is to increase gradually the kind and amount of food while decreasing the number of feedings to three meals plus nourishing snacks. This period is optimal for the establishment of proper food habits at home, and therefore there is a significant need for nutritional education of mothers. The nutritional needs of the growing child vary during spurts of growth. The kind and size of food servings should be adjusted with age, stage of development, appetite, and outside influences such as play and school activities.

Adolescence

The unique nutritional needs of adolescence are determined primarily by the building of new body tissues and the emotional changes attending maturation. In general, the growing adolescent requires a high-calorie intake, an abundance of good-quality protein, and liberal amounts of minerals and vitamins. Because of the onset of menstruation, adolescent girls have specific needs for iron, protein, and other nutrients essential for blood formation. Nutrition education should be focused on preventing or correcting the poor eating habits of adolescence, such as inappropriate or excessive snacking and a tendency to eat foods with empty calories.

Adulthood

With respect to dietary needs, adulthood refers to the years between ages 21 and 65. Proper nutrition is important in adulthood because it is the longest period of the life cycle and possibly the peak productive years. Ideally, one should reach adulthood with a wide range of familiarity with, and acceptance of, different foods. An adult tends to resist changes in his food habits; hence, proper training in both food selection and regularity of eating is important as early in life as possible. One aim of good nutrition throughout adulthood is the maintenance of desirable body weight. It is recommended that the daily caloric intake be reduced with increasing age in proportion to the decrease in basal metabolic rate (BMR) and physical activity.

The Elderly

Physiological changes specific to the elderly present problems that contribute to nutritional inadequacy. These include poor dentition or loss of teeth; loss of appetite; reduced secretion of digestive enzymes; lack of neuromuscular coordination; reduced cellular, circulatory, and excretory functions; hormonal changes; and a tendency to develop osteoporosis, pernicious anemia, and other disorders. In addition to the physiological conditions that affect nutrition, there are socioeconomic and psychological ones such as boredom, inactivity, lack of interest in the environment, anxiety, faulty eating habits that resist change, and economic insecurity. Consideration of these influences is important in planning for the nutritional care of the elderly.

ENERGY REQUIREMENTS

The energy value of foods is of considerable interest in today's calorie-conscious society. The word *calories* is the term most commonly used to denote the heat energy available in food. *Calorie* is defined as the amount of energy needed to raise the temperature of 1 kg of water 1 degree C. A more accurate term to use is kilocalorie (k cal) inasmuch as the energy value of foods is 1,000 times the value of the calorie unit used by the physical scientist. The calories in food come from carbohydrate, protein provides about 4 k cal, whereas fat is a more concetrated source of energy and provides about 9 *k cal/gm*.

The energy needs of a person take precedence over all other needs. In addition to growth requirements during childhood, pregnancy, and lactation, there are three determinants of a person's total energy requirements: (1) basal metabolism, (2) physical activity, and (3) specific dynamic action of food.

Basal Energy Needs

Basal metabolism is the amount of energy required to maintain basal metabolic processes, which are the maintenance functions for which the body requires energy. These include the functioning of vital organs and glands, blood circulation, respiration, GI concentrations, cell metabolism, and maintenance of body temperature. The energy needs for basal metabolism constitute about 50 to 75 percent of the total daily caloric requirements for many people, especially those engaged in sedentary activities. The standard basal energy requirement is approximately 1 k cal/kg body weight per hour. Each person has his own basal energy requirement that depends on this BMR, which is the speed at which his body expends energy per unit of time. The rate is influenced by age, body composition, activity of endocrine glands, state of nutrition, rate of growth, and pregnancy or lactation.

At birth, the BMR is relatively high and continues to rise until about the age of 2 years. From this age on, there is a slow reduction in rate throughout life. The BMR declines about 2 percent per decade during adult life. This drop in BMR means that a person needs fewer calories to maintain body functions as he grows older. A gradual weight gain will result if a person continues to eat the same amount of food throughout his life.

Body composition also influences basal metabolic needs. More energy is needed for the metabolic activities in muscle and glandular tissues than in fatty tissue. As a group, women have a metabolic rate about 5 to 10 percent slower than men, even when of the same weight and height. Women have more fat and are less muscular than men, and fat is less metabolically active than muscle. During the menstrual cycle, the BMR fluctuates by an average of 360 kcal/day between its highest point before menstruation and its lowest point about 1 week before ovulation (Solomon, 1982). Two endocrine glands secrete hormones that have important influences on the BMR. The adrenal gland secretes adrenalin during periods of stress and high emotion, causing an acceleration in BMR. Thyroxine, an iodine-containing hormone secreted by the thyroid gland, has a more direct effect on BMR; an increased or decreased secretion of this hormone will result in a higher or lower BMR. People who live in cold climates average a rate about 20 percent higher than people in warm climates presumably because of the increased secretion of thyroxine in cold climates. When thyroxine is secreted at a normal rate, most people will require 1 kcal/kg body weight/hour to meet basal needs.

Other influences on BMR are noted under varying conditions. Some illnesses, such as those accompanied by fever or an infection, increase the BMR about 7 percent for each degree F rise in body temperature, or 13 percent for each degree C. In instances of malnutrition and starvation, the rate is lowered because the body seeks optimal utilization of calories ingested by reducing its basal metabolic rate.

Physical Activity

Next to basal metabolic needs, physical activity is the greatest single determinant of energy needs. The actual number of calories needed per day depends on body weight, the intensity of the activity, and the duration of the activity. Table 33.3 lists the energy requirements per day for various activities.

Specific Dynamic Action

Energy is required for the digestion and conversion of food to nutrients needed for cell metabolism. This is referred to as *specific dynamic action* (SDA). It varies with the type and amount of food eaten. Pure protein requires about 30 percent of its potential energy for the body to use it. The specific dynamic effect of fat is less, at 13 percent; carbohydrate is even much less, at 5 to 6 percent. On mixed diets, such as those typically consumed, the extra energy needed for the specific dynamic action of food is about 10 percent of the calories needed for basal metabolism and activity.

NUTRITION AND SPORTS

Athletes are individuals whose energy and nutrient needs vary considerably depending on the type, intensity, frequency, and duration of the sport; age, sex, and weight of the athlete participating in a sport can double or triple the individual's daily energy requirements, as shown in Table 33.4. An athlete's appetite usually increases correspondingly to support the need for additional calories, although very active athletes often have problems consuming enough energy food to meet their energy needs.

Even though each athlete has his own energy and nutrient needs, some nutritional concerns are common to all. An athlete's goal is to attain the weight and body composition that will best enhance athletic performance. Excess body fat hinders performance, and most athletes compete best when body fat is between 8 and 10 percent of body weight (male), and 12 and 14 percent of body weight (female). The percentages are considerably less than those of normal, well-nourished males and females who average 15 percent and

TABLE 33.3 ENERGY REQUIRED FOR VARIOUS ACTIVITIES

Activity	Amount (k cal/kg/day)	Increase Over Basal (%)
Basal or standard	25	
Minimal (bed rest)	27.5	10
Very light (typist)	30–35	20–40
Light (student, teacher, nurse)	35–40	40–60
Moderate (homemaker)	40–45	60–80
Hard (carpenter, house-maid at hard work)	45–50	80–100
Severe (farmer, dancer)	50–70	100–180
Very severe (athlete in training, lumberman)	75	200

Source: Krause, MV, Mahan, LK: Food, Nutrition and Diet Therapy, 7 ed. Philadelphia, W.B. Saunders Co. 1984, p. 393.

TABLE 33.4 DAILY ENERGY REQUIREMENTS OF VARIOUS SPORTS ACTIVITIES EXPRESSED AS CALORIES*

3000–4000		3000–5000	3000–6000	4000–6000
400-yd dash	Baseball	800-yd run	13 mile run	6 mile run
Swimming, 50- and 100-yd	Discus	1- and 2-mile runs	Football	Marathon
	Shot-put	Swimming, over 100 yd	Basketball	Running
Diving	Javelin	Wrestling	Ice hockey	Cross country running
Hurdle	Hammer throw	Most gymnastics	Lacrosse	Cross country skiing
Pole vault	Ski jumping	Downhill, slalom skiing	Gymnastics, all around	Soccer
Long jump	Golf		Fencing	

*Assumes similar body weight and size among male participants. Female athletes require approximately 10% fewer calories.
From: Kris-Etherton, PM: Nutrition, exercise and athletic performance, *Food Nutr News* 57 (3):13, 1985.

20 percent body fat respectively. Extra body weight may be advantageous in some high body contact sports, while a lower body weight is beneficial in sports such as gymnastics and sprint running.

The aim of any weight gain or weight loss program is to enhance performance and to meet any weight standards for competition in certain categories of sports such as boxing and wrestling. For effective weight gain an athlete should gain muscle and lose fat. Isometric exercise and an increase in calorie intake promote muscle weight gain; an increase in activity and a decrease in calorie intake promote a weight loss.

Carbohydrates should provide 50 to 55 percent of the total calories in an athlete's diet, while 10 to 20 percent from protein intake of 1 to 1.5 gm/kg body weight is enough to maintain nitrogen balance even in athletics who are still growing. A higher intake of protein, up to 2 gm/kg body weight may be needed during the early stages of training and again when the athlete is training intensively to gain strength and muscle mass. Protein and vitamin supplements are not needed (Short, 1983). The large amounts of calories eaten by athletes, if obtained from a variety of foods, will provide enough protein, vitamins, and minerals.

Complex carbohydrate foods, like starches, should be the major source of calories because carbohydrate can be stored in the body as muscle glycogen which provides the fuel used during intensive and continuous activities. The level of glycogen stored in muscle affects an athlete's endurance, and an athlete can perform two to three times longer on a high carbohydrate diet.

Starchy foods should be eaten several days before any event that requires heavy and continuing activity of more than 1 hour, and for endurance events demanding heavy work lasting 3 hours or more, such as long distance running and marathon racing, Carbohydrate loading can increase the normal storage of muscle glycogen by as much as 2.5 times (Sherman 1984).

Carbohydrate loading is accomplished by ingestion of complex carbohydrates (not sugar) as the source of at least 70 percent of the total calories. This is done for 3 days before the event, while the athlete simultaneously reduces most training activities. On the day of the event, a meal containing about 500 kcal should be taken 3 to 4 hours before the competition to provide the liver with an additional glycogen reserve for maintaining blood glucose levels. The precompetition meal should be low in fat and protein because they delay gastric emptying and may cause gastric distress during competition.

Athletes should be well hydrated before an event. A water loss equal to 2 percent to 3 percent body weight can impair performance, and a loss in excess of 5 percent can lead to serious dehydration. To replenish water loss, an athlete should drink 2 cups of fluid for each pound of weight loss during competition, or 5 to 8 oz of fluid for every 10 to 15 minutes of continuous activity. The American College of Sports Medicine recommends the use of fluids that contain small amounts of sugar (less than 2.5 percent) and electrolytes (10 mEq sodium and 5 mEq potassium).

When there is excessive sweating, the ideal fluid replacement is plain chilled water, which is absorbed faster and helps bring down body temperature (Wilmore, 1984). Salt tablets are not needed. A well-balanced diet contains enough salt to replace the salt lost through sweat, and too much salt draws water into the GI tract and causes cramping, nausea, vomiting, and dehydration.

OBESITY AND WEIGHT CONTROL

Obesity is a recognized public health problem of growing concern. It is estimated that approximately 30 percent of the population in the US is excessively overweight as a result of imbalances between calorie intake and calorie expenditure. Obesity creates a health hazard by reducing life expectancy and increasing the risk of such diseases as diabetes mellitus, hypertension, atherosclerosis, and congestive heart failure. It also increases surgical risk and complicates pregnancy, arthritis, and respiratory difficulties such as emphysema and chronic bronchitis.

Overweight is a condition in which there is an excessive deposit of fat, or adipose tissue. The condition may be either slight (overweight) or gross (obesity). A weight that is 10 percent above the ideal or desirable weight is indicative of obesity. A person's weight at age 25 is considered desirable for that person throughout adulthood.

There are several ways to determine body fatness. The most common method is to compare a person's weight against a standard weight/height table. The most widely used table is one published by the Metropolitan Life Insurance Company, which gives a range of weight according to body frame and height. An adaptation of the 1983 Metropolitan weight standard is presented in Table 33.5. Another quick method for determining desirable body weight is:

1. For women, allow 100 lb for the first 5 feet of height and add 5 lb for each additional inch.
2. For men, allow 110 lb for the first 5 feet of height and add 5 lb for each additional inch.
3. Allow a range of 10 percent above or below the calculated weight to accommodate individual differences.

Obesity generally results from any combination of increased caloric intake or decreased energy expenditure. Calories in excess of those needed for energy are stored as body fat. Several factors influence obesity. In some cultures, body fatness is considered desirable and is associated with affluence and good health. Every person's pattern of food consumption is shaped by a variety of pressures, both external and internal, to which he is constantly subjected. Poor food habits and family dietary patterns such as large serving portions, poorly planned meals high in fat and starch, calorie-packed convenience foods, and overindulgence in snacks can lead to excessive weight. Genetic influence, metabolic abnormality, and emotional and psychological influences also affect weight. Some people eat to satisfy an inner drive. Overindulgence in food can be a substitute for love, security, and satisfaction, or it can compensate for feelings of frustration and depression.

Many fad reducing diets have been introduced, ranging from starvation and formula diets to chemically defined diets. These diets promise a quick and easy way to reduce and are generally high in protein and low in

TABLE 33.5 RECOMMENDED WEIGHT IN RELATION TO HEIGHT*

Height inches	Men	Weight Women
		lb
58		113
59		116
60		119
61	128	122
62	130	125
63	132	128
64	135	131
65	138	134
66	141	137
67	144	140
68	147	143
69	150	146
70	153	149
71	157	
72	161	
73	165	

Adapted from the 1983 Metropolitan Height and Weight Tables based on 1979 Build Study.
*Weights represent the midpoint for a person of medium frame, in bare feet and without clothing.

carbohydrates, but *calories are calories.* Just as 1 gm of carbohydrate furnishes 4 calories, so does 1 gm of protein. Fat supplies 9 calories/gm. Any food, regardless of type, will result in weight gain if too much of it is consumed.

There are dangers associated with fad diets. Clinical abnormalities such as hypertension, electrolyte imbalances, anemia, and hyperlipidemia have been observed. Weight lost quickly is also regained rather quickly when customary eating habits are resumed.

The safest and best way to lose weight is to adopt a regimen of exercise and a diet that is low in calories, yet adequate in essential nutrients. A loss of 2 lb/week is generally recommended. To achieve this, 1,000 calories per day should be subtracted daily. It is important to provide emotional support and encouragement as well as good nutrition education to a person who is dieting. The process of re-education is difficult and entails a change in behavior as well as a change in dietary habits. Through techniques such as behavior modification, a person can gain insight into what infuences his eating habits or eating response so that the end result is weight loss, new eating habits, and maintenance of the reduced weight.

Eating Disorders

Anorexia Nervosa

Anorexia nervosa is a state of emaciation that is the result of deliberate self-imposed starvation. It is most often seen in adolescents and young adults of both sexes but is 10 times more frequent in young women. The classical description of a person with anorexia nervosa is "skeleton only clad with skin." The anorexic has a disturbed body image and takes pride in a skeletal appearance, which is not seen as abnormal by the person.

At the onset, the person may intend to lose only a few pounds; but dieting soon takes control and becomes an obsession (Schwartz, 1981). The anorectic has an intense fear of gaining weight, develops bizarre food habits, avoids "fattening" foods, complains of feeling full after only a few bites of food, and often refuses to eat even though preoccupied with food and eating. Some individuals may give in to episodes of binge-eating, but these are followed by self-induced vomiting and periods of starvation that eventually lead to a 25 percent weight loss (Crisp, 1980). To become extremely thin, the anorectic will also exercise to the point of exhaustion.

Anorexia nervosa may range from a mild condition that requires no intervention to very serious forms that require hospitalization and may lead to death (Lucas, 1983). Treatment is through a comprehensive approach that combines nutritional repletion and psychological management of the patient and the family. The goal of the dietary therapy should be gradual weight gain through normal eating. A nasogastric tube or parenteral feeding may be needed to prevent death in extreme cases of starvation.

The most important element is to motivate and encourage the patient to eat. Several forms of psychotherapy may be tried, including behavior modification and the use of psychotropic drugs.

Bulimia

Bulimia is a syndrome characterized by binging/gorging followed by vomiting/purging. Bulimarexia is the term applied to a binge/purge episode followed by starvation. It affects women a bit older than those afflicted by anorexia nervosa, and as many as 20 percent of college women are estimated to have this disorder (Halmi, 1981).

Bulimics compulsively overeat and then resort to vomiting and purging to keep their weight down. Most are secretive about the binge/purge episodes, which are usually accompanied by feelings of depression and low self-esteem. Foods consumed during a binge are high in calories, although an individual's ideas abut quantities may be distorted. The bulimic who practices self-induced vomiting as the primary means of weight control usually vomits a number of times each day. This persistent vomiting over a period of months or years carries serious side effects including a disturbed electrolyte balance and damage to teeth from continual exposure to acid vomitus.

Unlike the anorectic who continues on a near-starvation diet even after becoming extremely thin, the bulimic compulsively overeats but resorts to purging to avoid gaining weight. A comparison of anorexia nervosa and bulimia is shown in Table 33.6. There are similarities between them, in that both are seen in perfectionists and those who have unrealistically high personal expectations, and both are characterized by obsession with food and weight.

The treatment of bulimia, like that of anorexia nervosa, requires psychotherapy and nutrition counseling. Bulimics who seek help are often referred to organizations for anorexia nervosa, because the conditions are related. Voluntary self-help groups which offer their members support and assistance and provide referrals for medical and psychological services are listed below:

American Anorexia Nervosa Association, Inc.
133 Cedar Lane, Teaneck, N.J. 07666

National Anorexia Aid Society
P.O. Box 29461, Columbus, OH 43229

Anorexia Nervosa and Associated Disorders
P.O. Box 271, Highland Park, IL 60035

Anorexia Nervosa and Related Eating Disorders
P.O. Box 1012, Grover City, CA 93433

Over Eaters Anonymous
2190 190th St, Torrance, CA 90504

HOSPITAL MALNUTRITION

Failure to eat for any reason, physical or emotional, contributes to malnutrition, which, in turn, influences the body's response to disease and injury. In previously well-nourished people who are hospitalized due to severe surgical or medical disorders, muscle tissue will break down if energy and nutrient requirements are not met during the stress of illness.

Kwashiorkor and marasmus are the two types of malnutrition reported to be most common in hospitalized patients.

Kwashiorkor is protein malnutrition characterized by muscle wasting, decreased serum albumin, and edema. It can occur even in obese patients, and there may be no apparent weight change because of the accompanying edema, which is usually confined to the lower limbs.

Maramus is a condition of extreme undernutrition, primarily caused by a diet that is low in both protein

TABLE 33.6 CHARACTERISTIC FEATURES OF ANOREXIA NERVOSA AND BULIMIA

Anorexia	Bulimia
Fear of being fat	Fear of being fat
Significant weight loss of 25% or more	Body weight usually within 10–15% of normal
Turns away from food as means of coping	Turns to food as means of coping
Often denies problems; may take pride in weight loss	Recognizes abnormal eating patterns
Maintains rigid control of eating	Alternates between binge eating and purging or vomiting
Difficulty in accurately assessing body size	Little difficulty in accurately assessing body size
Some or all of the following symptoms	Some or all of the following symptoms
Amenorrhea	Eating pattern alternates between binges and fasts
Lanugo (growth of fine hair especially on the arms and back)	Secretive eating during a binge
Low blood pressure and slow pulse	Use of vomiting, laxatives, and diuretics to control weight
Periods of overactivity or excessive exercise, despite fatigue	Depressed mood and self-deprecating thoughts following a binge
Decreased consumption of high calorie foods	Consumption of high calorie foods during a binge

and calories. There is marked wasting of muscles and loss of subcutaneous fat; body weight is only 60 percent or less of expected weight. Symptoms of vitamin deficiencies, anemia, and diarrhea often are associated. Marasmus is reported to affect 25 to 50 percent of medical/surgical patients whose illness has required hospitalization for 2 weeks or more. Patients with chronic diseases that interfere with adequate food intake may also develop marasmus unless they have careful nutritional care.

Many standard hospital practices contribute to malnutrition. Most have their roots in long-standing ignorance about the importance of nutritional support during the stress of illness. Examples of such practices are: (1) failure to record height and weight; (2) failure to observe patient's food intake; (3) withholding meals because of diagnostic testing; (4) prolonged use of glucose and saline IV feedings; (5) use of tube feedings in inadequate amounts; (6) failure to recognize increased nutritional needs resulting from injury or illness; and (7) delay in nutritional support until the patient is in an advanced state of depletion.

The nurse plays a key role in preventing hospital malnutrition because of her unique opportunity to maintain constant surveillance of the patient's state of nutrition. The observation and recording of the patient's food and fluid intake are important aspects of nursing care.

TUBE AND PARENTERAL FEEDING

A patient who is unable to take adequate nutrients by mouth is fed either by tube or by total parenteral alimentation.

Tube Feeding

In tube feeding, a thick liquid formula is given via a tube that enters the stomach through the esophagus (nasogastric tube) or through a surgical incision made in the abdominal wall (gastrostomy tube).

Tube feeding is indicated for patients who are unable to consume food orally for reasons such as physical impairment from facial injuries; radical surgery; neurological impairment including paralysis and unconsciousness; and mental disturbances such as anorexia nervosa and depression (Fig. 33.1). The route of administration may be by nasogastric, esophagostomy, gastrostomy, or jejunostomy tube. The size of the tube is determined by the type of formula to be given. The formula is prepared in a blender, because of its thick consistency; a number 14 or 16 French tube is used. Commercial products (Sustacal, Ensure, Meritene) will flow through a number 10 French tube; defined formula or elemental diets (Vivonex, Flexical) will flow through a number 8 tube. As a general rule, the smallest tube through which the prescribed formula will flow freely should be selected to minimize problems of patient discomfort and diarrhea that are commonly associated with rapid introduction of the feeding.

In the first few days, the tube feeding should be diluted to at least half strength, and not more than 100 ml should be given at one time. The feedings are gradually increased to full strength and amount within 4 to 5 days. This enables the patient to develop tolerance to the osmolality of the formula. Gradual administration of the formula is especially important for those patients who are debilitated, those with gastrointestinal disorders, those being fed by gastrostomy or jejunostomy tube, and those whose GI tracts have been without food for a long period of time. The stomach contents should be suctioned before a new feeding is administered to ensure that there is only minimal residue from the previous feeding. Any stomach contents removed by suction are usually mixed with the fresh formula so that the patient will not lose electrolytes.

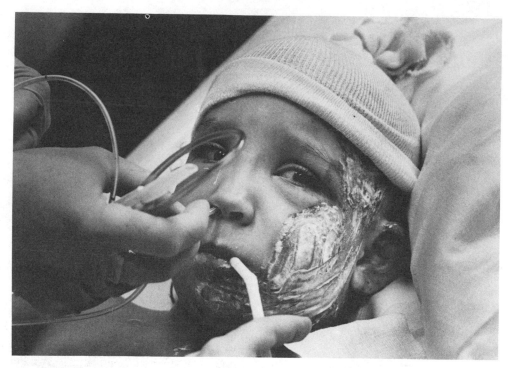

Figure 33.1 *Many severely burned patients cannot take enough food by mouth to provide the high-calorie, high-protein diet needed for healing extensive burns. Renee is being asked to swallow water through a straw to facilitate passage of a nasogastric tube. This tube remained in place during much of Renee's hospitalization because tube feedings were needed to supplement the amount of food she was able to eat.*

PROCEDURE 33.1

Giving a Tube Feeding*

SUMMARY OF ESSENTIAL NURSING ACTIONS

1. Make certain that tube is in stomach before giving feeding.
2. If stomach contents are aspirated before feeding to determine amount remaining from previous feeding, return aspirated contents to stomach to prevent disruption of electrolyte balance.
3. Warm feeding to room temperature.
4. Give feeding slowly and without undue pressure.
   - Suspend container about 12 inches above patient's head.

- Allow fluid to flow by gravity.
- Regulate flow so that a single batch feeding requires 15–20 minutes.
5. Rinse tube with 15–30 ml water.
6. Clamp tube unless against agency policy.
7. Detach tube from container and cover end of tube with gauze square and a rubber band.

*See inside front cover.

Diarrhea is the most common problem associated with tube feeding; other problems are abdominal cramps, stomach distention, nausea, and vomiting. These problems may be caused by feeding too much or too quickly, cold feedings, a formula that is highly concentrated, or excessive lactose in the formula. Continuous-drip administration of the feeding at about 80 to 120 ml/hour is ideal. If feeding is given in batches, 250 to 350 ml should be given at a slow rate in not less than 15 to 20 minutes.

Pour about 50 ml of water into the tube before and after feeding to prevent hypertonic dehydration from solute overload, to wash any of the feeding remaining in the tube into the stomach, and to rinse the tube. Abdominal cramping may be reduced by giving the feeding at room temperature or by warming a cold formula in hot water. If diarrhea continues even with slow administration of dilute formula, it may be due to lactose intolerance, which may be transitory or permanent. A lactose-free formula such as Isocal or Ensure may be tried. The addition of applesauce or pectin to the formula may also help bring the diarrhea under control. Unused formula should be refrigerated and used within 24 hours because of the danger of bacterial contamination.

The nurse should record the *actual* intake, any vomiting or diarrhea, and any signs of edema, dehydration, or inadequate feeding. Assessment of hydration is particularly important in comatose and weak patients who are unable to communicate their thirst. A condition called *tube feeding syndrome,* characterized by hypernatremia, increased blood urea nitrogen, and dehydration has been reported in tube-fed patients who are not given enough water. The amount of water needed is increased when there is water loss due to fever, perspiration, or fistula drainage, or to a concentrated formula that is high in protein. When the patient begins to resume eating by mouth, there should be some overlap between tube and oral feeding for several days, to allow the patient to adapt to eating once again and to prevent inadequate intake. The patient should be weighed regularly (at least twice a week) while on tube feeding.

Parenteral Feeding

When a patient is unable to absorb tube feedings, essential nutrients can be given directly into his bloodstream. *Total parenteral nutrition* (TPN, total parenteral alimentation, intravenous hyperalimentation) involves the administration of a *highly concentrated* solution of glucose, nitrogen, and other nutrients directly into the superior vena cava, where it is quickly diluted by the flowing blood. Parenterally administered glucose provides a maximum of 600 kcal/day, whereas total parenteral nutrition can supply enough calories and protein to ensure adequate anabolism—up to 3,000 kcal or more per day if necessary. TNP is usually managed in the hospital, though some patients have been taught to manage long-term hyperalimentation at home.

The TPN Solution

The TPN solution contains glucose, amino acids, a small amount of fat, electrolytes, vitamins, and minerals. At the usual strength, the formula provides about 1,000 kcal and 42 gm protein/L. Four liters per day is the maximum most patients can tolerate. Some patients receiving TPN still feel hungry and may be able to take some food orally. When TPN is no longer needed, it is important to decrease the amount infused gradually to prevent hypoglycemic shock. Oral intake should be well established and should increase as the TPN decreases.

NUTRITION AND STRESS

Selye describes stress as the nonspecific response to any demand made on the body. Many stimuli such as physical trauma, drugs, keen competition, and psychological shock can exert marked effects on the body, which will attempt to regain and preserve homeostasis. Hospitalized patients are subjected to stress ranging in degree from mild to severe.

Nutrition plays a critical part in determining the speed with which a patient recovers from a stressful situation. The stress of starvation promotes other manifestations of disease such as the development of ulcers and changes in the gastrointestinal mucosa. Emotional stress increases the need for vitamin C. Environmental stress influences the body's use of nutrients. Infections precipitate malnutrition in people whose diets are of borderline adequacy. An understanding of the metabolic effects produced by stress is important in the planning of nutritional support of patients experiencing infections, fever, injury or trauma, burns, surgery, and cancer.

Infections

Outbreaks of such diseases as typhus, cholera, and dysentery have been common during periods of famine. Pulmonary tuberculosis increases among populations that are chronically hungry. Epidemics and famine occur together because malnutrition lowers resistance to infection.

Infectious diseases increase both anabolism and catabolism, and disrupt normal nutrition. The interaction between malnutrition and infection is cyclic, in that infection interferes with normal nutrition, and malnutrition lowers resistance to infections.

Nitrogen balance is disturbed during acute infections and nitrogen is excreted in the urine because of the loss of protein. Protein depletion is particularly aggravated by vomiting or diarrhea from any cause. Infections also interfere with the manufacture of red cells by the bone marrow, causing a shortened life-span of those cells. The resulting syndrome, called *anemia of infection,* does not respond to the administration of iron, folic acid, or vitamin B_{12}.

Fever

Fever accelerates all metabolic processes and contributes to the wasting of body nitrogen and concomitant loss of energy. Fever increases calorie expenditure significantly, even when the patient is on bed rest. Basal metabolism is increased by 13 percent for each degree centigrade rise in body temperature above normal (7 percent for each degree Fahrenheit). The increase may be as much as 40 percent in a patient whose temperature is 40 degrees C (104 degrees F). A series of chills can raise a patient's daily calorie requirement to as much as 5,000 kcal. If the patient is restless or delirious, the total energy need is increased further by 10 percent to 30 percent. Catabolism is also increased; unless adequate protein is provided in the diet, negative nitrogen balance may result. Fever affects water requirements and electrolytes largely because of the increased evaporation and hyperventilation, so increased water intake is required to prevent dehydration.

The patient with fever needs more calories, protein, water, and possibly more vitamins and minerals. The diet must provide 3,000 kcal or more, and up to 1.5 gm protein/kg body weight to restore nitrogen losses. Soft, bland, easily digested foods are usually tolerated more rapidly, and food should be offered frequently, at 2- or 3-hour intervals, because most patients with an elevated temperature have poor appetites.

Injury

Trauma produces significant alterations in metabolism, many of which are mediated by hormones. The catabolic hormones, adrenalin and the glucocorticoids, are secreted in excessively large amounts, resulting in tissue breakdown and increased energy needs.

Nitrogen loss following trauma is the same as that caused by the stress response to infections and fever. Tissue breakdown is due to an increased secretion of cortical hormones by the adrenal glands. The rapid mobilization of protein is due to the increased energy demands during the hypermetabolic period of the response to major injury or trauma, which places a greater stress on endogenous (internal) energy sources. Glycogen stores are rapidly mobilized from liver and muscle reserves, and the resultant decrease in liver and muscle glycogen can induce a hypoglycemic reaction. Prolonged protein breakdown harms the immune system, eventually leading to poor wound healing and wound separation.

The blood-glucose level may remain high, and the glucose tolerance test may give results similar to those seen in diabetics, despite normal or increased insulin secretion. Injected insulin does not produce the expected decline in blood sugar, and glucose does not have its usual protein-sparing action. The immobilization and prolonged bed rest often necessary in severe injuries make further demands on the body, resulting in (1) decrease in muscle mass with loss of nitrogen, potassium, and sulfur; (2) decrease in bone with loss of calcium and phosphorus into the urine and consequent danger of osteoporosis and renal stone formation; and (3) pressure ulcers (bed sores).

The nutritional needs of the body after injury and trauma include increased calories, proteins, minerals, and vitamins, especially vitamin C. Food must be provided in a form and consistency that the patient can tolerate, and it should be attractively served to encourage the patient to eat. He may need emotional and social support.

Surgery

The patient's nutritional state will influence his metabolic response to surgery and his ability to survive stress. The tissue breakdown, nitrogen loss, and increased demand on energy follow the same patterns as the stress response to injury and trauma. In elective surgery, every effort should be made to correct preoperative nutritional deficits in protein, calories, vitamins, and minerals. Patients in a poor nutritional status have a longer recovery and are more likely to develop decubitus ulcers during prolonged bed rest. These ulcers may develop within a very short period of time if proper nursing care is not instituted along with nutritional care.

If the patient is obese, preoperative weight reduction is desirable because obesity increases the stress on the cardiovascular system during surgery. Excessive abdominal adipose tissue may also give rise to difficulties in suturing and wound healing. Patients who are malnourished need to receive 30 to 50 percent more protein. Because patients vary in the length of time needed before they begin to improve, their nutritional status should be evaluated every 7 days after nutritional support is initiated, in order to determine if they are ready for surgery. A patient who shows no improvement within 14 days may be suffering from sepsis (Buzby, 1982).

A diet that is high in calories, protein, vitamins, and minerals should be provided. Vitamin C is required for collagen formation and is necessary in wound healing. Vitamin A is also important for wound healing because it helps prevent gastric ulceration due to the stress of surgery, and functions in epithelial cell regeneration. Vitamin K is needed for blood clotting, and the B vitamins are essential for metabolism. Minerals, especially zinc, also help in wound healing. Special foods and supplemental feedings may be necessary if the patient is unable to eat adequately.

Burns

A patient with extensive burns requires the highest level of nutritional support. There is massive loss of protein from the burn site; and fluid and electrolytes, especially potassium and sodium, are lost through the exudate. Additional tissue destruction and nitrogen loss continue during the catabolic period that follows. The metabolic demands of infection, shock, or fever further increase the requirements for nutrients, and the energy needs may increase by 40% to 100% after burns.

The first priority in the initial treatment of a burn patient is fluid and electrolyte replacement. The loss of fluid generally slows after the first postburn day. The patient should be encouraged to eat, but other methods of feeding may be needed because the patient may be anorexic or find it difficult to swallow. Tube feeding or total parenteral feeding may be given. In extreme cases, oral, tube, and IV feedings may all be employed concurrently. The patient should be advanced to a high-protein, high-calorie diet by mouth as soon as this is feasible; and soft-to-regular food consistency will probably be tolerated well by the second week.

The need for protein may vary from 2 to 4 gm/kg body weight/day, depending on the extent of burn—*three to five* times the normal adult need for protein. From 3,500 to 5,000 kcal is needed to meet the demand for energy and to spare protein for wound healing and tissue regeneration, which also requires vitamins A and C. The B vitamins—thiamin, niacin, and riboflavin—are needed to form the enzymes necessary to metabolize the extra carbohydrate and protein. Healing is enhanced by zinc, and therapeutic doses of iron will alleviate anemia. Continuous support and encouragement are necessary to motivate the patient to eat all the food he requires.

Cancer

Malignant diseases influence nutritional status because they give rise to anorexia and dysguesia (impaired sense of taste). The cancer itself may cause increased catabolism with increased energy expenditure; and cancer treatment by surgery, radiation or chemotherapy creates other nutritional problems. Consequently, there is decreased resistance to infection, impaired gastrointestinal functioning, and fluid and electrolyte abnormalities.

After radical surgery of the head and neck, the patient may find chewing and swallowing easier from a reclining position, although liquids are swallowed with difficulty. Pureed foods are usually well tolerated. Resection of the GI tract produces malabsorption, often accompanied by the *dumping syndrome* (nausea, dizziness, and abdominal cramps after a meal). Pancreatectomy results in maldigestion and malabsorption owing to loss of pancreatic digestive enzymes, and causes diabetes mellitus owing to the lack of insulin. Bowel resection will cause serious long-term problems of water and electrolyte balance.

Radiation and chemotherapy often cause nausea and vomiting. If nausea occurs in the morning, offer the patient dry toast or crackers before he gets out of bed. The aroma of hot foods, greasy foods, and spicy foods aggravates nausea. Serving food at room temperature, or cooler, and cold foods, such as sherbet, cottage cheese, fruit, and a sandwich, are better accepted. Lemons and dill pickles may curb nausea, and ice pops are often tolerated when a patient cannot tolerate other foods. Loss of body fluids along with weight loss is a major nutritional concern when nausea and vomiting are severe. If oral feeding is not adequate, tube feeding should be instituted to sustain nutrition; if tube feeding is not possible, then total parenteral nutrition should be considered.

The senses of taste and smell are impaired during chemotherapy and radiation of the head and neck, leading to a condition described as *mouth blindness* or *taste blindness*. Foods may seem to have little taste or may taste unpleasant. Some patients may develop an aversion to meats, chocolate, and sweets of any kind. Having the patient drink fluids with meals may be helpful. If the patient does not like red meat such as beef, substitute chicken or fish; if he avoids all meats, offer eggs, cottage cheese, and other dairy products. Do not offer foods or beverages that the patient finds offensive. Learning how to deal with mouth blindness requires experimentation and observation of the patient's responses to various foods.

Decreased salivation makes the mouth dry, affects the taste of food, and makes chewing and swallowing more difficult. The patient may find that sucking hard candy, having an ice pop, and eating very sweet or tart foods may stimulate production of saliva. Foods that are soft and smooth, such as mashed potato, custard, and finely chopped or pureed foods, are easier to chew and swallow, especially when the mouth is sore and dry. Providing adequate quantities of fluids and food lubricants, such as gravy and sauce, is very helpful. Artificial saliva may be given if the mouth is very dry. Avoid offering sour foods high in acid if there is ulceration of the oral mucosa, because they are extremely irritating.

Cancer patients often complain they are less and less able to eat as the day progresses, and many feel at their best in the morning. Therefore, a big breakfast may be well tolerated, followed by small frequent meals through the rest of the day. Emphasizing the pleasurable aspects of eating and providing foods that are palatable to the patient will encourage the patient to eat and enjoy his meals.

ASSESSING NUTRITIONAL STATUS

Nutritional status is the overall state resulting from the consumption of food and the use of nutrients—the balance between nutrient intake and nutrient requirement. Any factor or condition that increases nutrient intake or decreases nutrient requirement results in a favorable or positive balance. Any factor or condition that decreases nutrient intake or increases nutrient requirement results in a negative balance. A person's nutritional status may be good, fair, or poor depending on the intake of dietary essentials, on the body's need for nutrients, and on the body's ability to use nutrients. The nutritional status is good when the essential nutrients—carbohydrates, proteins, fats, vitamins, minerals, and water—are supplied; the status is poor when the intake of essential nutrients is inadequate to meet the body's needs.

Assessment of nutritional status involves knowledge of the person's weight and height, dietary history and intake data, pertinent laboratory data, medication therapy, and clinical signs and symptoms that may indicate a nutritional deficiency state. The major focus of a nutritional assessment is to identify a patient who is at high risk of becoming malnourished and is likely to require nutritional intervention. High-risk patients include: (1) patients who are grossly overweight or grossly underweight; (2) patients with prior maldigestion, malabsorption, or inadequate nutrient intake; (3) patients with increased metabolic requirements due to fever, infection, trauma, burns, and hyperthyroidism; (4) patients with external losses such as draining fistulas, wounds, blood loss, and severe vomiting; and (5) patients who have been, or will be, unable to consume adequate amounts of food for 10 days (Butterworth and Blackburn, 1975).

Height and Weight

Measurement of height and weight is a useful indicator of nutritional status, particularly in growing children. In adults, regular weight measurements are especially important when there is chronic illness. A recent weight loss in a person whose weight had been normal indicates that he is not able to meet his nutritional requirements. In a hospitalized patient, rapid weight loss is a reliable index of change in protein nutritional status, as it usually reflects the use of protein for energy.

Height and weight measurements are compared to a standard (See Table 33.3). Ten percent above or below the standard is within the normal range.

Dietary History

A dietary history is done to identify the various influences on nutritional status. The patient or a member of his family may be interviewed; a questionnaire completed by the patient or a family member is also useful. Skillful questioning may reveal significant information about the patient and his food consumption patterns. Dietary informatin may vary from an estimate of food intake to a detailed history including: (1) description of recent food consumption patterns, eating habits, and meal composition; (2) circumstances of food purchase, storage, and preparation in the home; (3) number of meals eaten each day and where eaten; (4) types and amounts of food eaten at each meal; (5) amounts and types of beverages consumed; and (6) food idiosyncracies and food allergies. Additional data may be needed, depending on the nature of the patient's illness.

The information thus gathered must be correlated with observation of the patient's food and fuid intake while he is hospitalized, in order to determine the need for nutritional intervention and dietary counseling.

Laboratory Data and Medication Regimen

Laboratory measurements may permit early detection of marginal nutritional deficiencies. The following nutritional studies are of value: serum protein and albumin, hemoglobin, hematocrit, iron or transferrin, plasma-bound iodine, glucose, electrolytes, blood urea nitrogen, cholesterol, and triglycerides. A review of the patient's medications is also important in relation to his nutritional status, because drugs interact with foods in many situations. For example, antacids destroy thiamin, mineral oil decreases the absorption of fat-soluble vitamins, antibiotics may lead to the malabsorption syndrome, and anticonvulsants increase the need for vitamin D. A more detailed discussion of the effect of drugs on nutrition is given at the end of this chapter.

Clinical Signs

Some signs of poor nutritional status may be readily observed; others may require more careful examination. The mouth may show cracks, fissures, or redness, indicating a riboflavin deficiency. The hair may lack luster and become depigmentated as a result of protein deficiency. An enlargement of the thyroid can indicate iodine deficiency. Dryness of the cornea and conjunctivae as well as corneal opacity are often associated with vitamin A deficiency. Skin pallor and "spoon-shaped" nails that show bands or lines may be the result of iron deficiency. Subcutaneous hemorrhage is indicative of a vitamin C deficiency in infants. Pitting edema of the legs may indicate a deficiency in either protein or thiamin. An emaciated patient who has lost muscle mass and subcutaneous fat is suffering from marasmus.

Any of these findings should be immediately reported to the physician. The dietitian should also be alerted, so that a detailed analysis of the patient's food intake can be done. These observations are recorded, together with such information as body temperature, food and fluid intake, stool frequency, urinary loses, chewing and swallowing ability, loss by suction tube and drainage, vomiting, and behavior patterns.

MOTIVATING AND ASSISTING PATIENTS TO EAT

Appetite is a desire for food. A lack of appetite (anorexia) frequently accompanies illness and may be caused by physical discomfort such as pain or by psychological distress such as anxiety or depression. Patients who are upset usually do not eat well. An unpleasant environment, an unattractive tray, unfamiliar foods, medications, and various therapies all depress the appetite.

Improving the patient's appetite generally involves determining the reason for the lack of appetite and then dealing with the problem. Some suggestions for motivating a patient to eat are:

- Provide food that the patient likes and with which he is familiar.
- Present food attractively and at the proper temperature. Be sure to keep hot foods hot and cold foods cold.
- Offer foods in amounts the patient can eat. Large servings often discourage a patient.
- Make the environment conducive to eating by keeping out of sight all objects that are unpleasant to look at, such as urinals, bedpans, dressing trays, irrigation sets, and dirty dishes.
- Avoid unpleasant or uncomfortable treatments, such as injections, enemas, and dressings, immediately before or after a meal.
- See that the patient is clean, dressed adequately, and in a comfortable position for eating.
- Reduce psychological stress. Help the patient overcome any fear of the unknown or anticipation of a forthcoming operation, test, or treatment by discussing it and clarifying misconceptions.
- Alleviate pain and discomfort as far as possible and see that the patient has rest before mealtime.
- Observe and understand the possible reason for the loss of taste or smell. Some illnesses alter or inhibit the taste sensation. For example, cancer increases the sweet-taste threshold. To such patients, conventionally sweetened foods are flavorless.

Adding large amounts of sugar to foods will not only make food taste good but will add needed calories.

Some patients may need assistance with eating because of weakness or physical restrictions, such as traction, a cast, or loss of strength in hand or arm. It may be necessary to assist the patient, by cutting meat, buttering bread, and seasoning food, or placing the food tray conveniently within reach. Special utensils are available that assist a patient to eat: straws for those who have difficulty drinking from a cup or glass; weighted cups and glasses that do not tip; forks and spoons that have wide handles; and plate guards. A patient who has limited use of his arm and hand should be encouraged to hold his bread or straw to make him feel somewhat competent and not completely dependent on others. Patients who are unable to feed themselves should be positioned and supported properly to make swallowing easier. It is best to have the patient in as nearly an upright position as possible.

The nurse should help the patient to devise a way to let her know when he is ready for the next spoonful of food. She should sit in a comfortable position and be relaxed when feeding a patient so that he does not feel rushed. It is best to ask the patient which food he wants to eat first and to serve the food at the preferred rate. The nurse should also avoid having to leave the patient after starting to feed him, for to do so could make him feel neglected. With a blind patient or one whose eyes are bandaged, the nurse should describe the food and orient the patient to its placement on the tray.

NUTRITION AND DRUGS

Interactions between food and drugs occur in two ways: (1) certain foods alter drug absorption and patient response; (2) certain drugs interfere with nutrient absorption and use.

Effects of Food on Drugs

Foods can alter the absorption and action of drugs in a number of ways:

- Dilutional effect
- Decreased or delayed absorption from the gut
- Alteration in drug solubility and speed of excretion
- Formation of insoluble compounds
- Drug destruction or reduction of activity
- Inhibition or reversal of drug action
- Potentiation

The presence of food in the stomach can affect drug absorption by altering the pH of the gastrointestinal tract. Transit time and gastric emptying of food are also affected, and this may alter the blood level of drugs.

Some foods contain natural or added chemicals that react with certain drugs to render them less effective. For example, the interaction between the tetracyclines and dairy products is well known; oral absorption of tetracycline is impaired by dairy products, as well as by other foods. An insoluble compound of food and drug is that of lincomycin (Lincocin) and the cyclamate salts of Sweeta, Sucaryl, and diet drinks. The resulting product cannot be absorbed, so the therapeutic activity of lincomycin is reduced to near zero.

Mixing drugs and food to mask a disagreeable taste can create a new set of problems. Alteration of pH, a common result of this practice, could inhibit drug absorption and stability. Certain drugs should not be given with milk (in addition to tetracycline) because of decreased absorption (as with potassium chloride solutions) or because of increased gastric irritation (as with bisacodyl [Dulcolax]). In the latter case, milk dissolves the tablet's enteric coating and thus causes the drug to be released in the stomach rather than in the intestine. Bisacodyl is irritating to the stomach so should be taken in a form that bypasses the stomach and is released in the small intestine.

Some foods contain active substances that can cause an effect similar to that of a given drug or that can interact with a drug to produce an unexpected effect or a countereffect. Natural substances known as goitrogens, found in cabbage, turnips, kale, and brussels sprouts can cause goiter by inhibiting the production of thyroid hormone. It is therefore advisable to restrict the intake of these foods in a patient who is taking thyroid preparations. Excessive consumption of foods high in vitamin K, such as liver and leafy green vegetables, may hinder the effectiveness of anticoagulants. Vitamin K, which promotes clotting, works in direct opposition to anticoagulants, which prevent clotting.

TABLE 33.7 GUIDELINES FOR DRUG ADMINISTRATION

Avoid the use of alcoholic beverages while taking these drugs

Sedatives, hypnotics and other CNS depressants like barbiturates; certain antihistamines, and tranquilizers that are potentiated by alcohol; also avoid with aspirin and other drugs that produce adverse reaction with alcohol, such as oral hypoglycemic agents and MAO inhibitors

Do not take with milk or milk products

Drugs that are inactivated by calcium and other constituents of milk

Do not take with fruit juices

Certain antimicrobials and other drugs that tend to be destroyed by the constituents of fruit juices

Do not take with antacids

Ferrous gluconate and ferrous sulfate which form insoluble iron compounds that are poorly absorbed in the presence of alkalies

Do not take with mineral oil

Fat-soluble vitamins A, D, E, K and preparations; sulfasuxidine and sulfathalidine; dioctyl sodium sulfosuccinate laxatives

Take on an empty stomach

Certain antimicrobials and other drugs that are inhibited by various food constituents

Take 1 to 3 hours before meals

Drugs that require precise timing before intake of food to obtain the desired gastrointestinal effects; or drugs that require a specific minimum time for absorption before food can be taken

Take immediately before, with, or immediately after meals

Drugs that are nauseating or irritating

Take with food (with meals or immediately after meals)

Oral hypoglycemics
Antidiabetics; chlorothiazide; phenytoin; reserpine; triamterene; metronidazole; nitrofurantoin; trimeprazine tartrate; prednisone and prednisolone; rauwolfia and its alkaloids; potassium salts and preparations

Take with plenty of water

Uricosuric drugs such as allopurinol to prevent formation of xanthine calculi and precipitation of urates

Take with orange juice, banana, and other foods high in potassium

Diuretics such as ethacrynic acid, furosemide, and hydrochlorothiazide; also with steroids (aldosterone and desoxycorticosterone) that tend to cause hypokalemia

Alcohol reduces the biological half-life of tolbutamide (Orinase), an oral hypoglycemic agent. This may explain the relatively high failure rate in treating with Orinase those diabetics who drink sizable quantities of alcohol. (See Table 33.7.)

Effects of Drugs on Nutrition

Just as some foods can affect the way drugs respond in the body, some drugs can affect the way the body uses food and specific nutrients. Certain drugs can impair nutritional status and can produce a nutritional deficiency disease. Drugs exert their effect by one of several mechanisms:

- Effect on appetite and taste sensation
- Direct damage to lining cells of small intestine
- Inactivation of enzyme systems
- Inactivation or binding of nutrients
- Nutrient destruction or failure of synthesis
- Increased nutrient excretion

Digitalis, phenformin, and the amphetamines impair appetite because of their effect on the CNS. Anticholinergics, such as atropine, cause dryness of the mouth and thus impair taste acuity. Taste sensation may be altered by certain drugs, including griseofulvin (an antifungal agent used to treat certain skin problems), lincomycin (used to treat systemic infections), and penicillamine (used in Wilson disease). These drugs alter taste sensations either by decreasing the sweet taste or by increasing the sour or bitter taste. Some drugs have an unpleasant taste and cause nausea, vomiting, and anorexia. Chloral hydrate, paraldehyde, potassium chloride liquids, and vitamin B-complex liquids are unpleasant and produce a salty-bitter taste.

Except for anti-infective agents, most of the drugs that impair the absorption and use of nutrients are given for long-term treatment; and as a result, some supposedly harmless drug therapy can result in malnutrition, especially in children, the elderly, those with poor diets, and the chronically ill. Nutrient depletion occurs gradually and could remain undetected unless clinical indicators of nutritional status are monitored. For example, long-term anticonvulsant therapy can lead to deficiencies of folic acid and vitamin D by increasing the turnover rate of these vitamins in the body. Diuretics, especially the thiazides, may cause potassium depletion. If the potassium loss is not corrected in patients taking digitalis, the heart may become more sensitive to the digitalis. People taking diuretics regularly should eat foods that are good sources of potassium, such as bananas, cantaloupes, and tomatoes.

Anti-infective agents such as tetracycline, erythromycin, and sulfonamides and the antituberculosis drug isoniazid have been reported to decrease folic acid use, decrease vitamin D synthesis, and impair the absorption of vitamin B_{12}, calcium, and magnesium. Cytotoxic drugs such as methotrexate and aminopterin antagonize folic acid and interfere with the absorption of vitamin B_{12}. Cholestyramine, a drug used in the treatment of abnormally high cholesterol levels, can cause the malabsorption syndrome by decreasing absorption of fats and the fat-soluble vitamins, vitamin B_{12}, electrolytes, and iron.

Long-term oral contraceptive therapy can deplete the body's store of certain vitamins, notably folic acid and vitamin B_6. Fortunately, the diet of most healthy women is sufficiently balanced and the vitamin depletion is usually not serious enough to cause overt symptoms. But poor women or those who live on snack foods or have unusual food habits are likely to develop folate deficiency. Antacids used over a long period of time in high doses may result in thiamin deficiency and alter the rate of absorption of nutrients that are dependent on specific ranges of pH. Chronic use of antacids can also cause phosphate depletion, which produces muscle weakness and vitamin D deficiency.

Health care professionals need to develop an awareness of the immediate and long-term metabolic effects of drugs on nutritional status. Instances of drug-related malnutrition will probably increase over the years as new drugs are introduced. It appears increasingly obvious that any long-term drug therapy demands periodic examination of the patient's state of nutrition to prevent the development of iatrogenic malnutrition (resulting from therapy). Table 33.8 lists the effects of drugs on nutrients.

MEGAVITAMIN THERAPY AND FOOD MYTHS

Vitamins and minerals are required in relatively small amounts when compared to the needs for the macronutrients—carbohydrate, protein, and fat. Because most nutrients are present in a wide variety of foods, many different diet patterns are nutritionally adequate, and a person who eats properly does not require supplements. "If some is good, more is better" does not apply to vitamin and mineral needs.

Although vitamin and mineral requirements can be met through consumption of a balanced diet consisting of a variety of foods, the sale and use of supplements have increased in recent years. Consumers are misled by the advertisements and sales promotions for vitamin supplements, special dietary foods, and food supple-

TABLE 33.8 EFFECTS OF DRUGS ON NUTRIENTS

Drug	Effects
Mineral oil	Decreased absorption of fat-soluble vitamins, calcium, and phosphate
Laxatives	Decreased absorption of all vitamins and minerals
Stool softeners	Fecal loss of fat and fat-soluble vitamins
Antacids	Destruction of thiamin Decreased absorption of iron phosphate folic acid, vitamins C, D, and B_{12}
Anti-infectives ("sulfas," penicillin, tetracyclines, neomycin)	Decreased bacterial synthesis of vitamin K Malabsorption of vitamin B_{12}, calcium, and iron Inactivation of vitamin B_6 Decreased utilization of folic acid Sulfonamides increase vitamin C excretion Malabsorption syndrome with neomycin
Anticonvulsants	Inhibition of folic acid and vitamin B_{12} activity Increased breakdown of vitamins D and K Impaired absorption of calcium
Antineoplastics (methotrexate and aminopterin)	Inhibition of folic acid Interference of absorption of vitamin B_{12}
Antiarthritics	Malabsorption of vitamin B_{12}, fat, and electrolytes Decrease disaccharidase activity Increased fecal nitrogen excretion
Salicylates (Aspirin)	Increased excretion of vitamin C Loss of iron by gastric hemorrhage Folic acid deficiency by competitive binding
Diuretics	Loss of potassium, magnesium, and calcium Inhibition of folic acid activity
Tuberculosis drugs (INH, PAS, Isoniazid)	Vitamin B_6 deficiency by inactivation and excretion Malabsorption of fat Impaired absorption of vitamin B_{12} and folic acid Depletion of niacin and pyridoxine
Cholesterol reducers (cholestyramine)	Interference with bile salts and fats Decreased absorption of fat-soluble vitamins, particularly A and D Decreased absorption of calcium, vitamin B_{12}, and folate
Corticosteroids	Tissue breakdown and loss in muscle protein Increased metabolism of vitamin D Increased requirement for vitamin B_6 Increased urinary excretion of zinc
Oral hypoglycemic agent	Malabsorption of vitamin B_{12}
Oral contraceptives	Increased requirement for vitamin B_6 and riboflavin Decreased absorption of folic acid Decreased serum vitamin B_{12} and vitamin C
Antiparkinson drugs	Increased need for vitamin B_6 and vitamin C Increased urinary excretion of Na and K

ments. Groups most vulnerable to sales promotions are the elderly, the pregnant, the sick, and the poor; and, unfortunately, these people are often least able to afford such products. That these supplements are usually of no benefit in relation to the claims made increases the severity of this problem.

Consumers need to be informed if they are to avoid being misled by advertising techniques. Approaches ranging from nutritional insurance to miracle cures are often used to promote products, and false claims are made to entice potential buyers. A common claim is that supplements will cure fatigue, give extra pep, or help tired, run-down feelings. Vitamins and minerals are not energy sources and have no beneficial effect in treating "tiredness." Self-medication with supplements poses a serious danger, as it may delay treatment for a serious underlying cause of fatigue or other symptom. Large doses of vitamins have been advocated for quick and dramatic treatment of certain diseases. These megadoses are often five to ten or more times the recommended daily intakes. Vitamin E is claimed to slow aging, aid people with heart conditions, cure muscular dystrophy, and enhance sexual abilities. High levels of nicotinic acid are prescribed for the treatment of schizophrenia by orthomolecular psychiatrists. Megadoses of vitamin C to cure or prevent the common cold are pushed. Choline, biotin, and pantothenic acid also are commonly sold, but deficiency symptoms resulting from inadequate amounts of these nutrients are rare or nonexistent. They are synthesized by the body and are present in many foods.

Studies have shown no beneficial effects from megadoses or from any miraculous properties attributed to vitamins and minerals. Supplementation is of benefit only in treating diseases resulting from a *deficiency* of a specific nutrient. Several nutrients are toxic if consumed in large amounts. This poses a concern in that the use of daily supplements in addition to the vitamins and minerals already present in food could result in consumption of amounts approaching toxic levels for some nutrients; although, except for the fat-soluble vitamins A and D, the vitamins are generally considered to be less toxic than the trace minerals.

Symptoms of excess vitamin A include anorexia, blurred vision, hair loss, muscle soreness after exercise, and general drying and flaking of the skin. Anorexia, vomiting, renal insufficiency, hypertension, and systolic heart murmur have been associated with excessive intake of vitamin D. Concern has also been raised over two of the water-soluble vitamins, folic acid and vitamin C. High levels of folacin, or folic acid, may mask vitamin B_{12} deficiency. Possible drawbacks of excess vitamin C intake include increased urinary oxalate and resultant urinary stone formation; GI tract disturbances such as nausea, vomiting, cramps, and diarrhea; potential problems owing to increased iron and decreased copper absorption; interference with heparin and other anticoagulants; and increased breakdown of red blood cells. Rebound scurvy has occurred in infants born to mothers who have been taking high doses of vitamin C and also in adults who suddenly discontinue megadoses of this vitamin.

Many orthomolecular psychiatrists prescribe large doses (up to 500 times the normal recommended use) of nicotinic acid, vitamin C, and vitamins B_6 and B_{12} in treating some mental illnesses. This is a dangerous practice. Present knowledge of vitamin toxicity is limited and includes only short-term effects of large doses. Much less is known about chronic toxicity in which effects develop slowly over time.

A much narrower range of tolerance exists between the normal and toxic levels for most of the trace minerals. The margin of safety varies among the trace elements. A disproportionate intake of a mineral may create imbalances among nutrients or may diminish absorption and use of other minerals. Iron is the primary mineral of concern in toxicity due to excess. Interference with copper, zinc, and manganese absorption may result. Young children are especially susceptible to iron toxicity. Excess iron can accumulate in the liver and cause liver damage.

Supplementation *may* be necessary in certain situations, such as decreased food intake owing to prolonged illness or in cases where nutrient needs are increased, as in pregnancy and lactation. Even in these circumstances, however, supplements should be used under the direction of a physician. Self-medication may postpone treatment for a more serious problem or pose a danger if certain nutrients are consumed in excess. In addition, supplementation "just to be sure" can prove costly in the long run. When dollars are scarce, the family may neglect to buy foods that will fill its basic needs, in order to purchase a "guaranteed cure." Education of the public in this area is needed. Although the Federal Food and Drug Administration is charged with the legal responsibility for controlling the safety of all food and drug products, it is unable to fulfill this role in all situations. For example, the Rogers-Proxmire Act (1976) prohibits the establishment of maximum limits of supplemental vitamins and minerals, except for those sold for the use of children less than 12 years old and for pregnant or lactating women. Control is further limited by the First Amendment to the Constitution, which protects many of those who use false claims to promote products.

PATIENT TEACHING

Two of the most important aspects of patient teaching related to nutrition are (1) the concept of self-care, and (2) the importance of starting nutrition education during childhood.

Every person must be helped to realize that proper eating habits based on sound knowledge and self-discipline are essential for optimal health, and that each adult is ultimately responsible for his own nutrition. In order to help individuals and families maintain good patterns or acquire better eating patterns, the nurse must be knowledgeable about the cultural and emotional aspects of nutrition, as well as the financial ones. Eating habits are usually well ingrained in an individual's lifestyle, and are often extremely difficult to modify.

Nutrition education should begin with the preschool child by discussing the reasons why certain snacks, such as raw carrot sticks, are offered and why the sugared cereals advertised on television are not good. Elementary school children can learn to read package labels, and to select a balanced diet when appropriate foods are available. It is important to help the child learn to cope with peer pressure, and how to incorporate fast foods into a balanced food plan.

Children who take an active role in determining what and how much they will eat are much more likely to demonstrate adequate control over their own nutrition as adults than are children who are passive and eat what is set in front of them without question.

RELATED ACTIVITIES

1. If you and your family have always followed a fairly consistent and unvaried pattern of meals, begin to broaden your awareness of new and different foods. Venture into as many "ethnic" eating places as possible, so that you will have some understanding of the foods that patients of different cultural backgrounds prefer and find satisfying. You may not enjoy the taste of some of these foods, but you will at least be familiar with the taste and appearance. Such knowledge will help you understand the food preferences of your patients.

2. Overeaters Anonymous is a major source of help for compulsive overeaters, as well as for persons afflicted with bulimia. Contact your local organization, explain your interest, and ask if they hold *open meetings* which you might attend. Regular meetings are closed to outsiders to maintain the anonymity of members, but meetings open to the public are often held several times a year.

SUGGESTED READINGS

——— (Nursing grand rounds). TPN: the only road home. *Nursing 82* 1982 Sept; 12(9):44–49.

Beal, Virginia: *Nutrition in the Life Span.* New York, Wiley, 1980.

Beck, Cornelia: Dining experiences of the institutionalized aged. *J. Gerontal Nurs* 1981 Feb; 7(2):104–107.

Borgen, Linda: Total parenteral nutrition in adults. *Am J Nurs* 1978 Feb; 78(2):224–228.

Ciseaux, Annie: Anorexia nervosa: a view from the mirror. *Am J Nurs* 1980 Aug; 80(8):1468–1470.

Claggett, Marilyn Smith: Anorexia nervosa: a behavioral approach. *Am J Nurs* 1980 Aug; 80(8):1471–1472.

Guiness, Roxanne: How to use the new small-bore feeding tubes. *Nursing 86* 1986 April; 16(4):51–56.

Hui, YH: *Human Nutrition and Diet Therapy.* Monterey, CA, Wadsworth Health Sciences, 1984.

Irwin, Margaret M, and Diana R Openbrier: Feeding ventilated patients—Safely. *Am J Nurs* 1985 May; 85(5):544–546.

Johnston, Patricia K: Getting enough to grow on (vegetarian diets). *Am J Nurs* 1984 March; 84(3):336–339. (Note correction on p.720 of June 1984 *Am J Nurs*).

Kadas, Nancy: The dysphagic patient: everyday care really counts. *RN* 1983 Nov; 46(11):38–41.

Loustau, Anne, and Kathryn A Lee: Dealing with the dangers of dysphagia. *Nursing 85* 1985 Feb; 15(2):47–50.

Marks, Roberta G: Anorexia and bulimia: eating habits that can kill. *RN* 1984 Jan; 47(1):44–47.

Metheny, Norma Milligan: 20 ways to prevent tube feeding complications. *Nursing 85* 1985 Jan; 15(1):47–50.

Munro-Black, Janet: The ABC's of total parenteral nutrition. *Nursing 84* 1984 Feb; 14(2):50–55.

Parker, Cherry: Helping patients live with food allergies. *Am J Nurs* 1980 Feb; 80(2):262–266.

Rodin, Judith: A sense of control. *Psych Today* 1984 Dec; 18(12):38–45.

Salmond, Susan Warner: How to assess the nutritional states of acutely ill patients. *Am J Nurs* 1980 May; 80(5):922–924.

Tymkiw, Genie: Obesity: a challenge for patient teaching. *Can Nurse* 1978 Nov; 74(10):42–44.

Veninga, Karen Smit: An easy recipe for assessing your patient's nutrition. *Nursing 82* 1982 Nov; 12(11):57–59.

When Your Client Has a Weight Problem (special feature). *Am J Nurs* 1981 March; 81(3):549–572.

——— White, Jane A, and Mary Ann Schroeder: Nursing assessment.

——— Kornguth, Mary Lewis: Nursing management.

——— Langford, Rae W: Teenagers and obesity.

——— Overeaters anonymous: a self-help group.

——— Miller, Barbara K: Jejunoileal bypass: A drastic weight control measure.

——— Mojzisik, Cathy M, and Edward W Martin: Gastric partitioning: The latest surgical means to control morbid obesity.

Wilhelm, Lana: Helping your patient 'settle in' with TPN. *Nursing 85* April; 15(4):60–65.

REFERENCES

Albanese, AA: *Nutrition for the Elderly.* New York, Alan Liss, 1980.

Butterfield CE and Blackburn GL: Hospital Malnutriton. *Nutri Today.* 10(2):8, 1975.

Buzby, GP: Preoperative nutritional support: Nutritional indications for delaying surgery. *Clinical Consultations in Nutritional Support.* Ross laboratories. 1982 21(2):1.

Crisp, AH: *Anorexia Nervosa: Let Me Be.* New York, Grunne and Stratton, 1980.

Halmi, Katherine A, et al: Binge-eating and vomiting: a survey of a college population. *Psychol Med.* 1981 11(4):697.

Krause, Marie V, and L Kathleen Mahan: *Food, Nurition, and Diet Therapy.* ed.7. Philadelphia, Saunders, 1984.

Kris-Etherton, PM: Nutrition, exercise and athletic performance. *Food Nutr News.* 1985 57(3):13.

Lucas, Alexander R: Anorexia nervosa. in Spittell, JA (ed.): *Clinical Medicine,* Vol.9, Philadelphia, Harper & Row, 1983.

Pennington, Jean AT and Helen Nichols Church: *Bowes and Church's Food Values of Portions Commonly Used.* ed.14. Philadelphia, Lippincott, 1985.

Schwartz, Donald and Thompson MG: Do anorectics get well? Current research and future needs. *Am J Psych.* 138(3):319, 1981.

Sherman, William M and David L Costil: The marathon: dietary manipulation to optimize performance. *Am J Sports Med.* 1984 12(1):44.

Short, Sally H, and Walter R. Short: Four year study of university athlete's dietary intake. *J Am Diet Assoc.* 1983 82(6):632.

Slavin, JL: Dietary fiber. *Dietetic Currents.* 1983 10(6):31.

Wilmore, Jack H and Beau J Freund: Nutritional enhancement of athletic performance. *Nutr Abs Rev.* 1984 54(1):1.

34

Elimination

Prerequisites and/or Suggested Preparation
A basic understanding of the anatomy and physiology of the colon, kidneys, ureters, bladder, and urethra, and concepts from physics related to fluid flow and osmotic pressure (Chapter 11) are prerequisite to understanding this chapter. Suggested preparation includes an understanding of Freud's concepts of the anal stage of personality development (Chapter 15).

Section One

Intestinal Elimination

Problems associated with elimination are usually both psychologically and physically difficult for everyone concerned. An individual's self-esteem, self-respect, and dignity are dependent upon that person's ability to control the elimination of his own body wastes, and any impairment of that control is frustrating and humiliating. The emotional aspects of a person's inability to manage his own urine and feces demand great sensitivity and understanding on the part of the nurse.

INFLUENCES ON BOWEL FUNCTION

Psychosocial Influences

The toilet training of children is usually culturally determined and often has a significant influence on future bowel habits. The timing, rigidity, and vigor with which it is done affect the child's attitudes toward both his body and his bowel movements. For example, toilet training in some families is literally a battle, a contest of wills between parent and child in which the child may rebel and seek to retain his feces with such vigor that he is constipated most of the time. The parent is likely to panic if the child does not have a bowel movement and may assault the child with frequent enemas. This action increases the child's rebellion and his drive to keep what seems to be rightfully his. He continues to refuse to defecate on demand and on schedule, and the vicious cycle continues. In contrast, the toddlers in some cultures run about in a relaxed milieu without diapers or pants of any kind until they have learned by imitation to defecate in a socially acceptable manner.

Another influence on bowel habits is the type and availability of toilet facilities, which range from pit privies and outhouses in underdeveloped areas, through public and communal toilet facilities, to homes with several bathrooms for a single family. Bowel function is also affected by a person's habits and by his attitude toward his body. Many people, for example, are deeply concerned and often preoccupied with their self-imposed goal of a daily bowel movement.

Physiological Influences

Bowel function is affected by diet, especially by the amount of fiber and fluid. Low fiber and low fluid in-

take predispose a person to constipation while adequate fiber shortens the passage time of fecal matter through the intestines and the feces retain enough fluid to keep them soft.

Bowel function is disrupted by irregular meals and increased stress. Decreased physical activity leads to decreased muscle tone in the muscles used for defecation. An abnormal position, such as lying in bed, makes defecation more difficult.

Disease affects bowel function by increasing or decreasing the motility of the GI tract and thereby alters the speed of peristalsis. An inflamed, irritated intestinal tract tends to produce diarrhea; an atonic condition of the colon with markedly decreased peristalsis produces constipation. Bowel function can also be disturbed by a mechanical obstruction such as a tumor or constricting adhesions. Damage to the nerves supplying the intestinal tract from a spinal cord injury affects bowel function, as do drugs that alter sympathetic and parasympathetic interaction. Finally, bowel function is depressed by the effects of anesthesia and by manipulation and handling of the intestines during abdominal surgery.

ASSESSMENTS

Bowel function is assessed through information provided by the patient, examination of the abdomen, observation of feces, and diagnostic tests.

Patient History

Information from the patient will reveal data related to his attitude and feelings about his bowel function, the frequency of bowel movements, and the presence or absence of pain, cramps, need to strain, or other discomfort. Information related to any *change* in bowel function is particularly significant. A change in bowel habits is one of the seven warning signs of cancer; a shift from regular, soft bowel movements to seemingly permanent constipation, for example, could indicate serious pathology.

In addition to collecting data on the physiology of a patient's bowel function, the nurse needs to assess the conditions under which the described bowel function occurs. It may be that one person's *apparently normal* pattern of two soft, formed bowel movements each day without discomfort or straining occurs only as a result of his taking a daily laxative, while another person's *apparently normal* pattern of a slightly hard, formed stool three times weekly only follows the thrice weekly enemas he has taken since childhood.

Examination of the Abdomen

The techniques of examination used most frequently by the nurse include inspection, auscultation, and palpation. Since palpation of the abdomen can stimulate peristaltic action and thereby distort the sounds heard by auscultation, *palpation* is always done last.

Inspection of the abdomen provides data related to contour, scars, visible masses, or hernias. The contour of the abdomen is described as rounded, flat, or sunken (scaphoid).

Auscultation of the abdomen is done to assess bowel sounds. The frequency or level of activity, intensity, and pitch vary with the contents and health of the intestines. Diarrhea or any other condition that increases peristalsis produces bowel sounds which are hyperactive and higher pitched than normal, and bowel sounds are often *absent* immediately after abdominal surgery or with advanced intestinal obstruction.

Palpation of the abdomen is done to locate areas of pain or tenderness, to detect masses or hernias, to determine the height of the uterus after delivery, and to check for the presence of a distended urinary bladder.

The prostate gland can be palpated through the anterior wall of the rectum, and palpation during a rectal examination will indicate the size, shape, and consistency of the prostate gland.

The cervix can also be palpated through the anterior wall of the rectum.

The location of any masses, pain, or tenderness is indicated by reference to the areas or quadrants of the abdomen (Fig. 34.1).

Observation of Feces

Feces are observed for consistency, shape, color, odor, and the presence of any unusual matter.

Consistency

The consistency of a normal stool is soft but formed. Very solid stool is described as *hard* or *constipated*. Stools which are softer than normal are described as *soft* when they are without any free water, *loose* when they are watery but with some solid matter, and *liquid* when they consist of colored fluid only.

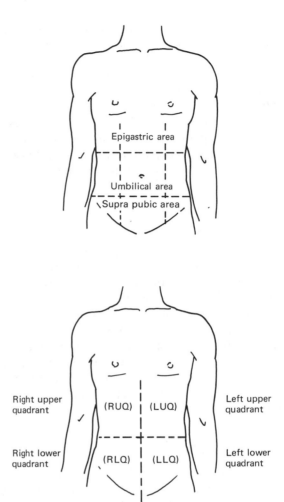

Figure 34.1 *Anatomical areas of the abdomen.*

Shape

Stool normally assumes the shape of the rectum; if some portion of the colon is constricted, by cancer for example, the stool may become pencil slim as it passes through the narrowed segment of intestine. Stool that is consistently small in diameter may be the result of serious pathology.

Color

Stool is normally colored brown by bilirubin derivatives and by the action of the bacteria normally found in the intestines. An absence of bile produces a very pale, putty-colored stool that is often referred to as a *clay-colored* stool and is usually associated with gallbladder or liver disease.

A dark, sticky, tarry stool may be the result of bleeding in the digestive tract and is created by the digestion of red blood cells from bleeding high in the gastrointestinal tract. Dark, digested blood is referred to as hidden, or *occult* blood. Visible red blood has escaped digestion and probably originated relatively low in the digestive tract. Streaks of fresh red blood on the outside of the stool indicate that the blood has been oozing from the walls of the rectum or from hemorrhoids at the anus.

Medications and food affect the color of feces. Iron or bismuth preparations (such as Pepto-Bismol) will turn fecal matter black, for example. If a person has eaten beets, the stools will be red, while food containing large amounts of chlorophyll will turn fecal matter green.

Unusual Matter

Feces should be observed for the presence of unusual or abnormal matter such as blood, mucus, worms, or undigested food. Both blood and mucus may be either mixed throughout the fecal matter or may have coated the outside of the stool as it passed through the intestines. Worms are not uncommon in this country, and are very common in some regions of the world. They are usually visible to the naked eye and range in size from pin worms, which resemble fine threads, to tapeworms, which are from $\frac{1}{8}$ to $\frac{1}{4}$ inch wide and from 5 to 20 feet long.

Diagnostic Tests

Diagnostic tests related to the intestinal tract include upper GI series (barium swallow), lower GI series (barium enema), gallbladder series, sigmoidoscopy, and proctoscopy (Chapter 17, Section 4). Other common diagnostic tests include chemical tests to detect occult blood and microscopic examinations for amebas and parasites. Tests for occult blood include orthotoluidine (Occultest), benzidine, and guaiac. The first two tests require that the person follow a meat-free diet for 3 days before the test, but the guaiac test does not involve a meat-free diet. Massive doses of vitamin C may cause a false-negative test. Many people refer to all tests for occult blood as guaiac tests and use the phrase *stool for guaiac* as a synonym for any or all of the tests for occult blood.

Most tests require only a small amount of fecal matter, although the laboratory may request the entire stool for some examinations. Unless the nurse is given other instructions, she should transfer a piece of stool about the size of a walnut from a clean, dry bedpan to a waterproof container by means of one or two tongue depressors. The patient should be cautioned not to urinate on the stool specimen, and to discard toilet paper elsewhere.

The solid matter from a diarrheal stool can be obtained by having the patient defecate onto a piece of newspaper in the bedpan or toilet. The newspaper absorbs the fluid and the solid matter can be removed with a tongue depressor and sent to the laboratory. Paper towels are not ordinarily used for this purpose because they often contain bismuth, which affects the chemical analysis of the stool.

Examination of fecal matter for some types of parasites and worms must be made while the stool is still warm, and any directions from the laboratory related to the collection and handling of the stool specimen must be followed exactly.

Careful medical asepsis must be observed to prevent the spread of disease to the nurse herself or the laboratory workers. Surgical asepsis may be indicated if the specimen is to be analyzed to detect a specific type of bacterium.

PROMOTION OF NORMAL BOWEL FUNCTION

Because adequate intestinal elimination is prerequisite for health, every person must assume responsibility for acquiring and maintaining a regular pattern of elimination. Many people do this without effort or difficulty but others need considerable assistance in doing so. There is seldom a single cause for problems related to intestinal elimination, but rather a complex interaction of diet, fluids, exercise, position, habits, and relaxation.

Diet and Fluid

A well-balanced diet and adequate fluid are two of the components of normal elimination. Adequate dietary fiber provides bulk, which helps keep the stool soft and which increases the speed of its passage through the intestines. This increased speed decreases the amount of water that can be reabsorbed by the large intestine, and the stool remains soft enough to be expelled without strain. A diet that lacks fiber is likely to produce small, hard pieces of fecal matter.

Nine to ten liters of water enter the intestines each day in the form of oral intake, saliva, gastric secretions, pancreatic juices, and bile, and a person's fluid intake must be adequate to sustain this level. This fluid liquifies the intestinal contents for movement through the intestines and for the absorption of nutrients and electrolytes. In health, almost all of this fluid is reabsorbed and only about 100 ml of water is excreted in feces.

Insufficient water and fiber give inadequate bulk, which slows the passage of food through the intestines, permitting increased reabsorption of water and thereby causing a very hard stool and constipation. A person who is constipated, therefore, should be helped to increase his intake of both fiber and fluid. The type of help needed may involve teaching him about the basic food groups, offering help in planning meals, or changing family food habits. Whole grain cereals, vegetables, fruit, and nuts are valuable sources of fiber.

Exercise

Normal defecation requires adequate strength in the abdominal and pelvic muscles. Patients who are weak and debilitated from severe illness or prolonged immobility may need to do conditioning exercises to strengthen the muscles of the abdomen and pelvic floor.

Position

The most physiologically effective position for defecation is a squatting position in which the pressure of the thighs against the abdomen increases the intra-abdominal pressure and thus aids expulsion of the stool. Most adults can achieve this position by leaning forward while sitting on the toilet, but children and short people may find it advisable to use a foot stool to raise their thighs when using the toilet. Some elderly people who find it difficult to rise from a low seat must use an elevated toilet seat to get off the toilet without assistance. A higher toilet seat often means that their feet barely touch the floor and they may therefore need to use a small box or foot stool to flex their knees and hips for effective defecation.

A patient confined to bed may be unable to defecate while lying flat in bed but may be able to do so in a more normal position, which can be achieved by raising both the head of the bed and the knee gatch if this is not contraindicated.

When a patient is helped onto a bedpan, the head of the bed should be elevated to an angle of 30 degrees to 40 degrees before he tries to get on the bedpan. If the bed is left flat, the patient will have to *hyperextend his back* to lift his hips high enough to get on the bedpan. This is both dangerous and uncomfortable for patients with arthritis or lower back problems, for example. On the other hand, if the head of the bed is elevated more than 40 degrees to 50 degrees, all of the patient's body weight will be over his pelvis and he will have to be lifted straight up to raise his hips enough to get on the bedpan. This is extremely difficult for a person with short or weak arms. The head of the bed should thus be raised high enough to prevent hyperextension of the spine and kept low enough to support the weight of the upper body while the patient raises his hips to get on the bedpan.

If the patient is unable to lift his hips off the bed, you will need to lower the head of the bed completely so that the bed is flat and you can help him roll onto and off the bedpan. With the bed flat, roll the patient onto his side, press the bedpan *firmly against his buttocks* and *down to into the mattress* at the same time, and roll him back onto the bedpan. Adjust the position of the bedpan until the patient is comfortable and elevate the head of the bed and the knee gatch unless it is contraindicated to do so. This method of positioning a bedpan is safe for the patient because there is little or no friction to injure the skin over his sacrum. *Never try to push, pull, shove, or otherwise force a bedpan under a patient.*

If the patient's skin is tender or he is very thin, protect his skin and make him comfortable by placing a folded towel over the rim of the bedpan. Even a washcloth offers some protection and will keep his skin from sticking to the bedpan in hot weather. Some patients need a special flat bedpan, often called a *fracture pan,* plus rather substantial padding such as a small, thin pillow for comfort and safety. Such a pillow or towel obviously should not be used for any other purpose.

Ensure as much comfort and privacy for the patient as possible and make certain that both the call bell and toilet paper are within reach before you leave the unit. Do not leave the patient on the bedpan longer than necessary.

To remove the bedpan, lower the head of the bed and the knee gatch; while holding the bedpan to keep it from spilling, roll the patient off the bedpan onto his side. Help the patient cleanse his rectal area and provide him with the articles he needs to wash his hands.

Throughout this entire process, touch only the *outside* of the bedpan; do *not* let your fingers touch the underside of the rim. Wash your hands thoroughly before you do anything else.

Habits and Patterns of Elimination

Each patient should be encouraged to use any techniques for maintaining bowel function that have proved helpful to him in the past, such as drinking a cup of hot water before breakfast or prune juice at night, or reading while using the toilet. Many of these measures are based on physiological processes and have a sound basis for their effectiveness. The practice of drinking warm fluids when one arises, for example, stimulates the gastrocolic reflex, which often initiates a desire to defecate.

Stress and tension can interfere with bowel function, especially in an already stressful hospital environment. Therefore, in addition to ensuring adequate privacy, it is important that the nurse provide enough time for the patient to have a bowel movement. Treatments and tests are sometimes scheduled so close that the patient

PROCEDURE 34.1

Giving and Removing a Bedpan*

SUMMARY OF ESSENTIAL NURSING ACTIONS

1. Make sure the bedpan is the appropriate size and shape for patient comfort and effective use.
   - Use a fracture pan for a small, thin, frail person.
   - Pad the rim of the pan as needed for comfort and to protect patient's skin.
2. If the patient *can raise buttocks* off the bed:
   - Raise the head of the bed 30–40 degrees.
   - Slide pan under patient as you help him raise buttocks off bed.
3. If the patient *cannot raise buttocks* off the bed:
   - Turn patient onto side, facing away from you.
   - Press bedpan against patient's buttocks and down into mattress at the same time.

*See inside front cover and page 677.

- Hold bedpan FIRMLY in position and roll patient over onto his back.
- Adjust position of bedpan until patient is comfortable.
4. Elevate head of bed until patient feels comfortable. Raise knee gatch of bed as needed to keep patient and bedpan from slipping.
5. Make sure signal cord and toilet paper are within reach.
6. When patient is ready, help him off the bedpan.
   - If patient cannot lift buttocks, hold bedpan *flat against the mattress* to prevent spilling as you roll the patient off the bedpan.
7. Cleanse the patient with toilet paper if help is needed.
8. Cover the bedpan and take it to be emptied.
9. Make provision for the patient to wash his hands.

---

has no relaxed, uninterrupted time for having a bowel movement. This situation can be very serious for a person with a neurological disorder who has succeeded in developing a satisfactory schedule of elimination at home, only to have it thoughtlessly disrupted during a hospitalization. This problem can be minimized if you make sure that the patient participates in all decision making and planning related to his care.

There is no right or normal pattern of bowel elimination, though frequencies ranging from once a week to three times a day are usually considered normal. When you assess bowel function, remember that the *consistency* of the stool is more important than its frequency.

ALTERATIONS IN BOWEL FUNCTION

In addition to the changes in bowel function that occur normally as a result of age, fluid intake, diet, stress, and daily routine, there are other changes, caused by illness, medication, treatment, and tests. Many specific causes of changes are described in detail in medical-surgical nursing texts; this chapter describes nursing care *in general* without mention of care related to specific pathological conditions. General aspects of bowel function include the nursing care of patients with constipation, impaction, diarrhea, incontinence, distention, and special problems such as hemorrhoids, worms, and ostomies.

Constipation

A person is considered constipated when fecal matter is passed in hard lumps and when, as a result, defecation is difficult or painful. Frequency of defecation is not necessarily a factor; a person who passes a soft, formed stool only twice a week is not constipated. On the other hand, a person would be considered constipated if his daily bowel movement consisted of small, hard lumps of fecal matter.

The treatment of constipation includes changes in diet and fluid intake, exercises to strengthen abdominal and pelvic muscles, and provision for adequate privacy and relaxation. Many of these measures require an extended period of time for an effect to be noticeable, so short-term measures such as drugs, suppositories, or enemas are used for more immediate relief of symptoms.

Laxatives and Cathartics

A drug used to promote evacuation of the bowel to relieve constipation or to prepare the colon for a diagnostic test is called a laxative or cathartic. A *laxative* is usually considered milder than a *cathartic,* and the term *purgative* is used to refer to a strong cathartic action.

Laxatives are habit forming, and dependence on them is difficult to break. They are effective and appropriate for occasional use, but every effort should be made to eliminate their habitual use. Some laxatives act rather quickly; others take up to 12 or 15 hours to act. It is important, therefore, to administer a laxative so that the resulting defecation will occur when it is convenient for the patient or appropriate for a prescribed test.

Laxatives in gum and candy form (such as Ex-Lax) can be dangerous if they are accessible to children. Such laxatives contain a tasteless drug (phenolphthalein), which can cause serious poisoning if taken in large doses.

Suppositories

A suppository is a slender, tapered stick of glycerin or other substance that melts at body temperature. Some suppositories release a drug as they melt and are used to produce a general, systemic effect, but others are used to stimulate defecation through mechanical pressure or chemical irritation of the nerve endings of the rectum.

A suppository usually works within 5 to 10 minutes and is often used during various phases of bowel training for people who must develop new patterns of elimination, such as after a spinal cord injury. The use of a suppository under the same conditions at the same time each day will often initiate a regular, predictable pattern of defecation.

Suppositories are made in two sizes, adult and infant; as with all drugs or health products, the label on the container should be read carefully. Most suppositories for bowel training are made of nonmedicated glycerin, but a moistened sliver of pure, mild castile soap can be substituted for a single occasion if glycerin suppository is not available.

Suppositories are kept refrigerated so they will be stiff enough to be inserted. The suppository must be inserted past the internal rectal sphincter, and a nonsterile glove or finger cot is used to protect the finger of the person inserting the suppository. It is not possible to insert an infant's suppository completely, so it is usually held in place by gently holding the baby's buttocks together for a few minutes to prevent premature expulsion.

Enemas

An enema is the administration of a warm solution into the rectum to stimulate peristalsis and cause defecation. Peristalsis is stimulated by mechanical pressure against the walls of the lower colon and rectum. This pressure can be created by the administration of a fairly large volume of fluid (500 to 1,000 ml).

TYPES. A *cleansing enema* involves the administration of enough fluid (up to 1,000 ml) to stimulate peristalsis and empty the lower bowel. Commonly used fluids include tap water, saline, or a soapsuds solution. A *tap-water enema* (TWE) does not irritate the mucosa of the intestine; but it must be given with caution because it is *hypotonic*. Water flows across a semipermeable membrane from the least concentrated (most dilute) solution to the more concentrated solution in an effort to equalize the two. Therefore, water from a TWE can pass from the intestines through the intestinal wall into blood vessels and interstitial spaces, and repeated enemas can cause water toxicity or circulatory overload in susceptible patients.

A *soapsuds enema* (SSE) increases the peristaltic stimulation of a tap-water enema because the soap irritates the lining of the lower intestine. A soapsuds enema (which should not have any suds) is prepared by adding approximately 5 ml of pure, liquid castile soap to 1,000 ml of warm water. Soap must be used with caution because it is irritating to the mucosa of the intestinal tract just as it is irritating to the conjunctiva, and household detergents should *never* be used. Many physicians do not permit the use of soapsuds enema before a proctocscopic or sigmoidoscopic examination because soap irritates the intestinal lining enough to distort the appearance of the mucosa.

For patients who cannot tolerate the large amounts of fluid needed for a tap water or soapsuds enema, a *hypertonic saline* enema is often used. Only 100 to 200 ml of fluid is needed because the hypertonic solution draws additional fluid into the intestines from the blood vessels and interstitial spaces by osmotic pressure. *Hypertonic saline enemas* are prepared commercially; because one of the first units was prepared by the C. B. Fleet Company, this type of enema is often referred to as a Fleet's Enema. A commercially prepared hypertonic enema is packaged in a squeeze bottle with a prelubricated tip, and the directions for administration are printed on the package.

The ease of administration and the relative patient comfort make the hypertonic enema popular for use despite the fact that it has several potential hazards. A hypertonic solution draws water from the tissues into the intestinal tract, and repeated hypertonic enemas can therefore contribute to dehydration and fluid imbalance. In addition, a hypertonic saline enema must be used with caution for a patient whose intake of salt is restricted, because enough salt can be absorbed by the intestinal mucosa to elevate the patient's serum sodium level.

If the fecal matter is very hard and cannot be passed without discomfort, pain, or excessive straining, an *oil-retention enema* is often given to soften the stool in preparation for a cleansing enema. The oil should be retained for several hours; therefore, the amount given is small (100 ml or less) so that peristalsis will not be stimulated and the patient will not feel the urge to expel the oil prematurely. Oil is given through a rectal tube with a small diameter connected to a small funnel, or by means of a commercially prepared unit consisting of an oil-filled squeeze bottle and a prelubricated tip. Olive oil is used most frequently, but any other pure vegetable oil can be substituted. The oil is heated to body temperature both for comfort and to avoid peristaltic stimulation by a cold liquid. The patient is instructed to retain the solution as long as possible. The bed should be protected against any possible leakage of oil.

EQUIPMENT. The equipment needed to give an enema consists either of a commercial squeeze container with a prelubricated tip, or a container for fluid with tubing, a regulating clamp, and rectal tube or tip. In addition, a bedpan, lubricant, toilet paper, and waterproof and absorbent materials to protect the bed are required.

ADMINISTRATION. Before giving an enema, allow enough fluid to run through the tubing to remove the air that would otherwise be forced into the rectum. Insert the lubricated tip about 2 in into the rectum, with the tip pointing toward the patient's umbilicus. Loosen the regulating clamp and, while you hold the container of fluid about 18 in above the patient's anus, let fluid enter the rectum slowly. An enema must be administered slowly because rapid administration stimulates peristalsis and promotes defecation before enough fluid can be administered to ensure good results.

A person with poor sphincter control may be unable to retain the enema fluid, and the enema must then be given on the bedpan or toilet. The person giving the enema can wear a disposable glove while holding the rectal tube in place.

If the patient complains of intestinal cramps, slow the flow of fluid by lowering the container or adjusting the regulating clamp. If necessary, stop the flow for a few minutes until the cramping sensation subsides. If the patient complains of being unable to hold the fluid any longer, slow or stop the flow and ask the patient to pant through his mouth. This reduces any tendency to expel the enema prematurely because the patient cannot pant and push down to expel the enema at the same time. The amount of fluid administered will vary from patient to patient. The first enema given postoperatively is usually about 300 to 500 ml, with the amount specified by the physician in most cases. Other enemas are usually 500 to 1,000 ml (1 pt. to 1 qt). A patient may find it very difficult to retain enema fluid, and care must be taken to keep him as comfortable as possible while trying to give an effective enema.

Most references still recommend that an enema be given with the patient lying on his left side even though

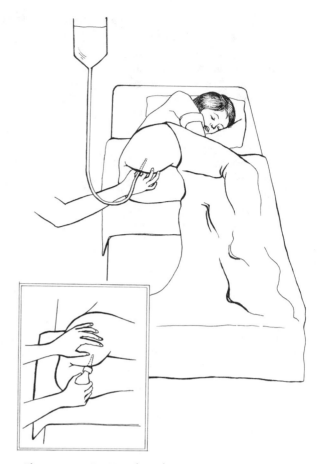

Figure 34.2 *Position for administration of an enema.*

there seems to be some doubt whether his position makes much difference in the effectiveness of the enema (Fig. 34.2). If a patient is to give himself an enema at home, it may not be feasible for him to lie down. Most people give themseves an enema in the bathroom. Although a young and agile person could lie down on the floor or in the bathtub, an *elderly person should not try to lie down,* especially in a small, cramped bathroom, because he may be unable to get up again, especially if he tries to hurry to expel the enema. An enema can be given while the patient is sitting on the toilet if it is given slowly enough for him to accept most of the fluid before peristaltic action stimulates defecation.

If a patient is directed to prepare himself at home for a diagnostic test such as a barium enema, he must be taught about the preparation needed. The phrase "enemas until clear" has little meaning for the patient unless he has been through the procedure before. If a person is, or has been, constipated, the returns of the first enema may consist of pieces of hard stool and clear water. The returns from the second and third enemas may consist of highly colored water mixed with soft

PROCEDURE 34.2

Giving an Enema*

SUMMARY OF ESSENTIAL NURSING ACTIONS

1. Prepare solution or use a commercially prepared enema of the prescribed amount and type.
   - If the temperature is not specified, warm the solution until it feels slightly warm against your wrist.
2. Expel the air from tubing and then clamp the tubing.
3. Position patient in accordance with his condition.
   - Position patient on side with upper hip flexed if feasible.
   - If patient is unable to retain fluid, position him comfortably on the bedpan.
4. Lubricate the tip of the rectal tube, separate the buttocks enough to *see the anus clearly.*
5. Insert the tip 2–4 inches for an adult, 1–2 inches for a child.
   - If the patient has hemorrhoids, insert the tip very gently and cautiously, or permit the patient to insert it himself.
6. Hold the rectal tip in place. (Wear a glove if the patient cannot retain the fluid.)
7. Hold or suspend the container of fluid 12–18 inches above the patient's rectum.

8. If the patient complains of abdominal cramps, or of a feeling that he must expel the fluid, clamp or pinch off the flow of fluid and ask the patient to take deep breaths or pant until the feeling passes.
9. Encourage the patient to retain the fluid as long as possible.
10. Help the patient onto the bedpan or commode, or into the bathroom. Make sure that toilet paper and signal cord are available.
11. Examine the expelled material before the bedpan is emptied or the toilet is flushed.
12. If the fluid is not expelled, it must be siphoned back.
    - Reinsert the rectal tip and allow more fluid to flow into the rectum.
    - WHILE THE FLUID IS STILL FLOWING, lower the container of fluid below the level of the rectal tip until the fluid flows back into the container.
    - Repeat as needed until all fluid has been siphoned back.
    - Remember that the equipment is now grossly contaminated with fecal matter, and unless it is disposable it must be thoroughly cleaned before reuse.

*See inside front cover and pages 679–680.

---

stool from higher in the intestines, while the fourth and fifth enemas may be clearer. "Enemas until clear" means that enemas are to be given until the returned fluid is clear (not cloudy or colored) and contains no fecal matter.

Fecal Impaction

A *fecal impaction* is a hardened mass of fecal matter that is wedged or impacted in a patient's rectum and which he cannot expel. This condition is caused by unrelieved

PROCEDURE 34.3

Removing a Fecal Impaction*

SUMMARY OF ESSENTIAL NURSING ACTIONS

1. Check agency policy and/or doctor's order before attempting the procedure.
2. Position patient on side with upper hip flexed.
3. Protect the bedding with a disposable pad under the patient's buttocks.
4. Place bedpan within reach to receive fecal matter.
5. Put on a clean (not sterile) glove, and lubricate your gloved index finger.
6. Separate the patient's buttocks until you can see the anus clearly.

7. Slowly and carefully insert your gloved finger and GENTLY try to loosen and break up the fecal mass.
8. The procedure is painful—DO NOT USE FORCE OR PRESSURE.
9. Remove the fecal matter a small piece at a time if possible.
10. Stop the procedure when the patient can tolerate no more or when no more pieces can be removed.
11. Assess the situation and decide whether to: (a) try again when peristaltic action may have moved more fecal matter closer to the anus, or (b) give an oil retention enema to soften the remaining fecal matter for easier removal.

*See inside front cover and pages 681–682.

constipation in people who are too sick, weak, or confused to expel the mass as it is forming. The longer fecal matter remains in the rectum, the more water is absorbed, and the harder and dryer the stool becomes.

The symptoms of a fecal impaction include *discomfort*, the *inability to defecate*, and *liquid stool* that trickles past the impaction. A fecal impaction should be suspected any time a previously constipated person or a person at risk of constipation suddenly begins to pass liquid stools.

Cleansing enemas and suppositories are usually not effective, and the impacted mass must often be removed digitally with a gloved finger, or with an instrument. An oil-retention enema is often given to try to soften the stool and to lubricate it. Then, a well-lubricated, gloved finger is inserted into the rectum, and the mass is manipulated *very slowly and very gently* in an effort to break up the impaction and dislodge the pieces. Once it is partially broken, a second oil-retention enema can be given to soften and lubricate the remaining mass for more comfortable removal. *The procedure is painful,* and it may not be possible to remove the impaction all at one time. Great caution and gentleness must be used throughout the procedure to avoid injury to the rectal mucosa and to minimize embarrassment. The removal of a fecal impaction can be dangerous during pregnancy and after rectal surgery, and should be done only under the direction of a physician.

Diarrhea

Diarrhea can be caused by infection, food poisoning, disease, stress, intolerance to a certain food, and antibiotics or other drugs. Severe diarrhea can be *life-threatening* to infants and debilitated people because fluids and electrolytes are lost. Nursing care of a patient with diarrhea includes assessing the patient and each liquid stool, giving skin care, and increasing fluids, and offering psychological support.

Assessment

Each stool should be examined for evidence of blood, shreds of mucus, pus, worms, or other unusual matter. When feasible, liquid stools should be measured and recorded as fluid output. The patient's abdomen should be palpated to detect areas of tenderness; and he should be asked about pain, cramps, or other discomfort and whether or not he knows or suspects what might have precipitated the diarrhea.

Skin Care

Meticulous skin care is needed to prevent breakdown of the skin, especially of infants, elderly people, debilitated patients who are already susceptible to skin irritation and injury. Toilet paper is often inadequate for thorough cleansing, and a warm, soapy washcloth is frequently needed. The anus and adjacent skin can quickly become irritated and sore, and should be protected with a coating of vaseline, zinc oxide, or other preparations such as those used to treat diaper rash.

Fluid Intake

Fluids should be forced by mouth unless the patient is nauseated and vomiting. If an adequate intake cannot be taken by mouth, fluids must be given parenterally. Parents should be taught that an infant can become dehydrated within a few hours or days, and that *severe or prolonged diarrhea can become a medical emergency*, especially if fluid intake is minimal. Many patients with diarrhea can tolerate a full liquid or a soft, bland diet. If the diarrhea is due to a disease such as dysentery or to the effects of medication, however, a modified diet may be necessary.

Psychological Support

A bout of diarrhea can be extremely disturbing, especially to a patient who must use a bedpan or a commode. Odors that spread throughout the bedside unit, the sounds of an explosive defecation of liquid stool, the spattering or soiling of the bedpan and possibly the bed linens, and the need to have another person empty and clean the bedpan (and possibly the patient's body) all contribute to a difficult situation for both nurse and patient.

The patient usually feels more secure if the bed is protected with both waterproof and absorbent pads, and he may want to keep the bedpan in the bed with him for easy accessibility. A room deodorizer, changes of linens and gowns as needed, and ample opportunity to wash and bathe will help the patient to feel fresh, clean, and socially acceptable.

If the patient must leave his unit for a treatment or test, he should know how to manage himself while away from his room. Sometimes the wheelchair or stretcher must be protected with absorbent pads, and the unit to which the patient is going should be alerted to a possible problem.

Incontinence

A patient is *incontinent* when he is unable to control his bowels or bladder. Defecation is usually easier to control than urination; many patients who are incontinent of feces are comatose or confused. Two top priorities for the care of a patient who is incontinent of feces are (1) protecting his skin, and (2) assessing his capabilities for bowel training.

Protection of Skin

Protection of the skin from feces when the patient is incontinent is important even though the necessary cleansing is usually unpleasant for both patient and nurse. If the patient is alert, he is likely to feel deeply embarrassed, and you will need to communicate considerable empathy and tact each time you clean the patient and his bed. The actual skin care is very similar to the care given to a patient with diarrhea.

Assessment of Capacity for Bowel Training

In addition to keeping the patient's skin clean and dry, it is important for you to study the patient's situation and analyze the conditions under which the patient is incontinent in order to determine the feasibility of bowel training. If, for example, an incontinent patient seems to defecate about one-half hour after lunch each day, it may be possible to offer the bedpan regularly at that time and to help the patient regain a regular pattern of bowel control. Some patients are incontinent because of neurological damage; others, because they are forgetful or unable to reach the call bell. Whatever the reason, it is often possible to combine a strict schedule with a specific stimulus, such as a suppository or hot drink, in order to help a patient regain control of his bowel function. The process of bowel training is complex, lengthy, and often discouraging for both patient and nurse, but the reward is very great—the restoration of a fellow human's sense of dignity and self-esteem.

Distention

Distention is the accumulation of gas (flatus) in the intestinal tract. It can be caused by an increased intake of air, by production of gas, or by a decreased expulsion of gas. Increased intake of air is caused by excessive swallowing of air when a patient is eating or using a drinking straw, by gum chewing, rapid intake of carbonated beverages, or any other condition in which air is repeatedly swallowed. Many foods, such as beans and cabbage, have been implicated as producers of large amounts of gas in susceptible people. Decreased expulsion of gas occurs whenever peristalsis is slowed, as the result of administration of drugs or an anesthetic, for example.

It has been suggested that, of the 7 to 10 L of gas that collects in the intestines each day, about 0.5 L is expelled and the rest is reabsorbed. A larger quantity is expelled when diarrhea or some other condition causes rapid peristalsis. When gas accumulates for any reason, the abdomen becomes distended and sounds hollow or drumlike (tympanites) when percussed. The condition is always uncomfortable and can be exceedingly painful.

Treatment of distention includes as much activity as possible plus the use of a *rectal tube* which stimulates peristalsis and keeps the sphincters open so that the accumulated gas can escape more easily. One end of a soft, rubber rectal tube is lubricated and inserted beyond the internal sphincter. The tube is usually taped to the patient's buttock to help keep it in place. The other end of the tube is placed in a small, waterproof container that is wrapped in absorbent material to catch any fecal matter that might be expelled. For maximal effect, a rectal tube is left in place for about 20 minutes. It is then removed and reinserted a short time later. If it is left in place indefinitely, the bowel adapts to its presence and peristalsis is affected only minimally. The process of insertion and removal is repeated until relief is obtained or until the physician orders another form of treatment.

Patients who can assume a knee-chest position sometimes find that this position makes it easier for the gas to rise toward the anus and be expelled. A heating pad set at the *lowest* temperature may offer some relief if it is not contraindicated by abdominal problems or the age of the patient. In general, almost any measure that *increases peristalsis* will tend to relieve distention.

Hemorrhoids

Hemorrhoids are engorged, distended veins around the anus. Internal hemorrhoids are located in the rectum; external hemorrhoids are visible around the anus. Hemorrhoids are caused by increased venous pressure as a result of portal hypertension, congestive heart failure, pregnancy, and straining during defecation. Hemorrhoids are extremely painful and can be incapacitating at times. Some hemorrhoids bleed easily, and any hard stool may be streaked with blood.

It is usually difficult to insert a thermometer, suppository, or rectal tube when a patient has large or painful hemorrhoids. The rectal area must be exposed in good light so that the nurse can try to separate the bulging, grapelike protrusions of vein and try to find a place through which she can gently insert the thermometer, enema tip, or suppository. Never try to *force* anything past hemorrhoids or try to insert it blindly.

Hemorrhoids are treated during the early stages of their development by preventing or relieving constipation through the regular use of stool softeners, and by the application of heat and astringents to relieve pain and discomfort. Severe hemorrhoids are treated surgically.

Worms

Worms are common in many parts of the world and in some sections of the United States. They are acquired through fecal matter on unwashed hands, by bare feet in contaminated water or soil, and by ingestion of infested, undercooked meat, especially pork. Prevention is based on improved sanitation and medical asepsis. Treatment includes the administration of a drug (an anthelmintic), which is specific for the type of worm involved.

Whipworms (roundworms) and pinworms are not uncommon in children. The worms cause restlessness, irritability, insomnia, anorexia, and sometimes convulsions. These worms are easily transferred from one person to another, and the patient will reinfect himself if his hands are not washed carefully after he uses the toilet. An infected person must not handle food.

Tapeworms cause pain, nausea, diarrhea, and anemia. Many segments of the worm may be passed in the stool, but until the head is passed, the worm will persist. All stool must be examined carefully to determine the effectiveness of treatment and to locate the head, which is about the size of the head of a pin with a long, threadlike neck.

Despite improved drug therapy for the treatment of worms, they continue to be a major health problem in many parts of the world because affected people become weak, debilitated, anemic, and more susceptible to a variety of other diseases.

Ostomies

Cancer and other diseases can create conditions in which fecal matter can no longer be passed through the rectum and an artificial opening must be created in the abdominal wall. This opening is called a *stoma* (ostomy) and may open into either the colon (colostomy) or the ileum (ileostomy).

The location of the stoma determines the consistency of the stool, which in turn determines to a large extent the method of caring for it (Fig. 34.3). Liquid fecal matter becomes more solid as water is absorbed during its passage through the large intestine. The farther the fecal matter passes, the more water is absorbed. Therefore, the location of the ostomy affects the amount of water that is absorbed from the fecal matter.

Stool from an *ileostomy* or a *colostomy in the ascending colon* will be liquid or very soft and will tend to drain at intervals throughout the day. A stoma in this location is kept covered with a plastic pouch or bag, which is attached to the skin with special adhesive. The bag is emptied, washed, and replaced once or twice a day. Meticulous skin care is needed to protect the adjacent skin from irritation and excoriation.

A colostomy in the *transverse colon* can produce a more solid, formed stool. The colostomy is usually ir-

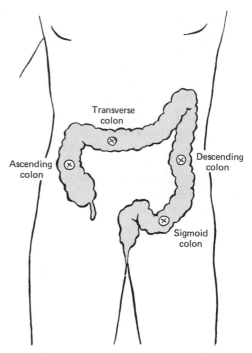

Figure 34.3 *Possible colostomy sites.*

rigated to produce a defecation at a predictable time each day, and the patient may or may not need to wear a bag. A colostomy *low in the descending colon* can produce a solid, formed stool at a scheduled time each day, and some patients are able to manage without a bag and with only an occasional irrigation.

A colostomy irrigation is similar to an enema. A small rectal tube or catheter is used to instill water through the stoma into the colon, and the return fluid is caught in a basin or drained into the toilet. The patient or a family member is taught to irrigate the ostomy before the patient is discharged from the hospital, using the same equipment that will be used at home.

Patient teaching includes information related to skin care, fluid intake, regulation of diet to control consistency of stools, control of odor, indications of electrolyte imbalance, and the establishment of a regular pattern of elimination.

Psychological support is essential as the patient and family try to adjust both to the disease that necessitated the ostomy and to the ostomy itself. The patient's body image is distorted, and both the patient and family may be in crisis for a time. Whenever possible, the patient needs the support of people who have experienced similar surgery. Contact with such people can be arranged through the local chapter of the American Cancer Society. Ostomy Club members can provide both psychological support and practical information about such concerns as new types of equipment, sexual relationships, clothing to conceal an ostomy bag, swimming, and managing an ostomy during a long day at work. Patients who are "loners" or who have never beloned to any kind of club may need encouragement and support to establish relationships with the people who can help them achieve a fairly normal life despite surgery that was initially overwhelming.

Section Two

Urinary Elimination

URINARY FUNCTION

A child's achievement of bladder control is often accompanied by words of praise and sighs of relief from those who are important in his life. This emotional involvement is likely to be much higher in cultures in which urinary control is the result of vigorous toilet training than it is in cultures in which control is achieved gradually as the expected result of normal growth and maturation. Regardless of the process involved, a person prizes his control of urinary elimination, and any subsequent loss of it is humiliating.

Loss of urinary control may be temporary or permanent, complete or partial. Its onset may be sudden or slow in coming, but being "wet" or having an "accident" is one of the most upsetting of all experiences.

Unfortunately, some causes of disturbed urinary function are more socially acceptable than others. For example, a young person who has lost control of his bladder as a result of a spinal cord injury is likely to receive understanding, support, and encouragement from the staff as he undergoes a bladder retraining program, whereas an elderly person who dribbles urine is often scolded, ignored, or diapered by his caretakers.

Age, disease, medication, fluid balance, infection, and stress can all affect urinary function, and the relative significance of each in a given patient situation can be determined only by careful nursing and medical assessments.

ASSESSMENTS

Urinary function is assessed on the basis of data obtained from the patient's history, examination of the abdomen, assessment of urine, and diagnostic tests.

Patient History

To obtain and *communicate* information related to a patient's urinary function, it is necessary to understand both the vocabulary of the patient and professional terminology. For example, when a small child is admitted to the hospital, it is important to ask his parents what words he uses to indicate a need to urinate. On the other hand, the nurse's ability to communicate effectively with professional colleagues involves an understanding of the appropriate *medical* terminology.

Examination of the Abdomen

When the patient has little or no urinary output, physical examination of the abdomen is important in dif-

Terms Used to Describe Urinary Function

- Anuria: Urinary output less than 100 ml in 24 hours; may be caused by kidney failure or by an obstruction in the urinary tract.
- Dysuria: Difficulty in urinating that may or may not be painful.
- Frequency: The need to void frequently, usually in small amounts. The symptoms of frequency and urgency often occur together as a result of irritation of the lower urinary tract.
- Hesitancy: Difficulty in starting the stream of urine; the flow may start and stop one or more times before the bladder is empty.
- Incontinence: Unintentional loss of urine.
- Micturition: Urination.
- Nocturia: Need to urinate more than once per night which wakens the person from a sound sleep (this is not the same as urination during the night by a person who is awake for some other reason).
- Oliguria: Small daily output of urine; may be caused by dehydration resulting from decreased fluid intake, fever, or disease.
- Polyuria: Unusually large output of urine; may be caused by an increased fluid intake, a diuretic medication, a diuretic drink such as beer, or disease such as diabetes.
- Residual urine: Urine remaining in the bladder after urination.
- Retention: The accumulation of urine in the bladder because of the bladder's inability to empty itself; may be caused by neurological dysfunction or by an obstruction.
- Retention with overflow: The passage of small amounts of urine from a full bladder which cannot empty itself.
- Suppression: The inability of the kidneys to secrete urine; may be life threatening.
- Urgency: A sudden, uncontrollable urge to urinate.
- Voiding or micturition: Urination.

ferentiating between *retention* and *suppression* of urine. If the patient's bladder is found to be distended, his kidneys are producing urine but he is unable to empty his bladder. If his bladder is not distended, his kidneys are producing very little urine.

When the bladder is *full,* physical examination of the area just above the symphysis pubis yields the following objective findings:

Inspection: the lower abdomen appears swollen.

Palpation: the area is tense and highly sensitive to touch.

Percussion: suprapubic *dullness,* not tympany, is heard.

Assessment of Urine

Data needed by the nurse as a basis for subsequent nursing action can be obtained by assessing the color, amount, specific gravity, and pH of the patient's urine.

Color

Urine is normally straw colored. Any deviation from a normal straw color should be recorded and its cause determined. You should take the initiative to measure the intake and output of any patient whose urine is either dark or pale. If urine is a very pale color it is usually dilute and if it is produced in large quantities, the specific gravity should be checked. Dark urine is often concentrated, and the patient's fluid intake should be increased without delay unless the dark color is known to be caused by a certain food or drug. Blood in the urine (hematuria) often produces red urine; the bile from obstructive jaundice turns the urine orange or a dark mahogany color.

Amount

The normal urinary output of an adult ranges from 1,000 to 1,500 ml/day. If a patient's urinary output is low and does not respond to an increased fluid intake, the physician should be notified at once. An output below 500 ml/day indicates an impairment of kidney function that could be life threatening.

Specific Gravity

Specific gravity is one indicator of the patient's state of hydration; it indicates the concentration of dissolved substances in the urine. The specific gravity of water is 1.000, and the normal range for urine is 1.010 to 1.025. Urine with a specific gravity below 1.010 is dilute; it may either reflect a high fluid intake or indicate that the kidneys are unable to concentrate the urine adequately. A specific gravity over 1.025 is concentrated and indicates inadequate hydration.

Specific gravity is measured with a urinometer, which consists of a small glass cylinder and a weighted glass float. A concentrated fluid has a high specific gravity and causes the float to rise; a dilute fluid allows it to sink. The urinometer is calibrated so that the level of the fluid is read as the specific gravity of the fluid.

pH

Urine is normally slightly acidic with a pH of 6.0. Urine varies throughout the day and is slightly more alkaline after a person has had a meal. Large amounts of meat and certain acidifying drugs cause the urine to be more acidic; a vegetarian diet causes it to be more alkaline. The growth of bacteria within the urinary tract is affected by the acidity of the urine, which the physician can alter by modifying the patient's diet.

Other Facts to Be Assessed

Urine is normally clear, and any *turbidity* (cloudiness) should be reported at once. Urine should contain no red or white blood cells, and no more than a trace of protein or glucose. Turbidity may indicate the presence of abnormal amounts of these substances or of pus or mucus.

The odor of fresh urine is distinctive and aromatic. An odor of ammonia is produced when urine is allowed to stand. This is caused by a breakdown of urea as the urine decomposes.

Diagnostic Tests of Kidney Function

The tests that are done most frequently are: routine urinalysis, 24-hour tests, culture and sensitivity, sugar and acetone, x-ray examinations, and the blood urea nitrogen (BUN) test.

Routine Urinalysis

The urine sample that is taken to the physician's office or submitted upon patient admission to the hospital is examined routinely and its color, specific gravity, pH, glucose, protein, red and white blood cells noted. This urinalysis is done at intervals throughout a patient's hospitalization; any abnormal findings indicate the need for further testing.

24-Hour Urine

All urine secreted in a 24-hour period is sometimes collected and analyzed to determine the total amount of a drug, dye, electrolyte, or other substance removed from the body by the kidneys in a 24-hour period. Such data contribute to the assessment of kidney function and subsequent diagnoses.

Composition of Urine

Color: amber
pH: slightly acidic (about 6.0)
Specific gravity: 1.003–1.035
Sugar: none
Acetone: none
White blood cells: none
Red blood cells: none
Protein: 10–100 mg/24 hours
Ketones: none
Urea: 20–40 gm/24 hours
Epithelial cells or casts: occasional

Sugar and Acetone

Glycosuria (glucose in the urine) occurs whenever the blood sugar is elevated above the kidney threshold. Acetone is found in the urine as a waste product of fat metabolism when available carbohydrates have been depleted during conditions such as dieting, dehydration, starvation, and diabetic acidosis.

The presence of sugar and acetone in the urine is detected by the use of reagents that produce a chemical reaction with the sugar or acetone in the urine. The chemical reaction is indicated by a color change on a tablet, paper tape, coated plastic strip, or dipstick, all of which have been impregnated with the chemical reagent. The intensity of the color change indicates the amount of sugar or acetone in the urine and is determined by comparing the color produced with a color chart supplied by the manufacturer of the testing materials. The reagent must be fresh and should not be used after the stated expiration date. Complete directions for use are supplied with each package of reagent and should be followed exactly.

These tests are used both in home and hospital to monitor a patient's progress and responses to therapy. The tests for glucose are used in mass screening programs for the detection of diabetes.

Occult Blood

Reagent tablets and strips containing orthotoluidine are used to determine the presence of occult (hidden) blood and hemoglobin in the urine.

Culture and Sensitivity

Urine is cultured to establish the presence of any microorganisms and to provide an accurate identification of the type and strain. Once the causative organism has been identified, it is then tested for sensitivity by being subjected to several antibiotics to determine which one is likely to be most effective in treating the infection.

Blood Urea Nitrogen

The blood urea nitrogen (BUN) test assesses kidney function by measuring the level of urea in the blood. Urea is normally excreted by the kidney but urea accumulates in the blood when renal blood flow and urine production are decreased. Blood urea nitrogen varies with diet, activity, and illness; a normal range is 10 to 20 mg/100 ml blood. An increase in the BUN can indicate impairment of kidney function. A patient with an elevated BUN may show signs of confusion and impaired memory, which can eventually be followed by unconsciousness and death.

X-Ray Examinations

Kidney function can be assessed by means of an intravenous pyelogram or a retrograde pyelogram in conjunction with a cystoscopic examination (Chapter 17, section 6).

Collection of Specimens

Whereas specimens of blood, gastric contents, spinal fluid, and other body fluids are usually collected by the physician or a laboratory technician, most urine samples are collected by the nursing staff. The accuracy of each test is affected by the techniques of collection, which must be precise and without error to ensure reliable results. Errors in the collection of urine specimens include improper labeling, contamination of a specimen that is to be cultured, and failure to note on the laboratory slip that the specimen might contain foreign matter from menstrual flow or vaginal discharge.

Random Sample

A *random specimen* is a single sample of urine that is collected in a clean container at any time without advance preparation. A urine sample for routine urinalysis is a random sample.

Fractional Sample

The term *fractional specimen*, as opposed to a 24-hour specimen, is applied to a urine sample that is obtained at a specified hour to be tested for glucose or ketone bodies (sugar and acetone). The specimens are collected regularly from one to four times daily and are referred to as *fractional urines* or by an older term, *partition urines*. Some patients are able to assume responsibility for obtaining the specimens just as they may have done at home; others are unable to do so, and collecting must be done by the nurse.

Double-Voided Specimen

The glucose level in the urine is often used to determine the next dose of insulin and must therefore reflect the *current* composition of urine, not the composition of urine which has accumulated in the bladder over a number of hours. Therefore, a *double-voided specimen* is commonly used. The patient is asked to empty his bladder about a half hour before the test is scheduled. He is allowed to drink water if he desires before the test specimen is collected, but this is not usually necessary because the kidneys normally produce at least 30 to 50 ml of urine per hour, and only 6 to 10 ml is needed for the test. The urine collected during the second voiding is a specimen of urine produced within the most recent half hour, and therefore indicates the *current* glucose level in the urine.

24-Hour Specimen

Collection of a 24-hour specimen usually begins at about 6 or 7 am, at which time the patient is asked to empty his bladder. This urine is discarded, the time is noted, and all urine produced during the next 24 hours is saved in one or more large containers. The urine should be refrigerated, or else a preservative should be added to it.

Every effort should be made to ensure that no urine is accidentally discarded or contaminated. All who might handle the urine (patient, family, and all staff) should know how to collect the urine and where to put it. The container should be clearly labeled, and signs should be posted near the toilet and in the utility room to indicate that a 24-hour urine collection is in progress. The patient must not contaminate the urine with feces, so the urine must be emptied before the bedpan is used for the bowel movement. Toilet paper should be kept out of the urine.

The patient should know the exact time the collection will end so that he can void as close to that time as possible. It does not matter if the latest voiding is 15 to 20 minutes before or after the hour as long as the *exact* time of voiding is recorded on the laboratory forms. The test results can be calculated precisely if the exact length of collection is known.

Clean-catch, or Midstream Specimen

Until recently, all urine for culture and sensitivity testing was collected by catheterization, but the risk of nosocomial infection from catheterization has increased so rapidly that specimens are rarely obtained by that method today. Research shows that a satisfactory specimen for culture and sensitivity tests can be obtained without catheterization if the genital area is cleansed thoroughly and if the first part of the specimen is discarded.

The equipment for a clean-catch specimen consists of a sterile collection container and materials for cleansing the area. The choice of a cleansing agent depends upon agency procedure and any possible allergies of the patient. Some people are allergic to iodine and therefore can not tolerate iodine-based preparations such as povidone (Betadine).

The male patient can be prepared for a clean-catch specimen without difficulty. To clean the urinary meatus, the patient or nurse grasps the shaft of the penis gently but firmly, retracts the foreskin if the patient has not been circumcised, and cleanses the head of the penis. The area is cleansed outward from the urinary meatus in concentric circles. With the foreskin still retracted, the patient starts to urinate into the toilet or urinal and then slips a sterile container under the stream. The initial voiding tends to flush out the urethra, and the subsequent urine is therefore uncontaminated with cells or secretions. The foreskin is replaced; the sterile container is carefully covered, labeled, and sent to the laboratory.

The process of collecting a clean-catch specimen from a female patient is somewhat more difficult. The labia minora must be separated and *kept separated* while the urinary meatus is cleansed with an antiseptic solution and while the specimen is being collected. Some patients are able to start to urinate into the toilet and then slip a sterile container under the stream; other patients find it easier to straddle two sterile containers on a low chair or stool, move the stream of urine from one container to the other, and then discard the first specimen. A patient who is confined to bed must start to urinate into the bedpan and then urinate into a sterile container, which usually must be held by the nurse. Contamination of the sterile specimen with menstrual blood or other discharge will render the specimen useless, and it is sometimes necessary to insert a tampon to protect the specimen from vaginal secretions.

Catheterized Specimen

Since the widespread acceptance of clean-catch specimens, a patient is seldom catheterized solely to obtain a urine specimen, except in an emergency. Most indwelling (retention) catheter systems have a specimen port or opening through which sterile urine samples can be obtained.

PROMOTION OF URINARY FUNCTION

Nursing Measures to Promote Normal Function

Sometimes a person with previously normal urinary function is unable to void despite having a full bladder. A patient may be unable to void after surgery because of the effects of anesthesia and physiological responses to the stress of surgery. Difficulty in voiding is compounded by the patient's discomfort and apprehensiveness.

If a bladder is allowed to fill beyond its normal capacity, the stretch receptors in the bladder wall become unresponsive, and the bladder becomes increasingly less able to empty itself. The patient begins to experience pain and discomfort; he becomes increasingly tense and less able to relax enough to urinate. Straining in an effort to urinate is not helpful because it tends to make more tense the already tight sphincters.

A patient's inability to void tends to invoke anxiety among the nursing staff, and as a result there is often considerable subtle (and not so subtle) pressure on the

patient through statements such as: "Have you gone yet?" "Do you want to try the urinal again?" "If you don't urinate by 6 PM, you'll have to be catheterized." The situation poses a very real quandary because it is dangerous to let the patient's bladder continue to fill, and yet catheterization subjects him to the risks of infection. Fortunately, there are a number of measures that have a high probability of success in helping the patient void.

Measures to Induce Voiding

First of all, a normal or nearly normal position is essential. Many patients are unable to urinate lying down and may be unable to do so even with the head of the bed raised. A male patient should be helped to stand to urinate even though he may need the support of several people to do so, unless this is contraindicated. If a female patient can stand and take a few steps, she can be helped out of bed and onto a bedside commode. If she cannot, it is often helpful to position her in a sitting position on the bedpan with her legs over the side of the bed and her feet resting on the floor or, if the bed cannot be lowered, supported on a chair or foot stool. If the patient is weak, she should not be left alone on the bedpan in this position. The nurse may need to obtain a physician's order in some situations to get the patient into a normal position, but the success that often follows justifies the time and energy expended.

In addition to being in a proper position, the patient needs to have as much privacy as possible, to be warm enough, and to be helped to relax. The patient should be encouraged to heed any sensation that has signaled a need to urinate in the past. Some people feel restless or notice a tingling or chilly sensation, for example. Such feelings are often referred to as a stimulus, or "call," and should not be ignored if it is important that the bladder be emptied.

The power of suggestion can be very strong, and in some instances it will help the patient to void. The sound and sensation of running water, for example, will often enable a patient to urinate. This can be accomplished by such measures as turning on a nearby water faucet, bringing a small basin filled with water for the patient to dabble his fingers in, or pouring a measured amount of warm water over the perineum. Some people find that the relaxation of a warm tub bath or shower bath creates a desire to void. If so, they should be taught to obey the urge and urinate at once, no matter how embarrassing or strange it may seem. Urine is sterile so it can't contaminate the bath water, and at that moment ability to empty the bladder without catheterization has top priority, even though under the circumstances it will be impossible to measure the amount voided.

It is important to take into account normal patterns of elimination when caring for a patient who seems to be unable to void. One patient, for example, was being watched closely after the surgical repair of a hernia. According to the staff, his "time would be up" at 2 pm. Fortunately, someone discovered from talking with the patient that he normally voided upon waking, again in the late afternoon, and at bedtime. Given this information, the staff waited, the patient voided spontaneously at his usual time, and catheterization was avoided.

Any suggestions made by the patient regarding measures that might help him void should be followed, if possible, whether it be a request to walk around a bit or for a diuretic drink ("just a few sips of beer"). Mild heat and gentle soothing massage or pressure just above the symphysis pubis may help, and diversions such as listening to music or reading coupled with a suggestion to relax and not try so hard may make it possible for the patient to urinate. Wrapping a warm, moist towel around his genitalia may help a male patient to void.

If nursing measures are unsuccessful, the physician may order a cholinergic drug. If all else fails, the patient must be catheterized.

Catheterization

Catheterization is the insertion of either a single-use catheter or a retention catheter into the patient's bladder through the urethra. A single-use catheter is left in place long enough to drain the bladder (about 5 minutes) and is then withdrawn. The procedure is repeated if indicated, and is termed intermittent catheterization. An indwelling or retention catheter is left in place. It is removed and replaced by a new one at regular intervals as specified by patient need or agency policy.

Purposes

Intermittent catheterization is done to empty a distended bladder, to check for the presence of residual urine after the patient has voided, or to obtain a sterile urine specimen when a clean-catch specimen cannot be obtained. An indwelling catheter is inserted to keep certain incontinent patients dry, to facilitate continual bladder drainage after injury to, or surgery on, the urinary tract; to splint the urethra or adjacent tissue to promote healing after urological surgery; and to permit accurate measurement of urinary output.

Hazards

Catheterization can be an important and necessary aspect of many diagnostic and therapeutic measures, but it is not without risk. Nearly half of all hospital-acquired infections originate in the urinary tract—almost as many as most other sites combined. The urinary tract is normally sterile, and it becomes infected quickly and easily whenever pathogens are introduced via the meatus. The lining of the urinary tract is continuous from the meatus and urethra through the bladder to the ureters and kidneys; the upward course of an infection is termed an *ascending infection*.

A urinary tract infection can cause the patient a longer hospitalization and increased medical expenses, absence from work, disrupted home life, pain, discomfort, and occasionally a life-threatening extension of the infection. Other hazards of catheterization include urethral irritation and damage to the bladder wall from the tip of the catheter.

Intermittent Catheterization

EQUIPMENT. Except for the catheter itself, all the equipment needed to catheterize a patient is usually found in a commercially prepared catheterization kit or on a catheterization tray which has been assembled and sterilized by the central supply department of the hospital. The catheter is selected on the basis of the patient's size and is added to the tray. The French system for indicating the size of a catheter is used, and catheters are sized by gauge. The larger the gauge number, the larger the catheter. Commonly used sizes are: 8 or 10 F for children, 14 to 16 F for adult women, and 16 to 20 F for adult men.

The catheterization tray or kit usually contains a sterile drape, a basin, a urine specimen container, and materials for cleaning the meatus. A package of sterile gloves is added by the nurse who will be wearing them. Additional nonsterile supplies include a newspaper or paper bag for waste, a disposable pad to protect the bed, a movable or adjustable light, and a bath blanket or extra sheet for draping.

GUIDELINES FOR CATHETERIZATION. Each school of nursing and hospital has its own prescribed catheterization procedure. The procedure that follows is merely a general overview or introduction to more specific guidelines and policies from other sources.

1. Check the physician's order and determine the purpose of the catheterization. Find out whether or not a urine sample should be taken for laboratory analysis.

2. Review the procedure and assemble the needed equipment.

3. Explain the procedure to the patient. If you will need assistance or supervision, tell the patient that a third person will be present and why this is necessary.

4. Ensure maximum privacy. Attach a sign to the door or bedside curtain as needed.

5. Position and drape the patient to permit full exposure of the urethral meatus.

   a. Position a male patient on his back with his legs extended. Cover his trunk with a patient gown of ample size, bath blanket, or extra sheet. Fold the top bedding down to his upper thighs to expose the penis, then cover it with a towel until you are ready to catheterize him.

   b. Position a female patient on her back with her knees flexed and wide apart. If she is unable to maintain this position, position her on her side in the Sims position, with the upper hip flexed sharply enough to expose the perineum and labia majora. Arrange the top sheet, gown, and extra sheet or bath blanket in such a way that the patient is completely covered.

6. Adjust the available light and obtain an extra lamp if needed. Move the patient, bed, or light until the genital area is well lighted. Unless you can see the meatus clearly, it is not possible to keep a catheter sterile during insertion. To attempt to do a catheterization in dim light is to deliberately subject the patient to the risk of infection from a contaminated catheter.

7. If your patient is female, separate the labia minora and locate the urinary meatus (Fig. 34.4). It may be difficult to identify if the perineum is swollen after childbirth or if there is any anatomical deviation. If the meatus is not visible, press a sterile gauze or cotton ball against the perineum over the vagina and gently pull downward. This movement is likely to reveal the meatus as a dimple above the vagina. If you cannot identify the meatus, do not try to catheterize the patient. Do not try to locate the meatus by poking and prodding with a catheter that has been contaminated by contact with the patient's perineal area. Make the patient comfortable and seek assistance from an experienced person.

8. Cleanse the area systematically.

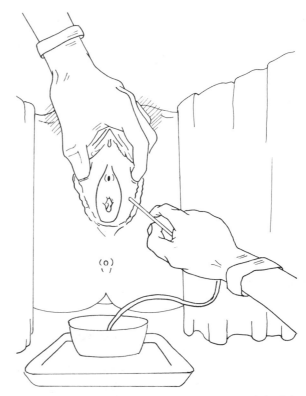

Figure 34.4 *Female catheterization. Separation of the labial folds is necessary to ensure adequate visualization of the urinary meatus.*

   a. If your patient is male, grasp the shaft of the penis, gently retract the foreskin if he has not been circumcised, and cleanse the head of the penis, working out from the meatus in concentric circles.

   b. If your patient is female, separate the labia with one hand and cleanse from front to back with the other one. Wipe down the center over the meatus, then down either side, using each cotton ball or sponge only once. If there is evidence of a vaginal discharge or menstrual flow, use a soapy wash cloth before cleansing with cotton balls. Keep the labia separated until you have inserted the catheter.

9. Lubricate the tip of the catheter and insert it into the urethra.

   a. For a male, hold the shaft of the penis at a right angle to the patient's body to straighten out the urethra (Fig. 34.5) and insert the catheter about 6 to 10 inches, until the urine starts to flow. If you feel a resistance against the catheter during insertion, twist it gently and ask the patient to push down a little as

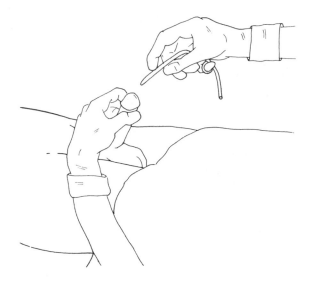

Figure 34.5 _Position of the male penis for catheterization._

if he were urinating. This will overcome any slight spasm of the urethra. If resistance continues, withdraw the catheter and seek qualified assistance. _Never use force_ to try to insert a catheter. To do so can be very painful and dangerous to the patient, because resistance may be caused by an enlarged prostate gland, a tumor, or some other unyielding obstruction.

b. For a female, keep the labia minora separated to avoid contaminating the catheter, and insert the catheter until the urine starts to flow, about 2 to 2½ in. If no urine flows and the patient is uncomfortable or in pain, move the catheter back or twist it a little

because it may have hit an obstruction or a fold of tissue.

If no urine flows following movement of the catheter, remove it and seek qualified assistance. If _no_ urine flows and the patient is _not_ uncomfortable, the catheter may be in the vagina. Withdraw the catheter and discard it. Locate the meatus and insert another sterile catheter. Some nurses routinely take a second catheter to the bedside for a female catheterization for use in the event the catheter becomes contaminated or is inserted into the vagina.

10. Collect urine in the sterile specimen container if a urine sample is needed, then collect the remainder in the sterile basin. Withdraw the catheter slowly to avoid friction and irritation. Leave the patient comfortable and the unit neat and clean. Tell the patient his urethra might be slightly edematous (swollen) after being catheterized, that he might find it a little difficult to urinate, and that for a few hours he may have a persistent feeling of wanting to void.

Indwelling Catheterization

An indwelling or retention catheter is often called a Foley catheter (a trade name), and it is inserted the same way as a single-use catheter. A retention catheter is kept in place by a balloon that is inflated _after_ the catheter has been placed in the bladder (Fig. 34.6).

Indwelling catheters are composed of either two or three tubes or compartments and are referred to as two or three _lumen_ catheters. One lumen carries urine from the bladder to the collection bag; another lumen carries water to and from the balloon when it is inflated or

---

PROCEDURE 34.4

Catheterizing a Patient*

SUMMARY OF ESSENTIAL NURSING ACTIONS

1. Determine whether or not you will need help to support or keep the patient in an effective position.
2. Arrange lights so that visibility is excellent.
3. Maintain surgical asepsis throughout the procedure.
   • Bring an extra catheter to the bedside if there is a possibility you might contaminate the first one.
4. Position and drape the patient.
5. Set up a sterile field and prepare your supplies.

6. Expose, cleanse, and assess the patient's perineal area. Locate the urinary meatus.
7. Lubricate the tip of the catheter, and insert it gently until the urine starts to flow—about 2 to 2½ inches for an adult female, and 6 to 8 inches for a male.
8. If an indwelling catheter is inserted, inflate the balloon in accordance with the manufacturer's directions.
9. Collect and label a specimen of urine as indicated.
10. Measure and record the amount of urine obtained.

*See inside front cover and pages 690–692.

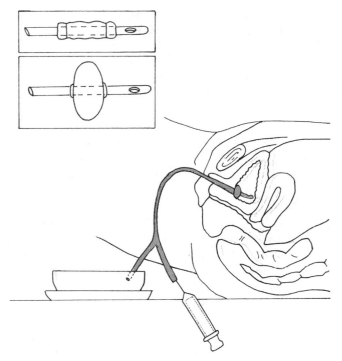

Figure 34.6 *Foley catheter in position with the balloon inflated. Insert shows the balloon before and after inflation.*

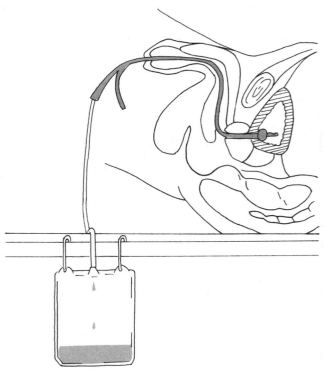

Figure 34.7 *Foley catheter in place and attached to a urinary drainage bag.*

deflated; and the third one is designed to carry medicine or an irrigating solution into the bladder.

The capacity of the balloon is marked on the catheter and on the package and is usually from 5 to 30 ml. The choice of balloon size is determined by the size of the urethra and sometimes by the activity of the patient. If an inflatable 5 ml balloon slips out of the bladder and down the urethra, a 10 ml balloon will be needed. If the patient is restless and tends to pull out a 5 or 10 ml balloon, a larger one is often tried, though damage to the urethra will be greater if he pulls out the larger one. It is sometimes necessary to restrain the patient's hands if he persists in pulling out an absolutely vital catheter. (See Chapter 26 for a discussion of the legal aspects of using restraints.)

An indwelling catheter is connected to a closed drainage system consisting of tubing and a plastic collection bag, which can be fastened to the frame of the patient's bed or wheelchair (Fig. 34.7). This drainage setup is referred to as *closed drainage* to differentiate it from earlier setups in which a length of tubing drained into an open glass container. A closed system minimizes contamination of the interior of the catheter, tubing, and collection bag and decreases the possibility of a nosocomial urinary tract infection.

INSERTION AND ATTACHMENT In addition to the equipment needed for inserting a single-use catheter, you

will need a syringe, needle, and fluid to inflate the balloon. The fluid, usually water or normal saline, must be *sterile* in order to protect the patient from infection should the balloon rupture or leak while in the bladder.

When the catheter has been inserted and you are certain that it is draining properly, inflate the balloon according to the manufacturer's directions. Gently pull on the catheter to see if the balloon is inflated enough to hold it in place. The catheter is then attached to the drainage system and taped in place.

The catheter of a female patient is taped to the inner aspect of her thigh with enough slack to prevent any pull by the balloon against the neck of the bladder when the patient moves about. The catheter of a male patient is taped to his abdomen to help to keep the penis extended and to help prevent pressure from the catheter on the penoscrotal angle (the angle formed between the penis and scrotum). This can be especially important for patients with paralysis and diminished sensation, such as quadriplegics and paraplegics.

PREVENTION OF INFECTION. Policies related to the use of indwelling catheters are determined by committees composed of people representing nursing, medicine, hospital administration, infection control, and the purchasing department in an effort to use the best equipment and the most effective techniques possible. Spe-

---

Guidelines for Preventing Urinary Tract Infections

WASH YOUR HANDS before you touch any part of the urinary drainage system. *Handwashing has proved to be the most significant of all efforts to reduce the incidence of infection.*

Cleanse the urinary meatus and the adjacent portion of the catheter with soap and water at least twice a day. Pull the catheter out slightly (about ½ inch), remove any crusts of mucoid discharge, and cleanse with an antiseptic solution if ordered. Apply an antibacterial cream to the meatus if ordered.

Prevent contamination of the drainage system. Read the manufacturer's directions and use the proper technique for draining the collection bag, obtaining urine specimens, and irrigating the bladder. Do not open the system unnecessarily. If the system must be opened (separated or disconnected), wipe all connections with alcohol before reattaching them, even though you have done everything possible to keep them sterile.

Prevent the backflow of urine. Keep the urine collection bag *lower than the patient's bladder* at all times to keep urine draining *away* from the bladder and to keep stagnant and possibly contaminated urine from flowing back to the bladder. Do not let urine collect in a sagging loop of tubing. Use appropriate holders and supports for the drainage bag when transporting the patient; do not place the bag on the abdomen of a patient on a stretcher.

---

cific measures taken to protect the patient will vary from institution to institution. The boxed guidelines which are listed above are basic to nearly all protocols and procedures.

MAINTAINING PATENCY. Until recently, it was considered necessary to irrigate an indwelling catheter at regular intervals to keep it patent and the urine flowing freely. Guidelines based on research studies now advocate minimal irrigation, only when necessary.

The terms *internal* and *external irrigation* refer to different ways of flushing out the drainage system. Proponents of an *internal* approach advocate a fluid intake of 2,000 to 3,000 ml/day, on the basis that a large volume of dilute urine is likely to keep the catheter and tubing from becoming plugged. If, however, a patient's urine is cloudy or bloody, or contains mucus, pus, or other sediment, it may be necessary to irrigate the catheter. The physician's order will designate the type and amount of irrigating fluid to be used.

The catheter and tubing should be changed only when it has been contaminated, when it is not draining well, or when it has developed an odor. The catheter and tubing should not be changed on the basis of time alone, because each interference with the system increases the risk of infection.

PROMOTING COMFORT. Both physical and psychological comfort are important aspects of the care of a patient with a long-term indwelling catheter. The patient and his family must be taught how to care for the catheter, both at home and when visiting or traveling. They should know that the physician should be notified if the patient experiences bladder pain or an elevated temperature, or if the urine becomes cloudy, bloody, scant, or foul smelling.

A normal sex life is possible with sensitive encouragement and planning. The nurse must often bring up the subject, either on the basis of cues from the patient or partner, or on the basis of experience with similar patient situations. A male patient is usually taught to remove his catheter for sexual intercourse and then replace it. A female patient is taught to push the tubing aside or tape it out of the way. Some patients who have been reluctant or unwilling to learn how to care for their catheters have been motivated to do so when satisfying sexual relationships seemed possible.

Self-catheterization

Many patients with permanent or long-term indwelling catheters have been taught to assume responsibility for their own catheters and to change them as needed, using sterile technique. Such people are *independent* with respect to their ability to take care of the catheter, but they are *dependent on the catheter* for leading a normal, active life.

This situation began to change when Jack Lapides, a urologist, discovered in the 1970's that people who were unable to void effectively could give up their indwelling catheters if they catheterized themselves at intervals throughout the day. His research showed that the key to an infection-free bladder is the *frequency* of catheterization, not necessarily the sterility of the technique.

He found that pressure on the walls of an overdistended bladder slows the circulation of blood through the walls of the bladder, and that this decrease in blood supply makes the bladder more susceptible to infection. Lapides discovered that frequent withdrawal of urine from the bladder (every 4 to 6 hours), whether by sterile or clean technique, decreases the susceptibility of the urinary tract to infection.

This technique is gaining wide acceptance by all age groups in a wide variety of nonhospital settings. Infection is not a problem with clean catheterization because, in general, the patient is in an environment free of most pathogenic organisms. Most of the bacteria of a normal household are nonpathogenic, and members of the family have developed resistance against most pathogenic organisms that might possibly be present.

Self-catheterization, also called clean catheterization, can be learned by almost anyone, including children after the age of about 6 years. The only requirement for the procedure is access to a bathroom. The patient carries a clean catheter in a clean plastic bag. He washes his hands, inserts the catheter, lets the urine drain into the toilet, washes the catheter, and replaces it in the clean plastic bag.

A male patient is able to locate his external urinary meatus without difficulty. A female patient is taught to use a mirror at first but is expected to learn to catheterize herself without it as soon as possible. She should not become dependent on a mirror because one might not always be available.

The advantages of clean catheterization include greater mobility and freedom at home, work, and school. Social life can be more relaxed and extensive, and a more normal sex life is possible without the presence of an indwelling catheter.

Clean catheterization is an important educational issue because large numbers of handicapped children are now attending public school. Many children who need to be catheterized are able to catheterize themselves, but a few are unable to do so because of spasticity, tremors, limited joint motion, or other problems. Legislation has been proposed that would require a school district to provide assistance for children who are unable to catheterize themselves.

DISTURBANCES OF URINARY FUNCTION

Three common disturbances of urinary function are retention, incontinence, and cystitis. Other conditions are described in detail in medical-surgical nursing texts.

Urinary Retention

Urinary retention is often the result of anesthesia, trauma, or an obstruction of the urethra, such as an enlarged prostate. Retention is characterized by an inability to void accompanied by sensations of pressure, discomfort, and tenderness over the bladder, which is palpable above the symphysis pubis. The discomfort of retention ranges from a sensation of pressure to extreme pain. Sensations of pressure and discomfort may result from a bladder that is slowly filling after anesthesia, while excruciating pain results from a badly distended bladder which may contain as much as 3,000 ml of urine or more.

When retention is suspected, it is important to note the last time the bladder was emptied, the amount of fluid intake since that time, the patient's normal pattern or schedule of voiding, and the height of the bladder. The latter is assessed by palpating the abdomen.

If nursing measures to promote normal voiding are not successful, the patient must be catheterized. The urine must be removed *slowly*, and as a rule, no more than 750 to 1,000 ml is removed at one time from a badly distended bladder. A complete or too rapid removal of urine could decompress the bladder faster than the blood flow through the walls of the bladder can be normalized, and the patient may experience chills, fever, light-headedness, and possibly shock.

Retention with overflow should be suspected whenever the patient's fluid intake is adequate, but he is passing only *small* amounts of normal urine. The fact that he is passing urine could be misleading if paralysis and diminished sensation, coma, or mental confusion prevents the patient from feeling the discomfort and pain of a full bladder.

Incontinence

Incontinence is the involuntary loss of urine after control had been achieved in childhood. Incontinence can involve a complete emptying of the bladder which soaks the patient's clothes or bedding, or it can involve a slow but rather constant dribbling of urine.

The causes of incontinence can be divided into those which result from changes in the structure or function of the urinary system, and those that are not directly related to urinary function. Causes of incontinence which are directly related to urinary function include infection, disease, local irritation, use of diuretics, and increased fluid intake.

Indirect causes of incontinence include:

Inability to reach the call bell or signal the nurse
Inability to walk to the bathroom (including being prevented by side rails raised on the bed)
Inability to reach the bedpan or urinal
Mental confusion
Unconsciousness

There are two additional types of incontinence: stress incontinence and urge incontinence. *Stress incontinence* occurs whenever the patient's intra-abdominal pressure is increased by laughing, vomiting, coughing, sneezing, or lifting. It is more common in women than men, probably because of their shorter urethras and because the musculature of the pelvic floor may have been weakened by numerous pregnancies or difficult labor.

Urge incontinence differs from stress incontinence in that the patient suddenly experiences an urge to urinate without any predisposing activity or stress. The patient is frequently unable to hold the urine until he can reach the bathroom and get his clothing out of the way. The cause of urge incontinence is usually related to neurological dysfunction.

Management of Incontinence

For many patients, families, and staff, incontinence is the worst of all possible conditions. Pain, dyspnea, and even dying can be borne with dignity, but the inability to control one's own excreta is seen as the ultimate humiliation. Great sensitivity and understanding are needed, therefore, by all who care for such a patient.

The first step in helping an incontinent patient is to determine the underlying cause. If incontinence has causes other than urinary dysfunction, it can sometimes be relieved rather quickly. If the cause of incontinence is related to urinary dysfunction, relief may be slower, but it can usually be accomplished. Whatever the cause, *incontinence must not be accepted as inevitable.*

Studies have found that *hope* and a *positive attitude* are major elements in the alleviation of incontinence. Adherence to a routine for urination, attention to fluid intake, encouragement, the wearing of street clothes, careful grooming, optimism, and patience have enabled many people to maintain or regain their self-esteem and their desired life-style. Diapers should *not* be used on a conscious patient, although disposable pads, pantie liners, and other protective devices designed for adults are useful when *requested* or *desired* by the patient. Such external protection is helpful when a person is traveling and when he is trying to maintain a normal social life.

CONDOM DRAINAGE. A male patient can be protected from dribbling urine by the use of a soft, flexible condom that fits over his penis and is attached by tubing to a small leg bag. The equipment is inexpensive and relatively easy to care for. The condom, tubing, and bag are washed once or twice daily and should be soaked in a weak vinegar solution periodically to control odors. Because the capacity of the leg bag is limited, the patient usually switches to a larger drainage bag beside the bed at night. The major problem associated with condom drainage is the need to protect the skin of the penis from excoriation or maceration due to long and continued contact with rubber and moisture.

PROTECTIVE MEASURES FOR FEMALE PATIENTS. There is no device comparable to condom drainage for women, and an acceptable solution to the problem of incontinence will depend on the ingenuity of patient and nurse, the wishes of the patient, and her financial resources or laundry services. A sanitary napkin and a waterproof shield offer enough protection for some women while others may need an adjustable panty with absorbency equal to that of a disposable diaper. Disposable protection is expensive for long-term use, and many women purchase or prepare a waterproof protector which holds a reusable washable liner.

Many patients are embarrassed to tell their family or the nursing staff about developing incontinence but welcome assistance in dealing with the problem once it has been acknowledged. The nurse will need to ask tactfully and gently about incontinence if she notices an odor of urine, or stained bedding or undergarments, or notes that a female patient is trying to cope by placing facial tissue or toilet tissue in her clothing to absorb dribbles of urine. Failure to take action to help an incontinent patient who needs assistance can demoralize that patient, whereas sensitive, professional assistance can maintain and improve the quality of the person's life.

Bladder Training

Bladder training is a complex process that requires knowledgeable participation of the patient and all who are involved in his care. It requires an adequate understanding of the patient's condition and aspirations, the setting of realistic goals, and a mutually agreed-upon approach to the problem. The process is long and often discouraging, and the success of any bladder-training program depends on the support, encouragement, and consistent reinforcement of all concerned.

Cystitis

Cystitis is inflammation of the urinary bladder and is often the result of a localized infection. Cystitis is characterized by pain and burning on urination, later by fever, sometimes accompanied by chills. Diagnosis is made by microscopic examination of the urine. Women and girls are susceptible to cystitis because their short urethras offer less protection from infection.

Causes of cystitis include failure to wash hands before touching the area around the urinary meatus and by contamination of the urethra with pathogens from a rectal or vaginal infection. A female patient should be taught to *wipe from front to back* (away from the urinary meatus) and to make sure that both she and her partner have clean hands before engaging in sexual activity. Some little girls are sensitive to the ingredients in various bubble baths and are likely to develop cystitis following even occasional usage.

Women and girls should be taught to wear underpants with an absorbent cotton crotch, to maintain a high fluid intake, and to empty the bladder frequently. Despite the demands of a busy schedule and the constraints of a work or school situation, the woman should obey the urge to urinate. A chronically full bladder contributes to the development of cystitis in susceptible women.

PATIENT TEACHING

Patient teaching related to *urinary* elimination should include information related to the prevention of cystitis, the home care of a patient with an indwelling catheter, and effective ways of helping an incontinent person. Every person responsible for the care of an elderly person should know that dark concentrated urine indicates an urgent need for a great fluid intake.

Patient teaching related to *intestinal* elimination should make certain that the patient and his family understand the importance of fluid, fiber and exercise, the dangers inherent in dependency on laxatives for adequate bowel function, and the hazards of severe or prolonged diarrhea to infants and elderly persons. In addition, each person should know how to give an enema safely in the event that one is needed during home care, or in preparation for a diagnostic test. Finally, young parents need a basic understanding of the process and ramifications of toilet training.

RELATED ACTIVITIES

1. In order to gain a broader perspective on the cultural and social aspects of elimination, ask a variety of people of different generations and cultural backgrounds about their toilet training practices and the outcomes. Some elderly people will remember that 50 to 60 years ago many public health nurses taught that toilet training should be started by the age of 6 weeks, while some young parents will be confident that toilet training can be accomplished in a *single day* "when the child is ready," between 2 and 3 years of age.

2. One way to appreciate the complexity of the emotional aspects of urinary elimination is to spend some thought on the following question: If you were the school nurse in an elementary school in which handicapped children were being mainstreamed into the public school system, what would you do to help the teacher of two new students who have problems with urinary elimination? Specifically, one child, age 8, is incontinent once or twice a week, and the other, age 7, may need assistance with her newly acquired

task of self-catheterization once a day. How would you proceed to help the teacher, the two children, and their classmates cope with the situation?

SUGGESTED READINGS

———— Update on treating acute diarrhea. *Am J Nurs* 1984 Aug; 84(8):1016.

Aman, Rose Anne: Treating the patient, not the constipation. *Am J Nurs.* 1980 Sept; 80(9):1634–1635.

Beber, Charles R: Freedom for the incontinent. *Am J Nurs* 1980 March; 80(3):482–484.

Bradshaw, Troy Wayne: Making male catheterization easier for both of you. *RN* 1983 Dec; 46(12):43–45.

Killion, Ann: Reducing the risk of infection from indwelling urethral catheters. *Nursing 82* 1982 May; 12(5):84–88.

Lerner, Judith, and Zafar Khan: *Mosby's Manual of Urologic Nursing.* St. Louis, Mosby, 1982.

McConnell, Edwina A: Assessing the bladder. *Nursing 85* 1985 Nov; 15(11):44–46.

Metheny, Norma: Renal stones and urinary ph. *Am J. Nurs* 1982 Sept; 82(9):1372–1375.

Oberle, Kathleen, and Anita Wildgrube: Intestinal helminths. *Can Nurse* 1981 Feb; 77(2):14–17.

Plantemoli, Lucille V: When the patient has a foley. *RN* 1984 March; 47(3):42–43.

Quinlan, Margo W: UTI: helping your patients control it once and for all. *RN* 1984 March; 47(3):38–42.

Schwalb, Robert B, and Bonnie-Dee Stiles: Preventing infection during pregnancy—and after. *RN* 1984 March; 47(3):4–45.

Sheahan, Sharon L, and John Patton Seabolt: Understanding urinary tract infection in women. *Nursing 82* 1982 Nov; 12(11):68–71.

Smith, Carole E: Detecting acute abdominal distension: what to look for, what to do. *Nursing 85* 1985 Sept; 15(9):34–39.

Sorrles, Alice J: Continuous ambulatory peritoneal dialysis. *Am J Nurs* 1979 Aug; 79(8):1400–1401.

Sugar, Elayne: Bladder control through biofeedback. *Am J Nurs* 1983 Aug; 83(8):1152–1154.

The Ostomy (continuing education feature). *Am J Nurs* 1985.

Part 1: Nov; 85(11):1241–1253.

———— Watt, Rosemary C: Why is it created?

———— Smith, Dorothy B: How is it managed?

———— Alterescu, Victor: What do you teach the patient?

Part 2: Dec; 85(12):1358–1367.

———— Boarini, Joy: What can go wrong?

———— Alterescu, Karen Burke: What about special procedures?

Vigliarolo, Diane: Managing bowel incontinence in children with meningomyelocele. *Am J Nurs* 1980 Jan; 80(1):105–107.

35

Rest and Sleep

Prerequisites and/or Suggested Preparation
There is no prerequisite preparation for this chapter.

REST

Rest can be defined either as the *intentional interruption of a given activity,* or as a *state of being.* The first definition refers to a deliberate attempt by an individual to refresh and revitalize himself. It is an active process and results in *active rest.* The second definition refers to *passive rest* in which the person's rest is dependent upon the efforts of other people, usually members of his family or the health care team. Passive rest is a state of reduced stress, and a time when a person can "let go" and relax between treatments or other activities.

Active Rest

Familiar names of periods of active rest include nap, coffee break, intermission, half time, day off, time out, and vacation. The individual deliberately chooses to engage in such an activity, although the period of active rest may involve the permission and planning of a group with which the individual is associated.

These periods of active rest vary in length from 5 or 10 minutes to several weeks, but in each case the intent is the same—to refresh, revitalize, and renew the individual so that he is ready and able to resume some purposeful activity. More specifically, active rest is characterized by the following outcomes:

- The individual gets his "second wind" or renewed strength
- The individual experiences a fresh outlook, increased motivation, and heightened enthusiasm
- It provides a transition from one type of activity to another
- The individual experiences a sense of increased mental and physical well-being
- When effectively used, active rest increases the quality of life by providing variety, stimulation, purpose, and improved health

---

Examples of Activities for Active Rest

Relaxation techniques; meditation; listening to music

Intellectual stimulation (reading, taking a school course, doing crossword puzzles or word games)

Physical activity (jogging, walking, organized sports, exercise programs)

Creative activities (knitting, gardening, woodworking)

Meeting personal needs (leisurely bath, shopping, napping)

Socialization (friends, church groups, clubs, volunteer work)

Prerequisites for Active Rest

The individual decides what use he will make of the opportunities for rest which are available, and therefore determines the outcome or effect on himself. For example, during an intermission, the conductor of a symphony or orchestra is free to relax with a few friends, mentally rehearse the rest of the concert program, doze for 5 min, or worry about his performance.

There are at least five conditions which are necessary for an individual to choose to engage in periods of active rest: (1) a conviction that rest is necessary and desirable; (2) adequate self-esteem; (3) freedom from guilt over resting; (4) the ability to set priorities; and (5) a history of success or past rewards for resting.

1. *Convictions about rest.* The individual must be convinced that adequate rest is essential to his optimal physical and mental well-being. In order to choose rest over some other activity, he must believe that rest is equally important to his health as nutrition, exercise, work, sleep, and other basic needs.

2. *Adequate self-esteem.* The individual must believe that he is a unique person who is valued for who he *is,* not for what he *does.* He must feel that he is worthy and important enough to justify periods of rest and relaxation in order to enhance his own creativity and well-being.

3. *Freedom from guilt.* The individual must have "come to terms" with his feelings and attitudes about what is expected of him by others and what he expects of himself. He must have learned to cope with the demands of everyday life, and be able to put the "shoulds and oughts" into proper perspective. The length and type of rest will vary greatly throughout the life cycle, depending upon the demands of each stage of development, but no matter what the type or how limited the period of rest may be, the individual should be able to enjoy it fully without feeling guilty about other things he might be doing.

4. *Ability to set priorities.* It is difficult to meet the other prerequisites for active rest unless one can effectively set priorities and goals for one's life. The individual must be able to provide some rational basis for answering questions such as "What do I want to achieve by the end of this week? This month? This year?" "What things do I absolutely, positively have to do today?" and "How many and what kind of 'time outs' or 'breaks' will be most effective in keeping me fit, alert, creative, and in good spirits?" Rest must be planned, just as meals and tasks are planned, and

the more hectic the pace, the greater the need to plan for rest.

5. *Past success with active rest.* A person is more likely to choose active rest as an activity if he has discovered that it "pays off." If 10-minute breaks or an afternoon off have proven beneficial in the past, that type of behavior will have been reinforced and will be more likely to be repeated.

Deterrents to Active Rest

Some people live out much of their lives without the benefits of adequate rest. The reasons are varied (Table 35.1) and in many situations, they seem impossible to overcome. Extensive teaching could make a significant difference, but many of these individuals and families are not in contact with the community health nurse or other source of information.

Nursing Interventions to Promote Active Rest

The primary types of nursing intervention are:

1. Teaching about the necessity and benefits of active rest
2. Promoting self-esteem and worth
3. Increasing ability to set priorities and problem solve
4. Modifying attitudes about rest
5. Teaching about relaxation skills and community resources

These interventions must be based upon a careful and ongoing assessment of the individual, the family, and community resources. In general, the goal is to

---

TABLE 35.1 FACTORS WHICH INHIBIT ACTIVE REST

Factor	Examples
Culture	Belief that work is good; idleness or play is bad (the "Protestant work ethic")
Knowledge	Lack of understanding of relationship between stress, mental and physical fatigue, and health.
Finances	Need to work overtime or hold a second job.
Personality	Tense, active, or compulsive; "workaholic."
Family demands	24-hour care of preschool, handicapped, disabled, sick, or aging family members.
Environment	Crowded, noisy, inadequate living conditions; lack of space, privacy, peace, quiet.

> ### Examples of Community Resources for Active Rest and Relaxation
>
> Ladies-Day-Out programs at YWCA, churches, and neighborhood centers. Low or no cost. Child care usually provided.
>
> Day care programs for adults so family members can run errands, shop, visit, or relax. Care by hour or day.
>
> Programs sponsored by local Department of Parks and Recreation. Low or no cost; varied.
>
> Respite Care programs developed to provide relief to families providing 24-hour home care to a sick, disabled or handicapped member. Volunteer or paid worker will give relief for a few hours, a day, or a weekend.

help the individual value, choose, and engage in some type of active rest on a regular basis. The kind of rest will vary, from reading for 10 to 15 min each day to square dancing once a week or exercising while watching a TV program, but in any case, the *criteria* will be the same. The proposed activity must:

- Seem desirable to the individual
- Be compatible with his culture and current attitudes
- Be affordable, in terms of both money and time
- Be practical in terms of living conditions
- Be realistic with respect to demands and expectations
- Have a high probability of maintaining or improving mental and physical well-being

Passive Rest

In a health care facility, the patient is unable to control his environment and the things that happen to him. It therefore becomes the responsibility of the staff to manage the situation in such a way that the patient's stress is reduced as much as possible. This state of reduced tension is a goal of nursing because it facilitates the healing process and the patient's recovery.

Prerequisites for Passive Rest

In order for a patient or other dependent person to rest between scheduled activities and treatments, there must be at least minimal satisfaction of his basic needs. He must feel safe, as physically comfortable as possible, psychologically secure, accepted and respected by the staff, and confident of his own worth and ability (Table 35.2).

TABLE 35.2 FACTORS WHICH PROMOTE PASSIVE REST

Factors	Examples
Safety	Staff appears competent and concerned; cleanliness and aseptic techniques are adequate (there seems to be no reason to fear nosocomial infection); all equipment works well. Call bell is answered promptly.
Physical comfort	Vigorous efforts are made to control pain, nausea, sleeplessness, itching, fever, constipation, and other discomforts. Time is scheduled for periods of inactivity and rest. Noise, glaring lights, and environmental odors are minimized.
Psychological security	Patient is well oriented to the unit; staff wear identifying tags and introduce themselves; patient knows routine and schedule; patient's fears, worries, and anxieties are identified and relieved. Privacy is maintained; embarrassment is averted.
Acceptance and respect	Staff demonstrate interest and concern for patient, address him by his preferred name, and anticipate his needs; personal possessions are respected; efforts are made to meet personal needs and preferred routines. Cultural differences, age, and stage of development are routinely taken into account.
Self-esteem	Patient is involved in all decision making; he is made aware of all his rights and options; patient teaching is done early and effectively; active efforts are made to enhance or maintain body image; patient is considered competent and capable of participating in own care.

SLEEP

A positive relationship between sleep and health or recovery from illness has been postulated and widely accepted for centuries, especially by lay people. Statements like "now try and get some rest" and "you'll feel better after a good night's sleep" acknowledge a person's need for adequate sleep and rest.

Researchers have not yet discovered the exact mechanisms by which sleep is beneficial, but the importance of sleep can be deduced from the effects of sleep deprivation, the universal complaints of people who feel that they have slept poorly, and the development of Sleep Disorders Centers across the country.

Sleep deprivation occurs when a person has been without sleep for a number of days or when his sleep has been repeatedly interrupted for several nights. The early symptoms of inadequate sleep are familiar to most people: fatigue, blurred vision, headache, and sleepiness. Some people become apathetic and listless; others become irritable and restless. After a while, speech becomes slurred and perception is distorted. A person becomes more sensitive to pain, and his coordination decreases. His ability to do his work or to perform ordinary tasks is often diminished. If sleep deprivation continues, the person may demonstrate behavior and personality changes. He may become depressed, confused, or disoriented; some people have experienced hallucinations. The effects of sleep deprivation are relatively consistent, regardless of the cause.

Prolonged loss of sleep can be caused by such diverse things as pressure to complete an important project, physical discomfort, or involvement in an emergency such as a fire or flood. An equally serious situation results when sleep is *repeatedly interrupted*. This occurs in an intensive care unit, for example, when the patient is subjected to an almost constant succession of treatments and tests, some of which occur only 15 to 20 minutes apart. In such a situation, the symptoms caused by interrupted sleep are sometimes referred to as intensive-care delirium. Similar but less intense reactions can occur in susceptible patients in a regular hospital unit unless the staff are skillful and creative in their efforts to ensure adequate sleep for each patient.

Stages of Sleep

Sleep is a cyclical process that usually occurs once in 24 hours for most adults. Within each 6- to 8-hour period of sleep, there are four to six sleep cycles of about 90 min each. Each of these 90-min cycles consists of two kinds of sleep: REM sleep and NREM (or non-REM) sleep. REM sleep is characterized by *rapid eye movements*; NREM sleep, by slow, rolling eye movements. Both kinds of sleep are essential for optimal health.

Researchers have discovered four distinct stages of NREM sleep that can be identified by their characteristic brain waves on an EEG (electroencephalogram). Stage 1 is a drowsy, relaxed period of transition between sleep and wakefulness. Stage 1 is brief, lasting from 1 to 7 minutes at the beginning and end of a night's sleep. The brain waves are small and shallow, and are known as alpha waves. The sleeper is easily aroused.

During stages 2 and 3, the EEG waves become larger, deeper, and slower. Muscles become more relaxed;

temperature and blood pressure are decreased; and the sleeper is more difficult to arouse.

In stage 4, brain waves are large and slow and are known as delta waves. Eye movements are large and slow and are known as delta waves. Eye movements are slow and rolling; the body is very relaxed; the sleeper rarely moves and is very hard to arouse. Stage 4 sleep is called deep sleep. Stage 4 sleep affects the healing processes of the body and also the level of blood cholesterol. Nighttime asthma attacks are less frequent during stage 4 than during other stages. Growth hormones are released during stage 4 sleep, especially during the early part of the night when the periods of stage 4 sleep are longer.

NREM sleep, especially stage 4, is called obligatory or essential sleep because it is necessary for physical health and well-being. When it is missed, it is made up before REM sleep is made up during the first few recovery nights.

REM sleep is often called paradoxical sleep because the skeletal muscles of the body seem virtually paralyzed while at the same time many body processes are accelerated. The brain waves are very active, resembling those of a person who is awake. Eye movements are rapid, and the eyes seem to dart about. The fine muscles of the face and neck may twitch. Dreams are exciting and dramatic, vital signs are increased, and adrenal hormones are released. Metabolic processes are accelerated, and the increased gastric secretions may result in episodes of pain for a patient with ulcers. When a heart attack occurs during the night, it is likely to occur during REM sleep.

REM sleep is believed to be related to a need for cerebral stimulation, especially in infants, and also to the functions of sorting and storing information, establishing relationships between new experiences and memory, and psychological coping. REM sleep restores a person *mentally* whereas stage 4 NREM restores one *physically*. REM dreams are vivid and emotional in contrast to NREM dreams, which are more realistic and factual.

The first REM sleep of the night is brief, and subsequent periods of REM sleep increase in length from about 10 minutes early in the night to as long as 30 minutes just before waking up in the morning. The total REM sleep per night is about 1½ to 2 hours. REM sleep is closely aligned with stage 2 sleep.

Both the total amount of sleep and the proportionate amount of REM sleep decrease with age. A newborn infant sleeps a total of 16 or 20 hours per day, whereas an elderly person often sleeps only 6 or 7 hours. The REM percentage of total sleep is approximately 50 percent for infants and drops to as little as 15 percent in old age.

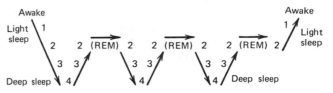

Figure 35.1 *Stages of sleep and sleep cycles.*

Progression through each sleep cycle is orderly, from light sleep to deep sleep and back to light sleep during each cycle. A stylized portrayal of this progression is shown in Fig. 35.1. When a person is awakened, he does not return to sleep at the same level at which he was interrupted. Instead, he starts a new cycle and moves in orderly fashion from light to deep sleep. Each cycle of REM plus NREM sleep takes approximately 90 minutes; and a person needs a minimum of 1½ hours of sleep between awakenings in order to include enough stage 4 sleep. If he is awakened frequently, he is constantly starting a new cycle and therefore either does not reach stage 4 or is able to remain there for only a short time before he is awakened again. With every sleep cycle that is cut short, it is the deep sleep (stage 4) that is missed.

ASSESSMENT OF SLEEP

A person usually concludes that he has had a good sleep if he feels refreshed when he awakens. In addition, he usually takes into consideration three aspects of sleep that affect its quantity and quality:

- Length of time needed to fall asleep
- Number of arousals or wakenings
- Duration of sleep

If one or more of these aspects are significantly altered, a person will usually deem his sleep inadequate and unsatisfactory. If it takes him longer than usual to fall asleep, if he is aroused more frequently than usual, or if his total sleep is less than he is used to, he will feel that he did not sleep well.

A patient's assessment of his night's sleep may differ from a night nurse's assessment. The nurse or attendant may have checked the patient several times and, if he was sleeping each time, concluded that he slept well that night. The assessments of a night nurse and the patient are likely to differ at times because the patient subconsciously includes in his assessment the effects of *inadequate stage 4 sleep* even though he cannot verbalize the effects he feels. A person's assessment of his own sleep is very personal and highly subjective. It transcends the judgment and opinions of other people, and it should be considered one of the most reliable sources of data about the satisfaction of the person's need for sleep.

VARIABLES THAT AFFECT SLEEP

There are 12 general categories that encompass a majority of the things that influence the quality and quantity of a person's sleep.

Age
The amount of sleep a person needs decreases as his age increases. An infant sleeps from 16 to 20 hours per day, depending on his personality and maturity. Children and adolescents need 10 to 12 hours of sleep, while the amount of sleep required by adults usually decreases slowly until old age.

Fatigue
A moderate amount of fatigue promotes sleep, especially if the fatigue is the result of satisfying work or enjoyable exercise. Exhaustive fatigue renders a person "too tired to sleep," and should be avoided whenever possible.

Circadian Rhythm
Circadian rhythms (circa = about, diem = day) are partially responsible for the daily fluctuations in a person's physical and mental processes. Every person has a daily cycle, with regularly recurring high and low points of energy and alertness. The low point, for most people, occurs during the early morning hours. Body temperature is lowest at this time and body processes are slowed, so a person's time for sleep should include this low point in his circadian rhythm.

Although most people are able to adjust to working an evening or night shift on a *longterm* basis, frequent changes are often unreasonable and unwise. Some hospitals assign nurses to rotating shifts, or require frequent random changes. It often takes 5 to 6 days to adjust to a different shift, thus frequent changes make an adequate adjustment impossible. As a result, both the well-being and the performance of the nurse are affected.

Morning people are alert and full of energy early in the day. They "run down" as the day progresses, and are ready for bed early in the evening. *Night people* awaken reluctantly and are unable to "get going" until late morning. After a slow start, they reach a peak of productivity late in the day and are full of energy and life well into the evening.

Some people experience great difficulty with schedules that do not fit their own circadian rhythms, especially during illness when treatment, tests, and procedures disrupt normal body rhythms.

Environment
Most people whose jobs require extensive travel develop an ability to obtain adequate sleep in whatever environment they find themselves. Other people find it difficult to sleep in strange surroundings.

Some of the environmental variables that can interfere with sleep are differences in light, sound, temperature, and the bed itself. For example, bright lights, instead of a familiar darkness, and city noises, instead of country sounds, are stressful to some people.

The effect of sleeping in a strange bed is intensified if the patient normally sleeps with another person. If a child has always slept with his brother or if a woman has never slept anywhere but in her own bed beside her husband for the past 45 years, sleep may be difficult because of the loss of a human source of comfort and reassurance during the night.

Stimulation
The activities that precede bedtime should provide moderate stimulation. Too little stimulation results in a boring and uneventful evening. This tends to foster drowsiness and napping during the evening which often results in subsequent wakefulness. On the other hand, intense stimulation of any kind makes it physically and psychologically difficult for a patient to settle down and fall asleep. For example, a scary bedtime story, a scolding or roughhousing before bedtime will make it difficult for a child to fall asleep. Similarly, bad news, too many visitors, or a painful procedure during the evening can make it difficult for a patient to fall asleep. Therefore, treatments, decisions, and problems should be dealt with as early as possible; and the evening should be interesting, relaxed, and reasonably quiet.

Bedtime Rituals
Seemingly old-fashioned rituals such as "wind the clock, put out the cat, check the weather, and lock the door" serve important functions in preparing a person for sleep. Routine activities that can be done almost without thinking enable the mind, body, and feelings to slow down, and such routines provide a transition from full wakefulness to sleeping. This kind of transition is especially important for a sick person because it serves as a punctuation point, marking the end of another day. Without a bedtime ritual, the days and nights seem to blend into one long blur of being in bed, with no clear-cut signal for nighttime sleep (Fig. 35.2).

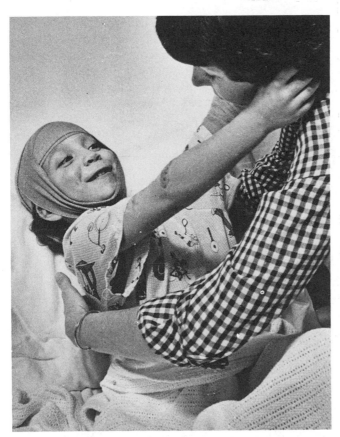

Figure 35.2 Bedtime rituals are important, and a good night hug is often even more essential in the hospital than it was at home.

Conditioning

Familiar objects in a familiar setting serve as stimuli for sleep, especially when coupled with bedtime rituals. A child connects his favorite toy, blanket, and crib with sleep; an adult associates his nightclothes, bed, bedroom, and alarm clock with sleep. Most people respond to such stimuli in fairly predictable ways.

Any significant alteration of stimuli will alter the response. A child who has always slept well may experience difficulty, for example, if his parents begin to put him to bed as a means of punishment. His crib or bed then becomes associated with feelings of anger, resentment, or guilt, none of which is conducive to sleep.

Emotional State

Any intense emotion can keep a person from sleeping. Fear, anxiety, joy, worry, or grief will prevent a person from relaxing enough to fall asleep. A number of commonly used phrases reflect the inner tension that pre-

vents relaxation. A person may say, for example, that he can't sleep because he feels "wound up," "up tight," or "tied up in knots."

One of the most significant aspects of promoting sleep, therefore, is the relief of any overwhelming or draining emotion through the technique of therapeutic communication or crisis intervention.

Physical Condition

Minimal physical comfort must be assured before restful sleep can take place. Nursing actions to relieve symptoms such as pain, nausea, chills, or itching must be among the first steps taken in preparing a person for sleep.

Drugs

A wide variety of drugs affect both the onset and duration of sleep. These drugs include stimulants, depressants, tranquilizers, sedatives, caffeine, and alcohol, as well as medications given to relieve pain, vomiting, or other discomforts. The relationship between the drug and sleep is determined by the age, size, and condition of the patient; the dose of the drug; and the time that has elapsed since the drug was taken.

Recent Sleep

A patient who, for some reason, has been heavily sedated for several days, a person who has slept around the clock to make up for missed sleep, or a person who has slept all day after working the night shift cannot be expected to fall asleep at his regular evening bedtime. On the other hand, a patient who slept poorly or was awakened early for a special treatment or test may find it very difficult to stay awake until his usual bedtime.

Motivation and Expectation

A person's ability to stay awake or wake up early can be affected by his motivation and desire to participate in some special event; in similar fashion, motivation can also promote sleep.

A strong, matter-of-fact *expectation* of sleep is an influential determinant of sleep, especially when it is coupled with appropriate activities such as an effective bedtime ritual and relaxation exercises or techniques.

MEETING THE PATIENT'S NEED FOR SLEEP

Assessments

The choice of nursing interventions to promote sleep should be based, in part, on the patient's description of his needs and desires. This information can be elicited by asking questions similar to the ones listed below.

- What is your normal pattern of sleep?
- What things may make it hard for you to fall asleep while you are here?
- What things do you do at home to get yourself ready for sleep?
- What can I do to help you sleep tonight?

The last question is perhaps the most important because it enables the patient to state his needs without fear of being considered fussy or demanding. Answers to the other questions provide a context for the last question and help the nurse to understand the basis for the patient's needs and desires.

Planning

Planning ways to meet a patient's need for rest and sleep includes the *management of daytime activities* as well as *careful scheduling of nighttime treatments and procedures*. Management of the patient's daytime activities includes the appropriate timing of both naps and exercise. A morning nap is usually preferable to an afternoon one because it is likely to be a continuation of REM sleep. It is a light sleep, and the patient wakens refreshed. An afternoon or evening nap is likely to include more NREM stage 4 sleep. It is a deep sleep; the patient feels groggy when he wakens; and nighttime sleep may be delayed.

Each patient should be kept busy enough during the day to prevent boredom, lethargy, and excessive napping—all of which tend to produce nighttime wakefulness. Moderate exercise and activity *during the day* promote nighttime sleep and tend to increase the amount of deep sleep; exercise just before bedtime is stimulating and can result in wakefulness. Overexertion and overtiredness also make it difficult to fall asleep.

Nighttime treatments and procedures must be scheduled carefully to permit adequate periods of sleep. Because each cycle of sleep lasts approximately 90 min, nighttime activities should, whenever possible, be *scheduled at least 90 min apart* to permit the patient to *complete* as many sleep cycles during the night as possible.

Sometimes, nursing activities are planned with little concern for the preexisting schedule and the patient's need for sleep. If, for example, the patient's vital signs are checked at 10 pm, 2 am, and 6 am and if a medication is scheduled for 11 pm, 3 am, and 7 am, the patient will be aroused six times within 9 hours. In all probability, one or the other of these activities could be rescheduled so that the times coincide and the patient will be awakened only three times.

It is important to identify the conditions that require a patient to be awakened, because there are many observations the nurse can make *without waking* a patient. She can determine, for example, that a sleeping patient's skin is cool, his respirations easy and regular, his catheter draining well, and his sleep quiet.

If there is another patient in the room, the procedures for both patients should be scheduled at the same time whenever possible to decrease the number of trips in and out of the room at night. If a "morning" and an "evening" person must share a room, the nurse may need to help them negotiate a reasonable compromise so that each gets adequate sleep and rest.

Nursing Interventions

The nursing actions that promote sleep are neither difficult nor necessarily time consuming, but they are often omitted by nurses who fail to recognize the importance of sleep as an integral part of the patient's overall therapy. The activities related to sleep are usually not accorded the importance attributed to prescribed treatments and procedures; hence a patient who seeks specific assistance in meeting his own needs may be labeled "fussy" or "demanding" by staff who are aware of the problems created by sleep deprivation.

Every effort should be made to permit the patient to get ready for bed at his usual time and in his usual way insofar as he is able, with the nurse doing for him those things he cannot do for himself. Some hospital units are short staffed in the evening, and it may be impossible for the nurse to meet the needs of each patient as fully as she would like. In such a situation, she and the patient will need to negotiate a set of mutually acceptable priorities, possibly using a direct approach such as: "We are really short staffed tonight, but I can spend about 10 minutes helping you get ready for sleep. What would be most helpful? What things are most important to you?" Most patients can understand and accept the realistic limitations of a heavy workload far better than they can tolerate what seems to be indifference or neglect by a nurse who gives no explanation of her behavior.

If a patient consistently needs more attention at bedtime than you are able to provide, it is often possible to enlist the aid of the patient's family or friends to make sure that important non-nursing needs which promote sleep are not neglected.

Four major objectives when preparing a patient for sleep are to:

- Maintain a near-normal bedtime routine
- Give care related to the patient's present condition
- Enhance feelings of safety and security
- Manage the immediate environment (Table 35.3)

TABLE 35.3 PREPARATION FOR SLEEP

Maintenance of Bedtime Routine and Rituals

Physical Preparation for Sleep

Hygiene (bath or shower as needed; care of teeth or dentures; put on night clothes).

Comfort (rub back, tighten linen, extra blanket as needed, light snack).

Psychological Preparation for Sleep

Child (rock him, sing to him, read a story, hear his prayers, get him a drink, and give him his usual bedtime toy).

Adult (Make it possible for him to listen to the news, read until sleepy, meditate, carry out relaxation techniques, pray, or read devotional materials).

Care Related to Present Condition

Relieve or minimize physical discomfort (pain, nausea, itching, cramps, other).

Check dressings, cast, traction, or other equipment.

Help patient assume as near-normal sleeping position as possible.

Promote Feelings of Safety and Security

Orient to night sounds, staff and routines.

Adjust night light, call bell, side rails as indicated.

Ask him if it is okay to touch him while asleep (some war veterans react with varying degrees of violent responses if touched while asleep).

Manage the Immediate Environment

Pull drapes as needed; adjust room temperature, ventilation.

Close door if desired by patient.

Control noise outside patient's room.

The Nursing Goal

It can be difficult to consistently and conscientiously try to meet a patient's need for sleep and rest if other staff seem unconcerned about it. The process of settling patients for the night has become increasingly haphazard in some places; it is often poorly planned, and assigned a low priority. Some health care workers do not understand that sleep is often the *most significant* component of the therapeutic regimen because it enables the body to use its own resources and energy toward its own restoration and healing.

It is very important to be able to separate your *reaction* to the numerous requests of the patient from your commitment to the *overall goal* of sleep. A patient on bed rest, for example, is likely to make half a dozen requests within a few minutes, ranging from "Will you

fill my hot-water bottle, please?" "I'd like to wash my face and hands" and "May I have an extra blanket?" to "I guess I'd better wear my socks tonight." and "Could I have my pain pills before you leave?" It is very easy to lose sight of your nursing objective and momentarily think of these activities as "catering to that fussy old lady in room 917" rather than as preparing a patient for 8 hours of restorative, healing therapy. Preparation of the patient for sleep should be as well planned and well executed as any other important treatment.

SLEEP DISORDERS

It is reported that up to one-third of the population has, or has had, a problem sleeping, and many of these people say that it is their most serious problem. The diagnosis and treatment of difficult disorders is usually done by specialists at a Sleep Disorder Center. (The name and location of such centers can be obtained from any chapter of the American Medical Association.)

Insomnia

Insomnia is the inability to fall asleep or a tendency to waken prematurely. It is a symptom, not a disease. The condition may be transient or chronic.

Insomnia results in sleep that is inadequate and unsatisfying either because the quality is poor or because the quantity is insufficient. The insomniac does not feel refreshed when he awakens.

Insomnia can be caused by physical conditions such as hypothyroidism, alcoholism, and chronic kidney disease. Depressed or anxious patients nearly always experience some degree of insomnia, but in many situations the cause of insomnia is not clear cut or readily apparent.

The treatment of insomnia is difficult. The usefulness of sleeping medications is *very limited* because such drugs do NOT relieve or treat the cause of insomnia and because prolonged usage will create a dangerous drug dependency. Effective treatment of insomnia includes

---

Types of Insomnia

- Initial: Inability to fall asleep, often because of worry or anxiety.
- Intermittent: Characterized by frequent and fairly lengthy arousals.
- Terminal: Person wakes up too early, is unable to go back to sleep; often associated with depression.

appropriate medical care for any underlying physical or psychological problem plus the development and maintenance of an effective routine to promote sleep. Such a routine includes:

- Adequate exercise during the day
- Minimal excitement during the evening
- A satisfying bedtime ritual

In addition, there are two specific rules or guidelines for insomniacs to follow.

1. An insomniac should get into bed only when he is sleepy, not when it is supposedly time to go to bed or when it seems as if he ought to go to bed.

An insomniac dreads the night and has a morbid fear of being unable to sleep. Lying awake in bed and trying to go to sleep while tossing, turning, and worrying creates stress and tension that in turn worsens the insomnia. The insomniac should be taught to pursue an interesting but relaxing pastime until he feels sleepy. If he does not have a suitable hobby, he should be encouraged to develop one that will occupy his attention each evening until he feels sleepy enough to go to bed. An insomniac may have such negative feelings about bedtime that it will be difficult to stimulate an interest in any such activity, but it is imperative that he learn *to relax in preparation for sleep*. It is also essential that he learn to stay up until he is sleepy enough to fall asleep, even if he must stay up for several hours past his desired bedtime. It is important for him to *associate going to bed with drowsiness and sleep* rather than with tossing, turning, and frustration.

2. If an insomniac cannot sleep, he should get up.

The insomniac should be taught that if he misjudged his readiness for sleep and finds himself still awake after 20 min or so, he should get up and pursue some relaxing activity. When he feels sleepy, he can try again to fall asleep.

If the insomniac has wakened very early in the morning and is unable to go back to sleep, he should get up promptly. If in the past he has occasionally been able to get drowsy and go back to sleep, he may choose to pursue a very quiet, restful activity in preparation for going back to bed. For many insomniacs, however, such an expectation is unrealistic, and they will find it more satisfying to engage in some activity that will give a sense of accomplishment, whether it be writing letters, cleaning the refrigerator, or balancing the checkbook. Staying in bed while awake gives no sense of accomplishment; it brings nothing other than a few more hours of frustration and tension. The association

between unpleasant feelings and his bed becomes stronger than ever for the insomniac, and he is no more rested than he would be had he gotten up when he awakened.

Insomnia and the Elderly Patient

Insomnia among the elderly presents a special set of problems, especially if the insomniac wants to walk about the house or nursing home. Some elderly people seem to have their days and nights mixed up; they get enough sleep in a 24-hour period, but they do so at unconventional times. If they live alone or are allowed to follow their inclinations, they might sleep until 2 or 3 pm, for example, and then stay up, off and on, until 3 am or later.

Insomnia in the elderly is caused by changes in lifestyle and living conditions, fewer obligations and a less definite schedule, physical ailments and discomfort, the need to urinate, and generally accepted expectations about sleep and aging.

The course of action that is taken with an elderly insomniac depends on the attitude of the family or staff and the safety of the patient. Unfortunately, the wishes of the patient are frequently disregarded.

In some situations a sharp distinction is made by the family or staff between walking in the daytime and walking at night. Patients are encouraged to walk about during the day; it is seen as something positive and beneficial, both physically and psychologically. On the other hand, walking around at night is called "wandering" and is often considered undesirable and negative, or a form of "senile" behavior. The fact of the matter is that walking about during the night may be a *physiological necessity* for a person who suffers from nighttime leg cramps, the "twitchy leg" syndrome, or poor circulation that causes numbness, tingling, or coldness in his feet and legs. No patient should be expected to lie in bed and endure such discomforts when some degree of relief can be obtained by walking about (within the limits of his own room, if necessary).

In some situations, any elderly patient who gets out of bed and "wanders" about during the night is physically restrained or is sedated heavily enough to keep him in bed. Both of these actions are taken in the name of "protecting the patient" from possible injury, but the use of either restraints or sedation is potentially hazardous. Most elderly people can be permitted to walk about at night, just as they do during the day, provided they are alert enough to respond to a few simple safety measures. At home, a gate at the top or bottom of the stairs may serve as an adequate reminder to stay on a designated floor. Street clothes or tailored nightclothes and slippers with good support will decrease the possibility of tripping and falling. An intercom will enable a family member to hear any unusual sounds or a call for help. If it seems dangerous for the elderly insomniac to use the stove in the night, a spigot-top thermos of hot water will permit him to safely fix a snack of cocoa or instant soup and crackers to relieve his hunger.

In nursing homes or group homes, it might be beneficial to modify the staffing patterns and employ more people at night. In other settings, concerned volunteers or nonprofessional personnel could supervise insomniac patients rather than having them restrained or sedated. As a rule, some safety measure can be devised for nearly any hazard that an elderly insomniac might encounter; with creative thinking and careful planning, an elderly person can be permitted the freedom and dignity to walk about when he is unable to sleep. Insomnia can be a devastating problem or it can be a problem that is made manageable by the concern and understanding of the family and staff.

Sleep Apnea

Sleep apnea is the cessation of breathing during REM sleep. Each episode may last from a few seconds to a minute or two, and may recur from a few times each hour to 500 to 600 times per night. Severe cases can be life threatening. The individual is unaware of these episodes and knows only that he wakes up during the night, and that he is very sleepy during the day.

There are two types of sleep apnea. *Central apnea* is caused by an absence of respiratory effort, and a temporary lack of movement of the diaphragm. It is treated by the use of drugs at night which will stimulate respiration.

Obstructive apnea is caused by a temporary collapse of the oropharyngeal airway. This is an exaggerated form of the normal muscle relaxation, which occurs during sleep. Obstructive sleep apnea is treated by surgery. A tracheostomy is done to provide an open airway during the night (it is covered or closed off during the day).

The individual with sleep apnea awakens with a loud snort when the carbon dioxide level in his blood rises enough to cause the resumption of respiration. The person with obstructive apnea may find himself sitting on the edge of the bed as a result of his body's effort to overcome the obstruction.

Sleep apnea should be suspected in persons who snore very heavily, who complain of sleeping poorly, and who are excessively sleepy during the day.

Hypersomnia

Hypersomnia is excessive daytime sleepiness. It can be caused by sleep apnea, narcolepsy, or severe depression. It can also be idiopathic or non-specific. Of nearly 4,000 patients treated over a 2-year-period at 11 sleep disorder centers, over 50 percent were afflicted with hypersomnia while approximately 30 percent had insomnia.

Narcolepsy is an uncontrollable desire to sleep, and is one of the most familiar forms of hypersomnia. There is no cure, and the condition is disabling because, among other things, it interferes with the ability to hold a job, drive a car, manage a career, or maintain social relationships. The individual may appear lazy and slow, uninterested in the world around him. The person may experience micro-sleeps of 1 to 3 seconds which may occur at the most unlikely times, or he may fall asleep for rather long periods. Narcolepsy is treated by medication, but optimal dosage levels are hard to establish. Adequate medical treatment and long-term supervision are essential.

Other Sleep Disorders

Somnambulism (sleepwalking) occurs during stage 4 NREM sleep and is most frequent in children. The child is difficult to arouse and usually does not remember the incident when he is wakened. It is important to protect the child from injury by locking the door to prevent access to the street and keeping a non-swimmer from the swimming pool, for example.

The sleep walker should be gently wakened, and escorted back to bed.

Nocturnal enuresis (bed-wetting) may be related to a limited bladder capacity, emotional problems, or unusually deep sleep. It usually occurs during stage 4 NREM sleep. Most children are dry all night by the age of 6 or 7, but enuresis may persist until the age of 10 or 12.

Treatment is often slow and frustrating. Any organic disease must be treated, and the physician may try to increase bladder capacity by medication. Moisture-sensitive alarms that awaken the child are available and have proven to be effective in correcting the problem.

Psychological support for the child and his family is essential; a matter-of-fact approach that avoids any suggestion of blame or punishment must be maintained. Parents need support and encouragement as they cope with wet bedding and nightclothes night after night and year after year. An older child must be helped to manage overnight visits to friends and relatives. He can be supplied both with a waterproof pad and absorbent pads to protect the mattress and with a plastic bag to bring wet things home in. He will need help in explaining his problem to friends and their parents, and in accepting a measure of responsibility for protecting the property of others, whether it be in a private home, a motel, or an overnight camp.

Other problems related to sleep include involuntary jerking of the legs (nocturnal myoclonus), "restless" legs, and nighttime leg cramps. *Nocturnal myoclonus* is characterized by rhythmical, repetitive movements during sleep which may be noticed first by a sleeping partner. *Restless legs* refers to a constant irresistible urge to move one's legs which prevents the individual from getting to sleep. *Nighttime leg cramps* are extremely painful, and are often treated with quinine.

PATIENT TEACHING

1. Every individual, starting at age 2 or 3, needs to learn the importance of active rest. Even small children can learn the value of taking "time out" when they are tired or things are not going well. Deliberate attempts should be made to initiate an ongoing program of active rest for each individual, especially those who tend to be harried and pressured with work. This teaching should start as early in life as possible because it often takes a long time to develop healthy attitudes and practices.

2. Patient teaching includes helping a person determine whether or not a sleeping problem is serious. Each individual and family needs to be able to differentiate between a sleep disorder that is temporary and frustrating, and a disorder that is chronic and disabling. If a serious problem is found to exist, the person should be referred to a specialist or to one of the many clinics which deal with sleep disorders.

RELATED ACTIVITIES

1. As an initial step toward understanding the importance of bedtime routines, examine your own routine for a week. You may not think that you have a routine, but careful analysis will undoubtably reveal at least a *minimal pattern*. For example, do you normally hang up your clothes? Brush your teeth? Feed your goldfish? Do your exercises? Say your prayers?

Many of these behaviors may seem unimportant to you, but *experiment with their omission*. For a week, deliberately *omit* or *do the reverse of* your usual behaviors, and note the degree of uncertainty or unsettledness you feel. Remember that you are young, healthy, in a familiar environment, and in control of the situation. Try

to imagine what a disrupted routine could mean to someone who is sick, very young or elderly, dependent, and away from home.

2. To increase your assessment skills and your empathy for the needs of future patients, ask at least two people in each of the major age groups (including the parents of two toddlers) to tell you the five bedtime activities that are most important to them. Try to identify the major similarities and differences between the various age groups.

SUGGESTED READINGS

Browman, Carl P, Michael G Sampson, Krishnareddy S Gujavarty, and Merrill M Mitler: The drowsy crowd. *Psych Today* 1982 Aug; 16(8):35–38.

Fabijan, Lucia, and Marie-Diane Gosselin: How to recognize sleep deprivation in your ICU patient and what to do about it. *Can Nurse* 1982 April; 78(4):20–23.

Goleman, Daniel: Staying up—the rebellion against sleep's gentle tyranny. *Psych Today* 1982 March; 24–35.

Gress, Lucille D, Sister Rose Therese Baker, and Ruth S. Hassanein: Nocturnal behavior of selected institutionalized adults. *J. Gerontal Nurs* 1981 Feb; 7(2):86–92.

Hayter, Jean: The rhythm of sleep. *Am J Nurs* 1980 March; 80(3):457–461.

Hopson, Janet L: The unraveling of insomnia. *Psych Today* 1986 June; 20(6):43–49.

Hoskins, Carol N: Chronobiology and health. *Nurs Outlook* 1981 Oct; 29(10):572–576.

McNeil, Barbara J, Karen P. Padrick, and Julie Wellman: "I didn't sleep a wink." *Am J Nurs* 1986 Jan; 86(1):26–27.

Melnechuk, Theodore: The dream machine. *Psych Today* 1983 Nov: 17(11):22–34.

Milne, Barbara: Sleep-wake disorders and what we can do about them. *Can Nurse* 1982 April; 78(4):24–27.

Natalini, John: The human body as a biological clock. *Am J Nurs* 1977 July; 77(7):1130–1132.

Thompson, Marcia J, and David W Harsha: Our rhythms still follow the African sun. *Psych Today* 1984 Jan; 18(1):50–54.

Tom, Cheryl K: Nursing assessment of biological rhythms. *Nurs Clin No Am* 1976 Dec; 11(12):621.

Walslebeen, Joyce: Sleep disorders. *Am J Nurs* 1982 June; 82(6):936–940.

Weaver, Terrie, and Richard P Millman: Broken sleep (sleep apnea). *Am J Nurs* 1986 Feb; 86(2):146–150.

36

Body Temperature

Prerequisites and/or Suggested Preparation
Knowledge of the sympathetic and parasympathetic nervous systems, and concepts from physics related to heat transfer (Chapter 11) are important for understanding this chapter.

Disease, trauma, or extreme environmental conditions can disrupt or overwhelm the body's normal regulatory processes and produce a life-threatening hyper- or hypothermia. The temperature of a victim of sunstroke may rise as high as 110 degrees F (45 degrees C), while a victim of accidental hyperthermia may have a temperature below 80 degrees F (26.4 degrees C). Some of these victims now escape death, however, because of new knowledge about the physiological effects of extreme body temperatures, and new techniques of raising or lowering a patient's body temperature.

BODY TEMPERATURE

Body temperature depends on the *balance* between heat production and heat loss. Body temperature will rise if the amount of heat produced by the body, or received from the environment, exceeds the amount of heat being lost. On the other hand, body temperature will fall if heat is lost from the body faster than it can be produced or received.

With respect to temperature regulation, the body can be considered as two interrelated parts, the core and the shell. The core contains those organs which produce heat and have life-sustaining functions—the heart, liver, brain, and kidneys. The function of the outer parts of the body (the skin, subcutaneous fat, skeletal muscles and peripheral blood vessels) is to either conserve or lose the heat that has been produced, depending upon the situation. During periods of vigorous exercise, however, the skeletal muscles become a major source of heat production.

HEAT PRODUCTION

Heat is produced by the metabolism of food and the subsequent release of energy. Many variables affect the rate of metabolism, including exercise, hormones, diet, illness, drugs, trauma, and fever. The rate of heat production (metabolic rate) is indicated by the number of calories burned per hour. The rate of heat production may be only 60 or 70 calories/hour when a person is completely quiet, relaxed, and healthy, but under other conditions it can be as high as 200 to 300 calories/hour. Any variable that increases the metabolic rate will increase body temperature if the amount of heat produced is greater than the amount lost. A high metabolic rate does not increase body temperature if there is a corresponding increase in the rate of heat loss.

In addition to the production of heat by metabolism, the body can absorb heat from the environment. The most significant sources are hot environmental air and the direct rays of the sun. Body temperature will rise if heat is absorbed from the environment faster than it can be lost.

HEAT LOSS

Heat is lost from the body when air currents carry heat away from the body, when the skin is in contact with a cold surface, and when sweat evaporates from the skin. The amount of heat lost depends upon the difference between body temperature and environmental temperature. The greater the difference between the two, the more heat will be lost from the body (Fig. 36.1).

Whenever the skin is moist, more heat is lost through the process of evaporation. When the skin is both moist and warmer than usual, the amount of heat lost by the body is increased significantly.

REGULATION OF BODY TEMPERATURE

Body temperature is usually maintained within a normal range by the interaction of the sympathetic and parasympathetic centers in the hypothalamus. Stimulation of the *sympathetic* center increases body heat, while stimulation of the *parasympathetic* center decreases body heat. Interaction between these two centers is reciprocal, so that when one is activated, the other is deactivated or depressed.

The interaction between the sympathetic and parasympathetic centers has been likened to the action of a thermostat on a furnace. When blood flowing through the hypothalamus is colder than the setting of the hypothalamic thermostat, the sympathetic system is stimulated to produce more heat. Heat production will continue until the body temperature exceeds the setting of the thermostat. The parasympathetic center then activates the mechanism for heat loss and inhibits further production of heat. When the blood becomes cooler than the setting of the hypothalamic thermostat, the sympathetic system is stimulated to produce heat, and the cycle of temperature regulation continues.

The setting of the body's thermostat is raised by *pyrogens*. These are substances, usually protein, that stimulate the hypothalamus to increase body temperature. Pyrogens are produced by bacterial and viral infections, trauma, neoplasms, incompatible blood transfusions, extensive radiation, and other kinds of cell destruction. When the hypothalamic thermostat has been reset by pyrogens, body temperature is raised to the level designated by the new setting and is then maintained at or near that setting until the situation that precipitated it has been corrected, at which time the thermostat is reset at a normal or near-normal level.

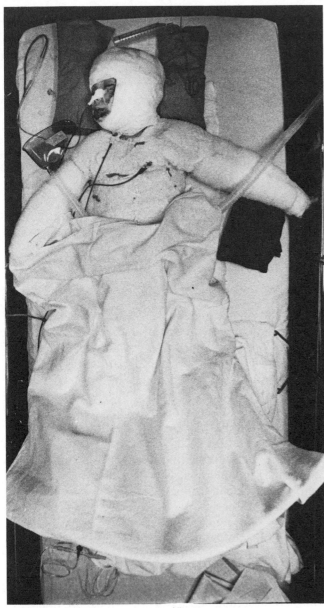

Figure 36.1 *Renee's bulky dressings served two purposes; they exerted enough pressure to help keep the fresh grafts in place and they protected her from a sudden drop in body temperature as she left the very warm operating room.*

Sympathetic Stimulation

When the sympathetic center of the hypothalamus is stimulated to increase body temperature, there are three immediate physiological responses:

1. The peripheral blood vessels constrict to reduce the amount of blood near the surface of the body, thereby decreasing the amount of heat that can be lost and conserving the amount of heat within the body.

2. There is an increase of muscular activity, either involuntary or voluntary. Both shivering and vigorous exercise such as rubbing oneself briskly or jumping up and down will greatly increase the production of heat.

3. Stimulation of the sympathetic center of the hypothalamus releases epinephrine and norepinephrine, which increase the rate of metabolism in all cells and thereby increase heat production.

Gooseflesh appears as a fourth response, but this phenomenon, although significant in lower animals, serves little purpose in humans. Piloerection (hair standing on end) in animals causes air to be trapped between the fur and the skin, giving a measure of insulation. The scarcity of hairs on human skin renders this response unimportant in the regulation of human body temperature.

Parasympathetic Stimulation

When body temperature *exceeds* the setting of the hypothalamic thermostat, the parasympathetic center is stimulated. The production of heat is inhibited, and the body prepares to lose heat in two ways.

1. The peripheral blood vessels *dilate*, bringing large amounts of blood to the surface of the body, where heat is lost both to the air and to any cool object in contact with the skin.

    The *internal* temperature of the body and of the blood is approximately 37 degrees C (98.6 degrees F), whereas *skin* temperature is only 34 degrees C (93 degrees F). When the blood vessels of the skin dilate and fill with warm blood, the *surface* temperature of the body is raised. Because environmental temperatures are usually much lower than body temperatures, large amounts of body heat are given off. Vasodilation of the peripheral blood vessels is, therefore, a major mechanism for increasing heat loss from the body.

2. Sweat glands are stimulated, and considerable heat is lost as sweat evaporates from the surface of the body.

VARIABLES THAT AFFECT REGULATION OF BODY TEMPERATURE

In health, the body temperature of a person is maintained within a narrow range that is *normal for that person*. Many variables cause fluctuations within this

TABLE 36.1 VARIABLES WHICH AFFECT BODY TEMPERATURE

Age	Infants and children: heat regulatory center is immature. Premature infants have virtually no subcutaneous fat or insulation from heat loss. Elderly people: Poor circulation and inactivity can seriously affect temperature control.
Circadian rhythm	Temperature *usually* peaks during late afternoon or evening; varies with the individual.
Hormones	Temperature affected by activity of adrenal glands, thyroid, and ovaries.
Environment	Extremes can cause heat exhaustion, sun stroke, frostbite, or hypothermia. May be fatal.
Clothing	Significant for persons lacking in judgment, persons ill-equipped for winter sports, and the poor.
Exercise	Important for elderly people in cool or cold homes. Should be minimized during hot, humid weather.
Position	Curled up, huddled up position minimizes heat loss but prolonged use promotes contractures and other problems related to immobility.
Drugs	May affect temperature directly (antipyretics) or indirectly (antibiotics, anticancer drugs).
Illness	Example: loss of skin from severe burns permits rapid heat loss; infection and trauma increase metabolic rate.

range as well as unhealthy deviations outside it. Such variables include age, circadian rhythm, hormones, environmental temperature, clothing, exercise, position, drugs, and illness (Table 36.1).

Age

Parents and other people who work with children are aware of the speed with which a fever can develop and then subside in a child. His body temperature is said to be *labile* (unstable). An infant's body temperature is labile partly because his heat regulatory center is immature and partly because he has less subcutaneous fat to insulate his body against environmental temperature changes.

The body temperature of adults and elderly people fluctuates more slowly than that of younger people, and recovery is slower after any disturbance in the control of body temperature.

Circadian Rhythm

Every person's body temperature fluctuates in accordance with his circadian rhythm. For most people, this results in a high point during the late afternoon or early evening. Therefore, if a patient's temperature is taken only once daily, it should be taken at the time of day when it is likely to be the highest.

Hormones

A number of hormones, such as those from the thyroid and adrenal glands, affect the regulation of body temperature. Some of the effects are general and diffuse; other are precise and specific, such as the change that occurs in women at the time of ovulation.

Environmental Temperature

When the environmental temperature is equal to or greater than body temperature, little or no heat is lost from the body, and even a slight increase in heat production will increase body temperature. High humidity further lessens the body's ability to lose heat because sweat is slow to evaporate when the air is already filled with moisture. Extremely high temperatures coupled with high humidity are especially hazardous for the very young and the elderly.

Very low environmental temperatures can result in accidental hypothermia, which is often fatal. One example of accidental hypothermia is immersion in an icy lake as the result of a boating accident. The victim often dies from hypothermia, not from drowning. Heat is lost more rapidly than it can be produced, and extreme vasoconstriction can prevent adequate oxygenation of body tissues, especially the brain.

During a blizzard, when below-freezing temperatures are accompanied by strong winds, the danger of hypothermia is increased because there is heat loss from both radiation and from convection as a result of the wind. Most weather reports include both the actual environmental temperature and the wind-chill factor. It is the latter that must be taken into account when dressing to go outside.

Clothing

Heat loss by radiation is minimized by trapping body heat between layers of clothing, thereby providing an insulating shield of warm air around the body. In some situations, a windproof outer garment is needed to prevent heat loss by convection.

In hot weather, heat loss is promoted by clothing which is porous and absorbent to promote the absorption and evaporation of sweat. Cotton is usually the fabric of choice. Synthetics such as nylon and dacron are nonabsorbent and nonporous. They feel cold and clammy when wet, do not absorb sweat, and do not let air circulate over the skin to promote the evaporation of sweat. (It is interesting that some groups of people do not use the word sweat in everyday conversation. As one elderly gentleman said, "Horses sweat, and men perspire, but ladies merely glow.")

A large body cast can markedly reduce heat loss. Efforts have to be made to maximize heat loss from other body surfaces to promote comfort and the control of body temperature.

Exercise

The hypothalamus is able to maintain a normal body temperature during periods of ordinary exercise; but heavy, violent, or unusual exercise can raise the body temperature 4 to 5 degrees F. The elevated temperature usually returns to normal 15 to 20 minutes after the exercise is stopped.

Position

The amount of heat lost from the body depends in part on the amount of body surface exposed to the air. To lose heat on a hot day, a person in bed instinctively throws back the covers and sprawls, spread-eagled, across the bed, with as much of his skin exposed as circumstances permit. To retain heat, a person instinctively curls up, almost in a fetal position, so that as little body surface as possible is exposed. This position is dangerous for elderly people who are confined to bed, because of the danger of contractures. The danger can be minimized by raising the temperature of the room or by adding blankets until the person stretches out and relaxes.

Drugs

An antipyretic (antifever) drug, such as aspirin or acetaminophen, reduces body temperature by direct action on the temperature-regulating mechanism of the body. Other drugs, such as antibiotics, reduce body temperature indirectly by attacking the infection that is causing the fever. Any drug that stimulates either the sympathetic or the parasympathetic nervous system has the potential for affecting body temperature.

Illness

The regulation of body temperature will be affected in varying degrees by the chemical and hormonal re-

sponses of the body to trauma, neoplasms, allergic reactions, bacterial or viral infections, burns, and other kinds of cell destruction.

ABNORMAL TEMPERATURES

An abnormal body temperature is usually caused by either (1) damage to the body's heat regulatory mechanism or (2) excessive demands on a healthy heat-regulatory system. In the first instance, the heat regulatory center may have been damaged or destroyed by neurological trauma or a lesion of the brain, for example. In the second instance, the temperature control mechanism is functional, and the patient's abnormal body temperature is a predictable physiological response to an intense stimulus.

The *extreme* range of temperature which could be compatible with life is considered to be 25 to 45 degrees C (77 to 113 degrees F).

Hypothermia

Hypothermia is defined as a core body temperature below 35 degrees C (95 degrees F). Hypothermia can be accidental, or it can be deliberate, controlled, and therapeutic. Accidental hypothermia most frequently results from prolonged exposure to snow, icy winds, or cold water, but it also affects elderly people living in cold houses or apartments. It is important for a community health nurse to teach elderly people, or those who are responsible for them, that an older person needs to maintain a room temperature of at least 70 degrees F, wear warm clothing, and keep active, even though housebound in winter. If the house or apartment is cold because of financial problems, the situation should be referred to the appropriate agency.

Intentional hypothermia is frequently used to lower the body's metabolic rate and its need for oxygen after certain types of brain injury, and during heart or brain surgery.

Regardless of the cause or type of hypothermia, the symptoms are similar (Table 36.2).

Treatment of accidental hypothermia is directed toward raising the body temperature as quickly as possible. Blankets, warm clothing, hot drinks, and all available sources of external heat are used. In a remote emergency setting, the only available source of heat may be the body of a rescuer. If so, the rescuer should remove the clothing from his upper body and lie as close to the victim as possible at once, because the later stages of hypothermia are progressive, and death is almost inevitable.

TABLE 36.2 MANIFESTATIONS OF HYPERTHERMIA

Core Temperature	Signs and Symptoms
35–37 degrees C (95–98 degrees F)	Cold, pale skin; alert and shivering; poor muscle coordination.
32–35 degrees C (90–95 degrees F)	Cold, waxy skin; slow slurred speech; lowered reasoning ability; confusion; slowed pulse and respiratory rate; no shivering; face may be pink and puffy.
30–32 degrees C (86–90 degrees F)	Muscle rigidity; stupor or unconsciousness; all vital signs diminished; dilated pupils; diminished reflexes.
Below 30 degrees C (Below 86 degrees F)	Fixed, dilated pupils; coma; vital signs barely detectable or undetectable; reflexes absent; body rigid; cyanotic.

Recent advances and research in the treatment of hypothermia have resulted in the near-miraculous survival of persons who were brought to emergency rooms with no clinical signs of life. The fact that hypothermia slows the body's metabolism and the brain's need for oxygen has made possible the survival of persons who had been under icy water for as long as 30 minutes. Every emergency room should be equipped with a *special thermometer* which will measure temperatures *below* 94 degrees F. and the temperature should be taken upon admission of every apparently dead person who exhibits any of the signs of hypothermia. It is now generally agreed that the only criterion for death from hypothermia is that resuscitation is still unsuccessful *after* rewarming of the body. In fact, an evolving adage is "A patient isn't dead until he's *warm* and dead."

The process of rewarming is complex and subject to many very serious physiological complications. Rewarming must be done slowly, no faster than 1 to 2 degrees per hr. Current techniques include (1) the inhalation of heated oxygen, (2) warm IV's, (3) warm gastric or peritoneal lavage, (4) exchange transfusions, and (5) warming the patient's blood by circulating it through machines outside his body.

Heat-Related Illnesses

In the US, the heat wave of 1980 killed over 1,200 people, and left others permanently affected. The very young and the very old are the most frequent victims of hot humid weather, but also at risk are people who are obese, have cardiovascular problems, or are taking certain drugs. Another factor which increases the risk of serious illness is poorly insulated housing without adequate ventilation or air conditioning. During a prolonged or severe heat wave, the prevention of heat-related deaths becomes both a professional and civic responsibility for all health care workers.

Heat Stroke

Heat stroke or sun stroke is an *emergency* that requires immediate hospitalization. It is often fatal. Heat stroke is caused by exposure to an excessively high environmental temperature. The victim's temperature-regulating mechanism fails, and he is unable to perspire. Symptoms include hyperthermia (a body temperature of 40.6 degrees C (105 degrees F) or higher; central nervous system involvement such as delirium, convulsions, or coma; and *hot, dry skin* because of failure of the sweating mechanisms of the body.

Treatment is directed toward the *immediate and rapid lowering* of the body temperature. Emergency measures include everything from pouring cool water over the victim to wrapping the victim in cool wet towels or using a gentle, fine spray from a garden hose until medical care is available.

Heat Exhaustion

Prolonged exposure to high temperatures can produce heat exhaustion, heat cramps, or both. The symptoms of heat exhaustion are related to its effect on the cardiovascular system, and they resemble the symptoms of shock: pale, cold, clammy skin; rapid, weak pulse; profuse perspiration, near-normal temperature; and generalized weakness. Cramps may occur in arms, legs, or abdomen if profuse sweating has caused a depletion of body fluid and sodium.

Treatment includes moving the victim to a cooler spot, giving fluids, and arranging for medical attention if needed. Salty tomato juice or broth can be given to replace salt and fluid lost by sweating. Plain salt water (1 tsp salt to 1 qt water) is less palatable but equally effective. A stimulant such as black coffee can be given as indicated.

Any person who perspires profusely should be taught to guard against heat exhaustion and heat cramps by slightly increasing his intake of salt during hot weather, unless such action is contraindicated by a health problem such as heart disease or hypertension that requires a low-salt diet.

Fever

Fever is the term used when an elevated body temperature is caused by illness or disease. When an elevated temperature is caused by strenuous exercise, or a very hot, humid environment, the condition is not usually described as a fever.

A fever can be caused by pryogens that act on the temperature-regulating centers of the hypothalamus. These pyrogens are produced by bacterial and viral infections, trauma, neoplasms, radiation, and other kinds of cellular damage and degeneration. A fever can also be caused by a head injury, a spinal cord injury, or a disease that results in damage to either the hypothalamus or the tracts leading to and from it. When the cause of a fever is not known, it is often designated as a fever of unknown origin (FUO).

Fever is considered a protective mechanism because it is frequently an early symptom of disease and prompts a person to seek medical attention. Fever may also make a person feel uncomfortable enough to seek the rest and sleep his body needs for its recovery.

The presence of a slight fever cannot be determined for a given person unless the *normal range* of temperatures for that person is known. This baseline information is especially critical when a diagnosis is being made. A temperature of 99.6 degrees F could be perfectly normal for one person and yet represent an elevation of 2 degrees F for another person whose usual body temperature is about 97.6 degrees F. When such baseline information is not available, a temperature over 37.8 degrees C (100 degrees F) is generally considered to signify a fever (pyrexia). A temperature over 40.6 degrees C (105 degrees F) is called hyperpyrexia (hyperthermia).

Types of Fever

INTERMITTENT. In an intermittent (quotidian) fever, the temperature is elevated each day but returns to normal or subnormal at some point during each day—usually in the early morning. An intermittent fever with *wide* fluctuations (up to 4 degrees F) within each 24-hour period is called a *septic* fever.

REMITTENT. In a remittent fever, the temperature is characterized by marked variations during each day but always remains above normal.

RELAPSING, OR RECURRENT. In a relapsing, or recurrent, fever, the temperature is normal for 1 or 2 days, then becomes elevated again for a period of time.

CONSTANT. In constant fever the temperature remains essentially without change for days or weeks.

Stages of Fever

A fever has three stages: onset, course, and termination. Each stage has its own symptoms and signs, based on the underlying physiology.

ONSET. The first stage, or onset, also called the invasion or chill phase, may be gradual or very sudden. Pyrogens have stimulated the hypothalamus to reset the body's thermostat at a higher level; and according to the new setting, the patient's body temperature is too low and he feels chilly. His body tries to produce more heat and to conserve existing heat.

Measures to produce more heat include increased muscular activity (shivering or a shaking chill) and increased cellular metabolism. Measures to conserve heat and prevent heat loss include vasoconstriction of peripheral blood vessels and the cessation or absence of sweating. As a result of these measures, body temperature begins to rise.

COURSE. The second stage, the course, includes the entire period of temperature elevation; it is the source of the saying "The fever must run its course." The course may last from a few hours or days to many weeks.

During this time, the temperature-regulating mechanism of the hypothalamus is functioning; it is merely set at a higher level. The temperature may fluctuate around the new higher level, or it may remain relatively constant. During the course of the fever, the patient may not complain of feeling hot if his temperature is only slightly elevated because his temperature corresponds to his current thermostat setting.

TERMINATION. During the last stage, termination, the disease processes usually have been arrested, either naturally or with the help of drugs such as antibiotics. In some cases, the disease has not been arrested, but the fever has been checked by an antipyretic drug, such as aspirin.

During this stage, the hypothalamic thermostat is reset at a lower level. The body temperature is now too high, according to the new setting, and the body tries to lose heat and cool itself. Measures to lose heat include vasodilation and sweating. As a result of these measures, the body temperature drops to the new setting. It may drop to normal very quickly (by *crisis*) or very slowly over a period of days or weeks (by *lysis*).

The point at which a high fever suddenly begins to fall is called the crisis. Before the widespread use of antibiotics, the physician and family would spend many hours at a patient's bedside waiting for "the fever to break" or "the crisis to pass" because, if it did, there was a possibility that the patient might survive. There is seldom such a dramatic turning point in the course of a fever today because antibiotics and other drugs are available to combat the cause of the fever and because a high fever can now be artificially lowered by a hypothermia machine or other cooling device.

Signs and Symptoms of Fever

Many individuals, especially children, have a characteristic response to a high fever. One child, for example, may typically become drowsy, lethargic, and apathetic. Another child may become bright-eyed, animated, and excitable. Parents and close associates often notice these signs and suspect the presence of a fever before they have touched the child's skin or heard him complain of feeling hot. Despite individual variations, however, there are a number of signs that are consistently present in a feverish patient:

- Skin becomes hot and flushed; may be dry or sweaty
- Metabolic rate increases 10 to 13% with each degree of fever
- Pulse rate increases 10 to 15 beats with each degree of fever
- Fluid balance is disrupted. Fluid loss is increased through sweating and often by vomiting and diarrhea; fluid intake may be decreased because of anorexia and nausea
- Neurological status may include headache, photophobia, malaise, restlessness or drowsiness, mental confusion, and delirium or convulsions

A body temperature over 41 degrees C (106 degrees F) is extremely dangerous, and brain damage or death often follows a temperature over 41.6 degrees C (107 degrees F). Death or brain damage results from the inactivation of essential enzymes, the destruction of cellular proteins by heat, or failure of the respiratory center.

Effects of a Fever

The physiological response of a patient to fever (his signs and symptoms) can be predicted with comparative accuracy. What cannot be predicted is the effect that these physiological changes will have on a given patient. Some patients will develop many complications, and others will develop none, *depending on the quality of nursing care each receives.*

Most of the secondary effects (complications) of a fever are *preventable,* and the occurrence of these effects indicates ineffective or negligent nursing care. Such symptoms of neglect include dark, concentrated urine; parched, cracked lips; a coated, swollen tongue; encrusted nostrils; poor skin turgor; weight loss; and debilitating weakness.

A person with a high fever is acutely ill and is experiencing extreme discomfort, both physical and psychological; but skillful nursing care can relieve his misery, prevent complications, and increase his chances for recovery.

NURSING CARE OF A PATIENT WITH FEVER

There are two aspects to the nursing care of a patient with a fever. One is related to the *cause* of the fever, and the other is related to the *effect* of the fever on the patient. Nursing care related to the various *causes* of a fever is included in all medical-surgical nursing texts; the emphasis here is on nursing care specific to the patient's *physiological responses* to the fever.

Nursing Care Related to Cause

Nursing care related to the cause of the fever requires, first of all, a knowledge of the underlying pathology. It is important to know, for example, whether a fever is caused by pressure on the hypothalamus, cell destruction from accidental radiation, or the accumulation of toxins from an infectious process.

Knowledge of the cause permits the nurse to maintain an appropriate type of asepsis. For example, strict *surgical* asepsis is required when a fever is the result of massive burns which have become infected, whereas careful *medical* asepsis is needed to protect others from a patient with scarlet fever.

Finally, nursing care includes participation in the treatment of the cause of the fever. Examples of such treatment include the administration of antibiotics for the treatment of an infection and the provision of dressing changes for burns or other kinds of trauma.

Measures to Decrease Heat Production

Nursing actions to decrease heat production are planned to minimize *basic* metabolic requirements and to avoid any *extra* metabolic requirements that would be created by exercise, emotional stress, and excitement. Both the patient and his family need to be taught the relationship between activity, heat production, and fever.

The family needs to learn how to assess and help to meet the needs of each particular patient, both at home and in the hospital, because there are no hard-and-fast rules they can follow.

Nursing Care Related to Physiological Responses

The nursing care of a patient with a fever has three major goals:

1. To decrease production or absorption of heat
2. To increase heat loss from the body
3. To minimize the effects of the fever and prevent complications

Suppose, for example, the mother of a preschool child is told to "keep him in bed for a few days until his temperature is normal." If the child, for hours on end, verbally and physically resisted being in bed during the day, these instructions could result in a steady *increase* in metabolic rate and a steady *increase* in heat production. The same child, however, if given a blanket and pillow, might fall asleep on the floor in front of the television set and sleep for several hours. (A cool or even a drafty floor is likely to be no more hazardous for the child than a fever sponge bath which might otherwise have to be given to reduce his body temperature.)

Measures taken to reduce the metabolic rate are determined by the extent of the fever and the characteristics and needs of the patient. Measures for promoting rest will be as varied as holding and rocking a small child, encouraging a family to use fast foods or frozen meals for a few days, or providing a feverish patient with a supply of relaxing "westerns" or "gothic" novels.

In some cultures, a person is expected to work for as long as he is able to get about. The idea of resting because of a fever would seem unreasonable, and the stress and energy required to try to rest could equal the energy required to do the work itself.

Because of individual needs and cultural differences. The question is not "How can I keep this person quiet or in bed?" but rather "What will help this patient decrease his metabolic rate as much as possible?"

Measures to Increase Heat Loss
Heat is lost from the body primarily by:

- The evaporation of moisture from the skin
- The use of currents of air to carry heat away from the body
- Contact between the skin and cold objects

These modes of heat loss (evaporation, convection, and conduction) form the basis for the nursing interventions which are used singly or in combination to reduce body temperature (Table 36.3).

FEVER SPONGE BATH. A fever sponge bath is often given for a fever over 102 degrees F. because it is a simple yet effective way to lower a patient's body temperature. It can be used in any setting and by almost any person with a minimum of instruction. Throughout the procedure, the patient's skin is repeatedly moistened with water, which is allowed to dry by evaporation. Because heat is required for the evaporation of a liquid, body heat evaporates the water, causing a drop in body temperature.

TABLE 36.3 WAYS TO INCREASE HEAT LOSS

Lower the temperature of the room; open the windows if necessary, even in the winter.

Increase the circulation of air in the room; use fans as needed.

Use loose cotton clothing and bedding.

In critical situations, remove as much of the patient's clothing as modesty permits; let air currents flow over his exposed body.

Use liberal applications of cold compresses or ice bags, especially over large blood vessels such as those in the groin or axilla. (Use ice with caution to prevent tissue damage.)

Give the patient a fever sponge bath (Procedure 36.1).

Use a hypothermia sheet or pad if available.

Apply a cool cloth to the patient's forehead for *comfort* (by itself, it does little to lower body temperature).

Although some agencies have detailed, written procedures for a fever sponge bath, the equipment and process are simple and uncomplicated. The basic equipment includes:

A basin or pan of water

A washcloth or its equivalent for moistening the skin

A towel or its equivalent to keep the bedding dry

Suggested Guidelines
1. Take the patient's temperature before you start the bath to get a basis for evaluating the effectiveness of the treatment.
2. Explain the treatment and the reasons for it to the patient and family. The patient may be reluctant and apprehensive. The treatment is often uncomfortable, and he may worry about its effect, perhaps remarking, "I'll probably catch cold or get pneumonia." Neither is likely, but either can be less dangerous than a prolonged high fever.
3. Use *tepid*, not cold, water. Cold water on the skin produces vasoconstriction, which conserves body heat and defeats the purpose of the treatment.
4. Carefully cover the patient's trunk and genitalia and completely expose his arms and legs. The localized application of cold compresses over the large blood vessels of the groin, axilla, and wrist is considered useful by some people. These compresses are changed whenever they have absorbed heat and have become warm.
5. Bathe the patient for a total of 25 to 30 minutes. Allow approximately 5 minutes for each arm and

leg and 5 to 10 minutes for the back and buttocks. Some nurses bathe one arm or leg for the allotted time and then bathe the next one. Others prefer to bathe all exposed surfaces in about half the allotted time and then repeat the process. There is a possibility that the latter is more effective because more body surface is moist for a greater percentage of the time, and more evaporation can thus take place.

6. Prevent or minimize shivering which would increase heat production. A hot-water bottle at the patient's feet increases his comfort and tends to avert shivering. If the patient starts to shiver, cover all limbs except the one you are bathing. Continue the fever sponge bath until the shivering has passed, because heat is being produced, not lost, as long as the patient is shivering.

7. At the conclusion of the procedure, blot or pat the skin dry. *Do not rub* the skin because friction stimulates the production of heat. Reclothe the patient; replace any damp linen; and leave him comfortable.

8. Take the patient's temperature in 15 to 20 minutes to evaluate the effect of the fever sponge bath. Repeat the procedure as needed.

In rare situations, it might be necessary to increase evaporation by covering the patient with a wet sheet and letting a fan blow across him. This process is very uncomfortable for a patient, and it increases the possibility of shivering. Occasionally, alcohol is added to the water used to bathe the patient. Evaporation is increased, but the fumes may produce nausea or vomiting, especially in children, unless there is adequate ven-

tilation. These measures should be used only in *emergency* situations because many patients are unable to tolerate such drastic action.

Measures To Minimize Adverse Effects

Many physicians and physiologists agree that the presence of a fever can be beneficial in some situations, but without proper supportive care, the adverse effects of a prolonged or high fever can be devastating to the patient. Supportive nursing care is focused on comfort, hydration, nutrition, skin, mouth and eye care, and safety.

COMFORT. The patient with a prolonged or high fever is physically and psychologically uncomfortable. He is restless, weak, and debilitated. The discomfort from his fever is diffuse, and there seems to be little he can do to get comfortable.

The patient is likely to feel generally miserable and irritable; he feels like the adult counterpart of a "fussy baby." Every effort should be made to decrease excitement, noise, confusion, and other excessive sensory stimulation. Quiet companionship and enough diversion to prevent boredom will help to make the patient's condition tolerable. Most patients, especially children, will have a shorter attention span than usual, and a fairly large variety of diversional activities may be needed throughout each day. People in contact with the patient will often need to make allowances for periods of irritability and frustration.

HYDRATION. The initial assessment of a patient's current state of hydration and fluid balance will affect the nurse's priorities. A patient who has been well cared for may need only a continuation of the nursing care he has

---

PROCEDURE 36.1

Giving a Fever Sponge Bath*

SUMMARY OF ESSENTIAL NURSING ACTIONS

1. Take patient's temperature *before* starting bath.
2. Reassure patient and family that he won't "catch cold" or "get pneumonia."
3. Use tepid (lukewarm) water.
4. Use enough towels to keep bed dry (usually one under each arm and leg, and under trunk.)
5. Apply heat to feet for comfort and to minimize shivering.
6. Expose arms and legs; leave uncovered.

7. Sponge all exposed surfaces; do NOT dry.
8. Sponge chest and back; do NOT dry.
9. Continue for 25–30 minutes, then blot or pat skin dry; use no friction.
10. Take patient's temperature after 15–20 minutes.

Note: Substitute a tepid tub bath if a child objects too strenuously to a fever sponge bath. Keep the child's arms and trunk wet as he plays in the cool water.

*See inside front cover and pages 719–720.

received to date, but a dehydrated patient will need extensive treatment. Dehydration occurs very quickly in children, and a dehydrated infant presents an acute medical emergency.

Accurate records of intake and output are essential; if oral intake is insufficient, *parenteral fluids will be needed.* The patient and family should be taught that dark, concentrated urine indicates that fluid intake is inadequate and must be increased. The amount of fluid needed will vary from 1,000 to 3,000 ml/day, depending on the age, size, and condition of the patient (Table 36.4).

Great ingenuity is often needed to ensure an adequate fluid intake for infants, children, and confused or resistant adults.

Unless contraindicated, broth is useful because it contributes to the fluid intake, and, since it is slightly salty, it replaces some of the salt lost through perspiration. It may also increase thirst, thereby stimulating the patient to drink more. Depending on age, individual preference, and possible dietary restrictions, a variety of fluids, such as lemonade, sherbet, beer, and soft drinks may be used.

Every patient over the age of 3 or 4 years should know his fluid intake goal for the day and should be taught to keep track of his progress toward that goal. Even a little child can understand, for example, a goal of 3 mugs of milk, 5 paper cups of juice, and 4 ice pops per day. (Some parents may need to be reassured that the possibility of dental cavities from soft drinks or ice pops is of secondary importance when possible dehydration is an immediate problem.)

NUTRITION. The old adage "Feed a cold and starve a fever" is *not* true; a prolonged or high fever greatly *increases* a patient's need for food. Even when a patient is physically inactive, a 4 to 5 degree elevation in body temperature can cause a 50% to 60% increase in his metabolic rate. Unfortunately, a patient's increased nutritional needs are often accompanied by a decreased interest in food. In addition to the problem of anorexia, an adequate food intake may be difficult because of nausea, vomiting, or bouts of coughing. A high-protein, high-carbohydrate diet is needed to promote heal-

ing, to meet the additional requirements of an increased rate of metabolism, and to prevent weight loss. Concentrated commercial food supplements may be needed for some patients, but imagination and ingenuity plus tempting food from home will enable most patients to meet their nutritional needs.

SKIN CARE. During periods of diaphoresis (perspiration), the patient should be bathed frequently. The sweat glands of the axillary and genital areas are especially active, and an offensive body odor can develop very quickly. In addition to cleansing baths, the patient may need a partial bath at intervals throughout the day to freshen his face, arms, and back, especially if the weather is hot and there is a plastic sheet on his bed.

If the patient is not perspiring and his skin is hot and dry, it must be kept supple with lotion to prevent cracking and abrasion. Lotions must be used in moderation, however, because excessive lotion and creams tend to insulate the body and prevent the loss of body heat.

MOUTH CARE. The patient with a fever requires two types of mouth care. First, the milk, eggs, and meat of his high-protein diet leave considerable debris on his teeth, and therefore his teeth or dentures should be cleaned *at least twice a day* to prevent the formation of a thick, foul coating called *sordes.*

The presence of sordes produces an offensive appearance, bad breath, and a decreased desire to eat. Vigorous, regular brushing plus mouthwash will prevent this condition and will give a fresh, clean taste that is conducive to eating.

The second aspect of mouth care is the prevention or treatment of parched, dry lips and tongue. Heat and dehydration can cause the mucous membranes of the mouth of a neglected patient to crack or split. Adequate hydration is the primary means of prevention and treatment, although some patients will require the extra protection of petroleum jelly, lotion, or one of the commercial sticks for lips. Proper mouth care is essential because, in addition to the need for comfort, a patient cannot eat enough to meet his nutritional needs if his lips and tongue are dry, cracked, and painful.

Fever blisters (herpes simplex) may appear on the lips of susceptible people. These lesions are caused by a virus and usually heal without scarring in about a week or two. The initial vesicle (blister) crusts over after several days and, unless it becomes secondarily infected, requires no treatment except relief of any local discomfort such as pain or itching. Analgesics and cortisone preparations are prescribed when the condition is severe.

TABLE 36.4 GOALS OF ADEQUATE HYDRATION

A patient's fluid intake must be large enough to:
  Eliminate the additional waste products resulting from his increased metabolism
  Eliminate the toxic by-products of infection or disease
  Compensate for fluids lost through increased perspiration
  Maintain good skin turgor
  Help prevent constipation

EYE CARE. A patient with a high fever may suffer from photophobia, and appropriate measures should be taken to relieve the discomfort. Some patients want the drapes drawn or the shades pulled down; others find a darkened room depressing and prefer to wear dark glasses or an eyeshade, or to keep a cloth over their eyes.

Any exudate (discharge) should be wiped from the patient's eyelids with a clean, wet washcloth or a moistened gauze pad.

SAFETY. A high fever is sometimes accompanied by delirium. As the patient is likely to be both frightened and physically active, a nurse or member of the family should remain with him whenever possible to help ensure his psychological comfort and physical safety. Side rails may be deemed necessary, depending on the patient's reaction to them and on agency policy. Side rails should be padded if the patient is thrashing about. Restraints are used only when absolutely necessary because a delirious patient tends to struggle against them, thereby increasing his metabolic rate and heat production.

Convulsions are not uncommon in children with high fevers; upon the child's admission the nurse should ask the parents whether or not the child has ever had a convulsion. If so, or if the nurse has reason to suspect that he might have one as a result of his present condition, she must make sure that a padded tongue depressor is in plain sight at the bedside, that the side rails are padded, and that the child is kept under close observation.

PATIENT TEACHING

Two of the most urgent areas for patient teaching are (1) how to care for a patient with a fever, and (2) how to prevent hypothermia, heat stroke, and heat exhaustion in elderly people. The first is important because of the increasing emphasis on self-care and the corresponding increase in the number of people who are cared for at home by their families.

The second aspect is important because the impact of greater numbers of elderly persons in our society is coupled with ever-increasing utility rates which makes it financially difficult for people on fixed incomes to heat their homes in winter and cool them adequately during exceptionally hot weather.

RELATED ACTIVITIES

Begin to collect information related to both hyper- and hypothermia in the elderly with the intention of preparing a short article for your local newspaper or newsletter during the next episode of extreme weather. Become knowledgeable about the physiological responses to both of these conditions, and even more importantly, concentrate on practical, realistic ways in which concerned citizens can combat the danger. Many groups such as churches, Rotary clubs, or the Chamber of Commerce would take action to prevent the tragic death of a senior citizen if they only knew of some way to help. People who live on the street present similar concerns for society.

SUGGESTED READINGS

Boyd, Linda T, Pamela Hastings Shurett, and Caroline Coburn: Heat and heat-related illnesses. *Am J Nurs* 1981 July; 81(7):1298–1302.

Davis-Sharts, Jean: Mechanisms and manifestations of fever. *Am J Nurs* 1978 Nov; 78(11):1874–1877.

DeLapp, Tina Davis: Accidental hypothermia. *Am J Nurs* 1983 Jan; 83(1):62–67.

DeLapp, Tina Davis: Taking the bite out of frostbite and other cold-weather injuries. *Am J Nurs* 1980 Jan; 80(1):56–60.

Griffin, Joyce P: Fever—when to leave it alone. *Nursing 86* 1986 Feb; 16(2):58–61.

Hayes, Karen Ballard: Dealing with heat injuries. *RN* 1984 July; 47(7);41–44.

LaVoy, Kathleen: Dealing with hypothermia and frostbite. *RN* 1985 Jan; 48(1):53–56.

Lipsky, Janice G: Saving the elderly from the killing cold. *Nursing 84* 1984 Feb; 14(2):42–43.

Muir, Bernice: *Pathophysiology: An Introduction to the Mechanisms of Disease.* New York, Wiley, 1980.

Price, Sylvia Anderson, and Lorrain McCarty Wilson: *Pathophysiology: Clinical Concepts of Disease Processes.* ed. 3. New York, McGraw Hill, 1986.

Smith, David S: Living death—don't let hypothermia fool you into a fatal mistake. *RN* 1983 Jan; 46(1):49–51.

Part Seven

Nursing Interventions in Specific Situations

37

Management of Pain

Prerequisites and/or Suggested Preparation
An understanding of the anatomy and physiology of the nervous system and concepts related to stress responses (Chapter 8) is prerequisite to this chapter.

PAIN

The relief of pain and suffering is one of the most significant of all nursing functions. Other activities such as the prevention of illness, the promotion of health, and contributions to the therapeutic regimen are important, but both patient and family often value above all else the nurse's ability to relieve pain and suffering. Pain is a major nursing concern, and is an emergency for many people who experience it. Virtually every person has experienced moderate to severe pain at some point in life and has known the quiet terror that accompanies it.

Some pain, such as that which follows a sprained ankle or an extracted tooth, is expected, self-limiting, and usually well tolerated by the patient. Other pain, such as that which is part of an uncertain diagnosis, terminal illness, or extensive surgery, is unknown, indeterminate, and difficult for most people to handle.

Nurses have been active in pain relief since nursing began, but recent research related to the nature and relief of pain has markedly increased the nurse's potential for relieving pain and suffering. The medical treatment of pain frequently consists of the use of drugs, surgical interruption of nerve pathways, nerve blocks, or other measures, and of these treatments, only drugs are used to relieve mild or moderate pain. Nursing, on the other hand, has a wide repertoire of techniques for relieving pain that can be used in any setting, without a physician's order, and for nearly any patient. These independent nursing actions include the use of heat or cold, physical or psychological distraction, positioning, massage, guided imagery, and other techniques.

Nursing research about effective pain relief suggests that the nurse must use an integrative approach which considers the biological, physical, and psychosocial responses of the person in pain. This broad view enlarges and extends the therapeutic options for treating an individual who suffers, and therefore, the more the nurse knows about the person, the meaning of his pain, and the factors contributing to the pain, the more effective she will be in promoting comfort and the relief of that pain.

The study of pain expanded during the '60s and '70s and has gradually evolved into a new medical specialty, *dolorology,* the science of pain. The International Association for the Study of Pain was founded in 1974 to foster research, promote education, and provide information about pain. A number of theories of pain have been advanced from time to time, and the gate control theory is currently favored.

Gate Control Theory

In 1965, Melzack and Wall made public their theory that certain cells in the horns of the spinal column function as gates that either permit or prevent the passage of pain impulses. The gate control theory of pain proposes that a mechanism in the spinal cord can alter the perception of pain by acting as a gate to allow an increase or decrease in the transmission of impulses. This mechanism can also be influenced by higher centers in the brain. Many factors, such as fear, an environment without adequate sensory stimulation, or tissue damage, can influence the gating process. Nursing care that reduces anxiety, provides adequate sensory input, removes noxious physical stimuli, or introduces cutaneous stimulation, as does rubbing the area, may decrease pain by closing the gate to at least some of the pain impulses.

Phantom pain which is perceived in a missing body part, such as an amputated leg, may demonstrate failure of the gating mechanisms since these pains probably originate higher in the spinal pathway.

NATURE OF PAIN

Pain is a protective mechanism that signals when certain body tissues are being injured or destroyed. Without pain, a person would receive no warning of tissue damage and might not seek medical care until his condition resulted in visible pathological changes. A person who cannot feel pain because of a spinal cord injury or other condition, for example, is extremely vulnerable to a variety of hazards.

Pain often persists until the offending condition is rectified and thereby prompts the individual to seek treatment. In many tissues, however, pain is felt only while tissue damage is being done and ceases after the tissue has been damaged (McCaffery, 1981).

Acute pain initiates the body's *stress response* which releases large amounts of adrenalin and cortisone, and precipitates the fight or flight reaction. The physiologic responses which follow are measurable and can be described as follows:

Heart rate and cardiac output are increased

Peripheral blood vessels constrict

Blood flow to brain, heart, and skeletal muscles is increased

Kidneys retain salt and water to maintain blood volume

Respiratory rate and lung expansion increase to meet demand for oxygen

Metabolism increases to release stored glycogen for energy

Pupils dilate and vision becomes more acute

Muscle tone is increased

These responses to acute pain are identical to the initial response of the body to any severe stressor; following this reaction, the body may enter the exhaustion phase if the stress is not relieved. Deep pain, for example, appears to exert a depressing effect which may cause nausea followed by inactivity and withdrawal. Severe pain is very apt to cause a sudden failure of the body's defense reactions, resulting in weakness, prostration, bradycardia, hypotension, pallor, sweating, and fainting. This is a protective biologic phenomenon when the pain cannot be escaped. A ruptured gastric ulcer and intestinal obstruction are examples of conditions of pain which cannot be warded off by accelerated coping responses.

Types of Pain

There are three major types of pain: pricking, burning, and aching. *Pricking pain* is felt when a sharp object such as a knife or needle penetrates the skin. It can also be felt when a large area of skin is intensely irritated. *Burning pain* is the type felt when the skin is burned. It can be excruciating and is the type most likely to cause intense suffering (Guyton, 1981).

An *aching pain* (deep pain) is usually more profuse and less well localized than superficial pain. It is not felt on the surface of the body, and people may describe deep pain in almost three-dimensional terms. Widespread aching, even of low intensity, can produce a sensation that is hard to tolerate.

Referred pain is the term used to describe pain that is felt in a part of the body other than the part that is causing the pain (Fig. 37.1). For example, the pain from an inflamed gallbladder is experienced over the tip of the right scapula, and pain from a myocardial infarction (heart attack) is felt down the inner aspect of the left arm. Referred pain provides important di-

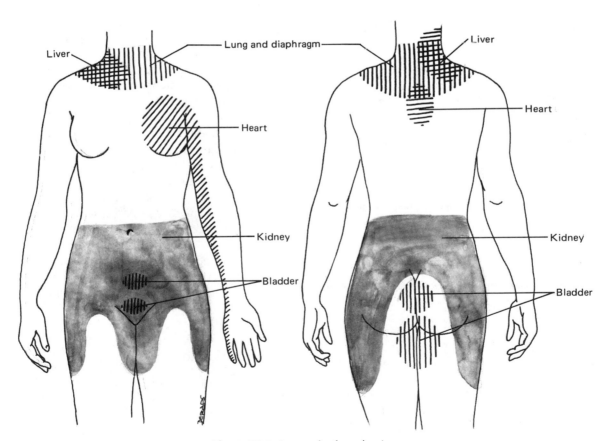

Figure 37.1 *Areas of referred pain.*

agnostic data, and therefore seemingly unrelated pains must be accurately reported and recorded. The patient often needs help in understanding why the pain is not where the problem is.

Referred pain is probably caused by the transmission of impulses from visceral pain fibers across a synapse in the spinal cord to pain fibers from the skin. Pain in an organ, therefore, can send impulses to the spinal cord, which are then conducted across a synapse to neurons from the skin, with the result that the person feels as if the pain originated on the surface of the body.

Phantom pain is pain that feels as if it were coming from an amputated limb. The pain, which appears soon after the amputation, can become a chronic problem, so it is not advisable to delay treatment in the hopes of a spontaneous recovery. The problem of phantom pain is complex, and any treatment of the problem that includes surgical or mechanical intervention is often slow and frustrating. The patient may need help in coping with problems of discouragement, depression, and anger, which are related both to the condition that necessitated the amputation and to his altered body image.

The words used to describe a given pain are significant because the patient's description is an important diagnostic aid. Many conditions produce a typical, characteristic pain which is described in similar terms by most patients.

Descriptions of Pain Associated With Selected Conditions

Condition	Description
Aneurysm	Bouncing, pounding
Bone injury	Deep, aching, boring
Muscle damage	Sore, aching
Colic	Cramping, gripping, twisting
Angina	Constricting, compressing, heavy
Peptic ulcer	Burning, sharp
Neuritis	Burning, stinging
Neuralgia	Sharp, cutting, paroxysmal

Duration and Timing

Pain is commonly categorized as either acute or chronic. *Acute pain* has been defined as the pain that accompanies an injury or illness and that usually subsides as the patient recovers. *Chronic pain* begins slowly, may become progressively worse, and may persist despite treatment. Examples of acute pain include the pain that follows a burn, a fracture, a scraped knee, or an operation. Examples of chronic pain include pain from ar-

thritis, advanced cancer, back problems, and persistent headaches. Some authorities state that the duration of acute pain is less than 6 months, whereas chronic pain may persist indefinitely.

Pain may occur or intensify at night for two reasons. Certain conditions may be aggravated by the increased parasympathetic activity which occurs during some parts of the sleep cycle, and a patient with a gastric ulcer or colic may experience pain during the night. Chronic pain is likely to intensify at night as the patient reacts to the quiet, darkness, absence of distractions, and periods of loneliness.

Perception of Pain

The point at which most people state that a stimulus is painful is remarkably consistent. For example, normal skin temperature is 43 degrees C, and the majority of people report pain when skin temperature reaches almost exactly 45 degrees C. Nearly everyone reports pain before a temperature of 47 degrees C is reached.

The *lowest intensity* of any stimulus that produces pain is called the *pain threshold* and is nearly the same for all people. As the intensity of a stimulus is increased during research, the subject can differentiate between degrees of intensity. Between the level of no pain at all and the most severe pain that can be differentiated, the average person can detect 22 distinct intensities. Each different level of intensity is called a *just noticeable difference* (JND) (Guyton, 1981).

A patient can assess the intensity of his pain and report it in a meaningful way but *only* if all parties use the same scale. The report of a patient who states his current pain is "terrible" may be misleading if he is comparing his current pain with the pain of tonsillitis (the only other pain he can remember), whereas another patient might compare the same pain with the pain of an extremely severe sunburn and describe it as "not too bad." The nurse can give the patient a graduated list of adjectives such as uncomfortable, moderate, and excruciating, or she can ask him to rank his present pain on a scale of 1 to 10, with 10 being the most severe.

Causes of Pain

Pain fibers are sensitive to thermal, mechanical, and chemical stimuli. Some pain fibers are sensitive to only one type of stimulus, but most of them are responsive to more than one. Thermal stimuli include contact of the skin with either extremely hot or extremely cold substances. Mechanical stimuli include such stressors as pressure, tension, stretching, and friction. Chemical stimuli include both chemicals foreign to the body and chemical substances released within the body by damaged tissue, such as histamine and proteolytic enzymes. Some chemicals actually damage nerve endings while other chemicals stimulate pain fibers without necessarily damaging them.

Tissue Ischemia

When the blood supply to a muscle is suddenly cut off, severe pain quickly results. The cause of pain from ischemia is not known, but is relieved by oxygenated blood. It is possible that chemicals are released by damaged cells and that pain is the result of chemical stimulation of pain fibers. Tissue ischemia accounts for the pain of a myocardial infarction and for the pain caused when an inflated BP cuff cuts off the blood flow in the arm.

Muscle Spasms

Muscle spasms probably cause pain by exerting mechanical pressure on pain fibers, by reducing blood flow through the area and creating tissue ischemia, and by releasing chemicals that stimulate nerve endings. The pain is relieved by relaxing the muscle enough to relieve the pressure and reestablish the blood flow through the area.

Transmission of Pain

Sensations of pain are transmitted from the injured tissue to the spinal cord and then to the brain by two pathways. Pricking pains are carried by small, fast type A fibers; burning and aching pain sensations are carried by larger, slower type C fibers. The fibers enter the spinal cord and carry pain sensations to the brainstem, thalamus, and cerebral cortex, where the pain is perceived and interpreted.

Responses to Pain

A person responds to a painful stimulus in accordance with the intensity of the stimulus, the integrity of the pathways, and his personal reaction, which is both physiological and psychological. This response to pain is highly individualized, and there is wide variation in responses to comparable levels of stimuli. This reaction to pain is called *pain tolerance*. It is important for members of the health care team to remember that, although the pain threshold is quite uniform from person to person, *pain tolerance varies widely.*

Pain is a stressor and the patient's usual coping mechanisms affect his behavioral response to pain. Collectively, these responses to pain are called *pain behav-*

iors and are especially significant in determining whether or not a patient can live a satisfying life in the face of chronic pain.

Effects of Pain

Pain, especially chronic pain, is one of the most disabling conditions a person can experience. Some people make relatively successful adaptations, but others are unable to do so and as a result they are burdened by innumerable related problems. Some of the problems engendered by prolonged and unrelieved pain are:

Problems arising from lack of activity or immobility, for instance, weakness, muscle atrophy, disuse osteoporosis, anorexia, constipation, boredom, and insomnia

Problems of decreased self-esteem, such as inability to hold a job or to maintain one's role within the family

Psychological problems such as depression, anxiety, hostility, irritability, dependence, or loneliness

Social problems such as altered interpersonal relationships, decreased social contacts, isolation, and loss of income

It is difficult to reverse a pattern of ineffective behavioral responses, especially if they have developed over a period of years. It is important, therefore, to provide appropriate nursing and medical intervention as early as possible in order to promote an optimal adaptation to the stress of living with chronic pain.

ASSESSMENT

The assessment of pain differs from most other assessments in two ways: (1) there are virtually no objective data that can be collected, and (2) the outcome is almost completely dependent on the nurse's acceptance of the patient's overall description of his pain. *Pain is whatever the experiencing person says it is, existing whenever he says it does* (McCaffery, 1979, p. 11). If you doubt or disbelieve the patient's statements, there can be no effective management of pain. You need not approve or condone any inappropriate pain behavior, but you must accept and believe that *his description of what he is feeling is accurate.*

Variables That Influence the Patient's Assessment

Each patient interprets personal pain on the basis of many variables, and this interpretation determines to a large extent the nature of his response to the pain. Some of the variables that influence an *assessment* of pain are:

- *Developmental stage.* The ability to understand explanations related to pain, to ask questions, and to follow directions related to pain relief
- *Integrity of the nervous system.* The level of consciousness; the ability to feel and interpret pain
- *Sociocultural variables.* Ethnic and cultural background, family and occupational roles, spiritual beliefs, sexual identity, and stereotypes of male and female responses to pain
- *Diagnosis and prognosis.* The nature of the condition causing the pain and an understanding of the probable outcome
- *Physical variables.* Fatigue, weakness, nausea
- *Psychological variables.* Fear, anxiety, discouragement, worry
- *Environmental variables.* Noise, confusion, excessively high or low room temperature, the unpredictability of the day's events

Each variable will influence the way a patient interprets and perceives his pain and must therefore be taken into account when you are trying to assess the patient's pain in preparation for your interventions. The com-

bined effect of these variables contributes to the meaning that pain has for that patient.

Pain History

The patient's verbal description of his pain provides the data needed for planning and evaluating nursing interventions. Some patients are initially reluctant to talk about their pain, but many others are willing and even anxious to discuss it in full detail. A structured interview guide may be helpful in obtaining a pain history from a person who does not volunteer, whereas a single sentence such as "Tell me about your pain," followed by a period of attentive listening, will elicit the necessary information from patients who are anxious to talk.

Observation

In addition to obtaining the patient's verbal description of his pain, you should note his nonverbal indications of pain. For example, fidgeting, handwringing, a flushed or pale face, rapid pulse, and pacing back and forth could all indicate the presence of pain. The patient may limit motion in part of his body by holding that part rigid (splinting).

Minimal mobility, reluctance to move about in bed, maintenance of a single position, and an altered or unusual posture are other possible indicators of pain. These nonverbal indications may or may not be accompanied by a verbal description of pain. Sometimes a patient not only fails to report his pain but may actually deny its presence. This might happen, for example, if the patient thought that knowledge of an unexpected return of pain might keep him from being discharged as scheduled.

MANAGEMENT OF PAIN

Throughout history, people have been subject to pain from injury and disease, and they have continually searched for new and better ways to relieve it. The focus of the search has usually centered on ways to block the sensations of pain, and for centuries, physicians and pharmacists have sought the perfect analgesic, one that would be effective, safe, and nonaddictive.

The pain research of the '60s and '70s concentrated on the *nature of pain* itself, not merely on efforts to block pain. Researchers began investigating transmission of pain impulses and the impact of pain on various structures of the brain as well as the mechanisms that relieve pain. Research on the meaning, interpretation,

---

Guide for Taking a Pain History

- *Location.* Where is the pain? (In addition to asking the patient where it hurts, ask him to point to the painful area. There may be a discrepancy between the two sites, and the area to which he points is likely to be the most accurate.)
- *Onset.* When and how did the pain begin?
- *Precipitating factors.* What precipitates the pain? What aggravates it?
- *Duration and timing.* When does the pain occur and how long does it last? Is it cyclical, regular, or random?
- *Quality.* What does the pain feel like?
- *Severity.* On a scale of 0–5 or 1–10, how severe is the pain?
- *Past occurrence.* When did the pain begin? Has it changed in any way? How often does it occur?
- *Past relief or treatment.* What measures have relieved the pain in the past? Do they still help? What other measures were tried but found unsuccessful?
- *Effects of pain.* How does the pain affect the patient's life? What is the effect, if any, on his appetite? Sleeping? Disposition? Ambulation? Work? Relaxation? Concentration?

and significance of pain is contributing to the development of new theories of pain and pain control.

Complicated or Prolonged Pain

There are at least three major types of facilities and approaches to the management of complex pain problems. First, a patient may be referred to a pain clinic, where a multidisciplinary team of specialists employ a variety of methods to diagnose and treat his particular problem. Pain clinics were rare until the 1970s and are now extensive enough to warrant the publication of a directory of pain clinics throughout the world. Pain clinics differ from one another in their approaches to the evaluation and treatment of pain. Most clinics deal mainly with chronic pain, on both inpatient and outpatient bases.

A second type of pain management is offered by hospice programs, which offer both inpatient and outpatient care to terminally ill patients. The care is supportive and palliative, with special emphasis on the relief of pain. Many of the patients have terminal cancer, and since the question of addiction is almost irrelevant at that point in the patient's life, opium derivatives are used liberally.

The most commonly used drugs are given orally in a mixture called a Brompton cocktail. The original mixture, used in England in Brompton Hospital, possibly as early as 1920, contained morphine, cocaine, gin, and honey. At present there are many formulas and variations in use. In England, either morphine or heroin is the narcotic analgesic. Heroin is illegal in the U.S., and so morphine is used, although methadone is being tried. Some hospices add additional drugs to reduce anxiety or relieve nausea and vomiting. The base of the cocktail is usually alcohol and a sweet flavoring syrup.

The hospice movement is growing rapidly as a result of the efforts of lay people as well as professional health care workers.

A third approach to the management of pain is the holistic health center, which focuses on the treatment of the whole person—body, mind, and spirit. Because pain is a complex phenomenon with both physiological and psychological components, a holistic approach often helps the person with complex, prolonged pain.

Medical Management

Whenever possible, the first medical intervention related to the relief of pain is diagnosis and treatment of the cause. In many situations, the pathophysiology is clearly defined, the diagnosis can be determined quickly, and treatment of the cause of the pain can be started promptly. In other situations, diagnosis may be a lengthy process, and analgesics and tranquilizers are used to control the pain until the cause can be determined.

Treatment of the underlying cause often relieves the pain rather quickly. For example, the pain that accompanies gallbladder disease or a hernia will be relieved by surgical treatment of the causative condition. The pain that accompanies angina or pleurisy is relieved by treating the disease with the appropriate vasodilator or antibiotic drug. Narcotic drugs may be needed for a day or so, but milder analgesics will soon suffice.

If the diagnosis indicates that the pain will be chronic, the physician will be very cautious about the types and amounts of drugs prescribed. Chronic pain control is fraught with many concerns, and the level of relief must be weighed against the problem of side effects and drug dependency when narcotics are often used.

The discovery in 1975 of two types of morphine-like compounds within the body, enkephalins and endorphins, has opened up new areas for study of pain control. *Enkephalins* are found mainly in the areas of the brain associated with pain control; *endorphins* are found in greatest abundance in the hypothalamus and the pituitary gland. It is presumed that these substances activate portions of the brain's analgesic system (Guyton, 1981). It also appears that endorphins inhibit the transmission of painful stimuli at various points along the CNS (Wilson and Elmassian, 1981, p. 722).

Further investigation may show that endorphins may be responsible in part for the effectiveness of various methods of pain relief such as the use of placebos and transcutaneous electric nerve stimulation (TENS).

Nonpharmacologic Management of Pain

Other kinds of medical treatment for persistent, prolonged, and intractable pain include:

Nerve blocks. Injections of various substances such as a local anesthetic close to a nerve to block transmission of pain impulses along that nerve.

Surgery. Surgical interruption of certain paths in the nervous system that relay pain impulses to the brain.

Dorsal-column stimulation. Electrical stimulation of the dorsal aspect of the spinal column by impulses from an implanted electronic device.

Acupuncture. The insertion of special needles into the body at specific locations and at prescribed depths and angles for anesthesia during surgery and for the relief of pain; needles are rotated manually or attached to a battery-operated pulsator.

Hypnosis. A method of relieving pain based on the

power of suggestion and carefully focused attention; useful in altering a person's reaction to pain.

Biofeedback. The use of instruments that give the patient information about his control over specific physiological functions and conditions that are normally involuntary. Some people can learn to assume varying degrees of self-control over pain.

TRANSCUTANEOUS ELECTRICAL NERVE STIMULATION (TENS). Another medical intervention that is currently used more frequently and for less difficult problems is TENS. This technique involves stimulation of the skin by a mild electric current through electrodes placed against the skin. Some stimulators are as small as a pack of cigarettes and can be used 24 hours a day. Other stimulators are used in a clinic setting three to five times a week. TENS is used primarily for chronic pain in adults and children, but its use for postoperative pain is being studied. The mechanism by which TENS relieves pain is not fully understood. A physician's prescription is needed for the sale or rental of a TENS unit.

Nursing Interventions

The nurse who is effective in caring for people in pain does not rely on a single approach to the treatment of pain. Skill in using a variety of interventions coupled with the philosophical belief that *pain can and should be controlled,* form the basis for the effective relief of pain.

Patient Teaching

One of the first and most significant interventions related to pain is patient teaching. Ignorance of the facts, lack of understanding, uncertainty, and doubt can increase the fear and anxiety that often accompany pain to an almost intolerable level.

A purposeful, planned teaching program that is instituted as soon as possible will help to avert an unmanageable level of anxiety and stress. When high anxiety is present, there is a tendency for a person to perceive a greater intensity of pain. The more a patient can learn about when pain is likely to occur, how to reduce it, and what to expect, the more in control of the pain he will be. The element of surprise is reduced and the patient feels less victimized.

A careful assessment of each patient will help to differentiate between patients who find considerable security in knowing as much as possible about their situations, and patients who find the details threatening. Depending on the patient's age, level of awareness, and personality, the following areas are likely to be of concern to him:

What is causing my pain? Something terrible, like cancer or AIDS?

Most people tend to fear the worst, and many live in near panic until a firm diagnosis is made. The patient needs to have a full and accurate understanding of his condition, proposed tests, planned treatment, and possible outcomes.

Is my pain going to get worse?

Many patients can tolerate considerable pain if they know what to expect in terms of duration, intensity, and quality of the pain. Precise answers are not possible, but you can advise a patient, for example, of the pain that usually follows most abdominal surgery, about the duration of the second stage of labor, or of the sore throat that follows a tonsillectomy.

What will I do if I can't stand the pain any longer?

Every person worries about losing self-control and being unable to cope. The patient needs to know what he can do to help himself, what kind of assistance is available, and how help can be summoned.

Nursing Interventions Related to the Causes of Pain

It is irresponsible for a nurse to ignore the *cause* of a patient's pain. This is especially true when she deals with problems of pain by administering a prescribed drug rather than by attending to factors related to the cause of pain.

AVOIDANCE OF PAINFUL STIMULI. Pain can often be averted by keeping painful stimuli from reaching the patient. If, for example, a patient experiences pain from his gastric ulcer about one-half hour before each scheduled mealtime, it is most beneficial to make sure that a portion of his meal is served *before* he experiences pain. If a patient with advanced bone cancer cringes in pain each time the bed is bumped or jarred, such pain should be *prevented* by hanging signs on the patient's door, bedside curtain, and the bed itself, reading: "Caution—Do not bump or jar bed. To do so causes intense pain." Such a sign will help reduce the number of occurrences caused by people simply unaware of the problem, such as the cleaning person, visitors, and laboratory technicians. It might also be necessary to rearrange the unit or to pad portions of the bed frame to prevent pain that follows each jolt and jar of the bed.

There are many ways pain can be prevented or minimized by careful scheduling of events, effective positioning of the patient, and avoidance of conditions (such as constipation or visits by an irritating acquaintance) that predictably precipitate pain for the patient.

REMOVAL OF SOURCE. Three causes of pain that are especially amenable to nursing intervention are ischemia, muscle spasm, and mechanical interference with body functions. These causes are often interrelated, and nursing care that affects one will also affect the others. The pain that results from ischemia can be lessened or even averted by any measures that increase the flow of oxygenated blood through the area. Appropriate exercise, enough heat to promote optimal vasodilation, avoidance of pressure against the walls of arteries which exerts a hindrance to arterial flow into the area and prevention of venous stasis are all examples of nursing measures to relieve ischemia.

Mechanical causes of pain can be minimized by avoiding positions and movements that exert pressure, create friction, or stretch, pull, or otherwise elongate body tissues. Examples of mechanical sources of pain are a distended bladder or bowel; an arm, leg, or neck twisted into poor position; compression of tissue against a hard surface; abrasion of skin from friction; and injury to tissue from a shearing force. Muscle spasms can be minimized by gentle handling of a body part, relaxation techniques that avert some muscle tension, and general reduction of stress.

Nursing Interventions Related to Relief of Pain

PAIN IN CHILDHOOD. Children are often allowed to suffer more pain than adults would tolerate, and pediatric nurses and doctors tend to underestimate a child's pain. This may be due to *misconceptions* that: (1) children experience pain differently than adults do, (2) they either do not feel, do not communicate, or do not remember pain, and (3) children are more likely than adults to have problems with narcotic dependency or respiratory depression from narcotic drugs (Fig. 37.2). Appropriate doses and careful monitoring for any possible side effects of analgesics make it feasible for the child to have full relief from pain.

Nursing management of the child in pain will vary according to the clinical situation and the individual child, but will center around three main activities:

- Providing adequate pain relief with appropriate analgesics and other selected strategies
- Sharing with colleagues the latest research related to pain relief in children
- Helping the child and his family cope with the pain experience

It is important for the nurse to demonstrate confidence in each measure used to relieve pain, and to assure the child and family that pain relief is a high priority in the overall treatment plan for the child. Pain

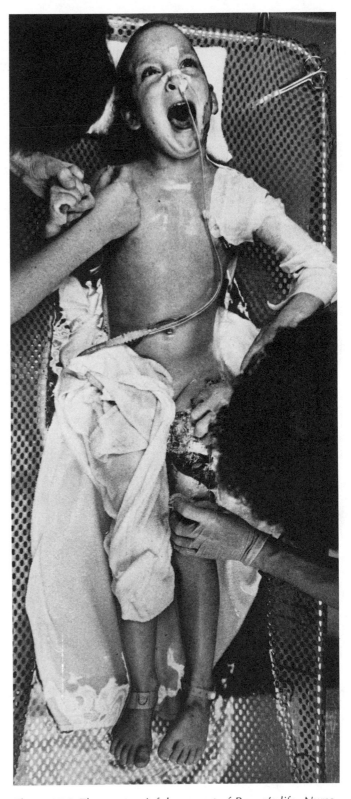

Figure 37.2 *The most painful moment of Renee's life. Nurse Debbie Nowack holds her hand as Bill Myers strips the blood-caked gauze from her thighs.*

associated with trauma can be especially difficult for a child because the injury is not only painful, but it limits the child's activities. Careful explanations and the presence of parents or other loved ones are also important aspects of any program of pain relief for a child.

REDUCTION OF FEAR AND ANXIETY. Fear, anxiety, and pain are so intricately interrelated that any measure that reduces fear and anxiety also reduces the perception of pain (McCaffery, 1979). Measures that accomplish this for a given patient are highly individualized and must be based on verbal and nonverbal input from the patient. Such measures include specific relaxation techniques, thorough patient teaching, emotional support and encouragement, spiritual guidance, a secure environment, and close physical contact.

Most of these nursing measures are an integral part of effective nursing, but specific relaxation techniques are not included in most nursing programs. These techniques include meditation, progressive relaxation exercises, self-hypnosis, transcendental meditation (TM), yoga, special breathing exercises, and many others. Some techniques such as TM and yoga require intensive practice by the patient over an extended period; others can be taught to the patient for immediate use. Most measures to promote relaxation are not new or unique but involve the conscious, deliberate use of interventions adopted from familiar activities. For example, the *infant-toddler technique* of relaxation (McCaffery, 1979) is essentially the same technique that mothers have used for centuries to relax and soothe a distraught infant: close physical contact with a rocking motion accompanied by the repetitive use of familiar and endearing terms, often in a singsong manner.

You will need to read widely on relaxation, select a few methods that seem consistent with your interests and aptitudes, and then develop skill in using them. You will need a repertoire of techniques to promote relaxation in patients of different ages and personalities who have various degrees of fear and anxiety.

DISTRACTION. Distraction from pain has been defined as "focusing attention on stimuli other than the pain sensation. . . . Attention to pain is sacrificed in favor of attention to other stimuli" (McCaffery, 1979, p 92). Distraction increases a person's tolerance for pain by diverting his attention away from the pain (Fig. 37.3). One of the most basic examples is that of talking with a patient throughout an uncomfortable procedure. Some patients, both adults and children, have already developed techniques of their own, such as counting, reciting poems, working puzzles, singing, knitting, playing cards, or any other activity that takes their minds off their pain.

Guidelines for Using Distraction to Relieve Pain

- *Distraction should be used in conjunction with other methods of pain relief.* It is usually not effective for long periods of time and therefore is used intermittently throughout the day.
- *The forms of distraction used must be consistent with the age and interests of the patient.* A TV comedy may be distracting for one patient; a game of chess, more effective for another.
- *Solitary forms of distraction are not helpful for some patients.* Many children, for example, are distracted from pain by a game of cards with another person but not by a game of solitaire.
- *Some people will use the same form of distraction for days on end; others need a variety of forms each day.*
- *Distraction that will be effective depends in part on its complexity and on the intensity of the pain.* A complicated diversion can be very effective with moderate pain, but it may be overwhelming when the pain is severe. The energy needed for the distraction cannot exceed the patient's energy and ability to concentrate.

It is important to realize that the effectiveness of distraction is not directly correlated with the intensity of the pain. Some patients with severe pain find relief through distraction; others with less pain do not find it very helpful. Therefore, staff and families should not assume that a person who can be distracted does not really have much pain. Although the intensity of the pain may be unchanged by distraction, the patient is temporarily less aware of it because he is not thinking about it as much.

If the concept of distraction is unfamiliar to the patient and family, it may take time and patience for it to become effective. It should be introduced as an adjunct form of pain relief, not as a substitute for a method on which he is currently dependent, such as analgesic drugs. His need for drugs may diminish as distraction becomes effective, but he is likely to reject distraction altogether if he fears that he might have to give up the relief he obtains from his medications.

CUTANEOUS STIMULATION. Cutaneous stimulation is the stimulation of the skin in an effort to relieve pain. Many explanations of this phenomenon have been set forth, and currently the gate control theory proposes that impulses generated by stimulation of the skin inhibit the transmission of pain impulses. The effects of cutaneous stimulation are highly variable and often unpredictable but have been beneficial to many patients. The techniques of cutaneous stimulation include the use of

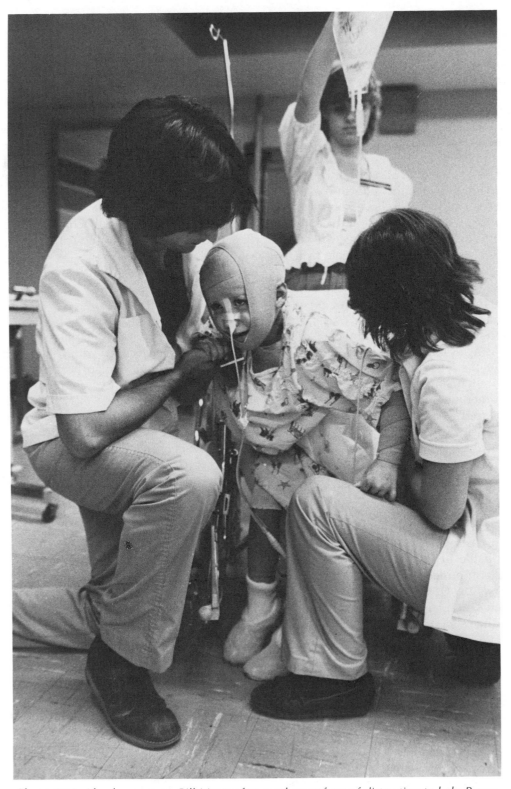

Figure 37.3 *After her surgery, Bill Myers often used some form of distraction to help Renee cope with her pain.*

massage, liniment, vibration, heat and cold, pressure, and electrical stimulation such as TENS.

Massage, especially the backrub, was used extensively in the past to promote comfort and relaxation. Early nursing textbooks emphasized the importance of the therapeutic effects of back massage, but in recent years, the art and science of massage has not been emphasized as a pain reliever in nursing. Health spas and athletic departments, however, have utilized the benefits of massage, and have employed masseurs and masseuses who participate in the treatment of clients and athletes. Massage is effective in the reduction of muscle tension and spasm, and pain is relieved by increasing blood and lymphatic flow and by using massage as a counterirritant. It is expected that massage will be used with increasing frequency for the relief of pain by nurses who seek alternatives to the use of analgesic drugs.

GUIDED IMAGERY. Imagery is the therapeutic use of images, or one's imagination, for healing or pain relief. The patient is taught to remember or imagine a significant situation, using as many of his five senses as possible. Imagery for the relief of pain often involves the recollection and reliving of a happy party, a day at the beach, or some other memorable event. This technique is sometimes referred to as *Waking Imagined Analgesic* (WIA).

Imagery is currently used with cancer patients for healing in conjunction with traditional methods of treatment. When used in this way, the patient creates for himself an *image of the healing that is taking place within his body*. A child, for example, might visualize his white blood cells as astronauts repelling the enemy (the cancer) with laser guns, and each treatment represents another battle in which the enemy is getting smaller and smaller. Considerable research is being done by persons such as Dr. O. C. Simonton to explore the ramifications and potential uses of imagery, both for healing and for the relief of pain.

STAYING POWER. Nurses are with the patient more frequently and for longer periods than any other health care workers and therefore have a unique opportunity either to relieve his pain or to help him learn to live with it. The care of a person in pain can be extremely difficult for the nurse as well as the patient, especially if the pain is intractable (not easily managed). It is not easy to give effective care to a patient who is frightened, angered, or depressed by severe and unrelenting pain. It is not easy to stand by the patient, to "hang in there" when nothing seems to be fully effective, and the nurse requires a special attribute known as *staying power* in order to do so. This characteristic makes it possible for a nurse to provide whatever physical and psychological comfort is possible by her presence, skill, and caring.

PATIENT TEACHING

The *patient* must learn that there are many ways in which he can participate in controlling his own pain, and *families* must learn ways to show compassion and support without letting the presence of pain dominate the life of the entire family. All persons involved with severe or chronic pain must know that even though it may not be possible to change the fact that pain is present, it is possible to change one's response to it, thereby creating a variety of new approaches to the problem.

RELATED ACTIVITIES

1. Read as widely as possible about the ways in which individuals have coped with pain. Lay literature will be especially helpful to you because first-hand, personal accounts of experiences with pain are usually rich in details which are often missing in professional literature. Try to read a number of books or articles written by parents who describe how they and their child coped with severe or chronic pain.

2. Encourage your patients to *talk about their pain*, and to describe the physical sensations and emotional responses which they are experiencing. "Textbook" descriptions can provide a basis for understanding the nature of pain, but it is the information which your patients share with you that will increase your sensitivity and skill in coping with pain.

SUGGESTED READINGS

Arrowsmith, Frances M, and Linda A Barile: Is it just a headache—or a warning? *RN* 1983 Oct; 46(10):29–32.

Beyerman, Kristine: Flawed perceptions about pain. *Am J Nurs* 1982 Feb; 82(2):302–304.

Booker, Jack E: Pain: it's all in your patient's head (or is it?) *Nursing 82* 1982 March; 12(3):47–51.

Bourbonnais, Frances: Pain assessment: development of a tool for the nurse and the patient. *J. Adv Nurs* 1981 July; 6(4):277–282.

Conway-Rutkowski, Barbara: Getting to the cause of headaches. *Am J Nurs* 1981 Oct; 81(10):1846–1849.

Graffam, Shirley: Congruence of nurse-patient expectations regarding nursing intervention in pain. *Nursing Leadership* 1981 June; 4(2):12–15.

Gramse, Carol Anne: For the control of severe pain: dorsal column stimulation. *Am J Nurs* 1978 June; 78(6):1022–1025.

Guyton, Arthur C: *Textbook of Medical Physiology.* ed. 6. Philadelphia, Saunders, 1981.

Hassett, James: Acupuncture is proving its points. *Psych Today* 1981 Dec; 14(12):81–89.

Heidrich, George, and Samuel Perry: Helping the patient in pain. *Am J Nurs* 1982 Dec; 82(12):1828–1833.

Jacox, Ada K: Assessing pain. *Am J Nurs* 1979 May; 11(5):895–900.

McCaffrey, Margo: Would you administer placebos for pain? *Nursing 82* 1982 Feb; 12(2):80–85.

McCaffery, Margo: When your patient's still in pain, don't just do something: SIT THERE. *Nursing 81* 1981 June; 11(6):58–61.

McCaffery, Margo: *Nursing Management of the Patient With Pain.* ed. 2. Philadelphia, Lippincott, 1979.

McGuire, Lora: 7 myths about pain relief. *RN* 1983 Dec; 46(12):30–31.

McGuire, Lora, Shayne Dizard, and Karen Panayotoff: Managing pain: in the young patient . . . in the elderly patient. *Nursing 82* 1982 Aug; 12(8):52–57.

McMahon, Margaret A, and Sr. Patricia Miller: Pain response: the influence of psycho-social-cultural factors. *Nurs Forum* 1978 17(1):58–71.

Melzak, Ronald: *The Puzzle of Pain.* New York, Basic Books, 1973.

Melzak, Ronald, and Patrick Wall: Pain mechanisms: A new theory. *Science* 1965; 150(11):971.

Meyer, Theresa M: TENS—relieving pain through electricity. *Nursing 82* 1982 Sept; 12(9):57–59.

Perry, Samuel W, and George Heidrich: Placebo response: myth and matter. *Am J Nurs* 1981 April; 81(4):720–725.

Sandroff, Ronni: When you must inflict pain on a patient, *RN* 1983 Jan; 46(1):35–39.

Vadurro, Judith F, and Priscilla A Butts: Reducing the anxiety and pain of childbirth through hypnosis. *Am J Nurs* 1982 April; 82(4):620–623.

West, B Anne: Understanding endorphins: our natural pain relief system. *Nursing 81* 1981 Feb; 11(2):50–53.

Wilson, Ronald W, and Bonnie J Elmassian: Endorphins. *Am J Nurs* 1981 April; 81(4):722–725.

38

Care of Wounds

Prerequisites and/or Suggested Preparation
The pathophysiology of inflammation, infection, and the healing process (Chapter 12), concepts related to body image (Chapter 24) and the principles of surgical asepsis (Chapter 27), are basic to understanding this chapter.

The cleansing and dressing of wounds has long been an important nursing activity and, although the advent of new materials such as non-stick dressings and stretch gauze bandages have simplified many procedures, the *significance* of the activity has not diminished. In many respects, the care of wounds is more critical than ever before because of the increasingly complex surgery that is being performed and because new strains of pathogenic organisms have increased the hazards of infection.

In this chapter, the word *wound* is used to designate an interruption in the continuity of muscle, skin, or bone. The term includes a variety of interruptions such as a surgical incision, severe burns, a gunshot wound, or an open pressure sore, for example. There are other types of tissue damage which are sometimes called wounds—bruises, sprains, or abscesses, for example—but this chapter is limited to the care of wounds that involve an intentional or accidental *severing or separation* of skin, muscle, or bone.

PSYCHOLOGICAL ASPECTS OF WOUND CARE

Some illnesses have little or no outward manifestation. No one can tell, for example, by looking at a person whether he has cancer, kidney trouble, diabetes, or hypertension. The onset of such a disease is gradual, and the patient is not faced with an immediate and obvious change in his body. A wound, on the other hand, elicits an immediate response, both from the person with the wound and from the person caring for him. These people may be parent and child, patient and nurse, or accident victim and passerby, but each one will have a psychological response to the wound.

Reactions of the Patient

It is not possible to predict how a person will react while a nurse is caring for his wound. The age and personality of the patient, the duration and nature of the wound, and the nurse's approach will affect the patient's reaction. Reactions to similar wounds will vary from patient to patient; but even more significantly, reactions will vary from day to day for a given patient.

While you are caring for a patient's wound, he may act irritable, critical, bossy, tearful, agitated, or resigned, or may exhibit any of a number of other behaviors. These outward manifestations of inner stress do not identify the source of the stress, and therefore you cannot base your response on the patient's overt behavior. To help the patient, you must determine the reason for his behavior.

First of all, do not presume to know the basis for a patient's behavior. Until you know what the wound and its care means to him, it is not possible to understand his reactions. Some possible responses of a patient to a wound and its care are:

Distress and anger ("Why me?")

Relief ("The surgery is over and I'm still alive!")

Denial of any negative feelings ("Doesn't the incision look great?")

Embarrassment ("I wish you didn't have to do this for me; it looks so awful.")

Guilt ("It's my own fault. I wouldn't be in this condition if only I had listened to the doctor, been more careful, acted more sensibly, etc., etc.")

Fear ("I don't know if I can stand the pain"; "This is going to take every penny we've got," etc.)

While you are caring for the patient's wound, it is important to listen for the *underlying message* of his verbal responses and observe his nonverbal responses carefully. These messages may be very different from the literal meaning of the words he is using. A patient's jovial and seemingly carefree attitude with many "humorous" references to the wound can be a defense against strong feelings of fear or revulsion.

Second, the degree to which you can help a patient depends on your ability to concentrate on caring for *the patient* rather than caring for his wound. A technician could be trained to dress a wound adequately, but the nurse is often the only person who helps the patient face his grief or anger so that he can adequately cope with the forthcoming stresses of convalescence or rehabilitation.

Reactions of the Nurse

Some wounds are easy to care for. A neat, clean incision following an appendectomy can, for example, be dressed with little or no psychological reaction within the nurse. On the other hand, the care of an open, draining, foul-smelling wound can be an ordeal for both patient and nurse. If an adult patient with massive burns cries with pain during each dressing change, or if a child screams with fear and must be both restrained and comforted, wound care can be as emotionally exhausting for the nurse as it is for the patient.

An honest acknowledgment of your own feelings is a first step in learning to function effectively. It is *not true* that "a good nurse can cope with anything; nothing bothers her." A good nurse can be nauseated by the odor of drainage from an infected wound as easily as anyone else. A good nurse may want to cry whenever the patient is hurt, whether physically by the debridement of necrotic tissue, for example, or psychologically by the knowledge that his surgery for cancer was done too late to effect cure.

ASSESSMENTS

Before you care for a patient's wound, you need to determine its nature and condition. Some data can be obtained from the Kardex and the patient's chart, but other information can be obtained only by examining the wound.

Data From the Kardex

Medical Orders

The physician's orders will often specify when, how, and by whom the wound will be dressed and treated. If the dressing itself is an essential part of the patient's treatment, the physician usually assumes responsibility for the care of the wound. A plastic surgeon, for example, will usually change the pressure dressing over newly grafted skin.

The physician's orders will indicate whether a dressing that becomes saturated with drainage should be changed by the nurse or reinforced with additional absorbent material until the physician can come to examine the wound.

Nursing Orders

The Kardex should indicate the preferred or usual way of caring for a patient's wound. The position of the patient, the equipment used, the sequence of actions, and patient preferences should be noted so that there is consistency and continuity of care. It is disconcerting for the patient to have a nurse devise a method of wound care that is safe but very different from the one with which he is familiar and which he may have helped to develop.

Data From the Chart

The admission notes or the operative notes will give the date of the patient's accident or surgery, the location and nature of the wound, and the types of sutures and drains, if any. The physician's progress notes and the nurse's notes should indicate the current condition of the wound and should describe the nature of any discharge, extent of healing, appearance of the surrounding tissue, any signs of infection, and other pertinent information.

Data From Examination of the Wound

Because the notations on the patient's chart were written at the time of the most recent dressing change, which might have been 12 to 24 hours earlier, the only reliable way to obtain current data about a wound is to actually *look at it*. It may not be feasible for you to examine the wound before you care for it, and if not, you will need to use information from the Kardex, the chart, and the patient to anticipate and predict the equipment and supplies you will need to care for the wound.

When the wound is exposed, the following aspects should be examined, recorded, and reported as needed: sutures, drains, drainage, healing, and signs of infection.

Sutures

The edges of an incision can be held together by sutures (stitches), metal clips, or adhesive butterfly tapes. *Internal sutures* are absorbable and therefore need not be removed. *Skin sutures* are usually made of black silk, nylon, or fine wire. Skin sutures or metal clips are removed in approximately 7 to 14 days, depending on the size and location of the incision or injury, the condition of the tissue, and the rate of healing.

Retention sutures extend across the incision and are inserted several inches beyond each side. They are used to reduce tension on the regular sutures of the skin and underlying tissue when there might be any unusual pull on the incision, from the weight of any extremely obese abdomen, for example.

Drains

A drain is inserted in a wound to remove an accumulation of normal body fluids, to promote drainage of purulent material from an infected wound, or to separate the edges of a deep wound so that it will heal from the deeper portion outward toward the surface. Drains can be made of hard rubber or plastic, like a catheter, or from soft rubber or latex, like a rubber glove. A *Penrose drain* is a soft rubber drain which usually has a large safety pin inserted crosswise through it to keep it from slipping down into the incision. A *cigarette drain* is a Penrose drain with a strip of gauze inside it to promote drainage. A drain is often removed by pulling it out a little more each day, although the physician may remove it all at once.

Some large wounds are packed with long strips of gauze that act like a wick or a drain. The gauze is often impregnated with iodoform or an antibiotic. Packing is usually removed after a few days, but drains can be left in place for longer periods.

Some drains, such as chest tubes, are attached to a suction machine. Other drains are attached to small, self-contained suction units, such as a Hemovac. These devices create a gentle suction which removes oozing drainage, such as blood from the site of a fractured hip.

Drainage

The discharge from a wound is described as *serous* (clear), *sanguineous* (bloody), *serosanguineous* (blood tinged), or *purulent* (thick and green or yellow). The amount of drainage is described either by measuring the quantity collected in the suction container, or by indicating the number of gauze pads that were saturated in a given time. An example of the latter might be "serosanguineous drainage soaked through three 4″ × 4″ gauze pads and one ABD (abdominal dressing) pad in 2 hours." When you assess the amount of drainage from a wound, be sure to look at the lower portion of the dressing and *under the patient's body.* Drainage can seep down from beneath the dressing and leave the upper portion dry, as if there was no drainage from the wound.

Some drainage is normal with certain types of wounds, but the physician should be notified at once if the amount seems excessive, if it is actually bloody rather than merely blood tinged, or if previously clear drainage is becoming purulent.

Sometimes there is drainage from a wound under a freshly applied cast, which soaks through and stains the cast. That area of the cast should be checked frequently, and after each check, the edges of the spot should be outlined with a waterproof pen or pencil, and the time and date written beside the outline. The physician should be kept informed of the rate of drainage because, if it continues, he may need to open the cast and assess the wound.

Healing

If the wound is *healing by first intention,* the edges of the incision will be aligned and approximated, and there will be only a thin line of scar tissue. There should be no sign of infection.

If the wound is *healing by second intention,* the edges of the wound are NOT together, and the wound heals gradually, filling in the granulation and scar tissue. There may be patches of *slough* (black necrotic tissue) that will loosen spontaneously or will be removed by the physician to uncover an area of living but unhealed tissue.

Dehiscence is an uncommon complication in which there is a spontaneous separation of the edges of a wound after surgery. It can occur when the patient's tissues are friable (easily torn) and fragile. *Evisceration* is the protrusion of the contents of a body cavity, usually the abdomen, through the separated edges of a wound.

Signs of Infection

The edges of an incision should be straight, even, approximated, and the same color as the surrounding skin. If the edges are rough, uneven, swollen, red and tender, the wound is probably infected. Other signs of infection are purulent drainage from the wound, pain or tenderness in the area of the wound, and an elevated body temperature.

DRESSINGS AND BANDAGES

A dressing consists of one or more layers of gauze, often covered with a thick, absorbent pad, and it is held in place by a bandage, a binder, or adhesive tape.

Dressings are applied to:

- Protect the wound from contamination by bacteria, dust, and dirt
- Absorb drainage and protect clothes and bedding
- Promote drainage via wicks, packing, and drains
- Keep ointment and medication on a wound
- Apply pressure to control bleeding

Bandages are used to keep dust and dirt out of a wound, to keep ointment on a wound, and to hold a dressing in place. Elastic bandages are used to immobilize a joint, to aid venous return from the legs, and to apply pressure to control bleeding or prevent swelling.

Some wounds are left uncovered to air-dry the surface and promote healing. A dry wound forms a scab and starts to heal more quickly than a moist one; a skinned knee that is uncovered tends to heal faster than one that is kept covered with adhesive bandages such as Band-Aids, for example. Some surgeons cover certain types of incisions with only thin layers of gauze applied loosely enough to let air circulate through and under the gauze. The decision to leave a wound uncovered or loosely covered is based on the location and nature of the wound and on the likelihood of infection. A *superficial wound* such as an abrasion or a shallow pressure ulcer, or an incision that does not penetrate a body cavity, can be left uncovered or lightly covered.

CHANGING A DRESSING

Pertinent details of wound care for each patient, such as the frequency and method or procedure, should be available on the Kardex. If the information is incomplete, the patient is an invaluable source of information. Ask him to describe the method that has been used and with which he is familiar. If it is feasible, you can then follow that procedure, using those principles of surgical asepsis which relate to the procedure.

Equipment

In some institutions, sterile dressing trays are purchased or prepared by the central supply department; in other agencies the nurse will need to assemble her equipment and supplies item by item. The sterile items commonly used to change a dressing include gauze squares (called sponges), absorbent pads, gloves or thumb forceps for handling sterile objects, scissors, antiseptic solution for cleansing the skin, medication, and cotton balls. In addition, the nurse will need adhesive tape, bandage, or a binder and also a newspaper or receptacle for the old dressing.

Preparation of the Patient

First explain the procedure to the patient as needed, and then pull the curtains around his bed to provide privacy and reduce air currents and possible contamination of the wound. Position the patient and make him comfortable and adjust the lighting as needed.

Depending on the patient's understanding of the procedure, tell him how he can help. Tell him not to sneeze, cough, or laugh across the wound and not to touch anything sterile. An infant or an irrational patient may need to be temporarily restrained (Fig. 38.1).

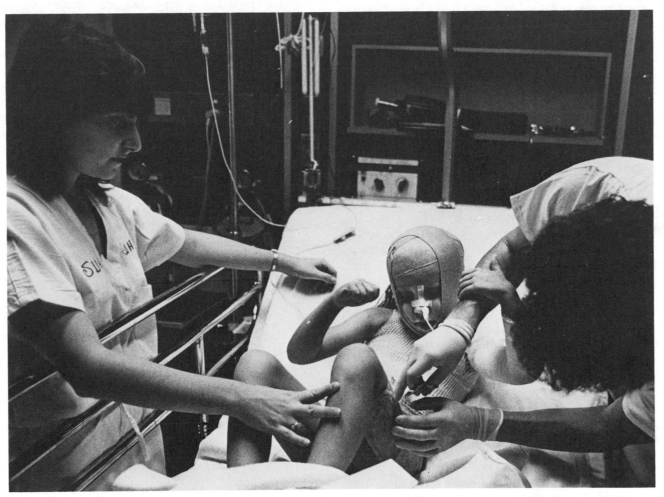

Figure 38.1 *Since the possibility of infection poses the greatest threat to Renee's recovery, sterile technique is used whenever her dressings are changed. Renee knows that she must not contaminate the sterile field, and therefore she keeps both hands well away from the dressing and the nurse's sterile gloves.*

Preparation of the Wound

Remove the bandage, adhesive tape, or binder to expose the dressing. A binder, if worn, should be unfastened and opened, or removed completely if it is soiled. A gauze bandage should be cut to one side of the wound to avoid running the bandage scissors over the wound. Collect the bandage in your hand as you cut it and drop it onto a newspaper or into a lined waste container.

Adhesive tape is removed by pulling each strip of tape *toward the incision* to avoid pulling on the incision. Tapes on the first side of the incision are automatically pulled toward the dressing, but the last half of the tape is often incorrectly removed by continued pulling in the same direction, which places considerable tension on the suture line.

If the outer layers of the dressing are *dry,* you can pick the dressing up with your fingers and drop it into the lined waste container or onto a newspaper. The dry gauze acts as a barrier between your fingers and the incision. If the dressing is wet with drainage, use forceps to pick it up and discard it. The forceps are then contaminated and cannot be used to pick up a sterile object.

If the innermost layer of the dressing is stuck, do *not* pull it loose. Carefully look under the dressing to see where it is stuck. If the dressing is adhering to an area of skin away from the wound, it may be possible to loosen it gently. If, however, the dressing is stuck to the wound, the underlying tissue will be damaged by pulling the dressing loose, and therefore you will have to *soak it off* with sterile water or hydrogen peroxide. This can be done by pouring the liquid over the dressing, by using a syringe to squirt liquid over the dressing, or by placing saturated gauze over the stuck gauze and letting the moisture soak through.

Should you ever encounter an eviscerated wound, wet some sterile gauze with sterile saline solution and quickly cover the area to keep the mucosa from drying out. Evisceration is frightening for both patient and nurse, and someone should stay with the patient while the physician is notified and the patient is prepared for surgery to repair the gaping wound.

Cleansing the Area

If the wound or incision is clean, with no evidence of fresh or dried drainage and no sign of infection, the nurse should *leave it alone,* apply a dry sterile dressing (DSD), and secure it. A wound should be touched as little as possible because each contact increases the possibility of accidental contamination and infection. If, however, there is fresh or dried drainage on the wound,

it must be cleaned off before the fresh dressing is applied.

The manner in which you cleanse the area depends on the location and type of wound, and the amount and type of drainage. If there is a small amount of drainage on or around the wound, you can probably clean the area with cotton balls and an antiseptic solution. If the fibers of the cotton balls catch on the sutures or skin clips it may be advisable to substitute 2-inch gauze squares for cleansing the area. If the wound and surrounding skin are covered with *copious drainage,* cotton balls may not suffice. You may need to start cleansing the area by washing the skin with a washcloth and soapy water, carefully keeping the washcloth several inches away from the incision or wound to avoid any possible contamination of the wound with bacteria from the skin. If the drainage is thick and purulent, minimize the spread of pathogens by using disposable materials such as soft paper or gauze squares. Moisten and soap them, one at a time, and cleanse the skin around the wound, discarding each gauze square or paper tissue after it has been used; do *not* put it back into the basin of water.

When the skin around the wound has been cleaned, cleanse the incision or wound. Pick up a cotton ball with your gloved hand or forceps, dip it into the sterile solution, and press it against the side of the container to remove any excess liquid. Make one stroke down the center of the incision (Fig. 38.2), or one small circular movement in the center of an irregular wound or puncture wound (Fig. 38.3). Discard that cotton ball, and repeat the process as many times as necessary, making only one stroke each time. The object is to move *away* from the incision with each stroke, or out in concentric circles from the central part of a wound.

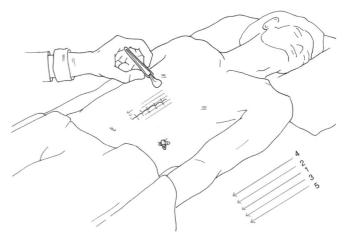

Figure 38.2 *A systematic pattern for the aseptic cleansing of a wound. The numbered arrows indicate the sequence of strokes.*

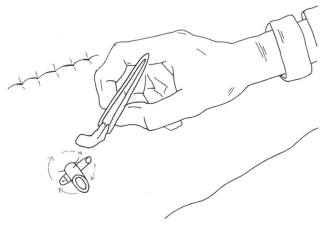

Figure 38.3 *Circular movement for cleaning around a puncture wound.*

This sequence of strokes is important because the incision or wound is considered cleaner than the surrounding skin. Even if the wound is infected, the skin may harbor other kinds of bacteria that could be transmitted to the wound. The skin around the wound protects the rest of the body from the pathogens in an infected wound.

Old adhesive marks can be removed with acetone. Keep the acetone away from the incision and rinse off the acetone with water or saline solution. Use mild soapy water and rinse well if the patient's skin is irritated. In the home, nail polish remover can be used if the patient is not sensitive to it and if it is thoroughly removed.

Dressing the Wound

If the skin is irritated from drainage, protect it from further irritation either by covering the clean skin with a thick, heavy ointment such as zinc oxide, or by laying a strip of gauze impregnated with petrolatum (vaseline gauze) along each side of the incision. Press the gauze down smoothly against the skin so that any drainage will run over the top of it.

The first layer of the new dressing should have a non-adherent surface such as Telfa or be made of a gauze mesh that is so fine that it will not stick to new granulation tissue. The gauze squares which are used for dressings are packaged both individually and in bulk. The commonly used sizes are 4 inches × 4 inches and 4 inches × 8 inches and are commonly referred to as 4 × 4s and 4 × 8s.

If the wound is draining, one or more thick, absorbent pads are placed over the gauze. Extra padding may be needed at the lower edge of the dressing or at the sides because the drainage will run down the sides of the patient's body when he is supine and down toward his feet when he is erect.

PROCEDURE 38.1

*Changing a Dressing**

SUMMARY OF ESSENTIAL NURSING ACTIONS

1. Check patient's chart and/or Kardex to determine the previous condition of the wound, the type and amounts of supplies needed, and any specific techniques which have proven helpful.
2. Assess the psychological aspects of the dressing change. (Is there an odor? Is the wound repulsive or extensive? Has the patient looked at the wound yet?)
3. Decide whether you need a prepackaged dressing tray, or whether you should merely assemble a few necessary items.
4. Prepare a sterile field as described in Procedure 25.
5. Maintain surgical asepsis at all times.
6. Gently and cautiously remove the old dressing.
   - Pull any adhesive strips TOWARD the incision or wound to avoid tension on the suture line or granulation tissue.
   - If the old dressing is stuck to the wound, loosen it by wetting the dressing with sterile water or saline.
7. Cleanse the skin gently but thoroughly.
   - Cleanse the area around a drain OUTWARD in ever enlarging concentric circles.
   - Cleanse the skin around an incision OUTWARD from the suture line.
   - Remove old adhesive with acetone as needed and rinse skin.
8. Apply any prescribed medication or protective ointment as needed.
9. Apply an appropriate dressing and secure it with adhesive, binder, or bandage.

*See inside front cover and pages 743–745.

PROCEDURE 38.2

*Irrigating a Wound**

SUMMARY OF ESSENTIAL NURSING ACTIONS

1. Check Kardex and/or patient's chart to determine the method which has been used.

2. Make sure that you have the correct quantity of the prescribed solution at the correct temperature.

3. Prepare the patient properly.
   - Position the patient so that the irrigating solution will flow by gravity from the wound into a curved basin placed against the body part.
   - Keep the bed dry with a towel or absorbent waterproof pad.

4. Maintain surgical asepsis throughout the procedure.

5. Remove and discard the old dressing.

6. Cleanse the area around the wound as necessary.

7. If the irrigating solution is irritating to the skin, protect the skin with sterile vaseline or other protective ointment.

8. If the wound is deep, gently insert the tip of the syringe or catheter into the wound.

9. Instill the irrigating solution into a deep wound, or flush it over a shallow wound, using slow, steady, and minimal to moderate pressure.

10. Allow irrigating fluid to drain from wound by gravity. DO NOT SUCTION THE FLUID BACK unless specifically ordered to do so!

11. Repeat actions 9 and 10 until the returning fluid is clear or the prescribed amount of solution has been used.

12. Dry the skin with sterile gauze and apply a sterile dressing.

13. Use your observations regarding the effect of the irrigation as a basis for determining the need for subsequent irrigations.

*See inside front cover and page 746.

Irrigating a Wound

In order for a wound to heal, it must be clean and free from purulent material and necrotic tissue. In many instances, the wound is cleansed by irrigating it to loosen and flush out the pus, drainage, and dead tissue. The solution to be used is prescribed by the physician, and will vary from sterile saline or solution of hydrogen peroxide to an antiseptic or antibiotic solution.

If the wound is shallow, such as a pressure sore or decubitus ulcer, the wound can be irrigated by means of a bulb syringe to squirt the irrigating fluid over the surface of the wound. If the wound is deep, such as an infected incision or stab wound, the tip of a catheter or the end of a rubber-tipped syringe must be inserted into the wound in order for the irrigating fluid to reach and cleanse the interior of the wound.

SECURING A DRESSING

The dressing is held in place by adhesive tape, bandage, or a binder, depending on the size and location of the dressing and the need for additional support.

Adhesive Tape

If the patient is allergic to adhesive tape, this fact should be noted in a prominent place on his chart. *Hypoaller-*

genic (nonallergic) tape is available and must be used for such patients because the blisters and subsequent excoriation from an allergic reaction are difficult to heal. If the area to be taped is covered with heavy hair, shaving the hair will increase adhesion of the tape and make its removal less painful.

Montgomery Straps

When a dressing must be changed frequently, Montgomery straps are used (Fig. 38.4). These are wide straps

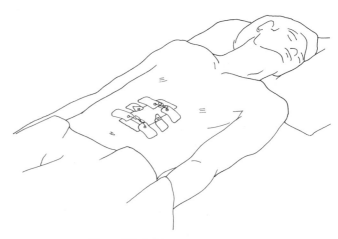

Figure 38.4 *Montgomery straps.*

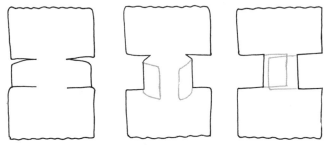

Figure 38.5 *Steps in preparing a butterfly closure for keeping the edges of a wound together.*

that can be bought commercially or fashioned by hand from wide adhesive tape. Each strip of tape is folded back on itself so that about a third of it is no longer sticky. A hole is made in the nonsticky end of each strap to make it possible to lace and unlace the straps to change the dressing without removing the adhesive tape each time. Tincture of benzoin is sometimes applied to the skin before the adhesive tape is applied to increase the adhesion of the tape and to protect the skin from irritation.

Butterfly Tapes

Butterfly tapes can be used instead of sutures to close a superficial wound. They can be purchased or are easily made by hand (Fig. 38.5). Two cuts are made on each side of a strip of tape. The middle section on each side between the cuts is then folded in to cover the center of the adhesive, forming a nonsticky bridge that does not adhere to the wound.

Bandages

Bandages are used alone to cover and protect a wound or to hold a dressing in place over a wound. Elastic (Ace) bandages are used to support or immobilize a joint or to give support to weakened or dilated veins in the legs. Bandage comes in rolls and is handled as shown in Fig. 38.6.

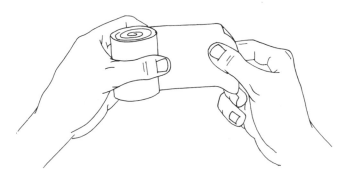

Figure 38.6 *Position for holding a roller bandage.*

Characteristics of Commonly Used Bandages

- *Gauze.* Inexpensive, but frays with use and cannot be reused. Has no stretch and is hard to use over irregularly shaped surfaces.
- *Muslin and cotton flannel.* Firm, durable, washable, and cheap. Can be made from strips of old sheets. Has little or no stretch.
- *Stretch gauze.* Easy to apply; assumes the contour of any body part; does not slip. Expensive; cannot be reused.
- *Stockinet.* Tubular knit fabric used to encase a body part. Heavy cotton jersey knit is used under a cast; loose stockinet is used to hold a dressing in place. Used as a head covering after brain surgery. Washable, durable.
- *Elastic bandage.* Expensive, durable, washable. Used for support, or for immobilization of a joint. Held in place by metal clips or safety pins.

Types of Bandages

The choice of fabric for a bandage depends on purpose, cost, durability, and the area to be bandaged.

Bandages are usually held in place by adhesive tape, although muslin and flannel bandages can be fastened with safety pins. Another way to secure a bandage is to split the end, tie the two end pieces in a single knot, wrap the two split ends in opposite directions around the bandaged part, and knot them securely.

A bandage that can be reused is rolled up as it is removed so that it is ready to be reapplied. If it is soiled and cannot be reused without being washed, it is carefully gathered up as it is removed so that it does not touch the floor or any other contaminated surface. Gauze bandages are removed by being cut off with bandage scissors. Do not cut the bandage section directly over the wound; the pressure of the scissors can be painful on the wound, and the scissors could slip and injure the wound.

Criteria for Effective Bandaging

A properly applied bandage is safe, effective, economical, and esthetically pleasing. A bandage should be durable, applied snugly enough so that it cannot slide off, and fastened securely. The width of the bandage used should be appropriate for the size of the body part to be bandaged. A 4 to 6 inch wide bandage is appropriate for an adult's thigh, for example, whereas a ½ to 1 inch wide bandage is suitable for a baby's hand. The bandage should be long enough to cover the area with a one-half width overlap on each turn. Excess length should be trimmed off rather than wrapped around the part because of the danger of creating excessive or uneven pressure. Safety depends on appropriate pressure, body alignment, and care of the skin.

PRESSURE AND TENSION. Pressure from a bandage must be evenly distributed. Each turn should overlap the preceding turn by a consistent amount, usually one-half the width of the bandage.

The tension of a stretch or elastic bandage should be even and moderate throughout. An elastic bandage should be snug enough to support the veins or joint, but *not* tight enough to restrict circulation. Because each turn overlaps the preceding one, the pressure from an elastic bandage is somewhat cumulative, and the bandage should be *stretched very little* as it is being applied. Circulation of the extremity should be checked soon after the bandage application, and at regular intervals thereafter.

BODY ALIGNMENT. If one or more joints are bandaged, care must be taken to bandage the joint in a position that is *safe and functional* for the patient. If a patient is susceptible to contracted joints, for example, his hands should probably be bandaged with his fingers extended to minimize the danger of contractures. Another patient's hands might well need to be bandaged with the fingers slightly flexed.

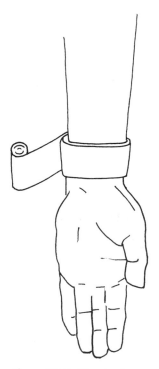

Figure 38.7 *Circular turns.*

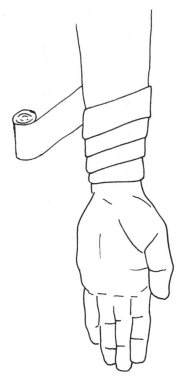

Figure 38.8 *Spiral turns.*

PROTECTION OF THE SKIN. Skin surfaces such as adjacent fingers or the folds of the axilla should be separated with gauze sponges or other absorbent fabric before bandages are applied. Skin surfaces that are in contact with each other are likely to become moist, and eventually macerated or excoriated.

If a bony prominence such as an ankle, scapula, or heel is bandaged, it should be padded to protect the skin against prolonged pressure from hard surfaces because the area will be covered and cannot be massaged to stimulate circulation.

Turns

There are five commonly used turns in bandaging: circular, spiral, spiral-reverse, figure-eight, and recurrent.

CIRCULAR. Nearly all bandaging begins and ends with two circular turns to anchor the end of the bandage. The second turn completely overlaps the first one (Fig. 38.7).

SPIRAL. The spiral turn is used around a body part that has a *consistent diameter* throughout its entire length, such as a child's forearm or lower leg. The first turn is angled upward from the circular anchoring turns, and all succeeding turns are parallel, with a one-half-width overlap (Fig. 38.8). Spiral turns can be combined with figure-eight turns around a joint such as the ankle.

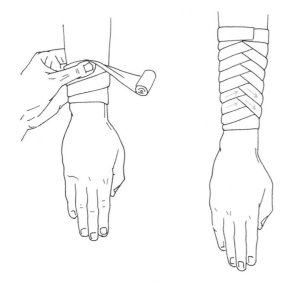

Figure 38.9 *Spiral-reverse turns.*

SPIRAL REVERSE. The spiral-reverse turn is used when the diameter of an extremity *increases rather quickly,* as on an adult thigh or forearm (Fig. 38.9). Spiral-reverse turns are often combined with figure-eight turns over a joint.

FIGURE EIGHT. The figure-eight turn is used to ensure a secure bandage over a joint (Fig. 38.10). If a leg, for example, is bandaged from ankle to groin with spiral or spiral-reverse turns, the turns over the knee would tend to shift and slip every time the knee was bent. A figure-eight turn permits some motion of the knee, ankle, hip, or elbow without disruption of the bandage.

RECURRENT. The distal portion of an extremity is difficult to bandage. The tip of a finger, the top of the head, or the stump of a leg following an amputation, for example, are rounded and hard to cover. The recurrent bandage is anchored securely and is then positioned on first one side and then the other of a center strip. These back-and-forth turns are overlapped by each succeeding turn (Fig. 38.11). Each strip of bandage is relatively long, and the turns are easily loosened, so they must be secured with spiral or spiral-reverse turns.

The advent of *stretch gauze,* such as Kling and Kerlex, has made it possible to bandage the end of an extremity without difficulty, using modified recurrent turns. The stretch gauze conforms to the shape of the part to be bandaged, and it does not slip.

Binders

In lieu of adhesive tape or bandages, a dressing can be held in place by a binder. Binders can be purchased commercially or sewn from muslin or cotton flannel and they are commonly applied over the abdomen, perineum, and breasts.

A *straight abdominal binder* is used to hold a dressing in place, to support a weak or pendulous abdomen, and to relieve tension and strain on an abdominal incision. Abdominal binders can be purchased in a variety of fabrics and sizes with adjustable Velcro tabs, or they can be sewn of muslin and fastened with safety pins.

A *scultetus (many-tailed) binder* serves the same purposes as a straight binder, but it conforms to the contour of the body and stays in place better (Fig. 38.12). The overlapping straps give firm, comfortable support. When you apply a scultetus binder, position it so that one of the two fully exposed straps is at the bottom and next to the patient's skin and is the first strap to be wrapped. If a strap that is partially covered by an overlapping strap is wrapped first, none of the tails will wrap smoothly.

A *T binder* is used to hold a rectal or perineal dressing in place (Fig. 38.13). T binders are made of muslin or cotton flannel and are fastened with safety pins. A double-T or split-T binder is used for a male patient and is

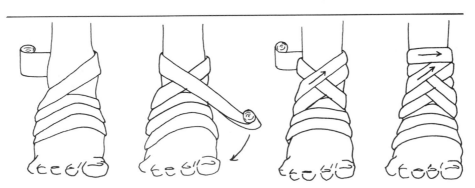

Figure 38.10 *Figure-eight turns.*

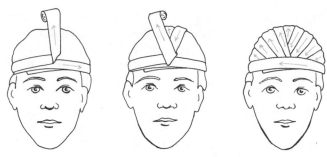

Figure 38.11 Recurrent bandage.

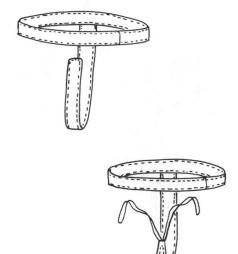

Figure 38.13 T binders.

positioned with a strap on each side of his scrotum. These T binders are occasionally hard to locate because some institutions seem to consider them outdated, but you should go to any length to obtain one for a male patient who needs it. Do not take the easy way out and give him an obviously feminine sanitary belt to hold his perineal dressing in place.

A *breast binder* is used most frequently to give support and apply pressure when a woman wants to dry up her breasts after childbirth. Most breast binders are straight and flat; small darts must be made with safety pins to support each breast and ensure a proper fit (Fig. 38.14).

Slings

A sling is used to limit movement of the patient's shoulder, elbow, or wrist and also to help support the weight of a cast. The *weight should be distributed across the patient's shoulders and back, not* around his neck (Fig. 38.15). Tying a sling around the neck is an easy and familiar method of application, but it can be both uncomfort-

able and dangerous for any person with a history of a stiff neck, arthritis, cervical injury, poor posture, or an unsteady gait.

The purpose of a sling determines its usage, and both nurse and patient should know the answers to questions such as: Should the sling be worn all day? At night? Can the sling be removed for bathing and dressing? If so, can the joints be extended, or should they remain flexed as if still in the sling?

If the sling is used to *promote healing* by immobilizing a joint, such as the elbow, the patient may be forbidden to extend his elbow when the sling is removed for bathing. If the sling is used *for comfort only*, the patient may be ordered by the physician to extend his elbow or to exercise his shoulder several times daily to maintain his range of motion.

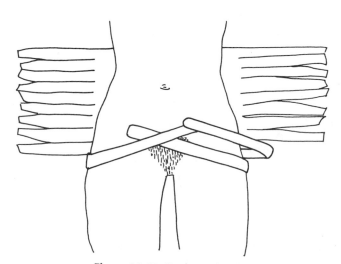

Figure 38.12 Scultetus binder.

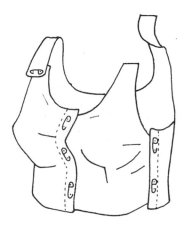

Figure 38.14 Breast binder.

Antiembolism stockings (often referred to by a trade name, T.E.D.) must be correctly fitted if they are to provide the proper comfort and support. Size is based on the circumference of the patient's calf and thigh, and stockings are available in both regular and long lengths. They are made in three styles: knee length, thigh length, and full length.

Elastic stockings should not be put on like ordinary stockings because, whenever the fabric is gathered up or bunched up, the *tension is greatly increased* and application is difficult and often painful. To apply an elastic stocking, reach into the stocking, grasp the center of the heel pocket, and turn the stocking inside out as far as the heel. Slip the foot and heel of the stocking onto the patient's foot, make sure the patient's heel is centered in the heel of the stocking, and then gradually work the stocking up over the ankle and calf. (Check the manufacturer's directions for details of application, especially for full-leg stockings with a waist belt.) Antiembolism stockings are removed for bathing and should be exchanged for clean ones whenever soiled or sweaty. The patient's circulation and skin should be checked each time the stockings are removed, and most brands have an opening on the underside of the foot that enables the nurse to pull the stocking back to check the circulation of the toes while the stocking is in place.

If the patient is to wear antiembolism stockings at home, make sure he knows how to put them on correctly, and that he is physically able to do so.

SPLINTS

A splint is a rigid device used to maintain a prescribed or desired position of a bone or joint. It can be made of metal, plastic, or plaster (Fig. 38.16). Some splints are inflatable; others, such as a cervical collar, are made

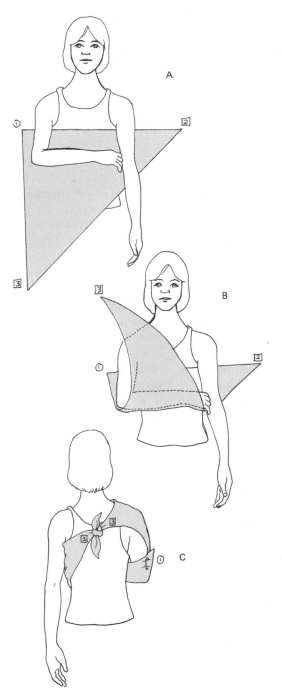

Figure 38.15 *Preferred method of applying a sling. Note that the weight of the arm is supported by the shoulder and back (c).*

Elastic Stockings

Elastic stockings (antiembolism stockings) are used in lieu of elastic bandages to promote venous return by supporting the veins in the legs. When used properly, they are easier to apply and are more comfortable, the pressure and support is more even, and they do not slip and wrinkle.

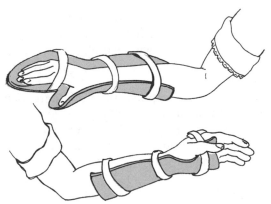

Figure 38.16 *Two types of splints. Top: patient's hand is immobilized. Bottom: patient has use of thumb and fingers; the wrist is immobilized.*

of a combination of materials. In an emergency, rolled up newspapers or magazines, a pillow folded lengthwise around an extremity, or pieces of wood will splint and protect a broken arm or leg.

Splints are used to:

Maintain the position of a bone after an accident to minimize the chances of further injury

Immobilize a bone or other tissue to promote healing

Relieve the pain of muscle spasms

Prevent or treat muscular contractions, such as foot drop or contractures of the fingers

Support weak muscles and permit various activities of daily living such as feeding and dressing oneself

Splints are used for these purposes with patients who have arthritis, cerebral palsy, muscular dystrophy, and injuries to the musculoskeletal system and nervous system.

The nursing care of a patient with a splint includes:

- Checking the circulation in the fingers or toes of the splinted extremity
- Examining the skin over bony prominences such as the malleolus of the ankle and the epicondyles of the elbow and then either adjusting the contour of the splint or using padding to relieve any areas of pressure
- Providing adequate skin care, including regular bathing
- Ensuring regular range of motion exercise when the splint is being used for a purpose other than immobilization and can be removed

CASTS

A cast is applied to maintain the position of a bone after a fracture has been reduced or set, once the broken ends of the bone have been aligned. A cast is also used to treat certain orthopedic conditions such as a club foot or scoliosis.

Before the cast is applied, the body part is encased in a length of tubular stockinet to protect the skin. Layers of wet gauze impregnated with plaster of Paris are then wrapped around the part until the cast has the desired strength and size. The wet cast *must be supported* on plastic-covered pillows to (1) maintain the normal body contours of the cast until it is dry and (2) keep the cast from flattening, breaking, or cracking while it is soft and wet. The cast will feel warm to the touch as the plaster crystallizes and dries. It takes 1 to 3 days for

a large cast to dry and the process cannot be speeded up very much because, if the outside dries too fast, the inner layers are sealed off and do not dry properly.

The edges of the cast must be finished off to protect the patient's skin from the irritation of rough edges and loose particles of plaster. This can be done by pulling the stockinet out and over each end of the cast, thereby covering up its edges.

The edges can also be finished by cutting oval petals of adhesive tape and overlapping them to cover the edges of the cast.

A cast is adjusted or removed by an electric cast cutter, which vibrates rapidly and causes the plaster to disintegrate along the cutting line. The process is noisy, and the patient needs to be reassured that the vibration cannot cut his skin.

Some casts, known as *bivalved casts,* are divided lengthwise into two parts so that first one half of the cast and then the other can be removed for examining or treating the underlying skin and tissue. One half of the cast is always in place to maintain the position of the body part. In some situations the body part is bandaged into the lower half of the cast, and the top half is left off for extended periods of time.

If drainage from a wound continues to seep through a cast or if the patient complains of localized pain under his cast, a window is cut into the cast to permit inspection of the wound or painful area. The window is not filled in with fresh plaster until the wound has ceased to drain or the pain has been relieved.

TRACTION

Traction is the pull exerted against the ends of a bone, usually to align a broken bone. Traction can be either *skeletal* (direct) or *skin* (indirect). Skeletal traction requires an attachment directly into the bone and perfect aseptic technique is needed to prevent infection at the point of entry into the bone. Skin traction is accomplished by attaching the traction apparatus to the skin, usually with wide strips of adhesive tape. Both skeletal and skin traction depend on weights and pulleys to exert the necessary pull on the affected bone. The physician specifies the weight to be used, such as 2, 5, or 10 lb, and it is essential for the prescribed weights to *hang free* (Fig. 38.17).

Some weights are heavy enough to pull the patient toward the foot of the bed; if this movement is not counteracted, the patient's feet will soon be pressed against the foot of the bed, or the weights will be resting on the floor. In either case, the prescribed pull of the traction is negated. A weight can exert no pull when it is resting on the floor; nor can traction be effective

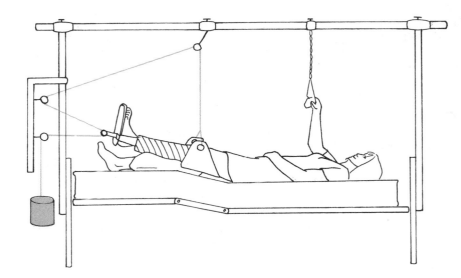

Figure 38.17 *Patient in traction. The weight must hang free at all times to exert the prescribed amount of traction.*

when the body part is braced against the foot of the bed. This situation can be prevented by checking the patient's position in bed at regular intervals and moving him toward the head of the bed as needed. It may also be necessary to shorten the weight cords, but unless you are knowledgeable about the principles of traction, this action should be taken only after consultation with the person who set up the traction apparatus. The interaction of weights and pulleys is complex and easily distorted by seemingly simple adjustments.

PATIENT TEACHING

Self-care often involves the care of a minor wound incurred at home or at work, or the care of a surgical wound after the patient's discharge from the hospital. In either case, the individual or his family needs to be taught the basic concepts of medical and surgical asepsis. An initial assessment of their current knowledge of both cleanliness and sterility plus an understanding of their available resources will provide the basis for a teaching plan which will be both realistic and effective. In some situations, the individual may have an extensive knowledge of asepsis, while in others, your teaching will have to start with an emphasis on frequent handwashing.

In order for teaching to be effective, you must know enough about the individual's environment and resources to help the person devise a plan of care which is realistic and acceptable. It is necessary to know, for example, whether he is financially able to purchase sterile dressings, or whether he must be taught to prepare a safe dressing by ironing a freshly washed piece of sheeting.

Each person who cares for a wound must know what to expect as the wound heals, the signs and symptoms of infection, what to do if possible complications arise, and under what circumstances he should contact the doctor.

RELATED ACTIVITIES

1. Begin to consider wounds from *two* points of view. First, study the clinical aspects of each situation, taking into account the pathophysiological processes involved, and the type and effect of the treatment being given. Second, try to imagine how the wound has affected, or will affect the individual, his family, and anyone else who is close to that person. How might you react if the wound were on your body or on the body of a person who is important to you?

2. Begin to develop your ability to help a patient or his family *talk* about a significant wound. Listen for cues which indicate whether they are ready and able to deal with their feelings, or whether they are still unable to do so.

Ask skilled practitioners how they help patients and families deal with their reactions to painful or disfiguring wounds. If you had been there, what would you have tried to do to help Renee, her brother, and her parents as they tried to deal with the psychological and physical aspects of her burns?

SUGGESTED READINGS

Bailey, Mary: Emergency! First aid for fractures. *Nursing 82* 1982 Nov; 12(11):72–81.

Bruno, Pauline: The nature of wound healing. *Nurs Clin North Am* 1979 Dec; 14(4):667–682.

Cohen, Stephen, and Gigi Viellion: Nursing care of a patient in traction. (programmed instruction) *Am J Nurs* 1979 Oct; 79(10):1771–1796.

Cuzzell, Janice Zeigler: Wound care forum: Artful solutions to chronic problems. *Am J Nurs* 1985 Feb; 85(2):162–166.

Davis, Judith, Lois Jedlicka, and Franklin Johnson: Sure-fire asepsis for your TPN patients. *RN* 1982 Dec; 45(12):39–41, 91.

Evers, Judith Anne, and Donna Werpachowski: Dealing with fractures. *RN* 1984 Nov; 47(11):53–57.

Farrell, Jane: Casts, your patients, and you—part 1: a review of basic procedures. *Nursing 78* 1978 Oct; 8(10):65–69.

Farrell, Jane: Casts, your patients, and you—part 2: a review of arm and leg cast procedures. *Nursing 78* 1978 Nov; 8(11):57–61.

Farrell, Jane: Casts, your patients, and you—part 3: a review of hip-spica procedures. *Nursing 78* 1978 Dec; 8(12):53–57.

Flynn, Margaret E: Promoting wound healing—influencing repair and recovery. *Am J Nurs* 1982 Oct; 82(10):1550–1558.

Flynn, Margaret E, and David T Rovee: Wound healing mechanisms. *Am J Nurs* 1982 Oct; 82(10):1545–1549.

Fritz, Carolyn P: Emergency! First aid for wounds. *Nursing 82* 1982 Oct; 12(10):68–75.

Meshelany, Cecelia: Post-op wound dressings. *RN* 1979 May; 42(5):22–23.

Neuberger, Geri Budesheim, and Joann Bell Reckling: A new look at wound care. *Nursing 85* 1985 Feb; 15(2):34–41.

Strange, Julie M: An expert's guide to tubes and drains. *RN* 1983 April; 46(4):35–42.

Welch, Lynne Brodie: "Relatively" painless wound debridement. *RN* 1983 Oct; 46(10):39–41.

39

Care of the Surgical Patient

Prerequisite and/or Suggested Preparation
This chapter, without prerequisite preparation, can provide a general overview of the care of a surgical patient, but full comprehension and understanding of this material *is dependent upon the content of Chapters 10, 12, 23, 27, 28, 29, 31 through 34, 37, and 38.*

Surgery is a major mode of medical therapy, and it is so commonplace that many people fail to realize that all surgery is serious, and that all operations are potentially life-threatening. Approximately 20 percent of all operations are unavoidable, such as those made necessary by trauma, hemorrhage, or appendicitis in which neither the doctor nor the patient has a choice. About 80 percent of all operations are elective—chosen by the patient based on medical advice.

Surgery is often classified as major or minor. *Minor surgery* results in little alteration in body structure or function, and represents little threat to life. Minor surgery is often performed in a surgeon's office or an outpatient surgical clinic. Local anesthesia is usually sufficient, but general anesthesia may be used. Though such surgery is regarded as minor, the operation often creates fear and anxiety for the patient and family, and is never without risk of unexpected complications.

Major surgery is usually performed under general anesthesia in a hospital setting, and results in extensive alteration of a body structure or function. Major surgery is always serious and is often life-threatening.

The *outcome* of a surgical procedure depends upon a variety of factors, including the:

- Physical and psychological condition of the patient
- Nature of the surgery
- Skill of the surgeon
- Competence of the anesthetist or anesthesiologist
- Adequacy of equipment and supplies
- Competence of operating room personnel

The interrelatedness of these factors makes it impossible to guarantee the outcome of any operation, and as a result, surgery is a stressful experience for the patient, family, and members of the health care team. Everyone is concerned about the risks of anesthesia, infection, equipment failure, and unexpected pathological findings, and in addition, the patient worries about pain, possible disfigurement, dependence on other people, a sense of powerlessness, changes in career and family roles, and the possibility of death. Many operations have an extremely low risk factor and a uniformly high rate of success, but until such an outcome is *certain,* some degree of stress is inevitable.

There are five types of surgery, which are not mutually exclusive and often overlap. These are categorized as follows:

- Diagnostic: to determine the cause of symptoms
- Curative: to remove a diseased organ or part
- Restorative: to correct a problem or strengthen a weak area

---

> ### Suffixes That Describe Common Surgical Procedures
>
> ectomy: removal of organ or gland; ex. appendectomy
> orrhaphy: repair by suturing; ex. herniorrhaphy
> ostomy: providing an opening or stoma; ex. colostomy
> oscopy: visually examining an organ or cavity; ex. laparoscopy
> plasty: cosmetic or plastic repair; ex. rhinoplasty

- Palliative: to relieve the intensity of pain and suffering even though the disease or problem cannot be cured
- Cosmetic: to improve the appearance (plastic surgery)
- Transplantation: to replace a dysfunctional organ or structure; may be either curative or restorative

Perioperative nursing is a relatively new term which includes all three phases of the care of a surgical patient: preoperative, intraoperative, and postoperative.

PREOPERATIVE ASSESSMENTS

Nursing History

It is imperative that the nurse obtain from the patient and/or his family the information which will provide a basis for individualized and relevant nursing care, both preoperatively and postoperatively. This information is referred to as the nursing history and is very different from the patient's medical history. The nursing history makes it possible for the nurse to plan nursing care which takes into account the patient's physical and psychological responses to the forthcoming surgery, and to use the patient's perceptions, expectations, and misconceptions as the foundation for patient teaching which will be needed.

Medical History

The patient's medical history provides information which may prove helpful in planning appropriate nursing interventions. A review of the patient's past illnesses and the reason for his seeking medical help often reveals conditions which could increase the risk of complications postoperatively if they were not taken into account. Information about medications and allergies is important because some drugs increase risks during and after surgery, and the regular use of any medication

TABLE 39.1 DRUGS WHICH AFFECT SURGICAL RISK

Type of Drug	Adverse Effect
Antibiotics	Untoward reaction if incompatible with anesthetic
Anticoagulants	Increase blood coagulation time
Depressants	Decrease central nervous system responses
Diuretics	Can create electrolyte imbalance, especially of potassium
Tranquilizers	Can cause hypotension, which contributes to shock

should be noted (Table 39.1). Allergies, especially medication allergies, should be noted on the front of the patient's chart and on the preoperative checklist.

Physical Assessment

Cardiovascular Assessment

Prior to surgery the patient's vital signs are taken and recorded. Surgery may be delayed or reconsidered if the *systolic* blood pressure is below 90 mm Hg or the *diastolic* pressure is above 120 mm Hg. The skin temperature, color, pulses, and sensation of the extremities are noted, with particular attention paid to evidence of ankle edema, cyanosis, or clubbing of the fingers. The patient is questioned about his history of smoking, drinking, and chest pain.

BLOOD STUDIES. The blood is typed and cross-matched in preparation for possible transfusions, and the following preoperative blood studies are usually done:

- WBC (white blood cell count)
- RBC, Hct (red blood cell count, hematocrit)
- Hgb (hemoglobin)
- Blood chemistry (sodium, potassium, chloride, blood glucose, CO_2 (carbon dioxide), and BUN (blood urea nitrogen)
- FBS (fasting blood sugar)
- Platelet count, bleeding and clotting time, and prothrombin time

An elevated WBC may be indicative of an inflammatory process, such as pneumonia or other infection, that would contraindicate surgery, while a decreased WBC may indicate bone marrow depression and an inability to fight infection, which might also contraindicate surgery. A low Hct may indicate overhydration, while a high Hct is indicative of dehydration.

EKG (or ECG). The condition of the heart, any cardiac arrhythmias, and myocardial damage are assessed by electrocardiography (an EKG, or ECG), which produces an electrocardiogram. These assessments are necessary for middle-aged and elderly persons as well as for those with suspected cardiac disease, diabetes, and hypertension.

Respiratory Assessment

The respiratory assessment includes the patient's history of smoking and asthma as well as information related to coughing, wheezing, shortness of breath, and difficulty breathing (dyspnea). The patient is examined for evidence of a barrel chest which is characteristic of emphysema, and his chest sounds are assessed by auscultation, palpation, and percussion.

A chest x-ray examination is routinely done in all surgical patients; it will often reveal an unsuspected pulmonary problem such as emphysema or bronchitis. Blood gases assess respiratory function (gas exchange), and tests of pulmonary function are done when there is evidence of respiratory deficiency.

Renal Assessment

The patient is examined for evidence of disturbed kidney function, such as periorbital edema, cloudy urine, ankle edema, and elevated blood pressure (hypertension). Preoperative urine studies usually include tests for the presence of bacteria, albumin, protein, sugar, acetone, pH, BUN, nonprotein nitrogen (NPN), specific gravity, creatinine, and electrolytes.

High-Risk Groups

Factors which increase the risks of surgery include old age, poor nutritional status, and substance abuse. Patients with defects in regulatory processes, such as the endocrine, cardiovascular, respiratory, and renal systems, are also at increased risk.

Age

Arteriosclerosis, hypertension, atherosclerosis, and cardiac defects place elderly patients at risk for complications after surgery. The lungs of older persons do not exchange oxygen and carbon dioxide as efficiently as those of younger persons, thus increasing the likelihood of pulmonary problems. There is also a loss of functioning renal tissue.

Nutritional Status

Patients who are malnourished may be in negative nitrogen balance; they do not have an adequate supply of the protein-sparing calories needed for effective healing. An obese patient is likely to have the following problems: (1) difficulty in moving and breathing deeply, which can lead to pulmonary complications; (2) longer time needed for surgery and longer exposure to the anesthetic, which can cause respiratory and circulatory problems; and (3) the poor blood supply in fatty tissues contributes to slower wound healing.

Substance Abuse

The alcohol abuser is often malnourished and anemic; his liver function is diminished, and this renders him less able to excrete medications, including anesthetics. The tobacco abuser is susceptible to pulmonary problems due to excessive respiratory tract secretions; these secretions increase when sedatives and muscle relaxants are administered.

PREOPERATIVE NURSING INTERVENTION

Management of Stress

Stress related to surgery is often briefer and more intense than stress related to some chronic or permanent conditions, and as a result, any necessary nursing interventions must be *prompt* and *vigorous*. Many surgical experiences are so brief that there is no time to "wait and see" how the patient and his family will manage. The nurse must take the initiative to assess the situation, and then quickly take action to support those who are *likely to need help* in coping with the stress of surgery. The nurse's assessments must be started as early as possible, and continued throughout the entire surgical experience as described in Chapter 8.

Preoperative Teaching

Preoperative teaching is an essential nursing intervention during this phase of perioperative care. Some hospitals have well-developed preoperative teaching programs, which utilize a variety of teaching methods including booklets, one-to-one examples, film strips, tapes, and closed circuit television programs. In many institutions, however, preoperative teaching is less effective than it could be because it is given low priority, done at an inappropriate time, or provided inconsistently.

Benefits

Many benefits to the patient result from good preoperative teaching. When the patient knows what to expect, he experiences less stress and anxiety which, in turn, results in less need for pain medication. Postoperative exercises may prevent complications and often facilitate an earlier discharge from the hospital. For example, respiratory exercises decrease respiratory complications such as pneumonia, and leg exercises coupled with early ambulation reduce circulatory problems such as phlebitis and thrombophlebitis.

Timing

Every principle of patient teaching (Chapter 14) is applicable to preoperative teaching; timing, however, is often of special importance. The patient may not be admitted to the hospital until the afternoon of the day before surgery, and a succession of events, such as admission procedures and examinations by the physician and anesthesiologist, make it difficult indeed to find adequate time for preoperative teaching. Some hospitals have resolved this problem by conducting preoperative teaching sessions at various scheduled times before the patient's admission. This teaching is often done on a group basis, although some departments schedule individual appointments. For example, the physical therapy department may require a preparatory session before admission of each patient who is scheduled to have a total hip replacement.

Most preoperative teaching deals with the surgical experience in general rather than with the details of a given surgical procedure; some hospitals have found it both possible and cost effective to conduct preoperative educational programs for groups in the community.

EMERGENCY SITUATIONS. When surgery must be done without delay, preoperative teaching takes on added significance. The nurse must take the initiative to provide the patient with the basic information he needs—information which will relieve his current stress and anxiety. The patient has neither time, capability, nor opportunity to obtain the information he needs, and the nurse has a moral and professional responsibility to act in his behalf. It takes only a few minutes to tell the patient what has been planned, where the surgery will take place, what mode of anesthesia and type of anesthetic will be used, where the patient will be taken after surgery, and what sensations he is likely to experience postoperatively.

Content of the Teaching

Preoperative teaching should encourage hope and a positive attitude, reinforce confidence in the health care system, and provide the patient with the knowledge and skills needed to contribute to his own recovery. The knowledge and skills needed in the immediate postoperative period are related to deep breathing, coughing, turning, leg exercises, and pain control.

DEEP BREATHING EXERCISES. In a patient under general anesthesia, the lungs do not ventilate properly, the cough reflex is suppressed, and mucus accumulates in the respiratory tract. All of these factors contribute to an increased risk of postoperative pulmonary complications so it is mandatory that the patient do deep breathing exercises. These exercises prevent hypoventilation, and improve lung expansion and oxygen delivery. Deep breathing exercises promote maximum gas exchange, prevent atelectasis, enhance circulation, loosen secretions, and force air below the lung secretions so that they can be coughed up. An incentive spirometer is often used to facilitate deep breathing.

COUGHING EXERCISES. A deep, productive cough is needed to remove accumulated respiratory tract secretions. The patient needs to understand the importance of coughing, and how to splint the incision when he coughs. Splinting is necessary because coughing causes discomfort; it is accomplished by placing an article such as a pillow or towel, or the hands, across the incision.

TURNING AND POSITIONING. Placing the patient in the Sims position will decrease tension on abdominal sutures; side-to-side and side-to-back turning should be done as well. Most surgical patients are able to cooperate and turn themselves, and, even though this may take longer, it promotes independence and self-care ability. Good posture and proper body mechanics after surgery can help to prevent complications such as pneumonia, improper drainage of cavities, contractures, circulatory impairment, and urinary or gastrointestinal difficulties.

LEG EXERCISES. Immobility during surgery predisposes the patient to thromboembolic complications. Leg exercises enhance venous return and thereby help to prevent thromboembolic and pulmonary complications.

The patient should be encouraged to flex his legs frequently and slowly, to move his feet, and to exercise his ankles by rotating his feet.

Healing of the surgical wound is more rapid if the patient begins to walk about very soon after surgery. Thus the patient is usually gotten out of bed the day or the night of the surgery. For the first few days he walks frequently but for short distances each time.

PAIN AND PAIN CONTROL. The patient needs to know that medication is available to relieve postsurgery discomfort. Usually it is given every 3 to 4 hours as necessary. In most hospitals, the patient must take the initiative to ask for any prescribed analgesic, and he must be prepared to do so. He should know that it is best to request medication before the pain becomes severe, because it is then less effective. For the first 48 hours after surgery, the patient should take pain medication so that he will be more willing and able to move, deep breathe, cough, ambulate, participate in self-care, and enjoy having visitors. Although not pain free, the patient will be able to rest; he will experience less anxiety and will have a more rapid recovery. Other pain relief measures include positioning, diversion, splinting, and relaxation exercises (Chapter 37).

Preparation for Surgery

Certain procedures are carried out routinely by the nurse for every patient undergoing surgery. These include: (1) obtaining informed consent; (2) providing necessary information; (3) assuring safety for the patient and his valuables; (4) preparing the skin; and (5) administering preoperative medication.

Informed Consent

The preoperative consent form is a legal document. It states that the patient understands the proposed surgical procedure and agrees to undergo it (Fig. 39.1).

ELEMENTS OF INFORMED CONSENT. Informed consent indicates that the patient has been given an explanation of the proposed procedure including the inherent risks, the benefits, and possible alternative treatments. The term means that the patient fully understands all aspects of his consent. This presumes that the patient was intellectually alert and capable, that he was not under undue stress, and that there were no barriers to communication. The patient must have had the opportunity to ask questions and the option to withdraw his consent at any time.

RESPONSIBILITY OF PHYSICIAN. It is the responsibility of the physician to provide the medical information a patient needs in order to make intelligent decisions and to give informed consent for the proposed procedure.

RESPONSIBILITY OF THE NURSE. The patient's signature must be witnessed (unless another notation is contained on the consent form). The nurse's signature identifies her as a witness to the patient's or family member's signature and does not imply that she has provided the patient with the necessary medical information. The nurse is, however, responsible for making sure that the patient understands what he has been told.

Information

In addition to preoperative teaching, the patient and his family need to know the time of surgery and where the patient will be taken in the immediate postoperative period. The family must know where they should wait for the surgeon, who usually meets with them briefly as soon as the surgery is over.

CONSENT TO OPERATE

1. I hereby authorize Dr. _____ and such physicians as may be selected by him to perform
   (Attending Physician)

   upon _____ the following procedure or operation:
   (state "myself" or name of patient)

   _____
   (state nature of procedure in laymans terms)

   _____

   _____

2. If any condition arises during the course of the operation calling, in the judgement of the operating surgeon, for procedures in addition to or different from those described, I further authorize the operating surgeon to alter the procedures as deemed advisable.

3. The benefits and purpose of the operation and the risks and discomforts involved have been fully explained to me. No guarantees have been made with respect to the results that may be obtained.

4. I understand that in addition to the risks explained to me, the possibility of other risks and consequences may arise. I have been advised that if I ask for any further information, it will be given me.

5. I have been advised of possible alternative procedures and they have been explained to me.

6. I consent to the administration of anesthesia and the use of such anesthetics as may be deemed advisable, under the supervision of an anesthesiologist.

7. I hereby authorize the release of any tissue removed to be used for scientific purposes after all necessary diagnostic tests have been completed. I understand that before any such specimens are made available, all identifying information will be removed.

8. For the purpose of medical education I consent to the photography and/or televising of the procedure to be performed provided my identity is not revealed.

9. I have read this entire document and understand its contents. In addition, I have been told that I am free to withdraw any portion of my consent.

10. I have either completed or crossed off any unacceptable statements prior to my signing.

_____ _____ _____
Date   (Time)   Signature of Patient

If consenting party is other than patient:

_____ _____ _____
Date   (Time)   Signature of Parent or Guardian

Witnesses:

_____ _____ _____
Date   (Time)   Signature of Witness

_____ _____ _____
Date   (Time)   Signature of Witness

Physician:

I have discussed the treatment described above with the patient or relative whose signature appears on this document.

_____ _____ _____
Date   (Time)   Physician's Signature

CROSS OUT ANY OF THE ABOVE PARAGRAPHS WHICH DO NOT APPLY AND INITIAL

Figure 39.1 Consent form for operation.

MEDICAL CENTER

<u>PRE-OP CHECKLIST</u>

Complete the Checklist for all Procedures scheduled in O.R., for Angiograms, Heart Catheterizations, Myelograms, Kidney Biopsies, and all procedures in G.I. lab.

1. Allergies: Chart Labeled _____
   No Known Allergies _____

2. Identification Bracelet On _____

3. Teds On _____
   Not Ordered _____

4. Voided: Time _____
   Amount _____

5. Nailpolish, Hairpins,
   Wigs, etc. Removed. _____

6. Pre-Op Medications
   Given and Charted _____

7. <u>Valuables Cared For:</u>   Location:

   Dentures _____ _____
   (Patient to wear dentures for
    Heart Catheterization)

   Glasses/Contacts _____ _____
   Prosthetic Devices _____ _____

   Rings/Medals:
   Removed _____ _____
   Taped On _____ _____

   Jewelry (watches, earrings)
   Removed _____ _____

8. For Heart Catheterization Patients:

   1. 5 lb. Sandbag with
      patient having heart
      catheterization _____
   2. Height _____
   3. Weight _____
   4. Coag/Hgb _____

Chart Assembled:
1. Intake and Output Record _____

2. Vital Signs Record _____

3. Medication Record _____

4. Physicians Orders _____

5. O.R. Permit _____

6. Disposal Permit _____

7. EKG Done____ Report on Chart _____
   (For Patient >40, good for 1 mo.)

8. Chest X-Ray Done _____
   Report on Chart _____
   (For Patient >40, good for 1 mo.)

9. Lab work in chart:

   SMA6_____ CBC_____ UA_____

   Blood: Typed and Screened _____

   Typed and X-matched _____

   Not Ordered _____

10. Addressograph plate with
    chart - _____

_____
Signature of Nurse Preparing
Patient for O.R.

Check List to Remain in Patient's
Record until discharge, then
destroyed.

Figure 39.2 Preoperative check list.

The nurse should also provide information about visiting hours, conveying it in such a way that visitors feel welcome. Communication of information to relatives during the course of the operation is important, and they, in turn, must be encouraged to approach the nurse with their questions or concerns.

Safety and Security

Because surgery takes the patient away from his room and renders him helpless for a period of time, it is necessary to assure that both the patient and his belongings are safe.

Measures used to protect the patient include: (1) removing nail polish, because the anesthesiologist and the surgeon check the color of the nailbeds which indicates the patient's state of oxygenation; and (2) keeping the patient NPO (nothing by mouth) for a period of time before the surgery to prevent vomiting and aspiration both during and following general anesthesia. In some hospitals an enema or a laxative is given, to decrease the possibility of contaminating the surgical area with feces, and to prevent the postoperative constipation which often follows general anesthesia due to decreased bowel motility.

The patient may return from surgery with drainage tubes in place; he needs to be told what to expect and needs to be warned of the possibility of bloody drainage. The nurse must also discuss the placement of chest tubes, catheters, nasogastric tubes, and so on, as well as postoperative monitoring that may be called for.

Before the patient is taken to the operating room, the nurse completes a preoperative check list (Fig. 39.2).

PREPARATION OF SKIN. It was long thought that unshaved skin in the surgical area increased the likelihood of postoperative infection, but research now indicates that the rate of wound infection in patients who are shaved before surgery is greater than in those who are not shaved. Shaving is sometimes done in the operating suite because there is less risk of infection when the interval between shaving and surgery is brief. The Centers for Disease Control recommends the use of clippers or a depilatory for removing hair, to reduce the nicking and cutting that leaves the skin vulnerable to bacterial growth.

CARE OF VALUABLES. To protect the patient's valuables from loss or breakage, it is recommended to the patient that he have a family member (or a friend) take all valuable items and unneeded cash home. Any articles the patient wishes to keep with him can be locked in the hospital safe on the day of surgery. The wedding ring is taped to the finger if the patient does not wish to take it off, but dentures, glasses, contact lenses, wigs, and prostheses must be removed prior to surgery.

TABLE 39.2 COMMON PREOPERATIVE MEDICATIONS

Drug	Example	Effect
Meperidine	Demerol	Analgesic when used alone; no sedative effect; may cause nausea/vomiting; antiemetic and sedative when given with promethazine (Phenergan); may depress respirations
Hydroxyzine	Vistaril	Prolongs and potentiates meperidine
Morphine		Analgesic and sedative; may cause nausea/vomiting; acts on respiratory center and depresses respirations
Atropine		Blocks vagal nerve response of decreased heart beat which occurs as reaction to some inhalation anesthetics; decreases respiratory tract secretions; may increase pulse rate, may be a danger to digitalized patients
Diazepam	Valium	Mild tranquilizer; helps patient relax, making induction of anesthesia easier; decreases stress and anxiety; relaxes skeletal muscles

Medication

The patient is often given a sedative on the evening before surgery to reduce apprehension and promote relaxation and sleep. Preoperative medications such as those listed in Table 39.2 are given on the morning of surgery.

A combination of drugs, such as morphine, atropine, and valium, is often given to produce a sedative, analgesic, and tranquilizing effect. Following such medication, the patient must be kept in bed with the side rails up to ensure his safety.

THE INTRAOPERATIVE PHASE

The intraoperative phase of surgical care begins when the patient is placed on the operating table and ends when he is transferred to the recovery room.

The Operating Room Team

The intraoperative team includes both "sterile" and "nonsterile" members. The sterile team usually includes the primary surgeon, assistants to the surgeon, and the scrub nurse or technician. The nonsterile team

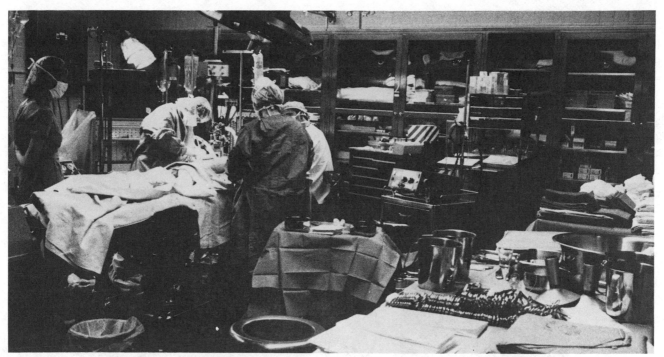

Figure 39.3 *As Renee's surgery progresses, the circulating nurse stands ready to attend to the many and varied needs of the surgical team.*

includes the anesthesiologist or anesthetist, the circulating nurse, and others such as technicians to operate monitoring devices or equipment, biomedical engineers, and a pathologist (Fig. 39.3).

Nursing responsibilities in the operating room are usually divided between the scrub nurse and the circulating nurse.

The Scrub Nurse

The role of the scrub nurse is frequently carried out by a trained technician or a practical (vocational) nurse. This person has the skill and knowledge to anticipate the surgeon's needs and assists him by providing sterile instruments and supplies throughout the operation. The scrub nurse also counts and disposes of soiled sponges and needles, and keeps track of all instruments used during the procedure.

The Circulating Nurse

The circulating nurse is responsible for the smooth running of the operating suite and makes sure that the needs of the surgeons and other sterile team members are met. The circulating nurse also:

- Helps to position and drape the patient
- Provides the scrub nurse with sterile supplies
- Disposes of soiled equipment and sponges, and keeps an accurate count of them
- Assists team members with regowning and regloving if technique is broken

Anesthesia

Anesthetic agents produce insensitivity to pain and other sensations and are administered to the patient throughout the surgical procedure. The goal is to provide analgesia (absence of pain) and skeletal muscle relaxation in the surgical area. Anesthetic agents are of two types: (1) general anesthetics, which are administered by intravenous infusion or inhalation; and (2) local anesthetics, which are applied topically or injected regionally.

General Anesthesia

A general anesthetic is administered by injection or inhalation, and produces loss of consciousness and decreased reflex movement (Fig. 39.4).

The patient who is given a general anesthetic passes through three of four stages:

- Stage one (early induction): from beginning of inhalation to loss of consciousness
- Stage two (delirium or excitement): no surgery performed at this point; dangerous stage; breathing irregular
- Stage three (surgical phase): begins when patient stops fighting and starts breathing regularly
- Stage four: medullary paralysis, respiratory arrest

The outcome of general anesthesia depends on the skill of the anesthesiologist, and the age, condition, and

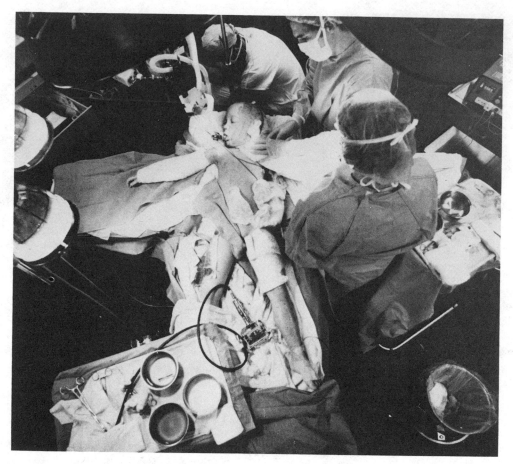

Figure 39.4 Renee's physiological responses to prolonged anesthesia, the loss of skin which normally serves as protection against infection, and pain will make her post-operative care complex and challenging.

preparation of the patient. Patients with cardiovascular, renal, or respiratory conditions are at high risk as are a pregnant woman and fetus. If the patient's stomach is full at the time of surgery, there is great likelihood that he will vomit and aspirate the vomit.

Local Anesthesia

When a local anesthetic is used, the patient is conscious, but pain and sensation are either decreased or absent in the surgical area. The three types of local anesthetics are: (1) topical, (2) infiltrated local nerve block, and (3) regional or central nerve block.

TOPICAL ANESTHETICS. Topical anesthetics, which are applied to the surface of the body, are used extensively for eye surgery, and also for hemorrhoidectomy, episiotomy, minor cuts, and burns. Systemic toxicity is rare, but local reactions are common, especially if the anesthetic is used for long periods of time on a patient who is allergic to it.

INFILTRATED LOCAL ANESTHETICS. This type of anesthetic is injected into the surgical area. Its effect is local, but

may be systemic if the agent is injected into a highly vascular area.

REGIONAL ANESTHETICS. Regional anesthetics are injected into the lower part of the spinal canal and produce analgesia in the lower part of the body. They are commonly known as *spinal, caudal, saddle,* or *epidural* anesthesia and are named for the respective areas into which they are injected.

POSTOPERATIVE CARE

The postoperative phase of surgical care includes both the immediate recovery period, which begins as soon as the operation is completed, and the postoperative convalescence period.

Care in the Recovery Room

If a general anesthetic has been given, the patient is usually taken to a *recovery room*, where care is provided by nurses who have received a report from the operating room team and who continually assess the patient's status. The care given depends on the surgery which was done and the patient's general response to the procedure and to the anesthetic.

Maintaining Respiration

An oropharyngeal or nasopharyngeal airway was inserted while the patient was in the operating room, and it is kept in place until the patient is awake and has regained the cough and swallowing reflexes. These airways are irritating and traumatizing, and the patient will often complain of having a sore throat postoperatively. Obstruction of the airway by accumulated secretions is prevented by suctioning and proper positioning.

Surgical patients often have decreased pulmonary expansion as a result of pain, obesity, lung disease, or drugs; therefore, oxygen may be administered in the recovery room, and deep breathing exercises should be encouraged as soon as the patient is conscious.

Maintaining Circulation

The most common cardiovascular complications in the immediate postoperative period are hypotension and cardiac arrhythmias. A *slight* decrease in blood pressure is common postoperatively, but careful assessment for early signs of *shock* is necessary. Prompt and vigorous treatment for shock can prevent damage to brain, heart, kidneys, and other vital organs. Vital signs are assessed every 15 minutes until stable, and then every 30 to 60 minutes.

Maintaining Fluid and Electrolyte Balance

Intravenous fluid is the primary means of maintaining postoperative fluid and electrolyte balance in the recovery room. Careful monitoring of intake and output is essential to prevent dehydration or overload.

Maintaining Safety and Comfort

Until the patient becomes responsive, safety measures are necessary, including keeping the bed side rails raised, turning the patient frequently, and maintaining good body alignment. Observation of the surgical site, equipment, and suction is also necessary.

Special attention should be given to signs of depression of the respiratory, circulatory, and central nervous systems. The nurse must also note the patient's fears and anxieties as he wakens from the anesthetic, and offer psychological support and reassurance. Careful explanations and orientation to time, place, and person are helpful.

Care in the Postoperative Unit

Patients who are acutely ill, or who require constant supervision and special care, are transferred to surgical intensive care units while other patients are transferred to a regular clinical unit, often the units they were in preoperatively. The patient is transferred from the recovery room to a postoperative unit when:

- Any postsurgical complications have been assessed and controlled
- Vital signs are stable
- Respiratory and circulatory functions are adequate
- The patient is awake and responsive
- Motor and sensory functions have returned following regional anesthesia

To prepare the postoperative unit, the nurse assembles any special equipment needed plus an IV pole, a stethoscope, and a sphygmomanometer. To prepare the postoperative bed, the nurse folds the top covers to the side or foot of the bed to ease the patient's transfer from the stretcher to the bed.

The initial assessment of each patient admitted to a postoperative unit includes:

- Level of consciousness
- Respiratory status
- Circulatory status
- Safety
- Dressings
- Nausea/vomiting
- Comfort
- Equipment and monitoring
- Needs of family members

Maintaining Respiration

Postoperative patients are at risk for pulmonary complications such as atelectasis and hypostatic pneumonia (inflammation of the lung). Atelectasis is a condition in which the bronchioles become blocked by secretions; the distal alveoli collapse when the existing air is absorbed, and hypoventilation results. The severity of the condition depends on the site of the blockage, and whether the entire lung or only one lobe is atelectatic.

Nurses are responsible for carefully assessing the patient's cough and chest expansion, and they use techniques of auscultation and percussion to monitor respiratory function. Nursing interventions to maintain pulmonary function include turning the patient frequently and promoting adequate ventilation by encouraging the patient to yawn, breathe deeply, cough, and use incentive spirometry as indicated.

Maintaining Circulation

Postoperatively, patients are at risk for thromboembolic complications such as phlebitis and the formation of emboli as a result of venous stasis which occurs both during and after surgery. A *previous history* of thromboembolic problems or congestive heart failure places the patient at risk as does the use of oral contraceptives. Immobility, obesity, and poor nutritional status increase the risk, especially for elderly patients and for those having abdominal, pelvic, and thoracic surgery.

Symptoms include discomfort in the legs, redness or tenderness along a vein, edema, and fever. Pain in the calf from dorsiflexion of the foot—the *Homans sign*—is an important indicator of possible thromboembolic problems. Nursing interventions are aimed at *preventing* problems, therefore, elastic stockings such as TEDS are used.

The nurse must teach the patient to:

- Sit with knees *uncrossed*
- Elevate feet on a stool when seated
- Avoid sitting for long periods
- Exercise legs and ankles at frequent intervals

The patient's legs should not be massaged or positioned with a pillow under the knees because massage could loosen a clot which has formed, and pressure against the back of the knee further decreases the already slowed circulation.

Maintaining Fluid and Electrolyte Balance

Large amounts of fluid are lost during surgery, not only from blood loss, but also from insensible fluid loss through the skin and lungs. The fluid and electrolyte balance is jeopardized because some body fluids are retained postoperatively for 24 to 48 hours as a result of the body's stress response to surgery, to the effect of anesthesia, and to stimulation of the antidiuretic hormone (ADH). Renal vasoconstriction and an increase in aldosterone lead to increased sodium retention and thus water retention. Overhydration is a special hazard for the elderly and the very young.

Assessment measures include observation for signs of both overhydration and dehydration, and nursing interventions are aimed at controlling or correcting these conditions. Tolerance for fluids is assessed at frequent intervals and ice chips or water are given by mouth as soon as peristalsis returns.

Maintaining Nutrition

Adequate protein is necessary for healing and for postoperative recovery, and it is important that the patient begin to ingest it orally as soon as possible. Protein-sparing foods are needed to prevent catabolism, which is usually the cause of both weight loss and negative nitrogen balance in the early postoperative period. Protein is essential to restore the nitrogen balance and provide the amino acids required for wound healing. Vitamin C is needed for healing.

Certain patients must be weighed daily, and special meals are planned by the dietitian to assure proper nutrition. Nursing interventions include providing a pleasant, relaxed environment for meals and encouraging physical activity to improve the appetite. It is important to provide small, frequent meals for those patients with a poor appetite and to offer high-protein foods, such as milkshakes and eggnogs, as indicated.

Maintaining Elimination

The nurse must make sure that both urinary and intestinal elimination are adequately maintained.

URINARY ELIMINATION. The amount of urinary output is often small the first postoperative day, possibly only 1500 cc or less for 24 hours. This decreased output results from loss of body fluid during surgery, increased insensible fluid loss, vomiting, GI suction, and increased secretion of ADH. Careful recording of intake and output is a vital measure for assessing urinary elimination. Balance is achieved when intake and output are equal.

To prevent urinary stasis, nursing interventions include encouraging voiding and forcing fluids (unless contraindicated). Discomfort, suprapubic distention, and a sensation of a full bladder are indicators of urinary retention, while fever, pain, and burning on urination suggest the presence of a urinary tract infection. If the patient does not void within 6 to 8 hours postoperatively, catheterization may be ordered; if repeated catheterization is necessary, an indwelling catheter is inserted.

BOWEL ELIMINATION. Peristalsis is decreased for 24 to 48 hrs postoperatively after general anesthesia, and especially after abdominal or pelvic surgery. Inactivity, a previous history of constipation, and the use of narcotics for the relief of pain all put the patient at risk for alterations in postoperative bowel elimination. When peristaltic activity returns, the patient will begin to pass flatus, and bowel sounds will be heard during abdominal assessment. The nurse must note the amount, color, and consistency of stools.

Physical activity, use of the bathroom as soon as possible, and fluid intake of 2,000 to 3,000 cc/day (unless contraindicated) are appropriate measures for maintaining bowel elimination. If the patient becomes constipated, prune juice and high fiber foods can be given, and the physician should be consulted if an order for a laxative or enema seems necessary.

Promoting Wound Healing

Promotion of wound healing is an important part of postoperative nursing care. The main complications related to wound healing are (1) infection; (2) dehiscence (separation of wound edges); and (3) evisceration (protrusion of the abdominal viscera through the incision).

INFECTION. A nosocomial (hospital acquired) infection is one of the most dreaded and most serious of all postoperative complications. These infections are extremely dangerous and can be life-threatening for two reasons: (1) many of them are caused by strains of organisms which have developed a resistance to most available antibiotics, and (2) the patient's surgery has opened and exposed hitherto protected areas of the body to invasion by microorganisms. As a result, certain areas of the patient's body are vulnerable to infection by organisms which are so virulent and resistant that they are virtually untreatable.

The danger of postoperative infection can be reduced by:

- Meticulous sterile technique in the operating room
- Scrupulous attention to the cleanliness of all equipment used postoperatively, such as drainage tubes and bottles, suction machines, and respirators
- Perfect technique when changing dressings and caring for the surgical incision
- Early detection of any signs of general or localized infection
- *Frequent and thorough handwashing*

EVISCERATION. This emergency situation is more likely to occur if the patient is:

- Malnourished
- Lacking in the protein-sparing foods necessary for healing
- Obese, and has increased pressure and tension on an abdominal incision

Abdominal binders may be comfortable to patients who are obese, but a binder can decrease respirations and should be used with care to avoid pulmonary complications.

If evisceration occurs, the physician must be notified immediately and the patient instructed to lie quietly and avoid coughing. Sterile wet saline compresses are applied to the exposed viscera, and vital signs are assessed. The nurse should offer reassurance and stay with the patient until the abdominal incision can be closed under local or general anesthesia.

Promoting Comfort

Physical discomforts after surgery include nausea, vomiting, abdominal distention, gas pains, and incisional pain.

NAUSEA AND VOMITING. Nausea and vomiting were serious complications with the older anesthetic agents, but these occur less often with the newer agents. Persistent vomiting may be due to pyloric obstruction, intestinal obstruction, or peritonitis. Nausea and vomiting tire the patient, put a strain on the incision, increase fluid loss, and may lead to aspiration. Nursing care measures include:

- Side-lying position to avoid aspiration
- No food or fluid until vomiting subsides
- Sips of water, ice chips, ginger ale, tea, dry toast, or crackers
- Good mouth care
- Antiemetic drugs if necessary

ABDOMINAL DISTENTION AND GAS PAINS. Abdominal distention results from an accumulation of gas in the intestines, handling of the bowel during surgery, and the swallowing of air. Gas pains are caused by contractions of the bowel as it attempts to move the accumulated gas along the intestinal tract. They persist until peristalsis returns and are frequently very uncomfortable. Distention is assessed by percussing the abdomen and by measuring abdominal girth. Having the patient take short, frequent walks and administering a rectal tube or an enema are effective interventions.

PAIN. Pain is common after surgical procedures, but it becomes less severe after 24 to 48 hours. The degree of pain depends on the extent of surgery, the pain threshold of the patient, and his response to pain. It is not possible to eliminate all surgical pain, but it can be reduced to the point that the patient is able to rest and engage in postoperative activities such as deep breathing, coughing, and ambulation. Reduction of stress and anxiety may also help to diminish the perception of pain.

Incisional pain can be decreased by offering such nursing measures as distraction, relaxation, and a change in position, and by administering analgesics, which are usually required on a regular basis for 12 to 48 hrs after major surgery.

Promoting Activity

Early ambulation aids postoperative recovery and prevents pulmonary and thromboembolic complications. This physical activity also reduces abdominal distention and accumulation of gas by promoting peristalsis. Before the patient ambulates, the nurse must assess his cardiovascular, respiratory, and motor status, as well as his level of alertness. Also, he must first dangle his legs over the side of the bed. This helps him resume the upright position without feeling discomfort. While he is dangling his legs, the nurse assesses his pulse and general condition. She may also find it necessary to adjust intravenous, nasogastric, or other tubes before the patient can ambulate with relative ease.

Planning for Discharge

Since the average hospitalization following major surgery is only 3 to 7 days, the family must be prepared to assume responsibility for the care required at home. Nursing responsibilities include making necessary arrangements for discharge, initiating referrals, contacting appropriate resource persons, and stressing the importance of follow-up examinations by the surgeon.

PATIENT TEACHING

In addition to the concepts included earlier in this chapter in the section on pre-operative teaching, it is important to emphasize the challenge presented by DRG's. In many instances, hospitalizations are shorter than ever before, and patients are being discharged soon after surgery without a period of convalescence in the hospital. The current expression is "They're going home quicker and sicker." This means that the patient and family require more extensive teaching within a shorter period of time. Assessments and teaching plans must be made as soon as possible after admission, and implemented without delay. Preparation for discharge and home care should be initiated as soon as the patient and family are psychologically ready to attend to that aspect of teaching.

RELATED ACTIVITIES

A good teacher is an effective translator, and patient teaching requires the nurse to be able to translate professional terminology into the language of the patient and family. In a few instances, this may be a foreign language, but more often than not, the nurse must translate essential material into the language of children, street people, persons who have a limited knowledge of anatomy and physiology, or people who are mentally retarded.

In preparation for these challenges, pick one treatment or procedure from each of your clinical assignments, and mentally plan how you would explain it to an eight year old. Decide what words you would use, and how you would evaluate the eight year old's understanding of your 'translation.' Whenever possible, actually give your explanation to a child or adolescent, and then ask for feedback to evaluate the effectiveness of your teaching.

SUGGESTED READINGS

Blackwell, Marian Willard, and Shirley A Roy: Surgical "routines" for profoundly retarded patients. *Am J Nurs* 1978 March; 78(3):402–404.

Blackwood, Sarah: Back to basics: The preop exam. *Am J Nurs* 1986 Jan; 86(1):39–44.

Brozenec, Sally: Caring for the postoperative patient with an abdominal drain. *Nursing 85* 1985 April; 15(4):55–57.

Cooper, Diane M, and Delores Schumann: Postsurgical nursing intervention as an adjunct to wound healing. *Nurs Clin North Am* 1979 Dec; 14(4):713–726.

Hewitt, Donna: Don't forget your preop patient's fears. *RN* 1984 Oct; 47(10):63–68.

McConnell, Edwina A: After surgery: how you can avoid the obvious—and not so obvious—hazards. *Nursing 83* 1983 Feb; 13(2):74–84.

Montanari, Joan: Documenting your postop assessment findings. *Nursing 85* 1985 Aug; 15(8):31–35.

Neuberger, Geri Budesheim, and Joann Bell Rickling: A new look at wound care. *Nursing 85* 1985 Feb; 15(2):34–41.

Patras, Angie Zaharopoulos: The operation's over, but the danger's not. *Nursing 82* 1982 Sept; 12(9):50–55.

Schumann, Delores: Preoperative measures to promote wound healing. *Nurs Clin North Am* 1979 Dec; 14(4):683–699.

Strange, Julie M: An expert's guide to tubes and drains. *RN* 1983 April; 46(4):35–42.

Watson, Sheila, and Patricia Hickey: Cancer surgery: help for the family in waiting. *Am J Nurs* 1984 May; 84(5):604–607.

40

Therapeutic Uses of Heat and Cold

Prerequisites and/or Suggested Preparation
A knowledge of the concepts of physics related to heat transfer (Chapter 11), the inflammatory process (Chapter 12), and the physiology of the skin, blood vessels, and automatic nervous system is necessary for understanding this chapter.

Like heat and cold themselves, the primary effects of heat and cold are diametrically opposed; thus, it would seem that the uses of heat and cold would be clear-cut and obvious. The choice is not that simple. Complicating variables as diverse as the patient's age and general condition, the condition of the body part to be treated, the purpose of the treatment, the method of application, the equipment available, and the patient's own family traditions of using heat and cold all make it necessary for a nurse to have a thorough understanding of the therapeutic uses of heat and cold.

A nurse may meet some resistance to any use of heat or cold if it is contrary to the patient's past experiences. ''But my mother always used to . . .'' is a common refrain. You will need to use tact as you explain that the circumstances may have been different, that knowledge and techniques have advanced, or that special equipment may not have been available to the patient's mother, without ever implying that the mother was wrong.

To many people, heat feels more comforting than cold, and unless they understand the body's physiological responses to heat and cold, these people naturally prefer to be treated with heat.

HEAT AND COLD

Heat can be measured precisely in terms of *intensity* (temperature) and in terms of *quantity* (calories or British thermal units). Cold is measured and described only in relative terms, such as lack of warmth. As molecular motion increases, the amount of heat present increases. As molecular motion decreases, the amount of heat present decreases, and the terms cool and cold come into use.

Common usage has provided recognizable terms to express varying degrees of warmth. Even without knowing the exact temperature of a substance, it may be perceived as being hot, warm, lukewarm or tepid, cool, or cold (Table 40.1).

The human body has special receptors to receive sensations of hot and cold, which, along with receptors for the perception of pain, make up the sensory end organs located in the skin. Cold receptors are eight to ten times more numerous than heat receptors, are more superficial, and are concentrated in the upper torso and the extremities. When stimulated, the receptors for heat and cold send impulses to the anterior hypothalamus, which serves as the body's thermostat. In turn, the hypothalamus forwards the impulses to the cerebral cortex for interpretation.

Despite the speed with which this complex transmission takes place, there are circumstances in which the body uses a shortcut in the spinal cord to trigger emergency responses. When the impulse being transmitted signals a threatening situation, the impulse is shunted, by way of an association neuron, from the sensory neuron to a motor neuron. This spinal cord reflexive response triggers defensive action without the need of cerebral interpretation. An example of this reflex action is the jerking away of one's hand upon accidental contact with a hot stove.

Even in nonthreatening situations, the time lapse from sensory receptor to the brain and back to the body part is only a few hundredths of a second. The physiological response of the body part is complex but *predictable*, and it is this predictability of response that permits the therapeutic use of heat and cold.

PHYSIOLOGICAL RESPONSES TO HEAT AND COLD

Initial Body Responses

Physiological responses to heat and cold are, for the most part, mirror images of one another. Heat causes *vasodilation* (dilation of blood vessels), resulting in a

TABLE 40.1 RANGES OF TEMPERATURE BY COLLOQUIAL DEFINITION AND METHOD OF APPLICATION

Term	Centigrade	Fahrenheit	Method of Application
Very cold	Below 15°	Below 59°	Ice bag; ice collar; chemical pack
Cold	15°–18°	59°–65°	Aqua K pad; cold compress
Cool	18°–27°	65°–80°	
Tepid	27°–37°	80°–98°	Alcohol bath; tepid water sponging
Skin	33.9°	93°	
Warm	37°–40°	98°–105°	Whirlpool bath; infrared, ultraviolet, or gooseneck (incandescent) lamps
Hot	40°–46°	105°–115°	Aqua K pad; hot water bag or chemical hot pack for young, debilitated, or aged; electric heating pad; hot soak; sitz (hip) bath; moist compress; heat cradle
Very hot	46°–52°	115°–125°	Hot water bag or chemical hot pack for adults

TABLE 40.2 THERAPEUTIC USES OF HEAT BASED ON PHYSIOLOGICAL RESPONSES

Physiological Responses to Heat	Therapeutic Application of Physiological Responses to Heat
Vasodilation Increased capillary surface Increased capillary permeability	Relief of swelling through absorption of fluids from tissues
Increased blood flow Increased metabolism of cells Increased supply of nutrients Increased waste removal	Relief of pain caused by deep congestion Healing of wounds Removal of toxins
Relaxation of muscles	Reduction of muscle spasm; sedation; relief of fatigue
Increased suppuration and phagocytosis Softening of exudates Intensified peristalsis Raised body temperature	Healing of wounds Decubitus ulcers Cleansing of wounds Elimination Warmth, comfort

TABLE 40.3 THERAPEUTIC USES OF COLD BASED ON PHYSIOLOGICAL RESPONSES

Physiological Responses to Cold	Therapeutic Application of Physiological Responses to Cold
Decreased blood flow Decreased capillary surface Increased viscosity of blood	Relief of pain by prevention of swelling and limitation of edema and inflammation Controlling hemorrhage Enhance clotting Early stages of burns
Decreased metabolism of cells Decreased sensitivity to pain	Prevention of gangrene Limitation of suppuration Aid in certain surgery Local anesthesia
Lowered body temperature	Reduce fever Comfort

reddened skin color. Cold causes *vasoconstriction* (constriction of the blood vessels), creating a pale bluish cast to the skin. Heat increases the metabolic action of cells, cold decreases it. Heat decreases the viscosity of the blood, and cold increases it.

Heat raises the temperature of the underlying tissues; increases the amount of capillary surface available for the osmotic transfer of bodily fluids; and increases blood flow, lymph flow, and motility of leukocytes. Cold lowers the temperature of the tissues; reduces the amount of fluid entering the tissues; and decreases blood flow, lymph flow, and motility of leukocytes. Heat increases capillary blood pressure and increases suppuration and inflammation. Cold decreases capillary blood pressure and reduces inflammation and suppuration. These effects are summarized in Tables 40.2 and 40.3.

Because of these predictable physiological effects, heat and cold should not be used for certain conditions because the effect would intensify or worsen the underlying condition. For example, *heat* should not be used in situations where there is a danger of hemorrhaging, in inflamed areas, in the presence of malignancy, or in cases of impaired lung, heart, or kidney function. *Cold* should not be used after the formation of edema, in treating the very fatigued patient, or in cases of disease or disorders resulting in impaired circulation, such as peripheral vascular disease, arteriosclerosis, diabetes, or certain neurological conditions.

Secondary Responses to Heat and Cold

The body tries to maintain a state of equilibrium (homeostasis) and consequently reacts after a period of time to reverse the initial effects of heat or cold. As a consequence, the continuous application of either heat or cold is self-defeating. As a general rule, treatments of heat or cold should be limited to a period of 20 to 30 minutes, and then discontinued for at least an hour's physiological recovery time, after which treatment may be repeated if so ordered or indicated.

Some secondary bodily responses occur in organs and body parts which are *remote* from the skin surface at the point of application. This phenomenon has been known for years and has often been depicted in cartoons that show a person soaking his feet to relieve the congestion of a chest cold. If the feet of a patient suffering from congestion of his abdominal organs are immersed in a warm bath, the increased flow of blood to the feet reduces the supply of blood available to the abdominal organs and brings about relief of deep congestion.

HEAT TRANSFER

The concepts and principles of *heat* transfer are used to explain the effects of both hot and cold applications, for there is *no transfer of cold*. The application of heat to a cooler surface causes a transfer of heat from the hotter surface to the cooler surface. The application of cold to a warmer surface does *not* cause a transfer of cold to the warmer surface. Instead, the warmer surface transfers some of its heat to the source of the cold. Thus, there is only heat transfer, either *to* the body part being treated, or *from* it.

Conduction as a means of heat transfer implies contact between the source of heat or cold and the body part being treated, as in the use of a hot-water bottle, an ice bag, or a hot or cold compress. *Convection* effects heat transfer by means of the movement of a liquid or gas. An example of this mechanism of heat transfer is the whirlpool bath, in which the body is immersed in warm, moving water.

Heat transfer by means of the *radiation* of invisible heat rays is the basis for the use of infrared, ultraviolet, or incandescent lamps. The radiant energy from these sources of invisible heat rays is transformed into heat in the superficial layers of skin.

VARIABLES THAT INFLUENCE EFFECTIVENESS OF HEAT AND COLD

Individual Tolerance and Condition of Patient

The ability to tolerate either heat or cold varies significantly from person to person and from one age group to another. The very young (those under 2 years of age), the debilitated, unconscious, paralyzed, or fatigued patient, and the elderly need special protection. Even among the normal population of adults, there are individual differences that must be taken into account.

General Condition

Shock or metabolic disorders, such as diabetes, increase the hazard of tissue damage. Impaired perception because of medication, mental impairment, or a lowered level of consciousness will alter a person's ability to describe his response to heat or cold, and may make it difficult to determine his potential for injury from the application of either heat or cold.

Condition of Specific Body Area

The *condition* of the body part to be treated is significant. The presence of inflammation, an open wound, internal pins or screws of metal, circulatory defects, or dependence upon a pacemaker will all determine the type of hot or cold application to be used and may even contraindicate any application at all. The size of the body area to be treated also affects the use of heat and cold, and a general rule of thumb is: the greater the area of the body to be treated, the more moderate the temperature of the application of heat must be. People with deeper skin pigmentation—brunettes and non-Caucasians—seem more tolerant of temperature extremes than do those with lighter skin tones, such as redheads and blondes.

Moisture

A major consideration in the choice of treatment method is the difference between moist heat or cold and dry

TABLE 40.4 MOIST VERSUS DRY HEAT

Quality or Characteristic	Moist Heat	Dry Heat
Penetration	More	Less
Drying of skin	Less	More
Loss of body fluids	Less	Greater
Skin maceration	More	Less
Potential for burning	More	Less

heat or cold. Because moisture is an excellent conductor of heat, it can enhance or intensify the effectiveness of treatment, and moist heat may be contraindicated by certain conditions in which such intensification could be dangerous. Moist applications of heat tend to soften crusts and exudates, to penetrate more deeply, and to have a more localized effect. They tend to reduce the amount of body fluid that can be lost through perspiration (diaphoresis) and are less likely to dry the skin.

Moist applications of cold do not require as low a temperature as dry applications of cold, and penetrate better than dry cold. Both hot and cold moist applications tend, however, to soften and wrinkle (macerate) the skin. With moist applications, dripping and spilling can create problems of discomfort for the patient. Soaks, sitz baths, and whirlpool baths require special attention to body posture and limb position in order to avoid cramping and constriction of circulation from pressure against the edge of the basin or tub. Some moist applications of heat permit the simultaneous administration of medication, cleansing of wounds, and comforting relief of pain. Dry heat from a heat lamp or heat cradle permits treatment of open or draining wounds, such as bedsores, the reduction of pain from poor circulation (ischemic pain) and muscle spasms, drying of large, plaster body casts, and treatment of burned areas where direct contact with the burned area is contraindicated (Table 40.4).

Duration of Treatment

The greatest amount of heat transfer is experienced during the initial contact with the source of heat or cold, when the *difference* in temperature between the two surfaces is greatest. There is a greater tolerance for extremes of either hot or cold when the duration of the application is brief. When a treatment is prolonged beyond the recommended time, the body's response may be exactly the opposite of the one desired and may thus nullify the effectiveness of the entire procedure.

Environmental Temperature

In warm or humid environments, heat is not lost from the body through evaporation to the same degree that it is in dry or cool circumstances. Little heat can be lost when the environmental temperature is equal to or greater than the body temperature. Conductive heat loss is greatest when the patient is in a cool, dry environment.

SAFETY MEASURES

The safety of the patient is your responsibility. No piece of equipment should be used without being thoroughly examined immediately before its use. Containers of fluid should be checked for possible leakage; electrical equipment for weakened, cracked, or loosened wires or connections; and for proper functioning. All appliances or equipment should be checked for accuracy of temperature settings. Solutions should be checked for proper temperature. Lamps should be checked for proper wattages and positioned at the optimal distance from the area to be treated.

Pins are not used with applications of heat because they can puncture the surface of a hot water bag, causing leakage. Pins could come in contact with the wiring of an electrical device, causing shock or a short circuit; and, being metal, they may conduct heat excessively. Sterile procedures should be followed when indicated. Provisions should be made for privacy, comfort, and modesty in keeping with the nature of the treatment.

Caution the patient about the hazards of lying atop or leaning against a source of heat because doing so *reduces air spaces* between him and the source of heat, and increases the likelihood of burns. Do not allow the patient to adjust the temperature control of an appliance; instruct him to use his call button to summon you to make any adjustments. Position the patient in such a way that he can move himself or the application if it is causing him discomfort or pain.

ASSESSMENTS

In addition to considering the variables mentioned above, an *ongoing assessment* is the responsibility of the nurse. Although the application of either heat or cold is often ordered by the physician, the person who administers the treatment is responsible for the patient's safety and is accountable for many of the problems that could arise. You are responsible for protecting the patient from burns, skin maceration, fainting, secondary bodily responses, or other adverse reactions to the treatment you administer.

Assessment Before Treatment

In addition to reading the patient's chart and observing his *general* condition plus any *specific* temporary con-

dition, you should ascertain his *level of sensation*. One method you can use to determine the patient's local sensory perception is to ask him to close his eyes, place your fingers on the surface to be treated, and ask him if he can feel your touch. Further distinctions may be made with the verbally capable patient by tracing a letter or shape on the body area to be treated and asking him to identify it. Discuss the procedure to be followed and the effects he may expect to experience, and encourage him to ask questions.

Assessments During Treatment

Within 5 or 10 minutes after starting any treatment, assess the patient's skin color, vital signs, and physical comfort. Encourage the patient to report any loss of sensation, unusual pain, or discomfort. The patient must be observed closely throughout the procedure, so that, in the event of an unfavorable reaction or accident, you can discontinue the procedure immediately.

After Treatment

At the end of the treatment, make the patient comfortable, position him for rest, take care of the equipment, and restore the patient's unit to order. Finally, chart the treatment, noting the type, location, duration, and temperature of the application, the condition of the body part, comments by the patient about any unusual sensations, and your own assessment of the effect of the treatment.

APPLICATION OF HEAT

Dry Heat

Hot-water Bottles
Hot-water bottles, so commonly used in self-care in the home, are actually far more dangerous than their comforting, homey image would indicate. In many hospitals, patients must sign a release form before a hot-water bottle may be used. Each agency has a policy regarding the maximum temperature for a hot water bottle. A thermometer should be used for testing the temperature of the hot water. If one is not available, test the temperature of the water on your wrist or forearm to make sure that it is not hot enough to burn the patient. The hazards inherent in the use of hot water can be minimized if the water is tested to the exact temperature recommended, if the bag is covered with a flannel or disposable cover for insulation and absorption of the patient's perspiration, and if the bag has been checked for leakage after being filled and thoroughly dried before its application. The bottle or bag

should be filled only half way, and the air should be expelled from the remaining space by lowering the opening to the level of the water before it is sealed. This keeps the bag limp for better conformity to the shape of the body part to which it will be applied. After use, the hot water bottle should be cleaned and then filled with air before it is stored, to prevent the interior surfaces from sticking together.

Electric Heating Pads

The *medium setting* for most heating pads (115 degrees to 126 degrees F) equals the temperature recommended for therapeutic use, so the high setting is frequently eliminated or rendered inoperative to prevent the controls from being moved to a dangerously high setting. As with a hot water bottle, a flannel cloth or cover is needed for insulation and absorption of perspiration. Pressure should not be used in conjunction with a heating pad, for pressure reduces the number of air spaces between the patient and the pad, thus eliminating the protective insulation of a layer of air and increasing the potential for burning.

Not only is there loss of air space when the patient lies or leans on the pad; blood vessels in the tissues are compressed, causing heat to accumulate because of the vessels' decreased ability to carry off the excess heat.

Infrared, Ultraviolet, and Incandescent Lamps

Infrared and ultraviolet lamps deliver invisible heat rays from beyond the red and violet ends of the spectrum, and are usually confined to use by the physical therapist. Infrared lamps are used primarily to stimulate circulation to a body part for the relief of ischemic pain and muscle spasms. Ultraviolet lamps are used in conjunction with pigmentation of the skin for production of vitamin D, and for bactericidal effects.

A flexible gooseneck lamp houses incandescent bulbs and can be used by the nurse in a variety of situations, including the home. Bulbs vary in wattage from 25 to 60. Recommended distances from bulb to body part depend on the wattage. Provide privacy by drawing the patient's bed curtains and draping the parts of the body which are not being treated; however, bedding or other fabric should *not* be draped over the lamp. Such draping creates a fire hazard and also intensifies the heat on the body part.

Chemical Packs

Chemical packs are fluid-filled plastic bags which become either hot or cold as a result of chemical activity. Each bag has two compartments, each containing a different chemical compound. These chemicals are combined and activated when the bag is squeezed. Once the chemicals have been combined, the bag usually

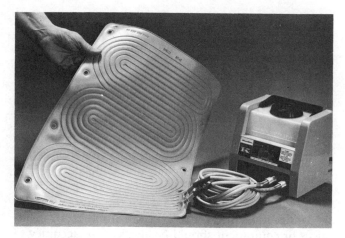

Figure 40.1 *Aqua K pad, used to administer heat to a body part.*

stays hot or cold for a considerable period of time, but the device cannot be reused. This feature of disposability increases the cost but greatly diminishes the incidence of cross-infection.

The nurse assesses whether the temperature of a chemical pack is tolerable by resting the bag against the inner aspect of her forearm, an area which is more sensitive than many other body parts. Like the hot water bottle and the electric heating pad, this appliance should be covered with flannel or other absorbent material to insulate and absorb perspiration.

Aqua K Pads

Aqua K pads (a trade name) are waterproof pads with hollow, parallel channels for the circulation of hot or cold water (Fig. 40.1). Inlet and outlet hoses are connected to a control unit with a small motor and a heating or cooling element. For optimum operation, the motor unit should be level with or higher than the treated part and the hoses should be kept free from kinks. The control unit may be set and locked at any desired temperature between no heat and 105 degrees F, making it possible to maintain a constant level of heat. Aqua K pads are available in a wide variety of sizes to fit the body part to be treated. The pad is covered in the usual manner for insulation and absorption of perspiration.

Heat Cradle

A Baker heat cradle is an arched frame of metal that contains a number of incandescent light bulbs. It may be equipped with a thermometer. The frame is not adjustable for distance from the body part to be treated, so control of the heat in this device depends on unscrewing one or more of the 25-watt bulbs to achieve the desired temperature. The construction of the cradle allows for safe draping with a sheet for privacy. Large cradles permit the treatment of large areas of the body, the drying of a body cast, or the treatment of burns.

Irritants and Counterirritants

The purpose of an *irritant* (rubefacient) is simply to bring about *hyperemia* (increased blood flow) on the surface of the treated body part. An irritating substance, contained in an ointment, poultice or plaster, is applied to the skin of the affected part, left for 20 minutes or other designated interval, and then washed off gently with warm water and soap.

An irritant becomes a *counterirritant*, when the reason for its application is to relieve congestion or pain in an underlying organ or structure. The underlying congestion or pain is relieved by redirection of blood from that area to the surface of the body. Of the poultices used in the past—linseed, flaxseed, and mustard—the mustard plaster has survived and is still used today. A simple mixture of dry mustard, flour, and warm (not hot) water is mixed according to the *age and condition* of the patient. Commercially prepared mustard plasters are also available. At the end of a treatment, the skin should appear reddened but *not blistered*. After bathing the area gently with warm water, dry the skin and soothe it with an application of petrolatum or olive oil.

Diathermy

Diathermy is the use of high-frequency electrical currents to provide deep heat within the tissues. The forms most commonly used by physical therapists are shortwave, ultrasound, and microwave. The nurse's function in preparing a patient for diathermy treatments includes removing from him anything made of metal, such as a ring, watch, or hearing aid. The nurse should also determine whether the patient has within or on his body any metal pins, screws, prostheses, or an implanted or external cardiac pacemaker. Metal exposed to diathermy reaches extremely high temperatures that will burn and may even be lethal, so this is a safety procedure of the utmost importance.

Moist Heat

Compresses and Packs

Hot *compresses* are squares of gauze or other moisture-retaining substances that are used to promote healing, relieve pain, and promote drainage. Hot compresses must be *sterile* when applied to areas vulnerable to infection, such as open wounds, surgical incisions, or sensitive areas such as the eye. Compresses need not be sterile when the skin is intact and the area is not vulnerable to infection.

Hot packs are large moist cloths applied to an area of the body more extensive than can be treated with the smaller compresses. Both compresses and packs are generally applied as hot as the patient can tolerate them, but additional caution is required with packs because a greater body surface is involved. The nurse must remember the principle: *the larger the area, the lower the temperature.*

Protection against burns is provided by covering the skin with an insulating coating of petrolatum. If there is an open would, sterile petrolatum is applied to the skin around the wound. You provide additional protection against burning by wringing the pack out to make it as dry as possible, and by shaking the pack slightly to dissipate some of the steam before applying it to the body surface.

PROCEDURE. In general, the procedure is the same for both compresses and packs. With clean hands, the nurse should assemble all equipment: solution as ordered (normal saline or antiseptic); petrolatum; dressings of the appropriate size and material; protection for the bed; a flannel bath blanket; a waterproof covering; tie tapes or a binder with pins; a dry, clean towel; a treatment thermometer; and a waterproof bag for disposing of soiled dressings. Sterile technique and sterile supplies are used as indicated.

After carefully identifying the patient, provide him with privacy, and expose the body part to be treated. Provide warmth for all other body parts, because the moist heat application will cause other parts of the body to feel chilly. Protect the bed from moisture and be sure the patient is comfortable and in good body alignment.

Heat the solution. Remove any dressings, cleanse the area and, where appropriate, spread a thin layer of petrolatum on intact skin surfaces. Because petrolatum is a poor conductor, it will serve as a form of insulation to help prevent burning. Compresses are usually immersed in a hot solution, but packs may be prepared by steaming rather than immersion. Wring out the compress or pack, using forceps to maintain sterility where indicated, and apply it to the designated area.

After a few seconds, lift the dressing to observe the skin for signs of complications such as pallor, extreme redness, or blotches. Be sure to ask the patient if he is experiencing pain or discomfort. As with any application of heat or cold, if you note complications or any undesired reaction, remove the application immediately, ensure the patient's safety, and report verbally to the charge nurse or physician. Also include any such incident in your charting.

Cover the compress or pack with a waterproof dressing and an insulating towel. Because moist heat dressings lose their heat quite rapidly, external heat in the form of a hot water bottle or waterproof heating pad may be used to maintain the heat needed for an effective treatment.

If the compress is causing no undue discomfort or complications, secure the dressing with tie tapes or a binder to prevent it from slipping or falling off.

Small hot *compresses* should be changed every 5 minutes, discarding soiled dressings in the container provided. Large *hot packs* may be left in place for as long as the temperature is maintained, usually about 20 to 30 minutes. Packs *without external heat* cool in from 10 to 15 minutes, however, and should be removed and replaced with another pack if continuous heat has been ordered.

When the treatment has been concluded, remove the final compress or pack. Dry the treated body part gently by patting it, not rubbing, because the skin has been softened by long exposure to moisture. Conclude the treatment by making patient comfortable and removing all equipment from the area. In your charting, be sure to report any exudate, the appearance of the wound, the type of solution used, and any statements of discomfort from the patient.

Soaks

The doctor's order will usually specify the body part to be soaked, the solution to be used, the temperature, duration, and frequency of the soak, and its purpose. Soaks are usually not sterile, but must be sterile if there is a break in the skin. Special care should be taken to avoid undue pressure of adjacent body parts against the edge of the tub or basin in order to prevent vascular constriction and muscle cramping. Position the limb comfortably to avoid muscle strain. Check the solution with a thermometer and maintain proper temperature by adding warmer solution from time to time. The addition of hot solution must be made with care to avoid burning the patient. After treatment, dry the treated part gently so as not to break the tender skin.

Sitz Baths

Sitz baths are a procedure whereby the patient's *perineal area and buttocks* are submerged in water in order to cleanse a wound, relieve pain, increase circulation, promote relaxation, or stimulate voiding. The temperature of a sitz bath ranges from 110 to 115 degrees F, (38 to 40 degrees C). The lower temperatures are used for cleansing; the higher ones for increasing circulation. A variety of tubs may be used including permanent fixtures, disposable plastic models, and portable tubs. Such tubs are preferred to a regular bathtub because the patient's legs should be kept out of the warm water to prevent vasodilation of the lower extremities. The edge of the tub should be padded for comfort and to prevent cutting off circulation to the patient's legs. Bath

blankets are used over the shoulders and legs to provide warmth and privacy.

The shift in blood supply from various parts of the body to the pelvis (perineal pooling) may cause the patient to feel weak or faint. If this occurs, assist him from the tub, dry him, and help him to lie flat until normal circulation is restored. Inform the physician of the patient's reaction.

Whirlpool Baths

Full-immersion whirlpool baths (given in a Hubbard tank) are helpful in relieving pain, promoting relaxation, and debriding burned tissue. The water is agitated by the injection of air, water, or both. Treatments are usually given in the physical therapy department, although some small home models are available.

APPLICATION OF COLD

Cold applications are used to prevent swelling, and relieve pain or itching. If cold is applied *immediately* to a sprain, bruise, or other injury, the resulting vasoconstriction will often prevent much of the swelling which would result from the inflammatory process. Once the area has become swollen and congested, however, heat rather than cold is applied in order to increase circulation through the tissues and promote removal of excess fluid and products of the inflammatory process.

Cold is used to relieve pain when the use of heat would cause pain by increasing circulation, congestion, or pressure *within a bony structure* as in the case of a toothache or headache. Cold is sometimes used to slow the inflammatory process when appendicitis is suspected, and the *preferred first aid* for a minor burn is immersion of the part in cold water.

It is important to change cold packs and compresses frequently in order to maintain coolness. An ice bag must be covered with flannel or terry cloth to protect the patient's skin from being injured, and must be used with caution if the patient has impaired circulation or diminished sensory function. Your assessment of the patient's reaction to the application of cold should take special note of mottling, skin maceration, extremes of color (redness, extreme paleness, or gray discoloration), blisters, or sensations of either burning or numbness. If any of these phenomena are observed, discontinue the treatment at once and immediately report your observations to the physician or charge nurse.

PATIENT TEACHING

Since the use of hot or cold applications to relieve pain or discomfort is a commonplace self-care activity, it is an important topic for patient teaching. Some of the most essential concepts include the following:

1. Hot or cold applications should be used with *great caution* on any person who has diminished pain perception, impaired circulation, an immature sensory system, or an inability to move away from heat or cold that is too intense.

2. Heat should not be used to relieve undiagnosed pain (such as abdominal pain which might be caused by appendicitis).

3. Cold applications are useful to *prevent* swelling from a sprain or strain, but once swelling has occurred, hot applications will improve circulation in the area and help to reduce the swelling.

4. The water in a hot water bottle should never be hot enough to burn or scald the patient if it should spring a leak or be pressed tightly against the person's skin.

5. An ice bag or hot water bottle should be covered with a towel or layer of flannel to provide an insulating layer of air between the hot or cold surface and the patient's skin.

RELATED ACTIVITIES

Increase your understanding of the *psychological* aspects of hot or cold applications by asking family and friends, both adults and children, how they react to heat and cold, and why. Ask them what they remember about the ways in which their parents used hot and cold applications within the home.

SUGGESTED READINGS

DeLapp, Tina Davis: Taking the bite out of frostbite and other cold-weather injuries. *Am J Nurs* 1980 Jan; 80(1):58–60.

Flitter, Hessel Howard, and Harold R Rowe: *An Introduction to Physics in Nursing.* ed.7. St. Louis, Mosby, 1976.

Fonger, Linda: Emergency! First aid for burns. *Nursing 82* 1982 Sept; 12(9):70–77.

Guyton, Arthur C: *Textbook of Medical Physiology.* ed. 6. Philadelphia, Saunders, 1980.

LaVoy, Kathleen: Dealing with hypothermia and frostbite. *RN* 1985 Jan; 48(1):53–56.

O'Dell, Ardis J: Hot packs for morning stiffness. *Am J Nurs* 1975 June; 75(6):986.

Petrello, Judith M: Temperature maintenance of hot moist compresses. *Am J Nurs* 1973 June; 73(6):1050.

Simpson, Carol F: Heat, cold, or both? (for arthritis). *Am J Nurs* 1983 Feb; 83(2):271–273.

Waterson, Marion: Hot and cold therapy. *Nursing 78* 1978 Oct; 8(10):46–49.

41

Administration of Drugs

Prerequisites and/or Suggested Preparation
A knowledge of the anatomy relevant to injection sites, and an understanding of sterile technique (Chapter 27) are prerequisite to this chapter.

DRUGS

In recent years, the phrase "using drugs" has carried a negative connotation that conjures up images ranging from experimentation with marijuana to cocaine addiction. Lay people and publications usually refer to the legitimate and appropriate use of drugs as taking "medicine" or "medications," reserving the word *drugs* for conditions of misuse and abuse or addiction. Within the context of health care, however, the terms drugs and medications are used interchangeably. The term *drug* is used most often in pharmacology texts and in reference to drug therapy in general, and the term *medication* is commonly used in reference to a specific patient or condition.

Technically, a drug is any substance used intentionally in the diagnosis, cure, relief, treatment, or prevention of disease. A drug is a substance other than food that is intended to affect the structure of body functions of humans or animals and that has been recognized by an official pharmaceutical standard such as the United States Pharmacopeia. Such recognized drugs range from the derivatives of herbs and barks that have been used for centuries to synthetic compounds that have only recently been approved by federal agencies for use on human subjects.

USES OF DRUGS

Although the most common use of drugs is in the treatment of disease, there are many other reasons for the administration of drugs. Some of these purposes are:

> *Prophylactic* (ex., fluorine to prevent cavities, or quinine to prevent malaria)
>
> *Diagnostic* (ex., radiopaque dyes)
>
> *Palliative* (ex., aspirin to reduce fever, or cough syrup to lessen a cough)
>
> *Substitutive* (ex., insulin, thyroid extract, or hormones)

Drug therapy is often the most significant component of a patient's health care, because for some pathological conditions such as hypertension or epilepsy, drug therapy is the primary means of control. The term *chemotherapy* currently refers to a specific type of drug therapy, namely, the use of drugs for the treatment of cancer.

Nonprescription, or over-the-counter (OTC), drugs are generally purchased by the public for a specific reason.

These reasons, which are usually *palliative* (giving relief of symptoms) include: to relax, to sleep, to reduce discomfort such as burning or itching, to relieve pain, to cure warts, to kill lice, to relieve constipation, and many others.

DRUG NAMES

Each drug has three or more names, each of which serves a different purpose.

The *chemical name* describes the drug's chemical formula. This name is rarely used by nurses. The *generic name* is assigned by the company that first produces the drug. It is usually an abbreviated and more pronounceable form of the chemical name.

The *official name* of a drug is the one that is listed in official publications, both national and international. The official name is usually the same as the generic name.

The *trade name* is the name assigned by each manufacturer of the drug. The trade name is capitalized when written and is also called the brand name, the common name, or the proprietary name.

Some drugs are manufactured by only one company and have only one trade name; other drugs are produced by several companies, each of which will assign its own brand name to the drug. These products are chemically identical and are usually interchangeable. Many agencies such as Medicare and the Veterans' Administration now require the use of generic names so that it is possible for the pharmacist to substitute one brand for another as needed to give the consumer the best possible service and price. If, however, the physician prescribes a specific brand name, the pharmacist may not substitute another brand, even though it is chemically identical.

DRUG SOURCES

Drugs are obtained from animal, vegetable, and mineral sources. Animal sources yield drugs such as cod liver oil, insulin, and thyroid preparations. Vegetable or plant sources yield drugs such as digitalis (from purple foxglove) and morphine (from the Oriental poppy). Mineral sources provide drugs such as calcium, aluminum (used in antacid preparations), and magnesium (used in cathartics).

The traditional sources of drugs now have greater historical interest than practical significance because increasing numbers of drugs are being synthesized, and dependence on plant and animal sources is decreasing.

DRUG STANDARDIZATION

Drugs from natural sources are subject to wide variations in purity and potency depending on the source (seeds, bark, leaves, other), the number of impurities present, and the process used to extract the active ingredient. Any such variations in strength and purity make precise dosage impossible, so over- or undermedication was not uncommon in the past.

The United States Pharmacopeia, first published in 1820, provides the official standards for the source, chemical composition, testing, physical properties, storage, dose, and dosage of all drugs prescribed in the United States. Most of the drugs are single drugs and are listed under their official names. This publication is revised every 5 years and supplements are issued at frequent intervals. The initials USP after the name of a drug indicate that the drug meets official standards of strength and purity. For example, every bottle of acetylsalicylic acid labeled "Aspirin U.S.P. 5 grains" meets the official standards for aspirin, whether it is the leading name brand or a cheaper product distributed by a large chain of drugstores.

A second official publication is the National Formulary (NF). First published in 1888, it became an official standard in 1906 and contains many formulas for drug mixtures. Other countries have their own official pharmacopeias, and the Pharmacopeia Internalis (PhI) was established by the World Health Organization in 1951.

LEGISLATION AND CONTROL

The major law regulating drugs in the United States is the Federal Food, Drug, and Cosmetic Act of 1938 and its amendments. Many of the provisions of this act are designed to ensure complete and accurate labeling. Labeling refers not only to the label of the container but also to all literature related to the drug. Some of the important provisions of this act are:

1. Statements on the label must not be false or misleading in any particular.
2. Drugs must not be dangerous to health when used in the dose or with the frequency prescribed, recommended, or suggested on the label.
3. The label must indicate the name and the business address of the manufacturer, packer, or distributor as well as an accurate statement of the contents.
4. The label must indicate quantitatively the presence of all habit-forming drugs, such as narcotics, hypnotics, or other habit-forming drugs or their derivatives. The label must also bear the statement: "Warning—May Be Habit Forming."

5. Labels must designate the presence of official drugs by their official names, and if nonofficial, they must bear the usual name of the drug or drugs, whether or not active.
6. The act requires that official drugs be packaged and labeled as specified by The Pharmacopeia of the United States, The National Formulary, or the Homeopathic Pharmacopoeia of the United States. Deviations in strength, quality, and purity are permitted, provided such deviations are clearly indicated on the label.
7. Labels must indicate the quantity, kind, and proportion of certain specified ingredients, including alcohol, bromides, atropine, hyoscine, digitalis, and a number of other drugs, the presence of which needs to be known for the safety of those for whom it is prescribed.
8. The label must bear adequate directions for use and adequate warning against unsafe use (a) by children and (b) in pathologic conditions.
9. The label must bear adequate warning against unsafe doses or methods or duration of administration or application in such manner and form as are necessary for the protection of the users.
10. New drugs may not be introduced into interstate commerce unless an application has been filed with the Food and Drug Administration and the application has been permitted to become effective. Adequate scientific evidence must be presented to show that the drug is safe for use under the conditions proposed for its use. The applicant does not have to prove the efficacy of the drug in order to obtain an effective application. During the time that the drug is under investigation by experts, the label of the drug must bear the statement: "Caution, New Drug—Limited by Federal Law to Investigational Use."

NOTE: When tests indicate that the requirements of the Food and Drug Administration have been met, the law permits a period of clinical testing by approved clinicians and clinical groups. Pertinent data are collected and submitted to the Food and Drug Administration for further evaluation. If the Administration is satisfied that the drug has therapeutic merit and is not unduly toxic, distribution and sale of the new drug are permitted. (Bergersen, 1979, pp. 21–22)

The Harrison Narcotic Act of 1914 was the first narcotic act passed by any nation to regulate the importation, manufacture, sale, and use of opium, cocaine, and their derivatives. This act was replaced in 1971 by the Controlled Substances Act, which was designed to provide increased research into, and prevention of, drug abuse and drug dependence; to treat and rehabilitate drug abusers and drug-dependent people, and to strengthen law enforcement in the field of drug abuse. The Controlled Substances Act also controls the manufacture, sale, and dispensing of narcotics and dangerous drugs. The act classifies drugs such as opium derivatives, barbiturates, amphetamines, and tranquilizers according to current medical use, the potential for abuse, and the degree of possible addiction and dependency. The act specifies whether a prescription must be written or whether the physician can give a prescription to the pharmacist over the telephone. It also specifies the number of times the prescription can be refilled and the type of verification needed by the pharmacist to make sure the prescription is valid (neither stolen nor forged).

Every nurse is responsible for her own actions when administering a drug, and violations of the Controlled Substances Act are punishable by a fine, imprisonment, or both plus revocation of the license to practice nursing. In the hospital, federal and state laws form the basis for institutional policies that include such precautions as the use of double locks (a locked container within a locked room or closet) for securing controlled substances, and the use of special forms and records. The dispensation of each dose must be recorded and signed, and any unused portion of a dose must be accounted for.

Controlled substances must be inventoried at the end of every shift by two persons; the medication nurse who is going off duty and the nurse who will replace her. Both nurses must indicate by their signatures that the drug count was correct.

All time limits must be rigidly obeyed. A narcotic order, for example, is valid for a designated number of hours, not days. After 48 to 72 hours, the order becomes invalid and must be rewritten by the physician.

DRUG CLASSIFICATION

A drug can be classified by its *effect on a system of the body* (such as a CNS depressant), in terms of the *symptoms it is expected to relieve* (as, for example, an anticonvulsant), or by the *effect that is desired* (as a tranquilizer). Regardless of the classification system used, there will be considerable overlap because a given condition can usually be treated by more than one drug and because a given drug may have several actions and can therefore be used to treat several conditions. For example, acetylsalicylic acid is used to reduce fever (by its antipyretic action), to reduce the inflammation of rheumatoid arthritis (through its anti-inflammatory action), and to relieve pain (by its analgesic action).

It is virtually impossible and highly impractical for nurses to try to memorize the specific details of each and every medication, partly because the number of drugs in current use is extensive and partly because additional drugs that have been proven safe and useful are added to the list almost every month. It is reasonable and necessary, therefore, to group drugs into categories that carry similar nursing responsibilities in order to condense excessive amounts of information into manageable units. There are, for example, numerous nursing considerations that are common to the care of all patients on anticoagulant therapy, regardless of the specific anticoagulant being used. Whenever a person's clotting mechanisms have been altered by drug therapy, he must be taught, for example, the ways in which his therapy intensifies the hazards of household or industrial accidents and emergency surgery, and that he must carry an appropriate medical identification card, bracelet, or tag.

STUDY OF DRUGS

Before giving any drug, the nurse must be familiar with the following data about that drug:

Generic and trade name
Normal dose or range of dose
Route of administration
Purpose or desired action
Common side effects
Contraindications (if any)
Special aspects of administration
Essential patient teaching

Name of Drug

Knowing the name of a drug one is about to give includes the ability to *pronounce and spell* both the generic and the trade names. This skill requires diligence to master if a nurse has difficulty spelling, but it must be done. The name of one drug may differ from the name of another by only one or two letters, as in *prednisone* and *prednisolone*. In some instances, a single letter will differentiate between a form that must be given orally and one that can be safely given intravenously, such as *Cedilanid* and *Cedilanid-D*.

If you are afflicted with a spelling problem, you will need to devise a system for learning to recognize the names of medications you administer, or that your patients are receiving, in order to ensure the patients' safety and to protect yourself from medication errors and possible malpractice. Whether it takes practice with medication flash cards or the use of a small pocket notebook, you must be able to identify correctly every medication with which you are involved.

Normal Dose or Range of Doses

Although the physician prescribes the drug, and the pharmacist dispenses the drug as ordered, the nurse who administers the drug to the patient shares the responsibility for making certain that the patient receives the correct dose. You therefore must *know the usual dose or range of doses* and be able to detect a dose that has obviously been prescribed in error.

Route of Administration

The choice of a route of administration is affected by the properties of the drug, by whether a local or systemic effect is desired, the physical and mental status of the patient, his age, and the nature of the health problem.

Routes for a Local Effect

A *local*, or *topical*, effect can be achieved by applying the drug to the patient's skin or mucous membranes.

SKIN. Methods of applying a drug to the skin include painting (with an antiseptic, for example), moist dressings, soaks, medicated baths, and inunction (rubbing in an ointment or liniment). The skin resists penetration of a drug, so there is little, if any, systemic effect. There are usually few side effects except for possible local irritation and localized allergic reaction. Absorption is increased, however, if the concentration of the drug is increased, if contact with the drug is prolonged, or if the patient has very thin skin.

MUCOUS MEMBRANES. Drugs can be applied to the mucous membranes of the mouth, nose, throat, eyes, vagina, urethra, and rectum. Methods of application include:

Inhalation: use of aerosol sprays or medicated steam.

Direct application of liquid: painting or swabbing the mouth or throat, gargling, and the use of eye drops or ointment.

Insertion into the body cavity or orifice: insertion of a medicated suppository into urethra, rectum, or vagina; placement of medicated packing or tampon into rectum or vagina.

Irrigation: flushing a body cavity (eye, ear, throat, rectum, vagina, or bladder) with medicated fluid. The fluid is not retained.

Instillation: placement of medicated fluid such as ear drops or nose drops into a body cavity. The fluid

is retained. Larger amounts are used in the rectum and bladder. Vaginal instillations are not done; the fluid cannot be retained because the vagina has no sphincter muscles.

Aqueous (not oily) solutions are well absorbed by mucous membranes, so certain drugs will also give a rapid *systemic* effect when absorbed. For example, a nitroglycerin tablet under the tongue produces an almost immediate effect on the cardiovascular system and quickly relieves an attack of angina pectoris; an aminophylline suppository placed in the rectum will quickly relieve many types of asthmatic attacks. Inhaling certain drugs can exert a significant systemic effect because of the enormous absorption surface of the lungs.

Mucous membranes differ in their sensitivity and rate of absorption. For example, if the concentration of a drug that is optimal for nose drops were considered normal or standard, a double-strength solution would be optimal for the oral mucosa, whereas only one-eighth to one-half strength should be used for the eye.

Routes for a Systemic Effect

The primary routes of administration for a *systemic* effect are those routes that involve the alimentary tract and parenteral routes (routes other than the alimentary tract). Routes involving the alimentary tract include sublingual, buccal, oral, and rectal administration.

SUBLINGUAL. In sublingual administration a tablet such as nitroglycerin is held under the tongue until it is completely dissolved. The advantage of this route is that it avoids the action of gastric and intestinal enzymes on the drug. The patient must be able to cooperate and keep from swallowing the tablet. He should also refrain from swallowing the saliva that contains the dissolved drug for as long as possible.

BUCCAL. Buccal administration requires a tablet to be held between the mucous membrane of the cheek and the teeth until it is dissolved. Only a few hormonal and enzyme preparations are given this way.

RECTAL. Rectal administration is used when the drug has an objectionable odor or taste, when the drug would be destroyed by gastrointestinal enzymes, or when the patient is nauseated, comatose, confused, or otherwise unable to take the drug orally. This route is often used in infants. The drug is given by retention enema or in a suppository that melts at body temperature. Absorption is slower and less predictable than when the drug is taken orally.

ORAL. Oral administration is the most convenient, comfortable, and economical method of drug administration. It is usually safer than injection because it avoids the danger of infection that is possible whenever the skin is punctured or broken. The drug action has a slower onset, is more prolonged, and is less potent than when the same drug is injected.

Oral administration is contraindicated when a patient is vomiting, has gastric or intestinal suction, is unable to swallow, or is unconscious. Oral administration may also be prohibited if the patient is NPO for tests or treatments.

Most drugs are absorbed from the small intestine, although some are absorbed from the stomach or large intestine. The site of absorption can be controlled by coating the tablet with a substance that will not dissolve in the stomach (called an enteric coating) or by using several types of coatings, some of which will dissolve in gastric acid while others are dissolved by enzymes throughout the intestines (called timed-release coating). Absorption is affected by the type and quantity of food in the intestinal tract as well as by the motility and pathology of the stomach and intestines. The disadvantages of oral drug administration are that some drugs have a bad odor, texture, or taste, and others discolor or damage teeth. Some drugs irritate the GI tract and can cause bleeding, nausea, vomiting, or diarrhea. Some drugs are destroyed and rendered inactive by gastric enzymes and cannot be given orally.

PARENTERAL ADMINISTRATION. Parenteral administration usually refers to the injection of a drug into subcutaneous tissue, muscle, or a vein. Drugs can also be injected into an artery, the spinal canal, the pleural cavity, the cardiac muscle, or the peritoneal cavity.

Drugs are given by injection when a rapid effect is needed, when the patient is unable to take the drug by mouth, when the drug would be destroyed by enzymes if taken orally, and when the drug is too irritating to be taken by mouth. The total dose can be smaller because *all* of the drug is absorbed; none of it is destroyed by digestive enzymes.

A major disadvantage of parenteral administration is that it is more dangerous than other routes because it is difficult to correct any error in medication, dose, technique, or choice of site. The drug is absorbed rapidly and cannot be recovered. (The length of time needed for blood to make one complete circuit of the arterial and venous systems of the body is less than half a minute.) The cost of administration is greater, and sterile technique is essential. Psychological and physical discomfort can be intense, especially for children and people on long-term parenteral therapy.

Purpose or Expected Action

A nurse needs to know why a drug was prescribed before she can plan appropriate supporting interven-

tions and before she can evaluate the effectiveness of the drug. For example, the nursing actions that should accompany the administration of chlorpromazine HCl (Thorazine) will be different depending on whether it is given to treat a mental or emotional condition, to treat hiccoughs, or for the relief of vomiting. It is not enough merely to administer a drug; the nurse must know its purpose so that subsequent nursing actions will enhance its intended effect.

Side Effects

To evaluate a patient's response to a drug, the nurse needs to be able to differentiate between symptoms that indicate that he is responding poorly to the drug and symptoms that are related to common and often unimportant side effects. For example, sufficiently large, yet safe, doses of aspirin will cause a person's ears to ring; atropine will make a patient's mouth dry. Usually, neither symptom is harmful, and in some situations the physician will intentionally increase the dose of a drug until such symptoms appear so he can assess the patient's tolerance for the drug.

It is important to be able to differentiate between side effects and dangerous toxic effects of various drugs. For example, a patient's complaint of discomfort (ringing) in his ears while taking aspirin is not usually cause for alarm, but a patient's complaint of changes in hearing while taking streptomycin sulfate is serious indeed because prolonged use of this drug can cause permanent deafness.

Contraindications

Although the physician prescribes the drugs for a patient, you must be knowledgeable about commonly encountered or obvious reasons for not administering a drug. Some drugs are incompatible and should not be taken concurrently. Some drugs will pass through the placenta to a fetus; you may know that a patient is pregnant while the physician may have forgotten to ask the patient if she is, or might be, pregnant. A patient may be treated by two specialists, neither of whom is aware that the patient is taking two sets of prescribed medications. In these and other situations you must assume a responsibility for working with both the physician and the patient to ensure the safety for prescribed medications.

Special Aspects of Administration

Some medications must be administered in special ways to ensure patient safety and comfort. For example, dilute hydrochloric acid that is prescribed for deficiencies for anemia or cancer of the stomach must be taken through a glass drinking tube to protect dental enamel.

Some medications should be taken with milk to minimize gastric irritation, whereas others are inactivated by milk and other foods, and must be taken on an empty stomach. A number of drugs are affected by diet, and the nurse is responsible for making sure that any necessary dietary adjustments are made. For example, certain diuretics create a need for an increased intake of potassium-rich foods.

SOURCES OF DRUG INFORMATION

It is unlikely that any one source will provide all the information a nurse seeks about a given drug. Such information will range from technical data about the drug to practical tips on ways to minimize the discomfort of unavoidable side effects.

Five of the most accessible and useful sources of drug information are a current pharmacology text, a copy of the Physician's Desk Reference (PDR), the pharmacist, material supplied by the manufacturer, and professional journals.

Pharmacology Textbooks

A reputable, current pharmacology text is an excellent source of basic drug information, but its use must be supplemented with other materials. No single text can include all details about each drug, and the information about new or controversial drugs may become outdated between editions whenever ongoing research discovers new effects, either beneficial or hazardous.

Physician's Desk Reference

The Physician's Desk Reference (PDR) is published yearly; a copy is often available on each nursing unit as well as in hospital, school, and agency libraries. The content is divided into five color-coded sections as follows:

Pink: alphabetic listing of drugs by brand name and manufacturer.

Blue: listing of drugs by therapeutic uses.

Yellow: generic and chemical name index.

White: information on the composition, action, uses, doses, administration, precautions, and contraindications of major drugs in current use.

Green: information on diagnostic drugs.

Literature from Manufacturers

When a PDR is not available, the same information can be obtained from the inserts, flyers, or brochures that most manufacturers supply with each of their products. If the hospital pharmacy prepares all drugs for patient use, this material may not accompany the drug to the nursing unit, but it can usually be obtained by a visit to the pharmacy and a request for the desired materials. This literature is usually very detailed, specific, complete, and accurate.

Pharmacist

Whenever the nurse needs *immediate* information about a drug or has been unable to find the answer to a question in any of the sources listed above, a phone call or visit to the pharmacist will provide the needed information.

Professional Journals

Some journals contain a monthly column on drugs in addition to special articles that describe the use of new or controversial drugs. Journal articles also present creative nursing approaches to the psychological and physical problems of chemotherapy.

PATIENT'S RESPONSE TO DRUG THERAPY

In general, drugs achieve their effects by influencing an existing process or mechanism within the body. Drugs can stimulate or depress the activity of cells (ex., CNS stimulants and depressants), stimulate or suppress the growth of cells (ex., anticancer drugs), and increase or decrease the production of hormones, enzymes, and other substances. Some drugs are chemically identical or similar to a specific substance in the body and can be used to supplement the body's natural resources (ex., insulin and estrogen).

Variables That Affect the Patient's Response

The response of a patient to a given drug is modified by a number of physiological and psychological variables that must be taken into account when drugs are prescribed and administered. These variables are: age, body size and structure, sex, physical condition, time and route of administration, individual differences, drug interactions, expectations, emotional status, and environment.

Age
Infants and small children are usually more sensitive to drugs than are older children and adults because, among other things, their mechanisms for using and excreting the drugs are immature. Aged people often have impaired physiological processes that interfere with

absorption, use, and excretion. They often exhibit idiosyncratic responses, some of which are the opposite of the intended effect. For example, some elderly people become agitated, excited, and unable to sleep when given a sedative such as phenobarbital.

Body Size and Structure
The adult dose of a drug is usually based on a "normal" body weight of about 70 kg (154 lb). If a patient weighs considerably more or less, the dose is usually changed accordingly, especially if the drug is potent. Adjustments in dose are also required for marked deviations in body mass. A very short, obese person weighing 150 lb is likely to respond to the average adult dose of some drugs differently from a very tall, lean person who also weighs 150 lb, because of differences in metabolism, especially of the fat cells.

Sex
Men and women respond differently to the administration of hormones such as testosterone. Certain drugs must be avoided or used with great caution during pregnancy to avoid injury to the fetus.

Physical Condition
Drugs are excreted by the lungs, kidneys, and liver. If one or more of these organs is diseased or injured, the excretion of drugs will be impaired, with potentially dangerous results.

The body's response to a drug is also affected by poor circulation, fluid and electrolyte imbalances such as dehydration and edema, nutritional and metabolic disorders, infection, fever, and pain. For example, a large dose of an analgesic such as morphine is needed and well tolerated by a patient in severe pain, whereas that same large dose would be very dangerous for that patient in the absence of severe pain.

Time and Route of Administration
The onset and effect of a drug that is taken orally is altered by the length of the interval between the administration of the drug and the closest meal. Time of administration is also important for patients with pronounced circadian rhythms.

A patient's response to a drug is affected by the speed with which the drug enters the bloodstream. Intravenous administration gives the fastest response; subcutaneous and intramuscular injections are slower; and oral administration is usually slowest of all.

Individual Differences
Some patients are allergic or otherwise unable to tolerate even a small dose of certain drugs. They may experience an exaggerated response to a drug, or a strange and unpredictable, idiosyncratic response. Other people exhibit virtually no response to the normal dose of a given drug.

Drug Interactions
Some drugs are purposely given together because each drug potentiates the effect of the other and gives an effect that is greater than would have been expected from simply combining the effects of each. This effect is termed *synergistic*. Other interactions are merely *additive*. On the other hand, some drugs are *antagonistic* in action. The possible effects of administering antagonistic drugs together are:

- Both drugs are inhibited, and neither drug is effective
- One drug is rendered ineffective by the other drug
- The interaction produces a dangerous or potentially fatal alteration in body function, such as respiratory arrest which can occur when alcohol and tranquilizers are taken together

Expectations
A drug is more likely to produce the desired response when the patient expects that it will relieve or at least ameliorate the symptoms for which it is taken than when the patient is convinced that the drug will not help him. Some patients welcome the administration of prescribed drugs, but other patients fight their use. The effectiveness of a placebo (an inactive substance given in lieu of a drug) is due in part to the patient's expectation that it will help him.

Emotional Status and Environment
High anxiety, apprehension, or panic can necessitate larger-than-usual doses of sedatives, tranquilizers, or analgesics to achieve even the minimal desired effect. The environmental milieu also affects a patient's response to drugs, especially those that are expected to modify his mood or CNS functioning. For example, the normal dose of a sedative would probably be ineffective in a stimulating or threatening environment.

Nontherapeutic Responses

Nontherapeutic drug reactions are usually undesirable—sometimes unexpected—responses. Some such reactions are merely annoying; others result in serious pathological conditions. Eight types of untoward, or nontherapeutic reactions are described below.

Side Effect
Any effect other than one that is desired and therapeutic is a *side effect*. Many side effects are harmless, such

as the temporary discoloration of urine by certain drugs; but others, such as drowsiness, are potentially dangerous if the person drives a car or works at a hazardous job. A side effect which is undesirable for one person can be therapeutic for another. Atropine, for example, causes a decrease in saliva. This condition is therapeutic during anesthesia and surgery but is an unpleasant side effect when atropine is taken for its antispasmodic effect.

Toxic Effect

A harmful or noxious effect of a drug is called a *toxic effect*. It can occur as the result of an accidental or intentional overdose of a prescribed drug, by the ingestion of a poisonous substance, or from a gradual, cumulative effect.

Cumulative Effect

A *cumulative effect* occurs whenever a drug is taken into the body more rapidly than it is being excreted. This can be caused either by an excessive intake of the drug or by faulty excretion. This effect may develop very slowly, like lead poisoning, or very quickly, as in alcohol intoxication.

Allergic Reaction

A drug allergy develops whenever the drug has acted as an antigen and stimulated the production of antibodies. When the patient next receives the drug, the antigen-antibody reaction provokes an allergic response, which may range from a minor skin rash to a fatal anaphylactic shock. Any person who has had even a mild allergic reaction should avoid that drug completely in the future, because subsequent reactions are likely to be much more severe. An example of such a drug is penicillin.

Idiosyncrasy

An *idiosyncrasy* is any unusual response to a drug, such as under-response, over-response, lack of response, a peculiar response, or any unpredictable or unexpected response.

Iatrogenic Disease

Some drugs that must be used over a long period of time can cause a drug-induced disease condition. Some of these *iatrogenic* (resulting from therapy) disease conditions are: malformation of a fetus, liver damage, kidney damage (especially of the glomeruli), skin eruptions, and serious blood dyscrasias (disorders).

Tolerance

Tolerance develops when a person requires increasingly large doses of a drug to achieve and maintain the de-

sired effect. Tolerance is evidenced during the process of addiction, for example, when a person no longer derives any satisfaction from small doses that were formerly adequate. Tolerance also develops with other drugs, as in nitroglycerin tolerance during the treatment of angina.

Dependence

The inclusive term *drug dependence* is replacing the terms *habituation* and *addiction*, which have been used in the past to describe various stages of drug abuse. The World Health Organization endorsed this change in terminology in 1964 and suggested the use of the terms *physical dependence* and *psychic dependence*. Physical dependence (addiction) is a physiological state in which a person experiences intense physical disturbances when the drug upon which he is dependent is withdrawn.

Psychic dependence (habituation) is a state in which a person relies on a drug for the relief of some discomfort or for an increased sense of well-being. The person will experience some degree of psychological discomfort, such as anxiety, if the drug is suddenly withdrawn, but no acute physical withdrawal symptoms. Psychic dependence often involves drugs such as sedatives, laxatives, and tranquilizers.

Because the characteristics and treatment of a drug-dependent state will vary with the drug used, the World Health Organization suggests that drug dependence be described by identifying the type of drug used, such as "physical dependence on opium derivatives" or "psychic dependence on diazepam (Valium)."

RESPONSIBILITIES FOR DRUG ADMINISTRATION

In most hospitals and institutions, there are four groups of people with a primary role in drug therapy, and each has well-defined responsibilities. The physician prescribes the drug; the pharmacist dispenses the drug; the nurse administers the drug and teaches the patient; and the patient notes and reports the effect the drug has on his body.

Responsibilities of the Physician

In a hospital or other institution, the physician writes his drug orders either on a designated page in each patient's chart or in the doctor's order book. In some situations a nurse is permitted to take a verbal order from a physician, either face to face or over the telephone, but she must obtain the physician's signature for that order within a designated time. The physician's drug orders are an integral part of the patient's record and become a permanent legal document.

In some states, nurse practitioners and other specially educated nurses are permitted to order certain drugs when acting within guidelines established by the physician.

Types of Drug Orders

Some of the common types of drug orders include:

A single dose to be given at once (a stat order)

A single dose to be given at a specified time, such as an order for preoperative sedation

Multiple doses for a limited time, such as q 4h × 10 days

Multiple doses to be given indefinitely, such as qd

Multiple doses to be administered as needed (a prn order), for example, q 4h prn for pain. (See Table 18.2 in Chapter 17, p. 326 for an explanation of abbreviations.)

A written order is needed to discontinue a current, valid medication order unless the hospital has an automatic stop policy for certain drugs. Such an automatic stop policy prevents the accidental or unintentional overuse of a drug by limiting the number of days or times it can be given without a written renewal order.

Drug Prescriptions

For a nonhospitalized patient, the physician writes a prescription that the patient takes to a pharmacist. A prescription is composed of the following parts:

Superscription: patient's name, address, age, and date plus the symbol R_x, which means "take thou."

Inscription: name of the drug, strength, and dose.

Subscription: directions to the pharmacist (usually the number of tablets or amount to be dispensed).

Signature ("write on the label"): directions to the patient, directions for refilling the prescription, and whether or not the label should include the name of the drug.

Personal data: signature of the physician and, if the drug is a controlled substance, the physician's registration number and address.

Responsibilities of the Pharmacist

The physician is responsible for the content of his written order or prescription, but the pharmacist is responsible for accuracy in filling the prescription and for correct labeling of the dispensed drug. The pharmacist is also responsible for verifying the validity of the prescription and for guarding against filling a forged or stolen prescription.

In hospitals, the nurse transcribes drug orders from the doctor's order book and requests the prescribed drugs from the pharmacy. The nurse is responsible for the accuracy of her transcription and the drug requisition, and thereby shares the pharmacist's responsibility for accurate dispensing of the prescribed drug.

Many systems have been devised to improve the administration of drugs within a hospital or other institution. Each system is designed to reduce the number of medication errors, minimize the expenditure of time and energy by the nurse and the pharmacist, and keep costs within reasonable limits. Four of these systems are: the stock supply system, the individual supply system, the unit dose system, and the self-medication system.

Stock Supply System

Under the stock supply system, all medications are stored in *bulk* containers in a medication room or closet. The drugs are dispensed and administered by nurses to patients on the unit.

Individual Supply System

Under the individual supply system, the drugs for each patient are stored in *individual* boxes or drawers in the medication closet. The drugs are dispensed and administered by nurses.

Unit Dose System

Small pharmacy substations are established throughout the hospital, and a pharmacist prepares each dose of medicine for each patient under a unit dose system. Some drugs are already individually packaged by the manufacturer. The pharmacist is able to foresee possible problems with incompatible drug interactions and to detect incorrect or unsafe dosages. If the pharmacist is responsible for medication on several nursing units, he may not be readily available for stat and prn orders, and appropriate contingency plans are needed.

Nurses administer the drugs and retain responsibility for related observations and nursing care. This system is likely to be used with increasing frequency as drug therapy becomes more complex and necessitates increasing input from the pharmacist.

Self-medication System

Some hospitals and institutions permit patients to assume responsibility for their own medications whenever possible, especially for those drugs that the patient was taking before admission and drugs that he must take at home after discharge.

Responsibilities of the Nurse

In the past, nursing responsibilities for drug therapy were often restricted to the *administration* of whatever drugs were ordered by the physician. Nurses are now expected to:

- Assess the patient to determine the need for, and the effect of, a given drug or type of drug
- Administer prescribed drugs or supervise their administration by others, such as LPNs or the family
- Safeguard the storage and access to drugs, especially controlled substances
- Integrate drug therapy into other aspects of patient care
- Enhance and potentiate the effect of prescribed drugs
- Teach the patient and family
- Serve as a role model for colleagues, patients, and the public with respect to the responsible use of drugs
- Participate in research, including the use of experimental drugs

These responsibilities require the nurse to have a sound knowledge of anatomy, physiology, pathology, and pharmacology. The nurse must be a highly competent practitioner who is often able to decrease a patient's need for drugs through the skillful use of appropriate nursing interventions.

You are legally responsible for your own actions and must therefore make certain that you administer all drugs safely and effectively.

Responsibilities Of the Patient

The patient is responsible for learning the essential facts about his medications, for taking the drugs as ordered and avoiding any misuse or abuse, for the safe storage of drugs in the home, and for the prompt reporting to the physician of any untoward effects.

ASSESSMENTS

There are two distinct aspects of assessment related to drug therapy: assessment of past use (the medication history), and assessment of the patient's present condition and an evaluation of the effectiveness of the drugs he is receiving.

Medication History

Drugs that the patient has been taking or is taking can account for some symptoms of his present physical or psychological condition and can affect his response to the drugs he is scheduled to receive. A medication history can contribute information that helps to make medical and nursing diagnoses accurate and that promotes the safety and effectiveness of drug therapy.

When taking a medication history, you must explain to the patient the purpose of the history, and you must appear nonjudgmental throughout the process, regardless of your inner feelings and responses. A patient is likely to withhold or alter information about drug use if he senses that you disagree or disapprove of his practices. Areas about which you are concerned can be explored and clarified during patient teaching at some later time.

Because many people do not consider as drugs some nonprescription medications and substances that they use regularly, the questions you ask must be specific and direct if you are to obtain a complete drug history. Some significant drugs that are often missed in a medication history are alcohol, birth control pills, antacids, caffeine, and illegal or nonsanctioned drugs such as marijuana. An example of a medication history is shown in Table 41.1.

Current Condition of Patient

Part of the ongoing assessment on each patient should be related to the drugs he is receiving. Even though

TABLE 41.1 MEDICATION HISTORY

Name _____ Age _____

Sex _____ Date _____

Current Health Problems:

TABLE 41.1 (Continued)

What medications are you now taking, or have you been taking, that were prescribed by your doctor?

	Medication	Dose	Frequency	Duration	Reason
1.					
2.					
3.					
4.					
5.					
6.					

Do you take any medicine, drug, home remedy, or other substances for any of the following conditions? If so, please explain.

Condition	Yes	No	Name of medicine or remedy
Acid indigestion			
Allergies			
Anemia			
Arthritis			
Bladder problems			
Blurred vision			
Colds			
Constipation			
Cough			
Depression			
Diarrhea			
Fainting			
Hay fever			
Headaches			
Hemorrhoids			
High blood pressure			
Insomnia			
Irritability			
Kidney problems			
Low back pain			
Menstrual problems			
Nerves			
Overeating			
Sinus trouble			
Skin problems			
Stress or tension			
Swollen ankles			
Upset stomach			
Vaginal discharge			
Other conditions:			
_____			
_____			

TABLE 41.1 (*Continued*)

Do you take or use any of the following drugs, medicines, or substances? If so, please indicate the amount and frequency.

	Yes	No	Amount, Frequency
Alcohol			
Appetite depressants			
Birth control pills			
Coffee			
Cola drinks			
Iron			
Marijuana			
Mood-changing drugs			
Tobacco			
Tranquilizers			
Vitamins			
Other:			

Are you allergic to any drug, food, dye, anesthetic, or other substance? _____ Yes _____ No
   If yes, please explain: _____

Have you ever had a strange or unexpected reaction to any medicine, drug, food, or other substance? _____ Yes _____ No
   If yes, please explain: _____

Are you now, or have you been, exposed to any chemical, solvent, fumes, or other substance that you feel might affect your health? _____ Yes _____ No
   If yes, please explain: _____

you may not be the person who administers the drugs to your patient, you are responsible for knowing the name, dose, and desired effect of each drug he receives. Your observations make it possible for the physician and medication nurse to plan and implement effective drug therapy. The questions which follow indicate the types of data to be collected.

Does the patient's medication history reveal or suggest any possible contraindications of which the physician may be unaware?

Is the prescribed route of administration appropriate for the patient at this time? For example, is the patient who had a local anesthetic for a bronchoscopy able to swallow yet?

Is the patient exhibiting any untoward effects that should be reported to the physician before another dose of the drug is given?

Does the drug seem to be effective, or should you consult with the physician about the patient's lack of response to the drug?

If the patient has a prn drug order, does he need the drug yet?

These questions suggest only a few of the many assessments that are relevant and essential to the implementation of a patient's drug therapy. Regardless of who administers the drugs, the nurse who cares for the patient is responsible for assessing the effect of his drugs. The assessments that must be made are determined in part by the purpose for which the drug was prescribed.

Knowledge of the patient's condition, the drugs he is receiving, and the desired effect of each are needed for the nurse to be able to identify side effects and untoward effects of his drugs. The medication nurse should indicate to the person caring for the patient what specific data she needs with respect to drugs she has given.

ADMINISTRATION OF DRUGS

General Guidelines

The following information, rules, and guidelines are applicable to *all* routes of drug administration.

Medicine Cards

As soon as possible after the physician writes a drug order for a patient, the nurse copies the order onto the medication section of that patient's Kardex and makes out a medication card or sheet that will be used each time the drug is prepared and administered.

At the beginning of each shift, the medication nurse or pharmacist checks the Kardex against the medicine cards to make sure that there is a proper medicine card for each drug ordered. This process is extremely important because drugs are often prepared and administered in accordance with the medicine cards.

The medication nurse reads down each patient's drug orders as they are listed on the Kardex and compares each order with the corresponding card. In doing so, the nurse:

- Becomes aware of any missing medicine cards that might have been inadvertently put into someone's uniform pocket and forgotten
- Notices any discrepancies between the doctor's order and the medicine card or medicine sheet
- Rewrites any card that is smudged, illegible, or otherwise unclear
- Checks the expiration time of any drug that was, or should have been, ordered for a specific period only
- Checks with the physician if any portion of an order is unclear, if the dose is outside the usual range, or if the route of administration is not appropriate

There are many opportunities for error in transcribing drug orders as each order is transferred from the doctor's order sheet to the Kardex to the medicine ticket. Ideally, each medicine ticket would be compared with the original order, but this is usually not practical. Therefore, responsibility for the accuracy of drug therapy on a given unit rests heavily on the person who copied the original drug order onto the Kardex and on the person who verifies the presence and accuracy of the medicine cards or medicine sheets at the beginning of each shift.

Advance Preparation

If a drug you are going to administer is unfamiliar to you, consult an appropriate reference or resource to determine the purpose and desired effect, usual dose, route of administration, contraindications, side effects, and any precautions or special nursing care that might be needed.

If the drug is to be given prn, check the patient's chart to make sure that someone has not already given it. Patients and families sometimes ask two or three nurses for the same medication if the patient is very uncomfortable and if the first nurse they asked has not yet brought the drug.

If the drug is being given for the first time or on the basis of a stat order, make sure that there is a clear and verifiable order for it. If you cannot read the physician's order, ask for clarification from an appropriate person (the physician, the head nurse, or the supervisor). If you should have any doubts about an order, report your concerns. If you question the safety of an order, *do not give the drug.* "The nurse may, and should, refuse to administer the drug as prescribed if she believes it will result in harm to the patient" (Asperheim and Eisenhauer, 1977, p. 38).

The Five "Rights"

The most fundamental goal of drug administration is to give *the right drug to the right patient in the right dose by the right route at the right time.*

RIGHT DRUG. To make sure the drug is the right one, compare the medicine ticket with the physician's written order or the Kardex. If the medicine ticket is correct, then compare the label of the drug container with the medicine ticket. The label and medicine ticket should be compared:

- When you take the drug from storage (when you take the labeled stock container from the shelf or the labeled container of medicine from the patient's individual supply box or drawer)
- When the amount of drug needed is removed
- When the labeled container is returned to storage

The nurse should respect and trust a patient's comments about his medication being "new" or "different" or being given in a different amount or by a different route. Any such indication of "differentness" might mean that his medication has been changed, but it could also mean that an error has been made. Withhold the drug until you have rechecked both the order and the preparation of the drug. Do *not* try to reassure the patient that everything is all right and insist that he take the medication you have prepared.

It is also important for the nurse to trust a patient's report that he cannot take a certain drug. The drug in question may be correct in terms of the physician's order, but it is not right for the patient if he knows from past experience or present symptoms that he should not be taking it.

RIGHT PATIENT. To make sure you have the right patient, follow two rules: (1) *Always check the patient's identification bracelet before giving a drug of any kind.* (2) *If the patient is able to respond, ask him to state his name.* Do *not* speak the patient's name and assume that a response from him means that he is the right patient. A person will usually acknowledge with a smile or nod any greeting that is addressed to him. If the name sounds wrong to him, he assumes that he simply heard it wrong because you were obviously speaking to him. This is especially true when a patient is dozing, talking with visitors, or distracted by pain or some other discomfort.

These two steps—checking the patient's ID band and asking him to state his name—cannot be overemphasized. They should be followed even when you know the patient well, because identification of the patient must be an integral part of every instance of drug administration. An analogy would be the action of stopping for a red light. A safe driver stops for each and every red light; he does not think about it and then conclude, "It looks safe; I guess I won't bother to stop this time." It takes only a second or two to identify each patient every time, but it can prevent an error that could be costly to both nurse and patient.

Special precautions should be taken when there are patients on the unit with the same or similar-sounding names. Medication cards and the Kardex should be flagged to alert the staff to this situation and its potential for error. If, for example, the medication nurse has been away from the unit for a few days and a nurse or family member tells her, "Mrs. Jones needs her pain medicine," an error is possible if she is rushed and forgets that a second patient named Mrs. Jones was just admitted.

RIGHT DOSE. Errors in dose are minimized when the unit system of drug administration is used and the drugs are prepared in the proper dose by the pharmacist or the manufacturer. Errors are most likely to occur when the dose needed is different from the strength or dose available and when the system of measurement used by the physician is different from the system of measurement used by the pharmacist or manufacturer. If, for example, the physician orders aspirin 0.6 gm (metric system) and the container from the pharmacy is labeled aspirin gr v (apothecary system), the number of tablets needed to give the required dose must be computed mathematically.

Many hospitals and institutions are using the metric system exclusively, but it may be many years before the apothecary and household systems of measurement have been given up completely.

Conversion tables are usually posted in each medication room, but you should be able to solve dose problems mathematically in case you find yourself without a conversion table. Tables of approximate equivalents are included in Appendix A.

If the drug dose for an infant or a child must be calculated, it is important to have a second person check the arithmetic because even a very small error in the dose could lead to a serious or fatal overdose. Whenever possible, pediatric doses are determined on the basis of data supplied by the manufacturer; but when this information is not available, the physician and pharmacist must calculate the dose before writing the drug order.

A number of formulas have been devised for calculating pediatric doses on the basis of age, weight, or body surface area. Of these three bases, age is likely to be the least reliable because a 1-year-old child could weigh 15, 20, or even 30 lb. Two 1-year-old infants, one of whose weight is double that of the other, should not receive equal doses.

A dose based on weight is usually safer. It is calculated by dividing the child's weight by 150 lb (the weight used as a basis for the usual adult dose) and multiplying by the usual adult dose:

$$\frac{\text{Child's weight} \times \text{adult dose}}{\text{Adult weight (150 lb)}} = \text{child's dose}$$

A more accurate dose is based on body surface area and involves the use of a nomogram, which is a graph that enables one to use a ruler or another straight edge to find the child's body surface area if one knows his height and weight.

RIGHT ROUTE. A serious error related to the route of administration is the injection of a substance that was never intended for parenteral administration. Injections may be prepared *only* from those tablets, powders, or liquids that are specially formulated for parenteral use. Injectable substances must be highly soluble and easily absorbed by the bloodstream; injections must *not* be prepared from drugs designed for other routes of administration. The injection of such substances can produce a local complication such as an abscess when given intramuscularly, or a dangerous or fatal systemic effect when given intravenously. If a preparation can be injected, it will be so labeled by the manufacturer. Therefore, *unless the label says "injectable," do not inject it without checking with the pharmacist or the PDR.*

RIGHT TIME. It is important to know why a drug was ordered to be given at certain times and whether or not any flexibility in timing is possible. For example, a drug ordered q 6h (every 6 hours) will be given four times a day, but the intent of the order is different from the order qid (4 times a day). The order q 6h means that the drug is to be given every 6 hours around the clock in order to maintain a consistent level of the drug in body fluids, and the patient will need to be wakened for at least one of the four doses. The order qid means that the daily dose is divided into four portions, which can be given during waking hours, usually near meals and at bedtime. Typical schedules are 8 am, 12, 4, and 8 pm, or 9 am, 1, 5, and 9 pm.

A drug that is ordered ac (before meals) is intended to be given on an empty stomach and should be given 30 to 60 minutes before a meal to allow time for optimal absorption. Absorption will be poor if the drug is swallowed at the beginning of a meal because the stomach will be empty for only a few minutes.

Because it is physically impossible for the medication nurse to administer simultaneously all the medications schedules for a given hour, priorities must be set so that those drugs that must take effect at a certain time are given with a very few minutes of the scheduled time. Insulin, for example, must be given at a precise interval before a meal, and an "on call" preoperative medication must be given whenever the OR nurse calls.

On a very busy unit, it is helpful to give medications to patients in the same order each time, so that the same patients always receive their scheduled medications first and others consistently receive theirs last. This maintains an equal time interval for each patient. If a patient's qid medications are scheduled for 8 am, 12, 4, and 8 pm and if the nurse starts at a different end of the corridor each time, he may receive the drug at 7:30 am, 12:30, 3:30, and 8 pm, making his 4-hour time intervals vary from 3 to 5 hours.

Timing is least important for drugs that are given qd (once a day) or qod (every other day), so whenever possible these should be scheduled for the least busy time of the day. A prn medication should be given whenever the nurse's assessments and clinical judgment indicate that the patient needs it. The patient should *not* have to ask for it each time. If a drug, such as an analgesic, is ordered q 3–4h prn, it can be given any time after 3 hours have elapsed. If your nursing assessment indicates that your patient needs an analgesic before 3 hours have elapsed, present your assessment findings to the physician and obtain a stat order if possible.

Additional Safety Measures

1. *You are responsible for the medications you administer;* therefore, administer only those drugs you prepared personally or that were prepared by the pharmacist.

2. Do whatever you can to decrease interruptions, noise, and confusion around you while you are preparing medications so that you can concentrate on the task at hand.

3. Do not prepare drugs from a container with a smudged, torn, or illegible label. A nurse cannot relabel medications; so return the container to the pharmacy for proper identification and labeling. In the patient's home, call the patient's pharmacy for identification of unlabeled prescription drugs.

4. Do not leave the medication closet or mobile medication cart unattended and unlocked for even a moment. Visitors, patients, staff, and other workers may be tempted by such easy access to drugs. If you are passing medications and are interrupted, take the tray of medications with you; do not leave it at a patient's bedside.

5. If you are unable to administer a prepared medication to a patient, lock it up in the medication closet until he is ready for it; do not leave it at his bedside. If the prepared drug cannot be administered at all, do not return it to a stock container. Instead, dispose of it in accordance with hospital policy. Unused portions of a controlled substance are usually labeled, signed by two persons, and returned to the pharmacy.

6. Do not use discolored or precipitated medications, or drugs that look or smell different than usual. Check the expiration date on each container and keep perishable drugs refrigerated as directed by the manufacturer.

Medication Errors

The nurse who makes a medication error has committed an unsafe act, but the greatest threat to patient safety comes from the nurse who fails to report her error or who is ignorant of the fact that an error was made. Virtually every error can be rectified *if* it is reported to the physician *at once.* Some errors are minor, and the physician may choose to take no remedial action. Other errors may require the administration of an antidote or the careful monitoring of vital signs. If the drug was injected, a tourniquet or ice pack may be ordered to slow absorption of the drug.

If you make a medication error, there are four things to be done. *First* of all, you are legally, professionally, and morally obligated to report it at once. *Second,* you must help to implement any measures that must be taken to counteract the effects of the drug. *Third,* you will be required to fill out an incident report describing what happened. The incident report is a legal record of the event, and in most situations one copy becomes part of the patient's record and one copy will be used by the committee responsible for patient safety. Information about the incident will probably be entered in your student or employee record.

Fourth, in fairness to yourself and to your future patients, it is important to reconstruct the event and discover the probable cause of the error. Some of these causes are inadequate work space, faulty transcription of drug orders, and failure of staff to use existing policies on the preparation and use of medicine tickets. Some causes might be personal, such as nervousness, fatigue from lack of sleep, lack of knowledge, and carelessness. If the causes were external, that information should be conveyed to the proper person. If the causes were internal and personal, that knowledge can lead you toward ways to prevent future errors.

Attitudes toward medication errors vary from one school or hospital to another. Some institutions analyze incident reports carefully in an effort to reduce errors and improve patient care. Others are harsh and punitive toward the individual nurse and may have a dismissal policy based on the number or frequency of medication errors. Threatening approaches make it harder for a nurse to acknowledge an error, while low numbers of reported errors make it difficult for the agency to analyze and deal with the problem in general.

Charting

Methods of recording the administration of medications range from merely initialing the appropriate space on a medication sheet to detailed charting in the nurse's notes. Because many hospitals and institutions assume that each medication was given as scheduled unless otherwise noted, the charting of omissions is especially important. Data related to the medication, such as the name, dose, and scheduled time of administration, should be noted, and the reasons for the omission should be clearly stated. Subsequent nursing and medical intervention depend on the reason for not giving the drug. Some of these reasons are:

Medication was not available

Patient refused the medication

Patient was showing signs of a nontherapeutic reaction

Patient was NPO for diagnostic test treatment

Drug was omitted because of error or oversight

Whenever a prn medication is given, it should be charted promptly, both to reduce the danger of the same medication being given twice and to let the staff know when the next dose can be given if the patient needs it.

All information related to the patient's response to his medications should be carefully documented to aid in evaluating the effectiveness of current therapy and in making decisions on future therapy.

Oral Administration

In addition to the preceding guidelines for drug administrations which are applicable to all routes of administration, there are additional guidelines that are *specific* to the oral route:

1. Pour tablets into an empty medicine cup or the cover of the bottle rather than into your hand so that extra tablets remain uncontaminated and can be returned to the original container. Do *not* pour them into a medicine cup containing other medications for the patient; the drugs may look alike, and it could be difficult to know for sure which tablet is the extra one and should be removed.

2. If the medication for a small child is not available in liquid form, the tablets may need to be crushed. One way to do this is to place the tablet between two spoons. A paper towel or similar object should be placed under the spoons before you crush the drug to catch any fragments of the tablet, which, if lost, would decrease the dose. The crushed tablet should be carefully mixed with a *small* amount of a palatable and compatible substance. It should not be mixed with the child's favorite food because the addition of medicine may alter the taste and could cause the child to avoid that food in the future.

3. Pour liquid drugs from the side of the bottle opposite the label so that liquid does not drip on the label and render it illegible. Hold the medicine glass or cup (made of clear plastic or glass) at eye level while you pour the drug to ensure accurate measurement. Wipe the rim of the bottle as needed before replacing the cap.

4. If a liquid medication is extremely unpalatable, give the patient an ice cube or a little crushed ice before and after he swallows the drug to numb his taste buds. Oily drugs can be made more palatable for some people if they are poured between layers of orange juice. Some liquids are more tolerable if mouthwash or a strong-tasting substance such as an olive is given as soon as the drug is swallowed.

5. Be sure that oral medications are swallowed. Do not leave them at the bedside for the patient to take later unless hospital policy permits or encourages self-administration of medications. Some patients save their oral medications, especially sedatives, for future use at home, and a depressed patient may hoard certain drugs until he has accumulated enough for a potentially fatal overdose.

PROCEDURE 41.1

Giving Oral Medications*

SUMMARY OF ESSENTIAL NURSING ACTIONS

1. Make sure that there is a valid, verifiable, understandable order for each medication you administer.
2. Give only those medications which you prepared personally or were prepared by the pharmacist.
3. Include all possible safety precautions when preparing medications.
   - CONCENTRATE on what you are doing. Minimize all distractions.
   - Check, double check, and triple check each label and drug order.
   - Know the normal dose or range of doses for each medication.
   - Know what each drug and solution should look like.
   - Do not leave medications unattended at any time.
4. Constantly strive to improve the efficiency and safety of your administration of drugs.

*See inside front cover and page 792.

- IDENTIFY EACH PATIENT.
  Ask each conscious patient to state his name.
  Check the identification bracelet of each unconscious patient.
- Remain with the patient until he swallows the medication unless there is a policy or an order permitting the patient to take his own medication.
- Make the drug as palatable as possible but check with the pharmacist before crushing coated tablets, emptying capsules, or mixing liquids.
- RESPECT STATEMENTS OF THE PATIENT regarding the medications he is being asked to take.
- Unless it is contraindicated, help each patient to assume an upright sitting position and provide an adequate amount of water for taking oral medications.

Parenteral Administration

An injection is rarely a routine event for a patient. Many people fear "shots," and military induction centers can document the saying that "strong men faint at the sight of a needle." The responses of children range from apprehension to panic. For persons in severe pain, the need for relief is often coupled with a dread of side effects and fear of possible addiction. The patient who states, "I feel like a pincushion," may be speaking symbolically or literally, because some patients receive so many injections during a serious illness that there seems to be no place for another one.

Equipment

The equipment and supplies used for an injection include the medicine ticket, the drug, a syringe and needle, a needle protector, and materials for cleansing the skin.

SYRINGE. Syringes range in size from a capacity of 1 ml to 50 ml, but syringes larger than 5 ml are rarely used for injections. A 2-ml syringe is adequate for most subcutaneous and intramuscular injections; a larger volume is very uncomfortable for the patient. Most hospitals and institutions use disposable plastic syringes, but glass syringes are less expensive for long-term use in the home.

Insulin syringes have a capacity of 1 ml and are calibrated in units. There is a syringe designed for use with each strength of insulin. For example, a syringe marked U100 is color-coded to match the color of the label of insulin that contains 100 unit/ml. It is possible, in an emergency, to measure insulin with a regular 2-ml syringe, but a person who is not proficient in arithmetic should never attempt to do so. Insulin is an extremely potent drug, and even a slight miscalculation can have serious consequences.

Tuberculin syringes also have a capacity of 1 ml, but they are long, slender, and calibrated in 0.01 ml. This

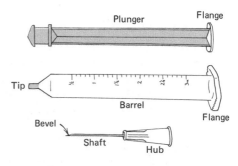

Figure 41.1 Syringe and needle. Shaded parts must be kept sterile.

fine calibration makes it possible to administer very small amounts of potent drugs such as those used for skin testing.

The outside of the barrel of the syringe and the handle of the plunger must, of necessity, be handled during the preparation and administration of an injection, but the inside and tip of the barrel and the shaft of the plunger must be kept sterile (Fig. 41.1).

NEEDLE. The needles that are commonly used for injections vary in length from ½ to 1½ inches and in diameter from 14 to 26 gauge (the larger the gauge, the smaller the diameter). A common size for a subcutaneous injection is 25 gauge, ⅝ inch; the needle for an intramuscular injection is larger and longer: 18 to 22 gauge, 1½ inches.

Some needles are made of surgical steel and can be used indefinitely. Other needles are disposable. Needles are usually packaged individually, to permit greater flexibility in selecting the right needle for a specific patient, although a syringe and needle may be packaged together if the size of the needle is relatively standard, like an insulin syringe and needle.

The hub of the needle will be handled while you are attaching it to the syringe, but the entire shaft of the needle must be kept sterile. The selection of a syringe usually depends on the size of the patient as well as on the characteristics of the drug. The *length* of the needle is determined by the size and weight of the patient and by whether the drug can be deposited in subcutaneous tissue or must be injected deep into a muscle. The *gauge* to be used depends on the viscosity of the fluid to be injected. A thin, watery, nonsticky solution can be injected easily through a fine-gauge needle (gauge 25 or 26), but a thicker, sticky solution requires a larger gauge needle (gauge 20 to 22).

OTHER EQUIPMENT. Disposable needles are packaged inside a plastic needle cover that can be used to keep the needle sterile en route to the patient's bedside. A reusable needle has no needle cover, and it must be kept sterile by being placed between layers of sterile gauze or being stuck into a large, sterile cotton ball.

An individually packaged alcohol swab, or a cotton ball and alcohol, will be needed to cleanse the injection site.

PREPARATION OF AN INJECTION FROM AN AMPULE

An ampule usually contains a single dose of drug in liquid form. It is made of glass, with a constricted neck that must be snapped off to permit access to the drug (Fig. 41.2*a*). Some ampules have a colored ring around the neck, which means that the ampule is prescored and the top is ready to be snapped off. Other ampules must be scratched at the constriction with a file before the top can be broken off.

Part of the liquid may have lodged above the neck of the ampule (Fig. 41.2*b*), and if so, it will be necessary to snap a finger against the top of the ampule to make the fluid flow down past the constriction so it can be withdrawn for injection (Fig. 41.2*c*). Before you break off the top of the ampule, wrap a sterile gauze square around the neck of the ampule to protect the fingers in case the glass should shatter, although this rarely happens. The gauze must be sterile because it will pass over the sterile drug when the top is broken and removed (Fig. 41.2*d*).

After the top of the ampule has been removed, two

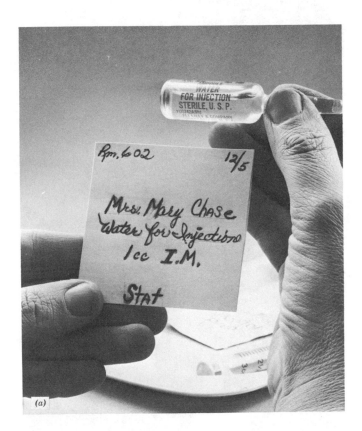

Figure 41.2 *Preparation of an injection from an ampule. (a) Ampule is compared with the medicine ticket. (b) Top of the ampule is checked for the presence of medication. (c) Top of the ampule is flicked to dislodge the medication. (d) Empty top is snapped off the ampule. (e) Position of hands for inserting the needle and inverting the ampule (the syringe is being held by the right hand). (f) Solution is withdrawn from the ampule. Note that the needle is centered in the opening so that the fluid will not trickle down the needle (see text for explanation).*

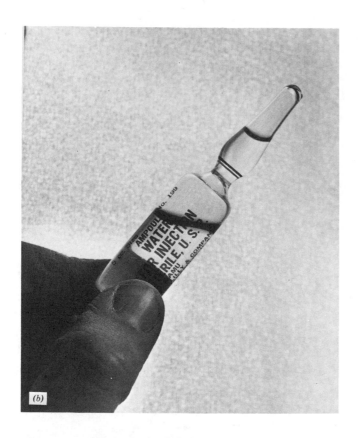

(b)

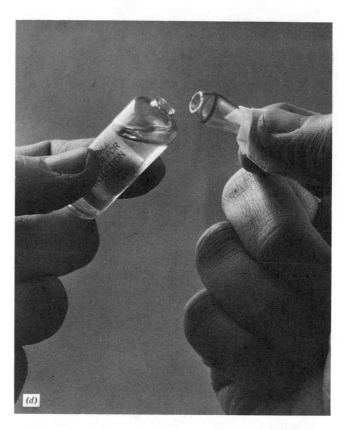

(d)

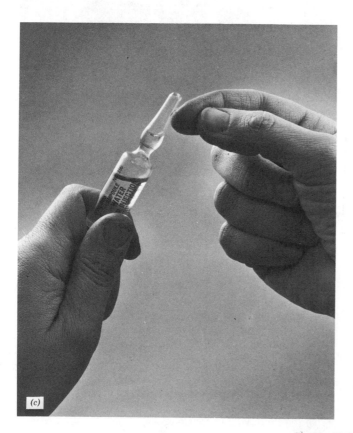

(c)

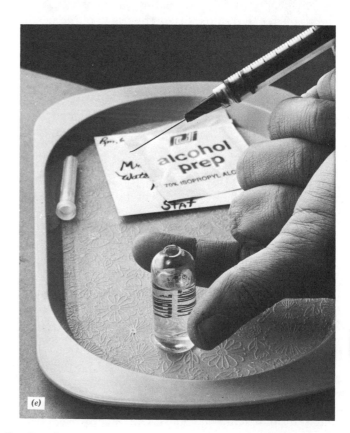

(e)

Figure 41.2 Continued

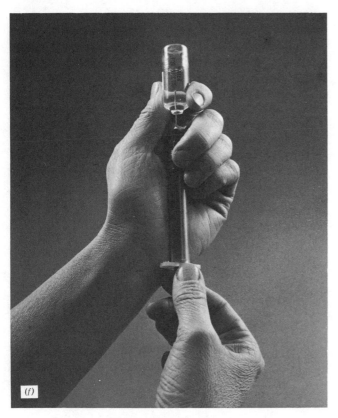

(f)

Figure 41.2 *Continued*

things must be done, in whatever sequence seems easier: the needle must be inserted into the center of the opening, and the ampule must be inverted (Fig. 41.2*e*). The ampule must be inverted to cause the fluid to flow toward the opening so it can be withdrawn by the needle. (If the needle happens to be long enough to *touch* the bottom of the ampule, it is possible to withdraw all the fluid without inverting the syringe.)

When the needle is *centered in the opening* of the inverted ampule, the fluid does not run out of the ampule because atmospheric pressure coupled with the surface tension of the fluid is sufficient to keep the fluid in place. The fluid *will* run out, however, if the needle touches the side of the opening. Some of the drug will trickle down the needle toward the syringe and will be lost.

It is important to keep the tip of the needle below the level of the fluid (Fig. 41.2*f*). If the tip of the needle is above the level of the fluid, air will be drawn into the syringe. If this happens, do *not* try to expel the air back into the ampule because the increased pressure within the ampule will blow the remaining fluid out of the opening and the drug will be lost.

If air enters the syringe, remove it by removing the needle from the ampule, holding the syringe with the needle pointed up so that the bubble of air will rise

toward the needle, then forcing the bubble of air into the atmosphere. Reinsert the needle into the ampule and withdraw the remaining drug. When the syringe has been filled, the needle is covered with a sterile needle protector, a sterile cotton ball, or sterile gauze.

PREPARATION OF AN INJECTION FROM A VIAL

A vial is a sealed glass container with a rubber insert in the top. It can contain either a single dose or multiple doses of a drug in either liquid or dry form. If the drug is not stable in solution, the vial will contain powdered drug, which must be dissolved in accordance with the directions on the label. The manufacturer specifies the type of solvent to be added, usually distilled water or normal saline, and indicates the amount to be added to produce the desired concentration of drug.

When the powder in a multiple-dose vial has been dissolved for injection, the vial must be labeled to indicate the resulting concentration so that subsequent users of that vial can calculate each dose accurately.

Before you attempt to withdraw fluid from a vial, you must inject air into the vial so that removal of the liquid does not create a partial vacuum and make withdrawal difficult (Figure 41.3e). The amount of air injected should equal the amount of fluid to be withdrawn. If you plan, for example, to remove 1 ml of fluid, inject 1 ml of air to replace the fluid. If too little air is injected, it will be difficult to withdraw the fluid. If too much air is injected, it will exert considerable pressure and will tend to force the plunger out of the syringe as you withdraw the fluid.

When several injections from a multiple-dose vial are prepared, a second needle can be inserted into the rubber insert to permit a constant intake of air, which will equalize the pressures inside and outside the vial as the fluid is withdrawn. (See Fig. 41.3.)

General Aspects of Parenteral Administration

SAFETY. Injections should be given in a site that is anatomically safe and in which the skin is free of irritation, inflammation, or infection. Drugs should not be injected into scar tissue or edematous tissue because absorption is poor and uneven from such sites.

The patient's skin should be cleansed with alcohol (70 percent rubbing alcohol is acceptable) or an antiseptic such as povidone-iodine (Betadine). Leave the alcohol sponge in place if there is a chance you will be unable to identify the cleansed site after you have looked away to pick up the syringe.

If the area to be injected is contaminated with urine or feces, or with dirt after a street accident, for example, the skin should be washed with soap and water before it is cleaned with alcohol, because the danger of infection is increased whenever contaminated skin is punctured. Cleansing with an alcohol sponge alone is not adequate.

The skin of some patients is hard to penetrate, and it is possible to bend a needle in the attempt. If a needle bends, it must be replaced with a new one. Do not try to straighten it and use it because additional stress on the needle could break it off.

If a needle does break off during an injection, mark the spot immediately with your pen or pencil. If for some reason you do not have a pen in your pocket, use the patient's call bell to summon help while you

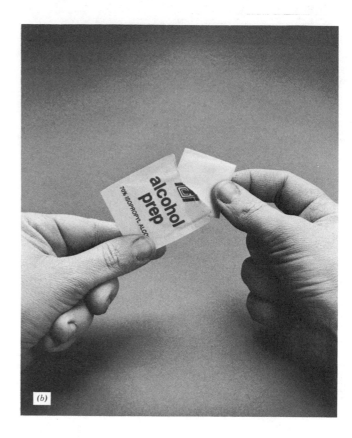

(b)

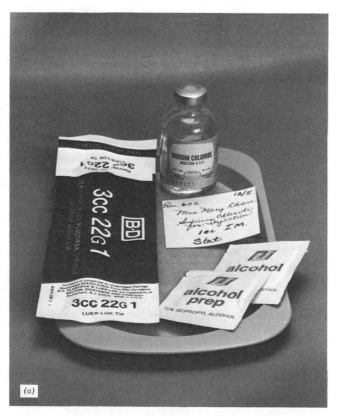

(a)

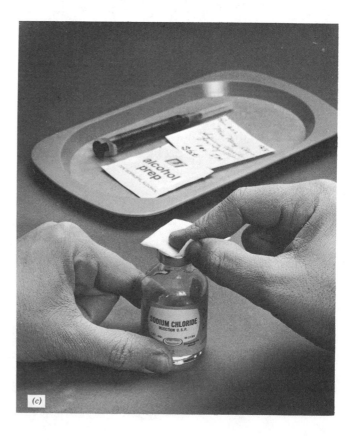

(c)

Figure 41.3 *Preparation of an injection from a vial. (a) Assemble equipment. (b) Remove one of the alcohol sponges from the package. (c) Clean the top of the vial with an alcohol sponge using a firm rotary motion. (d) Remove the needle protector and save it for later use. Note that the alcohol sponge was left on top of the vial to keep the top sterile. (e) Inject air into the vial in an amount equal to the amount of fluid to be withdrawn (see text for explanation). (f) Invert the vial and position the tip of the needle below the surface of the fluid and withdraw the desired amount of medication. (g) Carefully replace the needle protector, keeping the needle sterile.*

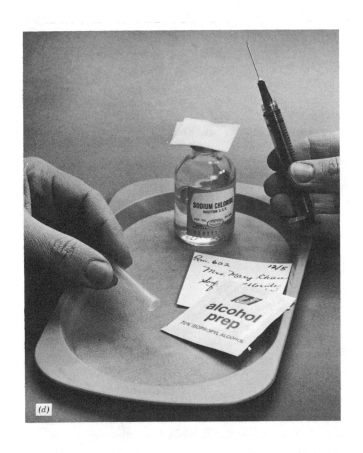

(d)

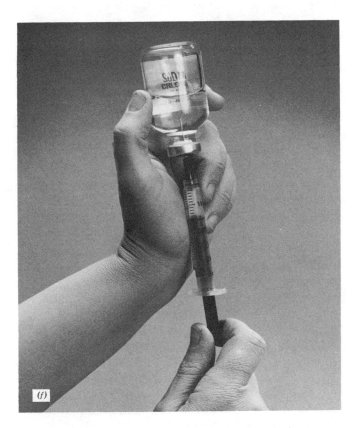

(f)

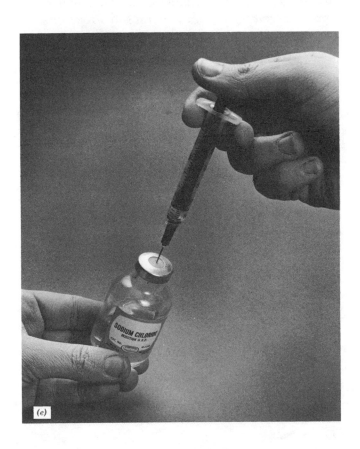

(e)

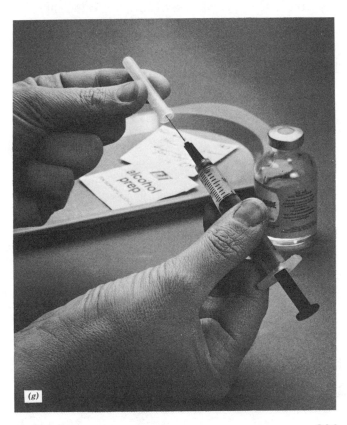

(g)

801

keep your finger at the site of the injection. Report the accident at once.

Before injecting a drug subcutaneously or intramuscularly, you must make certain that the needle has not penetrated a blood vessel. Therefore, before you inject a drug, it is necessary to *aspirate*. To do this, gently pull back on the plunger for about a second. If the needle is in a blood vessel, blood will enter the syringe at once; a forceful or prolonged pull on the plunger is not necessary. If blood appears in the syringe, do not inject the drug because it would be injected intravenously. Withdraw the needle and use a different site, being sure to aspirate again before you inject in the second site.

COMFORT. A patient can be made more comfortable during an injection by the use of faultless technique, proper positioning, diversion, and analgesia.

Faultless technique requires that the needle be sharp, free from burrs, and of the smallest suitable gauge. Disposable single-use needles are usually sharp and smooth, but the bevel of a reusable needle may have become roughened with use. You can test a sterile needle for burrs and roughness by drawing it across a sterile cotton ball or sterile gauze. If it catches and pulls the fibers, obtain another needle. In the home, you can test a reusable needle by drawing it across the back of your hand *before* it is sterilized. If it scratches your skin, remove the burr by drawing the needle across a fine pumice stone several times. During the injection, the syringe should be held like a dart or pencil and injected quickly and smoothly.

Positioning is important for comfort during an intramuscular injection because injection into a tense, taut muscle is painful, whereas injection into a relaxed muscle is sometimes scarcely felt. Effective positioning for each of the common intramuscular sites is described along with site selection later in this chapter.

Diversion can be provided in innumerable ways; it includes such diverse activities as asking the patient to focus his attention on a certain object, to think of something pleasant, or to whistle. A child can be diverted by telling him a joke or asking him to count. For many a patient, it is enough to just keep talking with him.

When you are giving an injection to a child, it may be advisable to have a second person distract him while you concentrate on injecting the drug. If the child struggles to avoid the injection, a third person may be needed to help hold him firmly but gently. Mechanical restraints should not be used except in extreme situations.

Analgesia may be needed for injections that are very painful. The area can be numbed with an ice cube or cold compress before and after the injection, or the physician may order a small amount of local anesthetic to be given with the injection.

Comfort and absorption will be increased by massage of the injected area for a few minutes unless this is contraindicated by the nature of the drug. *Firm pressure* should be exerted against the skin and underlying muscle as you move your fingertips in a rotary movement. Merely rubbing the skin does *not* promote comfort and absorption.

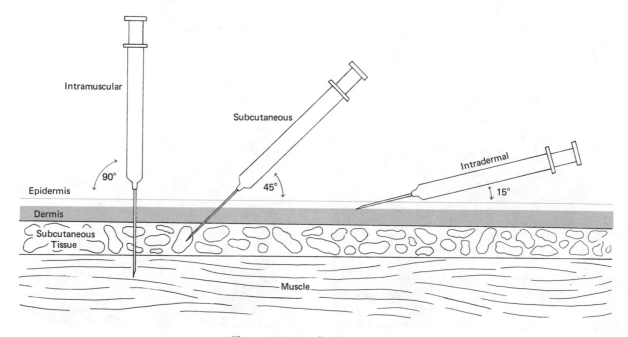

Figure 41.4 *Angles for injection.*

Types of Injections

INTRADERMAL INJECTIONS. Extremely potent or potentially hazardous substances such as those used for allergy testing are injected intradermally because adsorption from the skin is slow. If the drug were absorbed rapidly, the patient could suffer a severe or fatal anaphylactic shock. The anterior portion of the forearm is used most commonly, although the upper back can be used when extensive testing is needed.

A *short, fine-gauge* needle (26 gauge, ⅜ inch, for example) is inserted between the layers of skin at a 0 degree to 15 degree angle (Fig. 41.4). When the needle is properly inserted, the bevel of the needle is visible under the skin and the injected fluid raises the upper layer of skin.

The possibility of a severe reaction is so great that many physicians do not permit others to inject their patients. The patient is usually observed closely for a number of minutes. The area of injection should *not* be massaged because to do so would alter the body's reaction to the test agent. Charting should include the precise location and exact time of administration because it is usually necessary to observe the injection site at specified intervals.

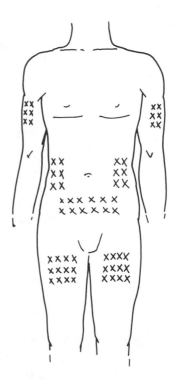

Figure 41.6 *Diagram for rotation of subcutaneous injection sites. Tissue damage occurs when medication, such as insulin, is injected repeatedly in the same site.*

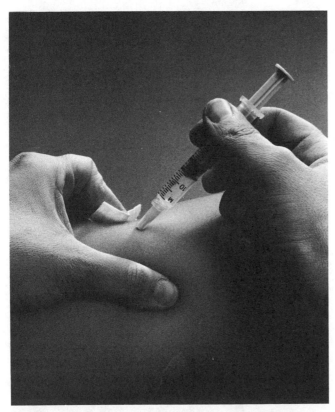

Figure 41.5 *Subcutaneous injection. Note the 45° angle. The left hand is lifting subcutaneous tissue away from the underlying muscle.*

SUBCUTANEOUS INJECTIONS. A subcutaneous (hypodermic) injection is given at a 45 degree to 60 degree angle into the loose tissue just under the skin (Fig. 41.5). Absorption is slower than by intramuscular injection, but subcutaneous injections are safer because there is less danger of striking a nerve or blood vessel with the needle. Some drugs are irritating to subcutaneous tissue and must, therefore, be given intramuscularly. Necrosis of the tissue can occur when an irritating drug is carelessly injected into subcutaneous tissue instead of deep into a muscle.

Insulin is administered subcutaneously, and because the drug is given once or twice daily over a number of years, it is important to *rotate the sites* to avoid the tissue damage that follows repeated injections in the same spot. A map or chart of the pattern of injection sites should be prepared and carefully followed (Fig. 41.6). Patients tend to use the front of their thighs almost exclusively and must be encouraged to use alternative sites such as the abdomen and upper arms.

INTRAMUSCULAR INJECTIONS. Drugs that are irritating to subcutaneous tissue or that must be given in fairly large amounts (over 2 ml) are given intramuscularly. Discomfort is reduced because there are relatively few nerve endings in muscles. Absorption is fairly rapid because muscles are more vascular than subcutaneous tissue. The risk of hitting a large blood vessel or nerve is greater than with a subcutaneous injection, and great caution must be exercised in selecting a site for injection. The complications of intramuscular injections include necrosis of tissue following the accidental injection of an irritating drug into subcutaneous tissue as a result of using too short a needle, accidental *intravenous* administration of a drug, and nerve injury, such as paralysis of a lower extremity following injury of the sciatic nerve.

An intramuscular injection is given at a 90 degree angle with a needle that is long enough to pass through the subcutaneous tissue and penetrate the underlying muscle (Fig. 41.7). A 1- to 1½-inch needle will suffice for some patients, but a 3-inch needle may be needed for an obese patient. Recent research indicates that many injections which are intended to be intramuscular never reach the muscle and are deposited in fat, and that more attention needs to be paid to the selection of an appropriate needle length.

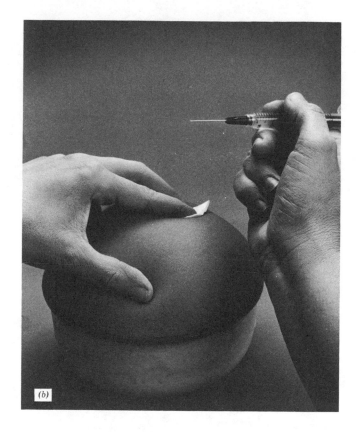

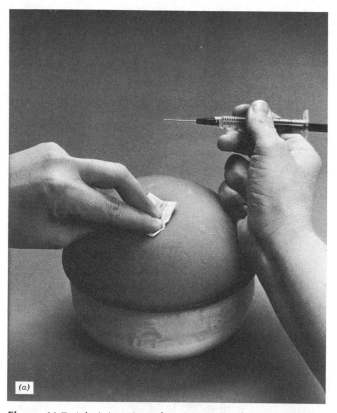

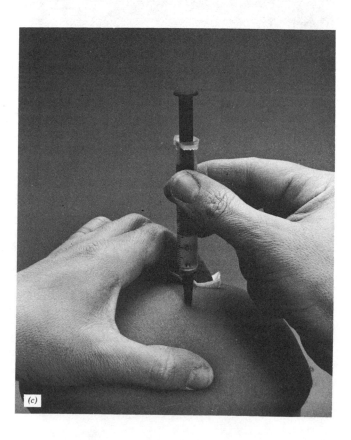

Figure 41.7 *Administration of an intramuscular injection. (a) Clean the site with an alcohol sponge using a firm circular motion. (b) Hold the skin taut while pressing down toward the underlying muscle. (c) Inject the needle at a 90° angle. Release pressure on the skin and transfer the syringe to that hand. (d) Pull back slightly and briefly on the plunger to determine whether or not the needle is in a blood vessel. (e) If no blood appears in the syringe, inject the medication slowly. (f) Apply pressure on the skin with an alcohol sponge while withdrawing the needle. Use the alcohol sponge to massage the injected area unless contraindicated.*

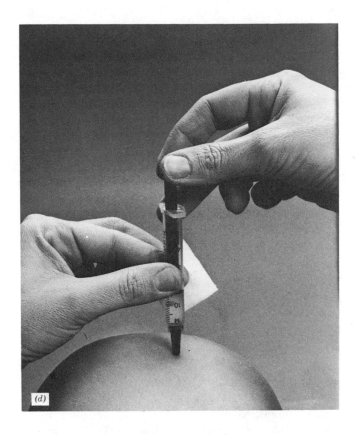

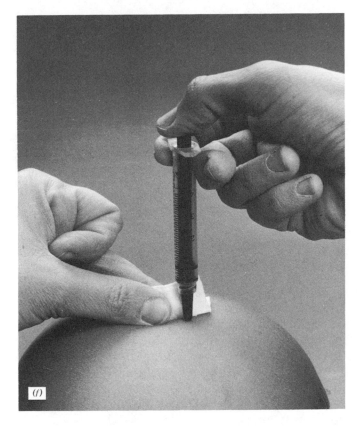

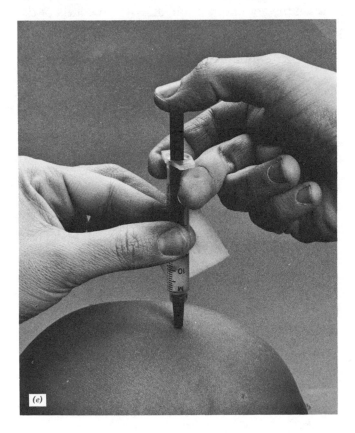

The skin over the injection site is usually pulled taut and pressed down to facilitate penetration of the muscle. It is sometimes necessary to grasp and *elevate* the muscle of a tiny infant or an extremely emaciated adult to prevent the needle from hitting the underlying bone even though a short needle is being used.

Aspiration is extremely important before an intramuscular injection because a muscle is more vascular than subcutaneous tissue, and there is a greater possibility of hitting a blood vessel, especially if the injection site is selected incorrectly.

SPECIAL TECHNIQUES. If a drug is known to be especially irritating to subcutaneous tissue, special techniques must be employed to avoid leaving traces of the drug as the needle passes through the subcutaneous tissue (Fig. 41.8).

First, the needle that was used to withdraw the drug from the vial or ampule should be wiped clean with a sterile cotton ball or sterile gauze sponge to remove all traces of the drug. If the drug is sticky, the needle should be replaced with a new one.

A second technique involves the use of an air lock. After the drug has been withdrawn from the vial or ampule, and before the injection is given, a small amount of air (approximately 0.2 ml) is drawn into the syringe. When the injection is given at the required 90 degree

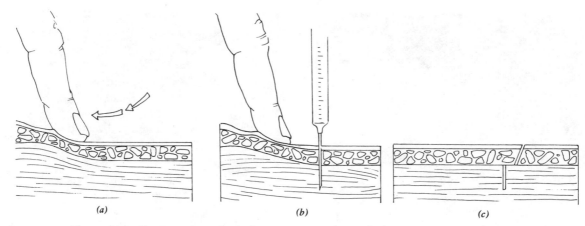

Figure 41.8 *The Z-track method of injection. (a) Skin pulled to one side and held there. (b) Needle in place. (c) Z-track sealed when the skin is released.*

angle, this air rises to the top of the syringe and follows the drug as it is injected. The air forces all the drug out of the needle so that none of it can be tracked back through the subcutaneous tissue as the needle is withdrawn. The injected air is absorbed by the muscle without difficulty. A *Z-track technique* is used in addition to an air lock for drugs that are especially irritating or that stain subcutaneous tissue and skin. Before you inject the needle, pull the skin and underlying tissue away from the intended point of injection and hold it there while the needle is inserted (Fig. 41.8a). If no blood enters the syringe during aspiration, inject the drug and the bubble of air from the air lock, wait for approximately 10 sec to permit the initial dispersion of the drug, and while still retracting the skin, withdraw the needle. When the skin and subcutaneous tissue are released, they return to their previous position. The track left by the needle in the subcutaneous tissue is thereby moved to one side, so no medication escapes from the muscle (Fig. 41.8c).

The process of aspirating for blood is more complex when this technique is used. Some nurses can handle the syringe and aspirate with one hand, while still holding the skin and tissue to one side with the other hand. If you cannot do so, continue to hold the skin and underlying tissue with your little and ring fingers and use your thumb and index finger to support the syringe while you aspirate with the other hand.

Intramuscular Site Selection
The choice of a site for an intramuscular injection depends on the volume of drug to be injected, the size of the patient's muscles, the accessibility of possible sites, and the number of times each potential site has been injected. The four most commonly used sites are the deltoid, dorsogluteal, ventrogluteal, and vastus lateralis muscles.

DELTOID. The deltoid muscle is a useful site when the volume of the drug is small and when other sites are inaccessible because of a body cast, dressings, or other obstructions. Accurate site selection is important because the area is small and is adjacent to significant blood vessels and the radial nerve. Accurate site selection is not possible if the patient merely pushes up his sleeve; the entire upper arm must be exposed for safe identification of the necessary landmarks. The deltoid site in the adult is a small rectangle that is bounded on the top by a line two fingers below the acromial process and on the bottom by a line drawn at the level of the axilla (Fig. 41.9). The width of the rectangle occupies the middle third of the side of the upper arm. The radial nerve curves around the lower edge of this rectangle.

The deltoid muscle is small and shallow in children and as a rule should not be used if another site is available. The deltoid muscle is relaxed for injection when the patient's arm is at his side.

DORSOGLUTEAL. The gluteus maximus and gluteus medius muscles constitute the traditional site of intramuscular injections. This is a potentially dangerous site because the sciatic nerve is located just below it, and there have been numerous incidents in which a patient's leg has been completely or partially paralyzed by damage to this nerve when the injection was given too low.

The dorsogluteal site is located above a diagonal line between the posterior superior iliac spine and the greater trochanter of the femur (Fig. 41.10). These landmarks are located by palpation. If the greater trochanter is obscured by large amounts of fat and subcutaneous tissue, it can sometimes be located by palpation while the patient flexes and extends his hip.

The above method for locating the dorsogluteal site replaces the older method of dividing the buttocks into quarters and using the outer aspect of the upper outer

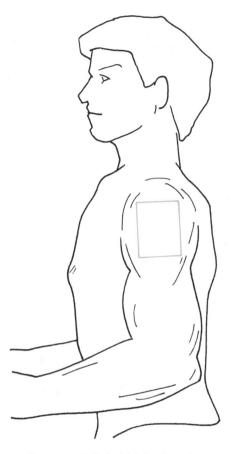

Figure 41.9 Deltoid injection site.

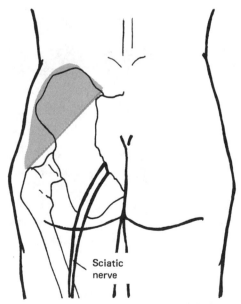

Figure 41.10 Dorsogluteal injection site (shaded area). Note that this site is safely above the sciatic nerve.

quadrant. The quadrant method is *unreliable* because flabby, sagging buttocks distort the gluteal folds and can lead to the selection of a site that is too low, with possible damage to the sciatic nerve.

The gluteal muscles are not well developed until a child has been walking for some time, and therefore, *the dorsogluteal site should not be used in infants and small children* except in an emergency when no other site can be used.

The patient should lie on his abdomen with his *toes pointed inward (internal rotation of the hips)* to relax the gluteal muscles before injection of the drug. If this is not possible, he can lie on his side with his hip and knee flexed. This site should not be used when the patient is standing because the gluteal muscles are contracted and tense when a person stands erect.

VENTROGLUTEAL. The ventrogluteal site uses the gluteus medius and minimus muscles, and because it is toward the front of the body, it is safely away from the sciatic nerve. To locate the site, place the palm of your hand over the patient's hips with your *thumb pointing toward his groin and lower abdomen.* Place your index finger over the anterior superior iliac spine and move your middle finger back along the iliac crest as far as possible. The V-shaped space between your fingers is the ventrogluteal site (Fig. 41.11).

This site is desirable because the muscle is deep enough for safety even if the patient is emaciated or an infant. No special positioning is needed to relax the muscle for injection, and the site is accessible for use whether the patient is lying on his side, back, or abdomen. It can also be used when a patient is sitting or standing, if the area is exposed enough for proper identification of the landmarks.

Some people find it difficult to remember which site is dorsal and which is ventral. It sometimes helps to associate the dorsogluteal site with the diagonal line between the posterior superior iliac spine and the greater trochanter, and to connect the ventrogluteal site with the **V** formed as the fingers touch the anterior superior iliac spine and the iliac crest.

VASTUS LATERALIS. The vastus lateralis is a long, thick muscle that extends the full length of the thigh and is relatively free of major nerves and blood vessels. It is the preferred site of injection in small children (Fig. 41.12).

The boundaries for an adult extend from a handbreadth above the knee to a handbreadth below the greater trochanter of the femur. The boundaries for a child mark the middle third of the distance from the knee to the greater trochanter (Figure 39.12). The width of the site in both children and adults extends from the

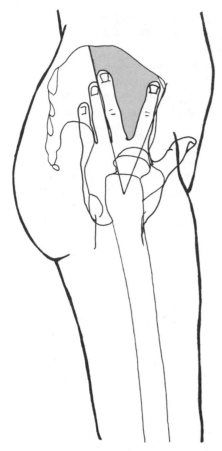

41.11 *Ventrogluteal injection site (shaded area between fingers).*

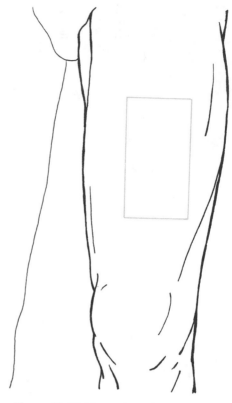

Figure 41.12 *Vastus lateralis injection site.*

midline of the top of the thigh to the midline of the outer side of the thigh.

The site is located and the injection is given with the patient lying on his back with his knees slightly flexed, or in a sitting position.

PROCEDURE 41.2

Giving an Injection*

SUMMARY OF ESSENTIAL NURSING ACTIONS

1. Check the medicine ticket for accuracy and validity.
2. Prepare the prescribed dose of drug using sterile technique.
3. Identify the patient.
4. Expose and select a safe and appropriate site.
5. Cleanse the skin thoroughly.
6. Inject the needle at the proper angle.
7. Aspirate for blood.

8. Inject the drug.
9. Apply pressure over the injection site and withdraw the needle.
10. Massage the area firmly.
11. Dispose of the needle properly.
   • Follow agency policy to prevent illegal possession or use of needles.

*See inside front cover and pages 796–808.

DRUG PROBLEMS OF THE ELDERLY PATIENT

Older people experience two major types of drug-related problems: those related to the *administration* of drugs and those related to the *physiological effects* of drugs.

Problems Related to Drug Administration

As a person ages, he becomes subject to an increasing number of chronic disease conditions, many of which must be treated with drugs. It is not uncommon, for example, for an elderly person to be taking medications for hypertension, glaucoma, a cardiac problem, arthritis, and constipation. The drugs used to treat these conditions are taken from one to four or five times daily, which can mean a total of 10 to 20 pills each day, plus additional drugs to treat an occasional cold, flu, or other ailment.

The task of taking multiple medications as prescribed is difficult enough for a younger person, and it can seem overwhelming to any elderly person who is hampered by poor vision, shaking hands, or a tendency toward forgetfulness. In addition, the side effects and interactions between drugs can compound the problem by causing restlessness, confusion, depression, or other disturbing conditions.

The nurse has two major goals when working with elderly patients, especially those who must assume partial or complete responsibility for taking multiple medications as prescribed. The first goal is to teach and encourage health practices that will decrease the number and dose of drugs as much as possible, and the second is to help the patient devise a safe, effective system of drug administration.

It may be difficult to establish health practices that will help an elderly person decrease the number or dose of his medications because health habits are hard to change. Examples of health practices that should be initiated or maintained include:

- Increased fluid intake and changes in diet to decrease constipation
- Decreased salt intake and loss of weight to help reduce hypertension
- Walking around the room each hour or elevating legs to improve circulation and help prevent swollen ankles
- ROM exercises to help delay stiffness from arthritis or immobility
- Regular exercise (even within a single room) and the avoidance of naps late in the day to prevent or relieve insomnia

The patient and family will sometimes feel that the benefits from such changes are not worth the effort involved. The task may be difficult and discouraging, and everyone involved in the patient's care must resist the temptation to rely on drugs to counter any complaints of discomfort. It often seems easier to reply, "Did you remember to take your pills?" than it is to help the patient *change his health habits* to minimize or alleviate his physical discomfort.

The goal of helping the patient to devise a safe system for taking those medications that must be taken may require considerable ingenuity. Systems that have been devised by nurses to help patients remember the scheduled time and date of each medication have included the use of little boxes or containers labeled with large, bold type; color-coded charts; and separate, labeled envelopes for every medication time (21 to 28 per week). As a rule, no one can devise an effective system *for* the patient; it is too difficult for an elderly person to unlearn his old patterns and to memorize a new one. The task is most likely to be successful when the nurse works *with* the patient to *increase the safety and effectiveness of the existing system.*

Problems Related to the Effects of Drugs

It is usually difficult to assess the effect of a given drug on an elderly person because the use of multiple drugs coupled with his altered physiological responses frequently produce responses that are unpredictable and often adverse. Metabolic changes and slowed circulation result in poor absorption of drugs. Changes in liver, kidney, and intestinal function cause decreased excretion of drugs. The prescribed intake of a drug combined with slow absorption and slow excretion can produce a cumulative toxicity that is often serious. Some toxic effects are missed and overlooked because symptoms such as depression, lethargy, confusion, or irritability are often attributed to senility rather than to drug toxicity. In some cases, additional drugs or increased doses of the very drugs that are causing the symptoms are prescribed in misdirected efforts to relieve the undiagnosed drug toxicity.

PATTERNS OF DRUG USE

The words *compliant* and *noncompliant* describe the manner in which a person follows a prescribed regimen of drug therapy. A person is said to be compliant (or in compliance) when he faithfully takes his prescribed medication in the right dose and at the right time. These terms are used most frequently in reference to long-term drug therapy for conditions such as diabetes, hypertension, and congestive heart failure.

Reasons for a patient's compliance can be hypothesized on the basis of his responses to other aspects of health care, but they cannot be known with certainty without direct input from the patient. Reasons for compliance are varied and include:

- Active effort to maintain or regain health
- Passivity (doing what the physician says without question)
- Fear of death if the disease is life-threatening
- Fear of displeasing or angering the physician, nurse, or family, and not knowing that it is possible to refuse a drug

Noncompliance refers to partial or complete failure to follow a prescribed drug regimen and involves the overuse, underuse, and misuse of prescribed drugs.

Overuse

A drug is *overused* when it is taken in doses greater than those prescribed, more frequently than prescribed, or for conditions that do not warrant the use of the drug. Reasons given by patients for overusing a drug include:

"If one tablet was good, I thought two would be better."

"I wanted to get well faster."

Possible Reasons for the UNDERUSE of Drugs

- Forgetfulness
- Lack of money or transportation to get prescriptions refilled
- The need to be seen by a physician before prescriptions can be refilled
- Religious or cultural beliefs that were not known or not taken into account when the drug was ordered
- Incompatibility of drug therapy with patient's usual lifestyle
- State of denial (in which the patient rejects the diagnosis and sees no reason to take the medications)
- Fear of physical or psychological dependency on drugs
- Fear of long-range side effects, such as cataracts after long-term cortisone therapy
- Belief that the condition has already been cured or relieved by the drug
- Dread of side effects such as the nausea and vomiting that follow each dose of some anticancer drugs

---

"I couldn't wait any longer—I was too uncomfortable."

"The medicine is too slow (or too weak)."

Drug overuse is fostered when drugs are offered too freely or are too accessible. Some patients have a very low tolerance for physical discomfort and find it easier to use drugs than to endure any type or degree of discomfort.

Underuse

A drug is *underused* when it is omitted, taken in reduced doses, or taken less frequently than prescribed. Possible underuse should be suspected whenever a patient's condition does not improve in response to a drug that is usually effective.

A patient should not be scolded or criticized until reasons for possible underuse have been explored and verified by the patient.

The nurse's role is to discover the reasons for the patient's underuse of prescribed drugs and then try to resolve the problem. For example, a patient who does not take his medication for hypertension because of distressing side effects should be encouraged to report his symptoms to his physician so that a different antihypertensive drug can be tried. A patient who dislikes the effects of his oral anticancer drug and decides to take only half the dose each day but to take it for twice as many days within each cycle of administration must be helped to understand that, although the total dose will be the same, a half-strength level of drug in his blood each day may be useless.

Misuse

The *misuse of prescribed drugs* involves such practices as saving prescribed drugs for future self-medication and sharing such drugs with other people. The *misuse of over-the-counter (OTC) drugs* occurs when nonprescription drugs are used indiscriminately or inappropriately.

Many minor conditions, such as head colds, superficial burns, and mild headaches, can be effectively treated with OTC drugs; and it is appropriate and practical for a person to do so. Intelligent self-medication saves money and frees a busy physician from treating a host of minor ailments.

Misuse of OTC drugs, on the other hand, can be hazardous indeed. For example, the cough that accompanies a cold can often be treated adequately and safely with an OTC cough syrup, but a persistent cough *could* be the result of a serious pathological condition; attempts to treat it with OTC remedies will only postpone proper diagnosis and therapy.

The hazards of self-medication can be decreased by teaching the public how to determine when self-medication is likely to be appropriate and safe and when it is inappropriate and unsafe. Every person should read the labels of OTC drugs carefully before purchasing them. Many drugs carry warnings, such as "Do not take unless ordered by your doctor if you have high blood pressure, thyroid problems, or diabetes." Other warnings are designed to protect children and pregnant women. Many OTC drugs contain a combination of ingredients; if a patient is hypersensitive to aspirin, for instance, there are a number of OTC drugs he should not take.

Abuse

Drug abuse refers to the persistent or excessive use of a chemical substance for nonmedical reasons. Drug abuse usually involves the use of controlled substances such as amphetamines, barbiturates, and opium derivatives, as well as substances such as alcohol, caffeine, and tobacco. As the drugs being abused were not usually prescribed as part of a therapeutic regimen, drug abuse is not commonly referred to as noncompliant behavior.

PATIENT TEACHING

There are two separate but related aspects to drug education: the *acquisition of factual information* about specific drugs and the *development of appropriate patterns of drug usage*. Neither aspect is more important than the other; and unless *both* are included, patient teaching cannot result in improved drug usage.

Teaching about Drugs

No matter how well-intentioned a patient may be, he cannot take medications safely and effectively if he has inadequate information about the drugs. He must acquire essentially the same information as a nurse, but in much less detail. He should know the name, appearance, dose, purpose, desired effect, possible side effects, route of administration, precautions, and contraindications for each drug he is taking.

The patient should be taught to ask questions such as:

- What is the purpose of this drug? What is it supposed to do?
- What are the side effects? Which ones would be serious enough to call the doctor about?
- Are there any foods, drugs, or other substances that I should avoid while taking this drug?

- How quickly will the drug take effect? How soon will I notice a difference in my condition?
- Are there any special directions or precautions to be observed while I am taking this drug?

This aspect of drug education is usually the easiest for both patient and nurse because it is factual, with few emotional overtones, and there are many ways to present the information. If the nurse's prior assessment of a patient indicates that he is literate, the necessary information can be written on 3 × 5 cards for him, or printed materials can be used. If literature supplied by the manufacturer is given to a patient, it is often advisable to underline or highlight the essential content. Some hospitals and nursing units have prepared printed information sheets for each of the most frequently prescribed drugs. The information can be studied and memorized by the patient and discussed by patient and nurse. The patient can be tested orally, or with paper and pencil, depending on his age and aptitude.

In addition to providing information about medications, you will need to assess each patient's knowledge of drug safety as well as that of the family.

Patient Teaching—Basic Rules of Drug Safety

1. Whenever possible, keep each drug in its original labeled container. If a drug must be transferred, the new container should be clearly and completely labeled.

2. Keep oral medications separate from external medications and other substances that should not be ingested.

3. Discard the unused portion of a drug that was prescribed for a specific illness. Do not save it for future self-medication. Discard drugs into the sink or toilet, not in the trash where children might find them.

4. Discard drugs when the expiration date is reached. If the container has no printed expiration date, ask the pharmacist about the length of the period of safe usage.

5. Refrigerate all drugs that require refrigeration.

6. Insist that all prescribed drugs have the *name of the drug on the label*. The identification of drugs by name decreases the likelihood that a wrong medication will be taken, and in the event of an overdose, it aids in emergency treatment.

7. Always read the label and identify the drug before you take it; do not take drugs in the dark. If anyone in the family has a tendency to do so, mark the container with an identification that can be felt, such as a strip of sandpaper or sticky tape.

8. Read and follow all instructions.

Teaching about Drug Usage

Variables to be considered when teaching a patient about drug usage include his feelings and beliefs about drugs, his perception of his role in drug therapy, and his current patterns of drug use.

Feelings and Beliefs

The attitude of a person toward the use of drugs will have evolved slowly throughout his entire life. Many older patients remember being given a distasteful "spring tonic" such as sulfur and molasses, for example, and a patient's current response to problems of constipation will be affected by the attitudes and practices of his parents toward intestinal elimination. The parents' use of drugs; the number and type of drugs in the family medicine chest; the patient's past experiences with drugs, both positive and negative; and many other factors influence a patient's attitudes toward drugs.

Some people view the use of medications as:

- A source of comfort and help, a sign that something is being done
- A sign of weakness; they believe "a person ought to be able to manage without pills"
- A dangerous practice that can lead to dependency and addiction
- An accepted part of everyday life; for them, the norm is: "Take two aspirin and go to bed"
- A welcome relief from suffering and discomfort; their attitude is: "If there is a pill for it, I'll take it!"

Conflicts, spoken or unspoken, can result whenever patient, nurse, physician, and family hold different views about the use of drugs.

The Patient's Role in Drug Therapy

A major goal of effective drug education is to help the patient develop an awareness of his own role in drug therapy. Depending on his age and competency, he must learn that many of his rights carry a concomitant responsibility and that he must assume an active role in this aspect of health care. This part of patient teaching is not easy; it is very hard for a person to learn to become involved in his own drug therapy, for example, if he has said for years, "I don't know what that medicine is for—it's just something the doctor told me to take."

PATIENT RIGHTS. In addition to relevant but general provisions of the Patient's Bill of Rights, a patient has rights that are specific to drug therapy. He should be taught that he has the right to:

- Be properly assessed and diagnosed before medications are prescribed and given to him
- Understand the relationship between his drug therapy and his overall plan of care
- Be warned about dangerous side effects or a potential for drug dependency so that he can give informed consent for the administration of a drug
- Refuse a medication (the term *doctor's order* does not mean that the patient can be ordered to take a given drug)
- Be informed and consent in writing to the use of experimental drugs
- Be given no unnecessary drugs
- Receive care that will minimize his need for drugs
- Be taught about his drugs in preparation for discharge or self-administration
- Be taught ways to reduce his need for drugs

PATIENT RESPONSIBILITIES. Each patient, in accordance with his capability, needs to learn effective ways to ensure the safety of himself and his family through the proper use and storage of drugs, and by carrying Medic Alert tags and wallet drug identification cards when needed. He must also learn to participate in his own drug therapy by asking questions, taking the prescribed medications as ordered, and reporting any untoward reactions to his physician.

RELATED ACTIVITIES

In preparation for teaching patients about drug usage, begin to examine your own feelings, beliefs, and practices related to drugs by considering the following questions:

- What is your earliest memory of taking medicine? How did you feel at the time about the incident?
- Under what circumstances do you take drugs rather than feel uncomfortable?
- Under what circumstances might you refuse to take a medication? Why might you do so?
- How do you react to a person who refuses to "take anything" to relieve his obvious discomfort or pain?
- What is your reaction to the sight of a shelf full of medicine in a person's kitchen?

It may be helpful to write a one-page statement of your beliefs about drug use based on your answers to the above questions. Such a statement may indicate which of your attitudes are likely to be therapeutic and which, if any, may warrant further exploration.

SUGGESTED READINGS

Allen, Marcia D: Drug therapy in the elderly. *Am J Nurs* 1980 Aug; 80(8):1474–1475.

Anderson, Kathy, and Carol Poole: Self-administered medication on a postpartum unit. *Am J Nurs* 1983 Aug; 83(8):1178–1180.

Brock, Anna M: Self-administration of drugs in the elderly. *Nurs Forum* 1979 July/Aug; 18(4):340–351.

Chaplin, Gail, Harriet Shull, and Paul C Welk III: How safe is the air-bubble technique for I.M. injections? *Nursing 85* 1985 Sept; 15(9):59.

Coyle, Nessa: Analgesics at the bedside. *Am J Nurs* 1979 Sept; 79(9):1554–1557.

Davis, Neil M, and Michael R Cohen: Learning from mistakes: 20 tips for avoiding medication errors. *Nursing82* 1982 March; 12(3):65–72.

Fonville, Ann McClung: Teaching patients to rotate injection sites. *Am J Nurs* 1978 May; 78(5):880–883.

Hudson, Margaret F, and Audrey S Rogers: Drugs and the older adult take special care. *Nursing 84* 1984 Aug; 14(8):47–51.

Leporati, Nina Chychula, and Lydia Helen Chychula: How you can really help the drug-abusing patient. *Nursing 82* 1982 June; 12(6):46–49.

Loebl, Suzanne, and George Spratto: *The Nurse's Drug Handbook.* New York, Wiley & Sons, 1986.

Long, Glenda: The effect of medication distribution systems on medication errors. *Nurs Res* 1982 May/June; 31(3):182–184, 191.

Milkman, Harvey, and Stanley Sunderwirth: The chemistry of craving. *Psych Today* 1983 Oct; 17(10):36–44.

Minion, Bernadine J: Truly caring for the patient who's an alcoholic. *Nursing 85* 1985 Aug; 15(8):55–56.

Mullen, Elaine M, and Michele Granholm: Drugs and the elderly patient. *J. Gerontal Nurs* 1981 Feb; 7(2):108–113.

Palmer, Dee Ann: Unit dose. *Am J Nurs* 1980 Nov; 80(11):2062–2063.

Slawson, Michelle: Thirty three drugs that discolor urine and stools. *RN* 1980 Jan; 43(1):51.

Spencer, Roberta, et al: *Clinical Pharmacology and Nursing Management.* ed.2. Philadelphia, Lippincott, 1986.

Winfrey, Audrey: Single dose I.M. injections: how much is too much? *Nursing 85* 1985 July; 15(7):38–39.

Wong, Donna L: Significance of dead space in syringes. *Am J Nurs* 1982 Aug; 82(8):1237.

42

Care of the Unconscious Patient

Care of the unconscious patient will be what you make it. It can be a depressing and frustrating experience, or it can be a quietly rewarding experience with many triumphs and satisfactions. The unconscious (deeply comatose) patient cannot be aroused, does not respond to pain or any other stimuli, and has no reflexes. The care of such a patient can be depressing if you look to the patient-nurse relationship as the source of your satisfaction and reward. A comatose patient is unable to communicate with you in any way, and some nurses find the day-after-day, or month-after-month, care of an unresponsive patient almost intolerable. The patient's family may be so preoccupied with their own needs that they may not seem to notice or appreciate your efforts. The staff may feel as you do, and as a result, it is possible to care for a comatose patient for days or weeks without hearing a single word of thanks, or appreciation of your efforts.

If, on the other hand, you are able to create an atmosphere of hope based on goals which are enthusiastically accepted by the family and other staff, your rewards will come from your *progress* toward those goals. The daily care of the patient will be physically and emotionally hard, and your interactions with the family may be difficult, but you will be able to say to yourself at the end of the day, "That's a good job well done!"

LEVELS OF CONSCIOUSNESS

Conditions of consciousness and unconsciousness extend along a continuum which ranges from normal alertness to deep coma. Movement along this continuum indicates whether the patient's condition is improving or worsening, and the nurse's ability to detect minute changes is basic to both medical and nursing diagnosis and treatment.

Consciousness has two components: (1) arousal (wakefulness), and (2) awareness of one's self and the environment. Arousal is a function of the reticular activating system (RAS) in the upper brain stem, while awareness is a function of the cerebral cortex. Consciousness is the result of normal interaction between these two parts of the central nervous system, the brain and the reticular activating system of the brain stem. An *altered* level of consciousness is the result of *disrupted* interaction between the cerebral hemispheres and the RAS.

An altered level of consciousness depends upon the location and severity of damage to the brain or brain stem. As would be expected, the greater the damage, the greater the impairment of consciousness will be. Of equal significance, the *lower* the site of injury, the greater the loss of consciousness.

The cerebral cortex is responsible for intellectual and emotional functions. Damage to these higher levels results in decreased alertness and confusion, but there may be minimal impact on vital functions such as respiration and temperature regulation. Injury to lower portions of the brain stem may render the patient unable to breathe, and he may require the permanent use of mechanical ventilation.

Descriptive Terms

Various terms have been used to describe levels of consciousness, none of which is precise enough to provide an accurate terminology for diagnosis, treatment, or research. The following descriptive terms are commonly used:

- *Conscious.* Alert; oriented to time, place, and person; interacts appropriately with the environment; thinks; responds to sensory stimuli.
- *Lethargic.* Somnolent; drowsy; makes sluggish responses; may be oriented when awake; can be aroused easily but drifts back to sleep.
- *Obtunded.* Sleeps much of the time but can be aroused; usually confused.
- *Stuporous.* Responds to vigorous and intense stimuli only; makes an appropriate response to a painful stimulus (withdraws or tries to push it away).
- *Semi-comatose (light coma).* No thinking; no feeling; no awareness of self or environment; motor responses to painful stimuli are inappropriate (serve no useful purpose).
- *Comatose (deep coma).* No responses; no reflexes; extremities flaccid; thermoregulatory mechanisms erratic; respiratory patterns irregular; EEG almost flat.

VEGETATIVE STATE. In addition to the traditional terms listed above, professional and lay person's often use the term *vegetative state* to describe an unresponsive level of consciousness. A patient in this condition is often awake, but is not aware of himself or his surroundings. His RAS is intact enough to permit arousal, but damage to his higher brain centers prohibits thought, perception, and awareness. His eyes may be open and may move, but they do not focus or follow a moving object. He may act restless at times in response to physical discomfort such as a fever or fecal impaction, but the response is nonspecific because the situation has no meaning for him. Periods of wakefulness and sleeping have no pattern and bear no relationship to day and night. A vegetative state may indicate progress from a coma toward a higher level of consciousness, or it may be a permanent condition.

The Locked-In Syndrome

The *locked-in syndrome* refers to a condition in which a fully conscious patient is imprisoned in a paralyzed body. He is awake and aware, but unable to communicate either verbally or through gestures because of severe damage in the brain stem to all motor pathways. This condition may be mistaken for a coma or a vegetative state, and in extreme situations, it can be distinguished from brain death only by the patient's normal brain waves (a normal EEG). The locked-in syndrome may be caused by a brain stem stroke, tumor, brain stem abscess, encephalitis, or amyotrophic lateral sclerosis (Lou Gehrig's disease). Depending upon the cause, the patient may remain mute and quadriplegic until death, although a few do regain a degree of understandable speech.

The possibility of locked-in syndrome makes it imperative that each unresponsive patient be assessed fully and regularly. Locked-in patients are alert, aware, and intelligent, and even though they may be unable to communicate normally, some of them are able to blink or move their eyes, and can communicate in response to yes-or-no questions. It is imperative that a locked-in patient not be treated as a comatose or vegetative patient because he hears, understands, and responds both mentally and emotionally to what is going on around him, and he should be helped to participate in planning his care and his future.

Table 42.1 GLASGOW COMA SCALE

Response	Behavior	Score
Eye-opening response	Opens eyes spontaneously, purposefully	4
	Opens eyes upon command to do so	3
	Opens eyes only in response to pain	2
	Does not open eyes at all	1
	Untestable (eyes bandaged or swollen shut	U
Verbal response	Fully responsive and oriented	5
	Confused regarding time, place, or person	4
	Responds with inappropriate words, phrases	3
	Makes unintelligible sounds; moans, groans	2
	Makes no speech sounds at all	1
	Untestable (tracheotomy; other intubation)	U
Motor response	Moves limbs upon command	5
	Moves limbs purposefully in response to pain	4
	Flexes arms in response to pain	3
	Extends arms in response to pain	2
	Does not move at all	1
	Untestable (limb immobilized by cast, etc.)	U

Glasgow Coma Scale

The adjectives which have been used to differentiate between various levels of consciousness are subject to the interpretation of both the observer/reporter, and the person receiving the report, and as a result, communication about an unconscious patient is imprecise and often misunderstood.

The Glasgow Coma Scale was developed at the University of Glasgow in 1974 in an effort to develop a uniform way of assessing and describing levels of consciousness. This scale assigns a numerical score to the type of responses made by the patient to specific stimuli. There are three categories of responses (eye-opening, verbal, and motor) which are scored separately, and then totaled to give an overall score. Total scores range from 3 to 15, and a score of 7 or less indicates a state of deep coma and a poor prognosis.

The total score will range from 3 to 14 if all responses are testable. The *higher* the score, the *higher* the level of brain function.

The advantages of the Glasgow Coma Scale are that it is *uniform* (the same rating is given by all observers), *quick* (numbers are used for charting and reporting), and *specific* enough to monitor fairly small changes in the patient's level of consciousness.

To use the Glasgow Coma Scale, determine whether or not a given response is testable, and then start with a mild or minimal stimulus. Since it is important to determine and record the patient's *best* score, it is necessary to start testing with the mildest stimulus possible. Use a normal tone of voice, repeating your questions or commands as necessary. If the patient does not respond to this verbal stimulus, call him by his first name, use a louder tone, even shout before you proceed to use a painful stimulus.

If the patient does not respond to loud, emphatic verbal commands, apply painful pressure. This can be done by pressing a blunt object such as a pen or pencil to the cuticle of the finger nail (the base of the nail where it meets the skin) or by pressing your finger in a circular motion over the patient's sternum. *Purposeful movements* in response to pain include withdrawal from the source of pain, or trying to push away the examiner's hand. It is important to apply the pain to a spot which the patient can reach; pinching the patient's calf or achilles tendon may not be a valid stimulus because the patient may be unable to reach those areas to try to brush the stimulus away.

When the patient's verbal responses are being tested, it is important to individualize and vary your questions, especially if assessments are repeated frequently. The patient who is asked repeatedly "What is your name?" and "Do you know what day this is?" may become annoyed and refuse to answer and thereby receive a lower and inaccurate score. Orientation to time, place, and person can be determined by asking about visitors, what was eaten at the previous meal, and what is likely to happen later in the day.

If the patient curses in response to a painful stimulus, further testing is needed to determine whether it is an appropriate verbal response (with a score of 5) or whether the patient can only utter single, inappropriate words (score of 3).

When you test *motor responses*, it is wise to avoid the command "Squeeze my hand" because it is difficult to differentiate between a grasp reflex and obeying the command. "Touch your chin" and "scratch your arm" are more useful commands.

An overall score of 14 indicates that the patient is fully conscious, while a patient with a score of 7 or below is usually considered to be in a coma. It is important to record the score for each subscale separately because different neurological conditions can yield the same overall score.

For example, the *total* scores of the following patients are identical, but the *different subscores* show that the nursing observations to be made and the nursing care to be given will vary, as will the medical diagnosis and treatment of each patient.

	Patient A	Patient B
Best eye-opening response	5	3
Best verbal response	1	2
Best motor response	2	3
Total score	8	8

Causes of Unconsciousness

Conditions which cause unconsciousness are either structural or metabolic/toxic in nature. *Structural* causes include all types of physical damage to the brain or brain stem such as a fractured skull, brain tumor, hemorrhage, contusion, and edema. *Metabolic/toxic* causes include conditions which interfere with normal brain metabolism such as anoxia, drug overdose, uremia, alcohol intoxication, hypoglycemia, electrolyte imbalance, and lead poisoning.

Structural damage is usually unilateral and localized initially, but if the condition is not treated, the effect becomes bilateral and generalized. Metabolic/toxic conditions affect the metabolism of the entire brain and brain stem, and the effects are not localized.

Types of Structural Lesions

Lesions* of the brain are categorized according to their location with respect to the tentorium. The *tentorium* is a tough fold of the dura which divides the cavity of the skull into anterior and middle fossae above, and the posterior fossa below. Lesions above the tentorium are called *supra*tentorial lesions while those below are called *infra*tentorial or *sub*tentorial. An opening in the tentorium accommodates various nerves, and is called the *tentorial notch* or *tentorial hiatus*.

Small, isolated lesions in one cerebral hemisphere do not cause unconsciousness as long as the ascending RAS and its connections to the cerebral cortex are intact. *Large* lesions, on the other hand, can press against the midline structures, and exert pressure on the opposite hemisphere. This bilateral pressure can cause unconsciousness by compressing the blood vessels and reducing the supply of oxygen to the brain. In addition to exerting pressure against the opposite hemisphere, a large supratentorial lesion can force cerebral tissue down through the tentorial notch and exert pressure on the upper brain stem. This is called *herniation of the brain* and is a dreaded complication of increased intercranial pressure.

Infratentorial lesions damage the brainstem and/or the RAS. It is possible for these lesions to cause herniation upward through the tentorial notch, and affect the cerebral hemispheres.

Increased Intracranial Pressure

The skull protects the brain from many types of injury, but its rigidity creates a dangerous situation whenever cerebral pressure is increased. Normal intracranial pressure ranges from 0 to 15 mm Hg with slight increases during activities such as coughing, sneezing, or strain-

---

*With reference to unconsciousness, the term *lesion* refers to any area of *pathologically altered tissue*. It refers to the area of involvement or damage, regardless of the cause or nature of the damage. This broad usage permits the use of the term *lesion* to refer to a wide variety of pathological conditions such as a localized tumor, a gunshot wound, generalized cerebral edema, or anoxia, and injury to the brain stem.

Causes of Increased Intracranial Pressure

- Increased amount of brain tissue: additional cells (brain tumor) or swollen, edematous cells
- Increased volume of cerebral spinal fluid: from impaired circulation or absorption of CSF
- Increased volume of cerebral blood: vasodilation, increased BP, or cerebral hemorrhage

ing at stool. Pressure in excess of 20 mm Hg is considered abnormal.

Intracranial pressure is determined by the space occupied by the contents of the skull which normally consists of brain tissue, cerebral blood, and cerebral spinal fluid. An increase in the amount of any of these components increases the intracranial pressure, since a larger volume occupies more space and exerts more pressure.

Effects of Increased Intracranial Pressure

The effects of increased intracranial pressure (IICP) constitute a vicious circle which perpetuates itself unless therapy is effective. Swelling (edema) is a normal part of the inflammatory response, and it occurs whenever any part of the brain is injured. Swelling of brain tissue increases intracranial pressure which compresses cerebral blood vessels which impairs circulation and reduces the amount of blood reaching the brain (ischemia). An inadequate blood supply results in lack of oxygen to the brain (hypoxia) which leads to an increase in CO_2 (hypercapnia). This imbalance produces more edema which increases intracranial pressure and impairs circulation even further.

The end result of increased IICP is physical damage to the brain or brain stem; herniation through the tentorial notch occurs, or there is metabolic damage as a result of insufficient oxygen and glucose. The brain makes up only 2 percent of an adult's body weight, but consumes 20 percent of the body's oxygen supply. The brain cannot store oxygen, and any interruption in the oxygen supply, whether from a heart attack or from increased intracranial pressure, leads to observable signs and symptoms within a matter of minutes. Glucose is the major source of fuel (energy) for the nervous system, and the supply must not be interrupted because the nervous system has no reserve stores of glycogen as the body does.

Medical Treatment

Increased intracranial pressure is treated by the use of hyperosmotic drugs to remove excess cerebral fluid, measures to reduce the volume of circulating blood, steroids, and hyperventilation to reduce the level of CO_2. In some situations, it is necessary to remove a section of skull bone (craniotomy) to relieve pressure from edema, or to permit removal of an accumulation of blood from a hemorrhage. Fluid intake is restricted, and the head of the bed is kept elevated at 30 degrees to promote the return of venous blood from the brain.

Intracranial pressure can be measured *directly* through a hollow device such as a cannula or catheter which has been inserted into the epidural space, subdural space, or ventricle. These measurements are potentially hazardous because of the danger of infection. IICP is monitored *indirectly* by careful observation and *early detection of changes* in the patient's pupils, LOC, and vital signs.

Nursing Responsibilities

There are four major types of nursing responsibilities related to the care of an unconscious patient: (1) making ongoing assessments of the patient's neurological status, (2) supporting and teaching the family, (3) maintaining your own energy and commitment to excellence, and (4) meeting the needs of the patient.

Assessment of Neurological Status

LEVEL OF CONSCIOUSNESS. The patient's LOC is assessed during the initial examination, and thereafter as often as indicated by his condition, sometimes as often as every 15 to 20 minutes. LOC is determined by the location of the damage to the brain and brain stem, and is important in both diagnosis and management of the condition. For example, momentary loss of consciousness, confusion, or headache is caused by involvement of the cerebral cortex and if treated effectively, is less dangerous than a brain stem lesion involving vital regulatory centers. Changes in LOC which indicate that lower centers are becoming involved point to a worsening condition, while changes in LOC which show some return of function of the next higher part of the CNS point to improvement.

The Glasgow Coma Scale is an efficient and effective tool for assessing level of consciousness when used correctly, but additional information should be sought at the time of the initial examination. Family members, friends, or others who might know should be asked: "How long has the patient been in this condition?" "What changes have been noted?" and "How rapidly have the changes occurred?"

PUPILLARY RESPONSES. The third cranial nerve (oculomotor) runs along the tentorial ridge, and responds to pressure by causing pupil dilation. Increased ICP exerts pressure on the nerve, and unilateral pupil dilation is important because it helps to determine which side of

---

Normal Pupillary Responses

- BRISK constriction in response to bright light
- CONSENSUAL reflex in response to light
- Pupils are in MIDPOSITION
- Pupils are CONJUGATE (move together)

the brain has been damaged. The *onset* (first appearance) of unilateral dilation is extremely significant because it signals increasing ICP and is a primary sign of impending herniation of the brain through the tentorial notch. Pupils which suddenly become *dilated and fixed* signal a medical emergency.

The presence or absence of reactive pupils helps to pinpoint the level of the lesion. For example, damage to the midbrain produces fixed pupils which do not react to light but which may fluctuate in size. Pupils that do react to light indicate a functioning midbrain. In a metabolic/toxic coma, the pupils may remain reactive until a terminal stage is reached.

OCULOCEPHALIC ("DOLL'S EYES") REFLEX. Eye movement of a comatose patient can be tested by rotating his head from side to side with his eyes open. The normal response (positive doll's eyes) is for both eyes to turn in the direction opposite the direction in which the head is rotated. When the neck is extended, the eyes turn down; when the neck is flexed, the eyes roll up. A normal response indicates a functioning brain stem.

If one or both eyes remain fixed, doll's eyes are absent (a negative response) which indicates pressure on the midbrain and upperpart of the brain stem.

This test cannot be done on a conscious person because he will control the movements of his eyes.

OCULOVESTIBULAR REFLEX (COLD CALORIC STIMULATION). Eye movement can be tested by instilling cold water into the ear canal of a comatose patient. The normal response is for the eyes to move toward the irrigated ear and implies some function of the brain stem. This test is never done until it has been determined that the tympanic membrane is intact.

This test is unnecessary if doll's eyes are present.

PHYSICAL EXAMINATION OF THE HEAD. During the initial examination of the patient, especially when the cause of coma is unknown, it is important to look for evidence of injury such as fresh or dried blood, a recent scar, a penetrating foreign object, or a depressed skull fracture.

The nose and ear canals should be inspected for evidence of bleeding or leakage of cerebrospinal fluid. Blood mixed with cerebrospinal fluid does not clot normally, so any unusual blood stains should be reported to the physician at once.

BREATHING PATTERNS. Patterns of expiration and inspiration are related to the location of the lesion or the extent of increasing intracranial pressure, and are therefore important diagnostic signs. The following patterns are significant:

- *Cheyne-Stokes breathing.* Alternating crescendos and decrescendos of depth of breathing (hyperpnea to apnea); associated with lesions in cerebrum and basal ganglia.
- *Central neurogenic hyperventilation.* Respirations which are regular, deep, and rapid (more than 24 per minute); associated with lesions in lower midbrain and middle pons area.
- *Apneusis.* Prolonged inspiration followed by a pause before a prolonged expiration; associated with extensive brain stem damage.
- *Cluster breathing.* Irregular spurts of breathing with periods of apnea; associated with damage to upper medulla.
- *Ataxic (Biot) breathing.* Completely irregular, unpredictable breathing which merits consideration of mechanical ventilation; associated with damage to medulla.
- *Other vital signs.* In addition to respiratory abnormalities, evidence of other pathological changes may appear. The patient's temperature may be unstable due to erratic functioning of his thermoregulatory mechanism. A severely increased intracranial pressure produces ischemia of the CNS which produces a marked increase in arterial blood pressure in an effort to overcome the high ICP and supply the brain cells with blood and oxygen.

MEETING THE NEEDS OF THE PATIENT

The needs of the unconscious patient are similar to those of any other patient—they vary only in degree and priority. For example, Maslow's hierarchy of needs is as applicable and relevant to the unconscious patient as it is to any other individual if the nursing emphasis is temporarily shifted toward the lower level needs. The unconscious patient requires concentrated efforts to meet his safety and physiologic needs, with less attention paid to his needs for esteem and respect.

Since the unconscious patient is completely unaware of his needs, he is totally dependent upon the nurse's ability to assess his condition, identify his needs, and take appropriate action. These aspects of nursing process must be done systematically because the patient can be in great jeopardy if any need is overlooked or neglected.

The assessment and care of an unconscious patient can be made systematic in a variety of ways such as following a head to toe sequence each time, doing an orderly review of body systems, or doing specific assessments at a given time each day. The material which follows has been organized to correspond with the sequence in which the basic content was presented in the preceding chapters of this text. The chapters related to physical care and comfort were organized as follows: safety, infection, sensory stimulation, physical activity, hygiene and grooming, fluid and electrolyte balance, respiration and circulation, nutrition, elimination, rest and sleep, and body temperature. This sequence of topics provides one of many possible ways to organize the assessment of needs and related nursing activities.

Regardless of the type of organization used, the nursing care of an unconscious patient is directed toward the following goals:

- The safety of the patient
- Maintenance and support of basic life functions
- Prevention of complications of the underlying cause of unconsciousness
- Prevention of complications related to immobility
- Maintenance of maximum potential for rehabilitation

Environmental Safety

Areas of Assessment Related to Safety

- Presence of side rails on bed
- Presence of identification bracelet or other means of positive identification
- Presence of protective mattress or pads, and bed boards if needed
- Condition and availability of monitors, equipment, and supplies
- Safety and stability of overhead equipment

Related Nursing Activities

Each nurse, upon entering the patient's unit, should automatically make a quick assessment of each factor which might pose a hazard to the patient by mentally asking questions such as: Is the bed in the proper position? Is the IV running at the proper rate? Is the suction machine plugged in and ready for use? Is the catheter free of kinks, and running well? Are emergency supplies available? Is a footboard or other device in place to protect the patient from footdrop? Is the unit free from clutter which might hinder the staff?

All unconscious patients are at risk of developing pressure ulcers, and therefore each bed should be equipped with a water or air mattress, alternating pressure pad, sheepskin pads, or other devices to protect the patient. It is only by careful attention to such environmental details that the patient can be protected from the dangers of which he is unaware.

Infection

Areas of Assessment Related to Infection

- Handwashing practices of staff
- Techniques of medical and surgical asepsis
- Condition of skin and mucous membranes
- Knowledge and understanding of family and visitors

Related Nursing Activities

An immobilized patient is vulnerable to infection, and since he is unable to call attention to obviously unsafe practices, each nurse must monitor her own performance and engage in a form of peer review of other staff. Every effort must be exerted to make sure that all staff, including aides and orderlies, realize that the skin and mucous membranes are the patient's first line of defense against infection, and that these surfaces must be kept intact at all cost.

Family members and other visitors must understand that the immune system of an unconscious patient may be depressed or otherwise altered, and that he should not be exposed to the "flu," colds, or other illnesses.

Sensory Stimulation

Areas of Assessment Related to Sensory Stimulation

- Condition of sensory organs (eyes, ears, nose, mouth, and skin)
- Amount of sensory stimulation (noise, lights, movement)

Related Nursing Activities

Care of the sensory organs of an unconscious patient is extremely important because they are the gateways to his mind. If any of these organs are damaged by inattention or neglect, any possible return to full awareness could be impaired.

EYES. An unconscious patient does not blink, so if the patient's eyes tend to remain open or partially open, you will need to protect the corneas from dryness. Dryness of the cornea leads to corneal ulceration and possible loss of vision. This can be prevented by lubricating each eye with commercially available artificial tears at regular intervals, and if necessary, by using eye pads to keep the eyes closed. Good nursing care makes it unnecessary for the physician to resort to the old practice of suturing the eyes shut to keep the corneas moist.

When you examine pupillary responses, it is important to position your fingers over the bone of the socket as you open the lids, and to avoid any pressure on the eyeball.

Strict medical asepsis must be maintained when the patient's face is washed; wipe the lids from the inner canthus toward the outer canthus (from the nose out toward the temple).

EARS. The ears should be observed as indicated for any evidence of leaking cerebrospinal fluid. They should be kept free from an accumulation of cerumen (ear wax) which could cause discomfort and impair the patient's ability to receive auditory stimuli.

If the patient normally wears a hearing aid, make sure that it is in place and functioning properly if he gives any sign of returning consciousness or responds in any fashion to the sounds around him. Make sure that the hearing aid is *adjusted properly* so that he is not distressed by excessive volume.

NOSE. The patient's sense of smell is affected by the condition of his nasal passageways and the mucous membranes of his nose. His nostrils should be kept clear and unobstructed, and should be lubricated as needed to counteract the irritation of a nasogastric tube or oxygen given by nasal cannula.

If the patient had a keen sense of smell and enjoyed a variety of aromas, it is sometimes possible to use that sense as a way of making contact with the patient. Some families bring the patient's favorite perfume or cologne, and believe that the patient is aware of it.

Each nostril should be checked regularly for the presence of leaking cerebrospinal fluid if such an assessment is warranted.

MOUTH. The mucous membranes of the mouth must be protected from dryness, irritation, and infection which can be caused by prolonged mouth breathing, inadequate cleansing, malnutrition, dehydration, chemotherapy, and the prolonged use of certain antibiotics. The mouth should be kept scrupulously clean and lubricated as often as necessary to keep the membranes moist. Either a soft toothbrush or a commercial substitute such as a sponge rubber toothette can be used to clean both the teeth and the tongue. Suction equipment should be ready for use, and a helper is usually needed to keep the patient's mouth open.

Examine the patient's mouth for lesions, bleeding gums, loosening teeth, or white patches which might indicate an infection such as thrush Candida albicans.

SKIN. Since an unconscious person is unable to communicate verbally, the possibility of non-verbal communication becomes increasingly important. It may be impossible to gauge the degree to which he is aware of the touch of a caring person, but in any instance, his awareness will be affected by the sensitivity of his skin.

Moist, supple, healthy skin is more sensitive to the touch than dry, scaly, or irritated skin, and equally important, healthy skin is more inviting to the touch of another person.

In addition to the care of an unconscious patient's sensory organs, it is important to monitor the quantity and quality of the sensory stimuli. Since feedback from the patient may be absent or minimal, the nurse will have to rely on her own professional judgment to evaluate the environmental stimuli.

Sound is the most important sensory stimulus because it is the sensation which is retained the longest as a patient loses consciousness or a coma deepens. There have been many documented instances in which a patient has regained consciousness and has reported the details of conversations which took place at his bedside while he was comatose.

Physical Activity

Areas of Assessment Related to Physical Activity

- Current range of motion
- Involuntary movements
- Usual position

Related Nursing Activities

One of the greatest tragedies in health care occurs when a patient awakens from a long coma with crippling deformities which could have been prevented. Examples of such deformities include footdrop and contractures of hips, knees, elbows, and fingers. Flexor muscles are stronger than extensor muscles, and if not counteracted, they soon pull an unconscious patient into a curled up fetal position.

Contractures can be prevented and joint flexibility preserved by putting each joint through its full range of motion three to four times a day. It is important that each joint be kept flexible: in addition to implications for future rehabilitation, joint flexibility is necessary for effective protective positioning. It is not possible to properly position a patient with multiple rigid, contracted joints!

Passive range of motion exercises provide an opportunity for family members to participate in the care of the patient. The exercises are easily learned, and they are so important that the family members are likely to view such involvement as a challenge rather than as a type of busy work.

The patient should be turned and repositioned every 2 hours in accordance with a preplanned sequence of positions. If the head of the bed must be kept elevated because of increased intracranial pressure, the prone position cannot be used because the position of the bed would hyperextend the patient's back.

If the patient is subject to involuntary movements or seizures, such movements must be carefully observed and charted; and to ensure his safety, pad the side rails of the bed and keep a padded tongue depressor at the bedside.

Hygiene And Grooming

Areas of Assessment Related to Hygiene and Grooming

- Condition of skin over bony prominences
- Condition of skin in deep folds such as the groin and under pendulous abdomen or breasts
- Condition of genitals
- Condition of hair and nails
- Presence of body odor

Related Nursing Activities

Hygiene and grooming are important for the unconscious patient for three reasons: (1) the skin must be maintained as an effective sensory organ; (2) the integrity of the skin must be maintained as a defense against infection; (3) the patient's appearance affects the care he receives.

The first two reasons are commonly taken into account by nursing personnel, but the significance of the patient's appearance is often underestimated. Humans are naturally drawn toward whatever is attractive and pleasing to them, and are turned away or repelled by whatever makes them feel uncomfortable or uneasy. It follows, therefore, that nurses and family members are affected by physical contact with a patient who is unclean and unkempt, with an unpleasant body odor. The appearance of an unconscious patient may be his only way of communicating with others, and that message should be "I am still a person, and I am worthy of your care and concern. I am still attractive and lovable."

SKIN. The daily bath provides an excellent opportunity for a complete head-to-toe inspection of every inch of the patient's skin. If the bath is delegated to a family member or non-professional member of the staff, that person should be taught to examine the skin over bony prominences such as the hips, ankles, heels, sacrum, elbows, back of the head, and ears for reddened areas which might indicate the start of a pressure sore. Deep folds of skin should be separated and cleansed, the skin should be assessed for dryness or excessive moisture, and the type of skin care adjusted accordingly. Rashes or breaks in the skin should be reported promptly.

GENITALS. Inadequate cleansing of the patient's genitals produces an offensive body odor, predisposes the patient to infection, and may result in discomfort which the patient is unable to communicate to you. These problems can be averted by the liberal use of warm water and soap and adequate visualization of the area by separating the labia, or lifting the scrotum and retracting the foreskin of the penis.

HAIR AND NAILS. The patient's hair should be shampooed regularly and kept free of tangles. The hair of a female patient should be styled as attractively as possible for the sake of the family, and the male patient should receive a shave and haircut as often as necessary.

Nails should be soaked for at least 15 to 20 minutes before you try to cut them; the podiatrist should cut the long curled nails of a patient who has previously been neglected.

Fluid and Electrolyte Balance

Areas of Assessment Related to Fluid and Electrolyte Balance
- Hydration of skin and mucous membranes
- Color, amount, and specific gravity of urine
- Laboratory values for electrolyes and blood gases
- Relationships between amount of fluid intake and output

Related Nursing Activities

An unconscious patient cannot tell you when he is thirsty, and is totally dependent upon you to watch for early signs of either dehydration or circulatory overload. The latter is especially dangerous if the patient has an increased intracranial pressure, because an increase in circulating blood volume will increase intracranial pressure even more.

It is essential, therefore, that careful attention be paid to the rate and amount of IV fluids, the dehydrating effects of diarrhea which might accompany tube feedings, and the effects of any treatment designed to reduce the patient's Pco_2 to reduce intracranial pressure.

Respiration and Circulation

Areas of Assessment Related to Respiration and Circulation
- Condition of airway; need for suctioning
- Rate, rhythm, and depth of respirations
- Heart and lung sounds heard on auscultation
- Pulse, blood pressure, and pulse pressure

- Adequacy of circulation in extremities
- Condition and functioning of equipment if mechanical ventilation is being used

Related Nursing Activities

Since the brain of an unconscious patient may already be ischemic and receiving inadequate oxygen, it is imperative that every effort be made to sustain the present level of oxygenation and prevent further deprivation. For example, the patient should be hyperoxygenated with an Ambu bag or other device *before* and after suctioning in order to compensate for the deprivation of O_2 during suctioning, and suction time should be limited to 15 seconds to minimize changes in blood gases. He should not be positioned flat on his back because his tongue could fall back and obstruct his airway, nor should he be positioned with his neck flexed when lying on his side.

If the patient has increased intracranial pressure, the head of the bed should be raised 20 to 30 degrees to promote venous return from the brain to the heart, he should not be placed in the Trendelenburg position, and the Valsalva maneuver (straining at stool) should be prevented whenever possible.

The patient's position should be changed every 2 hours to prevent pressure sores and to prevent pooling of secretions in the lungs. Side-lying positions provide an excellent opportunity for auscultating the upper lung on first one side and then the other.

Patterns of respiration are related to the location and extent of damage to the brain and brain stem, and it is imperative that the patient's respiratory pattern be assessed frequently enough to detect any change as soon as it occurs.

The frequency of taking vital signs is determined by the stability of the patient's condition, but during a period of increasing intercranial pressure, they should be taken frequently enough to detect a sudden rise in blood pressure, widening pulse pressure, and bradycardia which indicate a worsening condition.

If the patient's breathing is being controlled by a mechanical ventilator (respirator), the nursing staff is responsible for checking it at regular intervals, and reporting any potential problems to the proper maintenance personnel.

Elimination

Areas of Assessment Related to Elimination

- Frequency and consistency of bowel movements; test all stools for the presence of blood.
- Condition of abdomen (bowel sounds, distention, rigidity)
- Amount, appearance, and specific gravity of urine

Related Nursing Activities

Immobility coupled with tube feedings predisposes the patient to either constipation or diarrhea. Untreated constipation can lead to a fecal impaction, and therefore must be prevented by the use of a stool softener, mild laxative, occasional enemas, or suppositories. These measures are also important because the Valsalva maneuver is dangerous if the intracranial pressure is increased.

Urinary output should be within normal limits, and in proportion to the amount of fluid intake. If fluid intake is being restricted because of increased ICP, urinary output will decrease.

An unconscious patient is likely to have an indwelling catheter inserted, and since a catheter is a potential source of infection, his urine should be observed carefully for signs of infection such as cloudiness, blood, or shreds of mucus. If a male patient is using external condom drainage instead of a catheter, his penis should be inspected frequently for any signs of irritation or maceration; the skin of a female patient who does not have a catheter inserted should be checked for the presence of rash and excoriation.

Nutrition

Areas of Assessment Related to Nutrition

- Weight
- Electrolyte balance
- Bowel function
- Condition of skin, hair, gums, and mucous membranes

Related Nursing Activities

An unconscious patient should be weighed regularly to determine the adequacy of his nutrition. If his weight was within normal limits at the onset of his present condition, efforts should be made to maintain that weight by adjusting the formula of his tube feedings or other parenteral nutrition. A sudden weight gain is likely to indicate the retention of body fluids (edema) rather than a metabolic weight gain.

In addition to analyzing the patient's weight loss or gain, you should assess his nutritional status through laboratory tests which detect nutritional deficiencies such as protein malnutrition and a negative nitrogen balance. This type of analysis is especially important if the coma is associated with severe injuries, burns, or a progressive degenerative disease.

Problems related to tube feedings include diarrhea or constipation, electrolyte imbalances, vomiting, aspiration, and retention of formula in the stomach. These problems can be averted by changing the rate, frequency, amount, and temperature of the feedings, by checking the position of the tube, changing the size of the tube, and by modifying the composition of formula.

Rest and Sleep

Areas of Assessment Related to Rest and Sleep
- Sequence and frequency of scheduled nursing care
- Signs of excessive sensory input

Related Nursing Activities

It might seem that an unconscious patient would have no needs related to rest and sleep, but every living organism seems to require appropriate periods of rest in accordance with its own biorhythms. An unconscious patient may have no period of true wakefulness which must be followed by sleep, but at a basic level, his physiologic processes require time for restoration. This need suggests that nursing care be carefully planned and efficiently implemented so that the patient experiences interludes of rest between his frequent changes of position, pupil checks, tube feedings, and other essential activities. He should not be subjected to "nonstop" nursing care any more than any other patient.

Some patients who seem to be regaining a degree of consciousness can be disturbed by the efforts of family and staff to provide adequate sensory stimulation. Such a patient may seem restless, uncomfortable, irritable, or combative, and careful analysis of his behavior might indicate that he is being barraged with stimuli all day long, and that he is in fact suffering from sensory overload. The patient's behavior usually changes when several periods of peace and quiet are scheduled in each day's routine.

Body Temperature

Areas of Assessment Related to Body Temperature
- Body temperature
- Signs of altered body temperature (shivering, restlessness)
- Functioning of hypothermia equipment if it is being used

Related Nursing Activities

If the thermoregulatory mechanisms of the brain and brain stem have been affected, the body temperature may be unstable. An elevated temperature accelerates most body processes, and would increase an elevated intracranial pressure. Antipyretic drugs are usually used in combination with a hypothermia blanket to lower the patient's temperature to a safe level. This reduction should be done slowly enough to prevent shivering which can also increase ICP.

MEETING THE NEEDS OF THE FAMILY

Coma can be harder for a family to cope with than many other equally serious conditions. The sight of a loved one lying in a coma is extremely stressful, and the stress increases whenever the coma lasts for yet another day.

Psychosocial needs

Reactions of the family are affected by the cause and duration of the coma, the age, condition, and prognosis of the patient, and the resources of the family. The cause of the coma is a significant determinant of family reaction because of associated emotional responses. The coma of an elderly person who has just slipped into unconsciousness elicits a very different reaction than a coma caused by an athletic accident, drug overdose, or criminal assault. Responses include denial, anger, grief, and guilt if the condition might have been prevented.

If a state of unconsciousness was an expected outcome of the patient's condition, the family may have anticipated the coma and be well prepared to deal with it. If the coma resulted from an acccident, or is an unexpected complication of the patient's condition, the family may be in a state of crisis. If so, the techniques of crisis intervention should be used to help them through this period. Some crisis intervention techniques are simple: the nurse should introduce herself as the one who will be caring for the patient give family members a phone number so they can be in direct communication with the caregivers. Another technique is keeping the immediate family informed of any and all changes in the patient's conditions; this helps to ensure their ability to relay messages to absent family members and friends. Frequent reporting to the family also gives them an opportunity to make more informed decisions about the patient's personal affairs and/or business matters. Mapping the family structure and writing it in the Kardex or on the nursing care plan alerts all staff to each member of the immediate family and may prevent the isolation of individual members. These efforts by the nurse help to stabilize the family's environment and allows them some time to meet their own needs. Attending to physical needs, resting, eating regularly, and finding some means of relaxation will help families to maintain their own integrity and well-being throughout this very difficult situation. It is not unusual for other family members to become ill, have accidents or unusual events occur during this period of time, a result of added stress. Encouraging the family members to take breaks from the hospital setting and to care for their own health are important nursing measures. When there is no family or the patient is not allowed family visotors, the role of the nurse may be even more intricate. Health care providers may be a part of the bonded group that surrounds the patient. Family or friends who have not been a recent part of the patient's life may arrive when the patient is in a coma. Such visitors may have an unsettling effect on other family members and upon the situation as a whole. Providing a waiting room area where they may talk together away from the bedside is often the best immediate solution to privacy. Confidentiality is probably best maintained throughout by designating only immediate family to discuss patient information with outside callers and friends. Whether the coma state is short-term or long-term, it will be marked by different emotional responses of each family member. Those responses will be determined in part by culture, religious beliefs, and by a value system partially influenced by past experience and by the meaning of the unconscious patient's life upon their own. A nurse specially educated in the area of crises intervention may also be assigned to the family during this period of time.

MEETING THE NEEDS OF THE NURSE

For many nurses, the care of an unconscious patient is psychologically one of the most difficult of all nursing assignments. Factors which make this care so difficult include:

> Uncertainty about the patient's prognosis
>
> Lack of feedback and absence of interaction with the patient
>
> Monotony if the patient is comatose for weeks, months, or years
>
> Ethical concerns if the patient is being kept alive by extraordinary measures
>
> Difficulty in challenging one's self to maintain high standards of excellence

When you are caring for an unconscious patient, it is imperative that you examine your feelings and be attentive to any indications that the task is becoming increasingly stressful. If such is the case, prompt attention to your needs will help to avert a major problem later on.

One of the most important ways to help yourself is to use an individualized set of outcome criteria to evaluate your care at regular intervals, and by doing so, give you a sense of accomplishment. The criteria may be those used by all the staff, or they may be a modified version which includes *your* goals for the patient. Whatever the source, the criteria must accurately portray what *you* are trying to accomplish so that you can

be both rewarded and challenged by each personal evaluation. If this is not done, you are likely to become frustrated and depressed because if you don't know what you are trying to accomplish, you will miss the satisfaction of noting your progress.

Another way to cope with the situation is to align yourself with a supportive person or group. An instructor, mentor, or experienced staff nurse can provide help and understanding, as can a group of nurses who share similar problems. It is important for you to *acknowledge* your need and seek the help you need because if you give the appearance of managing well no one is likely to seek you out and offer to help.

A third type of help may be invaluable if you are troubled about any legal, ethical, or moral aspects of the situation. Some situations are exceedingly complex, especially when there is conflict between the family and professional persons regarding care of the patient, and a hospital chaplain, lawyer, or your own pastor may be able to help you sort out the troublesome issues involved.

If problems are acknowledged as soon as they are identified, and if appropriate help is sought promptly, it is usually possible to cope with the stress effectively enough to give excellent care to an unconscious patient over an extended period of time.

FAMILY TEACHING

Every person caring for the patient should talk to him throughout each procedure as if he were conscious, giving a full explanation of each activity. Family members and friends should be taught to converse with the patient by mentioning the weather, describing activities at home, and bringing news of relatives and friends. Some families make tape recordings of familiar sounds at home and in the community which can be played when they are unable to visit. Visitors and staff must be careful not to carry on conversations in low tones at the bedside, because a jumble of indistinct sounds is not an appropriate stimulus for the patient. In general, each sound which reaches the patient's ear should be potentially meaningful.

RELATED ACTIVITIES

1. Talk with people who have experienced an altered level of consciousness and read newspaper reports or magazine accounts of people who are or have been unconscious. It is important to study the people and the circumstances which could influence your reactions if you were caring for the patient. You may

care for an unconscious child who has been a victim of abuse, an older person whose condition has changed suddenly after a long history of chronic disease, or someone who has been in an accident or suffered an act of violence. Each situation will be vastly different and it will evoke an array of feelings within you. The culture and religious values of the family will have an impact as well. You can not know the variety of changing factors which will impinge upon such serious circumstances but you can define some of your personal reactions to what people tell you or what you read about.

2. Define what you believe to be the rights of a comatose person. When the patient can not speak for himself how will you speak for him? Ethical issues associated with the meaning of life and measures to extend life are important ones and are associated with the comatose state. It is important to remember that the longer the unconsciousness continues the more critical the concern will be for the survival of the patient.

SUGGESTED READINGS

————Nursing Grand Rounds. Overcoming acute complications in the unconscious patient. *Nursing 84* 1984 May; 14(5):42–45.

Coma: (continuing education feature) *Am J Nurs* 1986 May; 86(5):541–556.

————Scherer, Pricilla: Assessment: the logic of coma. 541–550.

————Hinkle, Janice L: Treating traumatic coma. 551–556.

Johnson, Laura K: If your patient has increased intracranial pressure, your goal should be: no surprises. *Nursing 83* 1983 June; 13(6):58–63.

Jones, Cathy: Glasgow Coma Scale: *Am J Nurs* 1979 Sept; 79(9):1551–1553.

Mauss-Clum, Nancy: Bringing the unconscious patient back safely. *Nursing 82* 1982 Aug; 12(8):34–42.

Stolarik, Anne: What the comatosed patient can tell you. *RN* 1985 April; 48(4):26–34.

Vernberg, Katherine, Janine Jagger, and John A Jane: The Glasgow Coma Scale: how do you rate? *Nurse Educator* 1983 Autumn; 8(3):33–37.

43

Care of the Dying Patient

Prerequisites and/or Suggested Preparation
The basic concepts of therapeutic communication (Chapter 9) and of psychological support related to crisis, loss, grief, anger, and depression (Chapter 24) are essential for understanding this chapter. In addition, Chapter 25 (spiritual needs) and Chapters 22 to 42 (meeting the physical needs of patients) are recommended.

The care of a patient who is dying presents one of the greatest challenges in all of nursing practice, and such care, when effective, represents one of the most significant accomplishments in nursing.

One reason that effective nursing intervention is important when a patient is dying is because everyone involved is in some degree of crisis. The family system has been thrown into imbalance but with help it can rebalance itself, regain its equilibrium, and in many cases, move on toward growth, improved mental health, and a higher level of functioning.

Effective intervention is possible, however, only when the nurse has explored and accepted her own feelings about death, when she is willing to risk the personal pain and hurt that is likely to accompany close involvement with death, and when she has the knowledge and skills for effective action.

An unprepared nurse who is reluctant to be involved can be of little help to either the patient or his family.

To give effective care to a patient and his family during a terminal illness, you must be *knowledgeable* about the phases of the process of dying, and *skilled* in your ability to intervene appropriately. In addition, it is necessary to be aware that many issues related to dying and death are controversial, such as the patient's right to die in the manner of his choice, the donation of organs after death, euthanasia, and the legal definition of death.

In general, these issues and others are related to two fundamental questions: (1) What can be done to help a person die well?, and (2) When is a person dead? These two questions are intricately interrelated but in this chapter they have been arbitrarily separated to permit discussion of the *process* of dying and the *event* of death as separate entities.

DYING AND DEATH

Over the centuries, dying has been described and defined in many ways and from many points of view. In the context of health care, a patient is acknowledged to be dying when one or more of the following conditions is present:

1. Nothing more can be done to save the patient's life.
2. The fact that nothing more can be done is recognized by medical and nursing personnel.
3. The fact that nothing more can be done is communicated to the patient and his family.
4. The patient realizes that he is dying.

Unfortunately, acknowledgement that the patient is dying does not ensure helpful patterns of communication. All too often a situation develops in which the patient is dying, and neither is able to talk to the other about it. Sometimes the staff knows that the patient is dying, but they do not talk with either the patient or family about dying and death, and do not help the patient and family talk with each other. Such inadequate interactions make the promotion of therapeutic communication during the process of dying a primary nursing goal.

PSYCHOLOGICAL ASPECTS OF DYING

The Phases of Dying

A dying person who is alert enough to be able to anticipate his own death grieves not only for the loss of his life but for the loss of everyone and everything that is important to him. The nature and type of these losses is highly personal, and based on individual differences and past experiences.

In addition to a person's individualized response, there is a series of responses that are relatively *constant from patient to patient*. These responses were identified by the research of Dr. Elizabeth Kubler-Ross; since their publication in 1969, they have provided a rational basis for effective nursing intervention with dying patients and their families.

Denial

During the denial phase, a person has no awareness, or no conscious access to his feelings about his forthcoming death. Almost every person experiences a period of shock and needs the phase of denial to serve as a buffer against reality in order to get himself ready and able to deal with impending death.

Denial is characterized by statements such as "No, not me!" or "It isn't true!" The patient may exhibit the following behaviors:

He may avoid the topic of dying or death.
He may speak of it with no emotional feeling or impact.
He may be able to talk realistically about dying and death for a time and then begin to contradict himself.

Anger

When the patient is no longer able to deny completely the fact that he is dying, the initial realization is painful. He may use anger to protect himself from other feelings

Kubler-Ross: Phases of Dying
• Denial
• Anger
• Bargaining
• Depression
• Acceptance

TABLE 43.1 WAYS OF EXPRESSING ANGER

Overt expression	Patient expresses anger directly to family, nurse, or other trusted person because he knows they will not abandon him if he does so.
Subtle expression	Patient is likely to withdraw and become emotionally inaccessible if he thinks that his caretakers will disapprove of his anger and take less care of him.
Indirect expression	Patient may become a "typical problem patient" who is uncooperative, complains a great deal, and never seems to be satisfied with any efforts to help him.
Passive-aggressive expression	Patient is neither cooperative nor aggressively uncooperative. He attempts to manipulate and control the situation by undermining the medical and nursing regimens. He will, for example, forget to take his prescribed medications, forget to collect necessary urine specimens, or fail to maintain a prescribed body position.

which he can't handle yet. This anger is often displaced or projected into other people or things. The anger phase often includes related feelings such as envy, rage, or resentment whenever the patient sees other people enjoying the things he is losing, such as obvious health, mobility, and a future on earth.

Anger results from a sense of powerlessness as the patient begins to realize that he is terminally ill, and it may be expressed in many ways, as shown in Table 43.1. The manner in which the patient expresses his anger is influenced by his trust and rapport with the people who are caring for him, and by the ways in which he has typically expressed (or failed to express) anger in the past.

Bargaining

The third phase of dying is usually a brief period during which the patient, having realized that he is terminally ill, attempts to postpone extreme discomfort, death, or both. Most bargains are made with God, and the patient asks for a reward for good behavior, often within a self-imposed deadline. For example, the patient may ask God to let him live long enough to go to a son's wedding or until a grandchild is born.

Many bargains are associated with guilt. The patient might say, for example, "I will go to church regularly if I can just live." The patient may be suffering from excessive guilt and fear of punishment, but he can be helped by appropriate nursing intervention.

Unless intervention is effective, most bargains, if seemingly met, elicit new bargains. For example, having seen a grandchild born, the patient will refocus on a daughter to be married soon and will bargain to live long enough to attend that wedding. Such a cycle of bargaining merely postpones the next psychological phases of dying.

Depression

When denial has given way to full realization by the patient that he is dying, there is a deep sense of losing all that is significant. This is characterized by the fourth phase of dying, an overwhelming depression. This depression may be of two types. The first type is a reac-

tion to what has *already been lost*, such as health, ability, body image, money, job status, and roles. The second type of depression is a preparation for the final phase of dying, which is acceptance. The patient grieves for *impending losses* and prepares for what lies ahead.

Acceptance

If the patient has had enough time and appropriate help, he usually has been able to work through his denial and subsequent realization of both past and impending losses and has come to a feeling of peace and quiet expectation.

This final phase of dying is not an unhappy phase but one that is almost devoid of feeling. Interest in the environment diminishes, and the patient may prefer to be alone or to have shorter visits from family and friends. Communication becomes less verbal and more nonverbal.

The patient is realistic about his impending death and seems at peace with the idea although traces of hope are present which may take the form of denial during periods of great suffering. Some degree of hope is essential throughout all the phases of dying; without it, the patient gives up and death is hastened.

Research has established the validity of these phases

as described by Kubler-Ross, but the following points must be emphasized:

- A given person may not go through all five phases, or may go through them in a different sequence.
- Different behaviors may express the same phase. For example, one patient may express denial of his dying by sleeping, whereas another may express denial by changing the topic at every mention of his condition.
- The patient, family, and staff may all go through these phases at different rates. For example, the patient may be denying his impending death while the family has progressed to the phase of anger, and the staff has accepted the coming death.
- Different phases require different interventions.

Assessments

In order to be effective, each nursing intervention must be appropriate for the current phase. Nursing assessments must be ongoing, so that all concerned persons are aware both of the patient's transition from one phase to another and of the overlapping of the phases. This awareness is important not only because the interventions are different for each phase but because people tend to respond differently to each phase. Some staff and families, for example, find the concept of *denial* difficult and have a tendency to pressure the patient to be ''realistic'' and ''face facts.'' Other people are frightened by outbursts of *anger* and attempt to make the patient control himself. Such inappropriate pressures are counterproductive and can be harmful to the patient; they can often be avoided if the behavior of the patient and the attitudes of the family and staff are accurately assessed in relation to the patient's phase of dying.

Nursing Interventions

In some respects, it is easier to assess the needs of a dying patient and his family when the relationship is relatively new, and there has been minimal personal involvement to date. It can be hard to assess needs objectively in a situation in which the nurse has cared for the patient over an extended period of time and has a deep personal commitment to both the patient and family. In the latter situation, both assessment and intervention are more complex because the nurse, as well as the patient and family, will be in crisis for a time and because everyone will be reacting to the phases of grief or dying, though perhaps at different rates. The effectiveness of nursing care will depend in part on the nurse's willingness to explore and accept her feelings

honestly and to promote open communication among herself, the patient and family, and others involved in the patient's care.

Interventions for Denial Phase

During the first phase of dying, it is important for the staff and family to understand the protective function of denial and to grant the patient adequate time to summon the strength needed to face his own death. At the same time, the nurse and family need to examine their own attitudes toward death and dying and to watch for any tendency toward behaviors that would prolong the denial phase of dying. It might, for example, seem easier, more comfortable, and ''nicer'' for all concerned if everyone were cheerful and brave, and did not acknowledge that the patient was dying. Such behavior does not help, or even permit, the patient to proceed to the next step of the task at hand, which is to die well, in comfort, and with dignity. Mutual denial, avoidance, and postponement of the next phase is neither helpful nor conducive to the mental health of patient, family, or staff.

The patient should be permitted to deny the reality of the fact that he is dying for as long as denial serves a protective, healthy function, but you should be alert for cues that this phase is ending and then respond appropriately. For example, the patient may begin to ask questions about his condition and prognosis. The questions may be tentative or indirect at first and should be answered gently but honestly to stimulate growth toward the next phase. A patient's questions and comments should not be dismissed lightly; nor should he be told, ''Now, don't worry yourself about that'' because such responses tend to block communication and discourage movement toward the next phase.

Interventions for Anger Phase

The second phase of dying is difficult for all concerned because the patient's expressions of anger tend to engender reactions of anger and frustration from staff and family. A typical response of the patient during the anger phase of dying is to call the nurses, family, or physicians ''no good'' or label them unhelpful or uncaring. This type of response often causes the family or staff to either withdraw from the patient or to retaliate in anger. There is a tendency to label an angry patient ungrateful and uncooperative, and both the family and staff may need considerable help in understanding that the patient's reactions are part of the process of dying and should not be taken personally.

Both patients and families may feel overwhelmed or guilty about the anger expressed during this phase, and such anger may be especially anxiety producing for people whose religion or culture considers the expression of anger to be wrong or inappropriate. It is important, therefore, to help the patient and his family understand at the beginning of this phase that *anger is a normal response* to immense loss and to the feelings of powerlessness experienced by a person who is unable to alter the fact that he is dying. They should know that anger is most likely to be directed at trusted people who the patient feels will not cease to care for him and that such anger must be expressed (within safe limits) if the patient is to progress toward the other phases of the process.

It is helpful to provide structure and order in the patient's care to help insure feelings of safety and security and to let the patient retain as much control over his life as possible to minimize his feelings of powerlessness.

Interventions Related to Bargaining

The third phase may pass unnoticed because the patient is likely to bargain in private, and it may recur at various times throughout the process. If the bargaining is based on guilt, repentance, and fear of retribution for past sins, real or imagined, the patient should be helped and encouraged to talk about them so that irrational fears and guilt can be relieved. In some cases it may help the patient to talk to a member of the clergy.

Interventions for Depression Phase

Most people feel disturbed, uneasy, and helpless in the presence of a deeply depressed person and oftentimes tend to avoid that person. The depression that precedes death is hard for families and staff to cope with because there is no way to relieve it.

Trying to cheer a person up is contraindicated at this time because the person has good reason to be sad and depressed. He is contemplating his great losses, without losing all hope as well.

Whenever the patient is grieving for *past* losses, such as his health, money, job, and position in the family, words are usually helpful. The nurse or family member should encourage and support the patient while he reviews and talks about his losses.

When the patient is grieving for *impending* losses and is beginning to accept his own impending death, the touch and silent presence of a nurse or a family member is often more helpful than words. It is hard for some family members to sit in silence with a dying person, but many are able to learn to do so when they learn that touching and being with the patient in silence are very important during this phase.

Interventions for Acceptance Phase

Patients who have had enough time and adequate help usually reach a phase of dying characterized by peace and a quiet, calm waiting for death. At this time, a patient's interest in his family and surroundings diminishes, and nursing interventions during this phase are designed to assure the patient that he is not alone and that he will not be rejected or left alone in the future despite his decreased interest in socialization.

The patient should not be pressured to maintain his social contacts, and his family and friends should be helped to understand if he prefers short visits, during which there may be little conversation. Finally, it is important during this phase to sustain the patient's sense of worth and importance, even though he is dying. For example, one woman who was dying from cancer of the face found some meaning for her death when a nurse helped her realize the change that her illness had brought in her family. They had learned to look past her facial disfigurement and respond to the person behind the face, and as a result they would look past the superficial aspects of other people in the future.

STAFF NEEDS AND PROBLEMS

Both professional and nonprofessional members of the health care team are likely to need assistance and emotional support as they try to interact effectively with dying patients. The areas in which assistance is often needed include knowledge and understanding of the dying process, communication skills, and intervention skills. Problems in these areas, coupled with fear or discomfort in caring for a dying person, lessen the likelihood of effective intervention. For example, it has been found that, though they are unaware of doing so, nurses who are uncomfortable with terminal illness are slower to answer the calls of dying patients.

Nurses who are fearful or uncomfortable with dying patients are unwilling to talk about dying and death and frequently *close off* the patient's attempts to discuss it by using techniques such as:

Changing the topic: "Let's talk about something more pleasant."

Reassurance: "You are doing just fine."

Fatalism: "Everyone is going to die, sooner or later."

Denial: "That can't be true."

Closing discussion: "I don't think things are nearly that bad."

Some nurses try to avoid discomfort by not getting deeply involved, by remaining aloof and distant, or by adopting a fatalistic attitude.

As the patient loses more and more control and life becomes increasingly tenuous, some staff become anxious and controlling and try to "manage" all aspects of the situation instead of concentrating on the needs of the patient. A nurse who tends to achieve satisfaction from "rescuing" patients may tend to make the patient feel more dependent and helpless so that she can "make things better." The nurse may find some satisfaction in feeling needed, but when the patient becomes angry or depressed, the situation worsens.

A nurse may experience a sense of conflict within herself when caring for a dying patient because her efforts to help the patient deal with approaching death may seem at odds with other efforts to prolong his life and foster hope. It is hard to be torn between a natural inclination to try to save a patient from death and at the same time try to help him die in comfort and with dignity.

Because of these and other problems, nurses who work in high-risk areas, such as intensive care and cancer units or in a geriatric care facility, will need ongoing support and assistance if they are to be effective in the care of dying patients and their families. As the staff invests more and more time and energy in the care of a dying patient, the staff will come to feel his death as a personal loss and react with varying degrees of anger, guilt, frustration, or depression. Such reactions can deplete a nurse's spirit and energy unless she is sustained and revitalized by adequate support and empathy. It helps to focus on the importance of helping a person to end his life well and of helping a family develop as a result of what could otherwise have been a devastating experience. When you elect to help a patient and family grow, you create a ripple effect that contributes to your own growth and touches the lives of numberless others.

PHYSICAL ASPECTS OF DYING

Physiological Changes as Death Approaches

Prior to death, changes are occurring in each cell, organ, and system of the body. These changes produce five major alterations in body function: (1) loss of muscle tone, (2) slowed peristalsis, (3) slowed circulation, (4) altered respiration, and (5) decreased sensation. The effects of these alterations are outlined in Table 43.2.

Physical Care as Death Approaches

The nursing care of a dying patient may require no new or different skills, but it does require the basic skills of nursing (both physical and psychological) to be used selectively and creatively. Nursing skills and techniques must be used selectively because there are times when something that you have always done or that "ought to be done" is not in the best interest of the dying

TABLE 43.2 SIGNS AND SYMPTOMS OF PHYSIOLOGICAL CHANGES PRIOR TO DEATH

Loss of muscle tone

Weakness, helplessness

Incontinence as a result of decreased sphincter control

Inability to maintain a protective or comfortable position without support

Decreased ability to swallow

Gradual loss of the gag reflex

Changed facial appearance (sagging jaw, flaccid lips and cheeks)

Diminished body movement

Slowed peristalsis

Decreased appetite or nausea

Increased flatus and distention

Constipation as a result of decreased bowel activity coupled with loss of muscle tone needed to expel feces

Inadequate intake of food and fluid

Dry mouth and slight fever caused by dehydration

Slowed circulation of blood

Extremities that look cyanotic and mottled

Extremities that feel cool, cold, or clammy even though body temperature may be slightly elevated

Possible perspiration; appearance of being too warm despite coldness of extremities; possible picking at bed clothes

Poor absorption of injected drugs because of decreased circulation

Altered respiration

Respirations are slow, labored, or irregular

Possible increased secretions in chest

Decreased sensation

Possible altered level of consciousness

Possible mental cloudiness (although some patients remain intellectually alert)

Some types of pain intensified; others gone

Vision possibly blurred; patient turning toward light; secretions on eyelids; conjunctiva possibly dry

Hearing is last sense to be affected

person. It is very difficult but necessary to try to differentiate between things done for the psychological comfort of yourself and the family and those needed to make the patient comfortable. For example, changing a wet sheet twice within 45 minutes may typify "good" nursing care to you and the family, who want to be sure that everything is done, but not necessarily to the

TABLE 43.3 GENERAL GOALS OF PHYSICAL CARE OF A DYING PATIENT

Maintain oral fluid intake as long as possible

Maintain at least minimal oral nutrition as long as possible

Position for optimal expansion of chest

Position for optimal drainage of mucus from mouth and throat

Prevent constipation and fecal impaction

Protect skin from urine and feces

Keep eyelids free of secretions

Protect conjunctiva of eyes from dryness

Keep mucous membranes of mouth moist and clean

Promote comfort

Relieve all pain

patient whose sensation is diminished, who does not notice the wet sheet, and who would rather you sat at the bedside for a few minutes and held his hand. *General* guidelines for care are listed in Table 43.3.

The duration of a patient's dying will vary from an hour or two to a number of days. Some patients gently slip away; others seem less ready to die. The period of terminal illness may have been long, hard, and painful, both psychologically and physically, but the person who has been well cared for, who is ready to die, and who knows he will not be left alone, dies quietly. Dr. Cecily Saunders, describing death in a hospice ward, writes:

It's always quiet, "It's as quiet as blowing a candle out," is how (the other) patients have described it to me . . . the end is always quiet and peaceful, and nearly always the patient is in a state of sleep or unconsciousness. The patient who dies fully conscious is rare, but a few do. (Pierson, 1969, p. 71)

The signs of imminent death include:

Dilated, fixed pupils

Faster, weaker pulse

Cheyne-Stokes respiration

Lowered blood pressure

Absent reflexes

Inability to move

As death approaches, the people responsible for the patient should know what to do when the patient dies. In most states, the patient must be certified dead by a physician who signs the death certificate and indicates the cause of death. If a person dies, or is expected to die, at home, the family's questions might include: Who should be called first, the doctor or the undertaker? How will the body be transported? Does the physician come to the house or go to the funeral parlor? The answers to these and other questions may vary with local practice and geographical location and should be determined in advance of the anticipated death and communicated to all involved.

Care of the Body

There are three factors which influence the care of the body after death: (1) the physiological changes that will occur, (2) the wishes of the family, and (3) legal requirements.

Care Related to Physiological Changes

The physical care of a dead body evokes a variety of responses in different people in different settings. A family member who has been caring for an elderly person who has quietly "slipped away" in his own bed may find the care of the body a natural and expected activity that gives a sense of completion and finality to the process of dying. On the other hand, a young hospital attendant who is callously directed to "take care of the body in room 310" may find the experience frightening and repulsive, especially if he has never seen or touched a dead person before.

Care of a body after death is especially difficult when the body is that of a child or a young person, when death was unexpected or caused by a needless accident or senseless violence, when the body is in poor condition because of a devastating illness, extensive trauma, or some delay between death and postmortem care, or when the caregiver has had little or no experience with death. Under such circumstances, the person giving care is faced with a triple challenge. Not only must he carry out a difficult task but in addition must cope with personal stress while considering the needs and responses of others.

Great care must be taken to make certain that the defense mechanisms and tension-relieving behaviors of the staff are not misinterpreted by other people. It can be devastating, for example, for a family member to overhear the laughter and rather crude jokes of staff who are trying to reduce their own stress to a manageable level. Denial in the form of laughter, carelessness, hurrying, or lack of response by the staff adds to the burden of those who care about the patient and is threatening to other patients who may be seriously or even terminally ill themselves. Careful attention and evidence of genuine concern, including nervousness and tears, can reassure others and help to refute the feeling that a hospital is an impersonal, hurtful place to be.

One of the initial tasks in caring for the body of a dead person is to make the body and the environment as esthetically acceptable as possible. If death was uneventful and uncomplicated, both the body and the unit may already be neat and clean. On the other hand, the body and the immediate environment may bear mute evidence of a long or intense struggle for life.

Remove all equipment and supplies and dispose of body wastes and soiled linen or dressings. This should be done quickly but carefully and in a manner that would not be distressing to anyone who enters the room at this time. For example, the body should not be exposed while you are working on it because the sight of a naked corpse could be distressing or offensive to people who enter the unit.

Wipe away all secretions and change dressings as needed. This is especially important if the patient had an infection because care must be taken to protect the mortician and others from the pathogenic organisms. It is not necessary to bathe the entire body; this will be done by the undertaker. Because muscle tone and body sphincters are relaxed at the time of death, there can be leakage of urine and feces, and absorbent pads should be used to prevent soiling the linen, stretcher, or other equipment.

The care and handling of the body is based on three physiological changes that occur soon after death: rigor mortis, livor mortis, and algor mortis. *Rigor mortis* (postmortem rigidity) is the stiffening of a dead body as the result of chemical changes within the muscle protein. The process occurs simultaneously in all muscles but it is first evident in small ones. It can be noticed first in the jaw and gradually becomes evident in the larger muscles of the arms and trunk and finally in the legs and thighs. Rigor mortis usually appears 2 to 3 hours after death and is completed in 6 to 8 hours.

Before rigor mortis is established, the body should be placed in a natural position, usually on the back with arms positioned beside the body or across the chest. The eyes should be closed. Dentures should be replaced if the lips and jaw have not yet become stiff. If any resistance is encountered, this task should be left for the mortician because any pressure on the lips and jaw can leave marks or indentations that cannot be removed and are often difficult to cover with makeup if the body is to be viewed.

The lower jaw should be supported in a normal position by placing a soft, folded towel or other soft material under the chin. The jaw should *not* be tied shut with strips of gauze or other fabric because the pressure over the cheeks and side of the face will leave disfiguring marks that the undertaker may not be able to remove or conceal. It is important to handle all body surfaces carefully but especially those areas of skin that are likely to be visible during the funeral. For example, it is important not to scratch the face with the comb or hairbrush because even small abrasions are permanent once the skin has lost its elasticity.

Livor mortis (postmortem lividity or postmortem hypostasis) occurs when the blood ceases to circulate and gravity pulls it toward the dependent parts of the body. The small capillaries become distended, and reddish-purple blotches begin to appear in 20 to 30 minutes. If a patient dies lying on his side, the body should promptly be placed in a supine position to prevent livor mortis on the underside of the face. One pillow is placed under the head to promote the drainage of blood and prevent any discoloration of the face. The blood in small blood vessels does not normally clot or coagulate after death, but the tissues do become permanently stained by hemolysis after 6 to 8 hr. The absence of extensive clotting enables the embalming fluid to reach all tissues and preserve them.

Algor mortis (postmortem cooling) is the loss of body heat after death. This occurs at a fairly predictable rate but is greatly influenced by environmental temperatures and exposure of the body.

Decomposition or putrefaction of the body causes serious problems when the body cannot be quickly refrigerated or embalmed after death. Following a large-scale disaster such as an earthquake, the dead must be buried as soon as possible to protect the living from disease or epidemics, and health care workers at the scene may be called upon to explain to the families the need for such haste.

Care Related to Family Wishes

If the family was present when the patient died, you may have determined by observation and conversation what some of their needs are likely to be. If their presence at the bedside was based on duty or other social pressure, they are likely to leave as soon as a physician has declared the patient dead. If, however, the family and friends are present because of love, concern, and caring, they may wish to be alone with the patient, to help prepare the body for the undertaker, or to conduct a religious or cultural ritual.

Although it seems obvious that no two families are alike, hospital personnel sometimes presume to know what a family needs or wants. In reality, one family may prefer to leave the room for a few minutes; another family may cluster more tightly than ever around the bed; a third may relieve their tension by arguing among themselves about whether to leave or stay.

Of primary importance is the fact that there are no "shoulds" or "oughts" in such a situation. Each family has its established patterns of interaction and ways of coping that may or may not seem desirable or appropriate to other people. Members of the family may need support and encouragement to do those things they want to do and they should not be urged or pressured toward a behavior that is deemed right or helpful by someone else. For example, family members who seldom, if ever, touch or embrace one another are not likely to want to touch the dead body. On the other hand, members of another family may find it satisfying to stroke and touch and kiss the body.

Between the two extremes are the people who would like to touch the body but either lack the courage or feel that it is not "proper." You can help by gently touching the body in a relatively casual way, such as brushing a lock of hair back from the face. Such an example of touching the body issues a nonverbal message to the family to do the same if they so desire.

If a person seems to be in a state of crisis and unable to leave the body, it may be helpful for you to gently remove that person's hands from the body as a first step in separation and leavetaking.

If members of the family are not present when the patient dies but arrive later, a quick but careful assessment must be made to determine their needs. Some people will seek detailed information about the patient's death; others will ask only a few questions. Some people who arrive after the death may give no indication of wanting to see the body and may prefer "to remember him as he was." Some people cry easily; some cry with permission; and others need nonverbal assurance that it is all right not to cry.

Some families are self-directed, competent, and financially able to manage; others are temporarily unable to decide what to do next. It may be necessary to contact the hospital social worker or chaplain, a local pastor, or relatives to help the family through the immediate crisis, especially if the death was unexpected. One young couple, for example, who were expecting their first baby had enough money for the hospitalization and delivery, but when the baby was born dead, they had no money to pay an undertaker. A sensitive nurse discovered their plight and contacted the social worker, who was able to help them.

Many older people have thought about their own dying and may have made plans for their deaths. The family should be encouraged to check the personal papers of the deceased for instructions and requests related to funeral arrangements. Such requests, if located in time, can personalize the funeral service and make it more meaningful for all concerned.

If this is the first death for a family, they may need an explanation of the role and function of the funeral director, or undertaker (see boxed material).

Care Related to Legal Requirements and Institutional Policies

A physician must certify the patient dead before anything can be done to the body. When this has been done and the family has left, the body is prepared for transport to the morgue or funeral home. The ankles are usually padded and tied together for ease in handling the body, which is then wrapped in a clean sheet or disposable shroud. Two labels are attached, one on the ankles and one on the shroud. Do not remove the hospital identification bracelet unless specified by hospital policy.

The body is taken to the morgue by stretcher in accordance with hospital policy, which usually has been designed to keep other patients from knowing that someone has died. Some hospitals close all doors up and down the corridor before the stretcher is taken from the patient's room, and some hospitals use a stretcher with a false bottom that conceals the body. Because it is usually not possible to tell from a distance that a person is dead, many hospitals merely place the body on a stretcher, arrange the sheets and a blanket to partially conceal the face and head, as if the patient were chilly, and take the stretcher down the hall and onto an empty elevator.

An autopsy (postmortem examination) is often done to determine the exact cause of death or to determine the effect on the body of a certain treatment. An autopsy is *required by law* under certain conditions, which include suicide, homicide, death within 24 hours of

---

Guidelines of Role and Responsibilities of the Funeral Director

- The funeral director can take charge and manage everything but should do so only when specifically requested to do so by the family.

- All arrangements should be made in accordance with family wishes and should permit as much participation as desired. For example, the parents of a little child may want to dress him for the last time.

- The undertaker is required by law to provide a detailed, *written* statement of all expenses before the funeral.

- It is both proper and appropriate to discuss such matters as costs and payment.

- If the undertaker is reluctant to meet the family's requests, they should ask whether the hindrance is based on state law, local custom, the undertaker's personal preference, or the funeral home policy. For example, in most states, the body need not be embalmed if buried within a specified time.

- The undertaker usually is experienced and knowledgeable about things that have proved helpful to other families.

- The funeral director prepares the death certificate, which is signed by the physician who pronounced the patient dead, and sends a copy to the local health department.

- The funeral director will write the obituaries based on material supplied by the family and send them to the newspapers.

admission to a hospital or in a jail, death from an unknown cause or in the absence of witnesses, or a suspicion of death by unlawful means.

Unless an autopsy is required by law, the next of kin decides whether or not one can or should be done. The nurse often helps to interpret and explain the physician's request for an autopsy and answers questions that may help the family decide whether or not to give their permission. The next of kin may want to consult with their clergyman or the hospital chaplain.

The autopsy is still the basis of all medical knowledge (Benton, 1978) and as such is an essential part of medical science and research. After the autopsy, specimens of tissue are saved for microscopic study. The organs are usually disposed of by incineration in the same manner as organs removed during surgery, although the family can request that the organs be preserved and buried with the body. After the body has been embalmed and prepared for viewing, no one can tell by looking at it that an autopsy was done.

ISSUES RELATED TO DYING AND DEATH

Definitions of Death

People need an accepted definition of death to guide them in the business of living. The physician must know when to cease his efforts; the family must know when to start mourning; and nurses must know when to change their roles and functions. The time of death can have serious implications for insurance, inheritance, business transactions, and other legal matters.

Uncertainty about the status of a dying person affects the nurse's perception of her work and the nature of the work itself. You are likely to respond quite differently when you believe you are helping a patient to die comfortably and peacefully than you do when you are caring for a patient who may already be clinically dead.

The task of supporting the family and helping them to grieve and mourn the pending loss is made incalculably more difficult when the status of the patient is uncertain and family members are in limbo. The family cannot complete the activities associated with death; neither can they proceed with the demands of daily living.

The need to define death and to know when death has occurred has characterized humans throughout history, and the ability to define death with accuracy has consistently eluded them. The passage from life to death is sometimes so gradual and slow that it is almost impossible to say at what moment death occurred. The *cessation of breathing* has always been accepted as an indicator of death; when breathing could not be seen,

its presence or absence was tested by holding a feather in front of the person's lips or nostrils. Following the discovery and understanding of the circulatory system, the *absence of a heartbeat* was accepted as an additional criterion of death. The cessation of breathing and the absence of a heartbeat, plus the disappearance of reflexes, came to serve as the criteria for death until medical technology made it possible to maintain heart and lung function indefinitely by artificial means. Questions related to death then assumed greater complexity. The question "Has the person stopped breathing yet?" became "If a person has stopped breathing and his heart has stopped beating, is he alive or dead when he is unconscious and a machine has assumed the function of his heart and lungs?"

In the normal course of events, if the heart fails to beat for approximately 5 minutes, the brain suffers irreversible damage and dies. Because the brain controls breathing, when the brain dies, the person dies. The phenomenon of brain death has been studied extensively, and many experts have suggested that an absence of brain waves indicates death despite the fact that heart and lung function can be maintained artificially. A normal brain produces a variety of levels of brain activity, and a flat line on the EEG indicates an absence of brain activity. A flat line can be caused by three conditions: a drug overdose, severe hypothermia, or death. In the absence of either of the first two conditions, it is presumed that a patient with a flat EEG line is dead.

In 1968, a committee of the Harvard Medical School published a set of criteria for defining death, as follows: (1) unreceptivity and unresponsivity, (2) no movement or breathing, (3) no reflexes, (4) flat electroencephalogram (Benton, 1978, p. 18). The Harvard criteria are frequently cited in legal proceedings, and form a basis for decisions about death by those who concur that the brain is indeed the center of human life. Even this definition is not without a degree of controversy, however. Some people state that, because human consciousness is centered in the cerebrum, only the cerebrum of the brain need be dead for the person to be considered dead. In other words, there might be minimal function in the brainstem of a legally dead person.

Controversy over definitions of death and protocol for making relevant decisions will continue for some time as concerned lawyers, judges, clergymen, patients, families, physicians, nurses, and citizens struggle to cope with age-old but ever-new questions of death. In simpler times, people were concerned about death because of the horror and fear of being buried alive, of inadvertently treating a living person as if he were dead. Now, some people find it equally abhorrent to treat a dead person as if he were alive, to continue to expend time, energy, money, equipment, caring, and love on a person who is rightfully dead. People today seek to define death partly for their own peace of mind and partly for practical reasons, such as the need to control an overwhelming technology and clarify public policy and legal responsibility. From these needs and interests has emerged the science of *thanatology*, the study of death.

Rights of the Patient and Family

Many people feel that a dying patient and his family lose virtually all control over the patient's destiny in a hospital setting, especially in an intensive care unit in a large medical center. The hospital team often seems more concerned with prolonging the patient's life through extraordinary means than it is with the wishes of the patient and his family. Death becomes a frightening, often impersonal, ordeal rather than a natural termination of life. In fact, many people believe that such measures do not even prolong life; they merely prolong the process of dying.

In an effort to protect themselves as best they can against the use of extraordinary measures when all reasonable hope of recovery has passed, many people prepare a *Living Will*. See boxed material.

In most states, a Living Will stands as a strong statement of the patient's beliefs and personal wishes, but many states now recognize the Living Will as a legal document. The strength of this document is based on

---

Living Will

To My Family, My Physician, My Lawyer

To Any Medical Facility in Whose Care I Happen to Be

To Any Individual Who May Be Responsible for My Health, Welfare, or Affairs:

Death is as much a reality as birth, growth, maturity and old age; it is the one certainty of life. If the time comes when I can no longer take part in decisions for my own future, let this statement stand as an expression of my wishes while I am still of sound mind. If the situation should arise in which there is no reasonable expectation of my recovery, I request that I be allowed to die and not be kept alive by artificial means or "heroic measures." I do not fear death itself as much as the indignities of deterioration, dependence, and hopeless pain. I therefore ask that medication be mercifully administered to me to alleviate suffering even though this may hasten the moment of death.

This request is made after careful consideration. I hope you who care for me will feel morally bound to follow its mandate. I recognize that this appears to place a heavy responsibility upon you, but it is with the intention of relieving you of such responsibility and of placing it upon myself in accordance with my strong convictions that this statement is made.

Signed _____   _____ Date _____

Witness _____ residing at _____

_____

Witness _____ residing at _____

_____

Copies of this request have been given to:

_____

_____

_____

_____

the premise that it was prepared while the patient was in reasonably good health, before a period of distress in which pain or despair could conceivably modify his desire to live. The patient should discuss the existence and contents of a Living Will with his family, physician, clergyman, and other significant people so that all will have a clear understanding of the patient's wishes. If the patient's physician does not accept the concept of a Living Will, the problem should be resolved between the patient and his physician well in advance of the patient's terminal illness.

It is important that family have an opportunity to fully understand the *implications* of a Living Will. It is one thing to agree to the concept of a person's Living Will in advance of a terminal illness, when the person is still relatively healthy, but it is quite a different matter at a later date to be faced with the realization that modern technology could keep the patient "alive" a while longer.

The presence or absence of a Living Will can help a family decide whether or not to ask the physician to write a "No Code" order (which means no resuscitative attempts in the event of cardiac arrest or respiratory failure).

Whenever a patient's death might be related to a crime or to illegal treatment, the decision to continue or suspend the use of life-support equipment is fraught with legal ramifications. The charges against an assailant may depend, for example, on whether it seems that the victim's death was caused by murder or manslaughter, or on whether the victim's death was caused by other factors than the assault, such as infection or removal of life-support equipment.

Need for Organ Transplants

The Uniform Anatomical Gift Act of 1978 has increased the frequency of organ transplantation, and the Uniform Donor Card is a legal document in all 50 states. Because a driver's license is one of the most accessible means of identification in the event of an accident or severe illness away from home, many states include a box on the license that can be checked to indicate that the person caring for the victim should check the reverse side of the license or look for a Uniform Donor Card. Instructions on the donor card direct that it should be kept with the driver's license.

Organ transplantation has become such an accepted mode of treatment that the demand for organs is far greater than the supply. In some states, legislation is pending, or has passed, which requires a physician to discuss the possibility of organ donations with each dying patient and/or his family.

Ethical and legal issues arise when a patient is being kept alive artificially and a selected patient is awaiting an organ transplant. The timing is often critical because some organs must be transplanted within a few hours after removal from the donor. There is no consensus as to who can make the decision to remove a brain-dead person from a life-support system, although there is agreement that the decision cannot be made by the physician whose patient needs the organ.

Euthanasia

Euthanasia originally meant "good death" but has come to mean "mercy killing" or causing the death of a person with an intent to prevent suffering. Proponents of euthanasia recognize varying forms.

Voluntary and direct. The patient terminates his own life, usually with an overdose of a medication that has been given to him.

Voluntary but indirect. The patient has given prior, specific consent for another person to terminate his life under certain circumstances.

Involuntary but direct. Death is accomplished by another person without specific request of patient.

Involuntary and indirect. The patient is allowed to die without a specific request from patient (Fletcher, 1973).

Other descriptions of euthanasia use the term *active* or *positive* to indicate acts of commission (mercy killing) and the term *passive* or *negative* to indicate acts of omission ("letting the patient go").

Advocates of euthanasia base their acceptance of it on the patient's inherent "right to die" or his "right to die with dignity," without interference, hindrance, or artificial delays. Opponents of euthanasia cite religious and legal considerations such as the Judeo-Christian commandment "Thou shalt not kill" and the commitment of physicians to preserve and prolong life.

VARIABLES WHICH INFLUENCE THE MANNER OF DYING AND DEATH

While the patient is dying, the nurse must be concerned with the reactions of the patient, the family, herself, and her colleagues. These reactions are affected by:

• Each person's age and stage of development
• Their religious and cultural beliefs
• Circumstances of the dying and death
• Availability of support and assistance
• Environment and surroundings

Age and Stage of Development

A person's perception of death is influenced by his age and developmental stage but is certainly not determined by it. Concepts of death tend to be fairly consistent for a given age group but stereotyped ideas of the relationships between age and death must be avoided. All 6-year-olds, for example, do not view death in the same way, nor do all elderly people. Some children are able to accept their own dying with equanimity (see box), whereas some elderly people are unable to do so.

People who are mentally retarded (developmentally disabled) must be carefully assessed to determine their concepts of death in order to plan appropriate interventions.

The age of the dying person has a significant impact on the reactions of the family and professional staff. People react quite differently to the death of a child than they do to the death of an elderly person or a young adult in the prime of his life.

Personal goals and expectations create different types of stressors for a dying patient. For example, some dying patients mourn an inability to complete a career. Others regret their inability to care for dependents or provide for loved ones.

Many dying people approach the problems of dying in a manner similar to the ways in which they have usually approached other problems in the past. Those coping skills and techniques that the patient has found effective in the past are likely to be used to cope with the stress of dying.

Religious and Cultural Beliefs

Some cultures value and encourage interaction between the dying patient and his family, friends and neighbors, while other cultures try to minimize the impact of death. The dying of some people is made more

---

Factors Influencing a Child's Reactions to Death

Age of child
Degree of emotional attachment to deceased
Availability of immediate surrogate for deceased
Previous experience with death, separation, loss
Familial/cultural attitudes toward death
Stability of child
Surrounding circumstances of death
Religious beliefs of family
Resultant changes in family structure

---

difficult by hospital policies and practices that keep family and friends at a distance.

Some cultures provide a reassuring and comforting framework of tradition and rituals related to dying and death; other cultures place great emphasis on individualism and require survivors to make their own decisions with minimal assistance and few traditions or guidelines. Not knowing what to do or what "ought to be done" increases the stress of the family.

Cultural traditions and rituals are important both to the dying person and to the next of kin, and the ability to incorporate traditional customs into the process of dying affects the behavior and perception of all involved.

The nature of a person's religious beliefs helps to determine whether the person thinks that death should be dreaded, welcomed, fought against, or responded to in some other way. Religious beliefs which affect a person's reaction to dying and death may include any of the following concepts of death:

The end point of biological life
The absence of all life
A place of darkness
A transition from one life to another
Another stage of personal development
Life in a different realm
The entry to eternal life

Circumstances of the Dying or Death

Reactions to a person's death are influenced by the cause and duration of his illness. For example, patients, family, and staff will perceive and experience death differently depending on whether it was caused by an assassin's bullet, environmental pollution by toxic wastes, cancer, an automobile accident, or nosocomial infection.

Some diseases cause a dying patient to become progressively weaker, less responsive, and more lethargic, while other conditions tend to make life increasingly unbearable. Treatment for extensive burns can be so painful that the patient often prays for release by death. Treatment for widespread cancer can be devastating, causing patient and family to wonder if death might not be preferable.

The expectedness of the death can be a major determinant of the way in which people react. A quick, unexpected death creates a crisis atmosphere for everyone; the death was not anticipated and people feel out of control. If an unexpected death occurs in a hospital, the staff and the institution are unsettled because the patient died in a place which focuses on the *prevention* of death, and some of the staff may be unable to help the family because of their own sense of loss or failure.

A death in the emergency room creates a unique situation which presents a special challenge to nursing and requires somewhat modified nursing interventions (see Table 43.4).

Death that follows an illness can result in reactions that are different from those of a sudden accidental death because the patient and family can be given psychological support even when the illness is brief. Even a short terminal illness can provide a number of opportunities for those involved to begin preparations for facing death. Patients seem to know when they are dying, even though many of them are supposedly "protected" from this knowledge by family or staff. A type of research study, done in retrospect and called a psychological autopsy, has shown that many patients gave numerous hints and signs prior to their deaths that indicated they knew they were going to die.

Whenever the duration of dying is long enough, the dying person goes through a process of grieving for his declining health, his ebbing life, and the loss of all that is significant to him on earth. The family engages in anticipatory grief, which is a reaction to a loss before it occurs. Anticipatory grief has been shown to be helpful in shortening the grief process for family and staff.

A patient's current phase of adaptation to dying, as outlined by Kubler-Ross, influences the manner of his dying and the reactions of those around him. Not all patients go through all phases, and some do not go through them in sequence. Misunderstandings and difficulties are likely to arise when the needs of patient and family conflict because they are in different stages of adaptation to the patient's dying.

During the time of dying, the stress of persons who are closely involved is compounded by nagging questions and uncertainties that surface from time to time. Examples of these concerns include questions such as:

- Is death really the certain outcome?
- Has everything been done that could be done?
- Is anyone to blame for the impending death?
- Has a type of death been predicted or anticipated?
- Has a time of death been estimated?
- Are there things to be done or preparations to be made at the moment?

Any death, no matter what the circumstances, affects all persons who are involved. Reactions to that involvement will vary widely, but the professional nurse is often the person who is best able to help survivors through this period of intense stress.

TABLE 43.4 CARING FOR THE BEREAVED FAMILY IN EMERGENCIES

Provide Privacy

Use area separate from regular waiting area but close to resuscitation area

Include comfort items: chairs, couch, ashtrays, phone, coffee

Make sure area is uncluttered and safe; remove dangerous objects to protect the occasional irrational grieving person

Assure that area protects family from open discussion of staff about the patient

Maintain Communication

Begin preparing family when seriousness of patient condition becomes evident

Keep family current about condition

Use simple instructions and provide clear, concise information

Help family accept reality of death by using word "dead" or "died"

Avoid interfering with family's pain as interference postpones grieving to less appropriate time and place; use minimal sedation; avoid "get hold of yourself" messages

Be aware of cultural differences in practices/ideas/values about death

Listen to cues from family about how they view the death

Draw on Resources

Family or friends: elicit information from less involved family member or close friend when possible

Hospital staff: find someone less involved in emergency (ex., ward clerk, student) to spend time with family who is alone

Community: police may be helpful in transporting family when they need to reach hospital quickly and safely

Information: have useful material available for family, e.g., pamphlets, addresses of support groups; offer to contact support group for family

Provide Support

Let family physician inform relatives of death when possible

Be present when physician tells family

Be aware of hospital and governmental procedures and regulations which must be followed

Use touch as an effective way to show caring and comfort

Do not be ashamed to show your own emotions

Seek support from other staff members who have dealt with a dying patient and family

Availability of Support and Assistance

The manner of dying is influenced by the availability of support and assistance. This is determined in part by the awareness of death that is held by patient, family, and staff. Four levels of awareness have been identified (Glaser and Strauss, 1965):

Closed awareness. The patient does not know he is dying; the staff and family are aware.

Suspicious awareness. The patient suspects that he is dying; the staff and family are aware (they may or may not know that the patient suspects that he is dying).

Mutual pretense. The patient, family, and staff all know that the patient is dying but pretend otherwise; they all act as if he were going to live.

Open awareness. The patient, family, and staff acknowledge that the patient is dying.

Communication and interpersonal relationships as well as medical and nursing care are affected by awareness that the patient is dying. Each level of awareness creates special interactions and encounters that are characteristic of that type of relationship. Each has its own advantages and disadvantages, its risks and securities. It is generally agreed that an open awareness is most helpful to all concerned, but it is also demanding, uncomfortable, and painful at times.

The levels of awareness of the patient and the people around him affect the care and support that can be offered to, or requested by, the patient. For example, the patient can expect and ask for different things when everyone acknowledges the fact that he is dying than he can when everyone is pretending that he will get well. Open awareness makes it possible for the patient to exercise his right to put his affairs in order and get ready for death in his own way. Every patient, regardless of age or condition, should be afforded this privilege.

Informing the Patient

As soon as the physician has diagnosed the patient as being terminally ill, the question of what and when to tell the patient becomes an issue. The physician is responsible for telling the patient about his illness and prognosis and usually does so, sooner or later. The timing of such information is influenced by that patient's condition, his verbalized curiosity, the wishes of the family, and input from the nursing staff. Some physicians state, "I'll tell him anything he wants to know, but he will have to ask. I'm not going to volunteer the information." Some families who feel unable to cope with dying often exert considerable pressure on the physician to withhold the information from the patient as long as possible.

Telling the patient that he is terminally ill is *not* usually a nursing responsibility, but you can encourage the patient to ask his physician for the information and clarification he seeks. You may want to stay with him while he questions the physician so that you can hear the explanation and help the patient understand and cope with the answers after the physician leaves.

Sources of Support

When it has been acknowledged that the patient is dying, family support and concern can be openly expressed,

---

The Dying Person's Bill of Rights*

I have the right to be treated as a living human being until I die.

I have the right to maintain a sense of hopefulness however changing its focus may be.

I have the right to be cared for by those who can maintain a sense of hopefulness, however changing this might be.

I have the right to express my feelings and emotions about my approaching death in my own way.

I have the right to participate in decisions concerning my care.

I have the right to expect continuing medical and nursing attention even though "cure" goals must be changed to "comfort" goals.

I have the right not to die alone.

I have the right to be free from pain.

I have the right to have my questions answered honestly.

I have the right not to be deceived.

I have the right to have help from and for my family in accepting my death.

I have the right to die in peace and dignity.

I have the right to retain my individuality and not be judged for my decisions which may be contrary to beliefs of others.

I have the right to discuss and enlarge my religious and/or spiritual experiences, whatever these may mean to others.

I have the right to expect that the sanctity of the human body will be respected after death.

I have the right to be cared for by caring, sensitive, knowledgeable people who will attempt to understand my needs and will be able to gain some satisfaction in helping me face my death.

*This Bill of Rights was created at a workshop, "The Terminally Ill Patient and the Helping Person," in Lansing, Michigan, sponsored by the Southwestern Michigan Inservice Education Council and conducted by Amelia J. Barbus, Associate Professor of Nursing, Wayne State University, Detroit.

although some families will need assistance in learning to do so. People who have never expressed their feelings openly in the past cannot suddenly begin to do so, especially under stressful circumstances; but they can often learn to do so with your example and encouragement.

In some situations, the Dying Person's Bill of Rights provides a useful basis for discussions among the patient, members of the family, and the staff. See boxed material.

The hospital chaplain is experienced in counseling dying patients, and when the patient's clergyman has been actively involved with the patient and family, he can be an additional support *if* he is kept informed of the patient's condition.

There are several types of organizations that have been developed, usually by lay people, for the mutual support of terminally ill patients and their families. One of the best known of these organizations, Make Today Count (MTC), was founded by Orville Kelly, a man in his forties who was terminally ill with cancer. There are chapters of the Make Today Count organization in many cities, and they can be located through the local office of the American Cancer Society. The philosophy and beliefs of this group are indicated by a set of suggestions that have been widely circulated through the newspapers and by cards placed in physicians' offices. See boxed material.

How to Live With Illness by Orville Kelly

1. Talk about the illness. If it's cancer call it cancer. You can't make life normal again by trying to hide what is wrong.
2. Accept death as part of life. It is!
3. Consider each day as another day of life, a gift from God to be enjoyed as fully as possible.
4. Realize that life is never going to be perfect. It wasn't before, and it won't be now.
5. Pray! It isn't a sign of weakness. It's a sign of strength.
6. Learn to live with your illness instead of considering yourself dying from it. We are all dying in some manner.
7. Put your friends and relatives at ease. If you don't want pity, don't ask for it.
8. Make all practical arrangements for funerals, wills, etc., and make certain your family understands them.
9. Set new goals; realize your limitations. Sometimes the simple things of life become the most enjoyable.
10. Discuss your problems with your family as they occur. Include the children if possible. After all, your problem is not an individual one. Have a good day . . . make it count.

Environment and Surroundings

One of the most important questions facing the dying person and his family is "Where shall death take place?" The question of where to live until death is not merely a question of physical location; the answer either reflects or dictates, to a large degree, the manner in which a person dies and the way in which his family responds.

Often the question is never voiced, either because it is too difficult or because the patient and family assume that there are no alternatives or choices to be made. Throughout most of the United States, there may be only two choices, home or hospital, but hospice programs are being developed in a number of cities.

Hospital

For some families, it is reassuring to place their dying loved one in a hospital where everything that can be done will be done. Other families find hospitalization necessary because they do not have the strength, energy, skill, space, or other resources to care for the patient at home. Sometimes hospitalization is necessary for financial reasons. For example, many insurance plans will pay hospital expenses but will not pay for the professional help needed by an elderly man to care for his dying wife at home.

Some hospitals are able to give care that is sensitive and concerned, and in some small towns the care is often personal and individualized. In a medical center, especially an intensive care unit, the care is likely to be technically skilled but routinized, impersonal, and often dehumanized. Many decisions must be made related to the use of equipment, life-support systems, and whether or not resuscitation should be attempted; and rightfully, the patient and family should be included in the decision making.

Home

Many dying patients desperately want to go home or stay at home with family, pets, and familiar surroundings, routines, and food. When trying to decide whether or not this is feasible, families tend to wonder first of all if they are emotionally and physically strong enough to manage, and second, if the care they can provide will be adequate. In some situations, only minimal discussion, preparation, and encouragement are needed to enable a family to care for the patient at home. Other times, thorough consideration of all the ramifications of such a decision and extensive preparation and support are essential (Table 43.5).

In addition to the normal support systems of the family, there are, in some communities, groups of lay people who have volunteered to help dying people and their families. These people are experienced in counseling and in providing psychological support and often spend many hours in a home as they help a dying person and his family to face the impending death. Information about such support groups can be obtained from the local cancer society.

Hospice

Dr. Cicely Saunders founded St. Christopher's Hospice in London in 1967 to care for dying patients. St. Christopher's has since become a prototype for similar institutions around the world that are characterized by highly personalized nursing care coupled with expert medical management. Patients at St. Christopher's and other hospices are assured almost complete relief of pain, virtually unlimited visitors, including children and pets, freedom to bring personal possessions and even items of furniture from home, and an opportunity to live life as fully as possible until the moment of death.

The hospice movement is based on the premise that dying is an integral part of life, not of death. Most hospices provide care for both inpatients and outpatients, and hospice teams provide the support that enables many patients to live out their lives at home.

DYING WELL

Interviews with dying people have indicated that most people want to be able to manage the events preceding their death in such a way that they can die in peace and dignity. This process is exemplified by the death of Sarah, an Alaskan Indian. Her story is told by Murray R. Trelease, who spent 8 years serving small Indian villages in the interior of Alaska as a parish priest.

TABLE 43.5 REQUIREMENTS FOR HOME CARE OF A DYING PATIENT

Desire of both patient and family for him to die at home.

Ready access to hospital facilities in an emergency.

Cooperation and support of the physician.

Supplemental nursing care for teaching, assessment.

Liaison with physician and hospital, and possibly some direct care.

Adequate equipment, drugs, and supplies.

Enough caregivers to permit each one to be free of direct care for an interval each day.

Effective communication between family, hospital, physician, nurse, pharmacist, and undertaker.

Adequate understanding of probable events and ways of managing complications such as hemorrhage, prolonged vomiting, difficulty in swallowing, or intractable pain.

The support of friends, neighbors, clergyman, relatives, or professional people during the dying and after the death.

A young member of a family would come to my cabin and ask me to come pray for grandma and bring Communion. And when I arrived the whole family and close friends would be there and we would have a service together. Within hours after that, the person would be dead. Sometimes the summons would originate with a member of the family and, occasionally, with a nurse stationed in a larger village. But most often it was the one dying who called everyone together. And I was told on several occasions that the dying person had spent the past few days making plans, telling the story of his life and praying for all the members of the family. There were as many variations on the theme as there were personalities. Some like to have a lot of people with them and others preferred just a favorite relative or to be alone. . . . I do not suggest that everyone waited for the priest to come and then died right away. But the majority who did not die suddenly die with some degree of planning, had some kind of formal service or celebration of prayers and hymns and farewells.

By far the most dramatic instance of timing and planning was the dying of Old Sarah. About two weeks before her death I received a radio message from Old Sarah summoning me to Arctic Village on a specific day. Nothing like this had happened to me before but I can remember thinking "she intends to die on that day." Dutifully I gathered three of her family in Fort Yukon and flew them to Arctic Village on the day designated. I was right about her intentions but wrong about the date. She had a son in another village and wished me to go and bring him to Arctic Village. She allowed enough time for me to bring in the last person. It was quite a company of people as was fitting for the undisputed matriarch of both the family and the community.

During the morning of the next day she prayed for all the members of her family. At noon we had a great celebration of the Eucharist in her cabin complete with all the hymns and prayers. Old Sarah loved every minute of it, joined in the prayers and the singing and was quite bright through the service. Then we all left and at six in the evening she died. For the next two days the entire village tuned out on the business of Sarah's funeral. Some of the women prepared her body and completely cleaned her cabin while others cooked vast quantities of food, much of which Sarah had bought for the occasion, for the workers. The mission house was turned into a carpentry shop for making the coffin and teams of men took turns picking and shoveling a grave in the frozen ground. All the village packed into the church for the service and accompanied the coffin to the graveyard, singing hymns while the grave was filled with dirt and placing hand-made crepe flowers on the mound before the final blessing. Then there was a great feast for all the village. The burial customs were similar to these in all the villages but never before or since in my experience were they planned and shared so much by the one who died. Old Sarah's dying was a priceless gift to all of us (Kubler-Ross, 1975, pp. 34–35).

PATIENT TEACHING

Two primary areas of teaching related to death and dying are (1) knowledge of the processes of dying and the nature of death itself, and (2) the communication between family and patient. With respect to the first, the patient and family need to know what to expect as the condition of the patient changes, that their feelings and responses are normal, what their options are, and what kinds of support and assistance are available to them. Some patients and families will accept and profit from some of the excellent books which are available for both children and adults. (See the bibliography for suggestions.)

Second, some families need to be taught the *importance* of clear, honest, and loving communication during the period of the patient's dying and at the time of his death. In addition, some families need to be taught *how* to communicate their feelings to each other, especially those of loss and grief. The assessment of their current ways of communicating must be thorough and accurate because your expectations and hopes for therapeutic communication within the family can not exceed the abilities and comfort of the patient and family. Role-modeling and subtle suggestions can help them to learn to express their ideas and feelings more easily, but the family and patient should not be pressured to interact with each other in ways that do not seem right or natural to them.

RELATED ACTIVITIES

Begin now to acquire a broad understanding of the ways in which people respond to dying and death.

1. Read as widely about dying and death as possible, especially personal accounts of a loved one's death. Note the reactions of the survivors, and look for helpful responses which you might use in your nursing practice.
2. Whenever appropriate ask people questions such as:

    "What did you talk to Grandma about when she was dying?"

    "What did the nurses do or say that was helpful when your sister died?"

    "When you are visiting patients in your role as hospital chaplain, how do you start and end the conversation?"

    "How do you keep going—working on a cancer unit with dying patients each day?"

Tell each person your reasons for asking the question and you will find that most people will be willing to share some part of their experiences with you in order to help you achieve the professional expertise you seek.

SUGGESTED READINGS

Benton, Richard G: *Death and Dying: Principles and Practices in Patient Care*, New York, D Van Nostrand, 1978.

deRamon, Pamela Babb: The final task: Life review for the dying patient. *Nursing 83* 1983 Feb; 13(2):44–49.

Dobihal, Shirley V: Hospice: enabling a patient to die at home. *Am J Nurs* 1980 Aug; 80(8):1448–1451.

Dolan, Marion B: If your patient wants to die at home. *Nursing 83* 1983 April; 13(4):50–55.

Dubree, Marilyn, and Ruth Vogelpohl: When hope dies—so might the patient. *Am J Nurs* 1980 Nov; 80(11):2046–2049.

Fassler, Joan: *My Grandpa Died Today*. New York, Behavioral Publications, 1971.

Geltman, Richard L, and Roberta Lyder Paige: Symptom management in hospice care. *Am J Nurs* 1983 Jan; 83(1):78–85.

Helm, Ann: Final arrangements: what you should know about living wills. *Nursing 85* 1985 Nov; 15(11):39–43.

Hime, Virginia H: Holistic dying: the role of the nurse clinician. *Top Clin Nurs* 1982 Jan; 3(4):45–54.

International Work Group in Death, Dying and Bereavement. Assumptions and principles underlying standards for terminal care. *Am J Nurs* 1979 Feb; 79(2):296–297.

Koff, Theodore H: *Hospice: A caring community*. Cambridge, MA, Winthrop Publishers, 1980.

Kubler-Ross, Elisabeth: *On Death and Dying*, New York, MacMillan, 1969.

——— *Death: The Final Stages of Growth*, Englewood Cliffs, NJ, Prentice-Hall, 1975.

Kubler-Ross, Elisabeth, and Warshaw, Mal: *To Live Until We Say Goodbye*, Englewood Cliffs, NJ, Prentice-Hall, 1978.

LeShan, Eda: *Learning to Say Goodbye*, New York, MacMillan, 1976.

Mandel, Henry R: Nurses' feelings about working with the dying. *Am J Nurs* 1981 June; 81(6):1194–1197.

Martinsen, Ida M: *Home Care for the Dying Child*, New York, Appleton-Century-Crofts, 1976.

Martinson, Ida M: Caring for the dying child. *Nurs Clin North Am* 1979 Sept; 14(3)467–474.

Mills, Gretchen Curtis: Books to help children understand death. *Am J Nurs* 1979 Feb; 79(2):291–295.

Papowitz, Louise: Life/Death/Life. *Am J Nurs* 1986 Apr; 86(4):416–421.

Seigel, Ronald K: Accounting for 'afterlife' experiences. *Psych Today* 1981 Jan; 15(1):65–75.

Smith, Mary L: When a child dies at home. *Nursing 82* 1982 Aug; 12(8):66–67.

Taylor, Phyllis B, and Marianne D Gideon: Holding out hope to your dying patient. *Nursing 82* 1982 Feb; 12(2):42–45.

Appendixes
Glossary
Index

Appendix A

Units of Measurement

METRIC UNITS

The metric system was developed by the French in the latter part of the eighteenth century. The basic unit is the meter (one ten-millionth of the then-supposed distance from the equator to the north pole).

The metric system is a decimal system, with prefixes that designate the various multiples or divisibles of 10. The prefixes that are most commonly used in medicine are:

Milli, which means one one-thousandth (0.001)
Centi, which means one one-hundredth (0.01)
Kilo, which means one thousand (1,000)

These prefixes may be affixed to any of the three basic units of measurement, which are:

Meter (m): the unit of length
Gram (gm): the unit of weight
Liter (L): the unit of volume

Therefore:

1 millimeter (mm) = 0.001 m
1 milligram (mg) = 0.001 gm
1 milliliter (ml) = 0.001 L
1 kilometer (km) = 1,000 m
1 kilogram (kg) = 1,000 gm
1 kiloliter (kl) = 1,000 L

Length

The meter (a little longer than a yard) and the kilometer (approximately 0.6 miles) are rarely used in medicine or nursing. The commonly used linear measures are:

1 centimeter (cm) = 0.01 m = approximately
0.4 in

Volume

The most frequently used measures of volume are the liter and the milliliter. These measures of volume are based on the meter, as are all the metric measures of both volume and weight.

The liter (approximately 1 qt) designates the volume of the cube that measures 10 cm on each side.

One liter contains 1,000 cubic centimeters (cc) (10 cm × 10 cm × 10 cm).

One liter also contains 1,000 ml. Therefore, 1 cc equals 1 ml.

Weight

The gram designates the weight of 1 ml of distilled water at 4°C. The most frequently used units of weight are:

1 kg = 1,000 gm (about 2.2 lb)
1 centigram (cg) = 0.01 gm
1 mg = 0.001 gm

Inasmuch as 1 ml (1 cc) of H_2O weighs 1 gm, milliliters (cubic centimeters) and grams may be used interchangeably to give an approximate measure of an *external* drug. For example: If you need 10 gm of salt to prepare a saline enema, you could measure 10 cc of salt more easily than you could find scales to weigh 10 gm of salt.

METRIC UNITS AND THEIR HOUSEHOLD EQUIVALENTS

Household measurement is very inaccurate, with wide variations in the size of teaspoons, tea cups, and so forth. The generally accepted household measures are:

60 drops (gtt) = 1 teaspoon (tsp or t)
3 t = 1 tablespoon (tbs or T)
12 T = 1 tea cup
16 T = 1 glass (or standard measuring cup)

The metric and household equivalents are as follows:

Metric Unit	Household Unit
5 cc	1 t
15 cc	1 T
180 cc	1 full tea cup
240 cc	1 full glass

(When fluids are served to a patient, the cup or glass is not usually completely filled. On the patient's intake record, the following values are often used.)

1 cup = 150 cc
1 glass = 180 or 200 cc

When starting to work in a new hospital, be sure to check on the accepted metric capacity of the glasses and cups that are used there.

APOTHECARY UNITS

In comparison with the precision of the metric system, there seems to be little rhyme or reason to the apothecary system of measurement. Fractional parts are not designated by prefixes, nor can their values be determined by calculation. They must be memorized.

The unit of weight is the *grain* (approximately the weight of a grain of wheat).

The unit of volume is the *minim* (approximately the amount of water that would weigh 1 grain).

Of the many units of measure in the apothecary system, you should know the following units, abbreviations, and equivalents.

Weight

60 grains (gr) = 1 dram (dr *or* ℨ)
8 drams (dr or ℨ) = 1 ounce (oz *or* ℥)

Volume

60 minims (min) = 1 fluid dram (fl dr *or* f ℨ)
8 fl dr = 1 fluid ounce (fl oz *or* f ℥)
16 fl oz = 1 pint (pt)
2 pt = 1 quart (qt)
4 qt = 1 gallon (gal)

In the apothecary system, the following rules are followed:

When the symbol or abbreviation is used, the quantity is written in lowercase Roman numerals and *follows* the symbol. Arabic numerals are used, however, in preference to large Roman numerals. For example:

5 gr = gr v
8 dr = ℨ viii

The quantity one-half may be indicated by the symbol *ss*:

1½ gr = gr iss
7½ gr = gr viiss

Other fractional parts are expressed as common fractions, for example, gr 1/250, gr 1/10.

When pint, quart, and gallon are written, the quantity is expressed in Arabic numbers. For example, 1½ pints or 7½ quarts.

APOTHECARY UNITS AND THEIR HOUSEHOLD EQUIVALENTS

1 drop = 1 minim (m i)
1 t = 1 dr (ℨ i)
1 T = ½ oz (℥ ss)
2 T = 1 oz (℥ i)
1 teacup = 6 oz (℥ vi)

1 glass or measuring cup = 8 oz (℥ viii)

2 measuring cups = 1 pt

MOST COMMONLY USED APPROXIMATE EQUIVALENTS

Metric	Apothecary	Household
0.06 gm	gr i	
0.06 cc	min i	1 drop
1.0 gm	gr xv	
1.0 cc	min xv	$\frac{1}{5}$ t
5 cc	(1 dr) ʒ i	1 t
15 cc	(1/2 oz) ʒ ss	1 T
30 cc	(1 oz) ʒ i	2 T
500 cc	(16 oz) ʒ 16	1 pt
1,000 cc	(32 oz) ʒ 32	1 qt

There are many discrepancies among these approximate equivalents. For example, 30 cc is the accepted equivalent for 1 oz (29.57 cc is the exact equivalent). Yet multiplying 5 cc per dram by 8 (℥ viii per ounce) results in an equivalent of 40 cc for 1 oz rather than the accepted equivalent of 30 cc = 1 oz.

Such discrepancies are inevitable when two systems are used whose equivalents are not exact. The discrepancies are within a 10% margin of error, however, which is usually acceptable in pharmacology.

COMMONLY USED METRIC UNITS AND THEIR APPROXIMATE APOTHECARY EQUIVALENTS

1 gm	1,000 mg	gr xv
0.6 gm	600 mg	gr x
0.5 gm	500 mg	gr viiss
0.3 gm	300 mg	gr v
0.2 gm	200 mg	gr iii
0.1 gm	100 mg	gr iss
0.06 gm	60 mg	gr i
0.05 gm	50 mg	gr 3/4
0.03 gm	30 mg	gr 1/2 *or* gr ss
0.02 gm	20 mg	gr 1/3
0.015 gm	15 mg	gr 1/4
0.016 gm	16 mg	gr 1/4
0.010 gm	10 mg	gr 1/6
0.008 gm	8 mg	gr 1/8
0.006 gm	6 mg	gr 1/10
0.005 gm	5 mg	gr 1/12
0.003 gm	3 mg	gr 1/20
0.002 gm	2 mg	gr 1/30
0.001 gm	1 mg	gr 1/60 = 1000 (mcg)
	0.6 gm	gr 1/100
	0.5 mg	gr 1/120
	0.4 mg	gr 1/150
	0.3 mg	gr 1/200
	0.25 mg	gr 1/250
	0.2 mg	gr 1/300
	0.15 mg	gr 1/400
	0.12 mg	gr 1/500
	0.1 mg	gr 1/600 = 100 mcg

Appendix B

Selected Abbreviations

aa	of each	CS	central supply dept.	exp lap	exploratory laparotomy
abd	abdomen	CSF	cerebrospinal fluid	ext	extract
ac	before meals	CTDB	cough, turn,	F	Fahrenheit
ad lib	ad desired		deep-breathe	FBS	fasting blood sugar
adm	admission	CV	cardiovascular	Fe	iron
AFB	acid-fast bacillus	CVA	(1) cerebral vascular	$FeSO_4$	ferrous sulfate
a.m.	morning		accident, (2) costal	Fr	French
amt	amount		vertebral angle	fld	fluid
anes	anesthesia	cysto	cystoscopy	ft	foot
aq	water	D & C	dilation and curettage	FUO	fever of undetermined
ASA	aspirin	D/C (DC)	discontinue		origin
ASHD	arteriosclerotic heart	def	defecate	fx	fracture
	disease	dept	department	gm	gram
ax	axillary	D_5S	5% dextrose (glucose) in	GB	gallbladder
Ba	barium		saline	GI	gastrointestinal
bid	twice a day	D_5W	5% dextrose (glucose) in	gr	grain
BM	bowel movement		water	GTT	glucose tolerance test
BMR	basal metabolism rate	diff	differential	gtt(s)	drop(s)
BP	blood pressure	dil	dilute	GU	genitourinary
BPH	benign prostatic	DOA	dead on arrival	Gyn	gynecology
	hypertrophy	DOE	dyspnea on exertion	h	hour
BRP	bathroom privileges	dr	dram	HCl	hydrocholoric acid
BSP	Bromosulfophthalein	DSD	dry sterile dressing	HCVD	hypertensive
BUN	blood urea nitrogen	dsg	dressing		cardiovascular disease
C	centigrade	DW	distilled water	Hg	mercury
c̄	with	Dx	diagnosis	Hgb	hemoglobin
Ca	(1) calcium, (2) cancer	ECG	electrocardiogram	HNP	herniated nucleus
C & S	culture and sensitivity	EEG	electroencephalogram		pulposus
cap(s)	capsule(s)	EENT	eye, ear, nose, and throat	HNV	has not voided
CBC	complete blood count	EKG	electrocardiogram	HO	house office
cc	cubic centimeter	elix	elixir	hs	at bedtime (hour of
cl	chlorine	ENT	ear, nose, throat		sleep)
cm	centimeter	ESR	erythrocyte	hct	hematocrit
CNS	central nervous system		sedimentation rate	H_2O	water
CO_2	carbon dioxide	exc	excision	H_2O_2	hydrogen peroxide

ia	if awake	**O₂**	oxygen	**Staph**	Staphylococcus
I & D	incision and drainage	**OU**	both eyes	**stat**	immediately
I & O	intake and output	**oz**	ounce	**Strep**	Streptococcus
IM	intramuscular	**P**	(1) pulse, (2) phosphorus	**STS**	serologiocal test for
inc	incontinent	**p̄**	after		syphillis
IPPB	intermittent positive	**PBI**	protein-bound iodine	**Sx**	symptom
	pressure breathing	**pc**	after meals	**T**	(1) temperature, (2)
IU	international unit	**per**	by		tablespoon
IV	intravenous	**pH**	hydrogen-ion	**t**	teaspoon
IVP	intravenous pyelogram		concentration	**TB**	tuberculosis
K	potassium	**PM**	post mortem	**tbc**	tuberculosis
KCl	potassium chloride	**p.m.**	afternoon	**tbsp**	tablespoon
kg	kilogram	**PO**	predominating organisms	**tid**	three times a day
KUB	kidney ureter bladder	**po**	by mouth	**tinct**	tincture
L	liter	**post-op**	after operation	**TLC**	tender loving care
lab	laboratory	**pre-op**	before operation	**TP**	total protein
lb	pound	**prn**	whenever necessary	**TPR**	temperature, pulse,
lg	large	**PSP**	phenolsulphonphtahlein		respiration
liq	liquid	**PT**	physiotherapy	**trach**	tracheotomy
LLL	left lower lobe	**pt**	pint	**tsp**	teaspoon
LLQ	left lower quadrant	**pulv**	to powder	**TV**	tidal volume
LP	lumbar puncture	**qd**	every day	**TWE**	tap water enema
LUL	left upper lobe	**qh**	every hour	**U**	unit
LUQ	left upper quadrant	**qid**	four times a day	**ung**	ointment
MOM	milk of magnesia	**qn**	every night	**URI**	upper respiratory
mEq	millequivalent	**qod**	every other day		infection
mg	milligram	**qs**	quantity sufficient	**VD**	venereal disease
MgSO₄	magnesium sulfate	**qt**	quart	**via**	by way of
MI	myocardial infarct	**q₂h**	every two hours	**VS**	vital signs
min	(1) minim, (2) minute	**R**	(1) rectal, (2) respiration	**Wass**	Wasserman
ml	milliliter	**RAI**	radioactive isotope	**WBC**	white blood cell (count)
mm	millimeter	**RBC**	red blood cell (*or* count)	**wt**	weight
mod	moderate	**Reg**	regular (diet)		
μg	microgram	**RLL**	right lower lobe		
Na	sodium	**RLQ**	right lower quadrant		
NaCl	sodium chloride	**RUL**	right upper lobe	*Other abbreviations often seen on charts:*	
NG (N/G)	nasogastric	**RUQ**	right upper quadrant		
no	number	**Rx**	(1) prescribed, (2) treated	**CC**	chief complaint
noc	night	**s̄**	without	**FH**	family history
NPN	nonprotein nitrogen	**sat**	saturate	**H & P**	history and physical
NPO	nothing by mouth	**sc**	subcutaneous	**LMD**	local medical doctor
NS	normal saline	**sed rate**	sedimentation rate	**LMP, or**	(on female chart) last
NTG	nitroglycerin	**SG**	specific gravity	**LNMP**	(normal) menstrual
O & P	ova and parasites	**sig**	to write		period
OB	obstetrics	**sm**	small	**PE**	physical examination
OD	right eye	**SOB**	short of breath	**PERLA**	pupils equal, react to light,
od	once daily	**sol**	solution		accommodate
on	once nightly	**SOS**	if necessary (one dose)	**PL**	present illness
OOB	out of bed	**SP**	suprapubic	**PTA**	prior to admission
op	operation	**spec**	specimen	**R/O**	rule out
OPD	outpatient department	**sp gr**	specific gravity	**ROS**	review of systems
OR	operating room	**SPP**	suprapubic	**UCHD**	usual childhood diseases
OS	left eye		prostatectomy	**WNWD**	well nourished, well
os	mouth	**SS**	soap solution		developed
OT	(1) old tuberculin, (2)	**s̄ s̄**	one-half		
	occupational therapy	**SSE**	soapsuds enema		

Appendix C

Artificial Respiration

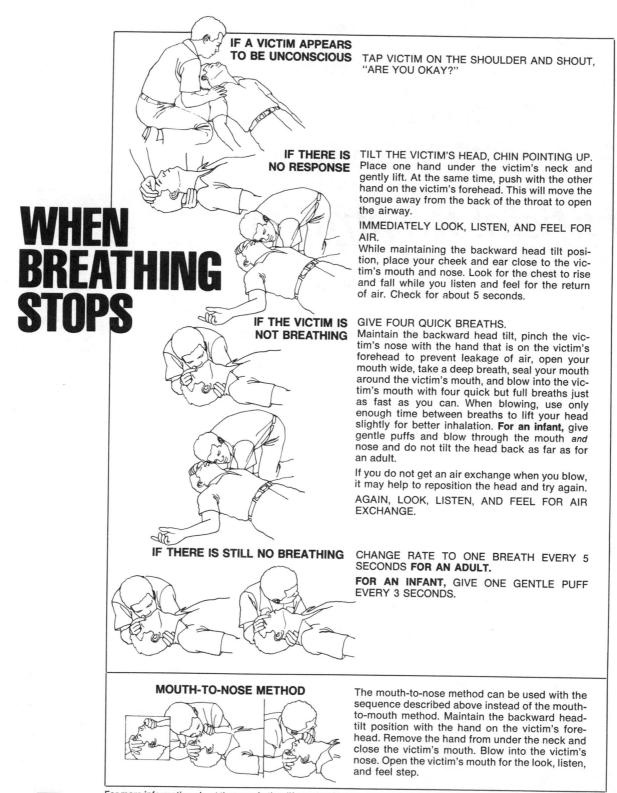

WHEN BREATHING STOPS

IF A VICTIM APPEARS TO BE UNCONSCIOUS TAP VICTIM ON THE SHOULDER AND SHOUT, "ARE YOU OKAY?"

IF THERE IS NO RESPONSE TILT THE VICTIM'S HEAD, CHIN POINTING UP. Place one hand under the victim's neck and gently lift. At the same time, push with the other hand on the victim's forehead. This will move the tongue away from the back of the throat to open the airway.

IMMEDIATELY LOOK, LISTEN, AND FEEL FOR AIR.
While maintaining the backward head tilt position, place your cheek and ear close to the victim's mouth and nose. Look for the chest to rise and fall while you listen and feel for the return of air. Check for about 5 seconds.

IF THE VICTIM IS NOT BREATHING GIVE FOUR QUICK BREATHS.
Maintain the backward head tilt, pinch the victim's nose with the hand that is on the victim's forehead to prevent leakage of air, open your mouth wide, take a deep breath, seal your mouth around the victim's mouth, and blow into the victim's mouth with four quick but full breaths just as fast as you can. When blowing, use only enough time between breaths to lift your head slightly for better inhalation. **For an infant,** give gentle puffs and blow through the mouth *and* nose and do not tilt the head back as far as for an adult.

If you do not get an air exchange when you blow, it may help to reposition the head and try again.
AGAIN, LOOK, LISTEN, AND FEEL FOR AIR EXCHANGE.

IF THERE IS STILL NO BREATHING CHANGE RATE TO ONE BREATH EVERY 5 SECONDS **FOR AN ADULT.**

FOR AN INFANT, GIVE ONE GENTLE PUFF EVERY 3 SECONDS.

MOUTH-TO-NOSE METHOD The mouth-to-nose method can be used with the sequence described above instead of the mouth-to-mouth method. Maintain the backward head-tilt position with the hand on the victim's forehead. Remove the hand from under the neck and close the victim's mouth. Blow into the victim's nose. Open the victim's mouth for the look, listen, and feel step.

For more information about these and other life-saving techniques, contact your Red Cross chapter for training.

AMERICAN RED CROSS   ARTIFICIAL RESPIRATION

Appendix D

CPR in Basic Life Support

CPR
IN BASIC LIFE SUPPORT
Place victim flat on his back on a hard surface.
If unconscious, open airway.
Neck lift, head tilt **or** Chin lift, head tilt

1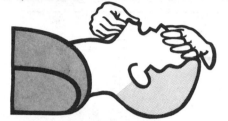

If not breathing, begin artificial breathing.

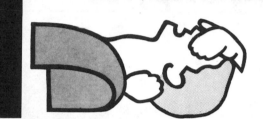

2

**4 quick full breaths.
If airway is blocked,
try back blows, abdominal or
chest thrusts and finger probe
until airway is open.**

Check carotid pulse.

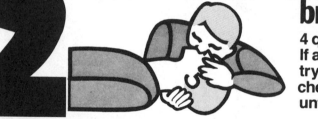

3

If pulse absent, begin artificial circulation. Depress sternum 1½" to 2".

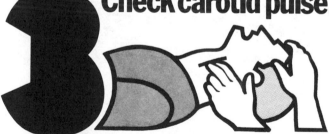

4

One Rescuer	Two Rescuers
15 compressions	5 compressions
rate 80 per min.	rate 60 per min.
2 quick breaths	1 breath

**CONTINUE UNINTERRUPTED UNTIL
ADVANCED LIFE SUPPORT IS AVAILABLE**

AMERICAN HEART ASSOCIATION
7320 GREENVILLE AVENUE, DALLAS, TEXAS 75231

77-006-AREV
77-50M
9-77-50M
© 1977 American Heart
Association

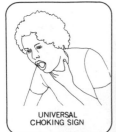

UNIVERSAL CHOKING SIGN

FIRST AID FOR
CHOKING

If victim can cough, speak, breathe ➡ *Do not interfere*

If victim __cannot__
cough
speak
breathe

Have someone call for help. Telephone : _____
                                                (Number)

⬇

TAKE ACTION: FOR CONSCIOUS VICTIM

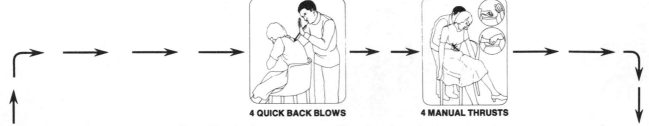

4 QUICK BACK BLOWS   **4 MANUAL THRUSTS**

Repeat steps until effective or until victim becomes unconscious.

TAKE ACTION: FOR UNCONSCIOUS VICTIM

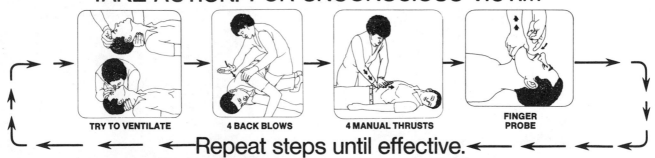

TRY TO VENTILATE   **4 BACK BLOWS**   **4 MANUAL THRUSTS**   **FINGER PROBE**

Repeat steps until effective.

Continue artificial ventilation or CPR, as indicated.

Everyone should learn how to perform the above first aid steps for choking
and how to give mouth-to-mouth and cardiopulmonary resuscitation. Call
your local Red Cross chapter for information on these and other first aid
techniques.

Caution: Abdominal thrusts may cause injury. Do not __practice__ on people.

AMERICAN RED CROSS

Poster 1030 (5-76)
(Sept. 1978 Prtg.)

31

Note: Back Blows have been eliminated from procedure.

Appendix E

Prefixes, Suffixes, and Combining Forms

The meaning of a medical term can often be figured out by analyzing the component parts of the word—the combining form and the prefix or suffix. For example: *bradycardia* brady (slow) + cardi (heart) = slow heart or slow pulse. *cholecystitis* chole (bile or gall) + cyst (bladder) + itis (inflammation of) = inflammation of the gall bladder.

COMBINING FORMS THAT DESIGNATE ORGANS AND BODY PARTS

Combining Form	Meaning
aden-	gland
angi-	vessel
arthr-	joint
aur-	ear
blephar-	eyelid
cardi-	heart
cephal-	head
cerebr-	brain
cervic-	neck
cheili-	lip
chol-	bile
cost-	rib
crani-	skull
cut-	skin
cyst-	bladder
cyt-	cell
dent-	tooth
derm-	skin
encephal-	brain
enter-	intestine
gingiv-	gums
gloss-	tongue
hem-	blood
hepat-	liver
hyster-	uterus
laryng-	windpipe
lip-	fat
lith-	stone
mamm-	breast
mast-	breast
mening-	membrane
my-	muscle
myel-	bone marrow; spinal cord
myring-	tympanic membrane (ear drum)
nephr-	kidney
neur-	nerve
oophor-	ovary
opt-	vision
ophthalm-	eye
orchi-	testicle
os-	mouth
ost-	bone
ot-	ear

pharyng-	throat
phleb-	vein
phren-	mind; midriff
pneumo-	lung
proct-	anus; rectum
pulmo-	lung
py-	pus
pyel-	pelvis; kidney pelvis
pylor-	pylorus
rhin-	nose
salping-	tube, especially fallopian tube
stom-	mouth; opening
thorac-	chest
trache-	windpipe
vas-	vessel
vesic-	bladder
viscer-	organ, especially abdominal

mega-	large; huge
necr-	corpse; dead tissue
neo-	new
olig-	small; few
path-	disease
peri-	around
poly-	many; much
pro-	in front of; forward
pyr-	fire; heat
retro-	backward; behind
semi-	half
sten-	narrow; contracted
supra-	above; beyond
tachy-	rapid; fast; swift
trans-	over; across

PREFIXES

Prefix	Meaning
a-, an-	without; not
ab-	away from; absent
ad-	near; toward
ante-	before (time or place)
anti-	against
bi-	two; life
brady-	slow
contra-	against; opposite
demi-	half
di-	two
dis-	apart
dors(al)	back
dys-	abnormal; difficult; bad
ect-	outside
end-	within
erythr-	red
ex-	away from; outside
hemi-	half
hyper-	above; excessive
hypo-	below; deficient
inter-	between; among
intra-	within
leuk-	white
mal-	ill; bad; poor; abnormal

SUFFIXES

Suffix	Meaning
-algia	pain
-asthenia	weakness
-cele	tumor; hernia; swelling
-centesis	tapping of puncture
-cid(e)	cut; kill
-ectomy	cutting out; excision
-emia	blood; blood products
-itis	inflammation of
-lysis	breaking down
-oid	like
-oma	tumor; swelling
-oscopy	examination
-osis	disease condition; chronic; increased
-ostomy	a mouth or surgical opening
-otomy	incision into
-path(y)	disease, suffering
-penia	deficiency; decrease
-phobia	persistent abnormal fear
-plasty	repair; surgical correction
-plegia	paralysis
-pnea	breathing
-ptosis	falling; downward displacement
-rhagia	excessive flow
-rhea	flow; discharge
-uria	condition of urine

Glossary

This glossary is intended to be a quick reference for words and for word usages specific to nursing. It is not a substitute for a medical dictionary.

Words whose meaning can be deduced from an analysis of the word are not included. For example, an *endoscope* is a lighted instrument for the direct examination of a body cavity, and *-scope* is the combining form of the word.

An otoscope is used to examine the ears.

An ophthalmoscope is used to examine the eyes.

A laryngoscope is used to examine the larynx.

A cystoscope is used to examine the bladder, and so on.

It would be repetitious to include every type of endoscope (scope) in a glossary. Therefore, the word *endoscope* is defined, but varieties of scopes are not included because such compound words can be deduced by an analysis of their prefixes and suffixes. Frequently used prefixes and suffixes are listed in Appendix E, which precedes this glossary.

Words used in this text which are not found in the glossary are those whose meanings can be determined from the meanings of their prefixes or suffixes, or words which appear in the index. Words not in common usage can be found in a medical dictionary.

Words and terms from the physical and social sciences are presumed to have been learned in other courses of study and are not repeated in this glossary.

abduction Movement of a body part *away* from the midline.

abrasion A scraping or rubbing away of a portion of skin or mucous membrane.

abscess A localized collection of pus.

acidosis A condition characterized by an excess of hydrogen ions in the extracellular body fluid compartment. The pH falls below 7.35.

adaptation Response of the body to a stressor; may be physiological, psychological, motor, or cognitive.

addiction An older term for physiological dependency on some drugs.

adduction Movement of a body part *toward* the midline.

afebrile Without a fever.

affective mode A mode of behavior or adaptation pertaining to, or resulting from, emotions or feeling.

AIDS Acquired immune deficiency syndrome; caused by a virus.

alarm reaction In the general adaptation syndrome, the first stage, which includes changes in the body when it is subjected to stressful stimuli.

alkalosis A condition characterized by a lack of hydrogen ions in the extracellular body fluid compartment. The pH usually exceeds 7.45.

alopecia Hair loss; baldness.

amblyopia Reduction or dimness of vision in an eye.

anabolism The metabolic process in which simple substances are synthesized into more complex compounds.

analgesic An agent that relieves pain; usually a drug.

anesthesia Partial or complete loss of sensation.

anesthetic An agent that produces insensibility to pain or touch; may be local or general in effect.

anion An ion that carries a negative electrical charge.

ankylosis Abnormal immobility and fixation of a joint.

anorexia   Lack or loss of appetite for food.

anoxia   Deficiency of oxygen.

antecubital   Pertaining to the anterior space at the bend of the elbow.

antenatal   Before birth.

antepartal   Before labor and delivery; prenatal.

antiemetic   A drug used to alleviate vomiting.

antipyretic   A fever-reducing agent; usually a drug.

antiseptic   A substance that inhibits the growth and development of microorganisms but does not necessarily kill them.

anuria   Absence of urine excretion from the body.

anxiety   Vague and ill-defined feelings of apprehension or uneasiness; different from fear.

apathy   Lack of interest in or feelings about persons, events, or situations.

Apgar Score   A numerical index of well-being applied to a newborn infant.

aphagia   Inability to swallow.

aphasia   Inability to express oneself properly through speech.

apical beat   Pulsation of the heart normally heard or felt in the fifth left intercostal space over the apex of the heart.

apical-radial pulse   The simultaneous measurement of the apical beat and the radial pulse by two people.

apnea   Cessation of breathing; usually temporary.

approximate   To bring the edges of an incision together.

arrhythmia   Irregular heart rhythm.

ascites   Excessive accumulation of fluid in the abdominal cavity.

asepsis   Freedom from infection.

  medical asepsis   Absence of pathogenic organisms; clean.

  surgical asepsis   Absence of all microorganisms; sterile.

aspiration   1. The drawing of material (usually vomitus) into the lungs on inspiration.   2. The withdrawing of a fluid by means of suction or syringe.

astigmatism   Eyes lack sharp focus and objects at a distance are blurred.

atelectasis   1. Incomplete expansion of the lungs at birth. 2. Collapse of the adult lung.

atony   Lack of normal muscle tone or strength.

at risk   A condition of increased susceptibility to a condition or disease.

atrophy   A wasting away; a diminution in the size of a cell, tissue, organ, or muscle.

auscultation   Listening for sounds, such as heart, chest, or bowel sounds.

auscultatory gap   Absence of systolic blood pressure sounds after initial sounds are heard. Sounds reappear after the silence, causing confusion over the actual systolic reading.

azotemia   An excess of urea or other nitrogenous products in the blood.

bacteriostatic   Inhibiting or retarding bacterial growth.

barium   A radiopaque substance administered orally or rectally before x-ray examination.

benign   Relatively mild; likely to have a favorable outcome (said of an illness); not malignant (said of a neoplasm).

bigeminal pulse   A pulse that consists of a pause every two beats.

biopsy   Removal of cells or a small piece of tissue for study and microscopic examination.

biorythm   Cyclic phenomena characteristic of life processes, for example, the menstrual cycle, circadian rhythm.

body image   The way a person thinks and feels about his body; basic to identity, with a profound effect on behavior.

bolus   A mass of food or drug, swallowed or injected intravenously.

bonding   The process by which mother and newborn infant develop a strong mutual attachment through repeated sensory contact. Psychological attachment or affiliation between a child and his parents and sibling, or among groups.

bowel sounds   Intestinal peristaltic action audible by stethoscope.

bradycardia   Slow heartbeat.

bulla   A large blister within or beneath the skin.

cachexia   General ill health, malnutrition, and wasting.

calculus   Stone; any abnormal concretion, usually composed of mineral salts.

calorie   Heat energy available in food; amount of energy needed to raise the temperature of 1 kilogram of water 1 degree C (kcal).

cancer   A large group of diseases characterized by uncontrolled growth and spread of abnormal cells.

carcinogen   Any substance which contributes to the causes of cancer.

carcinoma   A form of cancer which arises in glandular and epithelial tissue.

carcinoma in situ   A stage in the growth of cancer when it is still confined to the tissue in which it began.

cannula   A tube for insertion into a body cavity; insertion is usually facilitated by a pointed trochar or obturator.

cardinal signs   Signs of the inflammatory process: (1) heat, (2) redness, (3) swelling, (4) pain, and (5) loss of mobility of body part.

carrier   One who harbors a specific pathogenic organism in the absence of discernible symptoms or signs of disease and who is potentially capable of spreading the organism to others.

catabolism   Process of continual breakdown of protein reserve.

cathartic   An agent that causes bowel evacuation.

catheter   A flexible tube for injecting or removing fluids from the body.

cation   An ion that carries a positive electrical charge.

cauterization   Destruction of tissue by a caustic agent, hot object, or electric current.

cellulitis   Inflammation of cellular tissue, especially the purulent inflammation of loose connective tissue.

cerumen   Ear wax.

chemotherapy   Chemical agents used for treatment of cancer.

Cheyne-Stokes respiration   Breathing characterized by rhythmic waxing and waning of respiration depth, with regularly recurring apneic periods; may be forerunner to death.

circadian Pertinent to events that occur at approximately 24-hour intervals, such as certain biological rhythms.

circumcision Surgical removal of the prepuce, or foreskin, of the penis.

circumduction Action or swing of limb, such as the arm, in such a manner that it describes a cone-shaped figure.

clean Contains no *pathogenic* microorganisms.

cognitive mode A mode of behavior or adaptation that involves the use of specific intellectual activities.

colostomy Artificial opening from the colon to the abdomen for the purpose of fecal elimination.

coma A state of profound unconsciousness from which the patient cannot be aroused, even by powerful stimuli.

comedo Blackhead.

commode A portable toilet.

compliance Behavior of a patient which follows a nursing or medical regimen.

compromised A lack of ability by the body to resist infection or to produce an adequate immune response.

condom drainage A sheath or cover to be worn over the penis for the purpose of draining urine into a collection bag.

confidentiality The protection of a patient's privacy through careful use of oral and written communication.

confinement Childbirth and postpartum period.

contact In communicable disease, one who has recently been exposed to a contagious disease.

contaminate 1. To touch a clean surface with an unsterile object. 2. To touch a clean surface with an object that might contain pathogenic organisms.

contract A working agreement or arrangement between the nurse and patient that establishes the mutual goals or limits of nursing care; may be written or arrived at through mutual verbal discussion.

contusion A bruise without a break in skin.

cradle (overbed) A frame placed over the body of a bed patient for application of heat or to protect injured parts from contact with bed covers.

crisis An individual reaction to a given event which is perceived as hazardous coupled with at least a temporary inability to meet the demands of the situation.

criteria A specific set of standards against which outcomes can be evaluated; a yardstick for measuring effectiveness of nursing action.

cross-injection Infection which is transferred from one patient to another.

crust A layer of solid matter formed by dried exudate or secretions.

cue Any verbal or nonverbal response from a patient or other person that indicates the need for intervention from the nurse.

cyanosis A bluish discoloration of the skin and mucous membranes caused by an increased amount of deoxygenated hemoglobin.

cyst A closed sac or pouch with a definite wall that contains fluid or semifluid.

cytology The science that deals with the study of living cells.

debilitation Generalized weakness and lack of strength.

decubitus ulcer A bedsore; a pressure sore.

defecation Evacuation of the bowels.

dehiscence Spontaneous separation of wound edges.

dehydration A condition in which there is a deficit of extracellular fluid followed by a deficit of intracellular fluid.

delirium A mental disturbance of relatively short duration, usually reflecting a toxic state, and marked by illusions, hallucinations, delusions, excitement, restlessness, and incoherence.

dependent nursing functions Actions legally ordered and directed by a physician.

depression A mental state characterized by dejection, lack of hope, and lowered self-esteem.

dialysis Passage of blood or urine through a semipermeable membrane to remove waste products.

diaphoresis Profuse sweating.

dicrotic pulse A double pulse.

diffusion Dispersion of dissolved substances throughout a gas or liquid until the particles are evenly distributed.

diplopia Double vision.

disease Literally, the lack of *ease*; a pathological condition of the body that presents a group of symptoms.

disinfectant A chemical that kills bacteria.

disorientation The loss of proper bearings, or a state of mental confusion as to time, place, or identity.

distal Farthest from the center, from a medial line, or from the trunk; opposed to *proximal.*

distention A condition in which the bladder is overfilled with urine or the intestines are filled with gas.

distress Potentially harmful stress.

distributive care Health care that is usually preventive (screening and early diagnosis); occurs in community settings.

diuresis Increased excretion of urine.

diuretic An agent that promotes urine secretion.

diurnal Pertaining to or occurring during the daytime, or period of day light.

dolorology The study of pain.

dorsal Directed toward or situated on the back surface.

dorsal recumbent position On the back with legs moderately flexed.

dorsiflexion Backward flexion, or bending, of the wrist or ankle.

dyspareunia Painful intercourse; usually in females.

dysphagia Difficulty in swallowing.

dysphasia Difficulty in using language.

dyspnea Labored or difficult breathing.

dysuria Difficulty or pain on urination.

ecchymosis Bleeding in the skin and mucous membranes, which appears blue, purplish, or yellowish brown.

edema A localized or generalized condition in which the body tissues contain an excessive amount of fluid; swelling.

edentulous Without teeth.

electrocardiogram A record of the electrical activity of the heart.

electroencephalograph A record of the electrical activity of the brain.

emaciation The state of being exremely thin; a wasted condition of the body.

embarrass To impede the function of; to obstruct.

embolism A mass of undissolved matter that has traveled through the blood or lymphatic system and lodged in another area of the body.

emesis Vomiting.

endoscopy A lighted tube for observing the inside of an organ or cavity.

enema Introduction of fluid into the rectum.

entropy Tending toward increasing disorder or disorganization.

epidemiology The study of incidence, distribution, environmental causes and control of a disease in a given population.

episodic care Fairly intense health care given during acute illness; may occur in the hospital setting.

epistaxis Nosebleed.

eructation Burping; belching.

erythema Redness of the skin.

eschar Necrotic tissue formed over a burned area, usually a thick, dry crust.

euphoria A state of well-being, elation.

eustress Beneficial stress.

euthanasia An easy, painless death.

evaluation The process of comparing the result of an activity with a set of standards in order to determine the effectiveness or worth of the activity.

eversion Turning outward.

evisceration Protrusion of internal body contents through the separated edges of a wound, usually abdominal.

excoriation Abrasion (scraping) of the epidermis by trauma, chemicals, burns, or other causes.

excreta Waste matter excreted from the body, including feces, urine, and perspiration.

expectoration The coughing up and spitting out of material from the lungs, bronchi, and trachea.

extension To straighten a joint; opposed to *flexion*.

extravasation Escape of fluids, such as blood, into the surrounding body tissue.

extrinsic factors Variables associated with patterns of health and disease related to an individual's lifestyle and environment.

exudate A fluid containing protein and cellular debris that has escaped from blood vesels into tissues or onto tissue surfaces, usually as a result of inflammation.

febrile Pertaining to a fever.

feces Stool; excreta.

feedback The portion of a system's output (or behavior) that is fed back into the system.

fetus The unborn child in the uterus from the end of the eighth week after fertilization until birth.

first intention healing Union by approximation of wound edges.

fissure 1. A cracklike sore. 2. A groove or natural division.

fistula An abnormal passage within the body.

flatulence Excessive formation of gases in the intestine.

flatus Gas or air expelled through the rectum.

flexion The act of bending; opposed to *extension*.

foreskin Prepuce; loose skin covering the end of the penis.

Fowler's position A semisitting position in which the head is elevated and the knees are flexed.

fracture Disruption in the continuity of bone.

frequency The number of occurrences per unit of population or time, for example, cases of disease per 100,000 population.

urinary frequency Many voidings in a short period of time.

gavage Feeding through a tube passed into the stomach.

general adaptation syndrome (GAS) The process of adaptation, described by Selye, consisting of three phases: alarm reaction, resistance phase, and stage of exhaustion.

general anesthetic An agent which produces an unconsious state characterized by decreased reflexes and insensitivity to pain.

General Resistance Response (GRR) The process of adaptation, described by Aron Antonovky, consisting of individual or group characteristics which promote effective tension management.

gingivitis Inflammation of the gums.

girth Circumference; may be measured around the chest, abdomen, extremity, or head, for example.

Glasgow Coma Scale A numerical scale for assessing and describing grades of impairment of consciousness. This evaluation tool was developed at the Institute of Neurological Sciences, Glasgow, Scotland, in 1974.

glycemia Sugar in the blood.

granulation tissue New tissue formed during healing process.

halitosis Offensive breath odor.

healing

   first-intention healing Union by approximation of wound edges.

   second-intention healing Union by growth of granulation tissue.

hematoma A localized collection of extravasated blood, usually clotted, in an organ, space, or tissue.

hemiplegia Paralysis of one side of the body.

hemoptysis Expectoration of blood from the respiratory tract.

hemorrhoid A mass of dilated, tortuous veins in the rectum or anus.

high risk group Specific population which has an increased susceptibility to a condition or disease.

holism Concept of man as a functioning whole.

holistic health A dynamic harmonious equilibrium of body, mind and spirit promoted by each individual in a way which contributes to health.

homeostasis State of equilibrium.

hospice The care of terminally ill people in a special facility or at home.

hyperalimentation A method of providing nutrients, especially protein, directly into a large vein, usually the subclavian.

hyperextension Extreme or abnormal straightening beyond a position of extension.

hyperopia Farsightedness.

hyperpyrexia   High fever or hyperthermia.

hyperresonance   Abnormal sound that can be heard when a structure contains more air than normal.

hyperthermia   Body temperature over 40.6°C (105°F).

hypertrophy   An increase in the size of an organ or structure caused by increased size of *existing* cells.

hyperventilation   An increase in deep and rapid respirations, which causes CO_2 to be blown off more rapidly than normal.

hypodermoclysis   The injection of fluids into the subcutaneous tissues.

hypostatic pneumonia   Pneumonia occurring in elderly, debilitated, or post-operative patients who constantly remain in the same position and do not fully expand their lungs.

hypothermia   Body temperature falls below 35°C (95°F).

hypoventilation   A decrease in respiration, usually resulting in an accumulation of CO_2.

hypovolemia   Diminished blood volume.

icterus   Pertains to yellowish color; jaundice.

immobility   Lack of movement.

immunology   A branch of science dealing with the body's mechanism of resistance to disease or a foreign substance.

impaction   Condition of being tightly wedged into a part, as hardened feces in the bowels.

incidence   Number of new cases of a disease in a population during a stated period.

incontinence   Inability to control excretory functions.

infarct   An area of tissue that dies from loss of blood supply.

infection   The state or condition in which the body or a part of it is invaded by a pathogenic agent (microorganism or virus) that, under favorable conditions, multiplies and produces effects that are injurious.

inflammation   Tissue reaction to injury.

informed consent   A decision to accept treatment based on knowledge of both the possible hazards and the benefits of treatment.

infusion   A liquid substance introduced into the body via a vein for therapeutic purposes.

input   Information, materials, or energy that enter a system.

intermittent fever   Fever in which the temperature rises each day but falls to normal at some time during the 24-hour period.

intermittent pulse   Periods of regular pulse rhythm alternating with irregular rhythm.

intractable pain   Pain that is resistant to cure, relief, or often, to control.

intrinsic factors   Variables associated with patterns of health and disease related to the individual himself and therefore unalterable.

inversion   A turning inward, inside out.

inward rotation   Rotation toward the midline of the body.

ischemia   A deficiency or lack of blood to the tissue resulting from functional constriction or actual obstruction of blood vessel.

jaundice   Yellowish color of the skin, sclera, and excretions.

knee-chest position   Face down with hips elevated, knees flexed, weight on chest and knees.

Kussmaul's breathing   Very deep, gasping respiration associated with severe diabetic acidosis and coma.

Kwashiorkor   A severe form of protein malnutrition found especially in children.

labor   Process of childbirth consisting of three stages:

  first stage   contraction begins and continues until cervix is fully dilated and effaced.

  second stage   expulsion or birth of baby.

  third stage   expulsion of placenta and remaining products of conception.

laceration   Irregular tear, a wound.

lateral   Pertaining to the side.

lavage   Washing out of a cavity, usually the stomach.

lesion   An area of pathologically altered tissue.

lethargy   Drowsiness or sleepiness.

license   A legal credential issued by state or governing agency to ensure the public of at least a minimal standard of performance.

licensure law   The legal specifications for obtaining, renewing, and revoking a professional license.

lithotomy position   On the back with the knees and hips sharply flexed.

local adaptation syndrome (LAS)   Local reaction that results from responses to certain physical and physiological stressors, for example, the inflammatory response.

local anesthetic   Agent used to block pain and sensation in operative area; patient is usually conscious.

lumen   The interior of a hollow tube, vessel, needle, or bowel.

maceration   The softening of tissue by prolonged contact with moisture.

macule   A discolored spot on the skin that is not raised above the surface.

malaise   A vague feeling of ill-health, bodily discomfort, or both.

malignant   Tending to harm, destroy, or kill.

maramus   Starvation occurring in children (mostly in urban populations) as a result of low protein, low calorie diets, and unsterile foods.

medical asepsis   Absence of *pathogenic* microorganisms; clean.

metastasis   Spread of disease from one body site to another. All malignant tumors are capable of metastasis.

metric   Of or relating to the decimal system of measures, especially the metric system.

micturition   Urination or voiding.

mitosis   Process of cell reproduction by which new cells are formed.

morbidity   State of being diseased.

morbidity rate   The number of cases of a specific disease in a specific period of time per unit of population.

mortality   The death of a person.

mortality rate   The death rate; the ratio of the number of deaths to a given population.

multiple causation theory   A concept of health and illness that recognizes that many factors interact in complex ways to promote health or foster illness.

myopia Nearsightedness.

necrosis Death of areas of tissue or bone surrounded by healthy tissue or bone.

negative nitrogen balance A state in which more protein is being excreted than is being consumed.

negentropy Tending toward increasing order or organization.

neonatal Pertaining to the first month after birth.

neonate An infant during the first four weeks of life.

neoplasm A benign or malignant expanding lesion composed of proliferating cells; a tumor.

neurogenic bladder A bladder that does not function with the usual nervous innervation; may sometimes be retrained to avoid incontinence.

nocturia Excessive urination at night.

nocturnal enuresis Bedwetting.

node (nodus) A knotlike mass of tissue or cells; a small knoblike protuberance or organ; a swelling.

nodule (nodulus) A small node; a very small knotlike mass of tissues or cells.

nosocomial Pertaining to or originating in a hospital.

nutrient Any substance in the diet which furnishes nourishment for the body.

objective sign Evidence of the patient's condition that can be detected by another person, for example, a rash.

obturator An instrument with a smooth tapered end used to facilitate the insertion of a tracheotomy tube.

oliguria Diminished amount of urine formation.

oncology The study of tumors; a branch of science concerned with cancer.

orifice The entrance or outlet of any body cavity.

orthopnea Difficulty breathing unless in an upright position.

orthostatic hypotension Drop in blood pressure that occurs upon assuming an erect position.

output

    fluid balance output Measurable fluid loss from the body, for example, urinary output.

    systems theory output Information, energy, or matter produced by the system.

outward rotation Rotation away from the midline of the body.

palliative Serving to relieve or alleviate without curing.

pallor Lack of color, paleness.

palpation Process of examination with the hands or fingers.

palpitation Subjective awareness of the sensation of one's own heartbeat.

papule Elevated area on the skin; a circumscribed and solid lesion.

paraplegia A paralysis of the lower part of the body.

parenteral nutrition Feeding other than by mouth; usually refers to hyperalimentation.

parturition Process of giving birth.

passive exercises Form of bodily exercise done to and for the patient by another person.

patent Wide open; evident; accessible; unobstructed.

pathogen A microorganism or substance capable of producing a disease.

pathogenesis Study of the origins of disease.

pathogenic Capable of producing disease.

pediculosis Infestation with lice.

percussion Act of striking a blow to cause a body surface to vibrate.

perinatal Time before and after birth; conception to 28 days after birth.

periodontal Pertaining to the tissue around a tooth.

perioperative Term used to denote surgical care of patient prior to, during, and after an operation.

peripheral Located at, or pertinent to, the periphery (outer part or surface of a body).

petechia A small, purplish, hemorrhagic spot on the skin.

phlebitis Inflammation of a vein.

plantar flexion The act of bending the ankle as if to press the sole of the foot down on the floor.

plaque A patch on the skin or on a mucous surface.

polydipsia Excessive thirst.

polyuria Excessive secretion of urine.

postnatal Occurring after birth, or pertaining to the period after birth (relates to the infant).

postpartum Occurring after childbirth or pertaining to the period following delivery or childbirth.

prenatal Before labor and delivery; antepartal.

presbyopia Form of farsightedness which accompanies aging.

pressure sore Bedsore; decubitus ulcer.

prevalence Amount of a specific disease in a population at a given point in time.

prodromal Indicating the onset of a disease.

prognosis A forecast of the probable course and outcome of a disorder.

prone position Lying face downward.

prophylaxis Preventive treatment.

prosthesis An artificial substitute for a missing body part.

proximal Nearest the point of attachment, center of the body, or point of reference.

pruritis Severe itching.

puerperium Postpartum period: the period occurring just after delivery and measured from the delivery of the placenta until the uterus returns to normal (about 6 weeks).

pulse deficit Difference between the apical and radial pulse rates.

pulse pressure The difference between the systolic and diastolic blood pressures.

puncture wound A penetrating wound made by a very slender object.

purulent Containing pus.

pus Liquid product of inflammation made up of cells (leukocytes), liquid, and cellular debris.

pustule A small elevation of skin that is filled with lymph or pus, for example, a pimple.

pyrexia A fever or a febrile condition.

pyrogenic Producing fever.

pyuria Pus in the urine.

quadrant One of four parts or quarters of the surface of the abdomen.

quadriplegia Paralysis affecting all four limbs.

quality assurance Process whereby the quality of health care is evaluated in terms of predefined standards.

radiation

therapeutic radiation Treating diseases, usually cancers, with external or internal ionizing radiation.

diagnostic radiation Use of x-rays to detect disease or deviation from normal.

radiopaque Able to be seen on x-ray film.

rale An abnormal sound heard on ausculation of the chest.

range of motion (ROM) Movement of joints through the full extent to which they can be moved.

reasonably prudent nurse A nurse who behaves in accordance with what is established as the standard of nursing practice in a local area or community.

referred pain Pain seeming to arise in an area other than its origin.

renal dialysis The removal from the blood of certain elements that the kidneys would remove if they were functioning properly.

residual urine Urine remaining in the bladder after urination.

resolution Effective completion of a stage or phase of development.

restraint A device that limits a person's physical activity.

retching Attempting to vomit when the stomach is empty.

retention of urine Inability to empty the bladder completely.

reverse, or protective, isolation Practices that seek to protect the highly susceptible person from potentially harmful pathogens.

rhonchus Rattling in the throat or bronchial tree, owing perhaps to partial obstruction.

rotation Process of turning on an axis.

salutogenesis Study of the origins of health.

sanguineous Bloody.

sarcoma A malignant tumor which arises in muscle, bone, and connective tissue.

scope A tubular, lighted instrument used to visualize the inside of body organs or cavities.

self care As described by Dorothea Orem: activities that individuals personally initiate and perform on their own behalf to maintain life, health, and well-being; it is an adult's personal contribution to his own health and well-being.

sensory deprivation Severe reduction in stimulation of the human senses.

sensory overload An excessive stimulation of the human senses.

sepsis Presence of pathogenic organisms.

serosanguineous Blood-tinged.

serous Clear; describing drainage or discharge from a wound.

shock A circulatory disturbance in which the blood pressure is inadequate to supply vital tissues and organs with blood.

Sims's position Side-lying, usually on the left side with the right knee drawn up.

smegma Secretions of the sebaceous glands, especially in the genitalia.

sordes An accumulation of crusts, secretions, and debris about the teeth and mouth.

spasm Sudden, violent, involuntary muscular contraction; may constrict a passageway.

speculum An instrument for opening or distending a body orifice or cavity to permit visual inspection.

stasis Stagnation of the normal flow of fluids, such as urine or blood.

steady state Tendency of an open system to remain in equilibrium while maintaining a continuous exchange of inputs and outputs.

stenosis Constriction or narrowing of a passage or orifice.

sterile Free from all microorganisms.

stertor Snoring, or laborious breathing.

stoma An artificial opening from the skin to a body organ.

stopcock A valve that regulates the flow of fluid through a tube.

strabismus A constant misalignment of the eyes.

stress A condition caused by the body's response or adaptation to either internal or external forces that have disturbed the body's balance.

stressor Any agent or event that causes an increase in the stress response.

stricture An abnormal narrowing of a duct or passage.

stridor A harsh, high-pitched respiratory sound.

stupor Lethargy, unresponsiveness.

subjective symptom Evidence of the patient's condition that can be described only by the patient, for example, pain.

supine Lying on the back, facing upward.

suppression Failure of the kidneys to produce urine.

suppuration The process of pus formation.

surgical asepsis Absence of *all* microorganisms; sterile.

syncopy A temporary loss of consciousness, for example, fainting.

syndrome A group of signs and symptoms that collectively indicate a particular disease or abnormal condition.

tachycardia Rapid heartbeat, usually defined as above 100 beats per minute in the adult.

tenesmus Ineffectual and painful straining at stool or in urinating.

teratogen Any chemical or substance causing abnormal development of the fetus.

terminal illness An illness from which recovery is not expected.

thanatology The study of death.

therapeutic communication A deliberative process that consciously structures an interaction in order to achieve a certain outcome.

therapeutic touch The use of hands to promote healing.

thrombus A clot in a blood vessel or the heart.

tinnitus A ringing sound in the ears.

tissue A collection of similarly specialized cells which perform specific functions. There are four basic types: epithelial, connective, muscle, and nervous tissue.

tonometer An instrument for measuring intraocular pressure.

tonus That partial, steady contraction of muscle that determines tonicity, or firmness.

total parenteral nutrition (TPN) A method of providing all necessary nutrients directly into a large vein (usually the subclavian) by way of a central or peripheral venous catheter.

trauma A wound or injury, whether physical or psychic.

tremor An involuntary trembling or quivering.

trendelenburg position On the back with head about 45° lower than feet.

trocar A sharply pointed instrument to pierce a cavity wall and permit the insertion of a cannula.

tumor An expanding lesion due to a progressive apparently uncontrolled proliferation of cells; a neoplasm. (May be benign or malignant.) A swelling of any nature.

turgor Normal tension or elasticity; usually pertains to skin.

ulcer An open sore or lesion of the skin or mucous membrane of the body.

unconsious Insensible; incapable of responding to sensory stimuli.

urgency A sudden almost uncontrollable urge to urinate.

urticaria A vascular reaction of the skin characterized by a transient appearance of slightly elevated patches and associated with severe itching.

varicosity A swollen or distended vein.

vasoconstriction A narrowing of the lumen of the blood vessels.

vasodilation A widening of the lumen of the blood vessels.

vertigo A sensation of rotation or movement of oneself or one's surroundings; dizziness.

vesicle A blister.

viable Capable of living.

vital signs Blood pressure, temperature, pulse, and respiration.

void To empty the bladder.

vomitus Material ejected from the stomach by vomiting.

walker A device used to assist a person in walking.

wheal A localized area of edema on the body surface, often with severe itching.

wheeze A whistling respiratory sound.

wound Any interruption in the continuity of muscle, skin, or bone.

Index